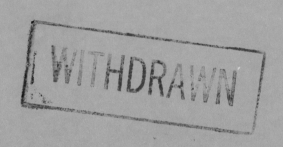

Dewhurst's Textbook of
Obstetrics & Gynaecology

This book is dedicated to my wife, Gill, and my children, Alastair, Nicholas and Timothy, and to the memory of Sir Jack Dewhurst.

Dewhurst's Textbook of Obstetrics & Gynaecology

EDITED BY

D. KEITH EDMONDS FRCOG, RRACOG

Consultant Obstetrician and Gynaecologist
Queen Charlotte's & Chelsea Hospital
London, UK

EIGHTH EDITION

WILEY-BLACKWELL

A John Wiley & Sons, Ltd., Publication

This edition first published 2012 © 2007, 1999, 1995, 1986, 1981, 1976 Blackwell Science; 1972 Blackwell Publishing Ltd; 2012 John Wiley and Sons, Ltd.

Wiley-Blackwell is an imprint of John Wiley & Sons, formed by the merger of Wiley's global Scientific, Technical and Medical business with Blackwell Publishing.

Registered office: John Wiley & Sons, Ltd, The Atrium, Southern Gate, Chichester, West Sussex, PO19 8SQ, UK

Editorial offices: 9600 Garsington Road, Oxford, OX4 2DQ, UK
The Atrium, Southern Gate, Chichester, West Sussex, PO19 8SQ, UK
111 River Street, Hoboken, NJ 07030-5774, USA

For details of our global editorial offices, for customer services and for information about how to apply for permission to reuse the copyright material in this book please see our website at www.wiley.com/wiley-blackwell

Library of Congress Cataloging-in-Publication Data

Dewhurst's textbook of obstetrics & gynaecology. – 8th ed. / edited by D. Keith Edmonds.
    p. ; cm.
Dewhurst's textbook of obstetrics and gynaecology
Textbook of obstetrics & gynaecology
Includes bibliographical references and index.
ISBN-13: 978-0-470-65457-6 (hardcover : alk. paper)
ISBN-10: 0-470-65457-0 (hardcover : alk. paper)
  1. Gynecology. 2. Obstetrics. I. Dewhurst, John, Sir, 1920– II. Edmonds, D. Keith. III. Title: Dewhurst's textbook of obstetrics and gynaecology. IV. Title: Textbook of obstetrics & gynaecology.
[DNLM: 1. Genital Diseases, Female. 2. Pregnancy Complications. WP 100]
RG101.D5573 2011
618–dc22

                                        2011011044

A catalogue record for this book is available from the British Library.

Wiley also publishes its books in a variety of electronic formats. Some content that appears in print may not be available in electronic books.

Set in 9.25 on 12 pt Palatino by Toppan Best-set Premedia Limited
Printed and bound in Malaysia by Vivar Printing Sdn Bhd

01 2012

Contents

Contributors

Sir Sabaratnam Arulkumaran PhD, FRCS, FRCOG
Professor and Head of Obstetrics and Gynaecology
Deputy Head of Clinical Sciences
St George's University of London
London, UK

George Attilakos MD, MRCOG
Consultant in Obstetrics and Fetal Medicine
Fetal Medicine Unit
University College London Hospitals NHS Foundation Trust
London, UK

Adam Balen MD, DSc, FRCOG
Professor of Reproductive Medicine and Surgery
Leeds Teaching Hospitals;
The Leeds Centre for Reproductive Medicine
Seacroft Hospital
Leeds, UK

Phillip Bennett BSc, PhD, MD, FRCOG
Professor of Obstetrics and Gynaecology
Imperial College London
London, UK

Sarah Blagden PhD, FRCP
Senior Lecturer in Medical Oncology
Ovarian Cancer Action Research Centre
Imperial College London Hammersmith Campus
London, UK

Tom Bourne PhD, FRCOG
Consultant Gynaecologist
Queen Charlotte's & Chelsea Hospital
Imperial College NHS Trust
London, UK

Janet Brennand MD, FRCOG
Consultant in Fetal and Maternal Medicine
Southern General Hospital;
Honorary Clinical Senior Lecturer
University of Glasgow
Glasgow, UK

Fiona Broughton Pipkin MA, Dphil,
FRCOG ad eundem
Professor of Perinatal Physiology
Department of Obstetrics and Gynaecology
City Hospital
Nottingham, UK

Sharon T. Cameron MD, FRCOG
Consultant Gynaecologist
NHS Lothian and Part-time Senior Lecturer
Department of Reproductive and Developmental Sciences
University of Edinburgh;
Chalmers Sexual and Reproductive Health Service
Royal Infirmary of Edinburgh
Edinburgh, UK

Linda Cardozo MD, FRCOG
Professor of Urogynaecology
Department of Urogynaecology
King's College Hospital
London, UK

Aaron B. Caughey MD, MPP, MPH, PhD
Professor and Chair
Department of Obstetrics and Gynaecology
Oregon Health & Science University
Portland, OR, USA

Peter Clark BSc, MD, FRCP, FRCPath
Consultant Haematologist and Honorary Reader
Department of Transfusion Medicine
Ninewells Hospital and Medical School
Dundee, UK

Hilary O.D. Critchley BSc, MD, FRCOG, FMedSci
MRC Centre for Reproductive Health
University of Edinburgh
The Queen's Medical Research Institute
Edinburgh, UK

Maureen Dalton FRCOG, FFFLM, FFSRH
Clinical Lead Adviser Peninsula SARCs (Exeter, Plymouth and Truro)
Consultant Obstetrician and Gyanecologist
Royal Devon and Exeter Hospital
Exeter, UK

John M. Davison BSc, MD, MSc, FRCOG
Institute of Cellular Medicine
Newcastle University
Newcastle upon Tyne, UK

Mandish K. Dhanjal BSc, MRCP, FRCOG
Consultant Obstetrician and Gynaecologist
Honorary Senior Lecturer
Queen Charlotte's & Chelsea Hospital
Imperial College Healthcare NHS Trust
London, UK

Claudine Domoney MBBChir, MRCOG
Consultant Obstetrician and Gynaecologist,
Chair of the Institute of Psychosexual Medicine
Chelsea and Westminster Hospital
London, UK

Anne Dornhorst DM, FRCPath, FRCP
Hammersmith Hospital
Imperial College Healthcare NHS Trust
London, UK

Alan Farthing MD, FRCOG
Consultant Gynaecologist
Imperial College NHS Trust
London, UK

Gillian Flett FRCOG, FFSRH, MIPM
Clinical Lead Sexual Health
Consultant Sexual and Reproductive Health
Centre for Sexual and Reproductive Health
Aberdeen, UK

Hani Gabra PhD, FRCP
Professor of Medical Oncology
Ovarian Cancer Action Research Centre
Imperial College London Hammersmith Campus
London, UK

Jason Gardosi MD, FRCSE, FRCOG
Honorary Professor of Maternal and Perinatal Health
University of Warwick;
Director
West Midlands Perinatal Institute
Birmingham, UK

Anna Glasier BSc, MD, DSc, FRCOG, FFPHC, OBE
Honorary Professor
University of Edinburgh Clinical Sciences and Community Health
Edinburgh;
School of Hygiene and Tropical Medicine
University of London
London, UK

Ian A. Greer MD, MFFP, FRCP, FRCOG
Consultant Obstetrician and Executive Pro-Vice-Chancellor
Faculty of Health and Life Sciences
University of Liverpool
Liverpool, UK

Mark Hamilton MD, FRCOG
Department of Obstetrics and Gynaecology
University of Aberdeen
Aberdeen Maternity Hospital
Aberdeen, UK

Andrew W. Horne PhD, MRCOG
MRC Centre for Reproductive Health
University of Edinburgh
The Queen's Medical Research Institute
Edinburgh, UK

Berthold Huppertz PhD
Professor of Cell Biology
Institute of Cell Biology, Histology and Embryology
Medical University of Graz
Graz, Austria

Davor Jurkovic MD, FRCOG
Consultant Gynaecologist
Pregnancy and Gynaecology Assessment Unit
King's College Hospital
London, UK

Sean Kehoe MA, MD, DCH, FRCOG, FHEA
Lead Gynaecological Oncologist
Oxford Gynaecological Cancer Centre
Churchill Hospital
Oxford, UK

Stephen Kennedy MA, MD, MRCOG
Professor of Reproductive Medicine and Head of Department
Nuffield Department of Obstetrics and Gynaecology;
Co-Director
Oxford Maternal and Perinatal Health Institute
Green Templeton College
University of Oxford;
Clinical Director Women's Services
Oxford Radcliffe Hospitals NHS Trust
The Women's Centre
Oxford, UK

Aradhana Khaund MD, MRCOG
Locum Consultant in Obstetrics and Gynaecology
Department of Obstetrics and Gynaecology
Southern General Hospital
South Glasgow University Hospitals
Glasgow, UK

Mark D. Kilby MD, FRCOG
Professor of Fetal Medicine
School of Clinical and Experimental Medicine
College of Medical and Dental Sciences
University of Birmingham;
Fetal Medicine Centre
Birmingham Women's Foundation Trust
Birmingham, UK

John C.P. Kingdom MD, FRCSC, FRCOG
Department of Obstetrics and Gynecology
Samuel Lunenfeld Research Institute
Mount Sinai Hospital
Toronto, Canada

Philippe Koninckx MD, PhD
Nuffield Department of Obstetrics and Gynaecology
University of Oxford
Oxford, UK;
Department of Obstetrics and Gynecology
University of Leuven
Leuven, Belgium

Sailesh Kumar FRCS, FRCOG, FRANZCOG, DPhil(Oxon), CMFM
Consultant and Senior Lecturer in Fetal Medicine, Obstetrics and Gynaecology
Queen Charlotte's & Chelsea Hospital
Imperial College London
London, UK

Stuart Lavery MBBS, MRCOG
Hammersmith Hospital
London, UK

William L. Ledger MA, DPhil, FRCOG, FRANZCOG
Professor and Head of Department of Obstetrics and Gynaecology
University of New South Wales
Royal Hospital for Women
Sydney, Australia

Christoph C. Lees MD, MRCOG
Consultant in Obstetrics and Fetal–Maternal Medicine
Lead, Fetal Medicine
The Rosie Hospital
Addenbrookes NHS Trust
Cambridge, UK

Bertie Leigh Hon FRCPCH, FRCOG ad eundem
Solicitor
Senior Partner Hempsons
Hempsons
London, UK

Fiona M. Lewis MD, FRCP
Wexham Park Hospital
Slough, UK;
St John's Institute of Dermatology
St Thomas' Hospital
London, UK

Andrés López Bernal MD, DPhil (Oxon)
School of Clinical Sciences
University of Bristol;
St Michael's Hospital
Bristol, UK

David M. Luesley MA, MD, FRCOG
Professor of Gyanecological Oncology
University of Birmingham
Birmingham, UK

Mary Ann Lumsden MD, FRCOG
Head of Section
Reproductive and Maternal Medicine
University of Glasgow
Royal Infirmary
Glasgow, UK

Andrew McCarthy FRCOG
Consultant Obstetrician
Imperial College Healthcare
London, UK

Sheila McLean LLB, MLitt, PhD, LLD (Edin),
LLD (Abertay, Dundee), FRSE, FRCGP, FBS, FMedSci,
FRCP (Ed), FRSA
Professor of Law and Ethics in Medicine
Institute of Law and Ethics in Medicine
University of Glasgow
Glasgow, UK

Adam Magos BSc, MB, BS, MD, FRCOG
Consultant Gynaecologist/Honorary Senior Lecturer
Royal Free Hospital
London, UK

Sallie M. Neill FRCP
St John's Institute of Dermatology
St Thomas's Hospital
London, UK

Catherine Nelson-Piercy MA, FRCP, FRCOG
Consultant Obstetric Physician
Professor of Obstetric Medicine
Guy's and St Thomas' Foundation Trust
Queen Charlotte's & Chelsea Hospital
London, UK

Jane E. Norman MD, FRCOG
Professor of Maternal and Fetal Health
MRC Centre for Reproductive Biology
University of Edinburgh
The Queen's Medical Research Centre
Edinburgh, UK

Errol R. Norwitz MD, DPhil (Oxon)
Department of Obstetrics
Gynecology and Reproductive Sciences Yale
New Haven Hospital
New Haven, CT, USA

P.M. Shaughn O'Brien DSc, MD, FRCOG
Professor of Obstetrics and Gynaecology
Keele University School of Medicine
Stoke on Trent, UK

Dick Oepkes MD, PhD
Department of Obstetrics
Leiden University Medical Centre
Leiden, Netherlands

Timothy G. Overton BSc, MRCGP, MD, FRCOG
Consultant in Obstetrics and Fetal Medicine
St Michael's Hospital
University Hospitals Bristol NHS Foundation Trust
Bristol, UK

Nick Panay BSc, MRCOG, MFSRH
Consultant Gynaecologist, Specialist in Reproductive Medicine
Queen Charlotte's & Chelsea Hospital;
Chelsea and Westminster Hospital
West London Menopause & PMS Centre;
Honorary Senior Lecturer
Imperial College London
London, UK

Sara Paterson-Brown FRCS, FRCOG
Consultant Obstetrician and Gynaecologist
Clinical Lead for Labour Ward and Maternity Risk
Queen Charlotte's & Chelsea Hospital
Imperial College NHS Healthcare Trust
London, UK

Felicity Plaat BA, MBBS, FRCA
Consultant Anaesthetist & Honorary Senior Lecturer
Queen Charlotte's & Chelsea Hospital
Imperial College School of Medicine
London, UK

Siobhan Quenby BSc, MBBS, MD, FRCOG
Professor of Obstetrics
Clinical Science Research Institute
University of Warwick
University Hospital – Walsgrave Campus
Coventry, UK

Dudley Robinson MD, FRCOG
Consultant Urogynaecologist/Honorary Senior Lecturer
Department of Urogynaecology
King's College Hospital
London, UK

Jonathan D.C. Ross MD, FRCP
Professor of Sexual Health and HIV
Whittall Street Clinic
Birmingham, UK

Glynn Russell MBChB, FCPSA, FRCP, FRCPCH
Division of Neonatology
Imperial College Healthcare NHS Trust
London, UK

Philip Savage PhD, FRCP
Consultant in Medical Oncology
Charing Cross Hospital
Imperial Hospitals NHS Trust
London, UK

Michael Seckl PhD, FRCP
Director
Charing Cross Gestational Trophoblastic Disease Centre and
Supraregional Tumour Masker Assay Service
Charing Cross Hospital
Imperial College NHS Healthcare Trust
London, UK

Mahmood I. Shafi MB, Bch, MD, DA, FRCOG
Consultant Gynaecological Surgeon and Oncologist
Addenbrookes Hospital
Cambridge, UK

Anthony R.B. Smith MD, FRCOG
The Warrell Unit
St Mary's Hospital
Manchester, UK

Gordon C.S. Smith MD, PhD
Department of Obstetrics and Gynaecology
The Rosie Hospital
Addenbrookes NHS Trust
Cambridge, UK

Maria C. Smith MD, MRCOG
Senior Lecturer/Consultant Obstetrician
Reproductive and Vascular Biology Group
Institute of Cellular Medicine
Newcastle University
Newcastle upon Tyne, UK

Catriona M. Stalder MBChB, MRCOG
Consultant Obstetrician & Gynaecologist
Queen Charlotte's & Chelsea Hospital
London, UK

Peter Stewart MA (Oxon), BMBCH (Oxon), FRCOG
Royal Hallamshire Hospital
Sheffield, UK

R. William Stones MD, FRCOG
The Puribai Kanji Jamal Professor and Chair
Department of Obstetrics and Gynaecology
Aga Khan University
Nairobi, Kenya

Allan Templeton CBE, MD, FRCOG, FRCP, FMedSci
University of Aberdeen
Aberdeen Maternity Hospital
Aberdeen, UK

Andrew J. Thompson BSc, MD, MRCOG
Consultant Obstetrician and Gynaecologist
Royal Alexandra Hospital
Paisley, UK

Geoffrey Trew MBBS, MRCOG
Hammersmith Hospital
London, UK

James J. Walker MD, FRCP, FRCOG, FRSM
Department of Obstetrics and Gynaecology
St James's University Hospital
Leeds, UK

Jason Waugh BSc (hons), MBBS, DA, MRCOG
Consultant Obstetrics and Maternal Medicine
Royal Victoria Infirmary
Newcastle upon Tyne, UK

Catherine Williamson MD
Institute of Reproductive and Developmental Biology
Imperial College London
London, UK

Ruwan C. Wimalasundera BSc, MBBS, MRCOG
Consultant Obstetrician & Lead for Fetal Medicine
Queen Charlotte's & Chelsea Hospital
Imperial College NHS Healthcare Trust
London, UK

Sarah Winfield BSc, MBBS, MRCOG
Consultant Obstetrician
Leeds Teaching Hospitals NHS Trust
Leeds, UK

Professor Sir John Dewhurst

Professor Sir John Dewhurst died on 1 December 2006. Jack, as he was known to all his colleagues, was a doyen amongst obstetricians and gynaecologists of the twentieth century. His reputation was internationally renowned and he became a worldwide expert in paediatric and adolescent gynaecology, for which he received due accolade. He was also an outstanding teacher of obstetrics and gynaecology, and, as such, this textbook, which he began in the 1970s, is testament to his dedication to the passing on of knowledge to others. In 1976 he became President of the Royal College of Obstetricians and Gynaecologists, a post he held for 3 years, for which he was subsequently knighted. He retired in 1986 after a long and distinguished career, but his legacy lives on and he will be remembered with great affection and professional respect by all who knew him.

Keith Edmonds
December 2011

Preface to the Eighth Edition

As I write this, it is almost 40 years since the 1st edition of *Dewhurst's Postgraduate Obstetrics and Gynaecology* was published. There are only a very few books that have stood the test of such longevity and it is a tribute to the concept that Jack Dewhurst had that the book continues now into its 8th edition. Jack's concept was to provide the postgraduate student with an advanced and integrated text for education and it is that philosophy which carries into this, the 8th, edition. No textbook can be totally comprehensive, and any postgraduate student reading this text we hope will be stimulated by the knowledge gained to go on and acquire further, more in-depth and specialist knowledge.

This edition has been redesigned with the hope that the readers will acquire knowledge in as quick and as comprehensive a way as possible. The specialty continues to develop and advance and gynaecology particularly is becoming increasingly a medical specialty and less of a surgical one. This of course is to the benefit of women as therapeutic advances offer them an increasing range of options to improve their quality of life. Obstetrics becomes increasingly focused on differentiating between the normal and the complicated pregnancy, with increasing emphasis on improved treatments for medically compromised mothers and fetuses and subsequently neonates. Again, quality of life is the overriding tenet as the practice of obstetrics and gynaecology improves worldwide.

It is still extremely sad that a quarter of a million women die every year worldwide as a result of childbirth and it is hoped that this volume will make some contribution towards improving these figures.

Many new authors have accepted the challenge to contribute to this edition and, along with those authors who have contributed in the past, I offer my sincere thanks for the time and effort they have put into constructing their chapters. We hope we have done this in a way that the reader will find intellectually challenging and rewarding.

Finally, I would like to thank my secretary, Liz Manson, who has been the tower of strength behind the production of this volume, and also the team at Blackwell Publishing, which has changed several times during the nidation of this edition but has never wavered in their endeavour to achieve the final vision.

Keith Edmonds
December 2011

Preface to the First Edition

Our purpose in writing this book has been to produce a comprehensive account of what the specialist in training in obstetrics and gynaecology must know. Unfortunately for him, he must now know a great deal, not only about his own subject, but about certain aspects of closely allied specialties such as endocrinology, biochemistry, cytogenetics, psychiatry, etc. Accordingly we have tried to offer the postgraduate student not only an advanced textbook in obstetrics and gynaecology but one which integrates the relevant aspects of other subjects which nowadays impinge more and more on the clinical field.

To achieve this aim within, we hope, a reasonable compass we have assumed some basic knowledge which the reader will have assimilated throughout his medical training, and we have taken matters on from there. Fundamental facts not in question are stated as briefly as is compatible with accuracy and clarity, and discussion is then devoted to more advanced aspects. We acknowledge that it is not possible even in this way to provide all the detail some readers may wish, so an appropriate bibliography is provided with each chapter. Wherever possible we have tried to give a positive opinion and our reasons for holding it, but to discuss nonetheless other important views; this we believe to be more helpful than a complete account of all possible opinions which may be held. We have chosen moreover to lay emphasis on fundamental aspects of the natural and the disease processes which are discussed; we believe concentration on these basic physiological and pathological features to be important to the proper training of a specialist. Clinical matters are, of course, dealt with in detail too, whenever theoretical discussion of them is rewarding. There are, however, some clinical aspects which cannot, at specialist level, be considered in theory with real benefit; examples of these are how to palpate a pregnant woman's abdomen and how to apply obstetric forceps. In general these matters are considered very briefly or perhaps not at all; this is not a book on *how* things are done, but on how correct treatment is chosen, what advantages one choice has over another, what complications are to be expected, etc. Practical matters, we believe, are better learnt in practice and with occasional reference to specialized textbooks devoted solely to them.

A word may be helpful about the manner in which the book is set out. We would willingly have followed the advice given to Alice when about to testify at the trial of the Knave of Hearts in Wonderland, 'Begin at the beginning, keep on until you come to the end and then stop'. But this advice is difficult to follow when attempting to find the beginning of complex subjects such as those to which this book is devoted. Does the beginning lie with fertilization; or with the events which lead up to it; or with the genital organs upon the correct function of which any pregnancy must depend; or does it lie somewhere else? And which direction must we follow then? The disorders of reproduction do not lie in a separate compartment from genital tract disease, but each is clearly associated with the other for at least part of a woman's life. Although we have attempted to integrate obstetrics with gynaecology and with their associated specialties, some separation is essential in writing about them, and the plan we have followed is broadly this – we begin with the female child *in utero*, follow her through childhood to puberty, through adolescence to maturity, through pregnancy to motherhood, through her reproductive years to the climacteric and into old age. Some events have had to be taken out of order, however, although reiteration has been avoided by indicating to the reader where in the book are to be found other sections dealing with different aspects of any subject under consideration. We hope that our efforts will provide a coherent, integrated account of the field we have attempted to cover which will be to the satisfaction of our readers.

Sir John Dewhurst
1972

Section 1

Obstetrics

Part 1
Basic Science

Chapter 1
Maternal Physiology

Fiona Broughton Pipkin
Department of Obstetrics and Gynaecology, City Hospital, Nottingham, UK

The physiological changes of pregnancy are strongly proactive, not reactive, with the luteal phase of every ovulatory menstrual cycle 'rehearsing' for pregnancy [1]. Most pregnancy-driven changes are qualitatively in place by the end of the first trimester, only maturing in magnitude thereafter. This chapter gives a brief overview of the major changes.

Maternal response to pregnancy

Normal pregnancy evokes a systemic inflammatory response, which includes the endothelium [2]. This may explain the greater risk of cardiovascular disease in later life of parous women in comparison with nulliparous women. Markers of oxidative 'stress' rise progressively throughout the first and second trimesters, but plasma concentrations of some endogenous antioxidants, such as superoxide dismutase, rise in parallel. The free radical superoxide is generated through a variety of pathways, including placental ones, but is more damaging when converted to the peroxide radical, a reaction catalysed by free iron in the plasma. Increasing concern is being expressed about over-supplementation with iron, especially in conjunction with vitamin C (which increases absorption) in pregnant women without evidence of iron deficiency and several studies have shown evidence of increased oxidative stress in such women [3]. Conversely, the low dietary selenium intake in women in the UK may predispose to lower activity of the antioxidant glutathione peroxidase and thioredoxin systems in pregnancy.

Immunology

Only two types of fetal tissue come into direct contact with maternal tissues: the villous trophoblast and the extravillous trophoblast. Villous trophoblast, which is a continuous syncytium, is bathed in maternal blood but seems to be immunologically inert and never expresses HLA class I or class II molecules. Extravillous trophoblast is directly in contact with maternal endometrial/decidual tissues and does not express the major T-cell ligands, HLA-A or HLA-B; the HLA class I molecules which are expressed are the trophoblast-specific HLA-G and HLA-C and HLA-E. The decidual uterine natural killer (NK) cells, the main type of decidual lymphocyte, differ from those in the systemic circulation. They express surface killer immunoglobulin-like receptors (KIRs), which bind to HLA-C and HLA-G on trophoblast. HLA-E and HLA-G are effectively monomorphic, but HLA-C is polymorphic, with two main groups, HLA-C1 and the HLA-C2. The KIRs are very highly polymorphic, but again fall into two main classes, KIR-A (non-activating) and KIR-B (multiply activating). Thus the very polymorphic KIR in maternal tissues and the polymorphic HLA-C in the fetus make up a potentially very variable receptor–ligand system.

The effect of this on implantation has been inferred from indirect evidence. Both recurrent miscarriage and pre-eclampsia are associated with poor trophoblast invasion. The maternal KIR genotype may be AA, AB or BB. Since the identifiable trophoblast HLA-C allotypes are HLA-C1 and HLA-C2, there are nine possible combinations. It has been shown that if the maternal KIR haplotype is AA, and the trophoblast expresses any HLA-C2, then the possibility of miscarriage or pre-eclampsia is significantly increased. However, even one KIR-B provides protection [4]. HLA-C2 is highly inhibitory to trophoblast migration, and thus appears to need 'activating KIR' to overcome it.

The uterus

The first-trimester human embryo appears to gain nutrients histiotrophically, from the endometrial glands. These glandular secretions are rich in carbohydrates, lipids and growth factors and can well support early growth while the conceptus is small [5]. The outer third of the myometrium, as well as the endometrium, is anatomically changed by pregnancy, and once a pregnancy has gone beyond the first trimester, these changes appear to be irreversible. The most striking change is in the spiral arteries, which undergo extensive remodelling. Extravillous trophoblast attacks these vessels as interstitial cells within the stroma, and as endovascular cells within the vascular lumen. In normal pregnancy, the summed effects are the conversion of these vessels into floppy thin-walled vessels that do not respond to vasoconstrictor stimuli, so allowing the maximum flow to reach the placenta. This remodelling is only completed in the early second trimester, but is impaired in both pre-eclampsia and normotensive intrauterine growth restriction.

The uterus must be maintained in quiescence until labour is initiated. The mechanisms responsible for this have not been fully elucidated, but include locally-generated nitric oxide, probably acting through cyclic GMP or voltage-gated potassium channels, while a number of hormones such as prostacyclin, prostaglandin (PG)E₂ and calcitonin gene-related peptide act through G_s receptors, and are relaxatory.

The cardiovascular system

There is a significant fall in total peripheral resistance by 6 weeks' gestation to a nadir of about 40% by midgestation, resulting in a fall in afterload. This is 'perceived' as circulatory underfilling, which activates the renin–angiotensin–aldosterone system and allows the necessary expansion of the plasma volume (PV) (Fig. 1.1) [6,7]. By the late third trimester, the PV has increased from its baseline by about 50% in a first pregnancy and 60% in a second or subsequent pregnancy. The bigger the expansion, the bigger, on average, the birthweight of the baby. The total extracellular fluid volume rises by about 16% by term, so the percentage rise in PV is disproportionate to the whole. The plasma osmolality falls by about 10 mosmol/kg as water is retained.

The heart rate rises synchronously, by 10–15 bpm, so the cardiac output begins to rise [8]. There is probably a fall in baroreflex sensitivity as pregnancy progresses, and heart rate variability falls. Stroke volume rises a little later in the first trimester. These two factors push the cardiac output up by 35–40% in a first pregnancy, and by about 50% in later pregnancies; it can rise by a further third in labour (Fig. 1.2). Table 1.1 summarizes the percentage changes in some cardiovascular variables during pregnancy.

Measuring systemic arterial blood pressure in pregnancy is notoriously difficult, but there is now broad con-

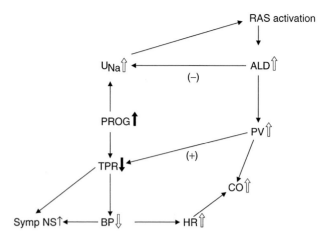

Fig. 1.1 Flow chart of the probable sequence of initial cardiovascular activation. ALD, aldosterone; BP, systemic arterial blood pressure; CO, cardiac output; HR, heart rate; PROG, progesterone; PV, plasma volume; RAS, renin–angiotensin system; Symp NS, sympathetic nervous system; TPR, total peripheral resistance; U_{Na}, urinary sodium excretion.

sensus that Korotkoff 5 should be used with auscultatory techniques [9]. However measured, there is a small fall in systolic, and a greater fall in diastolic, blood pressure during the first half of pregnancy, resulting in an increased pulse pressure. The blood pressure then rises steadily, in parallel with an increase in peripheral sympathetic activity, and even in normotensive women there may be some late overshoot of non-pregnant values. Supine hypotension occurs in about 8% of women in late gestation as the uterus falls back onto the inferior vena cava, reducing venous return.

The pressor response to angiotensin II is reduced in normal pregnancy but is unchanged to noradrenaline. The reduced sensitivity to angiotensin II presumably protects against the potentially pressor levels of angiotensin II found in normal pregnancy and is associated with lower receptor density; plasma noradrenaline is not increased in normal pregnancy. Pregnancy does not alter the response of intramyometrial arteries to a variety of vasoconstrictors. Nitric oxide may modulate myogenic tone and flow-mediated responses in the resistance vasculature of the uterine circulation in normal pregnancy.

The venous pressure in the lower circulation rises, for both mechanical and hydrodynamic reasons. The pulmonary circulation is able to absorb high rates of flow without an increase in pressure so pressure in the right ventricle, and the pulmonary arteries and capillaries, does not change. Pulmonary resistance falls in early pregnancy, and does not change thereafter. There is progressive venodilatation and rises in venous distensibility and capacitance throughout a normal pregnancy, possibly because of increased local nitric oxide synthesis.

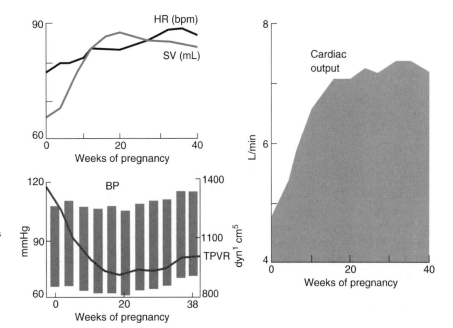

Fig. 1.2 Major haemodynamic changes associated with normal human pregnancy. The marked augmentation of cardiac output results from asynchronous increases in both heart rate (HR) and stroke volume (SV). Despite the increases in cardiac output, blood pressure (BP) decreases for most of pregnancy. This implies a very substantial reduction in total peripheral vascular resistance (TPVR).

Table 1.1 Percentage changes in some cardiovascular variables during pregnancy.

	First trimester	Second trimester	Third trimester
Heart rate (bpm)	+11	+13	+16
Stroke volume (mL)	+31	+29	+27
Cardiac output (L/min)	+45	+47	+48
Systolic blood pressure (mmHg)	−1	+1	+6
Diastolic blood pressure (mmHg)	−6	−3	+7
MPAP (mmHg)	+5	+5	+5
Total peripheral resistance (resistance units)	−27	−27	−29

MPAP, mean pulmonary artery pressure. Data are derived from studies in which pre-conception values were determined. The mean values shown are those at the end of each trimester and are thus not necessarily the maxima. Note that most changes are near maximal by the end of the first trimester.
Source: data from Robson *et al*. [8].

The respiratory system

Tidal volume rises by about 30% in early pregnancy to 40–50% above non-pregnant values by term, with a fall in expiratory reserve and residual volume (Fig. 1.3) [10]. Neither forced expiratory volume in 1 s (FEV_1) nor peak expiratory flow rate are affected by pregnancy, even in women with asthma. The rise in tidal volume is largely driven by progesterone, which appears to decrease the threshold and increase the sensitivity of the medulla oblongata to carbon dioxide. Respiratory rate does not change, so the minute ventilation rises by a similar amount. This over-breathing begins in every luteal phase; the P_{CO_2} is lowest in early gestation. Progesterone also increases erythrocyte carbonic anhydrase concentration, which will also lower P_{CO_2}. Carbon dioxide production rises sharply during the third trimester, as fetal metabolism increases. The fall in maternal P_{CO_2} allows more efficient placental transfer of carbon dioxide from the fetus, which has a P_{CO_2} of around 55 mmHg (7.3 kPa). The fall in P_{CO_2} results in a fall in plasma bicarbonate concentration (to about 18–22 mmol/L compared with the normal of 24–28 mmol/L), which contributes to the fall in plasma osmolality; the peripheral venous pH rises slightly (Table 1.2 and Fig. 1.4).

The increased alveolar ventilation results in a much smaller proportional rise in P_{O_2} from about 96.7 to 101.8 mmHg (12.9–13.6 kPa). This increase is offset by the rightward shift of the maternal oxyhaemoglobin dissociation curve caused by an increase in 2,3-diphosphoglycerate (2,3-DPG) in the erythrocytes. This facilitates oxygen unloading to the fetus, which has both a much lower P_{O_2} (25–30 mmHg, 3.3–4.0 kPa) and a marked leftward shift of the oxyhaemoglobin dissociation curve, due to the lower sensitivity of fetal haemoglobin to 2,3-DPG.

There is an increase of about 16% in oxygen consumption by term due to increasing maternal and fetal demands. Since the increase in oxygen-carrying capacity of the blood (see section Haematology) is about 18%, there is

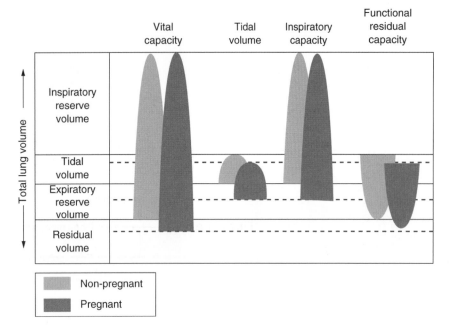

Fig. 1.3 Alterations in lung volumes associated with normal human pregnancy. In general terms, inspiratory reserve and tidal volumes increase at the expense of expiratory reserve and residual volumes.

Table 1.2 The influence of pregnancy on some respiratory variables.

	Non-pregnant	Pregnant – term
PO_2 (mmHg)	93 (12.5 kPa)	102 (13.6 kPa)
O_2 consumption (mL/min)	200	250
PCO_2 (mmHg)	35–40 (4.7–5.3 kPa)	30 (4.0 kPa)
Venous pH	7.35	7.38

Table 1.3 Although the increases in resting cardiac output and minute ventilation are of the same order of magnitude in pregnancy, there is less spare capacity for increases in cardiac output on moderate exercise than for increases in respiration.

	Resting	Exercise
Cardiac output	+33% (4.5–6 L/min)	+167% (up to 12 L/min)
Minute ventilation	+40% (7.5–10.5 L/min)	+1000% (up to ~80 L/min)

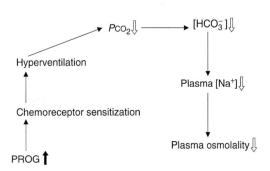

Fig. 1.4 Flow chart of the effects of over-breathing. HCO_3^-, bicarbonate; Na^+, sodium; PCO_2, carbon dioxide tension; PROG, progesterone.

actually a fall in arteriovenous oxygen difference. Pulmonary blood flow, of course, rises in parallel with cardiac output and enhances gas transfer.

Pregnancy places greater demands on the cardiovascular than the respiratory system [11]. This is shown in the response to moderate exercise (Table 1.3).

Haematology

The circulating red cell mass rises by 20–30% during pregnancy, with increases in both cell number and size. It rises more in women with multiple pregnancies, and substantially more with iron supplementation (~29% compared with 17%). Serum iron concentration falls, the absorption of iron from the gut rises and iron-binding capacity rises in a normal pregnancy, since there is increased synthesis of the β_1-globulin, transferrin. Plasma folate concentration halves by term, because of greater renal clearance, although red cell folate concentrations fall less. In the late 1990s, one-fifth of the female population aged 16–64 in the UK were estimated to have serum ferritin levels below 15 µg/L, indicative of low irons stores [12]; a similar survey appears not to have been undertaken since then (UK Scientific Advisory Committee on Nutrition Report

2008). Pregnant adolescents seem to be at particular risk of iron deficiency. Even relatively mild maternal anaemia is associated with increased placental weight/birthweight ratios and decreased birthweight. However, inappropriate supplementation can itself be associated with pregnancy problems (see above) [13]. Erythropoietin rises in pregnancy, more so if iron supplementation is not taken (55% compared with 25%) but the changes in red cell mass antedate this; human placental lactogen may stimulate haematopoiesis.

Pro rata, the PV increases more than the red cell mass, which leads to a fall in the various concentration measures that incorporate the PV, such as the haematocrit, haemoglobin concentration and red cell count. The fall in packed cell volume from about 36% in early pregnancy to about 32% in the third trimester is a sign of normal plasma volume expansion.

The total white cell count rises, mainly because of increased polymorphonuclear leucocytes. Neutrophil numbers rise with oestrogen concentrations and peak at about 33 weeks, stabilizing after that until labour and the early puerperium, when they rise sharply. Their phagocytic function increases during gestation. T and B lymphocyte counts do not change but their function is suppressed, making pregnant women more susceptible to viral infections, malaria and leprosy. The uterine NK cells express receptors that recognize the otherwise anomalous combination of human lymphocyte antigens (HLA-C, -E and -G) expressed by the invasive cytotrophoblasts. This is likely to be central to the maternal recognition of the conceptus [14] (see above).

Platelet count and platelet volume are largely unchanged in most pregnant women, although their survival is reduced. Platelet reactivity is increased in the second and third trimesters and does not return to normal until about 12 weeks after delivery.

Coagulation

Continuing low-grade coagulopathy is a feature of normal pregnancy [15]. Several of the potent procoagulatory factors rise from at least the end of the first trimester (Fig. 1.5). For example, factors VII, VIII and X all rise, and absolute plasma fibrinogen doubles, while antithrombin III, an inhibitor of coagulation, falls. The erythrocyte sedimentation rate rises early in pregnancy due to the increase in fibrinogen and other physiological changes. Protein C, which inactivates factors V and VIII, is probably unchanged in pregnancy, but concentrations of protein S, one of its cofactors, fall during the first two trimesters. An estimated 5–10% of the total circulating fibrinogen is consumed during placental separation, and thromboembolism is one of the main causes of maternal death in the UK. Plasma fibrinolytic activity is decreased during pregnancy and labour, but returns to non-pregnant values within an hour of delivery of the

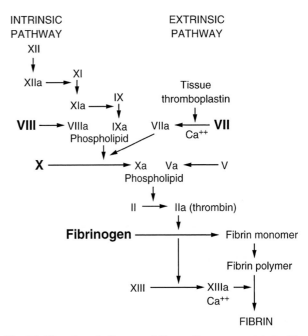

Fig. 1.5 Alterations in the coagulation pathways associated with human pregnancy. Factors which increase during normal pregnancy are in bold type. Modified from Letsky EA. The haematological system. In: Chamberlain G, Broughton Pipkin F (eds) *Clinical Physiology in Obstetrics*, 3rd edn. Oxford: Blackwell Science, 1998: 71–110.

Table 1.4 Percentage changes in some coagulation (upper) and fibrinolytic variables and fibronectin levels are expressed from postpartum data in the same women. The mean values shown are those at the end of each trimester and are thus not necessarily the maxima. Note the very large rise in PAI-2 (placental type PAI) and TAT III complexes in the first trimester.

	First trimester	Second trimester	Third trimester
PAI-1 (mg/mL)	−10	+68	+183
PAI-2 (mg/mL)	+732	+1804	+6554
t-PA (mg/mL)	−24	−19	+63
Protein C (% activity)	−12	+10	+9
AT III (% activity)	−21	−14	−10
TAT III	+362	+638	+785
Fibronectin (mg/L)	+3	−12	+53

PAI, plasminogen activator inhibitor; t-PA, tissue plasminogen activator antigen; AT III, antithrombin III; TAT III, thrombin–antithrombin III complex.
Source: Data from Halligan *et al.* [16].

placenta, suggesting strongly that the control of fibrinolysis during pregnancy is significantly affected by placentally derived mediators. Table 1.4 summarizes changes in some coagulation and fibrinolytic variables during pregnancy.

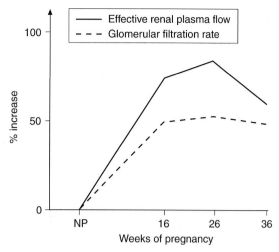

Fig. 1.6 The changes in renal function during pregnancy are largely complete by the end of the first trimester and are thus proactive not reactive to the demands of pregnancy. The filtration fraction falls during the first trimester but begins to return to non-pregnant levels during the third trimester. (Reproduced from Bayliss and Davison [17], with permission.)

The renal system

The kidneys increase in size in pregnancy mainly because renal parenchymal volume rises by about 70% with marked dilatation of the calyces, renal pelvis and ureters in most women [17]. Ureteric tone does not decrease, but bladder tone does. The effective renal plasma flow (ERPF) is increased by at least 6 weeks' gestation and rises to some 80% by mid-pregnancy falling thereafter to about 65% above non-pregnant values (Fig. 1.6). This increase is proportionally greater than the increase in cardiac output, presumably reflecting specific vasodilatation, probably via increased renal prostacyclin synthesis. The glomerular filtration rate (GFR) also increases, by about 45% by the ninth week, only rising thereafter by another 5–10%, but this is largely maintained to term, so the filtration fraction falls during the first trimester, is stable during the second, and rises towards non-pregnant values thereafter. However, these major increments do not exhaust the renal reserve. The differential changes in ERPF and GFR in late pregnancy suggest a mechanism acting preferentially at the efferent arterioles, possibly through angiotensin II.

The filtered load of metabolites therefore increases markedly, and reabsorptive mechanisms frequently do not keep up (e.g. glucose and amino acids; see below). These changes have profound effects on the concentrations of certain plasma metabolites and electrolytes and 'normal' laboratory reference ranges may thus be inappropriate in pregnancy. For example, plasma creatinine concentration falls significantly by the fourth week of gestation and continues to fall to mid-pregnancy, to below 50 mmol/L, but creatinine clearance begins to fall during the last couple of months of pregnancy, so plasma creatinine concentration rises again.

Total body water rises by about 20% during pregnancy (~8.5 L) with a very sharp fall in plasma osmolality between weeks 4 and 6 after conception, possibly through the actions of human chorionic gonadotrophin (hCG). The volume-sensing arginine vasopressin release mechanisms evidently adjust as pregnancy progresses. As well as water present in the fetus, amniotic fluid, placenta and maternal tissues, there is also oedema fluid and increased hydration of the connective tissue ground substance with laxity and swelling of connective tissue.

The pregnant woman accumulates some 950 mmol of sodium in the face of high circulating concentrations of progesterone, which competes with aldosterone at the distal tubule. The potentially natriuretic prostacyclin also rises markedly, with a small rise in atrial natriuretic peptide (ANP). This stimulates the renin–angiotensin system, with increased synthesis and release of aldosterone from the first trimester. The raised plasma prolactin may also contribute to sodium retention. It is assumed that glomerulotubular balance must also change in pregnancy to allow the sodium retention that actually occurs. There is a fall of some 4–5 mmol/L in plasma sodium by term, but plasma chloride does not change. Curiously, some 350 mmol of potassium are also retained during pregnancy, in the face of the much-increased GFR, substantially raised aldosterone concentrations and a relatively alkaline urine. Renal tubular potassium reabsorption evidently adjusts appropriately to the increased filtered potassium load.

Serum uric acid concentration falls by about one-quarter in early pregnancy, with an increase in its fractional excretion secondary to a decrease in net tubular reabsorption. The kidney excretes a progressively smaller proportion of the filtered uric acid, so some rise in serum uric acid concentration during the second half of pregnancy is normal. A similar pattern is seen in relation to urea, which is also partly reabsorbed in the nephron.

Glucose excretion may rise 10-fold as the greater filtered load exceeds the proximal tubular T_{max} for glucose (~1.6–1.9 mmol/min). If the urine of pregnant women is tested sufficiently often, glycosuria will be detected in 50%. The excretion of most amino acids increases, which is curious since these are used by the fetus to synthesize protein. The pattern of excretion is not constant, and differs between individual amino acids. Excretion of the water-soluble vitamins is also increased. The mechanism for all these is inadequate tubular reabsorption in the face of a 50% rise in GFR.

Urinary calcium excretion is also twofold to threefold higher in normal pregnancy than in the non-pregnant woman, even though tubular reabsorption is enhanced, presumably under the influence of the increased concentrations of 1,25-dihydroxyvitamin D. To counter this, intestinal absorption doubles by 24 weeks, after which it stabilizes. Renal bicarbonate reabsorption and hydrogen ion excretion appear to be unaltered during pregnancy. Although pregnant women can acidify their urine, it is usually mildly alkaline.

Total protein and albumin excretion both rise during pregnancy, to at least 36 weeks, due to the increased GFR, and changes in both glomerular and tubular function. Thus in late pregnancy, an upper limit of normal of 200 mg total protein excretion per 24-hour collection is accepted. The assessment of proteinuria in pregnancy using dipsticks has been shown to give highly variable data.

The gastrointestinal system

Taste often alters very early in pregnancy. The whole intestinal tract has decreased motility during the first two trimesters, with increased absorption of water and salt, tending to increase constipation. Heartburn is common as a result of increased intragastric pressure. Hepatic synthesis of albumin, plasma globulin and fibrinogen increases, the latter two sufficiently to give increased plasma concentrations despite the increase in PV. Total hepatic synthesis of globulin increases under oestrogen stimulation, so the hormone-binding globulins rise. There is decreased hepatic extraction of circulating amino acids.

The gallbladder increases in size and empties more slowly during pregnancy but the secretion of bile is unchanged. Cholestasis is almost physiological in pregnancy and may be associated with generalized pruritus but only rarely produces jaundice.

Energy requirements

The energy cost of pregnancy includes 'stored' energy in maternal and fetal tissues, and the greater energy expenditure needed for maintenance and physical activity. The weight gained during pregnancy arises from the products of conception, the increased size of maternal tissues such as the uterus and breasts, and the greater maternal fat stores. The basal metabolic rate has risen by about 5% by the end of pregnancy in a woman of normal weight [18]. The average weight gain over pregnancy in a woman of normal body mass index (BMI) is about 12.5 kg. The average weight gain from pre-pregnancy values at 6–18 months after delivery is 1–2 kg, but in about one-fifth of women can be 5 kg or more [19]. Obese women usually put on less weight during pregnancy, but retain more post partum. A 5-year follow-up of nearly 3000 women found that parous women gained 2–3 kg more than nulliparous women during this time. They also had significantly greater increases in waist/hip ratio, an independent risk factor for future cardiovascular disease [20].

Carbohydrates/insulin resistance

Pregnancy is hyperlipidaemic and glucosuric. Although neither the absorption of glucose from the gut nor the half-life of insulin seem to change, and the insulin response is well-maintained, by 6–12 weeks' gestation fasting plasma glucose concentrations have fallen by 0.11 mmol/L, and by the end of the first trimester the increase in blood glucose following a carbohydrate load is less than outside pregnancy [21]. This increased sensitivity stimulates glycogen synthesis and storage, deposition of fat and transport of amino acids into cells. The uptake of amino acids by the mother for gluconeogenesis may also be enhanced. After mid-pregnancy, resistance to the action of insulin develops progressively and plasma glucose concentrations rise, though remaining below non-pregnant levels (Fig. 1.7). Glucose crosses the placenta readily and the fetus uses glucose as its primary energy substrate, so this rise is presumably beneficial to the fetus. Fetal and maternal glucose concentrations are significantly correlated.

The insulin resistance is presumably largely endocrine-driven, possibly via increased cortisol or human placental lactogen. Plasma leptin concentrations are directly correlated with insulin resistance during pregnancy [22] while concentrations of glucagons and the catecholamines are unaltered. Adiponectin concentrations fall in pregnancy and are negatively correlated with fasting insulin concentrations and white fat mass. Adiponectin concentrations are also low in other insulin-resistant states, but whether this is cause or effect is still uncertain.

Lipids

Total plasma cholesterol falls early in pregnancy, reaching its lowest point at 6–8 weeks, but then rises to term. There is a striking increase in circulating free fatty acids and complex lipids in pregnancy, with approximately three-fold increases in very low density lipoprotein (VLDL) triglycerides and a 50% increase in VLDL cholesterol by 36 weeks [23], which is probably driven by oestrogens. High-density lipoprotein (HDL) cholesterol is also increased. Birthweight and placental weight are directly related to maternal VLDL triglyceride levels at term. The hyperlipidaemia of normal pregnancy is not atherogenic because the pattern of increase is not that of atherogenesis, although pregnancy can unmask pathological hyperlipidaemia.

Lipids undergo peroxidation in all tissues as part of normal cellular function. Excess production of lipid can result in oxidative stress, with damage to the cell membrane. During normal pregnancy, increases in plasma lipid peroxides appear by the second trimester in step with the general rise in lipids and may taper off later in gestation [24]. As the peroxide levels rise so do those of vitamin E and some other antioxidants; this rise is proportionately greater than that of peroxides so

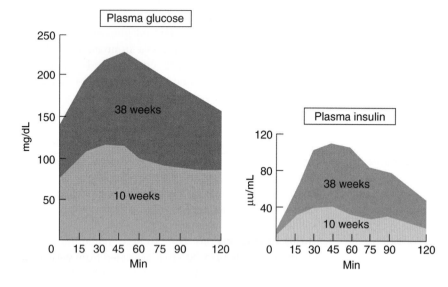

Fig. 1.7 Responses in normal pregnant women to a 50-g oral glucose load during early and late pregnancy. During early pregnancy there is a normal plasma insulin response with a relative reduction in plasma glucose concentrations compared with the non-pregnant state. In contrast, during late pregnancy plasma glucose concentrations reach higher levels after a delay despite a considerably enhanced insulin response, a pattern which could be explained by relative resistance to insulin.

physiological activities are protected. Lipid peroxidation is also active in the placenta, increasing with gestation. Since the placenta contains high concentrations of unsaturated fats under conditions of low Pao_2, antioxidants such as vitamin A, the carotenoids and provitamin A carotenoids are required to protect both mother and fetus from free radical activity.

Early in pregnancy fat is deposited but from mid-pregnancy it is also used as a source of energy, mainly by the mother so that glucose is available for the growing fetus [25] and to provide energy stores for the high metabolic demands of late pregnancy and lactation. The accurate measurement of pregnancy-related fat deposition is technically difficult, but total accretion is estimated at about 2–6 kg. The absorption of fat from the intestine is not directly altered during pregnancy. The hormone leptin acts as a sensor alerting the brain to the extent of body fat stores. Concentrations rise threefold during pregnancy and are directly correlated with total body fat; they are not related to the basal metabolic rate during gestation. Recent animal studies suggest that the hypothalamus, which contains the appetite-regulating centres, is desensitized to the effects of leptin in pregnancy. This allows the mother to eat more than she otherwise would consider doing, with consequent fat deposition.

Endocrine systems

The placenta is a powerhouse of hormone production from the beginning of gestation and challenges the mother's autonomy.

Placental hormones

hCG is the signal for pregnancy, but indirect effects, such as the oestrogen-driven increased hepatic synthesis of the binding globulins for thyroxine, corticosteroids and the sex steroids, also affect the mother's endocrinological function. The fetoplacental unit synthesizes very large amounts of oestrogens and progesterone, both probably being concerned with uterine growth and quiescence and with mammary gland development. However, they also stimulate synthesis of a variety of other important hormones. Oestrogens stimulate both the synthesis of vascular endothelial growth factor (VEGF) and its tyrosine kinase receptors and angiogenesis; the two are linked. VEGF appears to interact with other placentally produced hormones and angiopoietin-2 as major players in the development of the villous capillary bed in early human pregnancy. The peroxisome proliferator-activated receptor-γ (PPARγ) is a member of the nuclear receptor superfamily and has an important role in modulating expression of numerous other genes. It is expressed in human villous and extravillous cytotrophoblast. PPARγ binds to, and is activated by, natural ligands such as eicosanoids, fatty acids and oxidized low-density lipoproteins. Studies in knockout mice have shown it to be essential for placental development.

The hypothalamus and pituitary gland

The pituitary gland increases in weight by 30% in first pregnancies and by 50% subsequently. The number of lactotrophs is increased and plasma prolactin begins to rise within a few days of conception and by term may be 10–20 times as high as in the non-pregnant woman; the secretion of other anterior pituitary hormones is unchanged or reduced. hCG and the gonadotrophins share a common α-subunit, and the rapidly rising hCG concentration suppresses secretion of both follicle-stimulating hormone and luteinizing hormone, thus inhibiting ovarian follicle development by a blunting of response to gonadotrophin-releasing hormone.

Thyroid-stimulating hormone (TSH) secretion responds normally to hypothalamic thyrotropin-releasing hormone (also synthesized in the placenta). Adrenocorticotrophic hormone (ACTH) concentrations rise during pregnancy, partly because of placental synthesis of ACTH and of a corticotrophin-releasing hormone and do not respond to normal control mechanisms.

The adrenal gland

Both the plasma total and the unbound cortisol and other corticosteroid concentrations rise in pregnancy, from about the end of the first trimester. Concentrations of cortisol-binding globulin double. Excess glucocorticoid exposure *in utero* appears to inhibit fetal growth in both animals and humans. However, the normal placenta synthesizes a pregnancy-specific 11β-hydroxysteroid dehydrogenase, which inhibits transfer of maternal cortisol. The marked rise in secretion of the mineralocorticoid aldosterone in pregnancy has already been mentioned. Synthesis of the weaker mineralocorticoid 11-deoxycorticosterone is also increased by the eighth week of pregnancy, and actually increases proportionally more than any other cortical steroid, possibly due to placental synthesis.

The measurement of plasma catecholamines has inherent difficulties, but there is now broad consensus that plasma catecholamine concentrations fall from the first to the third trimester. There is some blunting of the rise in noradrenaline (reflecting mainly sympathetic nerve activity) seen on standing and isometric exercise in pregnancy, but the adrenaline response (predominantly adrenal) is unaltered [26].

The thyroid gland

hCG may suppress TSH in early pregnancy because they share a common α-subunit. The thyroid remains normally responsive to stimulation by TSH and suppression by triiodothyronine (T3). There is a threefold rise in the thyroid's clearance of iodine, allowing the absolute iodine uptake to remain within the non-pregnant range. Thyroid-binding globulin concentrations double during pregnancy, but other thyroid-binding proteins do not increase. Overall, free plasma T3 and thyroxine (T4) concentrations remain at the same levels as outside pregnancy (although total levels are raised), and most pregnant women are euthyroid. Free T4 may fall in late gestation [27].

Calcitonin, another thyroid hormone, rises during the first trimester, peaks in the second and falls thereafter, although the changes are not large. It may contribute to the regulation of 1,25-dihydroxyvitamin D.

The parathyroid glands and calcium metabolism

Calcium homeostasis changes markedly in pregnancy [28,29]. Maternal total plasma calcium falls because albumin concentration falls, but unbound ionized calcium is unchanged. Synthesis of 1,25-dihydroxycholecalciferol increases, promoting enhanced gastrointestinal calcium absorption. Parathyroid hormone (PTH) regulates the synthesis of 1,25-dihydroxyvitamin D in the proximal convoluted tubule. There is a fall in intact PTH during pregnancy but a doubling of 1,25-dihydroxyvitamin D; PTH-related protein (PTHrP) is also present in the maternal circulation. The main sources of PTHrP are the fetal parathyroid gland and the placenta. It is presumably placentally derived PTHrP that is transferred into the maternal circulation and affects calcium homeostasis by acting through the PTH receptor.

Renal hormones

The renin–angiotensin system is activated from very early in pregnancy (see section on the cardiovascular system above). A vasodilator component to the renin–angiotensin system has recently been described in which angiotensin 1–7 is the agonist; angiotensin 1–7 rises during pregnancy and may stimulate release of both nitric oxide and prostacyclin. Synthesis of erythropoietin appears to be stimulated by hCG; its concentration rises from the first trimester, peaking in mid-gestation and falling somewhat thereafter. Prostacyclin is a potent vasodilator, synthesized mainly in the renal endothelium. Concentrations begin to rise rapidly by 8–10 weeks of gestation, being fourfold higher than non-pregnant values by the end of the first trimester.

The pancreas

The size of the islets of Langerhans and the number of β cells increase during pregnancy, as does the number of receptor sites for insulin. The functions of the pancreas in pregnancy are considered above.

The endothelium

The endothelium synthesizes a variety of hormones, both vasodilator (e.g. prostacyclin, VEGF-A, nitric oxide) and vasoconstrictor (e.g. endothelin-1). The vasodilators are mostly upregulated in pregnancy, and allow the early fall in total peripheral resistance. Interestingly, although the lipid profile in pregnancy appears to be atherogenic, endothelial function in normal pregnancy, as assessed by flow-mediated dilatation, is not impaired. This may be due to the increased oestradiol concentrations, which upregulate endothelial nitric oxide synthase.

Conclusion

This chapter attempts to outline the physiology of normal pregnancy. The changes mostly begin very early indeed, and it may be that two of the major problems of pregnancy, intrauterine growth retardation and pre-eclampsia, are initiated even before the woman knows that she is pregnant. Better understanding of the mechanisms of very early normal pregnancy adaptation may help us to understand the abnormal.

Summary box 1.1

- Each ovulatory menstrual cycle prepares the potential mother for the physiological changes of pregnancy. Progesterone is the prime mover, and before conception initiates such changes as increased tidal volume, heart rate and glomerular filtration rate, as well as endometrial priming. These changes are proactive, not reactive, and in normal pregnancy are greater than physiologically necessary.
- Early pregnancy is associated with a systemic inflammatory response. The mother's immune response is altered to allow implantation and placentation and the remodelling of the spiral arteries.
- Total peripheral resistance falls very early, followed by the blood pressure; plasma volume and cardiac output rise. Alveolar ventilation and oxygen-carrying capacity increase more than oxygen consumption. Even normal pregnancy is associated with low-grade coagulopathy.
- Renal filtration increases very early. The rise in filtered sodium load activates the renin–angiotensin system, allowing sodium retention and the increased plasma volume. Plasma concentrations of various analytes are reduced both because of increased filtration and plasma volume expansion. Aminoaciduria and glycosuria are common.
- The average weight gain over pregnancy in a woman of normal BMI is about 12.5 kg. Some of this is usually retained after delivery. Pregnancy is associated with insulin resistance and hyperlipidaemia; there is considerable fat deposition.
- The placenta is a powerhouse of hormone and cytokine synthesis, modifying the mother's physiology for the demands of pregnancy.

References

1 Chapman AB, Zamudio S, Woodmansee W *et al*. Systemic and renal hemodynamic changes in the luteal phase of the menstrual cycle mimic early pregnancy. *Am J Physiol* 1997;273: F777–F782.

2 Redman CWG, Sargent IL. Placental stress and pre-eclampsia: a revised view. *Placenta* 2009;30(Suppl 1):38–42.

3 Milman N. Iron and pregnancy: a delicate balance. *Ann Haematol* 2006;85:559–565.

4 Moffett A, Hiby SE. How does the maternal immune system contribute to the development of pre-eclampsia? *Placenta* 2007;28(Suppl. 1):S51–S56.

5 Burton GJ, Jauniaux E, Charnock-Jones DS. Human early placental development: potential roles of the endometrial glands. *Placenta* 2007;28(Suppl 1):S64–S69.

6 Chapman AB, Abraham WT, Zamudio S *et al*. Temporal relationships between hormonal and hemodynamic changes in early human pregnancy. *Kidney Int* 1998;54:2056–2063.

7 Ganzevoort W, Rep A, Bonsel GJ, de Vries JI, Wolf H. Plasma volume and blood pressure regulation in hypertensive pregnancy. *J Hypertension* 2004;22:1235–1242.

8 Robson SC, Hunter S, Boys RJ, Dunlop W. Serial study of factors influencing changes in cardiac output during human pregnancy. *Am J Physiol* 1989;256:H1060–H1065.

9 de Swiet M, Shennan A. Blood pressure measurement in pregnancy. *Br J Obstet Gynaecol* 1996;103:862–863.

10 de Swiet M. The respiratory system. In: Chamberlain G, Broughton Pipkin F (eds) *Clinical Physiology in Obstetrics*, 3rd edn. Oxford: Blackwell Science, 1998: 111–128.

11 Bessinger RC, McMurray RG, Hackney AC. Substrate utilisation and hormonal responses to moderate intensity exercise during pregnancy and after delivery. *Am J Obstet Gynecol* 2002; 86:757–764.

12 Heath AL, Fairweather-Tait SJ. Clinical implications of changes in the modern diet: iron intake, absorption and status. *Best Pract Res Clin Haematol* 2002;15:225–241.

13 Scholl TO. Iron status during pregnancy: setting the stage for mother and infant. *Am J Clin Nutr* 2005;81:1218S–1222S.

14 Apps R, Murphy SP, Fernando R, Gardner L, Ahad T, Moffett A. Human leucocyte antigen (HLA) expression of primary trophoblast cells and placental cell lines, determined using single antigen beads to characterise allotype specificities of anti-HLA antibodies. *Immunology* 2009;127:26–39.

15 Brenner B. Haemostatic changes in pregnancy. *Thromb Res* 2004;114:409–414.

16 Halligan A, Bonnar J, Sheppard B, Darling M, Walshe J. Haemostatic, fibrinolytic and endothelial variables in normal pregnancies and pre-eclampsia. *Br J Obstet Gynaecol* 1994;101: 488–492.

17 Bayliss C, Davison JM. The urinary system. In: Chamberlain G, Broughton Pipkin F (eds) *Clinical Physiology in Obstetrics*, 3rd edn. Oxford: Blackwell Science, 1998: 263–307.

18 Butte NF, King JC. Energy requirements during pregnancy and lactation. *Public Health Nutrition* 2005;8:1010–1027.

19 Gunderson EP, Abrams B, Selvin S. Does the pattern of postpartum weight change differ according to pregravid body size? *Int J Obes Relat Metab Disord* 2001;25:853–862.

20 Gunderson EP. Childbearing and obesity in women: weight before, during, and after pregnancy. *Obstet Gynecol Clin North Am* 2009;36:317–332.

21 Butte NF. Carbohydrate and lipid metabolism in pregnancy: normal compared with gestational diabetes mellitus. *Am J Clin Nutr* 2000;71(5 Suppl):1256S–1261S.

22 Eriksson B, Löf M, Olausson H, Forsum E. Body fat, insulin resistance, energy expenditure and serum concentrations of leptin, adiponectin and resistin before, during and after pregnancy in healthy Swedish women. *Br J Nutr* 2010;103:50–57.

23 Herrera E, Ortega H, Alvino G, Giovannini N, Amusquivar E, Cetin I. Relationship between plasma fatty acid profile and antioxidant vitamins during normal pregnancy. *Eur J Clin Nutr* 2004;58:1231–1238.

24 Poston L, Raijmakers MT. Trophoblast oxidative stress, antioxidants and pregnancy outcome: a review. *Placenta* 2004;25(Suppl A):S72–S78.

25 Kopp-Hoolihan LE, van Loan MD, Wong WW, King JC. Longitudinal assessment of energy balance in well-nourished, pregnant women. *Am J Clin Nutr* 1999;69:697–704.

26 Barron WM, Mujais SK, Zinaman M, Bravo EL, Lindheimer MD. Plasma catecholamine responses to physiologic stimuli in normal human pregnancy. *Am J Obstet Gynecol* 1986;154: 80–84.

27 Ramsay ID. The thyroid gland. In: Chamberlain G, Broughton Pipkin F (eds) *Clinical Physiology in Obstetrics*, 3rd edn. Oxford: Blackwell Science, 1998: 374–384.

28 Prentice A. Maternal calcium metabolism and bone mineral status. *Am J Clin Nutr* 2000;71(5 Suppl):1312S–1316S.

29 Haig D. Evolutionary conflicts in pregnancy and calcium metabolism: a review. *Placenta* 2004;25(Suppl A):S10–S15.

Further reading

Broughton Pipkin F. Maternal physiology. In: Chamberlain G, Steer P (eds) *Turnbull's Obstetrics*, 3rd edn. London: Churchill Livingstone, 2001.

Chamberlain G, Broughton Pipkin F (eds) *Clinical Physiology in Obstetrics*, 3rd edn. Oxford: Blackwell Science, 1998.

Chapter 2
The Placenta and Fetal Membranes

Berthold Huppertz[1] and John C.P. Kingdom[2]
[1]Institute of Cell Biology, Histology and Embryology, Medical University of Graz, Graz, Austria
[2]Department of Obstetrics and Gynaecology, Samuel Lunenfeld Research Institute, Mount Sinai Hospital, Toronto, Canada

The placenta was already recognized and venerated by the early Egyptians, while it was the Greek physician Diogenes of Apollonia (*c.* 480 BC) who first ascribed the function of fetal nutrition to the organ. Aristotle (384 to 322 BC) reported that the chorion membranes fully enclose the fetus, but it was only in 1559 during the Renaissance that Realdus Columbus introduced the term 'placenta', derived from the Latin for a flat cake.

Structural characteristics of the human placenta

Placental shape

On the gross anatomic level, the placenta of eutherian animals can be classified according to the physical interactions between fetal and maternal tissues [1]. Such interactions may be restricted to specific sites or may be found covering the whole surface of the chorionic sac and the inner uterine surface. On this gross anatomical level, the human placenta is classified as a *discoidal* placenta, confining interactions to a more or less circular area (Fig. 2.1a).

Materno-fetal interdigitations

The next level of classification is based on the interdigitations between maternal and fetal tissues. In the human placenta maternal and fetal tissues are arranged is such a way that there are three-dimensional tree-like structures called *villous trees* of fetal tissues that float in a lake of maternal blood [1]. Like the knots and branches of a tree, the fetal tissues repeatedly branch into smaller and slender villi (Fig. 2.1b).

Materno-fetal barrier

On the level of interactions between uterine and fetal tissues, the human displays an invasive type of implantation and placentation [1]. The uterine epithelium is penetrated, and invasion of fetal cells into maternal tissues results in erosion into maternal vessels leading to bathing of placental villi in the mother's blood. An epithelial layer termed *villous trophoblast*, which comes into direct contact with maternal blood and which builds the placental barrier between maternal and fetal tissues, covers placental villi (Fig. 2.1c).

This type of placentation is termed *haemomonochorial* since on the maternal side there is only blood and no longer blood vessels (haemo) and on the fetal side there is only one layer of trophoblast (monochorial) between maternal blood and the fetal capillaries (Fig. 2.1c).

Vascular arrangement

It is not only the thickness and exact histological nature of the placental barrier that defines the rate of diffusional exchange. Another important determinant is the direction of blood flows of mother and fetus in relation to each other. The vascular arrangement of the human placenta cannot be clearly defined due to the branching of the villous trees into all directions and a respective maternal blood flow somehow bypassing these branches. Therefore, this unpredictable and variable flow pattern has been termed *multivillous flow* (Fig. 2.1d) [1].

Summary box 2.1

- The human placenta is a discoidal placenta.
- The interdigitations between maternal and fetal tissues are arranged as tree-like structures called villous trees, which are surrounded by a multivillous flow of maternal blood.
- The villous trophoblast builds the placental barrier between maternal blood and fetal tissues (haemomonochorial placentation).

Macroscopic features of the term placenta

Measures

The placenta at term displays a round disc-like appearance, with insertion of the umbilical cord in a slightly

---

Dewhurst's Textbook of Obstetrics & Gynaecology, Eighth Edition. Edited by D. Keith Edmonds.
© 2012 John Wiley and Sons, Ltd. Published 2012 by John Wiley and Sons, Ltd.

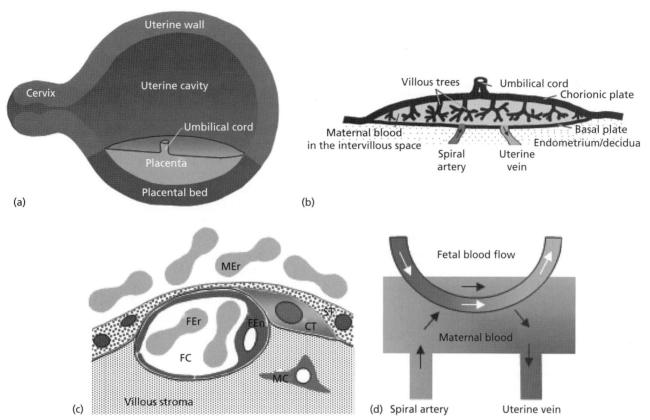

Fig. 2.1 Schematic representation of the structural characteristics of the human placenta. (a) The human placenta displays a discoidal shape. (b) The materno-fetal interdigitations are arranged in villous trees bathing in maternal blood that floats through the intervillous space. (c) The hemochorial type of placentation results in a materno-fetal barrier composed of villous trophoblast in direct contact with maternal blood. (d) Fetal and maternal blood flows are arranged in a multivillous flow. CT, cytotrophoblast; FC, fetal capillary; FEn, fetal endothelium; FEr, fetal erythrocyte; MC, mesenchymal cells; MEr, maternal erythrocyte; ST, syncytiotrophoblast.

eccentric position on the fetal side of the placenta [1]. The average measures of a delivered placenta at term are as follows: diameter 22 cm, central thickness 2.5 cm, and weight 450–500 g. However, one has to keep in mind that these data may vary considerably due to the mode of delivery, especially content versus loss of maternal and/ or fetal blood.

Tissue arrangements

On the fetal side of the placenta, the avascular *amnion* covers the *chorionic plate*. Underneath the amnion, chorionic vessels continue with those of the umbilical cord and are arranged in a star-like pattern. At the other end, these vessels continue with those of the villous trees where the capillary system between arteries and veins is located. The villous trees originate from the chorionic plate and float in a lake of maternal blood [1]. On the maternal side of the placenta, the *basal plate* is located (Fig. 2.1b). It is an artificial surface generated by separation of the placenta from the uterine wall during delivery. The basal plate is a colourful mixture of fetal trophoblasts and maternal cells of the decidua, all of which are embedded in trophoblast-secreted matrix-type fibrinoid, decidual extracellular matrices, and fibrin-type fibrinoid. At the placental margin, chorionic plate and basal plate fuse with each other, thereby closing the intervillous space and generating the *fetal membranes* or *chorion laeve*.

Summary box 2.2

The layers of a delivered placenta from the fetal to the maternal side comprise:

- avascular amnion (epithelium and mesenchyme)
- vascularized chorionic plate (mesenchyme with blood vessels)
- villous trees directly connected to the chorionic plate
- maternal blood in the intervillous space surrounding the villous trees
- basal plate with a mixture of fetal and maternal cells.

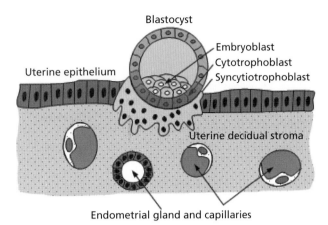

Fig. 2.2 During implantation of the blastocyst, trophoblast cells in direct contact with maternal tissues syncytially fuse and give rise to the syncytiotrophoblast. Only this multinucleated tissue is able to penetrate the uterine epithelium and to implant the developing embryo.

Placental development

Trophoblast lineage

At the transition between morula and blastocyst, the trophoblast lineage is the first to differentiate from the inner cell mass, the embryoblast (Fig. 2.2) [2]. Only after attachment of the blastocyst to the endometrial epithelium does further differentiation of the trophoblast occur. Exact knowledge of the processes in the human is still lacking, but it is anticipated that at this stage the first syncytial fusion of trophoblasts takes place. Fusion of those trophoblasts in direct contact with maternal tissues as well as the embryoblast generates the very first syncytiotrophoblast and only this layer is able to penetrate the uterine epithelium (Fig. 2.2).

Prelacunar stage

At day 7–8 post conception, the blastocyst has completely crossed the epithelium and is embedded within the endometrium. The developing embryo is completely surrounded by the growing placenta, which at this stage consists of the two fundamental subtypes of the trophoblast. The multinucleated syncytiotrophoblast is in direct contact with maternal tissues, while the mononucleated cytotrophoblast as the stem cell layer of the trophoblast is directed towards the embryo.

All the differentiation and developmental stages of the placenta described so far take place before fluid-filled spaces within the syncytiotrophoblast can be detected. This is why this stage is termed 'prelacunar' [1].

Lacunar stage

At day 8–9 post conception, the syncytiotrophoblast generates a number of fluid-filled spaces within its mass.

These spaces flow together forming larger lacunae (*lacunar stage*), and are finally separated by parts of the syncytiotrophoblast (trabeculae) that cross the syncytial mass from the embryonic to the maternal side [1].

At the end of this stage, at day 12 post conception, the process of implantation is completed. The developing embryo with its surrounding extraembryonic tissues is totally embedded in the endometrium, and the syncytiotrophoblast surrounds the whole surface of the conceptus. Mesenchymal cells derived from the embryo spread over the inner surface of the trophoblast (the extraembryonic mesoderm), thus generating a new combination of trophoblast and mesoderm, termed *chorion*.

The development of the lacunar system subdivides the placenta into its three compartments.
1 The embryonically oriented part of the trophoblast together with extraembryonic mesoderm will develop into the *chorionic plate*.
2 The trabeculae will become the *anchoring villi*, while the growing branches will develop into *floating villi*. The lacunae surrounding the villi will turn into the *intervillous space*.
3 The maternally oriented part of the trophoblast together with components of maternal decidual tissues will develop into the *basal plate*.

Early villous stage

Starting on day 12 post conception, proliferation of cytotrophoblast pushes trophoblasts to penetrate the syncytial trabeculae, reaching the maternal side of the syncytiotrophoblast by day 14. Further proliferation of trophoblasts inside the trabeculae (day 13) stretches the trabeculae resulting in the development of syncytial side branches filled with cytotrophoblasts (primary villi) [1].

Shortly after, the mesenchymal cells from the extraembryonic mesoderm follow the cytotrophoblast and penetrate the trabeculae and the primary villi, thus generating *secondary villi* with a mesenchymal core. At this stage, there is always a complete cytotrophoblast layer between penetrating mesenchyme and syncytiotrophoblast.

Around day 20–21, vascularization (development of new vessels from haemangioblastic precursor cells) within the villous mesenchyme gives rise to the formation of first placental vessels (*tertiary villi*). Only later will the connection to the vessel system of the embryo proper be established via the umbilical cord.

The villi are organized in villous trees that cluster together into a series of spherical units known as lobules or placentomes. Each placentome originates from the chorionic plate by a thick villous trunk stemming from a trabecula. Continuous branching of the main trunk results in daughter villi mostly freely ending in the intervillous space, the floating villi.

Trophoblastic cell columns

During penetration of the syncytial trabeculae, the cytotrophoblasts reach the maternal endometrial tissues while the following mesenchymal cells do not penetrate to the tips of the trabeculae. At the tips of the anchoring villi multiple layers of cytotrophoblasts develop, referred to as trophoblastic *cell columns* (Fig. 2.3) [1,3]. Only those cytotrophoblasts remain as proliferative stem cells that are in direct contact with the basement membrane separating trophoblast from mesenchyme of the anchoring villi.

Subtypes of extravillous trophoblast

The formation of cell columns does not result in a complete layer of a trophoblastic shell but rather is mostly organized as separated columns from which extravillous trophoblasts invade into maternal uterine tissues (Fig. 2.3) [1]. All these cells migrate as interstitial trophoblast into the endometrial stroma [4], while a subset of the interstitial trophoblast further penetrates the wall of the uterine spiral arteries (*intramural trophoblast*), finally reaching the vessels' lumen (*endovascular trophoblast*) (Fig. 2.3) [5]. Another subset of the interstitial trophoblast penetrates the walls of uterine glands, finally opening such glands towards the intervillous space (*endoglandular trophoblast*) (Fig. 2.4) [6]. Some of the interstitial trophoblasts fuse and generate the *multinucleated trophoblast giant cells* (Fig. 2.4) at the boundary between endometrium and myometrium.

Plugging of spiral arteries

The invasion of extravillous trophoblasts is the ultimate means of transforming maternal vessels into large-bore conduits that enable adequate supply of oxygen and nutrients to the placenta [1,7]. However, free transfer of maternal blood to the intervillous space is only established at the end of the first trimester of pregnancy [8]. Before the free transfer of maternal blood can occur, the extent of invasion and thus the number of endovascular trophoblasts is so great that the trophoblasts aggregate within the vessel lumina and plug the distal segments of the spiral arteries (Fig. 2.3). Hence, before 10–12 weeks of gestation, the intervillous space contains mostly glandular secretion products from the eroded uterine glands together with a plasma filtrate that is free of maternal blood cells (*histiotrophic nutrition*) (Fig. 2.3) [8,9].

The reason for such a paradoxical plugging of already eroded and transformed arteries may be because the lack of blood cells keeps the placenta and the embryo in a low-oxygen environment of less than 20 mmHg in the first trimester of pregnancy. This low-oxygen environment may be necessary to reduce formation of free

Fig. 2.3 Schematic representation of the developing embryo and its surrounding tissues at about 8–10 weeks of pregnancy. The amnionic cavity with the embryo inside is marked off by the amnion that has already contacted the chorion. From the chorion, villous trees protrude into the intervillous space where some villi have direct contact with the basal plate (anchoring villi). At these sites trophoblastic cell columns are the source for all extravillous trophoblast cells invading maternal tissues. Interstitial trophoblast cells derived from these columns invade endometrium and myometrium, while a subset of these cells penetrates the spiral arteries first as intramural and then as endovascular trophoblast cells. Onset of maternal blood flow into the placenta starts in the upper regions of the placenta (the abembryonic pole) where development is slightly delayed. The local high concentrations of oxygen contribute to the regression of villi at the abembryonic pole. This in turn leads to the formation of the smooth chorion, the fetal membranes.

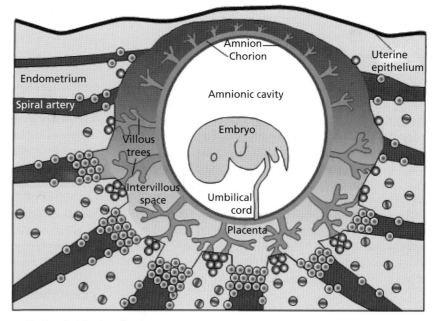

- ◉ Trophoblastic cell column
- ◉ Interstitial trophoblast
- ◉ Intramural/endovascular trophoblast

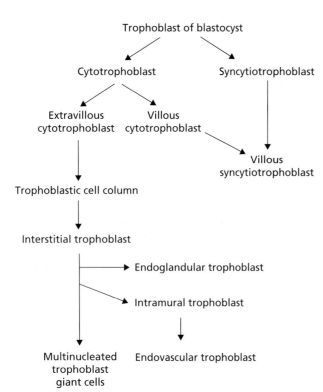

Fig. 2.4 Trophoblast differentiation and subtypes. The trophoblast lineage is the first to develop at the blastocyst stage. From this stage onwards, further differentiation leads to the generation of the syncytiotrophoblast and subsequently to the two main trophoblast types of placental villi, villous cytotrophoblast and villous syncytiotrophoblast. The trophoblast cells that start to invade maternal tissues are termed extravillous trophoblast. From the interstitital trophoblast all other subtypes of extravillous trophoblast develop.

Summary box 2.3

- Blastocyst stage: differentiation of the trophoblast lineage.
- Day 7–8 post conception: prelacunar stage of placental development.
- Day 8–9 post conception: lacunar stage of placental development.
- Day 12 post conception: implantation completed, embryo completely surrounded by placenta.
- Day 14 post conception: differentiation of extravillous trophoblast.
- Day 20 post conception: development of placental vessels and blood cells independent of vessel development in the embryo proper.
- First trimester: histiotrophic nutrition.
- Second and third trimester: haemotrophic nutrition.

radicals that affect the growing embryo in this critical stage of tissue and organ development [10,11].

Onset of maternal blood flow

At the end of the first trimester the trophoblastic plugs become pervious and maternal blood cells enter the inter-villous space, establishing the first arterial blood flow to the placenta (*haemotrophic nutrition*) [8,11]. The inflow starts in those upper parts of the placenta that are closer to the endometrial epithelium (the *abembryonic pole* of the placenta) (Fig. 2.3). These sites are characterized by a slight delay in development since the deeper parts at the *embryonic pole* have been the first to develop directly after implantation (Fig. 2.3). Therefore, at these upper sites the plugs inside the vessels contain fewer cells, enabling blood cells to penetrate the plugs earlier, and thus blood flow starts at these sites first. Here the placental villi degenerate in larger parts and the chorion becomes secondarily smooth. The regression leads to the formation of the fetal membrane or chorion laeve. The remaining part of the placenta develops into the *chorion frondosum*, the definitive disc-shaped placenta.

Basic structure of villi

Villous trophoblast

The branches of the syncytial trabeculae are the forerunners of the placental villi. Throughout gestation the syncytial cover remains and forms the placental barrier between maternal blood floating in the intervillous space and the fetal vessels within the mesenchymal core of the villi [1].

Villous cytotrophoblast

The layer of mononucleated villous *cytotrophoblast* cells is the basal layer of the villous trophoblast compartment resting on the basal lamina underneath the multi-nucleated layer of syncytiotrophoblast (see Fig. 2.1c) [1]. Villous cytotrophoblasts are a heterogeneous population: a subset proliferate throughout gestation (in contrast to the mouse, which terminally differentiates its chorionic trophoblast in mid-gestation), some exhibit a progenitor status because they can be induced to differentiate along the extravillous pathway, while others are in varying stages of differentiation, preparing for syncytial fusion directed by the transcription factor GCM1 (glial cell missing-1) [12,13]. The number of villous cytotrophoblasts continuously increases during pregnancy, from about 1×10^9 at 13–16 weeks to about 6×10^9 at 37–41 weeks of gestation. These cells are gradually dispersed into a discontinuous layer in the third trimester due to the rapid expansion and specialization of the peripheral placental villi responsible for gas and nutrient exchange.

Villous cytotrophoblasts do not normally come into direct contact with maternal blood, unless focal damage occurs to the overlying syncytiotrophoblast: if focal areas of syncytiotrophoblast are lost, for example due to focal necrosis, the deficit is filled with *fibrin-type fibrinoid* (a maternal blood clot product) that covers the exposed cytotrophoblasts [14].

Syncytiotrophoblast

The *syncytiotrophoblast* is a multinucleated layer without lateral cell borders, hence there is a single syncytiotrophoblast covering all villi of a single placenta [1]. Microvilli on its apical surface provide amplification of the surface (sevenfold) and are in direct contact with the maternal blood floating within the intervillous space (see Fig. 2.1c). Growth and maintenance of the syncytiotrophoblast is dependent on the fusion with the underlying cytotrophoblasts, since syncytial nuclei do not proliferate.

Within the syncytiotrophoblast the incorporated nuclei first exhibit a large and ovoid shape, while during maturation they become smaller and denser. Finally, they display envelope convolution, increased packing density and increased heterochromatinization [15]. These are the typical features of apoptosis, a physiological process in the normal placenta.

Syncytial fusion by far exceeds the needs for growth of the placental villi. Continuous syncytial fusion brings new cellular material into the syncytiotrophoblast including proteins like Bcl-2 and Mcl-1 that focally retard apoptosis [16]. Although a subset of syncytial nuclei is capable of RNA transcription in normal pregnancy [17], syncytial fusion remains critical for maintaining the functional and structural integrity of the syncytiotrophoblast, for example secretion of hormones such as chorionic gonadotrophin and the surface expression of energy-dependent transporters for the uptake of molecules such as glucose or amino acids. Consequently, the nuclei that are incorporated into the syncytiotrophoblast remain within this layer for at least 3–4 weeks. Then, the older nuclei accumulate and are packed into protrusions of the apical membrane known as *syncytial kots* [15].

Trophoblast turnover

Like every epithelium, the villous trophoblast exhibits the phenomenon of continuous turnover comprising [1]:

1 proliferation of a subset of cytotrophoblast progenitor cells;

2 differentiation of post-proliferative mononucleated daughter cells (2–3 days);

3 syncytial fusion of finally differentiated cells with the overlying syncytiotrophoblast;

4 further differentiation and maturation within the syncytiotrophoblast (3–4 weeks);

5 ageing and late apoptosis at specific sites of the syncytiotrophoblast;

6 packing of old material into syncytial knots; and finally

7 extrusion of membrane-sealed apoptotic corpuscles (syncytial knots) into the maternal circulation.

The majority of apoptotic syncytial knots are extruded from the syncytiotrophoblast surface into the maternal circulation [16]. In pathological pregnancies the molecular control of trophoblast differentiation is altered. In cases of severe early-onset intrauterine growth restriction

(IUGR) this physiology is likely disturbed in favour of greater apoptotic shedding, while in cases of pre-eclampsia this physiology is disturbed in favour of both greater apoptotic shedding and the release of necrotic and aponecrotic material into the maternal circulation [15,18].

Trophoblast release

Throughout gestation, syncytial knots are released into the maternal circulation and are mostly lodged in the capillary bed of the lung [19–21]. Hence, they can be found in uterine vein blood but not in arterial or peripheral venous blood of a pregnant woman. It has been estimated that in late gestation up to 150 000 such corpuscles or 2–3 g of trophoblast material can enter the maternal circulation each day [1].

Current knowledge places the multinucleated syncytial knots as products generated by apoptotic mechanisms [15,20]. As such, they are surrounded by a tightly sealed plasma membrane not releasing any content into the maternal blood. Hence, induction of an inflammatory response in the mother is not a normal feature of pregnancy. However, during placental pathologies with a disturbed trophoblast turnover such as pre-eclampsia, the release of syncytiotrophoblast material is altered [20,22,23]. This necrotic or aponecrotic release of trophoblast material could contribute to the endothelial damage typical of pre-eclampsia [19,20,22,23].

Villous stroma

The stromal villous core comprises the population of fixed and moving connective tissue cells, including:
- mesenchymal cells and fibroblasts in different stages of differentiation up to myofibroblasts [24];
- placental macrophages (Hofbauer cells); and
- placental vessels with smooth muscle cells and endothelial cells [1].

Oxygen as regulator of villous development

There is increasing recognition of the role that oxidative stress inside the placenta plays in the pathophysiology of pregnancy disorders ranging from miscarriage to pre-eclampsia [1,8,10,11,25,26]. During the first trimester, villous trophoblast is well adapted to low oxygen, and it appears that trophoblast is more susceptible to raised oxygen rather than low oxygen [20,27]. Hence, during the first trimester if the abembryonic part of the placenta is oxygenated by onset of maternal blood flow, villi display increased evidence of oxidative stress, become avascular and finally regress. These physiological changes result in the formation of the smooth chorion, the chorion laeve (see Fig. 2.3).

If such early onset of maternal blood flow and consequently early onset of oxygenation also occurs in the embryonic part of the placenta, damage to the whole placenta will result. The most severe cases are missed miscarriages, while less severe cases may continue but may lead to pathologies such as pre-eclampsia and IUGR [8,11]. It is becoming increasingly evident that the aetiology of pre-eclampsia involves increased oxidative stress, mostly without changes in the extravillous subset of trophoblast [28]. Recent data point to hyperoxic changes or to the occurrence of fluctuating oxygen concentrations [20,29].

Summary box 2.4

Villous trophoblast as the outermost epithelial layer of placental villi
- Cytotrophoblast: progenitor cells to maintain the syncytiotrophoblast throughout pregnancy.
- Syncytiotrophoblast: multinucleated, in direct contact with maternal blood.
- Syncytiotrophoblast: shedding of apoptotic material into maternal blood, at the end of gestation about 3 g daily.
- Pre-eclampsia: quantity and quality of syncytial shedding are altered. More fragments are released, mostly owing to necrosis and aponecrosis.

Villous stroma
- Mesenchymal cells and fibroblasts.
- Macrophages (Hofbauer cells).
- Vessels with media and endothelium.

Fetal membranes

During early embryonic development, the *amnionic cavity* increases in size and finally surrounds and encases the complete embryo. Fluid accumulation within the amnionic cavity leads to complete separation of the embryo from surrounding extraembryonic tissues, leaving only the developing umbilical cord as the connection between placenta and embryo. The amnionic mesenchyme comes into direct contact with the chorionic mesoderm lining the inner surface of the chorionic sac (see Fig. 2.3). Both tissue layers do not fuse, and it remains that amnion and chorion can easily slide against each other [1,30].

As described above, it is only at the implantation/embryonic pole that the definitive placenta develops. Owing to regression of villi, most of the surface of the chorionic sac (about 70%) develops in such a way that the early chorionic plate, together with the amnion, remnants of villi and the covering decidual tissues (*capsular decidua*), fuse and form a multilayered compact structure termed the chorion laeve or fetal membranes.

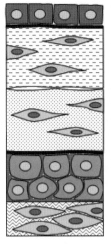

Amnionic epithelium (resting on a basement membrane)

Amnionic mesoderm (avascular; separated from the chorionic mesoderm by slender, fluid filled clefts)

Chorionic mesoderm (vascular; separated from extravillous trophoblast by a basement membrane)

Extravillous trophoblast (embedded in self-secreted matrix-type fibrinoid)

Capsular decidua (decidualized endometrial stroma in the chorion laeve)

Fig. 2.5 Layers of the fetal membranes. The amnionic epithelium is a simple epithelium that secretes and resorbs the amnionic fluid. The two layers of connective tissues (amnionic and chorionic mesoderm) are separated by fluid-filled clefts. The extravillous trophoblast of the fetal membranes displays a non-invasive phenotype and is embedded in a self-secreted matrix, termed matrix-type fibrinoid. Finally, on the maternal side, the fetal membranes are covered by the capsular decidua of maternal origin.

Layers of the chorion laeve

The layers of the chorion laeve, from the fetal to the maternal side, are as follows (Fig. 2.5).

1 *Amnionic epithelium.* A single cuboideal epithelium secreting and resorbing the amnionic fluid and involved in removal of carbon dioxide and pH regulation [31].

2 *Amnionic mesoderm.* A thin layer of avascular connective tissue separated from the amnionic epithelium by a basement membrane.

3 *Chorionic mesoderm.* This second layer of connective tissue is separated from the amnionic mesoderm by slender fluid-filled clefts. It is continuous with the connective tissue of the chorionic plate, which contains the branching vessels to and from the umbilical and villous vessels.

4 *Extravillous trophoblast of the fetal membranes.* This specific type of extravillous trophoblast does not display invasive properties and is separated from the chorionic mesoderm by a basement membrane.

5 *Capsular decidua.* This layer of maternal cells is directly attached to the extravillous trophoblast. At the end of the implantation process, the decidua closes again over the developing embryo, generating the capsular decidua. During the early second trimester, the capsular decidua comes into direct contact with the opposite wall of the uterus, causing obliteration of the uterine cavity.

Characteristics of the chorion laeve

After separation from the uterine wall, the fetal membranes have a mean thickness of about 200–300 µm at term [1]. The presence of the capsular decidua on the outer surface of the fetal membranes after delivery indicates that separation of the membranes takes place between maternal tissues rather than along the materno-fetal interface. Owing to the absence of vascular structures inside the connective tissues of the fetal membranes, all paraplacental exchange between fetal membranes and fetus has to pass the amnionic fluid.

Summary box 2.5

Layers of the fetal membrane, the chorion laeve
- Amnionic epithelium.
- Amnionic mesoderm.
- Chorionic mesoderm.
- Extravillous trophoblast.
- Decidua caspularis (maternal tissues).

Ultrasound

Using ultrasound just a few days after the expected menstrual period, a gestational sac with a diameter of 2–3 mm can be detected within the uterine endometrium. Developmental changes in the structure and organization of the placenta and membranes can be seen by ultrasound [32]. Minor anatomical variations, such as cysts and lakes, can readily be distinguished from lesions that destroy functioning villous tissue, such as infarcts and intervillous thrombi. Small placentas typically have eccentric cords, due to chorionic regression, and can have progressive parenchymal lesions, features typical of early-onset IUGR [33]. It is important to document placental location and cord insertion. Pathological placental invasion (placenta percreta) may be suspected by ultrasound, and can be confirmed by magnetic resonance imaging (MRI) [34].

Doppler ultrasound

Pulsed and colour Doppler ultrasound are valuable techniques for placental assessment. Umbilical cord flow can be visualized at 7–8 weeks, though end-diastolic flow (EDF) is not established until 14 weeks. Early-onset IUGR may be characterized by absent EDF in the umbilical arteries even by 22 weeks [33], associated with small malformed placentas and defective angiogenesis in the gas-exchanging terminal placental villi [35]. A major role for

Doppler ultrasound in placental assessment is determining maternal flow in the uterine arteries [36]. This screening test is performed either at the 18–20 week anatomical ultrasound or at a separate 22-week visit [37]. Integration of placental ultrasound, uterine artery Doppler and first- and second-trimester biochemistry screening tests (PAPP-A, hCG, PP13 and AFP) is an effective way of screening for serious placental insufficiency syndromes before they threaten fetal viability, thereby directing care to a high-risk pregnancy unit [38,39].

Pregnancies with multiparameter placental dysfunction in the 19–22 week window exhibit a 40% positive predictive value of delivery before 32 weeks due to clinical complications of placental insufficiency (IUGR, pre-eclampsia, abruption, stillbirth). Placental villous infarction complicates over 60% of such cases yet maternal thrombophilia is rare [38]. Since the normal healthy placenta expresses surface anticoagulant proteins, abnormal formation of the placenta may be the underlying cause of multifocal placental infarction. If this is the case, placental function testing in subsequent pregnancies may be a better determinant of future risk than maternal thrombophilia screening in the non-pregnant period.

Colour power Doppler

Colour power angiography (CPA) is an extented application in Doppler ultrasound and velocimetry. CPA can be used to map the vasculature within the placenta when combined with three-dimensional reconstruction (Fig. 2.6). This technique is able to identify red blood cells in vessels with a diameter of more than 200 µm [40]. Because the technique is three-dimensional, it can also be used to measure the proximal uterine arteries and therefore determine uterine artery blood flow rather than the descriptive assessment of the flow velocity waveform used in current practice.

Summary box 2.6

Ultrasound (including Doppler and colour power Doppler ultrasound)
- Week 3: visualization of the gestational sac.
- Week 7–8: visualization of blood flow in the umbilical cord.
- Week 13 until delivery: visualization of placental vessels with diameter larger than 200 µm.
- Week 14: establishment of EDF in the umbilical arteries.
- Week 18–22: screening of uterine arteries for pathological flow patterns.
- Week 22: early-onset IUGR can be predicted by absent EDF in the umbilical arteries.

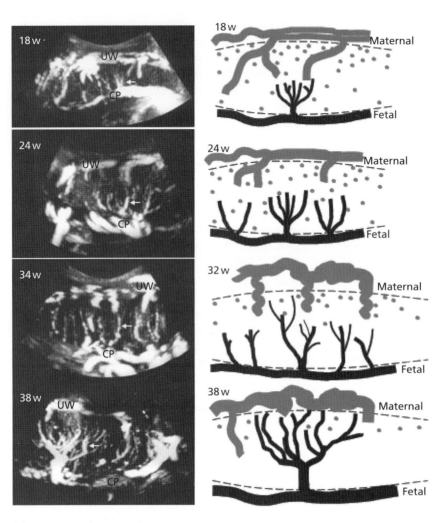

Fig. 2.6 Development of placental blood flow. Left column: Typical three-dimensional power Doppler scans from placentas of normal pregnant women at weeks 18, 24, 34 and 38. The flow signals within placental villi (white arrows) increase in extent, intensity, width and height with advancing pregnancy. At term (38 weeks) tree-like structures can be visualized. Since only anterior placentas have been used for these scans, the uterine wall (UW) is always at the top of the scan while the chorionic plate (CP) is always at the bottom of the scan. (Courtesy of Justin Konje, Leicester, UK.) Right column: Synoptic view of characteristic features of placental blood flow throughout pregnancy as depicted by three-dimensional power Doppler. (Adapted from drawings of Peter Kaufmann, Aachen, Germany.)

References

1 Benirschke K, Kaufmann P, Baergen R. *Pathology of the Human Placenta*. New York: Springer, 2006.

2 Hemberger M. Genetic–epigenetic intersection in trophoblast differentiation: implications for extraembryonic tissue function. *Epigenetics* 2010;5:24–29.

3 Kemp B, Kertschanska S, Kadyrov M, Rath W, Kaufmann P, Huppertz B. Invasive depth of extravillous trophoblast correlates with cellular phenotype: a comparison of intra- and extrauterine implantation sites. *Histochem Cell Biol* 2002;117:401–414.

4 Kurman RJ, Main CS, Chen HC. Intermediate trophoblast: a distinctive form of trophoblast with specific morphological, biochemical and functional features. *Placenta* 1984;5:349–369.

5 Kaufmann P, Black S, Huppertz B. Endovascular trophoblast invasion: implications for the pathogenesis of intrauterine growth retardation and preeclampsia. *Biol Reprod* 2003;69:1–7.

6 Moser G, Gauster M, Orendi K, Glasner A, Theuerkauf R, Huppertz B. Endoglandular trophoblast, an alternative route of trophoblast invasion? Analysis with novel confrontation co-culture models. *Hum Reprod* 2010;25:1127–1136.

7 Pijnenborg R, Bland JM, Robertson WB, Brosens I. Uteroplacental arterial changes related to interstitial trophoblast migration in early human pregnancy. *Placenta* 1983;4:397–413.

8 Jauniaux E, Watson AL, Hempstock J, Bao YP, Skepper JN, Burton GJ. Onset of maternal arterial bloodflow and placental oxidative stress: a possible factor in human early pregnancy failure. *Am J Pathol* 2000;157:2111–2122.

9 Burton GJ, Jauniaux E, Charnock-Jones DS. Human early placental development: potential roles of the endometrial glands. *Placenta* 2007;28(Suppl A):S64–S69.

10 Burton GJ, Hempstock J, Jauniaux E. Oxygen, early embryonic metabolism and free radical-mediated embryopathies. *Reprod BioMed Online* 2003;6:84–96.

11 Jauniaux E, Hempstock J, Greenwold N, Burton GJ. Trophoblastic oxidative stress in relation to temporal and regional differences in maternal placental blood flow in normal and abnormal early pregnancies. *Am J Pathol* 2003;162:115–125.

12 Baczyk D, Dunk C, Huppertz B *et al*. Bi-potential behaviour of cytotrophoblasts in first trimester chorionic villi. *Placenta* 2006;27:367–374.

13 Baczyk D, Drewlo S, Proctor L, Dunk C, Lye S, Kingdom J. Glial cell missing-1 transcription factor is required for the dif-

ferentiation of the human trophoblast. *Cell Death Differ* 2009;16: 719–727.

14 Kaufmann P, Huppertz B, Frank HG. The fibrinoids of the human placenta: origin, composition and functional relevance. *Ann Anat* 1996;178:485–501.

15 Huppertz B. IFPA Award in Placentology Lecture. Biology of the placental syncytiotrophoblast: myths and facts. *Placenta* 2010;31(Suppl):S75–S81.

16 Huppertz B, Kadyrov M, Kingdom JC. Apoptosis and its role in the trophoblast. *Am J Obstet Gynecol* 2006;195:29–39.

17 Ellery PM, Cindrova-Davies T, Jauniaux E, Ferguson-Smith AC, Burton GJ. Evidence for transcriptional activity in the syncytiotrophoblast of the human placenta. *Placenta* 2009;30:329–334.

18 Goswami D, Tannetta DS, Magee LA *et al*. Excess syncytiotrophoblast microparticle shedding is a feature of early-onset pre-eclampsia, but not normotensive intrauterine growth restriction. *Placenta* 2006;27:56–61.

19 Huppertz B, Tews DS, Kaufmann P. Apoptosis and syncytial fusion in human placental trophoblast and skeletal muscle. *Int Rev Cytol* 2001;205:215–253.

20 Huppertz B, Kingdom J. Apoptosis in the trophoblast: role of apoptosis in placental morphogenesis. *J Soc Gynecol Investig* 2004;11:353–362.

21 Iklé FA. Trophoblastzellen im strömenden Blut. *Schweiz Med Wochenschr* 1961;91:934–945.

22 Johansen M, Redman CW, Wilkins T, Sargent IL. Trophoblast deportation in human pregnancy: its relevance for pre-eclampsia. *Placenta* 1999;20:531–539.

23 Redman CWG, Sargent IL. Placental debris, oxidative stress and pre-eclampsia. *Placenta* 2000;21:597–602.

24 Graf R, Matejevic D, Schuppan D, Neudeck H, Shakibaei M, Vetter K. Molecular anatomy of the perivascular sheath in human placental stem villi: the contractile apparatus and its association to the extracellular matrix. *Cell Tissue Res* 1997;290: 601–607.

25 Burton GJ, Jauniaux E, Charnock-Jones DS. The influence of the intrauterine environment on human placental development. *Int J Dev Biol* 2010;54:303–312.

26 Kingdom JCP, Kaufmann P. Oxygen and placental villous development: origins of fetal hypoxia. *Placenta* 1997;18:613–621.

27 Zamudio S. The placenta at high altitude. *High Altitude Med Biol* 2003;4:171–191.

28 Huppertz B. Placental origins of preeclampsia: challenging the current hypothesis. *Hypertension* 2008;51:970–975.

29 Burton GJ, Woods AW, Jauniaux E, Kingdom JC. Rheological and physiological consequences of conversion of the maternal spiral arteries for uteroplacental blood flow during human pregnancy. *Placenta* 2009;30:473–482.

30 Menon R, Fortunato SJ. The role of matrix degrading enzymes and apoptosis in rupture of membranes. *J Soc Gynecol Investig* 2004;11:427–437.

31 Schmidt W. The amniotic fluid compartment: the fetal habitat. *Adv Anat Embryol Cell Biol* 1992;127:1–100.

32 Alkazaleh F, Viero S, Kingdom JCP. The placenta. In: Rumak CM, Wilson SR, Charboneau JW (eds) *Obstetric Ultrasound*, 4th edn. Philadelphia: Elsevier Mosby, 2004.

33 Proctor LK, Toal M, Keating S *et al*. Placental size and the prediction of severe early-onset intrauterine growth restriction in women with low pregnancy-associated plasma protein-A. *Ultrasound Obstet Gynecol* 2009;34:274–282.

34 Warshak CR, Eskander R, Hull AD *et al*. Accuracy of ultrasonography and magnetic resonance imaging in the diagnosis of placenta accreta. *Obstet Gynecol* 2006;108:573–581.

35 Krebs C, Macara LM, Leiser R, Bowman AW, Greer IA, Kingdom JC. Intrauterine growth restriction with absent end-diastolic flow velocity in the umbilical artery is associated with maldevelopment of the placental terminal villous tree. *Am J Obstet Gynecol* 1996;175:1534–1542.

36 Jauniaux E, Jurkovic D, Campbell S, Hustin J. Doppler ultrasound features of the developing placental circulations: correlation with anatomic findings. *Am J Obstet Gynecol* 1992;166: 585–587.

37 Alkazaleh F, Reister F, Kingdom JCP. Doppler ultrasound. In: Rumak CM, Wilson SR, Charboneau JW (eds) *Obstetric Ultrasound*, 4th edn. Philadelphia: Elsevier Mosby, 2004.

38 Toal M, Keating S, Machin G *et al*. Determinants of adverse perinatal outcome in high-risk women with abnormal uterine artery Doppler images. *Am J Obstet Gynecol* 2008;198:330.e1–7.

39 Costa SL, Proctor L, Dodd JM *et al*. Screening for placental insufficiency in high-risk pregnancies: is earlier better? *Placenta* 2008;29:1034–1040.

40 Konje JC, Huppertz B, Bell SC, Taylor DJ, Kaufmann P. 3-dimensional colour power angiography for staging human placental development. *Lancet* 2003;362:1199–1201.

41 Mayhew TM, Leach L, McGee R, Ismail WW, Myklebust R, Lammiman MJ. Proliferation, differentiation and apoptosis in villous trophoblast at 13–41 weeks of gestation (including observations on annulate lamellae and nuclear pore complexes. *Placenta* 1999;20:407–422.

42 Burton GJ, Jauniaux E. Placental oxidative stress: from miscarriage to preeclampsia. *J Soc Gynecol Investig* 2004;11:342–352.

43 Chaddha V, Viero S, Huppertz B, Kingdom J. Developmental biology of the placenta and the origins of placental insufficiency. *Semin Fetal Neonat Med* 2004;9:357–369.

44 Dugoff L. First- and second-trimester maternal serum markers for aneuploidy and adverse obstetric outcomes. *Obstet Gynecol* 2010;115:1052–1061.

Further reading

Structural characteristics of the placenta, see [1]

Definition of fibrinoid, see [14]

Trophoblast and its changes during pre-eclampsia, see [28]

Detailed descriptions of pathologies and their impact on macroscopic features of the placenta, see [1]

Classification of villi and the types of villi, see [1]

Stereological parameters of the growing placenta, see [41]

Syncytial fusion and the involvement of apoptosis, see [19, 20]

Impact of oxygen on placental development and placental-related disorders of pregnancy, see [42]

Composition and characteristics of fetal membranes, see [31]

Rupture of fetal membranes, see [30]

Placental assessment by ultrasound, see [43]

Placental Doppler, see [32, 36, 37]

Developmental placental pathology, see [1, 43]

Placental biochemistry in clinical practice, see [44]

Role of a placenta clinic, see www.mountsinai.on.ca/care/placenta-clinic

Chapter 3
Normal Fetal Growth

Jason Gardosi
West Midlands Perinatal Institute, Birmingham, UK

Developments in ultrasound imaging techniques and analysis of large databases has improved our understanding of normal fetal growth and maturation. Such an understanding is of immediate relevance for the assessment of fetal well-being at any stage of pregnancy.

Length of pregnancy

In any large database, the distribution of the length of pregnancy is skewed because babies are more likely to be born preterm than post-term, and at a wider range of gestations in the preterm period. Thus neither the mean nor median but the mode is the best measure to denote the typical length of pregnancy (Fig. 3.1).

Starting from the time of conception, the typical length of gestation, and the fetal age at the end of pregnancy, is 266 days or 38 weeks (i.e. 'conceptual age'). In most (but not all) cases, conception occurs in mid-cycle, and thus 2 weeks are added to denote menstrual age. By convention, gestational age is also expressed in this manner: the formulae used for dating pregnancies by ultrasound, to determine the length of pregnancy at any point and the expected date of delivery (EDD), also add a standard 2 weeks to derive 'gestational age'. The typical length of pregnancy is 280 days or 40.0 weeks; term is conventionally denoted as 37–42 weeks, preterm as less than 37.0 weeks and post-term as more than 42.0 weeks. However, these cut-offs may be varied for the purpose of looking at specific issues. For example, prematurity less than 34 weeks denotes babies that are more likely to require some form of special care; and limits of 290 days or more (EDD + 10) or even 287 days or more (41.0 weeks) have been used to study the effects of post-term pregnancy or for protocols to induce post-term pregnancy.

> **Summary box 3.1**
>
> - The typical (modal) length of pregnancy is 280 days (40.0 weeks) from the first day of last menstrual period (gestational age), or 266 days (38.0 weeks) from the date of conception (conceptional age).
> - 'Term' is defined as 37.0–42.0 weeks gestational age (259–294 days), although post-term is sometimes also defined as ≥290 days (EDD + 10).

Determination of gestational age

Accurate dating of pregnancy is important for a number of reasons, each of them constituting milestones which are more important than the prediction of the actual EDD itself.

1 *Antenatal screening.* Values of serum tests for chromosomal abnormalities (e.g. Down's syndrome), such as pregnancy-associated plasma protein A (PAPP-A), human chorionic gonadotrophin (hCG) or oestriol, are strongly related to gestational age and may give false readings if the 'dates' are wrong. As a result, it may be overlooked that the pregnancy is at risk, or false positives are produced, which can lead to unnecessary invasive diagnostic procedures such as chorionic villous sampling or amniocentesis.

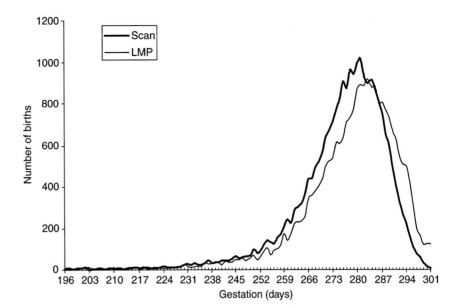

Fig. 3.1 Frequency distribution of gestational age at birth (*N* = 24 524 pregnancies) in Nottingham, 1988–1995, which had a record of the last menstrual period (LMP) and an ultrasound dating scan. The graph shows a general left shift associated with ultrasound dates.

2 *Estimating fetal viability at extreme prematurity.* Between say 23 and 28 weeks, the chance of a baby's survival is heavily dependent on the gestational age [1] and inaccurate dates may lead to wrong advice to the parents and inappropriate management.

3 *Post-term pregnancy.* Prolonged gestation is associated with a rise in perinatal morbidity and mortality. The reasons for this are not well understood, but it has become established practice to offer induction of labour in pregnancies that go beyond 290–294 days.

Before the advent of ultrasound, the menstrual age was used to determine gestational dates and the EDD. However, dating by menstrual history has several problems [2]. Firstly, the last menstrual period (LMP) may not be accurately remembered in a substantial proportion of cases. Secondly, dating by LMP assumes that conception occurred in mid-cycle, whereas it may have occurred earlier or (more likely) later. If the usual length of a woman's cycle tends to be longer, say 35 instead of 28 days, then an adjustment needs to be made by adding 7 days to the EDD. This is often not done, but even if it is, it represents an approximation only, as the actual length of the follicular phase at the beginning of that pregnancy is not known.

Dating by ultrasound has made the determination of gestational age more precise. The ultrasound scan dating can be done on the basis of the fetal crown–rump length (CRL), which is reliable between 7 and 12 weeks, or in the second trimester between say 15 and 22 weeks by the biparietal diameter (BPD) or the head circumference (HC). There are few studies which have compared whether first or second trimester measurement is more accurate in routine practice. Between 13 and 15 weeks,

dating by ultrasound can be less accurate, as the fetus flexes, making CRL difficult, while it may be too early for an accurate measurement of the head (BPD or HC).

Ultrasound measurement can also have error, but this error is smaller than that of LMP. Based on studies from pregnancies achieved with assisted reproduction techniques, i.e. where the exact date of conception was known, the error of routine scan dating by ultrasound was normally distributed and had a standard deviation of ±4, which means a 95% confidence interval of –8 to +8 days [3]. In contrast, LMP dating error is heavily skewed towards overestimation of the true gestational age, with a 95% confidence interval of –9 to +27 days [4].

One manifestation of such a tendency to overestimation is that many pregnancies which are post-term by LMP dates and considered in need for induction of labour are in fact not post-term if ultrasound dates are used. About three-quarters of 'post-term' (>294 days) pregnancies by LMP are not post-term by ultrasound (11.3 to 3.6%) [5]. This would suggest that many 'post-term' pregnancies in clinical practice, as well as in studies in the literature, prior to routine dating by ultrasound were in fact not post-term but misdated.

As an ultrasound scan is performed in most pregnancies in the UK at some stage in the first half of pregnancy, it is now recommended that gestation dates should preferentially be determined by ultrasound [2]. In many units, protocols have evolved whereby LMP is used unless it has a discrepancy of greater than 7, 10 or 14 days from the dates by ultrasound. However, this is not based on any evidence; in fact, even within 14, 10 or even 7 day cut-offs, scan dates are known to be more accurate than LMP dates in predicting the actual date of delivery [5].

Small for gestational age and intrauterine growth restriction

The traditional method of denoting a small baby as being below 2500 g, or 1500 g, does not distinguish between smallness due to short gestation and smallness due to intrauterine growth restriction (IUGR).

The terms 'small for gestational age' (SGA), 'average for gestational age' and 'large for gestational age' are therefore preferred, which adjusts the limit for the average at the respective gestational age. Traditionally, the 10th and 90th centiles respectively are used, although the 5th and 95th, or the 3rd and 97th (equivalent to ±2 standard deviations) can also be applied. However, SGA is not synonymous with IUGR, as it includes pathological as well as constitutional smallness.

Increasingly, it has become apparent that birthweight and fetal growth vary with a number of factors, apart from gestational age. These factors can be physiological (constitutional) or pathological.

Physiological factors include birth order (parity), maternal characteristics such as height, weight and ethnic origin, and fetal gender [6]. Coefficients have been derived to allow the normal birthweight ranges to be adjusted [6], from which growth curves can then also be derived (see below) [7]. In practice, well-dated birthweight databases with sufficient details about maternal characteristics and pregnancy outcome are used to derive the coefficients needed to adjust for constitutional variation.

Ultimately, the rate of significant pathological SGA should mirror the risk of adverse outcome. However, applying population centiles to small mothers results in a disproportionately large number of SGA babies which is not related to an increased risk of adverse outcome [8]. Conversely, population centiles underestimate the number of SGA babies in big mothers. In contrast, when the standard for growth/birthweight is adjusted for maternal variables, the rate of SGA corresponds very closely to that of perinatal mortality. This is illustrated in

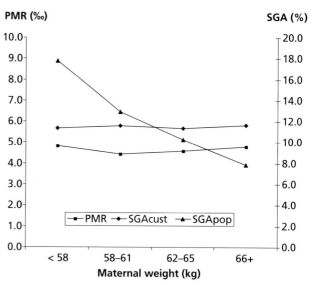

Fig. 3.2 Perinatal mortality rate (PMR) and smallness for gestational age (SGA) by customised (SGAcust) and population-based centiles (SGApop), according to maternal weights within normal body mass index (BMI 20–24.9). *t* test for difference of slopes: PMR vs. SGAcust, *P* = 0.743; PMR vs. SGApop, *P* < 0.001.

Fig. 3.2, which compares symmetrically small and large mothers (i.e. body mass index within normal range).

Pathological factors affecting growth include smoking, alcohol, social class and deprivation, multiple pregnancy, and pregnancy complications such as placental failure and related underlying conditions associated with hypertensive diseases in pregnancy, antepartum haemorrhage and diabetes (see Chapters 11 and 13). Although they clearly affect growth, such variables should *not* be adjusted for, as the standard needs to reflect the optimal growth potential of the fetus. For example, it is well established that maternal smoking adversely affects fetal growth; however the standard or norm should not be adjusted downwards if a mother smokes, but instead 'optimized' as if the mother did *not* smoke, to allow better detection of the fetus that is affected.

Adjustment of the standard for constitutional factors not only improves detection but also allows a better understanding of how pathology affects growth. For example, smoking is known to be associated with a birthweight deficit that can be quite substantial by the end of pregnancy, even after adjusting for different constitutional characteristics of mothers who smoke (e.g. they are on average shorter). The birthweight deficit at term is also dose dependent: compared with non-smokers, mothers who admit at the booking visit to smoking one to nine cigarettes a day have babies which weigh on average 153 g less at term; 10–20 cigarettes a day, 215 g less; and 20+ cigarettes a day, 246 g less [7].

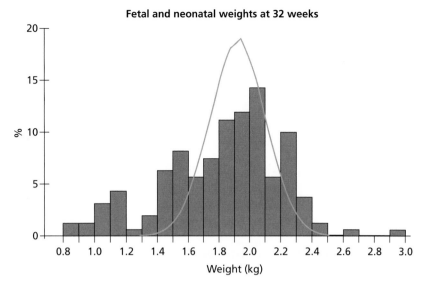

Fetal and neonatal weights at 32 weeks

Fig. 3.3 Ultrasound versus birthweight standard at 32 weeks' gestation. The line shows ultrasound weight estimations derived from pregnancies which have proceeded to normal term delivery. The curve is characterized by a relatively narrow normal distribution. The histogram shows birthweights of babies born at this same, preterm gestation in a dataset of approximately 40 000 cases in the Midlands. The distribution shows a lower median, a wider range and negative skewness.

Summary box 3.3

- SGA is not synonymous with IUGR, as it includes constitutional as well as pathological smallness.
- Adjusting for constitutional factors improves the association between SGA and pathology, making it a more useful clinical measure.
- Babies that are only constitutionally small do not have an increased risk of adverse outcome.

Fetal weight gain

In the first half of pregnancy, the fetus develops its organ systems and grows mainly by cell division. In the second half, most growth occurs by increase in cell size.

Determination of what is 'normal' is essential for the identification of abnormal growth in day-to-day clinical practice. Imaging techniques have allowed us to get a better understanding of normal fetal growth. These include two-dimensional and three-dimensional ultrasound as well as assessment of Doppler flow (see Chapter 18).

Previously, 'normal growth' was inferred from birthweight curves, which showed wide ranges especially at early (preterm) gestations, and flattening of the curve at term. A marked terminal flattening of the curve is evident in some birthweight standards still in widespread use [9]. However, this is an artefact due to misdating: because LMP error is more likely to overestimate rather than underestimate true gestational age, as shown above, the birthweights in many cases end up being plotted at later gestations than they should be, producing the erroneous impression of a flattening of fetal growth at term.

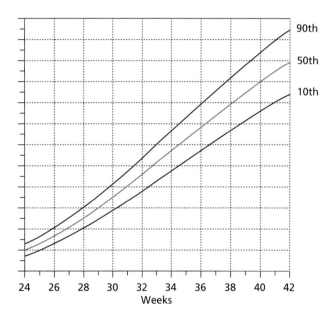

Fig. 3.4 Fetal growth curves derived from longitudinal ultrasound scans of normal pregnancies, showing a normal distribution and no flattening at term.

Many birthweight curves also show a depression or negative skewness at preterm gestations. This is associated with the known fact that many premature births, including those following spontaneous onset of labour, are of babies whose growth was restricted *in utero* [10,11]. In contrast, ultrasound curves based on fetuses which continue growth until normal term delivery show no such skewness [12–14] (Figs 3.3 and 3.4).

The dynamics of growth in normal pregnancy can be studied by converting the weight-for-gestation curve into a 'proportionality' curve, where term weight in normal pregnancies equates to 100%. As Fig. 3.4 shows, half of

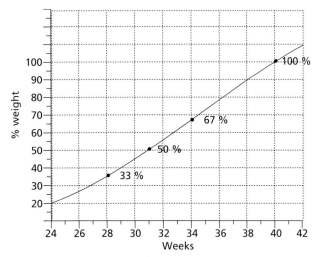

Fig. 3.5 'Proportionality' fetal growth curve. The line represents an equation derived from an *in utero* weight curve, transformed into a percent term weight versus gestation curve for any predicted term (280 day) birthweight point. % weight = $299.1 - 31.85GA + 1.094GA^2 - 0.01055GA^3$.

this weight should be expected to be reached at 31 weeks, and one-third and two-thirds should be reached by 28 and 34 weeks, respectively (Fig. 3.5).

Such proportionality curves can be used to project backwards the predicted, individually adjusted birthweight end-point. The constitutional variables affecting growth can result in an infinite number of combinations, which require calculation by computer software, such as GROW (Gestation Related Optimal Weight software; www.gestation.net), to produce individually adjusted or 'customised' norms for fetal growth in each pregnancy (Fig. 3.6). Thus 'normal' growth is not an 'average' for the population, but one that defines the optimal growth that a fetus can achieve, i.e. the 'growth potential' of each baby.

A number of studies have shown that standards for normal birthweight and growth adjusted for constitutional variation are better than local population norms to separate physiological and pathological smallness.

Customised standards improve detection of pathologically small babies in high- and low-risk populations [15,16]. Smallness defined by customised standards were also more strongly associated with adverse pregnancy outcome such as stillbirth, neonatal death or low Apgar scores [17,18] and were more closely linked with a number of pathological indicators such as abnormal antenatal Doppler, Caesarean section for fetal distress, admission to the neonatal unit and prolonged hospital stay [19].

Significantly, each of the studies showed that babies considered small only by the (unadjusted) population method do not have an increased risk of adverse pregnancy outcome. In the general population, up to one-third of babies are false-positively small when general rather than individually adjusted norms for fetal growth are used, which can result in many unnecessary investigations and parental anxiety. Conversely, about one-third of babies who should be suspected to be at risk are missed.

In population subgroups such as minority ethnic groups, application of an unadjusted population standard results in even more false positives and false negatives. The individual or customised method to determine normal fetal growth is recommended by guidelines of the Royal College of Obstetricians and Gynaecologists [20].

Summary box 3.4

- Curves to define normal fetal growth should be derived from ultrasound rather than birthweight standards, as preterm births are not normal and have a high association with abnormal growth.
- 'Normal' growth is not an average for the population, but one that defines the optimal growth that each fetus can achieve, i.e. its 'growth potential', adjusted for constitutional factors and free from any pathological influences.
- Use of unadjusted population centiles results in many babies within subgroups of the population (e.g. ethnic groups, high body mass index) being falsely categorized as normal or small.

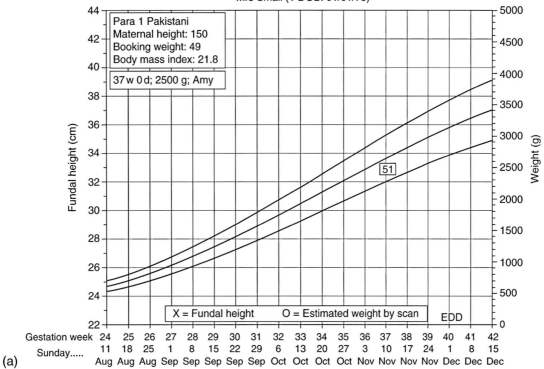

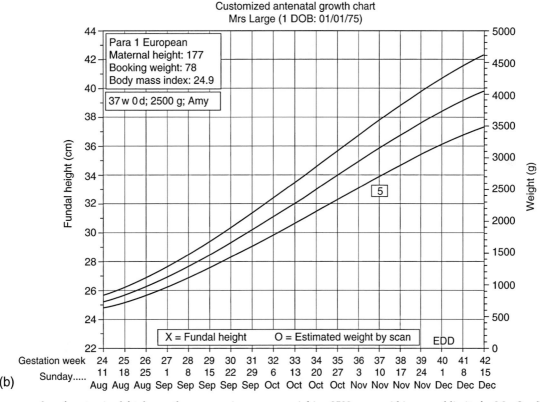

Fig. 3.6 Two examples of customized fetal growth curves, using GROW.exe version 5.11 (www.gestation.net). The charts can be used to calculate previous baby weights and ultrasound estimated fetal weight(s) in the current pregnancy. Serial fundal height measurements can also be plotted. The graphs are adjusted to predict the optimal curve for each pregnancy, based on the variables entered (maternal height, weight, parity and ethnic origin). In the example, a baby born at 37.0 weeks weighing 2500 g was within normal limits for Mrs Small (51st centile) but was growth restricted for Mrs Large (5th centile), as the latter's predicted optimal growth curve is steeper. The pregnancy details entered are shown on the top left, together with the (computer) calculated body mass index (BMI). The horizontal axis shows the day and month of each gestation week, calculated by the software on the basis of the EDD.

References

1 Draper ES, Manktelow B, Field DJ, James D. Prediction of survival for preterm births by weight and gestational age: retrospective population based study. *BMJ* 1999;319:1093–1097.

2 Gardosi J, Geirsson R. Routine ultrasound is the method of choice for dating pregnancy. *Br J Obstet Gynaecol* 1998;105:933–936.

3 Mul T, Mongelli M, Gardosi J. A comparative analysis of second-trimester ultrasound dating formulae in pregnancies conceived with artificial reproductive techniques. *Ultrasound Obstet Gynecol* 1996;8:397–402.

4 Gardosi J, Mongelli M. Risk assessment adjusted for gestational age in maternal serum screening for Down's syndrome. *BMJ* 1993;306:1509.

5 Mongelli M, Wilcox M, Gardosi J. Estimating the date of confinement: ultrasonographic biometry versus certain menstrual dates. *Am J Obstet Gynecol* 1996;174:278–281.

6 Gardosi J, Chang A, Kalyan B, Sahota D, Symonds EM. Customised antenatal growth charts. *Lancet* 1992;339:283–287.

7 Gardosi J, Mongelli M, Wilcox M, Chang A. An adjustable fetal weight standard. *Ultrasound Obstet Gynecol* 1995;6:168–174.

8 Gardosi J, Clausson B, Francis A. The value of customised centiles in assessing perinatal mortality risk associated with parity and maternal size. *BJOG* 2009;116:1356–1363.

9 Alexander GA, Himes JH, Kaufman RB, Mor J, Kogan M. A United States national reference for fetal growth. *Obstet Gynecol* 1996;87:163–168.

10 Tamura RK, Sabbagha RE, Depp R *et al*. Diminished growth in fetuses born preterm after spontaneous labour or rupture of membranes. *Am J Obstet Gynecol* 1984;148:1105–1110.

11 Gardosi J. Prematurity and fetal growth restriction. *Early Hum Dev* 2005;81:43–49.

12 Gardosi J. Ultrasound biometry and fetal growth restriction. *Fetal Maternal Med Rev* 2002;13:249–259.

13 Gallivan S, Robson SC, Chang TC, Vaughan J, Spencer JAD. An investigation of fetal growth using serial ultrasound data. *Ultrasound Obstet Gynecol* 1993;3:109–114.

14 Marsal K, Persson P-H, Larsen T *et al*. Intrauterine growth curves based on ultrasonically estimated foetal weights. *Acta Paediatr* 1996;85:843–848.

15 de Jong CLD, Gardosi J, Dekker GA, Colenbrander GJ, van Geijn HP. Application of a customised birthweight standard in the assessment of perinatal outcome in a high risk population. *Br J Obstet Gynaecol* 1998;105:531–535.

16 de Jong CLD, Francis A, Van Geijn HP, Gardosi J. Customised fetal weight limits for antenatal detection of fetal growth restriction. *Ultrasound Obstet Gynecol* 2000;15:36–40.

17 Clausson B, Gardosi J, Francis A, Cnattingius S. Perinatal outcome in SGA births defined by customised versus population-based birthweight standards. *BJOG* 2001;108:830–834.

18 McCowan L, Harding JE, Stewart AW. Customised birthweight centiles predict SGA pregnancies with perinatal morbidity. *BJOG* 2005;112:1026–1033.

19 Gardosi J, Francis A. Adverse pregnancy outcome and association with smallness for gestational age birthweight by customized and population based percentiles. *Am J Obstet Gynecol* 2009;201:28.e1–8.

20 Royal College of Obstetricians and Gynaecologists. *The investigation and management of the small-for-gestational age fetus*. RCOG Green-top Guideline No. 31, 2002. Available at www.rcog.org.uk/files/rcog-corp/uploaded-files/GT31SmallGestationalAgeFetus.pdf

Part 2
Normal Pregnancy

Chapter 4
Pre-conception Counselling

Mandish K. Dhanjal
Queen Charlotte's & Chelsea Hospital, London, UK

A woman who enters pregnancy in a good state of health with a healthy diet and well-controlled medical disease is more likely to have a healthy pregnancy and a good outcome than a woman who enters pregnancy with an unhealthy lifestyle and uncontrolled medical disease. Pre-conception or pre-pregnancy counselling involves seeing women several months prior to conception in order to discuss and modify lifestyle choices and assess and improve medical health before pregnancy. There is currently no UK guidance on pre-conception counselling, although the National Institute for Health and Clinical Excellence (NICE) has identified it as an important area in their antenatal guidelines [1].

Purpose of pre-conception counselling

All women considering having a baby should see their general practitioner (GP), and a specialist in pre-pregnancy counselling if they have a medical disease, prior to conceiving. The purpose of this consultation is to:
• inform the woman and her partner of general advice, and advice about lifestyle behaviours including exercise, diet, smoking and drinking;
• detect any medical issues that will impact on pregnancy and advise if pregnancy should not be contemplated at present;
• assess any known medical conditions and optimize the state of the disease, in particular adjusting medications;
• discuss how the above may impact on the pregnancy, fetus and the mother;
• identify couples who are at risk of having babies with genetic disorders and refer them for genetic advice before they embark on pregnancy; and
• discuss contraception if it is considered that pregnancy is not advisable at present or if the woman prefers not to get pregnant yet.
Broadly, for any medical condition, there should be a discussion about whether becoming pregnant has risks for the mother or fetus.

• Mother: disease exacerbation (antenatally or postnatally), maternal mortality.
• Fetus: malformations (genetic, teratogens), *in utero* growth restriction, preterm delivery, stillbirth, neonatal morbidity and mortality.

Pre-pregnancy counselling will inform women of their risks, empowering them to make an informed decision whether or not to proceed with pregnancy. It will allow planning or prevention of pregnancy, and access to the appropriate multidisciplinary specialized services if necessary.

> **Summary box 4.1**
>
> • All women should have pre-conception counselling to inform them of their own health and the health of their fetus in pregnancy, empowering them to make an informed decision whether or not to proceed with pregnancy.
> • It allows planning or prevention of pregnancy, and access to the appropriate multidisciplinary specialized services if necessary.

Who needs pre-conception counselling?

All women will benefit from the general advice offered by GPs. The last report of the confidential enquiry into maternal deaths specifically recommended that pre-conception counselling be provided for women of childbearing age with pre-existing serious medical or mental health conditions that may be aggravated by pregnancy, in particular the commoner conditions including epilepsy, diabetes, congenital or known acquired cardiac disease, autoimmune disorders, obesity with body mass index (BMI) of 30 or more, and severe pre-existing or past mental illness [2]. The recommendation especially applies to women prior to having assisted reproduction and other fertility treatments.

Dewhurst's Textbook of Obstetrics & Gynaecology, Eighth Edition. Edited by D. Keith Edmonds.
© 2012 John Wiley and Sons, Ltd. Published 2012 by John Wiley and Sons, Ltd.

Timing of pre-conception counselling

This should ideally take place 3–6 months prior to conceiving; however, few women are motivated enough to see a doctor prior to getting pregnant, even if they have a medical illness. Dedicated pre-pregnancy clinics or pre-pregnancy health check clinics would be ideal, but very few health authorities offer this service. Additionally it is estimated that 25–40% of pregnancies are unplanned. Pre-conception advice should therefore occur opportunistically when women attend their GP or their specialist for contraception, review of their medical disease or if they are referred to infertility clinics.

The average age of first sexual intercourse is 16 years and 0.78% of girls under the age of 16 years in the UK get pregnant [3]. The UK has the highest teenage pregnancy rate in western Europe and the USA has the highest rate in the Western World. Some medical conditions, such as complex congenital heart disease, would necessitate a discussion about pregnancy during adolescence (12–15 years old) depending on the degree of maturity of the child. This is not to encourage pregnancy in these teenagers, but to educate them of the risks that unintended pregnancy may hold for them.

Implicit in any discussion is the need for adequate contraception (see Chapter 40).

Healthcare professionals who should undertake pre-conception counselling

GPs are best placed to do this as they have a long-term relationship with their patients and will usually be seeing them for contraceptive advice and for other medical conditions. Specialists also have a role, particularly diabetologists, neurologists and cardiologists who will be seeing adolescents and women of reproductive age for regular checks of their diabetes, epilepsy or heart disease. Pre-conception counselling is vital in these groups as it can directly influence pregnancy outcome. Unfortunately some specialists may be reluctant to discuss the implications of medical disease and the associated medications in pregnancy because they are not up to date with current specific advice on pregnancy.

Maternal medicine specialists and obstetric physicians are ideally placed to offer pre-conception advice. They are well informed as to the effects of various medical diseases in pregnancy and are aware of the implications of drug use in pregnancy. Many will have dedicated pre-conception clinics in tertiary care. Many maternal medicine specialists will also be able to offer detailed contraceptive advice and in many instances are able to administer long-acting contraceptives, avoiding delay in gaining effective contraception.

Table 4.1 Foods that can affect the fetus in very early pregnancy.

Food	Risk of containing	Fetal risk in early pregnancy
Unpasteurized milk Soft mould-ripened cheeses (e.g. Camembert, Brie, blue-veined cheese) Pâté (including vegetable pâté) Uncooked or under-cooked ready made meals Raw shellfish (e.g. oysters)	Listeria	Miscarriage
Uncooked or cured meat (e.g. salami)	Toxoplasma	Fetal CNS defects
Liver and liver products	Excess vitamin A	Cranial–neural crest tissue defects
Shark, swordfish and marlin	Methylmercury	Fetal CNS defects

CNS, central nervous system.

General pre-conception advice

Diet

Women intending to conceive should be encouraged to eat fruit, vegetables, starchy foods (bread, pasta, rice and potatoes), protein (lean meat, fish, beans and lentils), fibre (wholegrain breads, fruit and vegetables) and dairy foods (pasteurized milk, yoghurt and hard, cottage or processed cheese) [1]. These will assist in increasing the stores of vitamins, iron and calcium.

The unpredictability regarding the exact moment a woman becomes pregnant leads to the recommendation that women trying to conceive should avoid the foods listed in Table 4.1, which may contain organisms or substances that can be harmful in early gestation. Even a planned pregnancy is not detected until 5–6 weeks of gestation, at which stage vulnerable organs, particularly the central nervous system, have already started developing and the neural tube is completely formed.

Vegetarians and vegans are at risk of nutritional deficiencies and may benefit from advice from a dietitian.

Women who have a heavy intake of caffeine should be advised to cut down before pregnancy. The Food Standards Agency recommends that pregnant women should limit their consumption of caffeine in pregnancy to 300 mg daily or less (four cups of coffee, eight cups of tea, or eight cans of cola) [1]. High caffeine intake mildly increases the risk of fetal growth restriction.

Supplements

Folic acid 0.4 mg daily should be recommended to all women trying to conceive and should be continued until

12 weeks' gestation along with an increase in folate-containing foods as this has been shown in randomized controlled trials to significantly reduce the incidence of fetal neural tube defects (NTDs) such as spina bifida and anencephaly [4]. A higher dose of folic acid (5 mg daily) is required in women:

• with a previous pregnancy affected by an NTD [5];
• who themselves are affected with an NTD;
• with a sibling or parent affected with an NTD;
• taking antifolate drugs (e.g. most antiepileptic agents and 5-aminosalicylate drugs used in inflammatory bowel disease); or
• with diabetes [6].

Some countries have fortified certain foods (e.g. flour, cereals) with folate in order to help protect those women who cannot afford medical supplementation and those who have an unplanned pregnancy [7]. There is some evidence that the risk of other congenital malformations may be reduced with folate and multivitamin supplementation [8].

Vitamin D can be beneficial for some women from the Indian subcontinent, Middle East and the Horn of Africa who, through a combination of diet (phytates in chapatti flour) and poor sun exposure, can be prone to vitamin D deficiency and osteomalacia that can present with muscle and bony pain [1]. A large World Health Organization trial has shown that if women who have low dietary intake of calcium are given calcium supplements, their risk of developing pre-eclampsia is halved [9].

Smoking

Women should be advised to stop smoking prior to pregnancy. They are usually aware of the risks to their own health of smoking, but are often less aware of the risks to the fetus, which include miscarriage, placental abruption, placenta praevia, premature rupture of membranes, preterm delivery, low birthweight, cleft lip and cleft palate, perinatal mortality, sudden infant death syndrome and impaired cognitive development [1]. Discussion of these risks often provides a strong motivation to pregnant women to stop smoking. It is estimated that if all pregnant women stopped smoking there would be a 10% reduction in fetal and infant deaths. Advice from the doctor, smoking cessation programmes and self-help manuals have been shown to help women stop smoking.

Alcohol

Women should limit alcohol intake to one to two standard units of alcohol per week as recommended by NICE as there is no evidence of fetal harm with this degree of consumption [1]. The dangers to the fetus of drinking alcohol in pregnancy occur with greater consumption, so that women who binge drink or drink heavily are at risk of subfertility, miscarriage, aneuploidy, structural congenital anomalies, fetal growth restriction, perinatal death and developmental delay [10]. Binge drinkers are more likely to have an unplanned pregnancy and hence may continue to drink erratically in the first trimester without knowing they are pregnant. Fetal alcohol syndrome occurs in 0.6 per 1000 live births (Canadian data) and is characterized by distinctive facial features, low birthweight, and behavioural and intellectual difficulties in later life. There is a further spectrum of fetal alcohol disorders [10]. Alcohol misuse can result in maternal ill health and is a significant cause of maternal death [2].

Body weight

Women should be advised to enter pregnancy with a normal BMI of 20–24.9 kg/m^2. Overweight women (BMI 25–29.9 kg/m^2) and obese women (BMI ≥30 kg/m^2) should lose weight by dieting and exercise before conceiving. They may require referral to a dietitian. They should be informed of the adverse pregnancy outcomes associated with obesity (Table 4.2) [11].

For women who are morbidly obese (obesity grade III) with a BMI of 40 kg/m^2 or more it is very difficult to achieve a normal BMI. In addition to referral to a dietitian, they should be assisted to lose weight by a variety of methods including prescription of weight reduction medication in a carefully supervised manner and referral for gastric surgery. They should strongly be advised to defer pregnancy until they have lost weight.

Women who are underweight (BMI <20 kg/m^2) may find it difficult to conceive due to anovulatory cycles. They have an increased chance of fetal intrauterine growth restriction.

Table 4.2 Risks of obesity to mother and her offspring.

Maternal risks of obesity
Subfertility
Miscarriage
Hypertensive disease
Gestational diabetes
Thromboembolism
Infection
Cardiac disease
Instrumental deliveries
Caesarean section
Postpartum haemorrhage
Maternal death

Risks to offspring of maternal obesity
Neural tube defects
Large for dates
Preterm delivery
Shoulder dystocia
Increase in birthweight
Neonatal hypoglycaemia
Offspring obese as children and adults

Summary box 4.2

Women should modify their diet, stop or reduce smoking and alcohol intake, aim to enter pregnancy with a normal BMI and take folic acid supplementation peri-conceptionally.

Advice regarding medications

It is a misconception that most drugs are harmful in pregnancy. Unfortunately this is an inaccurate belief held by the public and many health professionals including doctors. Many women will discontinue vital medications as soon as they realize they are pregnant and risk a flare of their disease, which will cause harm to them and their babies.

Women with medical diseases on treatment should have a discussion regarding the safety profile of the medications in pregnancy, before they conceive. There are valid concerns about the safety of some drugs in pregnancy, but most commonly used medications have good safety data and can continue to be taken in pregnancy. Even if a drug is known to have a risk of teratogenicity, the consequences of discontinuing it may be worse than the effects of taking it, justifying continuation of therapy (e.g. antiepileptic drugs). The smallest effective dose should be used. If a drug with a better safety profile is available, it should be used instead.

Drugs that are harmful to the fetus may have an effect depending on the time of exposure.
• Pre-embryonic stage (0–14 days after conception): can result in miscarriage, e.g. methotrexate, misoprostol, mifepristone, thalidomide, retinoids.
• First trimester: affect organogenesis resulting in congenital malformation (teratogen), e.g. antiepileptic drugs, angiotensin-converting enzyme (ACE) inhibitors, warfarin.
• Second and third trimester: can cause growth restriction, affect neuropsychological behaviour (e.g. high-dose sodium valproate), or have toxic effect on fetal tissues (e.g. ACE inhibitors, tetracycline).

It is important to know when harmful drugs carry a risk of fetal harm as use of an individual drug at a different stage in pregnancy may have no effect on the fetus, for example a teratogen will bear the risk of congenital malformation with first trimester use, but may be safe to use thereafter if required. A list of known teratogens and drugs that are safe to use in pregnancy is shown in Table 4.3.

Table 4.3 Drug safety in pregnancy.

Drugs that are harmful in pregnancy
NSAIDs (except low-dose aspirin)
Warfarin
Tetracycline, doxycycline, ciprofloxacin
Paroxetine
ACE inhibitors, angiotensin receptor blockers
Statins
Retinoids

Drugs that can be used in pregnancy (if clinically necessary: benefits outweigh risks)
Analgesics (paracetamol, codeine)
Antacids, ranitidine, omeprazole
Most antibiotics (avoid trimethoprim in first trimester and at term)
Most antidepressants (some SSRIs, tricyclic antidepressants)
Antihypertensives: methyldopa, nifedipine, labetolol, doxazosin, prazosin, hydralazine
Antiemetics (cyclizine, promethazine, prochlorperazine, metoclopramide, domperidone)
Antihistamines
Beta-agonists
Inhaled steroids
Hormones (insulin, thyroxine)
Laxatives
Low-dose aspirin

ACE, angiotensin-converting enzyme; NSAID, non-steroidal anti-inflammatory drug; SSRI, selective serotonin reuptake inhibitor.

Summary box 4.3

• Most commonly used medications have good safety data and can continue to be taken in pregnancy in the smallest effective dose.
• Inform women of any risks to pregnancy of medications they are taking.
• Change teratogenic medications before pregnancy if possible (may not be appropriate with some known teratogens (e.g. antiepileptic drugs).

Advice related to maternal age

Delaying childbirth is associated with worsening reproductive outcomes, with more infertility, miscarriage and medical comorbidity and an increase in maternal and fetal morbidity and mortality.

Table 4.4 shows the dramatic decline in fertility and rise in miscarriage rate in women over the age of 40 years [12]. The fertility rate is taken from 10 different populations that did not use contraception between the seventeenth and twentieth centuries. This provides the best approximation of the ability of women to conceive. In current times, the fertility rate in older women is increasing as many older women resort to assisted reproductive

Table 4.4 Risk of infertility and spontaneous miscarriage with age [12].

Maternal age (years)	Fertility rate per 1000 married women	Spontaneous miscarriages (%)
20–24	470	11
25–29	440	12
30–34	400	15
35–39	330	25
40–44	190	51
≥45	40	93

Table 4.5 Risk of pregnancy-specific diseases with age [14].

Pregnancy-related disease	Maternal age	
	20–29 years	>40 years
Pre-eclampsia	3.4%	5.4%
Gestational diabetes	1.7%	7%

Table 4.6 Risk of Down's syndrome (trisomy 21) with maternal age.

Maternal age (years)	Risk of chromosomal abnormality	Risk of Down's syndrome
15–24	1 in 500	1 in 1500
25–29	1 in 385	1 in 1100
35	1 in 178	1 in 350
40	1 in 63	1 in 100
45	1 in 18	1 in 25

technologies (ART) (see Chapter 46) such as *in vitro* fertilisation in order to conceive. The risks of ART include an increased incidence of ovarian hyperstimulation syndrome and multiple pregnancies, which further compounds all maternal age-related risks.

The risk of pre-existing hypertension, obesity, diabetes, ischaemic heart disease and cancer all increase with age and are twofold to fivefold greater in women over the age of 40 compared with women in their twenties [13]. These risks need to be put into context, as the absolute incidences of these diseases are low. Table 4.5 shows how the risks of pre-eclampsia and gestational diabetes increase with maternal age. Maternal death in women over 40 years of age, although rare, is triple that of women in their early twenties [2].

Chromosomal abnormalities increase dramatically with increasing maternal age (Table 4.6). Women should

be informed of these risks and advised that prenatal diagnosis, both screening and definitive testing, is available in pregnancy (see Chapter 17). The option of termination of pregnancy or continuation of pregnancy in the event of an affected fetus should be discussed.

Older mothers have poorer uterine contractility and a higher incidence of assisted vaginal deliveries and caesarean sections compared with younger mothers. The babies of older mothers are more likely to be of low birth weight and the stillbirth rate at all gestations is higher. At 41 weeks' gestation, the risk of a stillbirth in women aged 35–39 years is nearly double that of a woman in her twenties. The risk rises to 3.5-fold higher in women over 40 years [15]. However, it is important to remember that the absolute risk of stillbirth is still small.

The Royal College of Obstetricians and Gynaecologists states that women who start a family in their twenties or complete it by age 35 years face significantly reduced risks. Women contemplating delaying pregnancy should be told the health consequences of this and advised that completion of childbearing in their twenties will vastly reduce their obstetric and medical risks. If they do delay pregnancy to their forties for whatever reason, they should be supported. The absolute risks to the mother remain small, although risks of miscarriage and aneuploidy are high.

Summary box 4.4

Delaying childbirth is associated with worsening reproductive outcomes, with more infertility, miscarriage, chromosomal abnormalities and medical comorbidity and an increase in maternal and fetal morbidity and mortality.

Genetic counselling

Couples who have had a previous child with a chromosomal abnormality, an inherited disease such as cystic fibrosis and Fanconi's anaemia, or with a family history of a genetic disorder should be referred for genetic counselling so that they can be informed of the risks of recurrence and whether prenatal diagnosis is available for detection of the disorder. In some cases pre-implantation genetic diagnosis is available (see Chapter 46).

Conditions where pregnancy is not recommended

There are some conditions where pregnancy is not recommended due to the high risks of maternal and fetal morbidity and mortality.
- Pulmonary arterial hypertension (mortality up to 40%).
- Severe systemic ventricular dysfunction.

- Previous peripartum cardiomyopathy with any residual impairment of left ventricular function.
- Severe left heart obstruction, e.g. aortic/mitral stenosis with valve area <1 cm^2.
- Marfan syndrome with aortic dilatation >4 cm.
- Diabetes with HbA$_{1c}$ >10%.
- Severe respiratory compromise, e.g. forced vital capacity <1 L.
- Breast cancer within last 2 years.
- Severe renal failure (creatinine >250 mmol/L).
- Recurrent uterine scar rupture.

The most effective contraceptive should be used in these circumstances. Other methods of having a family including surrogacy and adoption should be discussed if pregnancy is not recommended. If maternal life expectancy is limited, discussion on the appropriateness of having a baby (by pregnancy, surrogacy or adoption) as well as issues of childcare in the event of maternal mortality or severe morbidity should be discussed.

Summary box 4.5

If pregnancy is not recommended due to severe maternal or fetal risks:
- Use the most effective contraceptive.
- Discuss surrogacy and adoption if maternal life expectancy is not severely limited.

Specific medical diseases

Pre-eclampsia

Women with a low dietary intake of calcium given calcium supplements at a dose of at least 1 g before and during pregnancy can halve their risk of developing pre-eclampsia [9]. Women who have had pre-eclampsia in a previous pregnancy have a 10% chance of recurrence. The recurrence is higher if the onset was early (<34 weeks' gestation), and in this group administration of low-dose aspirin from early pregnancy is associated with reduced risks of developing pre-eclampsia [16]. Women should be advised to start aspirin as soon as their pregnancy test is positive. They should not take it before conception as this may increase their risk of luteinized unruptured follicle syndrome, which can lead to female subfertility.

Hypertension

Women with pre-existing hypertension should have had secondary causes excluded and an assessment made of end-organ damage in those with long-standing hypertension. Their current drug treatment and blood pressure control needs to be reviewed, with replacement of teratogenic drugs (e.g. ACE inhibitors, angiotensin receptor blockers) with safer agents [17].

Diabetes

Many international guidelines exist on pre-conception care of women with diabetes, the latest being from NICE [18] and the American Diabetes Association [19]. Pre-pregnancy control of diabetes directly influences miscarriage and congenital malformation rates. NICE recommends weight reduction for women with a BMI over 27 kg/m^2, monitoring metabolic control and achieving an HbA$_{1c}$ target of less than 6.1% before conception to help reduce these risks. The woman and her partner should be taught about awareness and management of hypoglycaemia. Pregnancy is not recommended in women with HbA$_{1c}$ over 10% and adequate contraception should be provided until target glucose and HbA$_{1c}$ levels are achieved. Women should take a higher dose of folic acid around conception as diabetes is associated with an increased incidence of NTDs. Pre-existing retinopathy can progress rapidly in pregnancy and should be treated before pregnancy [18].

Renal impairment

Women with renal disease should be advised to conceive when their degree of renal impairment is mild to moderate. Delaying pregnancy may result in further loss of renal function. A pregnancy in these circumstances not only increases the risk of pre-eclampsia, fetal growth restriction and preterm delivery, but also the chances of accelerating the onset of end-stage renal failure.

Cardiac disease

Women with cardiac disease should have a risk assessment, with full history, examination and investigations as appropriate (e.g. ECG, echocardiogram, MRI). The effects of the cardiac disease on pregnancy and the effects of the pregnancy on the cardiac disease should be assessed, particularly the risk of deterioration, effect of treatment or intervention in pregnancy in event of deterioration, and fetal and maternal mortality risk. Some cardiac conditions may require surgical correction prior to pregnancy, for example severe mitral stenosis requiring valvuloplasty or valve replacement. Other conditions may require planning of alteration of anticoagulation in early pregnancy (e.g. metal heart valves). Some conditions have such a high maternal mortality associated with them that pregnancy is not recommended (e.g. pulmonary arterial hypertension). A decision should be reached whether pregnancy should be contemplated, delayed or avoided, with adequate contraceptive advice [20].

The long-term prognosis following pregnancy is important. Despite one successful pregnancy, some conditions have a high recurrence risk (e.g. peripartum cardiomyopathy) and others can deteriorate with age, increasing the risk to future pregnancies. Referral should be made to a geneticist where there is a family history of heart disease with features suggesting an underlying genetic or chromosomal abnormality.

Previous poor obstetric history

Women who have had a previous traumatic delivery or adverse pregnancy outcome may benefit from a discussion with an obstetrician prior to conception. They should all have had a debrief following the delivery, but may have unresolved issues or uncertainties regarding the risks of another pregnancy. This visit would allow plans for frequency of antenatal care, requirements for fetal surveillance and delivery plans to be discussed, allowing couples to make an informed decision prior to contemplating further pregnancy.

References

1 National Collaborating Centre for Women's and Children's Health. *Antenatal Care: Routine Care for the Healthy Pregnant Woman*. Available at www.nice.org.uk/guidance/index.jsp?action=download&o=40145.

2 Lewis G (ed.) *Saving Mothers' Lives: Reviewing Maternal Deaths to Make Motherhood Safer 2003–2005. The Seventh Report on Confidential Enquiries into Maternal Deaths in the United Kingdom*. London: The Confidential Enquiry into Maternal and Child Health, 2007. Available at: www.cmace.org.uk/getattachment/26dae364-1fc9-4a29-a6cb-afb3f251f8f7/Saving-Mothers'-Lives-2003-2005-(Full-report).aspx

3 Office for National Statistics. Teenage pregnancy statistics 2010. Available at: www.dcsf.gov.uk/everychildmatters/healthandwellbeing/teenagepregnancy/statistics/statistics/ Accessed May 2010.

4 Lumley J, Watson L, Watson M, Bower C. Periconceptional supplementation with folate and/or multivitamins for preventing neural tube defects. *Cochrane Database Syst Rev* 2001;(3):CD001056.

5 MRC Vitamin Study Research Group. Prevention of neural tube defects: results of the Medical Research Council Vitamin Study. *Lancet* 1991;338:131–137.

6 Mahmud M, Mazza D. Preconception care of women with diabetes: a review of current guideline recommendations. *BMC Womens Health* 2010;10:5.

7 Centres for Disease Control and Prevention. Trends in wheat-flour fortification with folic acid and iron: worldwide, 2004 and 2007. *MMWR* 2008;57:8–10.

8 Czeizel AE. The primary prevention of birth defects: multivitamins or folic acid? *Int J Med Sci* 2004;11:50–61.

9 Villar J, Abdel-Aleem H, Merialdi M *et al*. World Health Organisation randomised trial of calcium supplementation among low calcium intake pregnant women. *Am J Obstet Gynecol* 2006;194:639–649.

10 Royal College of Obstetricians and Gynaecologists. Statement no. 5. Alcohol consumption and the outcomes of pregnancy. Available at www.rcog.org.uk/files/rcog-corp/uploaded-files/RCOGStatement5AlcoholPregnancy2006.pdf. Accessed May 2010.

11 Lee CY, Koren G. Maternal obesity: effects on pregnancy and the role of pre-conception counselling. *J Obstet Gynaecol* 2010;30:101–106.

12 Heffner LJ. Advanced maternal age: how old is too old? *N Engl J Med* 2004;351:1927–1929.

13 Dhanjal MK. The older mother and medical disorders in pregnancy. In: Bewley S, Ledger W, Dimitrios N (eds) *Reproductive Ageing*. London: RCOG Press, 2009.

14 Gilbert WM, Nesbitt TS, Danielsen B. Childbearing beyond age 40: pregnancy outcome in 24 032 cases. *Obstet Gynecol* 1999;93:9–14.

15 Reddy UM, Ko CW, Willinger M. Maternal age and the risk of stillbirth throughout pregnancy in the United States. *Am J Obstet Gynecol* 2006;195:764–770.

16 Duley L, Henderson-Smart DJ, Meher S, King JF. Antiplatelet agents for preventing pre-eclampsia and its complications. *Cochrane Database Syst Rev* 2007;(2):CD004659.

17 Cooper WO, Hernandez-Diaz S, Arbogast PG *et al*. Major congenital malformations after first-trimester exposure to ACE inhibitors. *N Engl J Med* 2006;354:2443–2451.

18 National Institute for Health and Clinical Excellence. *Diabetes in Pregnancy: Management of Diabetes and its Complications from Pre-conception to the Postnatal Period*. Clinical Guideline 63. Available at: www.nice.org.uk/nicemedia/pdf/CG063Guidance.pdf

19 American Diabetes Association. Standards of medical care in diabetes: 2009. *Diabetes Care* 2009;32(Suppl 1):S13–S61.

20 Adamson DL, Dhanjal MK, Nelson-Piercy C, Collis R. Cardiac disease in pregnancy. In: Greer IA, Nelson-Piercy C, Walters B (eds) *Maternal Medicine*. London: Elsevier Health Sciences, 2007.

Chapter 5
Antenatal Care

George Attilakos[1] and Timothy G. Overton[2]
[1]Fetal Medicine Unit, University College London Hospital NHS Foundation Trust, London, UK
[2]St Michael's Hospital, University Hospitals Bristol NHS Foundation Trust, Bristol, UK

The care of pregnant women presents a unique challenge to modern medicine. Most women will progress through pregnancy in an uncomplicated fashion and deliver a healthy infant requiring little medical or midwifery intervention. Unfortunately, a significant number will have medical problems that will complicate their pregnancy or develop such serious conditions that the lives of both themselves and their unborn child will be threatened. In 1928, a pregnant woman faced a 1 in 290 chance of dying from an obstetric complication related to the pregnancy; the most recent Confidential Enquiry into Maternal and Child Health put this figure at 1 in 21 416 [1]. Undoubtedly, good antenatal care has made a significant contribution to this reduction. The current challenge of antenatal care is to identify those women who will require specialist support and help while allowing uncomplicated pregnancies to progress with minimal interference. The antenatal period also allows the opportunity for women, especially those in their first pregnancy, to receive information from a variety of healthcare professionals regarding pregnancy, childbirth and parenthood.

Aims of antenatal care

Antenatal education

Provision of information

Women and their husbands/partners have the right to be involved in all decisions regarding their antenatal care. They need to be able to make informed decisions concerning where they will be seen, who will undertake their care, which screening tests to have and where they plan to give birth. Women must have access to evidence-based information in a format they can understand. Current evidence suggests that insufficient written information is available especially at the beginning of pregnancy and information provided can be misleading or inaccurate. *The Pregnancy Book* [2] provides information on the developing fetus, antenatal care and classes, rights and benefits as well as a list of useful organizations. Many leaflets have been produced by the Midwives Information and Resource Service (MIDIRS) that help women to make informed objective decisions during pregnancy. The Royal College of Obstetricians and Gynaecologists has also produced many pregnancy-related patient information leaflets, most of them accompanying the relevant 'Green-top Guidelines' for clinicians. Written information is particularly important to help women understand the purpose of screening tests and the options that are available and to advise on lifestyle considerations including dietary recommendations. Available information needs to be provided at first contact and must take into account cultural and language barriers. Local services should endeavour to provide information that is understandable to those whose first language is not English and to those with physical, cognitive and sensory disabilities. Translators will be frequently required in clinics with an ethnic mix.

Couples should also be offered the opportunity to attend antenatal classes. Ideally such classes should discuss physiological and psychological changes during pregnancy, fetal development, labour and childbirth and how to care for the newborn baby. Evidence shows a greater acquisition of knowledge in women who have attended such classes compared with those that have not.

Lifestyle concerns

At an early stage in the pregnancy women require lifestyle advice, including information on diet and food, work during pregnancy and social aspects, for example smoking, alcohol, exercise and sexual activity.

Women should be advised of the benefits of eating a balanced diet that contains plenty of fruit and vegetables, starchy foods such as pasta, bread, rice and potatoes, protein, fibre and dairy foods. They should be informed of foods that could put their fetus at risk. Listeriosis is caused by the bacterium *Listeria monocytogenes* which can present with a mild flu-like illness but is associated with miscarriage, stillbirth and severe illness in the newborn. Contaminated food is the usual source including

Dewhurst's Textbook of Obstetrics & Gynaecology, Eighth Edition. Edited by D. Keith Edmonds.
© 2012 John Wiley and Sons, Ltd. Published 2012 by John Wiley and Sons, Ltd.

unpasteurized milk, ripened soft cheeses and pâté. Toxoplasmosis contracted through contact with infected cat litter or undercooked meat can lead to permanent neurological and visual problems in the newborn if the mother contracts the infection during pregnancy. (Salmonella food poisoning has not been shown to have adverse fetal effects.) To reduce the risk, pregnant women should be advised to thoroughly wash all fruits and vegetables before eating and to cook all meats thoroughly, including ready-prepared chilled meats. Written information from the UK Food Standards Agency (*Eating While you are Pregnant*) can also be helpful. For example, the Food Standards Agency advises women to reduce the consumption of caffeine to 200 mg/day (equivalent to two mugs of instant coffee), because of its association with low birthweight and miscarriage.

Women who have not had a baby with spina bifida should be advised to take folic acid 400 µg/day from pre-conception until 12 weeks of gestation to reduce the chance of fetal neural tube defects (NTDs). However, research has failed to show the efficacy of this strategy in analysing the population incidence of NTDs. This may be due to inadequate pre-conceptual intake of folate and/or poor compliance. Suggestions of adding folate to certain foods (e.g. flour) to ensure population compliance remain debatable. Current evidence does not support routine iron supplementation for all pregnant women and can be associated with some unpleasant side effects such as constipation. However, any woman who is iron deficient must be encouraged to take iron therapy prior to the onset of labour as any excess blood loss at delivery will increase maternal morbidity. The intake of vitamin A (liver and liver products) should be limited in pregnancy to approximately 700 mg/day because of fetal teratogenicity.

Because alcohol passes freely across the placenta, women should be advised not to drink excessively during pregnancy. The current UK advice for pregnant women is to avoid alcohol consumption in the first 3 months of pregnancy and, if they choose to drink alcohol, to limit their consumption to one to two units once or twice per week. Binge drinking and continuous heavy drinking causes the fetal alcohol syndrome, characterized by low birthweight, a specific facies, and intellectual and behavioural difficulties later in life.

Approximately 27% of women are smokers at the time of birth of their baby. Smoking is significantly associated with a number of adverse outcomes in pregnancy, including an increased risk of perinatal mortality, placental abruption, preterm delivery, preterm premature rupture of the membranes, placenta praevia and low birthweight. While there is evidence to suggest that smoking may decrease the incidence of pre-eclampsia, this must be balanced against the far greater number of negative associations. Although there is mixed evidence for the effectiveness of smoking cessation programmes, women should be encouraged to use local NHS Stop Smoking services and the NHS pregnancy smoking helpline [3]. Pregnant women who are unable to stop smoking should be informed of the benefits of reducing the number of cigarettes they smoke. A 50% reduction can significantly reduce the fetal nicotine concentration and is associated with an increase in the birthweight.

Women who use recreational drugs must be advised to stop or be directed to rehabilitation programmes. Evidence shows adverse effects on the fetus and its subsequent development.

Continuing moderate exercise in pregnancy or regular sexual intercourse does not appear to be associated with any adverse outcomes. Certain physical activity should be avoided such as contact sports which may cause unexpected abdominal trauma. Scuba diving should also be avoided because of the risk of fetal decompression disease and an increased risk of birth defects.

Physically demanding work, particularly those jobs with prolonged periods of standing, may be associated with poorer outcomes such as preterm birth, hypertension and pre-eclampsia and small-for-gestational-age babies but the evidence is weak and employment per se has not been associated with increased risks in pregnancy. Women require information regarding their employment rights in pregnancy and healthcare professionals need to be aware of the current legislation.

Help for the socially disadvantaged and single mothers must be organized and ideally a one-to-one midwife allocated to support these women. The midwife should be able to liaise with other social services to ensure the best environment for the mother and her newborn child. Similar individual help is needed for pregnant teenagers and midwife programmes need to provide appropriate support for these vulnerable mothers.

Common symptoms in pregnancy

It is common for pregnant women to experience unpleasant symptoms in pregnancy caused by the normal physiological changes. However, these symptoms can be quite debilitating and lead to anxiety. It is important that healthcare professionals are aware of such symptoms, can advise appropriate treatment and know when to initiate further investigations.

Extreme tiredness is one of the first symptoms of pregnancy and affects almost all women. It lasts for approximately 12–14 weeks and then resolves in the majority.

Nausea and vomiting in pregnancy is one of the commonest early symptoms. While it is thought that this may be caused by rising levels of human chorionic gonadotrophin (hCG), the evidence for this is conflicting. Hyperemesis gravidarum, where fluid and electrolyte imbalance and nutritional deficiency occur, is far less common, complicating approximately 3.5 per 1000 pregnancies. Nausea and vomiting in pregnancy varies in severity but usually presents within 8 weeks of the last menstrual period. Cessation of symptoms is reported by most by about 16 weeks. Various non-medical treatments have been advocated including ginger, vitamins B_6 and B_{12}, and P6 acupressure. There is evidence for the effectiveness of each of these but concerns about the safety of vitamin B_6 (pyridoxine) remains and there are limited data on the safety of vitamin B_{12} (cyanocobalamin). Antihistamines (prochlorperazine, promethazine) and metoclopramide appear to be the pharmacological agents of choice, as they reduce nausea and are safe in relation to teratogenicity, although they are associated with drowsiness [4].

Constipation complicates approximately one-third of pregnancies, usually decreasing in severity with advancing gestation. It is thought to be related in part to poor dietary fibre intake and reduction in gut motility caused by rising levels of progesterone. Diet modification with bran and wheat fibre supplementation helps, as well as increasing daily fluid intake.

Heartburn is also a common symptom in pregnancy but, unlike constipation, occurs more frequently as the pregnancy progresses. It is estimated to complicate one-fifth of pregnancies in the first trimester rising to three-quarters by the third trimester. It is due to the increasing pressure caused by the enlarging uterus combined with the hormonal changes that lead to gastro-oesophageal reflux. It is important to distinguish this symptom from the epigastric pain associated with pre-eclampsia which will usually be associated with hypertension and proteinuria. Symptoms can be improved by simple lifestyle modifications such as maintaining an upright posture especially after meals, lying propped up in bed, eating small frequent meals and avoiding fatty foods. Antacids (especially Gaviscon), histamine H_2-receptor antagonists and proton-pump inhibitors are all effective, although it is recommended that the latter be used only when other treatments have failed because of their unproven safety in pregnancy.

Haemorrhoids are experienced by 1 in 10 women in the last trimester of pregnancy. There is little evidence for either the beneficial effects of topical creams in pregnancy or indeed their safety. Diet modification may help and in extreme circumstances surgical treatment considered, although this is unusual since the haemorrhoids often resolve after delivery.

Varicose veins occur frequently in pregnancy. They do not cause harm and while compression stockings may help symptoms they unfortunately do not prevent varicose veins from appearing.

The nature of physiological vaginal discharge changes in pregnancy. However, if it becomes itchy, malodorous or is associated with pain on micturition, it may be due to an underlying infection such as trichomoniasis, bacterial vaginosis or candidiasis. Appropriate investigations and treatment should be instigated.

Backache is another potentially debilitating symptom, with an estimated prevalence of up to 61% in pregnancy. There is limited research on effective interventions for backache, but massage therapy, exercise in water and back care classes may be helpful in symptom relief.

Screening for maternal complications

Anaemia

Maternal iron requirements increase in pregnancy because of the demands of the developing fetus, the formation of the placenta and the increase in the maternal red cell mass. With an increase in the maternal plasma volume of up to 50% there is a physiological drop in the haemoglobin (Hb) concentration during pregnancy. It is generally recommended that an Hb level below 11 g/dL up to 12 weeks' gestation or less than 10.5 g/dL at 28 weeks signifies anaemia and warrants further investigation. A low Hb (8.5–10.5 g/dL) may be associated with preterm labour and low birthweight. Routine screening should be performed at the booking visit and at 28 weeks' gestation. While there are many causes of anaemia, including thalassaemia and sickle cell disease, iron deficiency remains the commonest. Serum ferritin is the best way of assessing maternal iron stores and if found to be low iron supplementation should be considered. Routine iron supplementation in women with a normal Hb in pregnancy has not been shown to improve maternal or fetal outcome and is currently not recommended.

Blood groups

Identifying the maternal blood group and screening for the presence of atypical antibodies is important in the prevention of haemolytic disease, particularly from rhesus alloimmunization. Routine antibody screening should take place at booking in all women and again at 28 weeks' gestation irrespective of their rhesus D (RhD) status. Detection of atypical antibodies should prompt referral to a specialist fetal medicine unit. In the UK, 15% of women are RhD negative and should be offered anti-D prophylaxis after potentially sensitizing events (e.g. amniocentesis or antepartum haemorrhage) and routinely at either 28 and 34 weeks' gestation or once at 32 weeks depending on the dosage of anti-D immunoglobulin used [3]. In the future, all RhD-negative women may have routine diagnosis of fetal RhD status by analysing free fetal DNA in the maternal plasma. This will allow targeted anti-D administration to women with RhD-positive fetuses, which will result in cost savings and allow many women to avoid an unnecessary blood product. A feasibility study has already been performed [5] and another UK study is currently ongoing.

Haemoglobinopathies

Screening for sickle cell disease and thalassaemias is important and each country will have a different screening strategy depending on the prevalence of these conditions. In the UK, this screening should be offered to all women as early as possible in pregnancy. If the regional sickle cell disease prevalence is high, laboratory screening should be offered. If the regional sickle cell disease prevalence is low, the initial screening should be based on the Family Origin Questionnaire.

Infection

Maternal blood should be taken early in pregnancy and with consent screened for hepatitis B, HIV, rubella and syphilis. Identification of women who are hepatitis B carriers can lead to a 95% reduction in mother-to-infant transmission following appropriate postnatal administration of vaccine and immunoglobulin to the baby. Women who are HIV positive can be offered treatment with antiretroviral drugs which, when combined with delivery by Caesarean section and avoidance of breast-feeding, can reduce the maternal transmission rates from approximately 25% to 1% [6]. Such women need to be managed by appropriate specialist teams. Rubella screening aims to detect those women who are susceptible to the virus, allowing postnatal vaccination to protect future pregnancies. All women who are rubella non-immune must be counselled to avoid contact with any infected person and if inadvertently they do, they must report the event to their midwife or doctor. Serial antibody levels will determine whether infection has occurred. Vaccination during pregnancy is contraindicated because the vaccine may be teratogenic. Although the incidence of infectious syphilis is low, there have been a number of recent outbreaks in England and Wales. Untreated syphilis is associated with congenital syphilis, neonatal death, stillbirth and preterm delivery. Following positive screening for syphilis, testing of a second specimen is required for confirmation. Interpretation of results can be difficult and referral to specialist genitourinary medicine clinics is recommended. Current evidence does not support routine screening for cytomegalovirus, hepatitis C, toxoplasmosis or group B *Streptococcus*.

Asymptomatic bacteriuria occurs in approximately 2–5% of pregnant women and when untreated is associated with pyelonephritis and preterm labour. Appropriate treatment will reduce the risk of preterm birth. Screening should be offered early in pregnancy by midstream urine culture.

Hypertensive disease

Chronic hypertension pre-dates pregnancy or appears in the first 20 weeks, whereas pregnancy-induced hypertension develops in the pregnancy, resolves after delivery and is not associated with proteinuria. Pre-eclampsia is defined as hypertension that is associated with proteinuria occurring after 20 weeks and resolving after birth. Pre-eclampsia occurs in 2–10% of pregnancies and is associated with both maternal and neonatal morbidity and mortality [7]. Risk factors include nulliparity, age 40 years and above, family history of pre-eclampsia, history of pre-eclampsia in a prior pregnancy, body mass index (BMI) greater than 35, multiple pregnancy and pre-existing diabetes or hypertension. Hypertension is often an early sign that pre-dates the development of serious maternal and fetal disease and should be assessed regularly in pregnancy. There is little evidence as to how frequently blood pressure should be checked and so it is important to identify risk factors for pre-eclampsia early in pregnancy. In the absence of these, blood pressure and urine analysis for protein should be measured at each routine antenatal visit and mothers should be warned of the advanced symptoms of pre-eclampsia (frontal headache, epigastric pain, vomiting and visual disturbances). However, when risk factors are present, more frequent blood pressure measurements and urine analyses should be considered.

Gestational diabetes

Currently there is little agreement as to the definition of gestational diabetes, whether we should routinely screen for it and how to diagnose and manage it. However, there has been increasing evidence that 'treating' gestational diabetes is more beneficial than expectant management [8]. Consequently, the National Institute for Health and Clinical Excellence (NICE) recently recommended screening for gestational diabetes using risk factors in a healthy population [3]. Women with risk factors should be tested for gestational diabetes using the 2-hour 75-g oral glucose tolerance test.

Psychiatric illness

The importance of psychiatric conditions related to pregnancy was highlighted in the 2000–2002 Confidential Enquiry into Maternal and Child Health [9]. A significant number of maternal deaths due to or associated with psychiatric causes were also reported in the most recent enquiry [1]. At booking, women should be asked about history of significant mental illness or previous psychiatric treatment. Family history of perinatal mental illness is also important. If mental illness is suspected, further referral for assessment should be made. Good communication, particularly with primary care, is paramount.

Placenta praevia

In approximately 1.5% of women the placenta will cover the os on the 20-week scan, but by delivery only 0.14% will have placenta praevia. Only those women whose placenta covers the os in the second trimester should be offered another scan at 32 weeks to check the placental position. If this is not clear on transabdominal scan, a transvaginal scan should be performed. There is no evidence for the effectiveness of a routine screening programme for vasa praevia at 20 weeks. However, the Society of Obstetricians and Gynaecologists of Canada advises that transvaginal ultrasound may be considered for all women at high risk for vasa praevia (e.g. low or velamentous cord insertion) [10].

Screening for fetal complications

Confirmation of fetal viability

All women should be offered a 'dating' scan. This is best performed between 10 and 13 weeks' gestation and the crown–rump length measured when the fetus is in a neutral position (i.e. not curled up or hyperextended). Current evidence shows that the estimated day of delivery predicted by ultrasound at this gestation will reduce the need for induction of labour at 41 weeks when compared with the due date predicted by the last menstrual period. In addition, a dating scan will improve the reliability of serum screening for Down's syndrome, diagnose multiple pregnancy and allow accurate determination of chorionicity and diagnose up to 80% of major fetal abnormalities. Women who present after 14 weeks' gestation should be offered a dating scan by ultrasound assessment of the biparietal diameter or head circumference.

Screening for Down's syndrome

Current recommendations from NICE advocate that all women in the UK are offered the combined screening test for Down's syndrome between 11 and 14 weeks' gestation. Those that book later should be offered serum screening between 15 and 20 weeks' gestation. The National Screening Committee further refined these guidelines in 2010, stating that the detection rate should be 90% for a screen positive rate of 2%. Because screening for Down's syndrome is a complex issue, healthcare professionals must have a clear understanding of the options available to their patients. Unbiased, evidence-based information must be given to the woman at the beginning of the pregnancy so that she has time to consider whether to opt for screening and the opportunity to clarify any areas of confusion before the deadline for the test passes. Recognizing the importance of this, NICE currently recommends that the first two antenatal appointments take place before 12 weeks' gestation to allow the woman adequate time to make an informed decision about whether to have screening. Following a 'screen positive' result the woman needs careful counselling to explain that the test result does not mean the fetus has Down's syndrome and to explain the options for further testing by either chorion villus sampling or amniocentesis. A positive screen test does not mean further testing is mandatory. Likewise, a woman with a 'screen negative' result must understand that the fetus may still have Down's syndrome (see 'Fetal medicine in clinical practice').

Screening for structural abnormalities

The identification of fetal structural abnormalities allows the opportunity for *in utero* therapy, planning for delivery, for example when the fetus has major congenital heart disease, parental preparation and the option of termination of pregnancy should a severe problem be diagnosed. Major structural anomalies are present in about 3% of fetuses screened at 20 weeks' gestation. Detection rates vary depending on the system examined, skill of the operator, time allowed for the scan and quality of the ultrasound equipment. Follow-up data are important for auditing the quality of the service. Women must appreciate the limitations of such scans. Local detection rates of various anomalies such as spina bifida, heart disease, facial clefting and the like should be made available. Written information should be given to women early in pregnancy explaining the nature and purpose of such scans, highlighting conditions that are not detected such as cerebral palsy and many genetic conditions. It is important to appreciate that the fetal anomaly scan is a screening test which women should opt for rather than have as a routine part of antenatal care without appropriate counselling (see 'Fetal medicine in clinical practice'). In 2010 the NHS Fetal Anomaly Screening Programme published a document for national standards and guidance for the mid-trimester fetal anomaly scan [11]. These standards set out the basis for the ultrasound screening service in England, describing what can and, importantly, what cannot be achieved.

Screening for fetal well-being

Each antenatal clinic attendance allows the opportunity to screen for fetal well-being. Auscultation for the fetal heart will confirm that the fetus is alive and can usually be detected from about 14 weeks of gestation. While hearing the fetal heart may be reassuring, there is no evidence of a clinical or predictive value. Likewise there is no evidence to support the use of routine cardiotocography in uncomplicated pregnancies. Physical examination of the abdomen by inspection and palpation will identify approximately 30% of small-for-gestational age fetuses [12]. Measurement of the symphysis–fundal height in centimetres starting at the uterine fundus and ending on the fixed point of the symphysis pubis has a sensitivity and specificity of approximately 27 and 88%, respectively, although serial measurements may improve accuracy. While evidence for the benefits of plotting serial symphysis–fundal height measurements is limited, it is recommended that women are offered estimation of fetal size at each antenatal visit; when there is concern, they should be referred for formal ultrasound assessment. Ultrasound assessment of fetal growth for a suspected large fetus is not recommended in a low-risk pregnancy.

Customized growth charts make adjustments for maternal height, weight, ethnicity and parity. However, there is no good-quality evidence that their use improves perinatal outcomes [3].

Traditionally, women have been advised to note the frequency of fetal movements in the third trimester. Although the evidence does not support formal counting of fetal movements to reduce the incidence of late fetal death, women who notice a reduction of fetal movements should contact their local hospital for further advice.

Organization of antenatal care

Antenatal care has been traditionally provided by a combination of general practitioners, community midwives, and hospital midwives and obstetricians. The balance has depended on the perceived normality of the pregnancy at booking. However, pregnancy and childbirth is to a certain extent an unpredictable process. The frequency of antenatal visits and appropriate carer must be planned carefully, allowing the opportunity for early detection of problems without becoming over-intrusive.

Who should provide the antenatal care?

A meta-analysis comparing pregnancy outcome in two groups of low-risk women, one with community-led antenatal care (midwife and general practitioner) and the other with hospital-led care did not show any differences in terms of preterm birth, Caesarean section, anaemia, antepartum haemorrhage, urinary tract infections and perinatal mortality. The first group had a lower rate of pregnancy-induced hypertension and pre-eclampsia, which could reflect a lower incidence or lower detection [13]. However, clear referral pathways need to be developed that allow appropriate referral to specialists when either fetal or maternal problems are detected.

There is little evidence regarding women's views on who should provide antenatal care. Unfortunately, care is usually provided by a number of different professionals often in different settings. Studies evaluating the impact of continuity of care do not generally separate the antenatal period from labour. The studies consistently show that with fewer caregivers women are better informed and prepared for labour, attend more antenatal classes, have fewer antenatal admissions to hospital and have higher satisfaction rates. Differences in clinical end-points such as Caesarean section rates, postpartum haemorrhage, admission to the neonatal unit and perinatal mortality are generally insignificant [3]. While it would

appear advantageous for women to be seen by the same midwife throughout pregnancy and childbirth, there are practical and economic considerations that need to be taken into account. Nevertheless, where possible, care should be provided by a small group of professionals.

Documentation of antenatal care

The antenatal record needs to document clearly the care the woman has received from all those involved. It will also serve as a legal document, a source of useful information for the woman and a mechanism of communication between different healthcare professionals. There is now good evidence that women should be allowed to carry their own notes. Women feel more in control of their pregnancy and do not lose the notes any more often than the hospital! In addition, useful information will be available to clinicians should the woman require emergency care while away from home. Many areas of the UK are endeavouring to work towards a standard format for the records. This would be of benefit to those women who move between hospitals so that caregivers would automatically be familiar with the style of the notes. If we are to move to an electronic patient record, there must be general agreement in a minimum dataset and a standard antenatal record would be a step in this direction.

Frequency and timing of antenatal visits

There has been little change in how frequently women are seen in pregnancy for the last 50 years. In 2003, NICE produced a clinical guideline entitled *Antenatal Care: Routine Care for the Healthy Pregnant Woman*, which was updated and revised in 2008 [3]. This document recognized the large amount of information that needs to be discussed at the beginning of pregnancy, particularly with regard to screening tests. The first appointment needs to be early in pregnancy, certainly before 12 weeks if possible. This initial appointment should be regarded as an opportunity for imparting general information about the pregnancy such as diet, smoking and folic acid supplementation. A crucial aim is to identify those women who will require additional care during the pregnancy (Table 5.1). A urine test should be sent for bacteriological screen and a dating ultrasound scan arranged. Sufficient time should be set aside for an impartial discussion of the screening tests available including those for anaemia, red-cell antibodies, syphilis, HIV, hepatitis and rubella. Because of the complexity of Down's syndrome, this too should be discussed in detail and supplemented with written information. Ideally another follow-up appointment should be arranged before the screening tests need to be performed to allow further questions and to arrange a time for the tests following maternal consent.

Table 5.1 Factors indicating the need for additional specialist care in pregnancy.

Conditions such as hypertension, cardiac or renal disease, endocrine, psychiatric or haematological disorders, epilepsy, diabetes, autoimmune disease, cancer or HIV
Factors that make the woman vulnerable (e.g. those who lack social support)
Age 40 years and older or 18 years and younger
BMI ≥35 or <18
Previous Caesarean section
Severe pre-eclampsia or eclampsia
Previous pre-eclampsia or eclampsia
Three or more miscarriages
Previous preterm birth or mid-trimester loss
Previous psychiatric illness or puerperal psychosis
Previous neonatal death or stillbirth
Previous baby with congenital anomaly
Previous small-for-gestational or large-for-gestational age baby
Family history of genetic disorder

Source: With kind permission of the National Collaborating Centre for Women's and Children's Health.

 Summary box 5.1

- The administration of folic acid 400 µg/day is recommended to reduce the incidence of NTDs.
- Women should be informed of the harmful effects of smoking in pregnancy.
- Nulliparous women require more antenatal appointments.
- Women with risk factors should be referred to specialist obstetric care.
- At booking, women should be asked about history of significant mental illness, previous psychiatric treatment or family history of perinatal mental illness.
- Dating scan should be performed between 10 and 13 weeks' gestation by measuring the crown–rump length.
- All women in the UK should be offered the combined screening test for Down's syndrome between 11 and 14 weeks' gestation.
- Antihistamines (prochlorperazine, promethazine) and metoclopramide appear to be the pharmacological agents of choice for nausea and vomiting in pregnancy.
- It is recommended that women are offered estimation of fetal size by symphysis–fundal height measurement at each antenatal visit; when there is suspicion of a small fetus, they are referred for formal ultrasound assessment.

The next appointment needs to be around 16 weeks' gestation to discuss the results of the screening tests. In addition, information about antenatal classes should be given and a plan of action made for the timing and frequency of future antenatal visits including who should see the woman. As with each antenatal visit, the blood pressure should be measured and the urine tested for protein. The 20-week anomaly scan should also be discussed and arranged and women should understand its limitations.

At each visit the symphysis–fundal height is plotted, the blood pressure measured and the urine tested for protein. At 28 weeks' gestation, blood should be taken for haemoglobin estimation and atypical red-cell antibodies. Anti-D prophylaxis should be offered to women who are rhesus negative. A follow-up appointment at 34 weeks will allow the opportunity to discuss these results. A second dose of anti-D should be offered at 34 weeks. At 36 weeks, the position of the baby needs to be checked and if there is uncertainty, an ultrasound scan arranged to exclude breech presentation. If a breech is confirmed, external cephalic version should be considered. For women who have not given birth by 41 weeks, both a membrane sweep and induction of labour should be discussed and offered. Additional appointments at 25, 31 and 40 weeks are proposed for nulliparous women.

In summary, a total of 10 appointments is recommended for nulliparous women and seven appointments for multiparous women, assuming they have uncomplicated pregnancies.

References

1 Centre for Maternal and Child Enquiries (CMACE). Saving Mothers' Lives: Reviewing Maternal Deaths to Make Motherhood Safer 2006–2008. The Eigth Report on Confidential Enquiries into Maternal Deaths in the United Kingdom. *BJOG* 2011; 118(Suppl 1):1–203.

2 National Health Service. *The Pregnancy Book*. London: Department of Health, 2009. Available at www.dh.gov.uk/en/Publicationsandstatistics/Publications/PublicationsPolicyAndGuidance/DH_107302. Accessed on 20 June 2010.

3 National Collaborating Centre for Women's and Children's Health. *Antenatal Care: Routine Care for the Healthy Pregnant Woman*. Available at www.nice.org.uk/guidance/index.jsp?action=download&o=40145.

4 Jewell D, Young G. Interventions for nausea and vomiting in early pregnancy. *Cochrane Database Syst Rev* 2003;(4):CD000145.

5 Finning K, Martin P, Summers J, Massey E, Poole G, Daniels G. Effect of high throughput RHD typing of fetal DNA in maternal plasma on use of anti-RhD immunoglobulin in RhD negative pregnant women: prospective feasibility study. *BMJ* 2008;336: 816–818.

6 Mandelbrot L, Le Chenadec J, Berrebi A *et al.* Perinatal HIV-1 transmission. Interaction between zidovudine prophylaxis and mode of delivery in the French perinatal cohort. *JAMA* 1998;280:55–60.

7 Sibai B, Dekker G, Kupferminc M. Pre-eclampsia. *Lancet* 2005;365:785–799.

8 Crowther CA, Hiller JE, Moss JR *et al.* Effect of treatment of gestational diabetes mellitus on pregnancy outcomes. *N Engl J Med* 2005;352:2477–2486.

9 Confidential Enquiry into Maternal and Child Health. *Why Mothers Die: 2000–2002*. London: RCOG Press, 2004.

10 Gagnon R, Morin L, Bly S *et al.* SOGC Clinical Practice Guideline: guidelines for the management of vasa previa. *Int J Gynaecol Obstet* 2010;108:85–89.

11 NHS Fetal Anomaly Screening Programme. *18 + 0 to 20 + 6 Weeks Fetal Anomaly Scan: National Standards and Guidance for England.* London: RCOG Press, 2010. Available at http://fetalanomaly.screening.nhs.uk/getdata.php?id=11218

12 Royal College of Obstetricians and Gynaecologists. *The Investigation and Management of the Small-for-gestational Age Fetus.* Green-top Guideline No. 31, 2002. Available at www.rcog.org.uk/files/rcog-corp/uploaded-files/GT31Small GestationalAgeFetus.pdf.

13 Villar J, Carroli G, Khan-Neelofur D, Piaggio G, Gülmezoglu M. Patterns of routine antenatal care for low-risk pregnancy. *Cochrane Database Syst Rev* 2001;(4):CD000934.

Part 3
Early Pregnancy Problems

Chapter 6
Spontaneous Miscarriage

Catriona M. Stalder
Queen Charlotte's & Chelsea Hospital, London, UK

Spontaneous miscarriage is an unfortunate outcome of early pregnancy. Despite its frequency, however, there is still scope for improvement in patient care as it remains responsible for considerable emotional and psychological trauma in patients. Recognizing and addressing this issue allows doctors to improve patient care. Part of this effort has involved the development of early pregnancy units providing dedicated care for these women. These units also improve clinical care from a diagnostic and management standpoint. In the UK, early pregnancy complications rarely result in maternal death. The most recent triennial report (2005–2007) reported one maternal death from spontaneous miscarriage although there were 18 direct deaths from maternal sepsis including deaths in early pregnancy [1].

With the advent of commercially available, sensitive and affordable pregnancy tests, women present at increasingly earlier points in pregnancy looking for reassurance and confirmation of viability. It is important that while their anxiety is recognized, we proceed along safe and familiar diagnostic pathways to avoid misdiagnosis. It is also important to recognize that pregnancy is a dynamic process and that a diagnosis of viability early in the first trimester does not necessarily signify that the pregnancy will continue, although if a fetal heart pulsation is detected at 6 weeks' gestation there is a 90% chance that the pregnancy will continue beyond the first trimester [2].

The rate of miscarriage varies depending on the gestation of pregnancy and maternal age. Up to 50% of early pregnancies will fail within 4 weeks from last menstrual period (LMP), so-called biochemical pregnancies. By 6 weeks' gestation, the rate is one in five pregnancies and by the second trimester the rate has fallen to 1 in 40 [3] (Fig. 6.1).

Definition

Spontaneous miscarriage is defined as the spontaneous loss of a pregnancy prior to viability, taken legally in the UK as a gestation date of 23 weeks 6 days. Beyond this, fetal demise is classified as stillbirth. First-trimester miscarriage occurs below 12 weeks' gestation and accounts for the majority. The overall rate is 20%. Second-trimester miscarriages are less common, accounting for 1–4% of all miscarriages [5]. While some second-trimester miscarriages can be explained as first-trimester losses where the diagnosis is made in the second trimester, nevertheless it seems likely that the causes are different.

The recent Royal College of Obstetricians and Gynaecologists (RCOG) guidelines of October 2006 have helped clarify the different definitions and terminology and how they have changed with a move away from the word 'abortion', which is firmly associated with therapeutic abortion among the general public (Table 6.1). The importance of accurately defining the different types of miscarriage is that it provides the bedrock upon which comparative research can be built, to better understand the relative benefits and outcomes of treatment options.

Terminology

The definitions in Table 6.2 can be seen to be a mixture of clinical and ultrasound-based diagnosis and are often suggested prospectively and confirmed retrospectively. Care must be taken when relying solely on a clinical diagnosis because this is often refuted by ultrasound. For example, in cases where the clinical picture suggests complete miscarriage, there will be ultrasound evidence of retained products in 45% of patients [6] though the clinical significance remains uncertain.

Aetiology

Although the causes of miscarriage in first and second trimester appear different, there is inevitably some overlap, in addition to the occasional situation where

Dewhurst's Textbook of Obstetrics & Gynaecology, Eighth Edition. Edited by D. Keith Edmonds.
© 2012 John Wiley and Sons, Ltd. Published 2012 by John Wiley and Sons, Ltd.

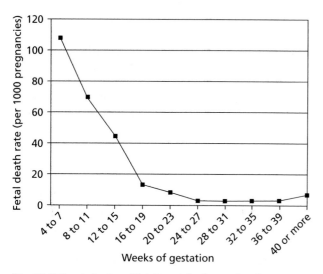

Fig. 6.1 Estimated rates of fetal mortality by weeks of gestation [4].

Table 6.1 Recommended terms for use in miscarriage.

Previous term	Recommended term
Spontaneous abortion	Miscarriage
Threatened abortion	Threatened miscarriage
Inevitable abortion	Inevitable miscarriage
Incomplete abortion	Incomplete miscarriage
Complete abortion	Complete miscarriage
Missed abortion/anembryonic pregnancy	Missed miscarriage/early fetal demise
Blighted ovum	Delayed/silent miscarriage
Septic abortion	Miscarriage with sepsis
Recurrent abortion	Recurrent miscarriage

diagnosis of a first-trimester miscarriage is delayed until the second trimester.

First-trimester miscarriage

Evidence suggests that a significant proportion of miscarriages result from chromosomal abnormalities. It is likely that abnormal implantation has a role to play in some cases and this is an area of current research. The frequency of chromosomally abnormal tissue among first-trimester miscarriages is 50–70% [7]. The following chromosomal abnormalities are associated with miscarriage.
• Trisomies: 68%, mainly trisomy 16, 21 and 22.
• Triploidy: 17.1%.
• Monosomy: 9.8% (XO, Turner's syndrome).
Other implicated causes of first-trimester miscarriage include the following:
• Maternal disease: antiphospholipid syndrome, diabetes, thyroid disease.

Table 6.2 Definitions of terms in common usage.

Term	Definition
Threatened miscarriage	Vaginal bleeding in the presence of a viable pregnancy
Inevitable miscarriage	Vaginal bleeding in the presence of an open cervical os and pregnancy-associated tissue still present*
Incomplete miscarriage	Vaginal bleeding that is ongoing where pregnancy tissue has already been passed but ultrasound suggests the presence of further products within the uterine cavity
Complete miscarriage	Clinical definition: cessation of bleeding and a closed cervix following miscarriage
	Ultrasound definition: an empty uterus with a falling hCG where an intrauterine pregnancy was previously confirmed
Missed miscarriage/early fetal demise	Miscarriage occurring in the absence of symptoms or minimal symptoms, where the pregnancy is still visible within the uterus
Recurrent miscarriage	Three or more consecutive early pregnancy losses
Biochemical pregnancy loss	Pregnancy not located on scan where there is/ has been a positive pregnancy test which then becomes negative
Empty sac	Sac with absent or minimal structures
Pregnancy of unknown location	Positive pregnancy test where the location of the pregnancy is not identifiable
Pregnancy of unknown viability	The presence of intrauterine structures, confirming the location of the pregnancy, but no fetal heart beat to confirm its viability†

* Extreme caution needs to be taken before making this diagnosis as it can be easy to mistake a parous os (external os open as a result of previous vaginal delivery) and the open cervix of inevitable miscarriage. It is a term probably best avoided.
† The RCOG Green-top Guideline No. 25 (October 2006) indicates a diagnosis of pregnancy of unknown viability in the presence of a gestation sac <20 mm in diameter with no obvious gestation sac or yolk sac or a fetal crown–rump length of <6 mm with no obvious fetal heart beat. This suggests that if the gestation sac is >20 mm or fetal pole >6–10 mm, then the diagnosis of miscarriage can be made but the data supporting this involve relatively small numbers of cases suggesting the need for caution and in general makes it advisable to rescan 7–10 days later to confirm the findings.

• Drugs: methotrexate, some antiepileptic drugs.
• Uterine abnormalities: the role of fibroids is uncertain but they may be implicated [5].
• Infection: varicella, rubella and other viral illnesses.

Second-trimester miscarriage

• Cervix: cervical injury from surgery, cone biopsy and large loop excision of the transformation zone [8].

- Infection: may occur with or without ruptured membranes. May be local to the genital tract or systemic.
- Thrombophilias.
- Uterine abnormalities: submucous fibroids and congenital distortion of the cavity (uterine septae) may be implicated.
- Chromosomal abnormalities: these too may not become apparent until the second trimester.

Diagnosis

 Summary box 6.1

It is important to recognize that pregnancy is a dynamic process and although at any point viability of a pregnancy can be confirmed, it does not necessarily imply that the pregnancy will continue.

Diagnosis is based on appropriate history-taking, examination and suitably directed diagnostic tests.

History-taking
- LMP: remember to confirm length of cycle, regularity, and use of contraception around time of conception, any of which can alter the presumed timing of ovulation (assumed as 15 days after LMP for the purpose of calculating gestation) and hence result in over- or underestimation of gestational age.
- Symptoms: pain and/or bleeding. It used to be taught that the presentation of one before the other helped differentiate between ectopic and intrauterine pregnancy but it is clear that this is not the case. The location and nature of the pain is also a poor prognostic indicator. Urinary frequency or diarrhoea can be subtle signs of peritoneal irritation due to intraperitoneal bleeding, associated with ectopic pregnancy.
- Past obstetric and gynaecological history may provide evidence of risk factors for other non-pregnancy-related causes of bleeding or indicate risk factors for ectopic pregnancy, such as sexually transmitted infection or pelvic inflammatory disease. It is important to ascertain the last smear date and any history of cervical abnormality/ colposcopic treatment.
- Past medical history: poorly controlled diabetes mellitus is known to be associated with miscarriage and other chronic illnesses may also be implicated, although these tend to be associated with reduced fertility (capacity to conceive) rather than fecundity (capacity to maintain a pregnancy).
- Medication: prescribed, non-prescribed and recreational.

Examination
General examination
A general examination to assess the immediate well-being of the patient is mandatory. Young women can mask blood loss and significant decompensation is a late sign; therefore attention should be given to the subtle sign of blood loss in addition to pulse and blood pressure, respiratory rate, pallor, reduced consciousness, and capillary return. Peritoneal distension may also result in bradycardia.

Abdominal palpation
- Determine the fundal height: the uterus generally becomes palpable above the pelvic brim at 12 weeks' gestation, although this will be affected by multiple pregnancy and the presence of uterine fibroids.
- Examine for evidence of other pelvic masses, which may explain the presence of pain (e.g. ovarian torsion, degenerating fibroids).
- Look for evidence of intra-abdominal bleeding or generalized tender distension of the abdomen.
- Confirm location of pain.

Vaginal examination
Vaginal examination will reveal whether the cervix is open or if products of conception are identifiable at the cervical os. If so, the relevant tissue should be removed and sent for histopathological diagnosis, as on rare occasions a decidual cast (in the presence of an ectopic pregnancy) can mimic products of conception. Products of conception cannot be confirmed on macroscopic inspection unless fetal parts are seen. Where there is a history of complete miscarriage, 45% of patients will show ultrasound evidence of retained products and up to 6% will have an ectopic pregnancy [9].

Speculum examination of the vagina is also a good opportunity to inspect the cervix and vagina to exclude local causes of blood loss in addition to the quantity of loss at presentation as patient description can be misleading.

Differential diagnosis (Table 6.3)
Hydatidiform mole is a relatively rare but important complication of pregnancy that should be considered in all cases of miscarriage and, where possible, tissue sent for histological confirmation of products of conception. It is clear, however, that in the presence of spontaneous miscarriage at home that this is not possible. It is likely that in these cases, where there is clinically significant molar change, women will present with ongoing bleeding and the diagnosis considered at this stage.

Diagnostic tools

Ultrasound
Ultrasound has progressed enormously since its first use in pregnancy in 1967. It has a pivotal role to play in

Table 6.3 Differential diagnosis.

	Uterine size*	Cervix	Blood loss	Pain
Threatened miscarriage	Equivalent to dates	Closed	Any	Variable
Incomplete miscarriage	Smaller than dates	Open	Usually heavy	Present
Complete miscarriage	Smaller than dates	Closed	Previously heavy, now settling	Previously present, now absent
Missed miscarriage	Variable	Closed	Variable	Variable

* Remember that the presence of fibroids may give a distorted assessment of uterine size.

diagnosis of miscarriage. However, care must be taken in diagnosing miscarriage on the basis of ultrasound findings alone because of natural variation in the appearance of structures and the inevitable uncertainty that surrounds dating. This is particularly relevant in the current climate of sensitive urinary pregnancy tests where women are presenting at increasingly early gestations, requesting reassurance scans; depending on the timing of presentation, it may be several weeks before a viable pregnancy can be visualized. Where there is any doubt, it is mandatory that a repeat scan is undertaken after a minimum of 7 days to confirm a suspicion of non-viable pregnancy.

The ultrasound landmarks visible on transvaginal scan are as follows.
• Week 5: visible gestation sac.
• Week 6: visible yolk sac.
• Week 6: visible embryo.
• Week 7: visible amnion.
Failure to identify these landmarks at the presumed gestational age may not necessarily indicate a miscarriage. Dating in early pregnancy is taken from the first day of LMP and conception presumed to have taken place on day 15. Clearly this leaves a large window for inaccuracy due to varying cycle lengths, delayed ovulation and inaccurate recall of menstrual dates.

Serum human chorionic gonadotrophin

There is little evidence to support the role of beta human chorionic gonadotrophin (β-hCG) in determining viability after the visualization of an intrauterine gestation sac and yolk sac, as considerable variation exists in the normal increase in β-hCG and occasionally falls are identified in the presence of subsequently viable pregnancy. Furthermore, the effect of twin pregnancy on β-hCG rise is uncertain.

β-hCG does have a role in managing pregnancies of unknown location as it is reported to rise exponentially in the early stages of pregnancy, with at least a 66% rise in 48 hours [10]. However, variation in this increase does not necessarily exclude viable pregnancy. Furthermore, it is important to recognize that tests are rarely exactly 48 hours apart due to timing of presentation and this will determine interpretation as well.

Progesterone

The main role of progesterone lies in the assistance it provides in determining the likely outcome of pregnancy of unknown location rather than in diagnosing miscarriage, although a progesterone level of less than 20 nmol/L suggests a non-viable pregnancy, a level above 60 nmol/L a live pregnancy (without determining its location) while values between 20 and 60 nmol/L are equivocable [11]. Its usefulness is further limited by the capacity of many laboratories to provide same day results. Progesterone levels assist in determining which patients are suitable for expectant management, in the case of pregnancy of unknown location and ectopic pregnancy. For example if an ectopic pregnancy is identified and the progesterone level is below 20 nmol/L, then expectant management is more likely to be successful than where the progesterone level is above 60 nmol/L. Where the pregnancy is known to be intrauterine, there is no role for monitoring progesterone levels.

Progesterone levels are also not valid where patients are taking exogenous progesterone as is often the case with assisted conception/recurrent miscarriage.

Summary box 6.2

• Ultrasound has a role to play, but caution must be excercised when diagnosing miscarriage on a single scan.
• Wide variation in normal levels of hCG at any gestation limits its use for assessment of viability.
• Progesterone levels do not correlate sufficiently well with viability to be a useful tool in diagnosing miscarriage.

Management

Management options fall into three groups: medical, surgical or expectant. Factors to be taken into account when discussing these options with patients include the following.
• Type of miscarriage: expectant management is less useful for delayed miscarriage and medical management appears to hold no benefit for the management of incomplete miscarriage [12].
• Gestation at which miscarriage is diagnosed: care needs to be taken where miscarriage is diagnosed at later

gestations (11 weeks and above where there is a missed miscarriage). These patients are at risk of heavier bleeding compared with earlier gestations and should be warned of such and possibly encouraged to consider surgical evacuation as the first line of treatment. If their preference is for medical evacuation, then this is more appropriately carried out in an inpatient setting.

- Facilities available at individual units: out-of-hours access to emergency care and advice in case of heavy bleeding with medical or expectant management. Capacity of units to offer inpatient medical management.
- Medical history: cardiac disease and sickle cell anaemia for example. The risks are increased in the presence of haemorrhage and so generally among these patients surgical evacuation, being associated with less blood loss, is the most appropriate choice.
- Patient choice.
- Cost.

Expectant management

Historically, women have been offered surgical management as the main treatment for miscarriage. However, the recognition of potentially serious risks associated with curettage has resulted in a move away from intervention and a wider choice of options being offered to women. Up to 85% of miscarriages will resolve spontaneously within 3 weeks of the diagnosis. The rate of success partly depends on the length of delay in intervention. There is also debate as to how to confirm the diagnosis of complete miscarriage, whether by ultrasound or symptoms. It seems likely that the best course to take involves both, rather than relying solely on a defined thickness of endometrium. Furthermore, the regularity and vascularity of the contents of the endometrial cavity are probably more important than the thickness alone. Again, the lack of agreement in defining completeness of a miscarriage hampers efforts to assess effectiveness of treatment options.

Patient satisfaction with expectant management depends on appropriate patient selection (earlier gestation, singleton pregnancy, social circumstances) and counselling. Patients should be made aware of what to anticipate (pain and bleeding), be given advice regarding analgesia and what to do with the tissue passed. The advice should be backed up with written information and contact details in case of concern or complications.

Surgical management

Surgical management involves evacuation of the uterus by dilatation and suction curettage ('evacuation of retained products of conception' is the term in general usage in the UK.) The procedure can be performed under general or local anaesthesia depending on local experience. Cervical dilatation can be assisted by cervical priming with a prostaglandin (e.g. misoprostol) a minimum of 1 hour prior to the procedure and is strongly recommended when the woman has not had a previous vaginal delivery [1]. This is believed to reduce the pressure required to dilate the cervix and hence risk of failure of the procedure, retained products and uterine perforation. Curettage is usually safe but it is important to counsel women about the associated risks. These include the risk of general anaesthesia (if relevant), the risk of infection or retained products (3–5%) and potential bleeding in association with this and the 0.5% risk of uterine perforation which could lead to other organ damage and the need to progress to laparoscopy or laparotomy in those circumstances. Patients should be reassured that in the presence of a uterine perforation and the absence of additional complications, the implications for future fertility are negligible. Asherman's syndrome, where intrauterine synechiae develop and interfere with conception, used to be said to arise from over-vigorous curettage. However, there is little supporting evidence for this.

Medical management

Medical management of miscarriage involves using uterotonic therapy, alone or in conjunction with antihormone therapy, to achieve evacuation of the uterine cavity.

Available uterotonic agents include gemeprost and misoprostol, both of which are prostaglandin (PG)E_1 analogues. Gemeprost is licensed for use in management of uterine evacuation. It requires refrigeration and is more expensive that misoprostol. Misoprostol is not licensed for gynaecological use, can be stored at room temperature and is significantly less costly. It can also be given orally as well as per vagina or rectum. Side effects include nausea, vomiting and diarrhoea, which can be problematic. There is no evidence to support the use of other uterotonics such as ergometrine, oxytocin or other prostaglandins in this situation. PGE_1 analogues can be used in conjunction with antihormone therapy: mifepristone, an antiprogesterone, can be used to sensitize the uterus to the effects of uterotonics and may improve complete evacuation rates. The effect of mifepristone is maximal 36–48 hours after treatment.

Overall, the success rate of medical management (72–93%) is similar to that of expectant management (75–85%) [13], but medical management has the advantage that patients can control the course of events by timing medication to allow the miscarriage to take place. However, success rates are dependent on how much time has elapsed following treatment: the longer the wait, the higher the success rate. Compared with surgical management, there is significantly more associated blood loss but no increased requirement for blood transfusion. Reassuringly, rates of infection between the three options are similar [14].

Summary box 6.3

- Expectant, medical and surgical management of miscarriage are all viable options in first-trimester miscarriage and the decision should be based on patient choice as well as clinical situation.
- The incidence of infection is not significantly higher in any management group.
- Blood loss is heaviest in medical and expectant management compared with surgical though with no increased risk of blood transfusion. This should be taken into account when counselling certain groups, for example patients with sickle cell anaemia, in whom blood loss should be kept to a minimum.

Rhesus status

Despite the absence of antigens on the surface of embryonic red blood cells until 12 weeks' gestation, there is concern regarding the possibility of sensitization of rhesus-negative women from early pregnancy events. Current guidelines from the British Blood Transfusion Society and the RCOG are quoted below.

Spontaneous miscarriage

Anti-D immunoglobulin should be given to all non-sensitized RhD-negative women who have a spontaneous miscarriage after 12 weeks of pregnancy. Published data on which to base recommendations in earlier miscarriages are scant. There is evidence that significant feto-maternal haemorrhage only occurs after curettage to remove products of conception but does not occur after complete spontaneous miscarriages [15,16]. Anti-D immunoglobulin should therefore be given when there has been an intervention to evacuate the uterus. On the other hand, the risk of immunization by spontaneous miscarriage before 12 weeks' gestation is negligible when there has been no instrumentation to evacuate the products of conception and anti-D immunoglobulin is not required in these circumstances.

Threatened miscarriage

Anti-D immunoglobulin should be given to all non-sensitized RhD-negative women with a threatened miscarriage after 12 weeks of pregnancy. Where bleeding continues intermittently after 12 weeks' gestation, anti-D immunoglobulin should be given at 6-weekly intervals. Evidence that women are sensitized after uterine bleeding in the first 12 weeks of pregnancy where the fetus is viable and the pregnancy continues is scant [17], though there are very rare examples. Against this background, routine administration of anti-D immunoglobulin cannot be recommended. However, it may be prudent to administer anti-D immunoglobulin where bleeding is heavy or repeated or where there is associated abdominal pain, particularly if these events occur as gestation approaches 12 weeks.

The recommended dose of anti-D immunoglobulin for miscarriage is 250 units before 20 weeks' gestation and 500 units after 20 weeks. It is further recommended that a Kleihauer test be performed to assess the quantity of feto-maternal haemorrhage after 20 weeks.

Summary box 6.4

Anti-D is required in the following circumstances for non-sensitized RhD-negative women:
- spontaneous miscarriage 12 weeks and beyond;
- miscarriage at any gestation where there has been intervention (medical or surgical) or if spontaneous where the bleeding is heavy or repeated;
- threatened miscarriage at 12 weeks and beyond – if repeat episodes, then anti-D should be repeated at 6-weekly intervals.

Psychology and counselling

Pregnancy loss at any gestation is an emotional time for women and it is important that counselling reflects that. The language used should be sensitive, avoiding terms such as pregnancy failure or abortion, which in layman's terms implies therapeutic abortion and has no place in terminology relating to miscarriage. Where possible, all information given should be supported by written material as, again, it is recognized that while we as doctors believe our counselling to have been thorough, in reality a distressed patient may take in very little and it is quite possible that any information given will need to be repeated before it is absorbed. Service provision should allow for that.

Post-traumatic stress disorder is a possibility. If psychological symptoms persist, patients should be encouraged to seek assistance.

Conclusion

Miscarriage is a frequent outcome of pregnancy. It is, for the most part, unavoidable. Therefore patient management should be focused on making the experience as bearable as possible by taking time over explanation and discussion of options to allow patients to feel supported and in control. Within the framework described, patients should be allowed to make choices best suited to them. Information should be backed up by written explanation.

References

1 Lewis G (ed.) *Saving Mothers' Lives 7th Report of the Confidential Enquiries into Maternal Deaths in the UK*. London: CEMACH, 2007.

2 Cashner KA, Christopher CR, Dysert GA. Spontaneous fetal loss after demonstration of a live fetus in the first trimester. *Obstet Gynecol* 1987;70:827–830.

3 Savitz DA, Hertz-Picciotto I, Poole C, Olshan AF. Epidemiologic measures of the course and outcome of pregnancy. *Epidemiol Rev* 2002;24:91–101.

4 French FE, Bierman JM. Probabilities of fetal mortality. *Public Health Rep* 1962;77:835–847.

5 Regan L, Rai R. Epidemiology and the medical causes of miscarriage. *Baillieres Best Pract Res Clin Obstet Gynaecol* 2000;14: 839–854.

6 Alcazar JL, Baldonado C, Laparte C. The reliability of transvaginal ultrasonography to detect retained tissue after spontaneous first trimester abortion clinically thought to be complete. *Ultrasound Obstet Gynecol* 1995;6:126–129.

7 Hassold T, Chen N, Funkhouser J *et al.* A cytogenetic study of 1000 spontaneous abortions. *Ann Hum Genet* 1980;44:151–178.

8 Kyrgiou M, Koliopoulos G, Martin-Hirsch P, Arbyn M, Prendiville W, Paraskevaidis E. Obstetric outcomes after conservative treatment for intraepithelial or early invasive cervical lesions: systematic review and meta-analysis. *Lancet* 2006;367: 489–498.

9 Condous G, Okaro E, Khalid A, Bourne T. Do we need to follow up complete miscarriages with serum human chorionic gonadotrophin levels? *BJOG* 2005;112:827–829.

10 Braunstein GD, Rasor J, Danzer H, Adler D, Wade ME. Serum human chorionic gonadotrophin levels throughout normal pregnancy. *Am J Obstet Gynecol* 1976;26:678–681.

11 Mol BW, Lijmer JG, Ankum WM, van der Veen F, Bossuyt PM. The accuracy of single serum progesterone measurement in the diagnosis of ectopic pregnancy: a meta-analysis. *Hum Reprod* 1998;13:3220–3227.

12 de Jonge ET, Makin JD, Manefeldt E, De Wet GH, Pattinson RC. Randomised clinical trial of medical evacuation and surgical curettage for incomplete miscarriage. *BMJ* 1995;311:662.

13 Nielson S, Hanlin H, Platz-Christensen J. Randomised trial comparing expectant with medical management for first trimester miscarriages. *Br J Obstet Gynaecol* 1999;106:804–807.

14 Trinder J, Brocklehurst P, Porter R, Read M, Vyas S, Smith L. Management of miscarriage: expectant, medical or surgical? Results of randomised controlled trial (miscarriage treatment (MIST) trial). *BMJ* 2006;332:1235–1240.

15 Royal College of Obstetricians and Gynaecologists. *Rh Prophylaxis, Anti-D Immunoglobulin*. Green-top Guideline No. 22, 2002. Available at: www.rcog.org.uk/womens-health/clinical-guidance/use-anti-d-immunoglobulin-rh-prophylaxis-green-top-22

16 Matthes CD, Matthews AE. Transplacental haemorrhages in spontaneous and induced abortion. *Lancet* 1969;i:694–695.

17 Ghosh, Murphy WG. Implementation of the rhesus prevention programme: a prospective study. *Scott Med J* 1994;39:147–149.

Chapter 7
Recurrent Miscarriage

Siobhan Quenby
Clinical Science Research Institute, University of Warwick, Coventry, UK

Definition

Recurrent miscarriage has several definitions. The Royal College of Obstetricians and Gynaecologists defines recurrent miscarriage as the loss of three or more consecutive pregnancies before viability [1]. The term therefore includes all pregnancy losses from the time of conception until 24 weeks of gestation [1]. However, advances in neonatal care have resulted in a small number of babies surviving birth before 24 weeks of gestation. Hence some late second-trimester miscarriages can also be considered as extreme preterm labour. At the other end of the spectrum is the issue of biochemical pregnancy losses. The European Society of Human Reproduction and Embryology defines biochemical losses as a transient positive pregnancy test without ultrasonic visualization of the pregnancy [2]. Miscarriage can be further classified, on ultrasound findings, into loss of an empty gestation sac (loss of pregnancy before 10 weeks' gestation) or loss of fetus (loss of a pregnancy after visualization of fetal heart activity) [2] (Table 7.1).

Despite attempts at standardization of definitions, some investigators consider women with two consecutive losses as recurrent miscarriage, as two losses have been found to increase the chance of a subsequent pregnancy ending in miscarriage [3].

Epidemiology

Approximately 15% of all pregnancies that can be visualized on ultrasound end in pregnancy loss [4]. Three or more losses affect 1–2% of women of reproductive age and two or more losses affect around 5% [4]. Despite extensive investigation of women with three or more miscarriages, the cause of recurrent pregnancy loss remains unknown in the majority of cases [5].

Advancing maternal age is associated with miscarriage. Age-related miscarriage rates are as follows: 12–19 years, 13%; 20–24 years, 11%; 25–29 years, 12%; 30–34 years, 15%; 35–39 years, 25%; 40–44 years, 51%; and 45 or more years, 93% [6]. This is because with increasing maternal age there is a decline in both the number and quality of the remaining oocytes.

An increasing number of previous miscarriages also adversely affects the risk of future miscarriage [5]. A history of a live birth followed by consecutive miscarriages does not reduce the risk of further miscarriage substantially [5]. Being both underweight and obese has been associated with recurrent miscarriage [7].

> **Summary box 7.1**
>
> - Recurrent miscarriage is defined as three consecutive pregnancy losses.
> - Miscarriages should be further classified on the basis of ultrasound findings into biochemical, empty gestation sac, fetal or second trimester.
> - In women with recurrent miscarriage, poor prognostic factors for further miscarriage include number of previous losses, maternal age and obesity.

Other associated factors and their management

Factors that have been associated with early recurrent miscarriage include parental and fetal chromosomal abnormalities [8,9], structural uterine abnormalities [10], antiphospholipid syndrome [11], some thrombophilias [12], autoimmune disease, and endocrinological disorders such as polycystic ovarian syndrome and untreated diabetes [13]. It is important to realize that many of these associations are weak and there are only a very few published observational studies that give prognostic implications for positive tests for conditions associated with recurrent miscarriage. Hence the evidence that many of the associated factors are causative is poor. There are even fewer high-quality large-scale randomized controlled trials showing that a treatment for women with recurrent

Dewhurst's Textbook of Obstetrics & Gynaecology, Eighth Edition. Edited by D. Keith Edmonds.
© 2012 John Wiley and Sons, Ltd. Published 2012 by John Wiley and Sons, Ltd.

Table 7.1 Classification of miscarriage.

Type of miscarriage	Gestation range (weeks)	Fetal heart activity	Ultrasound findings
First trimester			
Biochemical	0–6	Never	Not visualized
Empty gestation sac	4–10	Never	Empty gestation sac or large sac with minimal structures without fetal heart activity
Fetal	6–12	Lost	Crown–rump length and fetal heart activity previously identified
Second trimester	12–24	Lost	Fetus identified of size equivalent to 12–24 weeks' gestation

miscarriage is effective at preventing a subsequent miscarriage. Ideally, evaluation of a couple with recurrent miscarriage would achieve the aim of guiding management options by finding contributory factors to the pregnancy losses, providing prognostic value in the subsequent pregnancy and directing treatment of proven benefit to improve live birth rates. This ideal has not been achieved by current research.

Structural genetic factors

Fetal chromosomal abnormality

Chromosomal abnormality in the miscarried pregnancy is the most common cause of early pregnancy loss, especially in older women. This accounts for up to 70% of early pregnancy losses, falling to only 20% when the pregnancy loss is between 13 and 20 weeks' gestation [8]. Defects are commonly trisomy, polyploidy or monosomy. Ideally, products of conception should be sent for karyotyping, as an abnormal fetal karyotype is diagnostic for the cause of miscarriage and is an important prognostic factor, suggesting a successful outcome of more than 75% in the next pregnancy [8]. However, this investigation is not perceived to be cost-effective.

Parental chromosomal abnormalities

Parental chromosomal abnormalities are found in about 2% of women with recurrent pregnancy loss, with the most common being a balanced reciprocal translocation [14]. Couples with balanced translocations are at risk of conceiving future children with unbalanced

translocation. Hence, when an abnormality is found, the couple can be referred to a clinical geneticist for counselling and offered prenatal diagnosis. However, a large case series of couples with recurrent miscarriage and balanced translocation have found the risk of unbalanced translocation in offspring to be less than 1% [15]. This 1% miscarriage rate is close to the miscarriage rate of normal pregnancies after invasive prenatal diagnosis. Observational studies of couples with recurrent miscarriage and balanced translocations have found live birth rates of over 70% in the subsequent pregnancy [15]. This 70% live birth rate is similar to that in couples with recurrent miscarriage without chromosomal abnormalities [4]. Thus, the cost-effectiveness of investigating parental karyotype has been questioned [14]. If balanced translocation is detected, supportive care with the option of invasive prenatal diagnosis is appropriate [1].

There was hope that pre-implantation genetic diagnosis (PGD) and assisted reproductive techniques (ART) would improve the live birth rate for women with recurrent miscarriage and balanced translocations. However, in practice PGD-ART has a series of disadvantages. Not all the cells in a four- or eight-cell embryo are genetically identical, so PGD is not a reliable measure of the pregnancy karyotype. The pregnancy rate and live birth rate from PGD-ART is lower than from natural conception [16]. Furthermore, natural conception involves the selection of normal oocytes, then the selection of normal pregnancy, allowing genetically abnormal pregnancies to miscarry. These natural selection steps are circumvented in PGD-ART, creating large numbers of abnormal embryos. However, consideration can be given to PGD where women have subfertility and recurrent miscarriage and a balanced translocation, as observational studies show that PGD-ART has better pregnancy outcomes, despite lower rates of embryo transfer and shorter time to a successful pregnancy [16].

 Summary box 7.2

- Recurrent miscarriage is associated with parental balanced translocations.
- In the presence of a balanced translocation couples still have a 70% live birth rate in a subsequent pregnancy.
- Only 1% of offspring from couples with balanced translocations have unbalanced translocations.
- Parental karyotyping is no longer thought to be cost-effective.

Anatomical factors

Congenital uterine anomaly

The prevalence of congenital uterine anomaly, such as septated, bicornuate or arcuate uterus, in the general population is about 6.7% but approximately 16.7% in women with recurrent miscarriage [10], though a direct causative link is uncertain due to the vast difference in criteria and techniques for diagnosing abnormal uterine morphology. Advances in hysteroscopic surgery mean that these malformations can be corrected using a resectoscope. Observational studies suggest that surgery (hysteroscopic metroplasty) may improve pregnancy outcome [17,18]. However, there have been no randomized controlled trials of this treatment so efficacy of intrauterine surgery has yet to be demonstrated [19].

Cervical weakness

Cervical weakness is a recognized contributing factor to second-trimester loss. The diagnosis of this condition can be based on history, resistance to Hegar dilators, or transvaginal sonographic assessment of the cervix in pregnancy. Treatment with cervical cerclage is associated with potential hazards related to the surgery and the risk of stimulating uterine contractions and hence should only be considered in women who are likely to benefit [1].

Transabdominal cerclage has been advocated as a treatment for second-trimester miscarriage and the prevention of early preterm labour in selected women with a previous failed transvaginal cerclage and/or a very short and scarred cervix [20,21]. A systematic review concluded that abdominal cerclage may be associated with a lower risk of perinatal death or delivery before 24 weeks of gestation and a higher risk of serious operative complications [21]. However, there have been no published randomized controlled trials of vaginal versus abdominal suture.

Acquired uterine anomaly

Acquired uterine abnormalities such as fibroids or intrauterine adhesions (Asherman's syndrome) have also been associated with recurrent miscarriage. The location, size and number of fibroids do not significantly influence postoperative pregnancy rates but observational studies report a trend towards lower pregnancy rates with larger fibroids in the submucous region [22]. Again there are no randomized controlled trials of hysteroscopic corrective treatment.

Summary box 7.3

- Recurrent miscarriage is associated with uterine structural abnormalities.
- Observational studies suggest that hysteroscopic surgery is effective.
- Hysteroscopic surgery has not been proven to be effective in randomized controlled trials.

Prothrombotic factors

Antiphospholipid syndrome

Antiphospholipid syndrome (APS) has a prevalence of 15% in women with first-trimester recurrent miscarriage and this, as well as a single second-trimester miscarriage, is one of the clinical components for diagnosis of the syndrome [11,23]. Treatment options including low-dose aspirin (LDA), heparin, prednisolone and intravenous immunoglobulin (IVIG) have been investigated. A systematic review showed that prednisolone and IVIG do not improve pregnancy outcomes and are associated with increased risk of diabetes and premature birth [24]. The same review concluded that LDA alone was not of significant benefit but a combination of LDA and unfractionated heparin reduced subsequent pregnancy loss by 54% [24]. Thus, LDA and heparin are the recommended treatment for women with recurrent miscarriage and APS [1]. In clinical practice, low-molecular-weight heparins are preferred as they have reduced risk of thrombocytopenia, only need once-daily administration and levels do not need to be monitored. However, low-molecular-weight heparin may not have the same effect in reducing risks of miscarriage in APS [24]. Even when treated, women with APS have high-risk pregnancies and should be monitored for complications in all three trimesters [1].

Thrombophilia

Some thrombophilias, factor V Leiden mutation, activated protein C resistance, prothrombin gene G20210A mutation and protein S deficiency have been significantly associated with recurrent miscarriage [12]. However, there is still controversy about the prognostic implications of positive tests. A full thrombophilia screen can produce abnormal results in 20% of women with uncomplicated obstetric histories. Thus it is uncertain if all women with early recurrent miscarriage should be screened for thrombophilia [25]. Treatment with LDA with or without low-molecular-weight heparin has been proposed as thromboprophylaxis to prevent putative placental infarcts or vascular thrombosis. Small initial studies suggest there may be beneficial effects with thromboprophylaxis in terms of improved live birth rates [26,27]. However, more recently, high-quality large randomized controlled trials failed to substantiate an improvement in live birth rate in women with either idiopathic or thrombophilia-associated recurrent miscarriage [28–31]. Thus, there is no evidence to support the use of LDA and heparin in the treatment of women with recurrent miscarriage without APS. However, thromboprophylaxis to prevent maternal thrombosis does need to be considered in women with multiple risk factors for this.

Summary box 7.4

- Recurrent miscarriage is associated with thrombophilia.
- In the presence of APS, aspirin and heparin are thought to be effective treatments.
- In the absence of APS, neither aspirin and heparin nor aspirin alone have been found to prevent miscarriage.

Endocrinological factors

Polycystic ovarian syndrome

There is an association between polycystic ovarian syndrome and recurrent miscarriage. The possible mechanisms for this are hyperandrogenism and insulin resistance [32]. However, the variation in criteria for diagnosing polycystic ovarian syndrome makes it difficult to assess the importance and the prognostic value of detecting it. Nevertheless, a simple, safe and cheap way to reduce pregnancy loss in obese women with polycystic ovarian syndrome is weight loss [33]. Small studies suggest there may be a role for metformin in reducing miscarriage rates, especially in the presence of an abnormal glucose tolerance test, and metformin is now regarded as having low risks to pregnancy [32,34]. However, a randomized controlled trial in infertile women indicated that clomifene is superior to metformin in achieving live births but made no difference to the rates of miscarriage [35].

Abnormalities of glucose metabolism and thyroid disorders

It is known that well-controlled thyroid disorders and diabetes are not risk factors for recurrent miscarriage. Thus national guidelines do not recommend routine screening in the absence of symptoms [1,25].

Immunological factors

Immunological mechanisms are thought to play a part in the success of pregnancy where the maternal immune system interacts with the allogeneically dissimilar embryo.

Antithyroid antibodies

The presence of antithyroid antibodies has been associated with a higher pregnancy loss rate, the underlying mechanisms of which are either autoimmune or mild thyroid insufficiency [13,36]. A small study suggested that women with recurrent miscarriage and antithyroid antibodies but normal thyroid function tests may benefit from levothyroxine treatment [37]. Further large-scale trials are needed to substantiate this finding.

Natural killer cells

Another immunological factor of interest involves the natural killer (NK) cells that can be found in the peripheral blood or endometrium. Both peripheral and uterine NK cells have been associated with recurrent miscarriage [38,39]. However, there is still considerable controversy in the exact role and function of NK cells in recurrent miscarriage and the prognostic value of increased numbers or function of these cells is uncertain [40]. A systematic review of 20 trials of various immunotherapies, such as paternal cell immunization, third-party-donor-cell immunization, trophoblast membrane infusion and intravenous immune globulin, showed no significant beneficial effect over placebo in improving live birth rates [41].

Idiopathic recurrent miscarriage

Tender loving care

Women with recurrent miscarriage are anxious and appreciate reassurance when they fall pregnant again. Three-quarters of these women with idiopathic recurrent miscarriage will achieve a live birth in the subsequent pregnancy with tender loving care involving regular reassurance scans and psychological support in a dedicated early pregnancy assessment unit [5,43].

Aspirin

Empirical use of aspirin is common. However, a recent systematic review showed no evidence of an improvement in live birth rates in women with recurrent miscarriage [43] and in a randomized controlled trail there was a trend towards aspirin increasing the chance of miscarriage [29,43].

Progesterone

Progesterone is needed for successful early pregnancy. A systematic review of progesterone supplementation found that it did not significantly reduce the risk of miscarriage [44]. A subgroup analysis on women with recurrent miscarriage found that it did show a significant decrease in the miscarriage rate but these studies were small and of poor quality. Further high-quality large-scale randomized controlled trials are needed.

Human chorionic gonadotrophin

A small randomized controlled trial of human chorionic gonadotrophin (hCG) found no benefit, but a subgroup analysis found an improved live birth rate with hCG in women with oligomenorrhoea [45].

Conclusions

The management of recurrent miscarriage is challenging because of lack of evidence-based effective treatments.

Couples with recurrent miscarriage can be offered investigations and supportive care. Empirical treatment in women with idiopathic recurrent miscarriage should be avoided and entry into high-quality and methodologically sound trials should be considered whenever possible in order to improve the evidence base for this distressing condition.

References

1 Royal College of Obstetricians and Gynaecologists. *The Investigation and Treatment of Couples with Recurrent Miscarriage.* Green-top Guideline No. 17, 2003. Available at: www.rcog.org.uk/files/rcog-corp/uploaded-files/GT17Recurrent Miscarriage2003.pdf

2 Farquharson RG, Jauniaux E, Exalto N. ESHRE Special Interest Group for Early Pregnancy (SIGEP). Updated and revised nomenclature for description of early pregnancy events. *Hum Reprod* 2005;20:3008–3011.

3 Bhattacharya S, Townend J, Bhattacharya S. Recurrent miscarriage: are three miscarriages one too many? Analysis of a Scottish population-based database of 151 021 pregnancies. *Eur J Obstet Gynecol Reprod Biol* 2010;150:24–27.

4 Wilcox AJ, Weinberg CR, O'Connor JF et al. Incidence of early loss of pregnancy. *N Engl J Med* 1988;319:189–194.

5 Quenby SM, Farquharson RG. Predicting recurring miscarriage: what is important? *Obstet Gynecol* 1993;82:132–138.

6 Nybo Anderson AM, Wohlfahrt J, Christens P, Olsen J, Melbye M. Maternal age and fetal loss: population based register linkage study. *BMJ* 2000;320:1708–1712.

7 Metwally M, Saravelos SH, Ledger WL, Li TC. Body mass index and risk of miscarriage in women with recurrent miscarriage. *Fertil Steril* 2010;94:290–295.

8 Hogge WA, Byrnes AL, Lanasa MC, Surti U. The clinical use of karyotyping spontaneous abortions. *Am J Obstet Gynecol* 2003;189:397–400; discussion 400–402.

9 Stephenson MD, Sierra S. Reproductive outcomes in recurrent pregnancy loss associated with a parental carrier of a structural chromosome rearrangement. *Hum Reprod* 2006;21:1076–1082.

10 Saravelos SH, Cocksedge KA, Li TC. Prevalence and diagnosis of congenital uterine anomalies in women with reproductive failure: a critical appraisal. *Hum Reprod Update* 2008;14:415–429.

11 Greaves M, Cohen H, Machin SJ, Mackie I. Guidelines on the investigation and management of the antiphospholipid syndrome. *Br J Haematol* 2000;109:704–715.

12 Rey E, Kahn SR, David M, Shrier I. Thrombophilic disorders and fetal loss: a meta-analysis. *Lancet* 2003;361:901–908.

13 Arredondo F, Noble LS. Endocrinology of recurrent pregnancy loss. *Semin Reprod Med* 2006;24:33–39.

14 Barber JC, Cockwell AE, Grant E et al. Is karyotyping couples experiencing recurrent miscarriage worth the cost? *BJOG* 2010;117:885–888.

15 Franssen MT, Korevaar JC, van der Veen F, Leschot NJ, Bossuyt PM, Goddijn M. Reproductive outcome after chromosome analysis in couples with two or more miscarriages: index [corrected]-control study. *BMJ* 2006;332:759–763.

16 Fischer J, Colls P, Escudero T, Munné S. Preimplantation genetic diagnosis (PGD) improves pregnancy outcome for translocation carriers with a history of recurrent losses. *Fertil Steril* 2010;94:283–289.

17 Valli E, Vaquero E, Lazzarin N et al. Hysteroscopic metroplasty improves gestational outcome in women with recurrent spontaneous abortion. *J Am Assoc Gynecol Laparosc* 2004;11:240–244.

18 Roy KK, Singla S, Baruah J, Kumar S, Sharma JB, Karmakar D. Reproductive outcome following hysteroscopic septal resection in patients with infertility and recurrent abortions. *Arch Gynecol Obstet* 2011;283:273–279.

19 Kowalik CR, Mol BW, Veersema S, Goddijn M. Critical appraisal regarding the effect on reproductive outcome of hysteroscopic metroplasty in patients with recurrent miscarriage. *Arch Gynecol Obstet* 2010;282:465.

20 Farquharson R, Topping J, Quenby S. Transabdominal cerclage: the significance of dual pathology and increased preterm delivery. *BJOG* 2005;112:1424–1426.

21 Zaveri V, Aghajafari F, Amankwah K, Hannah M. Abdominal versus vaginal cerclage after a failed transvaginal cerclage: a systematic review. *Am J Obstet Gynecol* 2002;187:868–872.

22 Yu D, Wong YM, Cheong Y et al. Asherman syndrome: one century later. *Fertil Steril* 2008;89:759–779.

23 Rai RS, Regan L, Clifford K et al. Antiphospholipid antibodies and beta 2-glycoprotein-I in 500 women with recurrent miscarriage: results of a comprehensive screening approach. *Hum Reprod* 1995;10:2001–2005.

24 Empson MB, Lassere M, Craig JC, Scott JR. Prevention of recurrent miscarriage for women with antiphospholipid antibody or lupus anticoagulant. *Cochrane Database Syst Rev* 2005;(2):CD002859.

25 American College of Obstetricians and Gynecologists. Management of recurrent pregnancy loss. ACOG practice bulletin, No. 24, February 2001. (Replaces Technical Bulletin Number 212, September 1995.) *Int J Gynaecol Obstet* 2002;78:179–190.

26 Brenner B, Bar J, Ellis M et al. Effects of enoxaparin on late pregnancy complications and neonatal outcome in women with recurrent pregnancy loss and thrombophilia: results from the Live-Enox study. *Fertil Steril* 2005;84:770–773.

27 Deligiannidis A, Parapanissiou E, Mavridis P et al. Thrombophilia and antithrombotic therapy in women with recurrent spontaneous abortions. *J Reprod Med* 2007;52:499–502.

28 Laskin CA, Spitzer KA, Clark CA et al. Low molecular weight heparin and aspirin for recurrent pregnancy loss: results from the randomised, controlled HepASA Trial. *J Rheumatol* 2009;36:279–287.

29 Kaandorp SP, Goddijn M, van der Post JA et al. Aspirin plus heparin or aspirin alone in women with recurrent miscarriage. *N Engl J Med* 2010;362:1586–1596.

30 Clark P, Walker ID, Langhorne P et al. SPIN: The Scottish Pregnancy Intervention Study: a multicentre randomised controlled trial of low molecular weight heparin and low dose aspirin in women with recurrent miscarriage. *Blood* 2010;115:4162–4167.

31 Visser J, Ulander VM, Helmerhorst FM et al. Thromboprophylaxis for recurrent miscarriage in women with or without thrombophilia. HABENOX: a randomised multicentre trial. *Thromb Haemost* 2011;105:295–301.

32 Cocksedge KA, Li TC, Saravelos SH, Metwally M. A reappraisal of the role of polycystic ovary syndrome in recurrent miscarriage. *Reprod Biomed Online* 2008;17:151–160.

33 Clark AM, Ledger W, Galletly C *et al.* Weight loss results in significant improvement in pregnancy and ovulation rates in anovulatory obese women. *Hum Reprod* 1995;10:2705–2712.

34 Zolghadri J, Tavana Z, Kazerooni T *et al.* Relationship between abnormal glucose tolerance test and history of previous recurrent miscarriages, and beneficial effect of metformin in these patients: a prospective clinical study. *Fertil Steril* 2008;90:727–730.

35 Legro RS, Barnhart HX, Schlaff WD *et al.* Clomiphene, metformin, or both for infertility in the polycystic ovary syndrome. *N Engl J Med* 2007;356:551–566.

36 Stagnaro-Green A, Glinoer D. Thyroid autoimmunity and the risk of miscarriage. *Best Pract Res Clin Endocrinol Metab* 2004;18:167–181.

37 Vaquero E, Lazzarin N, De Carolis C *et al.* Mild thyroid abnormalities and recurrent spontaneous abortion: diagnostic and therapeutical approach. *Am J Reprod Immunol* 2000;43:204–208.

38 Dosiou C, Giudice LC. Natural killer cells in pregnancy and recurrent pregnancy loss: endocrine and immunologic perspectives. *Endocr Rev* 2005;26:44–62.

39 Quenby S, Nik H, Innes B *et al.* Uterine natural killer cells and angiogenesis in recurrent reproductive failure. *Hum Reprod* 2009;24:45–54.

40 Tuckerman E, Laird SM, Prakash A, Li TC. Prognostic value of the measurement of uterine natural killer cells in the endometrium of women with recurrent miscarriage. *Hum Reprod* 2007;22:2208–2213.

41 Porter TF, LaCoursiere Y, Scott JR. Immunotherapy for recurrent miscarriage. *Cochrane Database Syst Rev* 2006;(2):CD000112.

42 Brigham SA, Conlon C, Farquharson RG. A longitudinal study of pregnancy outcome following idiopathic recurrent miscarriage. *Hum Reprod* 1999;14:2868–2871.

43 Kaandorp S, Di Nisio M, Goddijn M, Middeldorp S. Aspirin or anticoagulants for treating recurrent miscarriage in women without antiphospholipid syndrome. *Cochrane Database Syst Rev* 2009;(1):CD004734.

44 Haas DM, Ramsey PS. Progestogen for preventing miscarriage. *Cochrane Database Syst Rev* 2008;(2):CD003511.

45 Quenby S, Farquharson RG. Human chorionic gonadotropin supplementation in recurring pregnancy loss: a controlled trial. *Fertil Steril* 1994;62:708–710.

Chapter 8
Gestational Trophoblast Tumours

Philip Savage and Michael Seckl
Charing Cross Hospital, London, UK

Gestational trophoblast tumours (GTT) arise from the cells of conception and form a range of related conditions, from the generally benign partial hydatidiform mole through to the aggressive malignancies of choriocarcinoma and placental site trophoblast tumours (PSTT). The combination of this unique biology, relative rarity and effective therapies makes trophoblast tumours an extremely interesting and important area of gynaecological and oncological care.

Despite the rarity of these illnesses, patients with molar pregnancies requiring additional treatment after evacuation can expect successful treatment outcomes, with overall cure rates for GTT approaching 100% [1]. For patients with choriocarcinoma and PSTT, using the treatments that have been established for over 25 years, the majority of patients can also be treated with a high expectation of cure with minimal long-term toxicity [2].

With the effectiveness of the current medical therapies, the main developments in trophoblast disease management in the UK are aimed at improving supportive care. These areas include strategies for ensuring human chorionic gonadotrophin (hCG) monitoring after molar pregnancies, improvements in pathology reporting and maintaining clinical awareness for the earlier diagnosis of choriocarcinoma and placental site tumours.

For nearly 40 years the UK has had centralized surveillance, follow-up and treatment facilities for GTT and much of the content of this chapter is based on the experience from the Trophoblast Tumour Centre at Charing Cross Hospital in London.

Classification, demographics and risk factors

The World Health Organization classification for GTT divides trophoblast tumours into premalignant partial and complete hydatidiform moles and the malignant diagnoses of invasive mole, choriocarcinoma and PSTT.

The reported incidence of molar pregnancies in Europe and North America is in the order of 0.2–1.5 per 1000 live births [3] and a recent study from the UK has indicated an overall incidence of one molar pregnancy per 591 viable conceptions for the period 2000–2009 [4]. Overall, partial molar pregnancies are more common than complete moles, with an approximate ratio of 60:40. Whilst there are some modest variations in the incidence of molar pregnancies based on race and geography, there are two clearly documented risk factors for an increased risk of molar pregnancy: the extremes of maternal age and a previous molar pregnancy.

The relative risk for molar pregnancies is highest at the extremes of the reproductive age group. The results from the recent England and Wales analysis, summarized in Table 8.1, indicate that there is a modest increased risk for younger teenagers, a relatively level risk for women aged 16–45 and then increasing risks after the age of 45 and particularly for those over the age of 50. Of interest the risk of partial molar pregnancy remains relatively unchanged across the age group, with most of the change in overall risk due to an increased incidence of complete molar pregnancies. In the 18–40 age group, complete moles make up about 40% of all molar pregnancies, but in the 45+ age group they account for over 90% of cases [4].

Premalignant pathology and presentation

Partial mole
The genetic origins of complete and partial molar pregnancies are demonstrated in Fig. 8.1. Partial moles are triploid with 69 chromosomes comprising two sets of paternal and one set of maternal chromosomes. Macroscopically and on ultrasound scanning during the first trimester partial mole will often resemble normal products of conception. The embryo can appear viable on an early ultrasound scan but becomes non-viable by week

Dewhurst's Textbook of Obstetrics & Gynaecology, Eighth Edition. Edited by D. Keith Edmonds.
© 2012 John Wiley and Sons, Ltd. Published 2012 by John Wiley and Sons, Ltd.

10–12. The histology of partial mole shows less swelling of the chorionic villi than in a complete mole and there may be only focal changes. As a result the diagnosis of partial mole can often be missed after a miscarriage or evacuation, unless the products are sent for expert pathological review.

Table 8.1 Risk of molar pregnancy compared with the number of viable conceptions at varying maternal ages in England and Wales.

Age	Per cent partial moles of viable conceptions	Per cent complete moles of viable conceptions	Overall risk of molar pregnancy
13	0.08	0.32	1 in 250
14	0.07	0.20	1 in 370
15	0.04	0.21	1 in 400
20	0.05	0.06	1 in 909
25	0.09	0.06	1 in 666
30	0.11	0.05	1 in 625
35	0.11	0.05	1 in 625
40	0.18	0.09	1 in 370
45	0.29	0.75	1 in 96
50+	0.59	16.2	1 in 6

Source: adapted from Savage *et al.* [4].

The clinical presentation of partial mole is most frequently via a failed pregnancy rather than irregular bleeding or by detection on routine ultrasound. The obstetric management is by suction evacuation and histological review; all patients with partial mole should be followed up by registration and serial hCG measurement.

Fortunately, partial mole rarely transforms into malignant disease, and there is an overall risk of 0.5–1% of patients requiring chemotherapy after a partial mole [5].

Complete mole

In complete moles the genetic material is totally male in origin, resulting from the fertilization of an 'empty' anucleate oocyte lacking maternal DNA. The chromosome complement is most commonly 46XX, which results from one X chromosome-carrying sperm that duplicates its DNA, or less frequently 46XY or 46XX from the presence of two separate sperm.

The clinical diagnosis of complete mole most often occurs as a result of first-trimester bleeding or an abnormal ultrasound. There is no fetal material and the histology shows the characteristic oedematous villous stroma. The textbook 'bunch of grapes' appearance is only seen in the second trimester and as most cases are diagnosed earlier, this is now rarely observed in UK practice. The typical macroscopic appearances of a complete mole are shown in Plate 8.1. Obstetric management is by suction

Normal conception

A single sperm with 23 chromosomes fertilizes an egg with 23 chromosomes

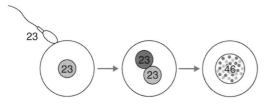

Complete mole

All 46 chromosomes are from the father
May involve one or two sperm

Monospermic complete mole

The paternal chromosomes double up

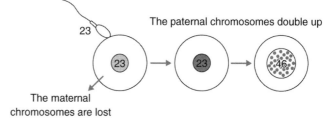

The maternal chromosomes are lost

Partial mole

Two sperms fertilize an egg
This results in a triploid conceptus with 69 chromosomes

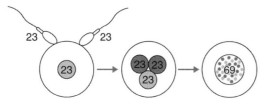

Dispermic complete mole

Fertilization by two sperm

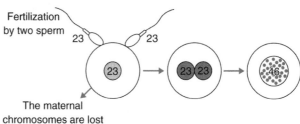

The maternal chromosomes are lost

Fig. 8.1 The genetic origin and structure of a normal conception, partial mole and complete molar pregnancy.

evacuation followed by registration and serial hCG measurement. Complete mole pregnancies have an appreciable risk of proceeding to invasive disease, with approximately 15% of patients with complete mole requiring chemotherapy.

Registration and surveillance

Overall 90% of patients with molar pregnancies will not need any additional treatment following their evacuation. In these patients the residual trophoblast tissue cells fail to proliferate and as the cells stop growing, the hCG levels return to normal. At present there is no effective prognostic method that allows accurate distinction between the patients who will develop invasive disease after evacuation and the majority who will not. As a result all patients with molar pregnancy should be registered for an hCG follow-up system. The use of this approach allows the early identification of patients whose disease is continuing to proliferate, while also allowing careful observation of patients with more slowly falling hCG levels, so minimizing unnecessary chemotherapy.

Patients taking part in an hCG surveillance programme have the need for additional treatment determined by the pattern of their hCG results. Table 8.2 shows the Charing Cross Hospital recommended indications for treatment. Those patients recovering from molar pregnancy enrolled in the surveillance service and who go on to require treatment have a cure rate approaching 100%, and over 95% will initially fall into the low-risk treatment group. Overall, from the 1400 patients registered annually approximately 8% receive chemotherapy.

Malignant pathology and presentation

Invasive mole (chorioadenoma destruens)

Invasive mole nearly always arises from a complete mole and is characterized by invasion of malignant cells into the myometrium, which can lead to perforation of the

uterus. Microscopically, invasive mole has a similar histological appearance as complete mole but is characterized by the ability to invade into the myometrium and local structures if untreated. Fortunately, the incidence of invasive mole in the UK has fallen substantially with the introduction of routine ultrasound, the early evacuation of complete moles and effective hCG surveillance, and is now rare.

Choriocarcinoma

Choriocarcinoma is histologically and clinically overtly malignant and presents the most frequent emergency medical problems in the management of trophoblast disease. The diagnosis often follows a complete mole when the patients are usually in a surveillance programme but can also arise in unsupervised patients after a non-molar abortion or term pregnancy. The clinical presentation of choriocarcinoma can be from the disease locally in the uterus leading to bleeding, or from distant metastases that can cause a wide variety of symptoms, with the lungs, central nervous system and liver the most frequent sites of distant disease.

The cases of choriocarcinoma presenting with symptoms from distant metastases can be diagnostically challenging. However, the combination of the gynaecological history and elevated serum hCG usually makes the diagnosis clear and so avoids biopsy, which can be hazardous due to the risk of severe haemorrhage as demonstrated following a liver biopsy in Fig. 8.2. On the occasions when choriocarcinoma pathology is available, the characteristic findings show the structure of the villous trophoblast but sheets of syncytiotrophoblast or cytotrophoblast cells, haemorrhage, necrosis and intravascular growth are common. The genetic profile of choriocarcinoma is a range of gross abnormalities without any specific characteristic patterns.

Table 8.2 The indications used at Charing Cross Hospital for initiating chemotherapy treatment in patients with gestational trophoblast tumours.

Raised hCG level 6 months after evacuation (even if falling)
hCG plateau in three consecutive serum samples
hCG >20 000 IU/L more than 4 weeks after evacuation
Rising hCG in two consecutive serum samples
Pulmonary, vulval or vaginal metastases unless the hCG level is falling
Heavy vaginal bleeding or gastrointestinal/intraperitoneal bleeding
Histological evidence of choriocarcinoma
Brain, liver, gastrointestinal metastases or lung metastases >2 cm on chest radiography

---

hCG, human choriocarcinoma.

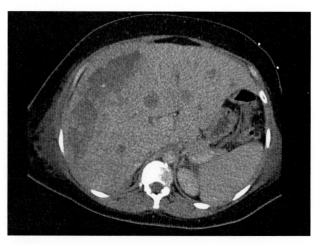

Fig. 8.2 CT scan of the abdomen in a patient with choriocarcinoma demonstrating multiple liver metastases and a large subcapsular haematoma secondary to a core biopsy.

Placental site trophoblast tumour

Placental site trophoblast tumour was originally described in 1976 [6] and is the rarest form of gestational trophoblast disease with four to six cases annually in the UK. PSTT most commonly follows a normal pregnancy but can also occur after a non-molar abortion or a molar pregnancy.

In contrast to the more common types of trophoblast disease, which characteristically present fairly soon after the index pregnancy, in PSTT the average interval between the prior pregnancy and presentation is 3.4 years. The most frequent presentations are amenorrhoea or abnormal bleeding. In nearly all cases the serum hCG level is elevated, but is characteristically lower for the volume of disease than in the other types of GTT. The tumour can arise after any type of pregnancy including complete and partial moles and is believed to be derived from the non-villous trophoblast. The pathology is characterized by intermediate trophoblastic cells with vacuolated cytoplasm, the expression of placental alkaline phosphatase and hCG, and the absence of cytotrophoblast and villi. The clinical presentation of PSTT can range from slow-growing disease limited to the uterus to metastatic disease, with lung and liver the most common sites of distant spread [7].

The role of hCG in trophoblast disease diagnosis and management

Produced predominantly by syncytiotrophoblast cells, hCG is a glycosylated heterodimer protein consisting of the α and β units held together by non-covalent bonds. In malignant disease a number of hCG variants can occur, including hyperglycosylated hCG, nicked hCG, hCG missing the β subunit C-terminal peptide and the free β subunit. With the potential exception of a few atypical cases of PSTT, hCG is constitutively expressed by all malignant trophoblast tumours.

The measurement of hCG allows estimation of tumour bulk, forms an important part of the assessment of the patient's disease risk and provides a simple method to follow the response to treatment. The hCG level can be measured by a variety of immunoassays but at present there is no internationally standardized assay and the various commercially available kits used in different hospitals can vary in their ability to detect different portions of partially degraded hCG molecules and so can give divergent results and occasional false negatives [8,9].

In the absence of tumour hCG production, the serum half-life of hCG is 24–36 hours; however, in the clinical situation total hCG levels characteristically show slower rates of fall as the tumour cells continue to produce some hCG as their number decreases with treatment.

Prognostic factors and treatment groups

Data from the early days of successful chemotherapy treatment for trophoblast disease show clearly that there is a relationship between the level of elevation of hCG at presentation, the presence of distant metastases and the reducing chances of cure with single-agent chemotherapy. This relationship and the impact on treatment choice and cure rate were first codified by the Bagshawe scoring system published in 1976 [10]. Subsequently there have been a number of revisions and parallel systems introduced that are broadly similar to this original. Table 8.3 shows the revised 2000 International Federation of Gynaecology and Obstetrics (FIGO) prognostic score. From assessment of these parameters, an estimate of the risk category can be obtained and patients offered initial treatment either with single-agent chemotherapy if their score is 6 or less or multiagent combination chemotherapy for scores of 7 and over [11].

Low-risk disease management

Over 90% women with molar pregnancies in the UK who require additional treatment following their initial evacuation fall into the low-risk treatment category as defined by the FIGO prognostic scoring system. The role of repeated uterine evacuation in the management of these

Table 8.3 The International Federation of Gynaecology and Obstetrics (FIGO) prognostic scoring system employed for assessing the intensity of the initial chemotherapy treatment.

Scores	0	1	2	4
Age (years)	<40	≥40	–	–
Antecedent pregnancy	Mole	Abortion	Term	–
Months from index pregnancy	<4	4–6	7–13	≥13
Pre-treatment hCG (IU/L)	<1000	1000–10000	1000–100000	>100000
Largest tumour size	<3cm	3–5cm	≥5cm	–
Site of metastases	Lung	Spleen, kidney	Gastrointestinal	Brain, liver
Number of metastases	–	1–4	5–8	>8
Previous chemotherapy	–	–	Single agent	Two or more drugs

patients has been a subject of uncertainty until recently. A number of recent studies looking at the impact of repeated evacuation in women with rising or static hCG levels following their first evacuation have suggested that a repeated procedure is rarely curative [12,13]. Based on these data, the current recommendation is that a repeated evacuation should only be considered if the hCG level is under 5000 IU/L and tissue is seen in the uterine cavity on ultrasound.

For patients meeting the FIGO standard for low-risk treatment, the most widely used protocol is methotrexate given intramuscularly with oral folinic acid rescue following the schedule shown in Table 8.4. The first course of treatment should be administered in hospital with the subsequent courses administered at home. However, patients with an hCG level above 10 000 IU/L often stay in for up to 3 weeks as they have a higher risk of bleeding, particularly as the tumour shrinks rapidly with the initial chemotherapy. Bleeding usually responds well to bed rest and less than 1% of low-risk patients require emergency interventions such as vaginal packing, embolization or hysterectomy.

The low-risk chemotherapy treatment is usually well tolerated without much major toxicity. Methotrexate does not cause alopecia or significant nausea and myelosuppression is extremely rare. Of the side effects that do occur, the most frequent problems are from pleural inflammation, mucositis and mild elevation of liver function tests. For low-risk patients with lung metastases visible on their chest radiographs, the policy at Charing Cross Hospital is to add central nervous system (CNS) prophylaxis with intrathecal methotrexate administration to minimize the risk of development of CNS disease.

Treatment is continued until normalization of the serum hCG level and then it is usual to continue treatment for another three cycles (6 weeks) to ensure eradication of any residual disease that is below the level of serological detection [1]. A typical example of the treatment graph for a patient successfully completing methotrexate chemotherapy is shown in Fig. 8.3.

An overview of the data for the 1990s indicates that 67% of patients in the low-risk group will only require treatment with the methotrexate protocol to successfully complete their therapy. Patients who have an inadequate response to methotrexate therapy as shown by an hCG plateau or rise have their treatment changed to second-line therapy. This may be either single-agent actinomycin D (0.5 mg for days 1–5 every 2 weeks if hCG is below 300 IU/L) or etoposide, methotrexate, actinomycin D, cyclophosphamide and vincristine (EMA/CO) combination chemotherapy if hCG is above 300 IU/L (Table 8.5).

An individual example of the pattern of hCG levels during the course of management is shown in Fig. 8.4. This demonstrates the rise in hCG that led to the

Table 8.4 The low-risk methotrexate and folinic acid chemotherapy treatment schedule.

Day 1	Methotrexate 50 mg i.m. at noon
Day 2	Folinic acid 15 mg p.o. at 6 p.m.
Day 3	Methotrexate 50 mg i.m. at noon
Day 4	Folinic acid 15 mg p.o. at 6 p.m.
Day 5	Methotrexate 50 mg i.m. at noon
Day 6	Folinic acid 15 mg p.o. at 6 p.m.
Day 7	Methotrexate 50 mg i.m. at noon
Day 8	Folinic acid 15 mg p.o. at 6 p.m.

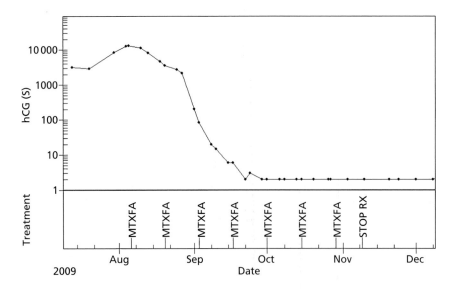

Fig. 8.3 The treatment and human chorionic gonadotrophin (hCG) graph of a low-risk patient with a gestational trophoblast tumour, successfully treated with methotrexate and folinic acid chemotherapy.

introduction of methotrexate chemotherapy; following this, the hCG initially falls but after two cycles appears to plateau. The introduction of second-line treatment with EMA/CO chemotherapy leads to a rapid fall in hCG to normal and the completion of chemotherapy after 6 weeks further treatment. Overall the survival in this group is nearly 100% and the sequential introduction of additional chemotherapy as necessary minimizes the potential long-term carcinogenic risks of excess treatment.

High-risk disease management

Historical data from treatment prior to the introduction of multiagent chemotherapy demonstrated that less than one-third of high-risk patients would be cured with single-agent therapy [14]. The introduction of combination chemotherapy treatments in the 1970s transformed this situation, and modern data indicate a cure rate for high-risk patients of 85–90% using EMA/CO chemotherapy [2,15]. This combination delivers a dose-intense treatment with the five chemotherapy agents, delivered in two

groups 1 week apart as shown in Table 8.5. This approach to chemotherapy, rather than the more usual 3 or 4 weekly cycles used in other malignancies, appears to be the most effective approach to this rapidly proliferating malignancy. Overall the EMA-CO regimen is well tolerated and serious or life-threatening toxicity is rare and the majority of patients tolerate treatment without any major problems.

However, these drugs are myelosuppressive and granulocyte colony-stimulating factor (G-CSF) support is frequently helpful. Fortunately, serious or life-threatening toxicity is rare and the majority of patients tolerate treatment without any major problems. As in the low-risk situation, treatment is continued for 6 weeks after the normalization of hCG. In selected patients the dose of etoposide can be reduced after the hCG falls to normal, to contain the total dose exposure and so minimize the potential risk of developing secondary malignancies. An example of a high-risk patient treated in this case with high-risk chemotherapy regimen is shown in Fig. 8.5, which demonstrates the resolution of extensive lung metastases and normalization of hCG levels in response to treatment.

Of the high-risk patients treated with EMA/CO, approximately 17% develop resistance to this combination and require a change to second-line drug treatment. In this situation, the EP/EMA or TE/TP regimens may be used, which incorporate cisplatin and additional etoposide into the combination along with paclitaxel in the TE/TP regimen. These treatments, combined with surgery mostly to the uterus for defined areas of drug-resistant disease, produce a cure rate approaching 90% in this relatively small group of patients [16,17]. We aim to minimize short-term infective risks and long-term bone toxicity by avoiding the routine use of dexamethasone in

Table 8.5 EMA/CO chemotherapy.

Week 1	
Day 1	Actinomycin D 0.5 mg i.v.
	Etoposide 100 mg/m² i.v.
	Methotrexate 300 mg/m² i.v.
Day 2	Actinomycin D 0.5 mg i.v.
	Etoposide 100 mg/m² i.v.
	Folinic acid 15 mg p.o. 12-hourly × 4 doses
	Starting 24 hours after commencing methotrexate
Week 2	
Day 8	Vincristine 1.4 mg/m² (maximum 2 mg)
	Cyclophosphamide 600 mg/m²

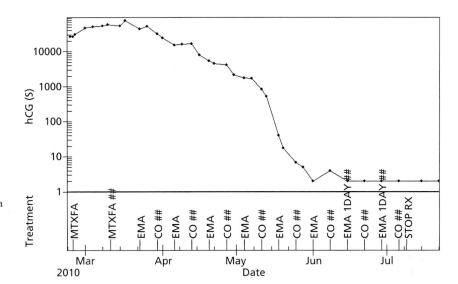

Fig. 8.4 The treatment and human chorionic gonadotrophin (hCG) graph of a low-risk patient with a gestational trophoblast tumour, initially treated with methotrexate and folinic acid chemotherapy, changing to EMA-CO treatment in response to an hCG plateau.

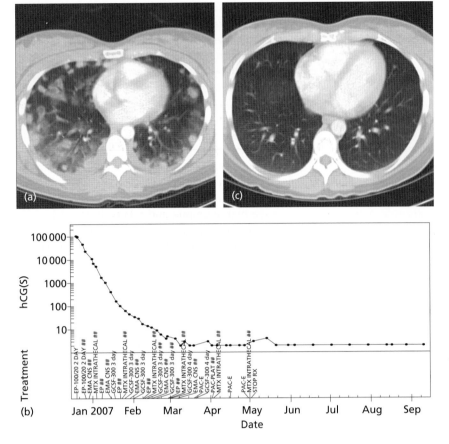

Fig. 8.5 The pre-treatment chest CT scan (a), treatment graph (b) and post-treatment CT scan (c) in a 29-year-old woman presenting with respiratory failure secondary to choriocarcinoma 2 months after the birth of a healthy child.

antiemetics, as this can be associated with both *Pneumocystis* infection and avascular necrosis of the femoral head.

Approximately 4% of patients presenting with trophoblast disease have cerebral metastases at the time of diagnosis. In contrast to most other malignancies, where cerebral metastases are associated with a very poor prognosis, trophoblast patients with CNS disease can routinely be cured of their disease. Treatment may include an initial surgical resection if the disease is superficial and then chemotherapy with modified EMA/CO containing a higher dose of methotrexate which enhances penetration into the CNS. This treatment, combined with intrathecal methotrexate administration, has produced a cure rate of 86% for patients with CNS disease who are fit enough at presentation to commence effective treatment [18].

Management of placental site trophoblast disease

The original description of PSTT suggested a relatively benign malignancy. However, further data demonstrated that this is a malignancy that can often metastasize but can frequently be cured with effective therapy.

The optimal management of PSTT depends on the staging. When disease is limited to the uterus, curative treatment can usually be achieved with hysterectomy alone. For patients with disseminated disease the recommended treatment is with EP/EMA chemotherapy, which is continued for 6–8 weeks after the normalization of the hCG level. Following successful chemotherapy treatment, hysterectomy is generally recommended as viable tumour cells may persist in the uterine wall. The data for patients with PSTT treated between 1976 and 2006 demonstrates a 100% cure rate for those presenting within 4 years of the antecedent pregnancy, but a poorer prognosis for those presenting after a longer interval [7].

Risk of relapse and late treatment complications

For the majority of patients with trophoblast disease who achieve a serological remission the outlook is very bright in terms of the very low risks of relapse, the high possibility of further successful pregnancies and only modest long-term health risks from the chemotherapy exposure. Once the hCG has fallen to normal, the risk of relapse is less than 2% for patients starting in the low-risk category and 8% for patients in the high-risk EMA/CO category

[19]. Generally, recurrences occur within the first 12 months after treatment. For the patients who initially had successful treatment and then relapse, treatment with further chemotherapy, and on occasion surgery to sites of disease, leads to cure in over 80% of cases. In contrast the outlook for the small number of patients who do not reach a normal hCG level with their first-line combination chemotherapy regimen is less good, with subsequent treatment leading to a cure rate of approximately 50% [19].

Subsequent fertility

Following chemotherapy treatment, fertility is usually maintained and regular menstrual periods restart 2–6 months after the completion of chemotherapy. However, chemotherapy treatment does bring the average age of the menopause forward, by approximately 1 year for those treated with methotrexate and 3 years for those treated with EMA/CO [20].

Further pregnancy should be deferred for 12 months after treatment to avoid any teratogenic effects on developing oocytes and to minimize the possible confusion from the rising hCG levels between a new pregnancy and disease relapse. The modest impact on future fertility is reflected in the data demonstrating that 83% of women wishing to conceive after chemotherapy treatment have been able to have at least one live birth. Despite the frequent long exposure to cytotoxic chemotherapy in the high-risk group, there does not appear to be any significant increase in fetal abnormalities [21].

Many patients after experiencing one molar pregnancy, and particularly those who require chemotherapy, are anxious about the problem occurring again in any subsequent pregnancy. While the data suggest that the risk of a further molar pregnancy is about 10-fold higher than in the normal population, this only equates to an approximate 1 in 70 risk [22]. This risk appears to be independent of chemotherapy exposure, being similar for those patients who required chemotherapy and those where the molar pregnancy was cured by evacuation alone.

Long-term toxicities

With the prolonged follow-up data available from the patients with trophoblast disease treated from the 1970s onwards, it is clear that exposure to combination chemotherapy carries some long-term health risks. Data from a study of 1377 patients treated at Charing Cross Hospital show that those receiving combination chemotherapy have enhanced risks of developing a second malignancy. From this series of patients, the overall relative risk (RR) was increased 1.5-fold and is particularly marked for myeloid leukaemia (RR 16.6), colon cancer (RR 4.6), breast cancer (RR 5.8) and melanoma (RR 3.41) [23]. This database is being updated and as the cohorts of treated patients get older, these risks may further increase. In contrast, the patients treated with single-agent methotrexate do not appear to have increased risks of second malignancies.

This long-term health concern from the use of combination chemotherapy reinforces the benefits derived from an effective surveillance programme that allows treatment to be commenced with single-agent methotrexate in the large majority of women with GTT after a molar pregnancy.

Personal and psychological issues

Despite the high cure rate and relatively low long-term toxicity from chemotherapy treatment, it is unsurprising that the diagnosis of a gestational tumour and particularly treatment with chemotherapy can result in a number of psychological sequelae.

The main areas that can lead to stress in the short term include the loss of the pregnancy, the impact of the 'cancer' diagnosis, the treatment process and the delay of future pregnancy. During chemotherapy treatment issues regarding potential side effects, emotional problems and fertility concerns are frequent and patients will benefit from the support of an experienced counsellor. A number of studies have shown that these concerns can remain for many years, with feelings regarding the wish for more children, a lack of control of fertility and an ongoing mourning for the lost pregnancy still frequently reported 5–10 years after successful treatment [24,25]. A number of surveys have demonstrated the wish of many patients to have more support throughout their diagnosis and treatment through counselling and other forms of support. With the rarity of the diagnosis, providing expert counselling close to home is likely to be challenging, but support in the form of the patients internet forum on www.mymolarpregnancy.co.uk has proved extremely useful to many patients in the UK and elsewhere.

Summary

All forms of GTT including molar pregnancies are rare and their aetiology, biology and responsiveness to treatment are very different from other form of malignancy.

Over 90% of molar pregnancies will be cured with the first evacuation and the cases that require chemotherapy are generally cured with very low toxicity treatment. Choriocarcinoma and PSTT, the rarer forms of GTT, can occur with a wide variety of presentations and a formal hCG measurement should be performed in all women with a new diagnosis of metastatic cancer.

In the UK there is a well-established centralized surveillance and treatment service that links all the obstetric and gynaecology teams in the UK with an effective registration, follow-up and expert treatment service. There is a 24-hour emergency advice and treatment service available in both major centres in the UK and they are always willing to give advice on any UK and overseas patient on request.

Summary box 8.1

- Molar pregnancies occur at an approximate rate of 1 per 500 viable conceptions for women in the UK. The risk of a molar pregnancy increases with maternal age: for women aged 45 the risk is 1 in 96; for women aged 50 and over the risk is 1 in 6.

- The risk of requiring chemotherapy treatment after the evacuation is approximately 15% for complete molar pregnancies and 1% for partial moles. Modern treatment produces cure rates of nearly 100% using primarily low-toxicity methotrexate chemotherapy.

- Choriocarcinoma is a rare diagnosis, with an incidence of 1 per 50 000–100 000 conceptions. The majority of cases occur after a normal pregnancy but the diagnosis can occur after a molar pregnancy or a miscarriage. The presenting symptoms and findings in choriocarcinoma can be varied and it is recommended that every women presenting with previously undiagnosed cancer should have a formal laboratory hCG check.

- The UK has a national service for the registration, surveillance and specialist treatment of gestational tumours. All patients with proven or suspected molar pregnancies should be registered and expert advice for emergency cases is available 24 hours a day.

References

1 McNeish IA, Strickland S, Holden L *et al.* Low-risk persistent gestational trophoblastic disease: outcome after initial treatment with low-dose methotrexate and folinic acid from 1992 to 2000. *J Clin Oncol* 2002;20:1838–1844.

2 Bower M, Newlands ES, Holden L, Bagshawe KD. EMA/CO for high-risk gestational trophoblastic tumours: results from a cohort of 272 patients. *J Clin Oncol* 1997;15:2636–2643.

3 Smith HO, Kim SJ. Epidemiology. In: Hancock BW, Newlands ES, Berkowitz RS, Cole LA (eds) *Gestational Trophoblastic Diseases*, 2nd edn. Sheffield: International Society for the Study of Trophoblastic Diseases, 2003.

4 Savage P, Williams J, Wong S-L, Short D *et al.* The demographics of molar pregnancies in England and Wales 2000–2009. *J Reprod Med* 2010;55:341–345.

5 Seckl MJ, Fisher RA, Salerno G *et al.* Choriocarcinoma and partial hydatidiform moles. *Lancet* 2000;356:36–39.

6 Kurman RJ, Scully RE, Norris HJ. Trophoblastic pseudotumor of the uterus. An exaggerated form of 'syncytial endometritis' simulating a malignant tumour. *Cancer* 1976;38:1214–1226.

7 Schmid P, Nagai Y, Agarwal R *et al.* Prognostic markers and long-term outcome of placental-site trophoblastic tumours: a retrospective observational study. *Lancet* 2009;374:48–55.

8 Cole LA, Shahabi S, Butler SA *et al.* Utility of commonly used commercial human chorionic gonadotropin immunoassays in the diagnosis and management of trophoblastic diseases. *Clin Chem* 2000;47:308–315.

9 Harvey RA, Mitchell HD, Stenman UH *et al.* Differences in total human chorionic gonadotropin immunoassay analytical specificity and ability to measure human chorionic gonadotropin in gestational trophoblastic disease and germ cell tumours. *J Reprod Med* 2010;55:285–295.

10 Bagshawe KD. Risk and prognostic factors in trophoblastic neoplasia. *Cancer* 1976;38:1373–1385.

11 FIGO Oncology Committee. FIGO staging for gestational trophoblastic neoplasia. *Int J Gynaecol Obstet* 2002;77:285–287.

12 van Trommel NE, Massuger LF, Verheijen RH *et al.* The curative effect of a second curettage in persistent trophoblastic disease: a retrospective cohort survey. *Gynecol Oncol* 2005;99:6–13.

13 Savage P, Seckl MJ. The role of repeat uterine evacuation in trophoblast disease. *Gynecol Oncol* 2005;99:251–252.

14 Bagshawe KD, Dent J, Newlands ES, Begent RH, Rustin GJ. The role of low-dose methotrexate and folinic acid in gestational trophoblastic tumours (GTT). *Br J Obstet Gynaecol* 1989;96:795–802.

15 Escobar PF, Lurain JR, Singh DK, Bozorgi K, Fishman DA. Treatment of high-risk gestational trophoblastic neoplasia with etoposide, methotrexate, actinomycin D, cyclophosphamide, and vincristine chemotherapy. *Gynecol Oncol* 2003;91:552–557.

16 Newlands ES, Mulholland PJ, Holden L, Seckl MJ, Rustin GJ. Etoposide and cisplatin/etoposide, methotrexate, and actinomycin D (EMA) chemotherapy for patients with high-risk gestational trophoblastic tumours refractory to EMA/cyclophosphamide and vincristine chemotherapy and patients presenting with metastatic placental site trophoblastic tumours. *J Clin Oncol* 2000;18:854–859.

17 Wang J, Short D, Sebire NJ *et al.* Salvage chemotherapy of relapsed or high-risk gestational trophoblastic neoplasia (GTN) with paclitaxel/cisplatin alternating with paclitaxel/etoposide (TP/TE). *Ann Oncol* 2008;19:1578–1583.

18 Newlands ES, Holden L, Seckl MJ, McNeish I, Strickland S, Rustin GJ. Management of brain metastases in patients with high-risk gestational trophoblastic tumours. *J Reprod Med* 2002;47:465–471.

19 Powles T, Savage PM, Stebbing J *et al.* A comparison of patients with relapsed and chemo-refractory gestational trophoblastic neoplasia. *Br J Cancer* 2007;96:732–737.

20 Bower M, Rustin GJ, Newlands ES *et al.* Chemotherapy for gestational trophoblastic tumours hastens menopause by 3 years. *Eur J Cancer* 1998;34:204–207.

21 Woolas RP, Bower M, Newlands ES *et al.* Influence of chemotherapy for gestational trophoblastic disease on subsequent pregnancy outcome. *Br J Obstet Gynaecol* 1998;105:1032–1035.

22 Bagshawe KD, Dent J, Webb J. Hydatidiform mole in England and Wales 1973–83. *Lancet* 1986;ii:673–677.

23 Rustin GJ, Newlands ES, Lutz JM *et al.* Combination but not single-agent methotrexate chemotherapy for gestational trophoblastic tumours increases the incidence of second tumours. *J Clin Oncol* 1996;14:2769–2773.

24 Wenzel L, Berkowitz R, Robinson S *et al.* The psychological, social, and sexual consequences of gestational trophoblastic disease. *Gynecol Oncol* 1992;46:74–81.

25 Wenzel L, Berkowitz RS, Newlands E *et al.* Quality of life after gestational trophoblastic disease. *J Reprod Med* 2002;47:387–394.

Further reading

Hancock BW, Newlands ES, Berkowitz RS, Cole LA (eds) *Gestational Trophoblastic Disease*, 2nd edn. Sheffield: International Society for the Study of Trophoblastic Diseases, 2003.

Royal College of Obstetricians and Gynaecologists. *The Management of Gestational Trophoblastic Neoplasia*. Green-top Guideline No. 38, 2010. Available at: www.rcog.org.uk/files/rcog-corp/GT38ManagementGestational0210.pdf

Soper JJ, Mutch DG, Schink JC. Diagnosis and treatment of gestational trophoblastic disease: American College of Obstetricians and Gynecologists Practice Bulletin No. 53. *Gynecol Oncol* 2004;93:575–585.

Websites

International Society for the Study of Trophoblastic Diseases (ISSTD): www.isstd.org/index.html

US hCG reference service: www.hcglab.com/

UK Hydatidiform Mole and Choriocarcinoma Information and Support Service: www.hmole-chorio.org.uk/

Chapter 9
Ectopic Pregnancy

Davor Jurkovic

King's College Hospital, London, UK

First descriptions of ectopic pregnancy in England date back to 1731 when Gifford described implantation of a pregnancy outside the uterine cavity. Charles Meigs provided particularly vivid descriptions of severe cases of ectopic pregnancy in the mid-nineteenth century, when ectopic pregnancy was considered to be a rare but universally fatal condition. With the improvements in surgical techniques at the turn of the twentieth century, ectopic pregnancy became curable [1]. However, it was still considered a very serious problem with high mortality rates. This perception has changed only recently with the increased ability to establish the diagnosis of ectopic pregnancy non-invasively in women with minimal clinical symptoms. Although there has been a massive increase in the incidence of ectopic pregnancy in recent years, the mortality of the disease has been static [2]. Therefore the main challenge in modern clinical practice is to identify and treat as early as possible cases of ectopic pregnancy with the potential to cause serious morbidity and death, and at the same time to minimize interventions in those destined to be resolved without causing any harm.

Epidemiology and aetiology

Over the past 30 years the incidence of ectopic pregnancy has increased in most industrialized countries. The incidence of ectopic pregnancy may be expressed in various ways, for example number of births, number of pregnancies or number of women of reproductive age may be used as a denominator. Because of difficulties in registering all pregnancies, the number of women aged 15–44 is often used as the denominator when comparing the figures from different populations. The reported annual incidence rates vary between 100 and 175 per 100000 women aged 15–44 [3]. In recent years a stabilization or even decline of ectopic rates has been noted in some countries such as Sweden and Finland. The incidence of ectopic pregnancy in the UK has changed little in recent years,

with 9.6 per 1000 pregnancies in 1991–1993 and 11.1 per 1000 pregnancies in 2003–2005 [2].

The perceived increase in the incidence of ectopic pregnancy may be due to a number of factors. The increase may be a true reflection of the larger number of cases in the population or a result of the improved sensitivity of diagnostic tests for ectopic pregnancy. In the past a significant number of ectopic pregnancies may have resolved spontaneously without being detected, which is less likely to occur in modern clinical practice. Therefore the increased incidence of ectopic pregnancy may be partly explained by the increased effectiveness of screening.

A number of factors have been identified that increase individual risk of ectopic implantation. An association between increased maternal age and ectopic pregnancy has been well documented in the past. The incidence of ectopic pregnancy is three times higher in women aged 35–44 compared with those in the age group 15–24 [4,5]. In recent years the age at first conception has increased, which may have contributed to the increased incidence.

The observed increase in incidence of ectopic pregnancy could also be attributed to an increase in risk factors such as sexually transmitted infections. A recent meta-analysis showed that the odds of having an ectopic pregnancy are significantly higher in women with a history of pelvic infection, multiple partners and early age of intercourse. Odds were particularly high in women with history of chlamydia infection [6]. Another study from Sweden also supports an association between ectopic pregnancy and preceding infection by chlamydia. These data showed that a surge in the incidence of ectopic pregnancy was preceded by a similar peak in the incidence of acute salpingitis 15 years earlier [7]. It has also been found that the reduction in the rate of chlamydia infection due to screening and treatment leads to concomitant decline in the incidence of ectopic pregnancy. However, the findings from epidemiological studies may have been confounded by other factors and they should

Dewhurst's Textbook of Obstetrics & Gynaecology, Eighth Edition. Edited by D. Keith Edmonds.
© 2012 John Wiley and Sons, Ltd. Published 2012 by John Wiley and Sons, Ltd.

Table 9.1 Risk factors for tubal ectopic pregnancy.

History of previous ectopic pregnancy
IUCD or sterilization failure
Pelvic inflammatory disease
Chlamydia infection
Early age of intercourse and multiple partners
History of infertility
Previous pelvic surgery
Increased maternal age
Cigarette smoking
Strenuous physical exercise
In utero diethylstilbestrol exposure

be interpreted with caution. It is possible that the temporal association between the incidence of chlamydia infection and ectopic pregnancy may actually be due to the changes in screening policies for chlamydia and continuous improvement of diagnostic methods for the detection of ectopic pregnancy.

All methods of contraception are effective in reducing the number of both intrauterine and extrauterine pregnancies. However, when pregnancies occur as a result of contraceptive failure, the risk of ectopic pregnancy is significantly increased in women who fall pregnant after tubal sterilization or while using the intrauterine contraceptive device (IUCD), but not in women conceiving due to the failure of oral hormonal contraception or barrier methods [8].

Other factors associated with an increased risk of ectopic pregnancy include previous pelvic surgery, history of infertility, *in utero* diethylstilbestrol exposure, strenuous physical exercise and cigarette smoking. The risk of ectopic pregnancy among black women and other ethnic minorities is 1.6 times higher than the risk among white women in the USA [4].

In women with previous ectopic pregnancy the risk of recurrent ectopic pregnancy is 12–18%. The future risk increases further with every successive occurrence [9,10] (Table 9.1).

 Summary box 9.1

- The incidence of ectopic pregnancy in the UK remains stable.
- The incidence of ectopic pregnancy increases with maternal age.
- A history of sexually transmitted disease increases the chance of ectopic pregnancy.
- All methods of contraception reduce the number of ectopic pregnancies.

Mortality

Ectopic pregnancy remains an important cause of maternal mortality worldwide. Figures from the USA show that the incidence of ectopic pregnancy increased fourfold between 1972 and 1987. At the same time the mortality has decreased nearly sixfold, from 19.6 to 3.4 per 10000 cases. However, the absolute number of deaths has decreased by less than half, from 47 to 30 cases per year [11]. In the UK both the number of ectopics and the number of deaths have been static in the last 12 years, with the mortality rate at 4 per 10000 pregnancies [2]. This trend has been maintained despite a massive expansion over the last decade in the services available to women with suspected early pregnancy complications. A possible explanation is that women with the most serious forms of ectopic pregnancy, such as interstitial ectopics, are typically asymptomatic until sudden rupture accompanied by massive internal bleeding occurs. The lack of early warning signs prevents women seeking the semi-elective services available to them.

Pathophysiology

Any abnormality in tubal morphology or function may lead to ectopic pregnancy. In normal pregnancy the egg is fertilized in the fallopian tube and the embryo is transported into the uterus. It is believed that the most important cause of ectopic pregnancy is damage to the tubal mucosa, which could obstruct embryo transport due to scarring. The other possibility is that a small defect in the mucosa attracts implantation in the fallopian tube [12]. The mucosal damage may be caused by infection or surgical trauma. However, evidence of tubal damage is lacking in many cases of ectopic pregnancy. In these women the cause of ectopic pregnancy may be dysfunction of tubal smooth muscle activity. In general, oestrogens stimulate tubal myoelectrial activity while progesterone has an inhibitory effect. An altered oestrogen/progesterone ratio may affect tubal motility in different ways. Abnormally high oestrogen levels may cause tubal spasm, which could block transport of the embryo towards the uterine cavity. This may be an explanation for increased rates of ectopics following ovarian hyperstimulation and postcoital oral contraception. Conversely, pharmacological doses of progesterone in women using progesterone-only contraception could cause complete tubal relaxation leading to retention of the fertilized egg within the tube [13]. Embryonic abnormalities have also been studied in an attempt to explain the occurrence of ectopics in the absence of tubal pathology and although the majority of tubal pregnancies are non-viable, the incidence of chromosomal defects is no higher than in samples obtained from intrauterine pregnancies [14].

Clinical presentation

The clinical presentation of ectopic pregnancy is very variable and reflects the biological potential of pregnancy to develop beyond a very early stage. This in turn is largely determined by the location of pregnancy within the tube. In general, more proximal implantation to the uterine cavity shows more advanced development. Ampullary ectopics, which represent 70% of all tubal ectopics, rarely develop beyond a very early stage and clinical symptoms of tubal abortion may be present as early as 5 weeks' gestation. On the other hand, one-third of interstitial tubal ectopics develop in a similar way to healthy intrauterine pregnancies with evidence of a live embryo on ultrasound examination. These pregnancies tend to be clinically silent until sudden rupture occurs [15].

Most ectopic pregnancies represent a form of early pregnancy failure and the first symptom is usually brown vaginal discharge, which starts soon after the missed menstrual period. However, the amount of bleeding varies and in some women it can be quite heavy. Passage of a decidual cast may sometimes lead to an erroneous diagnosis of miscarriage. Abdominal pain is usually a late feature in the clinical presentation of ectopic pregnancy. The localization of pain is not specific and it is not unusual for women to complain of pain on the side contralateral to the ectopic. Some women may complain of period-like pain or upper abdominal discomfort. The pain is usually caused by tubal miscarriage and bleeding through the fimbrial end of the tube into the peritoneal cavity. The pain varies in intensity and does not necessarily reflect the volume of blood lost inside the abdominal cavity. About 10–20% of ectopic pregnancies present without bleeding [16]. In a significant proportion of these cases a viable embryo is detected on ultrasound scan, which increases the risk of rupture. Pain associated with rupture tends to be more intense, with signs of peritonism on abdominal palpation. Severe rupture sometimes presents with nausea, vomiting and diarrhoea, which may resemble a gastrointestinal disorder. This confusing picture may cause delay in the diagnosis of ectopic pregnancy. Indeed this misdiagnosis was made in more than one-third of women who have died from ectopic pregnancy in the UK since 1998 [2]. However, significant intra-abdominal bleeding can be recognized by the typical signs of haemorrhagic shock, including pallor, tachycardia, hypotension and oliguria.

Women with suspected early pregnancy complications have traditionally been subjected to vaginal examination including speculum and bimanual palpation. Speculum examination has very little value in the detection of ectopic pregnancy. It may help to diagnose miscarriage by visualization of the products of conception within the cervix or vagina. Although this reduces the chance of an ectopic, it does not eliminate the possibility of a heterotopic pregnancy.

Palpation of pelvic organs is also of limited diagnostic value. Most ectopic pregnancies are very small and cannot be felt on palpation. The assessment of uterine size is rarely helpful and cervical excitation is not a specific sign of an ectopic [17]. Internal examination is unpleasant for women and is often uncomfortable even in those with normal intrauterine pregnancies. One could also argue that the application of significant pressure on a tube swollen with an ectopic pregnancy during such an examination could facilitate tubal rupture and complicate the further management of ectopic pregnancy. In modern clinical practice where ultrasound diagnostic facilities are readily available, vaginal examination in women with suspected ectopic pregnancy is of little value and it should not be routinely employed.

> ### Summary box 9.2
>
> - Symptoms of ectopic pregnancy vary depending on the location of the pregnancy within the tube.
> - The most common symptom is brown vaginal discharge.
> - Abdominal pain is a late symptom due to intraperitoneal bleeding.

Diagnosis

Surgery

Traditionally, the diagnosis of ectopic pregnancy was made at surgery and then confirmed on histological examination following salpingectomy. At laparoscopy an unruptured ectopic pregnancy typically presents as a well-defined swelling in the fallopian tube [18] (Fig. 9.1). The diagnosis may be difficult in the presence of extensive pelvic adhesions, which impair visualization of the tubes. Anecdotal cases of false-positive and false-negative laparoscopic findings have been reported, but no formal assessment of the accuracy of laparoscopy in the diagnosis of ectopic pregnancy has been published. Some authors have advocated the use of dilatation and curettage in the diagnosis of ectopic pregnancy. The presence of chorionic villi helps to provide some reassurance since the incidence of heterotopic pregnancy is relatively low, but as mentioned previously it does not exclude an ectopic. However, the majority of women with absent villi on curettage do not have ectopic pregnancies on subsequent laparoscopy and therefore the diagnostic value of curettage is very limited [19].

Ultrasound

With the advent of diagnostic ultrasound and the increasing use of conservative treatment, the diagnosis of ectopic

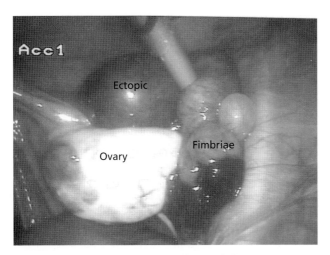

Fig. 9.1 A laparoscopic view of an isthmic tubal ectopic pregnancy with bleeding from the fimbrial end of the tube. (Courtesy of Dr E. Saridogan, University College Hospital, London.)

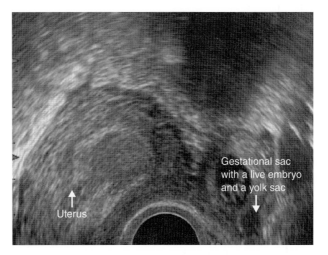

Fig. 9.2 An ultrasound image of a tubal ectopic gestational sac left of the uterus, which contained a live embryo and a yolk sac.

pregnancy is increasingly made without the help of surgery. The sensitivity of ultrasound examination in the diagnosis of ectopic pregnancy depends on the quality of ultrasound equipment and the experience and skill of the operator. With the use of transabdominal ultrasound, direct visualization of ectopic pregnancy is rarely possible. The only value of transabdominal ultrasound is therefore the detection of an intrauterine pregnancy in women with clinical suspicion of an ectopic. Even the diagnosis of intrauterine pregnancy is difficult to make with confidence until 6–7 weeks' gestation. In addition, it is almost impossible to differentiate between interstitial ectopics and intrauterine pregnancies on transabdominal scan. For these reasons transabdominal ultrasound should not be routinely used in women with a clinical suspicion of ectopic pregnancy.

Transvaginal scanning provides much clearer images of pelvic structures in comparison to transabdominal scanning. By using the transvaginal approach it is possible to palpate pelvic organs under visual control, which enables assessment of their mobility and helps to establish the source of pelvic pain. Gentle pressure applied with the tip of the probe may be used to see whether the suspected tubal ectopic moves separately from the ovary. This 'sliding organs' sign helps to avoid false-positive diagnosis of ectopic pregnancy in women with a prominent corpus luteum on ultrasound [20,21]. In experienced hands, transvaginal ultrasound will detect 75–80% of clinically significant tubal ectopics at the initial examination [22]. The remaining 20–25% can be detected on follow-up visits and ultrasound should rarely fail to visualize an ectopic preoperatively. The reported sensitivity of preoperative ultrasound examination (including follow-up scans) is 87.0–99.0% with a specificity of 94.0–99.9% [22,23]. However, the majority of these studies included follow-up ultrasound examinations, so not all ectopic pregnancies were visualized on the initial transvaginal ultrasound scan. Some women would initially have had an inconclusive transvaginal ultrasound examination and would have been classified as 'pregnancy of unknown location'.

The morphology of ectopic pregnancy can be classified into five categories: gestational sac with a live embryo (Fig. 9.2), sac with an embryo but no heart rate, sac containing a yolk sac, an empty gestational sac and solid tubal swelling. The first three morphological types are very specific and enable a conclusive diagnosis of an ectopic to be made. The potential for false-positive diagnosis is higher when the sac is empty or in cases with an inhomogeneous tubal swelling [23,24].

The presence of free fluid in the pouch of Douglas is a frequent finding in women with normal intrauterine pregnancies and it should not be used to diagnose an ectopic. However, the presence of blood clots is important and is a common finding in ruptured ectopics. Blood clots appear hyperechoic and irregular on the scan and they may be mistaken for bowel loops. Checking for the presence of peristalsis helps in the differential diagnosis.

In women with ectopic pregnancy, bleeding within the uterine cavity may resemble an early intrauterine pregnancy ('pseudosac'). The distinction between a pseudosac and a true gestational sac may be difficult on transabdominal scan. Therefore a transvaginal scan should be performed in all women at risk of ectopic pregnancy and with an empty sac on transabdominal scan, in order to differentiate between the two using the criteria listed in Table 9.2 (see also Figs 9.3 and 9.4).

In women with intrauterine pregnancy on the scan, the possibility of heterotopic pregnancy should be excluded. This is particularly the case in women who conceived

Table 9.2 Differential diagnosis between early intrauterine gestational sac and pseudosac.

	Early gestational sac	Pseudosac
Location	Below the midline echo buried into the endometrium	Along the cavity line, between endometrial layers
Shape	Steady, usually round	May change during scan, usually ovoid
Borders	Double ring	Single layer
Colour flow pattern	High peripheral flow	Avascular

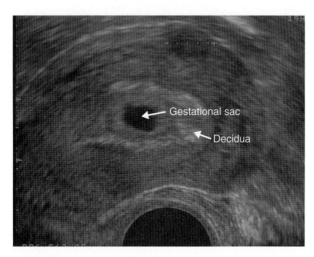

Fig. 9.3 A longitudinal section through the uterus showing a normal early intrauterine pregnancy at 5 weeks' gestation. The sac is surrounded by a well-defined layer of trophoblast tissue and thick decidua.

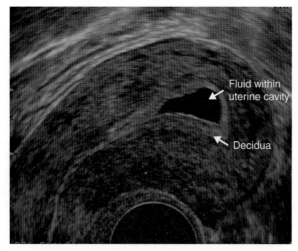

Fig. 9.4 Uterine cavity distended with fluid resembling an intrauterine pregnancy (pseudosac) in a woman with a tubal ectopic pregnancy.

after stimulation of ovulation or *in vitro* fertilization. In symptomatic women with spontaneous pregnancies it is helpful to examine the number of corpora lutea. If more than one corpus is present, a concomitant ectopic needs to be excluded.

Summary box 9.3

- Transabdominal ultrasound has a limited role in the diagnosis of ectopic pregnancy.
- Transvaginal scanning is the imaging modality of first choice.
- Transvaginal ultrasound can detect 75–80% of ectopic pregnancies on the initial examination and the remaining 20–25% will be detected during follow up.

Biochemical measurements

Serum human chorionic gonadotrophin

Serum human chorionic gonadotrophin (hCG) measurements have traditionally been used as a secondary investigation in women with suspected ectopic pregnancy in whom ultrasound examination has failed to identify an intrauterine or ectopic pregnancy. With the use of transabdominal ultrasound, a normal pregnancy could be seen in most cases when serum hCG exceeds 6500 IU/L (Third International Reference 75/537, World Health Organization) [25]. With transvaginal ultrasound this threshold can be lowered to 1000 IU/L [26]. These observations have helped to introduce the concept of 'discriminatory hCG zone' above which a normal intrauterine pregnancy should be detectable on ultrasound scan. However, the concept of discriminatory zone is often misinterpreted in clinical practice. There are many clinicians who assume that in the absence of a visible intrauterine pregnancy on ultrasound scan, serum hCG reading below a predefined level equals normal intrauterine pregnancy and that a reading above that level is diagnostic of an ectopic [27]. This is clearly not the case as hCG levels are often high in the aftermath of a complete miscarriage because of its long clearance half-time of 24–36 hours. It has also been shown that more than 50% of ectopics, which are detectable on the scan, present with hCG levels below 1000 IU/L [28,29]. In view of this, the concept of a discriminatory zone is of limited value in clinical practice and is only useful in assessing asymptomatic women with uncertain menstrual dates.

Abnormally slow rise in serum hCG has also been used to diagnose ectopic pregnancy. In normal early pregnancy the hCG doubling time is 1.4 days before 5 weeks' gestation and 2.4 days from then until 7 weeks' gestation. A prolonged hCG doubling time is an indicator of an abnormal pregnancy. However, it cannot discriminate between intrauterine miscarriages and ectopics. It has also been shown that in about 10% of ectopic pregnancies, serum hCG increases at a normal rate [28].

The use of hCG to select patients for expectant, medical and surgical management of ectopic pregnancy and to assess the efficacy of treatment at follow-up visits is discussed later.

Progesterone

Progesterone production from the corpus luteum is dependent on the slope of hCG increase in early pregnancy. The half-life of progesterone clearance is only 2 hours compared with 24–36 hours for serum hCG [30]. As a result serum progesterone levels will respond quickly to any decrease in hCG production. Measurement of progesterone can therefore be used as a bioassay of early pregnancy viability. Serum progesterone below 20 nmol/L reflects fast decreasing hCG levels and can be used to diagnose spontaneously resolving pregnancies with a sensitivity of 94% and specificity of 91% [28]. Progesterone levels above 60 nmol/L indicate a normal increase in hCG levels, but values between 20 and 60 nmol/L are strongly associated with abnormal pregnancies. In clinical practice serum progesterone measurements are particularly useful in women with a non-diagnostic ultrasound scan. Although the majority of these women have failed intrauterine pregnancies, they are usually followed up with serial hCG measurement because of the fear of missing potentially significant ectopic pregnancies. The routine measurement of serum progesterone can reliably diagnose pregnancies in regression and can reduce by 50–60% the need for follow-up scans and serial hCG measurements in pregnant women with non-diagnostic scan findings [28,31].

Management

Surgery

Surgery has been traditionally used for both the diagnosis and treatment of ectopic pregnancy. In the second half of the twentieth century laparoscopy was mostly used as a diagnostic tool and open surgery was used to treat ectopic pregnancy. With recent advances in operative laparoscopy, the minimally invasive approach has also become accepted as the method of choice to treat most tubal ectopic pregnancies. There are important advantages of laparoscopic over open surgery, including less postoperative pain, shorter hospital stay and faster resumption of social activity [32]. However, the future reproductive outcomes following laparoscopic or open surgery are not significantly different. Although the rate of recurrent ectopics is slightly lower following laparoscopic surgery, the rate of subsequent intrauterine pregnancies appears to be similar [33].

It remains unclear whether laparoscopic salpingotomy with tubal conservation offers any advantage over salpingectomy. Laparoscopic salpingotomy is usually a longer operation, with a higher risk of intraoperative and postoperative bleeding. In addition there is a 10–15% risk of persistent trophoblast following salpingotomy, which may require further surgical or medical treatment. However, data from observational studies indicate that tubal conservation results in slightly higher rates of subsequent intrauterine pregnancy [34]. Until this finding is tested in a prospective randomized trial, the choice between removal of the tube and tubal conservation should be made depending on the circumstances in each individual case. At present there is a consensus that tubal conservation should be attempted if a woman desires further pregnancies and there is evidence of contralateral tubal damage at laparoscopy. In the presence of a healthy contralateral tube, salpingectomy may be performed with the patient's consent [33].

Medical management

Medical management of ectopic pregnancy has grown in popularity in recent years following several observational studies that reported success rates in excess of 90% using single-dose systemic methotrexate [35]. However, the diagnosis of ectopic pregnancy was based in many cases on monitoring the dynamics of serum hCG and progesterone, rather than on direct visualization of the ectopic on ultrasound or at laparoscopy. It is therefore possible that in a significant number of cases intrauterine miscarriages were misdiagnosed as ectopics, contributing to the high success rates. Nevertheless, there are some obvious attractions of medical treatment such as the option to manage patients on an outpatient basis and avoidance of surgery. However, due to the need for prolonged follow-up and the increased failure rate in women presenting with higher initial hCG measurements, medical treatment is only cost-effective in ectopics with serum hCG below 1500 IU/L [36].

Selection criteria for treatment with methotrexate are usually strict and are listed in Table 9.3. Two randomized trials that compared methotrexate to surgery showed that only one-third of all tubal ectopics satisfied these criteria and were suitable for medical treatment, with success rates between 65 and 82% [37,38]. The overall contribution of methotrexate to successful treatment of tubal ectopics was between 23 and 30% while all other women required surgery. The other problem with methotrexate is the risk of tubal rupture and blood transfusion, which occurred significantly more often in women receiving methotrexate compared with those who had surgery, emphasizing the need for very close follow-up [37]. There is also a risk of side effects such as gastritis, stomatitis, alopecia, headaches, nausea and vomiting. Disturbances

Table 9.3 Selection criteria for conservative management of tubal ectopic pregnancy.

Minimal clinical symptoms
Certain ultrasound diagnosis of ectopic
No evidence of embryonic cardiac activity
Size <5cm
No evidence of haematoperitoneum on ultrasound scan
Low serum hCG (methotrexate <3000IU/L; expectant <1500IU/L)

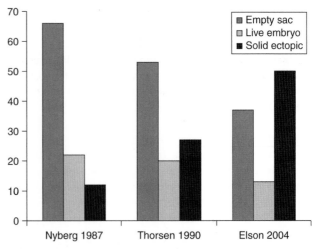

Fig. 9.5 Relative frequencies of different morphological types of ectopic pregnancy detected on ultrasound scan in the last two decades. The proportion of more severe forms such as live ectopics and well-formed gestational sacs is decreasing, while the proportion of mild forms such as small solid ectopics is increasing. This finding reflects the ability of modern equipment to detect tubal ectopics, rather than the change in the nature of the condition.

in hepatic and renal function and leucopenia or thrombocytopenia may also occur.

In view of this, the overall role of methotrexate in the management of ectopic pregnancy is limited, but may be offered on an individual basis to highly motivated women with small unruptured ectopics and a serum hCG level of 1500–3000 IU/L who are likely to comply with well-organized follow-up.

Expectant management

Expectant management has important advantages over medical treatment as it follows the natural history of the disease and is free from the serious side effects of methotrexate. The progress of ectopic pregnancy is easier to monitor as serum hCG measurements accurately reflect trophoblastic activity of the ectopic pregnancy, with rising levels indicating an increased risk of rupture. This is different from medical treatment, which is characterized by an initial rise in serum hCG following administration of methotrexate in cases with both successful and unsuccessful outcomes. Therefore with medical treatment it is often impossible to be confident about the probability of successful treatment for up to a week following injection, which increases the risk of adverse outcomes in comparison to expectant management.

Expectant management requires prolonged follow-up and may cause anxiety to both women and their carers. However, the main limiting factor in the use of expectant management is the relatively high failure rate and the inability to identify with accuracy the cases likely to fail this type of management. To minimize the risk of failure many authors have used very strict selection criteria for expectant management, such as initial hCG level below 250 IU/L [39]. The use of these strict selection criteria has resulted in relatively high success rates, sometimes reaching 70–80% [40,41]. However, only a small minority of ectopics were considered suitable for expectant management, resulting in a low overall contribution to successful management of tubal ectopics of only 7–25%. Recent studies have shown that by using more liberal selection criteria for expectant management up to 40% of all tubal ectopics may resolve spontaneously on expectant treatment [18]. This observation also reflects the increased

sensitivity of modern ultrasound equipment, which enables detection of very small ectopics (Fig. 9.5). It is very likely that a large proportion of these small ectopics went undiagnosed in the past and were treated as early intrauterine miscarriages. However, the sensitivity of equipment will probably improve further in the future and it is imperative for modern practice to continue efforts to refine the selection criteria for expectant management of tubal ectopics.

According to the current literature the success of expectant management may be determined by the serum hCG levels at the initial presentation. In general, if hCG is less than 1500 IU/L and the ectopic pregnancy is clearly visible on ultrasound scan, the success of expectant management is 60–70% [18]. The addition of the serum progesterone and morphological features of ectopics on ultrasound scan enable further refinement in the prediction of the likely success of expectant management.

Long-term fertility outcomes in women treated expectantly are similar to those in women treated by conservative surgery or medically. Several authors have examined reproductive outcomes in women with ectopic pregnancies following successful expectant management compared with those who required surgery. They found no significant differences in the ipsilateral tubal patency rates and the rates of subsequent intrauterine and extrauterine pregnancy [42]. Therefore the main advantage of expectant management is avoidance of any intervention, rather than improvement in the reproductive outcomes.

Fertility after tubal ectopic pregnancy

Intrauterine pregnancy rates following ectopic pregnancy range between 50 and 70% [42]. Recurrent ectopic pregnancies occur in 6–16% of women with previous history of ectopics [43] and these women should be offered early scans in all future pregnancies to detect recurrent ectopics before complications can occur.

Summary box 9.4

- Tubal ectopic pregnancy can be managed surgically or medically.
- Strict criteria need to be observed to choose a medical route.
- Methotrexate is the medical treatment of choice.
- Intrauterine pregnancy rates after ectopic pregnancy are 50–70%.
- Recurrent ectopic pregnancy rates of 6–16% can be expected in women with a history of ectopic pregnancy.

Non-tubal ectopics

Interstitial ectopics

The implantation of the conceptus in the proximal portion of the fallopian tube, which is within the muscular wall of the uterus, is called an interstitial pregnancy. The incidence of interstitial ectopic is 1 in 2500–5000 live births and accounts for 2–6% of all ectopic pregnancies [44]. Risk factors predisposing to an interstitial pregnancy are the same as those for tubal ectopics and include previous ectopic pregnancy (40.6%), assisted reproduction treatment (37.5%) and sexually transmitted infections (25%) [45]. A unique predisposing factor to interstitial pregnancy is previous ipsilateral salpingectomy. Maternal morbidity associated with interstitial pregnancy is still high, and the maternal mortality rate of this form of ectopic pregnancy is about 2–2.5% [2].

Interstitial pregnancy remains the most difficult type of ectopic to diagnose preoperatively. This is partly due to lack of any symptoms prior to sudden rupture. In modern clinical practice the diagnosis of interstitial pregnancy should be made non-invasively using transvaginal ultrasound. The diagnosis is based on visualization of the interstitial tube adjoining the lateral aspect of the uterine cavity and the gestational sac, and the presence of a continuous myometrial layer surrounding the chorionic sac [46] (Figs 9.6 and 9.7).

Ruptured interstitial pregnancy usually presents dramatically with severe intra-abdominal bleeding, which requires urgent surgery. Haemostasis can usually be achieved by removing the pregnancy tissue and suturing the rupture site. However, in cases of extreme bleeding a cornual resection or in rare cases a hysterectomy may be necessary to arrest the bleeding.

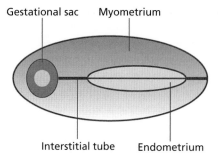

Fig. 9.6 Schematic illustration of interstitial pregnancy.

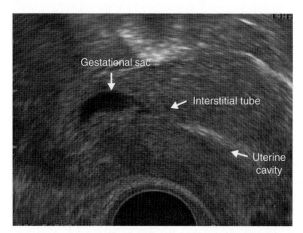

Fig. 9.7 An oblique section through the uterus showing an empty uterine cavity and the interstitial portion of the tube adjoining the cavity and an ectopic sac. The sac is completely surrounded by a myometrial mantle, which is typical of interstitial pregnancy.

Earlier non-invasive ultrasound diagnosis prior to the rupture facilitates the use of laparoscopic surgery for the treatment of interstitial ectopic pregnancy. Various procedures have been described including laparoscopic cornual resection, cornuostomy or salpingotomy [47]. Intramyometrial vasopressin injection and suture-loop tourniquet through broad ligament have been used to reduce intraoperative blood loss.

Unruptured interstitial pregnancy less than 12 weeks in size can be managed conservatively. Medical treatment with methotrexate should be given to all women with rising serum hCG on follow-up visit. Good results have been reported with both systemic and local methotrexate [48,49]. However, in viable interstitial pregnancies local injection under ultrasound guidance is preferable as it enables fetocide to be carried out at the same time, which increases the success rate of medical treatment. Small interstitial pregnancies with declining serum hCG levels can be managed expectantly without any intervention.

Apart from the side effects of methotrexate, the main disadvantage of conservative treatment is the time taken

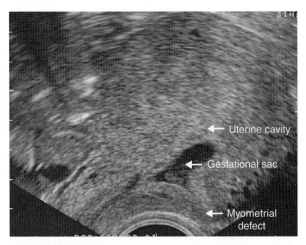

Fig. 9.8 A 7 weeks' Caesarean scar pregnancy with the gestational sac herniating into the myometrial defect.

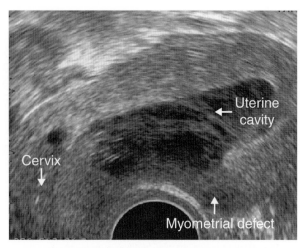

Fig. 9.9 An anterior myometrial defect is clearly visible following evacuation of a Caesarean pregnancy.

for the pregnancy to be fully absorbed; in larger pregnancies this may take up to a year.

Pregnancies located below the internal os: cervical and Caesarean scar ectopics

Cervical pregnancy is defined as the implantation of the conceptus within the cervix, below the level of the internal os. Caesarean scar pregnancy is a novel entity that refers to a pregnancy implanted into a deficient uterine scar following previous lower segment Caesarean section [50]. Prior to the introduction of high-resolution transvaginal scanning, the distinction between cervical and Caesarean scar pregnancies was not possible. In older literature 33% of 'cervical' pregnancies occurred in women with a history of previous Caesarean section, which indicates that scar pregnancies probably account for a significant number of ectopics below the level of the internal os [51].

The common characteristic of both cervical and Caesarean scar pregnancies is implantation into myometrial defects following previous intrauterine surgery (Fig. 9.8). In the case of cervical pregnancy, implantation is usually into the false passage that occurred during previous attempts at cervical dilatation. As a result of myometrial involvement, surgical evacuation of cervical or Caesarean ectopics often results in serious haemorrhage. The bleeding tends to be more severe with increasing gestation. Pregnancies below the internal os are often viable and it is not unusual for Caesarean ectopics to progress to full term. In these cases women usually develop placenta praevia/accreta, which is often complicated by severe postpartum haemorrhage and peripartum hysterectomy [52].

An attempt to remove cervical or Caesarean section pregnancy is likely to cause severe vaginal bleeding, and hysterectomy rates of 40% have been described when dilatation and curettage was attempted without preoperative diagnosis of cervical pregnancy [53]. Various methods directed at reducing the bleeding from the implantation site have been used in conjunction with dilatation and curettage, including insertion of a Foley catheter into the cervix, intracervical vasopressin injection, cervical Shirodkar cerclage, transvaginal ligation of the cervical branches of uterine arteries or angiographic uterine artery embolization. The use of any of these methods in conjunction with dilatation and curettage reduces the risk of hysterectomy to less than 5% (Fig. 9.9).

Similar to other types of ectopic pregnancy, medical treatment with methotrexate or expectant management can be used in smaller non-viable cervical pregnancies. Although conservative management is successful in some cases, it is associated with prolonged vaginal bleeding that may last for many months and there is also a risk of infection and sepsis. For these reasons surgery should be used in preference for cervical/Caesarean scar ectopics except in very small cases on non-viable pregnancies which can be managed expectantly [54].

The risk of recurrence of cervical/Caesarean ectopics is low, and provided the next pregnancy is located normally within the uterine cavity, it is likely to be uncomplicated [54].

Ovarian pregnancy

Ovarian pregnancy is defined as the implantation of the conceptus on the surface of the ovary or inside the ovary, away from the fallopian tubes. There are no direct risk factors associated with primary ovarian pregnancy, although there are reports of associations with the use of IUCDs, pelvic inflammatory disease and assisted conception [55]. Chance might also have played a role in some cases, as recurrent cases of ovarian pregnancy have rarely been reported.

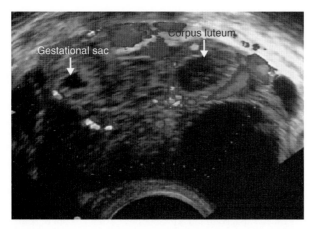

Fig. 9.10 A case of ovarian pregnancy diagnosed on ultrasound scan. The gestational sac with a distinctive trophoblastic ring is seen lateral to a cystic corpus luteum.

The diagnosis of ovarian pregnancy is rarely achieved preoperatively, so most women are treated surgically as the diagnosis is reached only at operation [56]. On ultrasound scan a small ovarian pregnancy can be seen implanted into the ovary next to the corpus luteum (Fig. 9.10).

Laparoscopy has emerged as the gold standard method for the management of most ovarian pregnancies. The technique of laparoscopic removal depends on the size and location of the pregnancy within the ovary, as well as the patient's haemodynamic status. Conservative laparoscopic surgery involves ovarian resection or aspiration of the pregnancy combined with coagulation of the implantation site using a thermocoagulator [57]. However, in cases with profuse intraoperative bleeding an oophorectomy or salpingo-oophorectomy may be necessary to achieve haemostasis.

Abdominal pregnancy

Abdominal pregnancy is a rarity that only a few gynaecologists will encounter during their professional career. Most abdominal pregnancies are the result of reimplantation of ruptured undiagnosed tubal ectopic pregnancies. With the increasing accuracy of first-trimester transvaginal scanning it is likely the prevalence of advanced abdominal pregnancy will decrease even further in the future. The clinical and ultrasound features of an early abdominal pregnancy are very similar to those of tubal ectopic pregnancy. However, viable abdominal pregnancies that progress beyond the first trimester are typically missed on routine transabdominal scanning. Abdominal pregnancy should be suspected in women with persistent abdominal pain later in pregnancy and in those who complain of painful fetal movements. In abdominal pregnancy it is often difficult to obtain clear images of the fetus due to overlying bowel loops, and there is often evidence of oligohydramnios and early intrauterine growth resriction. Perinatal mortality is high (>40%) and the incidence of fetal malformations is also increased [58].

In women with clinical suspicion of abdominal pregnancy a transvaginal scan should be performed to assess the uterus and establish the continuity between the cervical canal, uterine cavity and gestational sac. If pregnancy is clearly outside the uterine cavity, the differential diagnosis includes abdominal pregnancy and pregnancy in an atretic non-communicating cornu of a unicornuate uterus. Visualization of both interstitial portions of the tubes favours the diagnosis of abdominal pregnancy.

Treatment of abdominal pregnancy is surgical. The timing of the intervention depends on clinical signs and the patient's symptoms. In advanced abdominal pregnancies accompanied by normal fetal development diagnosed in the late second trimester, termination of pregnancy may be delayed for a few weeks until the fetus reaches viability. At surgery the gestational sac should be opened carefully avoiding disruption of the placenta. The fetus should be removed, the cord cut short and the placenta left *in situ* [59]. Any attempt to remove the placenta may result in massive uncontrollable haemorrhage. Adjuvant treatment with methotrexate is not necessary and the residual placental tissue will absorb slowly over a period of many months, sometimes a few years. The placental tissue left *in situ* may become infected and lead to the formation of a pelvic abscess, which may require drainage.

Conclusions

Improvements in non-invasive diagnosis of ectopic pregnancy have led to substantial changes in the management of this common condition. Nowadays women diagnosed with ectopic pregnancy typically present with mild symptoms, either because the diagnosis is made early in the natural history of disease before rupture occurs or because ectopic pregnancy is already failing. The ability to determine the potential of ectopic pregnancy to do harm can be used to offer women different management options, ranging from expectant management to surgery. Even when surgery is required, the operation can usually be performed semi-electively using a minimally invasive approach. Despite these major improvements, there is no room for complacency as the mortality rates of ectopic pregnancy have remained stubbornly constant for the last two decades. The main future challenge is therefore to devise strategies that lead to further reduction in the mortality of ectopics. Additional efforts are also required to refine selection criteria for conservative management of ectopics, in particular for expectant management. Tubal conservation at surgery also remains an important issue and efforts should continue to improve surgical techniques of salpingotomy in order to minimize iatrogenic damage to the tube and preserve future fertility.

References

1 Tait RL. Five cases of extrauterine pregnancy operated upon at the time of rupture. *Br Med J* 1884;1:1250.

2 Lewis G (ed.) *Saving Mothers' Lives: Reviewing Maternal Deaths to Make Motherhood Safer 2003–2005. The Seventh Report on Confidential Enquiries into Maternal Deaths in the United Kingdom.* London: The Confidential Enquiry into Maternal and Child Health, 2007. Available at www.cmace.org.uk/getattachment/26dae364-1fc9-4a29-a6cb-afb3f251f8f7/Saving-Mothers'-Lives-2003-2005-(Full-report).aspx

3 Coste J, Bouyer J, Ughetto S *et al.* Ectopic pregnancy is again on the increase. Recent trends in the incidence of ectopic pregnancies in France (1992–2002). *Hum Reprod* 2004;19:2014–2018.

4 Egger M, Low N, Davey Smith G, Lindblom B, Herrmann B. Screening for chlamydial infections and the risk of ectopic pregnancy in a county in Sweden: ecological analysis. *BMJ* 1998;316:1776–1780.

5 Goldner T, Lawson H, Xia Z, Atrash H. Surveillance for ectopic pregnancy: United States, 1970–1989. *MMWR CDC Surveill Summ* 1993;42:73–85.

6 Westrom L, Bengtsson LPH, Mardh PA. Incidence, trends and risks of ectopic pregnancy in a population of women. *BMJ* 1981;282:15–18.

7 Ankum WM, Mol BWJ, Van der Veen F, Bossuyt PMM. Risk-factors for ectopic pregnancy: a meta-analysis. *Fertil Steril* 1996;65:1093–1099.

8 Bjartling C, Osser S, Persson K. The frequency of salpingitis and ectopic pregnancy as epidemiologic markers of *Chlamydia trachomatis. Acta Obstet Gynecol Scand* 2000;79:123–128.

9 Mol BW, Ankum WM, Bossuyt PM, Van der Veen F. Contraception and the risk of ectopic pregnancy: a meta-analysis. *Contraception* 1995;52:337–341.

10 Bouyer J, Job-Spira N, Pouly JL *et al.* Fertility after ectopic pregnancy: results of the first three years of the Auvergne Registry. *Contracept Fertil Sex* 1996;24:475–481.

11 Maymon R, Shulman A, Halperin R, Michell A, Bukovsky I. Ectopic pregnancy and laparoscopy: review of 197 patients treated by salpingectomy or salpingotomy. *Eur J Obstet Gynecol Reprod Biol* 1995;62:61–67.

12 Cartwright PS. Incidence, epidemiology, risk factors and etiology. In: Stovall TG, Ling FW (eds) *Extrauterine Pregnancy. Clinical Diagnosis and Management.* New York: McGraw-Hill, 1993:27–64.

13 Vasquez G, Winston RML, Brosens IA. Tubal mucosa and ectopic pregnancy. *Br J Obstet Gynaecol* 1983;90:468.

14 Pulkkinen MO, Talo A. Tubal physiologic consideration in ectopic pregnancy. *Clin Obstet Gynecol* 1987;30:164.

15 Coste J, Fernandez H, Joye N. Role of chromosome abnormalities in ectopic pregnancy. *Fertil Steril* 2000;74:1259–1260.

16 Hafner T, Aslam N, Ross JA, Zosmer N, Jurkovic D. The effectiveness of non-surgical management of early interstitial pregnancy: a report of ten cases and review of the literature. *Ultrasound Obstet Gynecol* 1999;13:131–136.

17 Elson J, Tailor A, Banerjee S, Salim R, Hillaby K, Jurkovic D. Expectant management of tubal ectopic pregnancy: prediction of successful outcome using decision tree analysis. *Ultrasound Obstet Gynecol* 2004;23:552–556.

18 Kitchin JD, Wein RM, Nunley WC. Ectopic pregnancy: current clinical trends. *Am J Obstet Gynecol* 1979;134:870.

19 Beck P, Broslovsky L, Gal D, Tancer ML. The role of laproscopy in the diagnosis of ectopic pregnancy. *Int J Gynaecol Obstet* 1984;22:307–309.

20 Lindahl B, Ahlgren M. Identification of chorion vili in abortion specimens. *Obstet Gynecol* 1986;67:79–81.

21 Timor-Tritsch IE, Yeh MN, Peisner DB, Lesser KB, Slavik TA. The use of transvaginal ultrasonography in the diagnosis of ectopic pregnancy. *Am J Obstet Gynecol* 1989;161:157–161.

22 Kirk E, Papageorghiou AT, Condous G, Tan L, Bora S, Bourne T. The diagnostic effectiveness of an initial transvaginal scan in detecting ectopic pregnancy. *Hum Reprod* 2007;22:2824–2828.

23 Condous G, Okaro E, Khalid A *et al.* The accuracy of transvaginal sonography for the diagnosis of ectopic pregnancy prior to surgery. *Hum Reprod* 2005;20:1404–1409.

24 Brown DL, Doubilet PM. Transvaginal sonography for diagnosing ectopic pregnancy. *J Ultrasound Med* 1994;13:259–266.

25 Kadar N, DeVore G, Romero R. Discriminatory hCG zone: its use in the sonographic evaluation for ectopic pregnancy. *Obstet Gynecol* 1981;58:156–161.

26 Cacciatore B, Stenman U-H, Ylostalo P. Diagnosis of ectopic pregnancy by vaginal ultrasonography in combination with a discriminatory serum hCG level of 1000 IU/L (IRP). *Br J Obstet Gynaecol* 1990;97:904–908.

27 Pisarska MD, Carson SA, Buster JE. Ectopic pregnancy. *Lancet* 1998;351:1115–1120.

28 Banerjee S, Aslam N, Woelfer B, Lawrence A, Elson J, Jurkovic D. Expectant management of early pregnancies of unknown location: a prospective evaluation of methods to predict spontaneous resolution of pregnancy. *BJOG* 2001;108:158–163.

29 Kirk E, Condous G, Van Calster B, Van Huffel S, Timmerman D, Bourne T. Rationalising the follow-up of pregnancies of unknown location. *Hum Reprod* 2007;22:1744–1750.

30 Fridstrom M, Garoff L, Sjoblom P, Hillens T. Human chorionic gonadotropin patterns in early pregnancy after assisted conception. *Acta Obstet Gynecol Scand* 1995;74:534–538.

31 Day A, Sawyer E, Mavrelos D, Tailor A, Helmy S, Jurkovic D. Use of serum progesterone measurements to reduce need for follow-up in women with pregnancies of unknown location. *Ultrasound Obstet Gynecol* 2009;33:704–710.

32 Grey D, Thorburn J, Lundorff P, Strandell A, Lindblom B. A cost-effectiveness study of a randomised trial of laparoscopy versus laparotomy for ectopic pregnancy. *Lancet* 1995;345:1139–1143.

33 Royal College of Obstetricians and Gynaecologists. *The Management of Tubal Pregnancy.* Green-top Guideline No. 21, 2004. Available at www.rcog.org.uk/files/rcog-corp/GTG21Tubal11022011.pdf

34 Bangsgaard N, Lund C, Ottensen B, Nillas I. Improved fertility following conservative surgical treatment of ectopic pregnancy. *BJOG* 2003;110:765–770.

35 Stovall TG, Ling FW. Single-dose methotrexate: an expanded clinical trial. *Am J Obstet Gynecol* 1993;168:1759–1765.

36 Sowter M, Farquhar C, Gudex G. An economic evaluation of single dose methotrexate and laparoscopic surgery for the treatment of unruptured ectopic pregnancy. *BJOG* 2001;108: 204–212.

37 Hajenius PJ, Engelsbel S, Mol BW *et al*. Randomised trial of systemic methotrexate versus laparoscopic salpingostomy in tubal pregnancy. *Lancet* 1997;350:774–779.

38 Sowter MC, Farquhar CM, Petrie KJ, Gudex G. A randomised trial comparing single dose systemic methotrexate and laparoscopic surgery for the treatment of unruptured tubal pregnancy. *BJOG* 2001;108:192–203.

39 Cacciatore B, Korhonen J, Stenman U-H, Ylostalo P. Transvaginal sonography and serum hCG in monitoring of presumed ectopic pregnancies selected for expectant management. *Ultrasound Obstet Gynecol* 1995;5: 297–300.

40 Ylostalo P, Cacciatore B, Sjoberg J, Kaaraianen M, Tenhunen A, Stenman U-H. Expectant management of ectopic pregnancy. *Obstet Gynecol* 1992;80:345–348.

41 Makinen JI, Kivijarvi AK, Irjala KMA. Success of non-surgical management of ectopic pregnancy. *Lancet* 1990;335:1099.

42 Strobelt N, Mariani E, Ferrari L, Trio D, Tiezzi A, Ghidini A. Fertility after ectopic pregnancy. *J Reprod Med* 2000;45: 803–807.

43 Dubuisson JB, Aubriot FX, Foulot H. Reproductive outcome after laparoscopic salpingectomy for tubal ectopic pregnancy. *Fertil Steril* 1990;53:1004–1007.

44 Bouyer J, Coste J, Fernandez H, Pouly JL, Job-Spira N. Sites of ectopic pregnancy: a 10 year population-based study of 1800 cases. *Hum Reprod* 2002;17:3224–3230.

45 Tulandi T, Al-Jaroudi D. Interstitial pregnancy: results generated from the society of reproductive surgeons registry. *Obstet Gynecol* 2004;103:47–50.

46 Ackerman TE, Levi CS, Dashefsky SM, Holt SC, Lindsay DJ. Interstitial line: sonographic finding in interstitial (cornual) ectopic pregnancy. *Radiology* 1993;189:83–87.

47 Lau S, Tulandi T. Conservative medical and surgical management of interstitial ectopic pregnancy. *Fertil Steril* 1999;72: 207–215.

48 Cassik P, Ofili-Yebovi D, Yazbek J, Lee C, Elson J, Jurkovic D. Factors influencing the success of conservative treatment of interstitial pregnancy. *Ultrasound Obstet Gynecol* 2005;26: 279–282.

49 Jermy K, Thomas J, Doo A, Bourne T. The conservative management of interstitial pregnancy. *BJOG* 2004;111:1283–1288.

50 Vial Y, Petignat P, Hohlfeld P. Pregnancy in a cesarean scar. *Ultrasound Obstet Gynecol* 2000;16:592–593.

51 Ushakov FB, Elchalal U, Aceman PJ, Schenker JG. Cervical pregnancy: past and future. *Obstet Gynecol Surv* 1996;52: 45–57.

52 Herman A, Weinraub Z, Avrech O, Maymon R, Ron-El R, Bukovsky Y. Follow up and outcome of isthmic pregnancy located in a previous caesarean section scar. *Br J Obstet Gynaecol* 1995;102:839–841.

53 Jurkovic D, Hacket E, Campbell S. Diagnosis and treatment of early cervical pregnancy: a review and a report of two cases treated conservatively. *Ultrasound Obstet Gynecol* 1996;8: 373–380.

54 Jurkovic D, Ben-Nagi J, Ofilli-Yebovi D, Sawyer E, Helmy S, Yazbek J. The efficacy of Shirodkar cervical suture in securing haemostasis following surgical evacuation of Cesarean scar ectopic pregnancy. *Ultrasound Obstet Gynecol* 2007;30: 95–100.

55 Raziel A, Golan A, Pansky M, Ron-El R, Bukovsky I, Caspi E. Ovarian pregnancy: a report of twenty cases in one institution. *Am J Obstet Gynecol* 1990;163:1182–1185.

56 Seinera P, Di Gregorio A, Arisio R, Decko A, Crana F. Ovarian pregnancy and operative laparoscopy: a report of eight cases. *Hum Reprod* 1997;12:608–610.

57 Morice P, Dubuisson JB, Chapron C, De Gayffier A, Mouelhi T. Laparoscopic treatment of ovarian pregnancy. *Gynecol Endocrinol* 1996;5:247–249.

58 Attapattu JAF, Menon S. Abdominal pregnancy. *Int J Gynaecol Obstet* 1993;43:51–55.

59 Martin JN Jr, Sessums JK, Martin RW, Pryor JA, Morrison JC. Abdominal pregnancy: current concepts of management. *Obstet Gynecol* 1988;71:549–557.

Chapter 10
Induced Abortion

Gillian Flett[1] and Allan Templeton[2]
[1]Centre for Sexual and Reproductive Health, Aberdeen, UK
[2]University of Aberdeen, Aberdeen Maternity Hospital, Aberdeen, UK

Induced abortion is one of the most commonly practised gynaecological procedures in the UK. Surgical abortion by vacuum aspiration or dilatation and curettage was the main method from the 1960s, with the introduction of vacuum aspiration and flexibile catheters forming the turning point in practice by reducing volume of blood loss and perforation risk. The late 1980s and 1990s saw exciting new developments in medical methods for early abortion and an improvement in medical methods for mid-trimester termination with the introduction of mifepristone, one of the most significant developments in fertility control of recent years. The result has been an ever-evolving extension of patient choice and a diversification in the provision of abortion services, with an emphasis on safety and efficacy, with widened opportunity for delivery outwith hospital settings. In 2009, 189 100 abortions were performed in England and Wales [1] and there were 13 005 abortions in Scotland [2], both rates showing a decrease on previous years for the first time. There is a clear link with deprivation and around one-quarter of women will have had a previous abortion. Around one in three British women will have had an abortion by the age of 45 [3]. In the UK, over 98% of abortions are undertaken on the grounds that the pregnancy threatens the mental or physical health of the woman or her children [1,2]. It is these abortions which form the focus for this chapter. A minority of abortions are undertaken because of fetal abnormality, multi-fetal pregnancy reduction and selective termination for abnormality and the special legal, ethical and service issues relating to these merit separate consideration.

The availability of NHS abortion provision varies considerably throughout the UK and improving timely access to quality abortion services remains a major sexual health priority. The closer alignment of abortion care with sexual healthcare has been advantageous in delivering an integrated care package, with improved sexual health risk assessment and testing, alongside improved and immediate provision of the full range of contraceptive methods, particularly the long-lasting implant and intra-uterine methods.

The law and abortion

The legal criteria surrounding abortion are specific to the country of practice. The abortion legislation in the UK is based on the 1967 Abortion Act [4] as amended by the Human Fertilisation and Embryology Act 1990 [5]. Amendments to the abortion law were considered during the passage of the Human Fertilisation and Embryology Bill in the parliamentary session 2007–2008. Members of Parliament were informed by a report from the cross-party Science and Technology Committee [6], which included updated information on fetal pain and viability, along with the Government response authored by the Department of Health [7], but these were not fully considered by the House and abortion statute remains unchanged. Before an abortion can proceed, a certificate must be signed by two medical practitioners authorizing the abortion and this certificate requires to be retained for a period of at least 3 years. A notification form, which is forwarded to the Chief Medical Officer (CMO) for the relevant country, must be signed by the doctor taking responsibility for the procedure, although with medical termination it is frequently members of the nursing team who administer the drugs that have been pre-prescribed by the doctor. Most abortions are undertaken on the statutory grounds C or D, which state that the pregnancy has not exceeded its 24th week and where continuance of the pregnancy would involve risks greater than if the pregnancy were terminated of injury to the physical or mental health of the woman or of the existing children of her family (Table 10.1).

It should be noted that the Abortion Act does not apply in Northern Ireland where grounds for abortion are very highly restricted. Following direction from an appeal

Dewhurst's Textbook of Obstetrics & Gynaecology, Eighth Edition. Edited by D. Keith Edmonds.
© 2012 John Wiley and Sons, Ltd. Published 2012 by John Wiley and Sons, Ltd.

Table 10.1 Statutory grounds for legal abortion in the UK.

A	The continuance of the pregnancy would involve risk to the life of the pregnant woman, greater than if the pregnancy were terminated
B	The termination is necessary to prevent grave permanent injury to the physical or mental health of the pregnant woman
C	The pregnancy has not exceeded its 24th week and the continuance of the pregnancy would involve risk, greater than if the pregnancy were terminated, of injury to the physical or mental health of the pregnant woman
D	The pregnancy has not exceeded its 24th week and the continuance of the pregnancy would involve risk, greater than if the pregnancy were terminated, of injury to the physical or mental health of the existing child(ren) of the family of the pregnant woman
E	There is a substantial risk that if the child were born it would suffer from such physical or mental abnormalities as to be seriously handicapped
F	To save the life of the pregnant woman
G	To prevent grave permanent injury to the physical or mental health of the pregnant woman

---

Summary box 10.1

- Abortion practice is governed by law with which practitioners must be familiar.
- Good communication, information provision and supportive counselling are essential.
- Abortion is a frequent and safe gynaecological procedure.
- Abortion has an association with intimate partner violence.
- Sexually transmitted infection (including HIV) risk assessment and testing is important.
- Provision of contraceptive advice and initiating the method at the time of abortion is an essential part of abortion care.

Counselling and pre-assessment for abortion

Gestation is a major determinant of the options available for abortion and a decision is usually reached by the woman in consultation with her medical carers and pregnancy counsellors. The abortion method chosen has to be acceptable to the woman as well as being safe and effective. Full guidelines on good practice for the care of women requesting induced abortion have been published by the Royal College of Obstetricians and Gynaecologists (RCOG, guideline update in progress 2010) [11]. Choice is an integral part of abortion care and provision of information, along with sensitive counselling, is essential to help the woman select an abortion method that is right for her and which will optimize the abortion experience. Increasingly, women are referred to dedicated abortion services offering care separately from other gynaecological patients but with the full support of a gynaecological service should that be required. There is strong evidence supporting a lower risk of complications for abortions undertaken at earlier gestations. Because of this, services need to be organized to offer arrangements which minimize unnecessary delay.

At the pre-assessment consultation, counselling and choice of procedure are likely to dominate, but it is also an opportunity to screen for any pre-existing medical conditions that might require cross-specialty liaison and, despite the sensitivities of abortion, it is unusual for a woman to withhold her permission for this to happen. Increasingly self-assessment questionnaires are used as part of the consultation. For serious medical conditions the risks of abortion are going to be lower than the risks of a continued pregnancy. The pre-assessment also provides an opportunity to enquire about previous contraceptive methods and to plan for intended use of contraception in the future. There should be routine enquiry about gender-based violence with appropriate support and information provided, recognizing the frequent association of domestic abuse with abortion, in particular repeat abortion [12]. It is usual to check the

hearing on a judicial review in 2004, guidance for professionals on the termination of pregnancy in Northern Ireland was published in 2009 [8] and up-to-date information on the issue is available on the Family Planning Association's website (www.fpa.org.uk/).

Doctors looking after women requesting abortion care should apply principles of good practice as described in the General Medical Council (GMC) document *Duties of a Doctor* [9]. There is a conscientious objection clause within the Abortion Act and the British Medical Association (BMA) has produced a useful overview on the legal and ethical position [10]. Where practitioners have a conscientious objection they should provide advice and organize the first steps for arranging an abortion, where the request meets the legal requirements. This would usually include prompt referral to another doctor as appropriate. Doctors and nurses can refuse to take part in an abortion but cannot refuse to take part in any emergency treatment.

Before an abortion proceeds, a clinician will certainly wish to be certain that all legal statute is fulfilled but it is also important to be sure that a woman has considered all her options carefully and is sure of her decision and gives informed consent. In recent years, sexual and reproductive health services and abortion providers have become more aware of the specific needs of young women and a competent young person can give her own consent, although supportive encouragement is given for the involvement of parents/carers and an assessment is always made to identify any child protection concerns.

body mass index and blood pressure for all patients. Patients opting for general anaesthetic surgical abortion will need auscultation of chest and heart. Although an idea of gestational age would have been gained from the menstrual history, it is well recognized that menstrual recall may be inaccurate and bimanual examination is very limited for assessing gestation. The greater accuracy of either abdominal or vaginal ultrasound, as relevant to the anticipated gestation, means that ultrasound is now, for most centres, routine practice. Viability and pregnancy location can also be confirmed. It is important that this scan is undertaken in a sensitive setting and manner and the patient is advised that it is not necessary for her to watch the ultrasound examination in progress. A full blood count is recommended if a pre-existing medical condition should indicate the possibility of anaemia, for example renal disease. A thalassaemia and sickle cell screen may also be relevant. It is also a useful opportunity to confirm immunity to rubella and to offer subsequent immunization if not immune. All patients have blood sent for confirmation of ABO and rhesus status with antibody screening. All unsensitized rhesus-negative women should be given anti-D prophylaxis.

Increasingly, centres include pre-test discussion and offer testing for human immunodeficiency virus (HIV), syphilis, hepatitis B and hepatitis C, but unless a policy for routine screening has been adopted and accepted, such testing remains on a selective basis and may be influenced by the personal history, sexual health risk assessment, recent testing history and population disease prevalence. Cervical screening is not essential to abortion care but again there is an opportunity to check that screening is up to date and, where it is not, opportunistic cervical screening can be offered. For all tests it is important to ensure that the result can be communicated to the woman and appropriate action taken on any abnormal result.

Screening for genital tract infection is helpful for identifying pathogens that increase the risk of post-abortion infection and pelvic inflammatory disease, as well as the long-term sequelae of tubal factor infertility and ectopic pregnancy. The most important infecting organisms are *Chlamydia trachomatis* and *Neisseria gonorrhoeae*. Bacterial vaginosis is also associated with increased infection risk. Control group data from trials of prophylactic antibiotics for abortion suggest that infection complications occur in up to 1 in 10 termination cases, but infection rate data vary widely. A full infection screen, including for sexually transmitted infections (STIs), allows the opportunity for patient follow-up and partner notification and treatment to avoid reinfection. Prophylactic antibiotics at the time of abortion are advocated by many and a meta-analysis by Sawaya *et al.* [13] showed a reduction in risk for subsequent infective morbidity of around 50%, with the protective effect also evident in the low-risk patient group.

However, that approach still leaves the women at risk from reinfection from unrecognized and untreated partners. A third, and possibly ideal, strategy would provide a prophylactic regimen effective against bacterial vaginosis and *Chlamydia* along with a full vaginal STI screen [14]. Prophylaxis and a 'screen and treat' policy have been compared in a randomized trial which concluded that universal prophylaxis is at least as effective as a policy of screen and treat in reducing the short-term infective complications of abortion and could be provided at lower direct cost [15], but the study did predate the introduction of the more sensitive nucleic acid amplification chlamydia and gonorrhoea tests.

The RCOG Guideline Development Group in the UK [11] recommended that all abortion services should adopt a strategy to reduce post-abortion infective problems and the very minimum recommendation is for antibiotic prophylaxis against *Chlamydia* and bacterial vaginosis. Metronidazole 1 g rectally at the time of abortion, or 800 mg oral metronidazole plus 1 g oral azithromycin post procedure, would be a suitable regimen. Azithromycin seems to be increasingly favoured over a 7-day course of doxycycline, where patient compliance can be more problematic. However, the evidence for specific prophylactic antibiotic regimens and timing remains limited.

Choosing the method of abortion

The determining factors in an individual woman's choice for medical or surgical abortion are complex. Some women see advantages in the surgical methods, which are simple and quick and associated with a relatively low risk of complication or failure. Medical methods are often favoured because they appear more physiological, like a miscarriage, and avoid the need for uterine instrumentation and share the advantages of low rates of complication and failure. Some women feel that they lack control when a surgical procedure is undertaken, whereas others specifically wish to remain unaware and have the procedure undertaken by their clinician. In 1991, the antiprogestogen mifepristone was licensed for termination up to 9 weeks' gestation and since then an extensive literature has built up to support the safety, efficacy and acceptability of the medical regimen for early first-trimester abortion [16–19]. In 1995 there was an extension of the licence to include pregnancies over 13 weeks' gestation. At present, the medical regimen is not licensed for use in women over 9 and up to 13 weeks' gestation and the majority of abortions at these gestations remain surgical. However, there is randomized trial evidence comparing medical and surgical abortion at 10–13 weeks' gestation confirming that the medical regimen is an effective alternative to surgery with high acceptability [20]. Increasing numbers of units now offer medical abortion

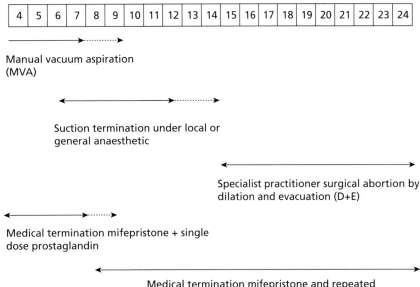

| 4 | 5 | 6 | 7 | 8 | 9 | 10 | 11 | 12 | 13 | 14 | 15 | 16 | 17 | 18 | 19 | 20 | 21 | 22 | 23 | 24 |

Manual vacuum aspiration
(MVA)

Suction termination under local or
general anaesthetic

Specialist practitioner surgical abortion by
dilation and evacuation (D+E)

Medical termination mifepristone + single
dose prostaglandin

Medical termination mifepristone and repeated
doses of prostaglandin

Fig. 10.1 Methods of abortion suitable at different gestations.

as an alternative choice at these gestations In our experience about half of women in the late first trimester opt for medical methods. While ideally abortion services should be able to offer a choice of recommended methods across all the gestation bands, the minimum recommended by the RCOG guideline is that a service should be able to offer abortion by one of the recommended methods in a particular gestation band (Fig. 10.1).

Scottish statistics indicate that 70% of all abortions are now medical and 81% are undertaken medically at gestations under 9 weeks [2]. Medical abortion has been slower in its introduction in England and Wales and there continues to be significant variation in its provision across health authorities. Interestingly, the introduction of medical abortion has not affected the overall abortion rate. That women value choice of method appropriate to the gestation of their pregnancy has been confirmed from patient surveys [21,22]. Both methods can be used for multiple pregnancy.

The RCOG guidelines recommend that conventional suction termination should be avoided at very early gestations under 7 weeks because the procedure is three times more likely to fail to remove the gestation sac than where the termination is performed between 7 and 12 weeks [23]. Although medical termination has been advocated at these very early gestations under 7 weeks, there is renewed interest in manual vacuum aspiration (MVA) under local anaesthesia, combined with ultrasound to confirm aspiration and using strict protocols to identify tissue and where necessary track subsequent β-human chorionic gonadotrophin (hCG) levels. The selection of medical or surgical method for later abortions beyond 15

weeks depends on the availability of healthcare personnel who are trained and willing to participate in late dilatation and evacuation (D+E). There are fewer abortions at these gestations and they tend to be undertaken within the specialist independent sector. It is the case that as gestational age increases the safety of second-trimester surgical abortion depends highly on the operator's skill and experience. Clinics and clinicians usually set the limits for operative care based on these considerations. Hysterotomy, with its high associated morbidity and mortality, has disappeared from practice.

Day-case care is recognized as a cost-effective model of service provision and a typical abortion service will be able to manage well over 90% of its patients on a day-care basis. Pre-existing medical problems, social factors, geographical distance and the possibility of a planned day case subsequently requiring overnight stay because of surgical or medical problems will, of course, influence the day-care rate. Those women undergoing a mid-trimester procedure in particular should be advised of the possible need for an overnight stay, although again this is for a minority, around 3% of mid-trimester procedures in practice.

Medical abortion in the first trimester

The anti-progestogen mifepristone is used in combination with prostaglandin doses to achieve medical abortion. There are few contraindications to medical termination, but include suspected ectopic pregnancy, where an intra-uterine device is in place and unable to be removed prior to abortion, chronic adrenal failure, long-term steroid use, haemorrhagic disorders, treatment with anticoagulants, known allergy to mifepristone or misoprostol, acute porphyria and breast-feeding women. Most anaemic women with a haemoglobin under 9.5 or 10 g/dL are also excluded, as transfusion rates for blood, although very low, are higher for medical than for surgical procedures. Medical abortion may have advantage in obese women where the cervix can be difficult to visualize, where fibroids may obstruct access to the uterine cavity and for some uterine anomalies. Because telephone interactions are more frequent for medical abortions, language skills and ability to understand have to be taken into account.

Medical abortions need to be performed in hospitals or premises registered for abortion. The patient attends briefly to take the mifepristone dose and attends subsequently for day-patient admission, usually 36–48 hours later. It is customary for legal reasons to supervise the swallowing of the mifepristone tablets, but side effects are trivial and the women can leave after 10 min. Women may bleed slightly in the 48 hours following the mifepristone dose and, particularly at early gestations, a very small number may miscarry. The route of prostaglandin administration and regimens vary, and have been refined to cause fewer side effects, be more cost-effective and to be more acceptable to staff and women. While it has been customary in this country for women to remain under supervision for 4–6 hours after prostaglandin administration, during which time the majority will have expelled the pregnancy (Table 10.2), more recently women have gone home after the misoprostol dose has been taken.

It must be noted that home self-administration of misoprostol has become the standard of care elsewhere in the world, such as the USA and increasingly in Sweden and France, for gestations up to 63 days. For supervised procedures the nursing staff confirm passage of the products. The amount of bleeding can be variable, but is often similar to a heavy period and increases with gestation. It is usual for women to have some lower abdominal cramp which will require administration of oral analgesia and a minority at later gestation might require opiate analgesia. The length of gestation influences the efficacy and complete abortion rate for the procedure, as well as complications, but this is more of an issue at 9–13 weeks' gestation. The risk of a continuing pregnancy, particularly in the 9–13 week gestation band, remains a problem, and those units undertaking medical abortions at these gestations are careful in counselling women regarding this. Where women pass only minimal or no products of conception, ultrasound should be carried out. An unrecognized ongoing pregnancy would be of particular concern because of the risk of fetal abnormality associated with misoprostol use. Surgical evacuation is required.

Table 10.2 Examples of medical regimens.

Up to 7 weeks (49 days) of gestation
*Mifepristone 200 mg orally followed 36–48 hours later by misoprostol 800 μg administered vaginally either by the woman or clinician (600 μg sublingually is a suitable alternative)

7–9 weeks (49–63 days) of gestation
If abortion has not occurred 4 hours after misoprostol administration, a second dose of 400 μg misoprostol may be administered vaginally or orally (depends on bleeding or preference). (This would be a 400-μg dose by sublingual administration where a sublingual regimen is being followed)

Other licensed regimen up to 9 weeks of gestation
Mifepristone 600 mg orally (200 mg also effective) followed 36–48 hours later by gemeprost 1 mg vaginally

9–13 weeks of gestation
*Mifepristone 200 mg orally followed 36–48 hours later by misoprostol 800 μg vaginally. A maximum of four further doses of misoprostol 400 μg may be administered at 3-hour intervals, vaginally or orally depending on amount of bleeding

Mid-trimester abortion (13–24 weeks of gestation)
*Mifepristone 200 mg orally followed 36–48 hours later by misoprostol 800 μg vaginally, then misoprostol 400 μg orally, at 3-hour intervals, to a maximum of four oral doses

Other licensed regimen
Mifepristone 600 mg orally (200 mg also effective) followed 36–48 hours later by gemeprost 1 mg vaginally every 3 hours, to a maximum of five pessaries (5 mg)

* These regimens are unlicensed.

Early medical abortion at gestations up to 9 weeks

Where mifepristone is available, single agents have been abandoned in favour of combined regimens of mifepristone plus prostaglandin. For many years a 600-mg dose of mifepristone was recommended for early medical abortion but lower-dose mifepristone (200 mg) is equally as effective and is also more economical. A Cochrane review concluded that the dose could be lowered to 200 mg without significantly decreasing efficacy and a multicentre trial conducted by the World Health Organization (WHO) further assessed the effect of reducing the dose of mifepristone [24,25]. In 2007 the 200-mg dose of mifepristone used in conjunction with a vaginal prostaglandin analogue was approved by the European Medicines Agency, applicable across the entire European Union. Although gemeprost is the conventional prostaglandin analogue used for abortion, it has the disadvantage of cost and is not stable at room temperature. The alternative prostaglandin analogue misoprostol is also effective and now the most frequently used in practice, having substituted gemeprost over the years. Misoprostol is more effective if administered vaginally rather than orally [26–28]. A large review of 2000 women undergoing medical abortion up to 63 days' gestation using mifepristone 200 mg followed by a single dose of misoprostol 800 μg given vaginally achieved a complete abortion rate of 97.5% [29]. It was noticed, however, that efficacy significantly decreased at gestations of 49 days or greater. A subsequent large case series has shown that mifepristone in combination with two doses, rather than a single dose of misoprostol abolishes this gestation effect [30]. There is current research interest in evaluating shorter time intervals between mifepristone and misoprostol.

Medical abortion in the late first trimester (9–13 weeks)

Data continue to accumulate for the high uptake, acceptability and efficacy of medical termination at 9–13 weeks and although still unlicensed at these gestations, it is likely to be offered as a choice for women undergoing abortion in many units. A randomized trial [31] comparing vacuum aspiration under general anaesthesia with medical abortion using a regimen of mifepristone 200 mg followed 36–48 hours later by up to five doses of misoprostol showed that complete abortion rates for women not requiring a second procedure were 94.6% in the medical group and 97.9% in the surgical group, which was not a statistically significant difference. The same group subsequently reported a consecutive series of 1076 women at 64–91 days of gestation managed using the same regimen. The complete abortion rate for the series was 95.8%, with an ongoing pregnancy rate of 1.5% and a clear gestation effect was apparent [32]. Other studies have been consistent with a 5–10% evacuation rate quoted. Local experience in Aberdeen would suggest that most patients abort after three doses of misoprostol but up to two further doses to a total of five doses will result in higher complete abortion rates and is worth trying while planning surgical evacuation later. In contrast to regimens up to 9 weeks, where home self-care is possible, women undergoing late first-trimester medical abortion have all been kept in a supervised and observed clinical environment for the procedure. In many ways late first-trimester abortions should be managed as second-trimester abortions.

Mid-trimester medical abortion

Mid-trimester medical abortion with mifepristone followed by prostaglandin has been shown to be safe and effective, with shorter induction to abortion intervals than previous methods with prostaglandin alone or supplemented by oxytocin infusion. Again randomized trial evidence supports use of a 200-mg mifepristone dose [33].

The induction abortion interval tends to be longer with increasing gestation [34] and reported cumulative experience suggests that 97% of women abort successfully on the day of treatment within five doses of misoprostol. A second or third day of treatment may be required to complete the termination medically and patients should be forewarned of this possibility. Surgical evacuation of the uterus is not required routinely following mid-trimester medical abortion and should only be undertaken where there is clinical evidence that the abortion is incomplete and this is likely to be required in less than 8% of cases [34]. Gentle suction evacuation of placental tissue is often possible without resort to general anaesthesia as the cervical os is wide open.

Analgesia requirements

Abdominal pain is a common accompaniment to medical abortion. Analgesia requirements have been reported to be higher for women of younger age, higher gestation and longer-induction abortion interval, while women with a previous live birth(s) are less likely to use analgesia [35]. In a series of over 4000 women undergoing medical abortion up to 22 weeks' gestation, 72% used analgesia, the majority (97%) using oral analgesia and only 2.3% requiring intramuscular opiate [35]. The role of pre-emptive analgesia use needs to be evaluated, although the RCOG Guideline Group took the view that requirements for analgesia vary and there was no benefit for routine administration of a prophylactic analgesic. However, it is important that a range of oral and parenteral analgesics are available to meet women's needs and many centres do use analgesia routinely.

Summary box 10.2

- Women value choice for the method of abortion.
- Medical abortion is a suitable alternative to surgical abortion, with high efficacy and patient acceptability.
- Mifepristone followed 36–48 hours later by a prostaglandin analogue, usually misoprostol, is highly effective for abortion.
- There is a clear gestation effect and after 49 days additional doses of prostaglandin are required.
- Misoprostol is more effective administered vaginally than orally, with sublingual and buccal administration being associated with more frequent side effects.

Surgical abortion

Surgical abortion is performed in either a hospital setting or dedicated facility in a designated clinic. General anaesthesia used to be standard practice in the UK, although use of local anaesthesia, paracervical block, with or without sedation, is increasingly being offered, the shorter recovery and observation period with local anaesthesia being a distinct advantage. Vacuum aspiration is the standard procedure, using a plastic cannula for aspiration with complete avoidance of sharp instruments within the uterus, thereby minimizing the risk of uterine damage. Suction termination may be safer under local anaesthesia, but studies comparing the safety of local and general anaesthesia have been observational or only partially randomized.

Many clinicians avoid surgical termination under 7 weeks' gestation because of the risk of failure to remove the pregnancy. However, with the increased sensitivity of pregnancy tests, many women now present at very early gestations, shortly after a first period has been missed. For these women, it is not acceptable to defer the abortion until a suitable gestation for surgery and their preference might not necessarily be for medical abortion; indeed, in certain circumstances, there could be contraindications to medical abortion. Suction abortions performed at less than 7 weeks' gestation are three times more likely to fail to remove the gestation sac than those performed between 7 and 12 weeks [23].

The 1990s saw renewed interested in MVA which had its origins in the 1960s in relation to the practice of 'menstrual extraction'. MVA can take longer than electronic vacuum procedures, especially as the gestation increases towards 9 weeks. For MVA, uterine evacuation is accomplished using a 4-, 5- or 6-mm flexible cannula attached to a 50-mL hand-held, manual vacuum syringe. It is less noisy than electronic aspiration, an advantage for awake patients. At early gestation, following cervical priming, it may be possible to directly pass the thin aspirating cannula without further dilatation, avoiding a cervical block. MVA had largely been abandoned after the legalization of abortion because of its failure rate, but modern protocols relying on high-resolution ultrasound before and after the procedure, careful immediate tissue inspection linked with hCG assay are effective. Although the technique is well established in the USA, there is renewed interested in introducing these early surgical abortion techniques in the UK, where they are ideally suited to early gestation and awake patients. Creinin and Edwards [36] report a continuing pregnancy rate of only 0.13%, but other series have reported 2.3% rates [37]; indeed, if conventional electronic suction abortion is the only method available within a service, the RCOG Guideline Group recommendation is to defer the procedure until the pregnancy has exceeded 7 weeks' gestation. It should be noted that there is no randomized trial evidence comparing MVA with medical termination at present.

Conventional suction abortion is appropriate at 7–15 weeks' gestation although, possibly reflecting the skill and experience of practitioners, many units adopt medical abortion at gestations above 12–13 weeks.

Cervical priming prior to surgical abortion reduces the complications of cervical injury, uterine perforation, haemorrhage and incomplete evacuation. Younger patient age is a risk factor for cervical damage, and increasing

Table 10.3 Cervical priming agents for surgical abortion

---

*Misoprostol 400 µg (two 200-µg tablets) administered vaginally or sublingually, either by the woman or clinician, 3 hours prior to surgery

Gemeprost 1 mg vaginally, 3 hours prior to surgery

Mifepristone 200 mg orally 36–48 hours prior to surgery

---

* This regimen is unlicensed.

gestation, particularly in multiparous women, is associated with uterine perforation. Mifepristone and the prostaglandin analogues gemeprost and misoprostol are effective cervical priming agents (Table 10.3). In the UK, gemeprost is the licensed preparation, although there is evidence that misoprostol is an effective lower-cost alternative and in practice is the most commonly used priming agent. The optimal time interval for misoprostol administration is at least 3 hours before surgery [38]. Mifepristone has also been shown to be an effective priming agent [39]. Mifepristone has higher efficacy than gemeprost and misoprostol when given 48 hours ahead of surgery, but mifepristone has the disadvantage of requiring administration 36–48 hours ahead of the abortion and there could be problems with preoperative bleeding. More recent work suggests that the sublingual route of administration of misoprostol is also effective for cervical priming, but is associated with an increased rate of gastrointestinal side effects, although it has the convenience of being able to be self-administered by the woman in advance of attending for the procedure, reducing time spent within the surgical facility [40].

Performing surgical abortion

Good technique is fundamental and aseptic technique should be observed, with careful and gentle instrumentation to avoid injury to cervix or uterus. The operation itself is straightforward with low complication rates but skill and experience are important so that serious complications are quickly recognized and remedied. Precise techniques vary among operators. After confirming the position, size and shape of the uterus by bimanual examination, it is usual to apply a vulsellum or tenaculum to the cervix and to dilate the cervix. The suction cannula should be positioned in the mid to upper fundus and when the operator is sure of correct placement, suction can be turned on. The cannula is gently rotated in a back and forth motion withdrawing only as far as the internal os until the flow of tissue and fluid has ceased and a gritty sensation is felt as the cannula moves against the wall of the contracted empty uterus.

Sometimes sponge or polyp forceps may be required to remove products from the cervical canal. Sharp curettage should be avoided. Because of low rates of haemorrhage, oxytocics are not routinely administered. The surgeon should ascertain that the major elements of the pregnancy are removed and are in keeping with the gestation of the pregnancy.

The risk of uterine perforation at the time of surgical abortion is of the order of 1–4 in 1000 from reports of large reviewed case series. The potential consequences resulting from visceral damage are so serious that if a perforation is suspected a laparoscopy should be undertaken as a minimum to confirm whether there is a perforation; certainly when there is any possibility or suspicion of bowel injury, formal surgical laparotomy should be undertaken. The advantages of cervical priming in reducing the risk of cervical injury have been outlined. Precise rates are difficult to state because of the varying definitions of cervical injury and variable data collection. Overall, the rate of cervical injury is not thought to be greater than 1% for first-trimester vacuum aspiration [11]. Cervical injury is more frequent and more serious with D+E in the second trimester. Failure to remove the pregnancy with ongoing pregnancy is a recognized association with surgical termination and the quoted failure rate is around 2.3 per 1000 surgical abortions [23]. The rate is increased for multiparous women, for abortions undertaken at less than 7 weeks' gestation, where small cannulas are used or in the presence of a uterine anomaly (usually unrecognized prior to abortion) or where the procedure is undertaken by an inexperienced clinician. Ultrasound is increasingly used in the operating room to confirm pregnancy evacuation and is useful when undertaking more challenging abortions to confirm safe access to the uterine cavity and guide the evacuation.

Surgical abortion after the first trimester

Late D+E is practised extensively in the USA and there are skilled practitioners in England, the Netherlands, France and parts of Australia. Otherwise, it is not widely performed and, for example, in Scotland mid-trimester terminations are almost exclusively undertaken using modern medical termination methods. D+E has not found favour among NHS gynaecologists in England, but is more widely used by the non-NHS providers. Conventional first-trimester surgical evacuation can be used up to 15 weeks' gestation, but thereafter specific techniques of cervical preparation and special instruments need to be used. More modern methods of aggressive cervical preparation, coupled with extensive clinical experience of the procedure, have improved safety. The use of real-time ultrasound scanning during the procedure can reduce the perforation rate. A retrospective cohort study compared complication rates of D+E and contemporary methods of medical abortion using misoprostol, but even excluding women in the medical group who had surgical evacuation of retained placental tissue, the complication rates were greater in the medical termination group compared with D+E (22% vs. 4%) [41]. Historically, it was felt that

D+E was a risk factor for subsequent adverse pregnancy outcome with pregnancy loss and preterm delivery. A recent retrospective case analysis suggests that this is not the case [42]. There has been no randomized controlled trial of late medical abortion and D+E and a pilot randomized controlled trial in the USA found that women declined randomization for the perceived advantages of D+E [43]. The procedure can really only be safely undertaken by gynaecologists who have been trained specifically in the technique and have an adequate clinical throughput to maintain their skills. The difficulty in comparing the two techniques is that medical abortion is associated with more minor complications but surgery can cause rare serious complications.

Summary box 10.3

- Cervical priming is important and optimally achieved with misoprostol 400 µg administered vaginally or sublingually 3 hours ahead of abortion.
- Aspiration abortion can be performed at very early gestation with meticulous tissue examination and appropriate follow-up arrangements to ensure complete evacuation of the pregnancy.
- Surgical skill and experience are important.
- Surgical abortion after 15 weeks requires additional specific training in the technique and sufficient caseload to maintain skills.

Future directions

Studies from the USA have reported high efficacy and acceptability of early medical abortion in home settings and home care is established in the USA. Evaluation in the context of a randomized trial has not occurred. A multicentre questionnaire survey, sponsored by the Family Planning Association, to assess women's views on the home administration of misoprostol for medical abortion indicated that there is acceptability and support for this approach [44]. Pilot work for home self-administration of misoprostol at early gestations up to 56 days has also confirmed feasibility and acceptability in a UK setting [45] and although further research is required, it is a development which could radically change the provision of abortion services and might have important cost implications and be relevant to shifting the balance of care away from hospital to community.

More recent research has focused on the time interval between mifepristone and misoprostol administration. Acceptability is higher for the shorter time intervals [46]. Only the non-oral routes have sufficient efficacy to be considered. Vaginal, sublingual and buccal routes have all been considered in different studies and investigations have examined various time intervals between administration of mifepristone and administration of misoprostol, i.e. within 15 min, after 6–8 hours and after 23–25 hours.

It is likely to be an area for further research and the acceptability of timing and dosing routes and dose frequency need to be examined in more depth against efficacy. What women feel are important factors will help refine medical options further to optimize individual care.

Complications and problems

Legal abortion in developed countries is extremely safe. Sadly, illegal unsafe abortion remains a major contributor to maternal mortality on a global basis. Complications do increase with older age, multiparity and increasing gestational age. Complications are usually categorized into those which occur immediately at the time of the procedure and those which arise subsequently. Most of the immediate complications have been discussed directly in relation to the medical and surgical procedures. The study of long-term complications is challenging and has been limited by data quality and the limitations of study design.

The most common complication to occur following termination is for the patient to present with problematic bleeding or pain and it is important for retained products and infection to be excluded. Ultrasound is extremely useful in helping to resolve the situation. Trials of prophylactic antibiotics for abortion do suggest a reduction in infective complications. Most infections tend to be polymicrobial and respond well to oral broad-spectrum antimicrobial therapy and aspiration of any confirmed retained products. However, clinicians should always be vigilant for rare infections associated with rapid multisystem deterioration as these serious infections are associated with cytotoxin release and can be rapidly fatal. The causitive organisms are certain strains of *Staphylococcus aureus*, group A *Streptococcus*, certain clostridial strains of *Clostridium perfringens* (formerly *welchii*) and *Clostridium sordellii*. The latter has been associated with a cluster of deaths in the USA but no European deaths have been reported and the precise aetiology remains under investigation.

Major reviews have been undertaken regarding subsequent risk for breast cancer after termination and the conclusion rebuts any causal relationship between induced abortion and subsequent increased risk for breast cancer [47,48]. Women often have concerns regarding their future reproductive health. Evidence continues to confirm that there is no proven association with subsequent ectopic pregnancy, placenta praevia or secondary infertility. Published literature regarding an association with preterm birth has been conflicting, with the earlier

studies suggesting no effect but more recent studies showing a positive link [49–51]. Studies are influenced by competing and confounding risks and, when retrospective, by selective recall on the part of the woman. Many women report a sense of relief following abortion while others report complex emotional feelings in the 2–3 weeks immediately afterwards, although these subsequently settle. Sadness is common and should be acknowledged as part of a normal response. Most services offer follow-up support counselling as required. Some studies suggest higher rates of psychiatric illness or self-harm among women who have previously had an abortion, but interpretation needs to be careful, as the situation may reflect a continuation of pre-existing conditions.

There is no convincing evidence that abortion is associated with major negative psychiatric sequelae [52] and psychological problems should always be viewed in the context of alternative outcomes for the pregnancy such as birth and child-rearing or adoption, which may have carried greater emotional risk.

Summary box 10.4

- Abortion is one of the safest clinical intervention procedures in medical practice.
- Complication rates increase with increasing gestation.
- Prophylactic antibiotics reduce post-abortion infection but the optimum regimen and timing remains unclear.
- Major haemorrhage is infrequent but requirement for transfusion, although infrequent, is more likely after medical abortion.
- Ultrasound has an important role in recognizing failed abortion and retained products for further management.
- Evaluating possible adverse long-term outcomes is difficult but, with the possible exception of a slightly increased risk of preterm labour in a subsequent pregnancy, there is no evidence to suggest significant adverse health outcomes.

Post-abortion follow-up

First and foremost it is important to offer contraceptive advice prior to discharge and to provide starter supplies or initiate the method immediately following termination. Women should also be given a written account of the symptoms that they could experience following abortion and which would require urgent medical consultation. A 24-hour telephone helpline number should be available if women have concerns about pain, bleeding or high temperatures. Urgent emergency gynaecology assessment and admission needs to be available to back up abortion services. It is usual practice to offer a 2-week follow-up appointment with either the abortion service or the referring clinician, but there is no proven benefit to follow-up [53]. In practice many women seem to default on this appointment.

The discharge letter on the day of termination should contain sufficient information about the procedure to allow another practitioner to deal with any complications. Counselling support should be available for any woman or partner who wishes this following termination and proactive support given for women who have a previous history of mental health problems. Women who experience particular difficulty after termination are often those who have been ambivalent prior to the procedure, who lack a supportive partner, who have a previous mental health problem or who have held strong opinions and considered abortion to be wrong.

Summary

Abortion is one of the most frequent but safest procedures in modern medicine. Complications and failure are not completely avoidable, but can be minimized by careful attention to detail at the pre-screening visit and with careful medical and surgical practice, based on the available published evidence and guidelines. It is important that the gestation is accurately assessed. If prophylactic antibiotics are not used, infection screening including for STIs should be undertaken. For surgical procedures, sound aseptic techniques should be employed. The clinicians involved should be experienced and comfortable with the procedures which they perform. There should be a high index of suspicion for possible complications and the patient must have good and easy access to clinical services for post-abortion advice and management of complications. Abortion is a necessary part of fertility control, but efforts aimed at improving utilization, accessibility and availability of emergency contraception and regular contraception should remain a sexual health priority.

References

1 Department of Health. Abortion Statistics, England and Wales: 2009. Available at: www.dh.gov.uk/en/Publicationsand statistics/Publications/PublicationsStatistics/DH_116039

2 Scottish Health Statistics Abortions 2010. ISD Scotland, Sexual Health, Abortions. Avalable at: www.isdscotland. org/isd/1918.html

3 Birth Control Trust. *Abortion Provision in Britain: How Services are Provided and How They Could Be Improved.* London: Birth Control Trust, 1997.

4 Abortion Act 1967. London: HMSO.

5 Human Fertilisation and Embryology Act 1990. London: HMSO.

6 House of Commons Science and Technology Committee (2007). *Scientific Developments Relating to the Abortion Act 1967.* Twelfth report of Session 2006–2007, Vol. 1. HC 1045-1. Available at: www.publications.parliament.uk/pa/cm200607/cmselect/cmsctech/1045/1045i.pdf

7 Department of Health. (2007) *Government Response to the Report from the House of Commons Science and Technology Committee on the Scientific Developments Relating to the Abortion Act 1967.* Available at: www.dh.gov.uk/en/Publicationsandstatistics/Publications/PublicationsPolicyAndGuidance/DH_080925

8 Department of Health, Social Services and Public Safety, Northern Ireland. *Guidance on the termination of pregnancy: the law and clinical practice in Northern Ireland.* March 2009. Available at: www.dhsspsni.gov.uk/hss-md-9-2009.pdf

9 General Medical Council. *Maintaining Good Medical Practice.* London: GMC, 1998.

10 British Medical Association. *The Law and Ethics of Abortion: BMA Views.* London: BMA, 1997 (revised 1999).

11 Royal College of Obstetricians and Gynaecologists. *The Care of Women Requesting Induced Abortion 2000, revised 2004.* Evidence-based Guideline No. 7. London: RCOG Press, 2004.

12 Aston G, Bewley S. Abortion and domestic violence. *Obstet Gynaecol* 2009;11:163–168.

13 Sawaya GF, Grady D, Kerlikowske K, Grimes DA. Antibiotics at the time of induced abortion: the case for universal prophylaxis on a meta-analysis. *Obstet Gynecol* 1996;87:884–890.

14 Blackwell AL, Thomas PD, Wereham K, Emery SJ. Health gains from screening for infection of the lower genital tract in women attending for termination of pregnancy. *Lancet* 1993;342:206–210.

15 Penney GC, Thomson M, Norman J *et al.* A randomised comparison of strategies for reducing infective complications of induced abortion. *Br J Obstet Gynaecol* 1998;105:599–604.

16 Spitz IM, Barden CW, Benton L, Robins A. Early pregnancy termination with mifepristone and misoprostol in the United States. *N Engl J Med* 1998;338:1241–1247.

17 Bartley J, Tong S, Everington D, Baird DT. Parity is major determinant of success rate in medical abortion: a retrospective analysis of 3161 consecutive cases of early medical abortion treated with reduced doses of mifepristone and vaginal gemeprost. *Contraception* 2000;62:297–303.

18 Ashok PW, Templeton A, Wagaarachchi PT, Flett GM. Factors affecting the outcome of early medical abortion: a review of 4132 consecutive cases. *BJOG* 2002;109:1281–1289.

19 Slade P, Heke S, Fletcher J, Stewart P. A comparison of medical and surgical termination of pregnancy: choice, emotional impact and satisfaction with care. *Br J Obstet Gynaecol* 1998;105:1288–1295.

20 Ashok PW, Kidd A, Flett GM, Fitzmaurice A, Graham W, Templeton A. A randomised comparison of medical abortion and surgical vacuum aspiration at 10–13 weeks gestation. *Hum Reprod* 2002;17:92–98.

21 Howie FL, Henshaw RC, Naagi SA *et al.* Medical abortion or vacuum aspiration? Two year follow up of a patient preference trial. *Br J Obstet Gynaecol* 1997;104:829–833.

22 Penney GC, Templeton A, Glazier A. Patients' views on abortion care in Scottish Hospitals. *Health Bull* 1994;52:431–438.

23 Kaunitz AM, Rovira EZ, Grimes DA, Schuz KF. Abortions that fail. *Obstet Gynecol* 1985;66:533–537.

24 Kulier R, Gulmezoglua AM, Hofmeyr GJ, Cheng LN, Campana A. Medical methods for first trimester abortion. *Cochrane Database Syst Rev* 2004;(2):CD002855.

25 World Health Organization Task Force on Post-Ovulatory Methods for Fertility Regulation. Lowering the doses of mifepristone and gemeprost for early abortion: a randomised controlled trial. *BJOG* 2001;108:738–742.

26 Grimes DA. Medical abortion in early pregnancy: a review of the evidence. *Obstet Gynecol* 1997;89:790–796.

27 el-Refaey H, Rajasekar D, Abdulla M, Calder L, Templeton A. Induction of abortion with mifepristone (RU486) and oral or vaginal misoprostol. *N Engl J Med* 1995;332:983–987.

28 el-Refaey H, Templeton A. Induction of abortion in the second trimester by a combination of misoprostol and mifepristone: a randomised comparison between two misoprostol regimes. *Hum Reprod* 1995;10:475–478.

29 Ashok PW, Penney GC, Flett GM, Templeton A. An effective regimen for early medical abortion: a report of 2000 consecutive cases. *Hum Reprod* 1998;13:2962–2965.

30 Ashok PW, Templeton A, Wagaarachchi PT, Flett GMM. Factors affecting the outcome of early medical abortion: a review of 4132 consecutive cases. *BJOG* 2002;109:1281–1289.

31 Ashok PW, Kidd A, Flett GMM, Fitzmaurice A, Graham W, Templeton A. A randomised comparison of medical abortion and surgical vacuum aspiration at 10–13 weeks of gestation. *Hum Reprod* 2002;17:92–98.

32 Hamoda H, Ashok PW, Flett GM, Templeton A. Uptake and efficacy of medical abortion over 9 and up to 13 weeks gestation: a review of 1076 consecutive cases. *Contraception* 2005;71:327–332.

33 Webster D, Penney GC, Templeton A. A comparison of 600 and 200 mg mifepristone prior to second trimester abortion with the prostaglandin misoprostol. *Br J Obstet Gynaecol* 1996;103:706–709.

34 Ashok PW, Templeton A, Wagaarachchi PT, Flett GM. Mid trimester medical termination of pregnancy: a review of 1002 consecutive cases. *Contraception* 2004;69:51–58.

35 Hamoda H, Ashok PW, Flett GM, Templeton A. Analgesia requirements and predictors of analgesia use for women undergoing medical abortion up to 22 weeks of gestation. *BJOG* 2004;111:996–1000.

36 Creinin MD, Edwards J. Early abortion: surgical and medical options. *Curr Probl Obstet Gynecol Fertil* 1997;20:6–32.

37 Paul ME, Mitchell CM, Rogers AJ, Fox MC, Lackie EG. Early surgical abortion; efficacy and safety. *Am J Obstet Gynecol* 2002;187:407–411.

38 Fong YF, Singh Kuldip, Prasad RNV. A comparative study using two dose regimens (200 µg and 400 µg) of vaginal misoprostol for preoperative cervical dilatation in first trimester nulliparae. *Br J Obstet Gynaecol* 1998;105:413–417.

39 Henshaw RC, Templeton AA. Pre-operative cervical preparation before 1st trimester vacuum aspiration; a randomised controlled comparison between gemeprost and mifepristone (RU486). *Br J Obstet Gynaecol* 1991;98:1025–1030.

40 Carbonell Esteve JL, Mari JM, Valero F *et al.* Sublingual versus vaginal misoprostol (400 µg) for cervical priming in first trimester abortion: a randomised trial. *Contraception* 2006;74:328–333.

41 Autry AM, Hayes EC, Jacobson GF, Kirby RS. A comparison of medical induction and dilatation in evacuation for second-trimester abortion. *Am J Obstet Gynecol* 2002;187:393–397.

42 Kalish RB, Chasen ST, Rosenzweig LB, Rashbaum WK, Chervenak FA. Impact of mid-trimester dilatation and evacuation on subsequent pregnancy outcome. *Am J Obstet Gynecol* 2002;187:882–885.

43 Grimes DA, Smith MS, Witham AD. Mifepristone and misoprostol versus dilatation and evacuation for midtrimester abortion: a pilot randomised controlled trial. *BJOG* 2004;111:148–153.

44 Hamoda H, Critchley HOD, Paterson K, Guthrie K, Rodger M, Penney GC. The acceptability of home medical abortion to women in UK settings. *BJOG* 2005;112:781–785.

45 Hamoda H, Ashok PW, Flett GMM, Templeton A. Home self-administration of misoprostol for medical abortion up to 56 days gestation. *J Fam Plann Reprod Health Care* 2005;31:189–192.

46 Schaff EA, Fielding SL, Westhoff C *et al.* Vaginal misoprostol administered 1, 2 or 3 days after mifepristone for early medical abortion: a randomised trial. *JAMA* 2000;284:1948–1953.

47 American College of Obstetrics and Gynecology Committee on Gynecology Practice. ACOG Committee Opinion. Induced abortion and breast cancer risk. *Int J Gynaecol Obstet* 2003;83:233–235.

48 Beral V, Bull D, Doll R, Peto R, Reeves G and Collaborative Group on Hormonal Factors in Breast Cancer. Breast cancer and abortion: collaborative reanalysis of data from 53 epidemiological studies, including 83 000 women with breast cancer from 16 countries. *Lancet* 2004;363:1007–1016.

49 Thorpe GM Jr, Hartmann KE, Shadigan E. Long-term physical and psychological health consequences of induced abortion: review of the evidence. *Obstet Gynecol Surv* 2002;58:67–79.

50 Henriet L, Kaminski M. Impact of induced abortions on subsequent pregnancy outcome: the 1995 French national perinatal survey. *BJOG* 2001;108:1036–1042.

51 Ancel PY, Lelong N, Papiernik E, Saurel-Cubizolles MJ, Kaminski M. History of induced abortion as a risk factor for preterm birth in European countries: results of the EUROPOP survey. *Human Reprod* 2004;19:734–740.

52 Charles VE, Polis CB, Sridhara SK, Blum RW. Abortion and long-term mental health outcomes: a systematic review of the evidence. *Contraception* 2008;78:436–450.

53 Grossman D, Ellertson C, Grimes DA, Walker D. Routine follow-visits after first-trimester induced abortion. *Obstet Gynecol* 2004;103:738–745.

Part 4
Maternal Medicine

Chapter 11
Hypertensive Disorders

Jason J.S. Waugh[1] and Maria C. Smith[2]
[1] Royal Victoria Infirmary, Newcastle upon Tyne, UK
[2] Reproductive and Vascular Biology Group, Institute of Cellular Medicine, Newcastle University, Newcastle upon Tyne, UK

Pre-eclampsia is an idiopathic disorder of pregnancy characterized by proteinuric hypertension. Recent estimates indicate that over 63000 women die worldwide each year because of pre-eclampsia and its complications, with 98% of these occurring in developing countries [1]. In the UK, pre-eclampsia is the second largest cause of both direct maternal death and perinatal loss, responsible for the death of six to nine women annually [2] and over 175 babies [3]. More than 10% of women will develop pre-eclampsia in their first pregnancy and although the overwhelming majority of these will have successful pregnancy outcomes, the condition can give rise to severe multisystem complications including cerebral haemorrhage, hepatic and renal dysfunction and respiratory compromise. The development of strategies to prevent and treat the disorder has been challenging due to an incomplete understanding of the underlying pathogenesis.

Pathophysiology

The pathogenesis of pre-eclampsia originates in the placenta. The disease can occur in the absence of fetal tissue (molar pregnancy) and manifestations of the disease will only resolve following delivery of the placenta. The blueprint for establishing pre-eclampsia is determined at the outset of pregnancy when placental trophoblast invades the maternal uterine spiral arteries at the time of implantation. In pregnancies destined to be complicated by pre-eclampsia, transformation of the spiral arteries is impaired, with suboptimal remodelling of small-capacitance constricted vessels into dilated large-capacitance conduits. The prevailing theory has been that the subsequent relative placental ischaemia causes release of vasoactive factors into the circulation which then give rise to endothelial-mediated end-organ damage and clinical manifestations of the disease. Scientific endeavours to determine these elusive vasoactive factors have largely been responsible for pre-eclampsia being known as the 'disease of theories'.

Several candidates have been considered in the role of a key circulating vasoactive factor, including interleukins, tumour necrosis factor (TNF)-α and components of the angiotensin pathway. Whilst all these elements are subject to modification in pre-eclamptic pregnancies, it has not been possible to demonstrate that any have an initiating role in the disease process. Pre-eclampsia is a disease of higher primates only and the lack of a clinically relevant animal model has been a significant research obstacle. The discovery of soluble fms-like tyrosine kinase (sFlt)-1 has been particularly exciting because it is the first candidate that has been demonstrated to cause a pre-eclampsia phenotype in an animal model [4].

sFlt-1 is variant of vascular endothelial growth factor receptor (VEGFR)-1, which has an extracellular ligand-binding domain but lacks the transmembrane and cytoplasmic domains. Circulating sFlt-1 is therefore able to competitively bind to VEGF and placental growth factor (PGF) and therefore reduce biologically active binding of these factors that usually promote angiogenesis and placentation. Women with pre-eclampsia have increased circulating levels of sFLT-1 and reduced circulating free VEGF and PGF. VEGF is important in maintaining normal fenestration of the glomerular endothelium [5,6] and it has been suggested that the early renal manifestations of pre-eclampsia may be a consequence of the particular sensitivity of the kidney to reduced levels of VEGF. In animals it has been shown that both VEGF and PGF must be reduced to cause a pre-eclampsia phenotype [4]. *In vitro* and *in vivo* studies [7] have shown that the hypoxic placenta produces increased levels of sFLt-1 and primate studies [8] indicate that this may be sufficient to produce a pre-eclampsia phenotype. Another factor in this story is endoglin (sEng), a modified form of the transforming growth factor (TGF)-β coreceptor. sEng is also increased in pre-eclampsia and has been shown to augment the effect of sFlt-1 and is particularly associated with hepatic endothelial damage [9]. Importantly, sFlt-1, PGF and sEng have been shown to be elevated in the serum of women destined to suffer pre-eclampsia several weeks in advance of clinically evident disease [10].

Summary box 11.1

- The pathogenesis of pre-eclampsia remains elusive but a greater scientific knowledge of the condition is emerging.
- Pre-eclampsia accounts for approximately 25% of all very low birthweight infants, a significant number of preterm births and has a high perinatal mortality.
- Pre-eclampsia is the second most frequent cause of direct maternal death.
- These deaths are avoidable as substandard care complicates 90% of these deaths.

An intriguing aspect of this hypothesis is its link to a potential explanation as to why smokers have a reduced incidence of pre-eclampsia. The combustible component of cigarette smoke induces haemoxidase (HO)-1. This is a stress response gene that has a cellular protective role, particularly against hypoxic injury. HO-1 degrades haem into biliverdin, carbon monoxide (CO) and free iron. Both biliverdin and CO have been demonstrated to reduce endothelial expression of sFlt-1 and sEng [11]. Appreciation of the potential role of the HO-1 pathway has led to the suggestion that pharmacological agents known to have HO-1 activity might be useful in ameliorating pre-eclampsia. Statins are widely used outside obstetrics to reduce serum lipids and forthcoming studies will evaluate whether their theoretical potential can be translated safely and usefully into pregnancy.

Defining hypertensive disease in pregnancy

There has always been considerable debate over the most appropriate definition of the hypertensive disorders in pregnancy. It has been recognized that there are benefits in having a broader clinical definition whilst retaining a very tight phenotypic research definition. Hypertension complicates 6–12% of all pregnancies [12], and includes two relatively benign conditions (chronic and gestational hypertension) and the more severe conditions of pre-eclampsia or eclampsia. Pre-eclampsia complicates 3–5% of all pregnancies, and is characterized by placental and maternal vascular dysfunction that may lead to adverse outcomes such as severe hypertension, stroke, seizure (eclampsia), renal and hepatic injury, haemorrhage, fetal growth restriction, or even death [13].

The diagnosis of pre-eclampsia, and hence the prediction of adverse events, is based on traditional but somewhat unreliable and non-specific clinical markers such as blood pressure, urine protein excretion, and symptoms. For example, more than 20% of women who have eclampsia will fail to meet the common diagnostic criteria of pre-eclampsia prior to their event, making the prediction of this adverse outcome extremely difficult [14].

Conversely, only 0.7–5.0% of women with classically defined pre-eclampsia will experience any composite adverse outcomes [15].

For this reason consistency is required both for clinical management and to allow the comparison of outcomes from clinical units/regions. The recently published NICE Clinical Guideline 107 [16] has defined management pathways for hypertension in pregnancy in the UK. The list below outlines the NICE definitions associated with hypertension in pregnancy used in this chapter.

- *Gestational hypertension*: new hypertension presenting after 20 weeks without significant proteinuria.
- *Pre-eclampsia*: new hypertension presenting after 20 weeks with significant proteinuria.
- *Chronic hypertension*: hypertension that is present at the booking visit or before 20 weeks or if the woman is already taking antihypertensive medication when referred to maternity services. It can be primary or secondary in aetiology.
- *Eclampsia*: a convulsive condition associated with pre-eclampsia.
- *HELLP syndrome*: haemolysis, elevated liver enzymes and low platelet count.
- *Severe pre-eclampsia*: pre-eclampsia with severe hypertension and/or with symptoms, and/or biochemical and/or haematological impairment.
- *Significant proteinuria*: defined as a urinary protein/creatinine ratio of greater than 30 mg/mmol or a validated 24-hour urine collection result showing greater than 300 mg protein.
- *Mild hypertension*: diastolic blood pressure 90–99 mmHg, systolic blood pressure 140–149 mmHg.
- *Moderate hypertension*: diastolic blood pressure 100–109 mmHg, systolic blood pressure 150–159 mmHg.
- *Severe hypertension*: diastolic blood pressure 110 mmHg or greater, systolic blood pressure 160 mmHg or greater.

Summary box 11.2

- Pre-eclampsia is a multisystem disease diagnosed by the characteristic appearance of gestational hypertension and gestational proteinuria.
- Gestational hypertension is a persistent *de novo* blood pressure >140/90 mmHg occurring after 20/40 gestation in pregnancy. On its own it carries little additional morbidity.
- Gestational proteinuria is a protein excretion above 300 mg per 24 hours (equivalent to a protein/creatinine ratio of 30 mg/mmol).
- There are errors associated with the measurement of both blood pressure and proteinuria in pregnancy which can be minimized by a combination of good technique and automated devices.
- All the above conditions can occur superimposed on chronic hypertension, making diagnosis difficult.
- Postnatal follow-up is essential to confirm the 'pregnancy diagnosis' and to advise about long-term risk.

Measuring blood pressure and proteinuria in pregnancy and pre-eclampsia

The errors associated with blood pressure measurement have been well described in both non-pregnant and pregnant populations. Care in taking these measurements will reduce false-positive and false-negative results and improve clinical care. Machine/device errors have led to strict validation protocols for automated blood pressure devices in specific populations and clinical settings [17] and the human errors inherent in manual readings have led to guidelines on the measurement of blood pressure with both manual and automated devices in clinical practice [18]. Digit preference (the practice of rounding the final digit of blood pressure to zero) occurs in the vast majority of antenatal measurements and simply taking care to avoid this will limit inaccurate diagnoses. Using a standard bladder in a sphygmomanometer cuff will systematically undercuff 25% of an average antenatal population. Having large cuffs available and using them will prevent the over-diagnosis of hypertension [19]. Keeping the rate of deflation to 2–3 mmHg/s will prevent over-diagnosis of diastolic hypertension, as will using Korotkoff 5, which is now universally recommended for diagnosing diastolic hypertension. Korotkoff 4 (the muffling of the sound) is less reproducible, and randomized controlled trials confirmed that it is safe to abandon it, except in those rare situations when the blood pressure approaches zero [20,21].

The reliable detection of proteinuria is essential in differentiating those pregnancies with pre-eclampsia from those with gestational or chronic hypertension and, in the process, identifying those pregnancies most prone to adverse outcome. The measurement of significant proteinuria, traditionally 300 mg excretion in a 24-hour period, is also prone to collection and measurement error. The collection of 24-hour urine samples is not practical as a routine test and so urine dipstick screening is employed as a first-line screening test with secondary tests employed to confirm positive dipstick diagnoses. Visual dipstick reading is unreliable [22] but the use of automated dipstick readers significantly improves the accuracy of dipstick testing and as such is recommended by NICE for use in pregnancy [23]. NICE also recommends that quantification of proteinuria should follow diagnosis. There are two methods that NICE supports. The first is the 24-hour urine protein estimation and this requires that an assessment of sample completeness is undertaken, with measurement of creatinine excretion being the most common. NICE also supports the use of the protein/creatinine ratio test. This test is done on a 'spot' urine sample and is therefore much quicker. This test has been shown in numerous studies to be comparable to the 24-hour urine protein estimation [24]. The threshold for defining

Table 11.1 Risk factors to identify women at increased risk of pre-eclampsia.

Any single high-risk factor
Hypertensive disease during a previous pregnancy
Chronic kidney disease
Autoimmune disease such as systemic lupus erythematosus or antiphospholipid syndrome
Type 1 or type 2 diabetes
Chronic hypertension

Or two or more moderate risk factors
First pregnancy
Age 40 years or older
Pregnancy interval of more than 10 years
Body mass index of 35 kg/m^2 or more at first visit
Family history of pre-eclampsia
Multiple pregnancy

significant proteinuria by this test is 30 mg protein/mmol creatinine.

Risk assessment and risk reduction

There have been attempts to screen the antenatal population for pre-eclampsia over the past 60 years, with over 100 potential biochemical, biophysical or epidemiological candidate tests. Despite not yet having a single universal test to apply, it is still possible to advise women regarding their risk of pre-eclampsia from their clinical history and some investigations.

NICE guidelines for routine antenatal care [25] emphasize that a woman's risk of pre-eclampsia should be evaluated. Several risk factors for pre-eclampsia are known and these have been incorporated into the NICE recommendations [26,27]. Table 11.1 outlines risk factors that should be identified at booking to identify women at risk of pre-eclampsia. Many of the risk factors listed in this table are modifiable and may lead to a reduction in risk either prior to or between pregnancies.

Individual risk is not a simple numerical addition. A family history of pre-eclampsia in a first-degree relative is significant and two relatives even more so, whilst exposure over time to paternal antigen through increased periods of cohabitation and non-barrier contraception can reduce risk as can prior miscarriage or termination of pregnancy. Pre-eclampsia is more common at the extremes of reproductive age and is increased further following IVF treatment, particularly with donor sperm. Other factors often associated with increasing age, such as obesity, gestational and pre-gestational diabetes, and any disease affecting the cardiovascular system are potent risk factors for pre-eclampsia. The relative risk for

Table 11.2 Relative risks of developing pre-eclampsia.

	Relative risk	Confidence intervals
Antiphospholipid syndrome	9.72	4.34–21.75
Previous history of pre-eclampsia	7.19	5.83–8.83
Pre-existing diabetes	3.56	2.54–4.99
Multiple pregnancy	2.93	2.04–4.21
Nulliparity	2.91	1.28–6.61
Family history	2.90	1.70–4.93
Raised BMI		
Before pregnancy	2.47	1.66–3.67
At booking	1.55	1.28–1.88
Age over 40	1.96	1.34–2.87
Raised diastolic blood pressure (>80 mmHg)	1.38	1.01–1.87

pre-eclampsia for some of these risk factors is shown in Table 11.2 [27].

Clearly, from the relative risks quoted, the majority of women who are high risk will still not develop pre-eclampsia whilst a considerable number of cases will arise *de novo* in the 'low-risk' population. Identifying women at risk will allow increase in surveillance and use of prophylactic therapies can be considered. If adequate preventive measures become available, then these screening test will become increasingly important. Tests that might be employed to screen the population (high or low risk) for pre-eclampsia centre on the identification of poor placental function, which is an almost universal prerequisite for the clinical condition. Doppler assessment of the maternal uterine circulation is considered to be a promising test. This test when 'positive' demonstrates the high resistance in the uterine arteries as well as a 'notch' apparent within the Doppler waveform. These two features have been used in isolation and combination to screen low- and high-risk populations. Early studies suggested that approximately one in five women who have an abnormal Doppler at 20 weeks' gestation will develop pre-eclampsia [28], and at 24 weeks' gestation the prediction value is greater. In 2008, NICE recommended that uterine artery Doppler screening should not be employed universally for low-risk women [25]. More recently NICE Clinical Guideline 107 recommended that this test should not be universally employed in high-risk women based on the relatively poor quality of the studies performed to date. However, it did recognize its potential and made a research recommendation regarding its use in the management of high-risk women.

No other biophysical test other than accurate measurement of blood pressure in the first trimester has either any clinical application or is practical enough to employ in clinical practice. Numerous haematological and biochemical markers have been used to both predict and evaluate pre-eclampsia. For example, in women who have chronic hypertension the measurement of uric acid and platelets can help in determining those who suffer superimposed pre-eclampsia; again the tests lack sensitivity and specificity [29]. Furthermore, very few of these markers have been independently evaluated for their ability to separately predict the timing or severity of specific adverse outcomes such as placental abruption, severe hypertension, neurological injury and fetal growth restriction. The reason for this is that the biomarkers previously studied were mostly generic indicators of vascular activation and dysfunction, which arise late in the pre-eclamptic disease process and which are not specific to pre-eclampsia or even to pregnancy.

As outlined previously, recent advances have identified a class of pregnancy-specific angiogenic and anti-angiogenic factors (e.g. PGF, VEGF) that are produced by the placenta and which closely correlate with the preclinical and clinical stages of pre-eclampsia [10,30–33]. Assays of these markers are currently under assessment as tools to predict and/or diagnose pre-eclampsia prior to the onset of clinical disease and significant morbidity. The FASTER trial of 2003 demonstrated that, when measured as part of the quadruple aneuploidy screen at 15–18 weeks' gestation, the odds ratios for the development of pre-eclampsia when inhibin-A and β human chorionic gonadotrophin (hCG) levels are above the 95th centile were 3.42 (95% CI 2.7 and 4.3) and 2.20 (95% CI 1.7 and 2.9), respectively [34].

In 2008, the Society of Obstetricians and Gynaecologists of Canada Genetics Committee, following systematic review, suggested that abnormal uterine artery Doppler in combination with an elevated α-fetoprotein (AFP), hCG and inhibin-A, or decreased pregnancy-associated plasma protein A (PAPP-A), identifies a group of women at increased risk of intrauterine growth restriction and pre-eclampsia. They also stated that multiple maternal serum screening markers at present should not be used for population-based screening as false-positive rates are high, sensitivities are low and no protocols have shown improved outcome [35].

Screening is important to focus resources on high-risk women as well as to identify those in whom prophylactic therapies might have some benefit. Aspirin and calcium have been found to have a beneficial effect whilst other agents, most recently antioxidants, have not proven useful. NICE Clinical Guideline 107 recommends low-dose aspirin therapy (75 mg/day) for all high-risk women from 12 weeks' gestation. Antiplatelet agents were associated with statistically significant reductions in the risk of pre-eclampsia in moderate-risk women and in high-risk women (moderate-risk women: 25 studies, $N = 28\,469$, RR 0.86, 95% CI 0.79–0.95; high-risk women: 18 studies, $N = 4121$, RR 0.75, 95% CI 0.66–0.85).

A meta-analysis using individual-patient data from 32 217 women and their 32 819 babies found a statistically significant reduction in risk of developing pre-eclampsia (RR 0.90, 95% CI 0.84–0.97). The data from this study suggest that one case of pre-eclampsia would be prevented for every 114 women treated with antiplatelet agents. In addition to the 10% reduction in pre-eclampsia in high-risk women receiving antiplatelet agents, there was a 10% reduction in preterm birth. No particular subgroup of women in the high-risk group was substantially more or less likely to benefit from antiplatelet agents. There was no statistically significant difference between women who started treatment before 20 weeks (RR 0.87, 95% CI 0.79–0.96) and those who started treatment after 20 weeks (RR 0.95, 95% CI 0.85–1.06; $P = 0.24$). Of importance there were no statistically significant differences between women receiving antiplatelet agents and those receiving placebo in the incidence of potential adverse effects such as antepartum haemorrhage, placental abruption or postpartum haemorrhage, but there was a reduction in the risk of preterm birth before 37 weeks (RR 0.93, 95% CI 0.89–0.98) [36].

Trials of calcium to prevent pre-eclampsia are more controversial. There is good evidence that in areas where the dietary intake of calcium is low, calcium supplementation reduces the risk of pre-eclampsia but this is also influenced by prior risk status. In studies conducted where dietary calcium intake is normal, supplementation was not found to be of benefit. No other intervention can be recommended, including magnesium, folic acid, antioxidants (vitamins C and E), fish oils or bed rest. Diet or lifestyle changes may be beneficial for general health and weight loss may reduce the prior risk of hypertensive disease but modifications such as a low-salt diet have no proven benefit.

Chronic hypertension

Women with chronic hypertension should receive prepregnancy care. This should aim to determine the severity and cause of the hypertension; review potentially teratogenic medications such as angiotensin-converting enzyme (ACE) inhibitors, angiotensin receptor blockers (three times the risk of congenital abnormality) and diuretics; inform women of the risk associated with pregnancy and of prophylactic strategies (all should receive low-dose aspirin in pregnancy); and to assess comorbidities such as renal impairment, obesity or coexistent diabetes.

The main risk is of superimposed pre-eclampsia, but even in its absence the perinatal mortality is increased. Drugs appropriate for treating hypertension in pregnancy include methyldopa, labetalol, nifedipine and hydralazine. Safety data on other antihypertensives are lacking but there are several where no association with congenital abnormality has been established and so they can be used when clinically indicated.

Blood pressure control should be tailored to the individual. Where the chronic hypertension is secondary to other disease then the care should be multidisciplinary with the appropriate physician aiming to keep blood pressure below 140/90 mmHg and often at lower limits. When the chronic hypertension is uncomplicated (usually essential) the target should be 150–155/80–100 mmHg [16].

There is a recognized risk of fetal growth restriction (FGR) in this group and so serial fetal biometry is recommended and women should be seen with increased frequency to maintain blood pressure control and to screen for pre-eclampsia. Delivery should be for either fetal indications or for poor hypertension control once corticosteroids for fetal lung maturity have been given if less than 34 weeks' gestation.

At term, NICE recommends delivery after 37 weeks when agreed with the individual, so long as blood pressure control is maintained. Following delivery blood pressure should be maintained below 140/90 mmHg and medication should be reviewed and optimized for both blood pressure control and breast-feeding.

Gestational hypertension

Gestational hypertension is relatively common and as such most units will assess women identified in the community in their day unit. Here, the first assessment is of proteinuria to identify those with pre-eclampsia. In the absence of proteinuria NICE Clinical Guideline 107 recommends an integrated package of care dependent on blood pressure.
- If blood pressure 140–149/90–99 mmHg, then review weekly and test for proteinuria only (as described above).
- If blood pressure 150–159/100–109 mmHg, then treat with labetalol as first line and target blood pressure is 140–150/80–100 mmHg. Check urea and electrolytes, liver function tests and full blood count once, then review twice weekly testing for proteinuria only.
- If blood pressure >160/>110 mmHg, then admit until below 159/109 mmHg and treat as above. When controlled review twice weekly as above. Test for proteinuria each visit and also retest bloods weekly.

The guideline also recognizes that the earlier the presentation, the greater the likelihood of progression to pre-eclampsia and the frequency of visits should be adjusted accordingly. Gestational hypertension does not require aspirin prophylaxis and patients do not require routine hospital admission if blood pressure is controlled.

Fetal monitoring is also controversial. The suspected small baby (from customized symphysis–fundal height measurment) should be investigated with fetal biometry. No benefit (reduction in perinatal mortality) has been shown in trials where additional monitoring is offered to women with gestational hypertension where FGR was absent. As such the generic advice given to all pregnant women regarding awareness of fetal movements is all that NICE Clinical Guideline 107 recommends.

A large randomized controlled trial, the HYPITAT study [37], compared delivery at term (by induction of labour) with conservative care for gestational hypertension and mild pre-eclampsia. This study showed a reduction in severe hypertension in pre-eclamptic women but not gestational hypertension and no neonatal benefits were noted. Following this NICE suggests that women are not induced prior to 37 weeks unless blood pressure is uncontrolled and beyond 37 weeks that time of delivery is a balanced judgement of risk agreed between the obstetrician and the woman.

It is imperative that women with gestational hypertension are followed up with a postnatal visit where their blood pressure is checked. Those who remain hypertensive require specialist review and a percentage of these women will be found to have chronic hypertension and they require cardiovascular risk assessment and advice.

Summary box 11.3

- Pre-eclampsia requires admission to hospital but gestational hypertension does not.
- Blood pressure of 140–149/90–99 mmHg does not require pharmacological treatment.
- Blood pressure of 150–159/100–109 mmHg requires treatment to achieve a target blood pressure of 130–149/80–99 mmHg.
- Blood pressure of ≥160/≥110 mmHg requires urgent treatment to achieve target blood pressure as above.

Pre-eclampsia

Pre-eclampsia is diagnosed when there is significant proteinuria in the presence of gestational hypertension. The relationship between the level of proteinuria and maternal and fetal complications is poor. One systematic review [38] found that there was an increased risk of stillbirth with proteinuria and a reduced likelihood of stillbirth in the absence of proteinuria (at a level of 5 g per 24 hours). Because of this NICE recommends that when pre-eclampsia has been diagnosed women should be admitted to hospital, blood pressure should be treated as for gestational hypertension and proteinuria does not need to be requantified. NICE recommends conservative care

up to 34 weeks' gestation with steroid administration for fetal lung maturity as well as individualized plans for fetal monitoring, recognizing the increased risk associated with coincident FGR. NICE recommends delivery with a stable blood pressure when hypertension is severe after 34 weeks and after 37 weeks when hypertension is mild or moderate. When women present late (after 37 weeks) they should be delivered after 24–48 hours of stabilization [37].

Planning delivery

Delivery of the placenta remains the only intervention which leads to resolution of both the clinical and biochemical manifestations of pre-eclampsia. Unfortunately, some women will initially deteriorate in the immediate postpartum period before the recovery phase and all the serious complications of pre-eclampsia can be encountered at this time. It is therefore important that women are delivered in an environment where they can be closely monitored and appropriately managed. In most cases this will be a consultant-led delivery facility able to provide continuing postnatal surveillance, although some women will require high dependency or intensive care particularly if systemic complications develop. The mode of delivery will depend upon gestation, severity of maternal disease, degree of fetal compromise as well as maternal and clinician preference.

Isolated controlled hypertension or mild pre-eclampsia

Women with treated hypertension or mild pre-eclampsia at term who labour spontaneously or following induction of labour should continue their antihypertensive medication and have their blood pressure monitored hourly. Haematological and biochemical parameters should only be checked in women who have not previously been under surveillance or in whom those investigations are not up to date [16]. Cardiotocography is recommended during active labour, particularly if there is any suspicion of FGR and labour attendants should be vigilant for signs of abruption. Providing hypertension remains well controlled there is no evidence to support routine limitation of the duration of second stage and many women should therefore be able to achieve delivery without instrumentation.

Active third-stage management is encouraged as women with pre-eclampsia will be less tolerant of postpartum haemorrhage. Ergometrine is associated with exacerbation of hypertension and should not be used routinely. Oxytocin is the recommended drug for routine management of the third stage in the UK and this also applies to hypertensive women. In the event of postpartum haemorrhage it should be remembered that pharmacological uterotonic alternatives to ergometrine such as misoprostol can also be associated with hypertension.

Severe pre-eclampsia

The diagnosis of severe pre-eclampsia is usually made along with a decision to deliver once the maternal condition has been stabilized. Women should be managed in a high-dependency environment by a multidisciplinary team of senior clinicians including high-risk midwifery staff, obstetricians and anaesthetists in a clinical setting where additional support can be obtained if needed from intensivists, nephrologists, haematologists, hepatologists, neurologists and neonatologists. Care is focused around careful fluid management, treatment of hypertension, prevention/treatment of eclamptic fits and prompt recognition and supportive management of any complications which arise prior to the recovery phase.

Treatment of hypertension

Uncontrolled hypertension, particularly persistent systolic pressures above 160 mmHg or mean arterial pressures sustained above 125 mmHg, lead to compromised cerebral autoregulation. The associated complications of cerebral haemorrhage and encephalopathy are the leading cause of maternal mortality in hypertensive pregnancies in the UK and it is for this reason that one of the key recommendations from the most recent CEMACE report [2] was that severe hypertension should be more actively controlled. The aim of treatment is to gradually reduce blood pressure and sustain levels in the region of 150/80–100 mmHg.

The most common antihypertensive agents used in the UK for acute management of hypertension in pregnancy are labetalol (α- and β-receptor blocker), hydralazine (α-receptor blocker) and calcium channel blockers (nifedipine). The available meta-analyses have failed to demonstrate that one agent is a more effective antihypertensive in this population and the choice of drug therefore depends upon the pharmacological profile and anticipated side effects in an individual clinical scenario. Labetalol can be administered by oral and intravenous routes, nifedipine is given orally and hydralazine is reserved for intravenous administration in UK obstetric practice. Prior to delivery it is important to prevent precipitous drops in blood pressure, which will be associated with a reduction in placental perfusion and can give rise to fetal distress particularly in growth-restricted babies. Rapid reduction in blood pressure is most commonly seen following hydralazine and this has led some clinicians to recommend a 500-mL bolus of colloid to be given before or at the same time as the first dose of hydralazine. It is currently unclear if this practice reduces the incidence of fetal compromise or if the practice is associated with any increased maternal morbidity especially fluid overload. Certainly there is no role for fluid preloading following delivery of the baby. Precipitous drops in blood pressure can also be a feature of nifedipine especially if they are coadministered with magnesium sulphate when potentiation of the vasodilative action can be problematic. Labetalol has therefore emerged as the first-line agent (in non-asthmatics) and is currently the only agent in this group to be licensed in the UK for the acute treatment of hypertension in pregnancy.

Prevention and treatment of eclamptic fits

Magnesium sulphate is the recommended drug to treat and prevent eclampsia. The Magpie (Magnesium Sulphate for Prevention of Eclampsia) trial [14] recruited 10 141 women with pre-eclampsia and randomized them to receive magnesium sulphate or placebo. The incidence of eclampsia was significantly lower in women who received magnesium sulphate. The greatest effect was seen in women who were at the highest risk: 63 women with severe pre-eclampsia needed to be treated to prevent a fit in contrast to 100 women with mild or moderate disease. No benefit was seen in other outcomes including maternal or neonatal morbidity or mortality.

Cochrane reviews have reported that magnesium sulphate is superior to diazepam or phenytoin for the treatment of eclampsia [39]. The incidence of recurrent maternal fits is reduced and improved neonatal outcomes, including reduced need for admission to special care baby unit or ventilation, are seen in women who delivered following magnesium sulphate.

The precise mechanisms by which magnesium sulphate acts to reduce cerebral irritability is unclear. It is a vasodilating agent and contributes to reduction of cerebral perfusion pressures but it also has other relevant properties including membrane stabilization. Magnesium sulphate is emerging as a potential agent to reduce rates of cerebral palsy in preterm infants, although the mechanism and optimal dose for this purpose remain unclear. These properties may contribute to improved neonatal outcomes in women who deliver preterm due to pre-eclampsia.

Magnesium is given intravenously as a 4-g loading dose over 5 min followed by an infusion of 1 g/hour which is usually maintained for 24 hours. Recurrent seizures should be treated with a further dose of 2–4 g over 5 min and diazepam should be reserved for use in women who continue to fit despite magnesium sulphate. The therapeutic range for magnesium plasma levels is 4–8 mg/dL; toxicity causes loss of deep tendon reflexes at 10 mg/dL and respiratory paralysis at 15 mg/dL. The drug is excreted in the urine and toxicity is therefore more likely in women who have renal manifestations of pre-eclampsia. Calcium gluconate 1 g (10 mL of 10% solution) over 2 min is administered to reverse magnesium toxicity with ventilatory support if required.

Summary box 11.4

- Magnesium sulphate is the drug of choice for the treatment of eclamptic seizures.
- Magnesium sulphate is the drug of choice for the prevention of eclamptic seizures.
- Over 25% of eclamptic seizures will occur postnatally.

Fluid management

The combination of vascular endothelial injury and the normal physiological fluid shifts during the early postpartum period make pre-eclamptic women particularly vulnerable to pulmonary oedema at this time. Six deaths were reported to the Confidential Enquiry into Maternal Deaths in the UK between 1994 and 1996 and in all women injudicious fluid management in pre-eclampsia was felt to be a significant contributory factor. Encouragingly, following recommendations made in that report for tighter fluid management there were no deaths in this group of patients in the following triennial report attributed to iatrogenic fluid overload.

The current recommended practice is to restrict fluid intake to 80 mL/hour until a postpartum diuresis is established. In women where there are ongoing losses or where persistent minimal urine output raises concerns about renal injury, invasive monitoring may help guide fluid replenishment whilst avoiding overload.

Anaesthetic issues

Both regional and general anaesthesia can be problematic in the pre-eclamptic patient. Epidural anaesthesia is often advocated for labouring pre-eclamptic women due to the belief that it will contribute to lowering of blood pressure by both reducing pain-associated anxiety and peripheral vasodilatation. Whilst there may be a modest antihypertensive effect there do not appear to be any significant improvements in maternal or fetal outcomes in women who have epidural anaesthesia for labour. As in the general obstetric population, epidural anaesthesia is associated with a longer second stage and increased incidence of instrumental delivery. There is therefore no evidence to recommend the routine use of epidural anaesthesia in labouring pre-eclamptic women and the diagnosis should not influence the woman's choice of analgesia for labour. An important exception to this is women who have severe pre-eclampsia with thrombocytopenia. A platelet count below 80×10^9/L is a contraindication to regional anaesthesia due to the increased risk of spinal haematoma.

General anaesthesia can be complicated by exacerbation of severe hypertension in response to intubation. Furthermore, laryngeal oedema can make intubation technically difficult and should only be undertaken by senior anaesthetic clinicians. The greatest risks are seen in women who have not been appropriately stabilized prior to anaesthesia.

Complications

Hepatic

Approximately 12% of women with severe pre-eclampsia will develop HELLP syndrome, characterized by haemolysis, elevated liver enzymes and low platelet count. Not all components are necessarily evident at presentation and the diagnosis is not necessarily associated with the most severe hypertensive presentations. Many affected women will be asymptomatic or will present with non-specific malaise and nausea, although a few will describe classical epigastric and right upper quadrant tenderness. The diagnosis is based on laboratory investigations including a blood film, platelet count and measurement of liver transaminases. Treatment is largely supportive. High-dose steroids have been used to try to hasten the recovery of thrombocytopenia but this has not been shown to be associated with any improved maternal outcomes and is not recommended.

Rarely, liver ischaemia can cause intrahepatic haemorrhage and subcapsular haematoma. This complication is associated with a significant risk of maternal mortality. Conservative management with ultrasound surveillance may be appropriate in the postpartum patient who is haemodynamically stable and where the haematoma is not expanding. Measures described to achieve haemostasis at laparotomy include compression, haemostatic sutures, application of topical coagulation agents, embolization or lobectomy.

Renal

Although glomerular capillary endotheliosis is a classical pathological feature of pre-eclampsia and relative oliguria is common in the early postpartum period, these features usually resolve spontaneously. Acute renal failure is a rare complication of pre-eclampsia, with an estimated incidence of 1 in 10 000–15 000 pregnancies. Obstetric haemorrhage is a much more common precipitating factor in this population. Treatment is supportive; meticulous fluid management along with a high-protein, low-potassium diet and daily electrolyte monitoring will usually be sufficient whilst awaiting spontaneous resolution. Dialysis is rarely required in women who do not have pre-existing renal pathology.

Neurological

Neurological sequelae of pre-eclampsia, other than fits, include cerebral haemorrhage, encephalopathy and temporary blindness (amaurosis). Disruption of cerebral autoregulation, increased perfusion pressures and increased vascular permeability are contributory factors but the aetiology is complicated by haemoconcentration predisposing to thrombosis and vasospasm associated with fits. Any focal neurological signs should be investigated with cranial imaging to exclude other pathologies but no specific treatment is recommended.

Postnatal management

One-third of women who have had pregnancy-induced hypertension or pre-eclampsia will sustain hypertension in the postnatal period and this increases to over 75% in women who have had preterm delivery triggered by maternal hypertensive disease. Poorly managed hypertension causes anxiety for the woman and her carers, delays discharge to the community and can occasionally put her at risk of significant complications. There is little evidence to inform clinicians when managing postpartum hypertension and until such evidence is available a pragmatic approach has been recommended [16]. Women should remain in hospital until they are asymptomatic, their blood pressure is stable within safe limits and their biochemical indices are resolving.

All women who have been prescribed antenatal antihypertensives should have these continued in the postnatal period. Women who have been given methyldopa should be changed to an alternative agent before the third postnatal day due to the association of methyldopa with postpartum depression. If the blood pressure is persistently below 140/90 mmHg, then reduce the dose. Most women will not require medication beyond 6 weeks. Commonly prescribed antihypertensive agents which have no known effects on breast-feeding infants include labetalol, atenolol, metoprolol, nifedipine, enalapril and captopril.

Women who have not previously been treated with antihypertensives should have their blood pressure monitored four times daily while an inpatient and should be treated if blood pressure is above 150/100 mmHg. Women in the community should have their blood pressure measured once between days 3 and 5 using a similar threshold for treatment. If medication is initiated, follow-up should be within 48 hours to ensure an appropriate response.

Over 25% of eclampsia will present in the postnatal period, often in women who have not been previously identified as having hypertensive disease [40]. Any woman describing severe headache or epigastric pain postnatally should have pre-eclampsia excluded. Women who have developed pre-eclampsia should be offered an obstetric review around 6 weeks after birth. This affords the opportunity to confirm that hypertension and proteinuria have resolved, or to arrange referral for further investigation if there are concerns about underlying pathology. Women should be made aware of their risk of developing pre-eclampsia in future pregnancies; overall the risk of recurrence is around 16% but this increases to 55% if they were delivered before 28 weeks' gestation due to hypertensive disease. This discussion should also identify any other modifiable risk factors which might be addressed prior to embarking on another pregnancy, for example weight management. Finally, women should be made aware of the emerging evidence that pre-eclampsia is thought to identify a group who are at increased risk of future cardiovascular morbidity [41]. It is hoped that this awareness will encourage modification of other lifestyle factors (e.g. smoking cessation) that may ameliorate this risk.

References

1 World Health Organization. *Trends in Maternal Mortality: 1990 to 2008*. Geneva: WHO, 2010. Available at: http://whqlibdoc.who.int/publications/2010/9789241500265_eng.pdf

2 Centre for Maternal and Child Enquiries. Saving Mothers Lives: Reviewing Maternal Deaths to Make Motherhood Safer: 2006–2008. The Eighth Report on Confidential Enquiries into Maternal Deaths in the United Kingdom. *BJOG* 2011;118(Suppl 1):1–203.

3 Centre for Maternal and Child Enquiries. *Perinatal Mortality 2008*. Available at: www.cemach.org.uk/getattachment/60bc0b7b-e304-4836-a5e7-26895c97ab20/Perinatal-Mortality-2008.aspx

4 Maynard SE, Min JY, Merchan J *et al*. Excess placental soluble fms-like tyrosine kinase 1 (sFlt1) may contribute to endothelial dysfunction, hypertension, and proteinuria in preeclampsia. *J Clin Invest* 2003;111:649–658.

5 Ballermann BJ. Glomerular endothelial cell differentiation. *Kidney Int* 2005;67:1668–1671.

6 Maharaj AS, Saint-Geniez M, Maldonado AE, D'Amore PA. Vascular endothelial growth factor localisation in the adult. *Am J Pathol* 2006;168:639–648.

7 Nevo O, Soleymanlou N, Wu Y *et al*. Increased expression of sFlt-1 in in vivo and in vitro models of human placental hypoxia is mediated by HIF-1. *Am J Physiol* 2006;291:R1085–R1093.

8 Makris A, Thornton C, Thompson J *et al*. Uteroplacental ischemia results in proteinuric hypertension and elevated sFLT-1. *Kidney Int* 2007;71:977–984.

9 Venkatesha S, Toporsian M, Lam C *et al*. Soluble endoglin contributes to the pathogenesis of preeclampsia. *Nat Med* 2006;12:642–649.

10 Levine RJ, Lam C, Qian C *et al*. Soluble endoglin and other circulating antiangiogenic factors in preeclampsia. *N Engl J Med* 2006;355:992–1005.

11 Cudmore M, Ahmad S, Al-Ani B *et al*. Negative regulation of soluble Flt-1 and soluble endoglin release by heme oxygenase-1. *Circulation* 2007;115:1789–1797.

12 Report of the National High Blood Pressure Education Program Working Group on High Blood Pressure in Pregnancy. *Am J Obstet Gynecol* 2000;183:S1–S22.

13 ACOG Committee on Practice Bulletins: Obstetrics. ACOG practice bulletin. Diagnosis and management of preeclampsia and eclampsia. *Obstet Gynecol* 2002;99:159–167.

14 Altman D, Carroli G, Duley L *et al.* Do women with pre-eclampsia, and their babies, benefit from magnesium sulphate? The Magpie Trial: a randomised placebo-controlled trial. *Lancet* 2002;359:1877–1890.

15 Menzies J, Magee LA, Li J *et al.* Instituting surveillance guidelines and adverse outcomes in preeclampsia. *Obstet Gynecol* 2007;110:121–127.

16 National Institute for Health and Clinical Excellence. *Hypertension in Pregnancy. The Management of Hypertensive Disorders During Pregnancy.* NICE Clinical Guideline 107, 2010. Available at: www.nice.org.uk/nicemedia/live/13098/50418/50418.pdf

17 O'Brien E, Petrie J, Littler W *et al.* An outline of the revised British Hypertension Society protocol for the evaluation of blood pressure measuring devices. *J Hypertens* 1993;11:677–679.

18 O'Brien E, Asmar R, Beilin L *et al.* European Society of Hypertension recommendations for conventional, ambulatory and home blood pressure measurement. *J Hypertens* 2003;21:821–848.

19 Shennan AH, Waugh JW. The measurement of blood pressure and proteinuria in pregnancy. In: Critchley H, Poston L, Walker J (eds) *Pre-eclampsia.* London: RCOG Press, 2003: 305–324.

20 Brown MA, Buddle ML, Farrell T, Davis G, Jones M. Randomised trial of management of hypertensive pregnancies by Korotkoff phase IV or phase V. *Lancet* 1998;352:777–781.

21 Shennan A, Gupta M, Halligan A, Taylor DJ, de Swiet M. Lack of reproducibility in pregnancy of Korotkoff phase IV as measured by mercury sphygmomanometry. *Lancet* 1996;347:139–142.

22 Waugh JJ, Clark TJ, Divakaran TG, Khan KS, Kilby MD. Accuracy of urinalysis dipstick techniques in predicting significant proteinuria in pregnancy. *Obstet Gynecol* 2004;103:769–777.

23 Waugh JJ, Bell SC, Kilby MD *et al.* Optimal bedside urinalysis for the detection of proteinuria in hypertensive pregnancy: a study of diagnostic accuracy. *BJOG* 2005;112:412–417.

24 Côté AM, Brown MA, Lam E *et al.* Diagnostic accuracy of urinary spot protein:creatinine ratio for proteinuria in hypertensive pregnant women: systematic review. *BMJ* 2008;336:1003–1006.

25 National Institute for Health and Clinical Excellence. *Antenatal Care: Routine Care for the Healthy Pregnant Woman.* NICE Clinical Guideline 62, 2008. Available at: http://guidance.nice.org.uk/CG62

26 Milne F, Redman C, Walker J *et al.* The pre-eclampsia community guideline (PRECOG): how to screen for and detect onset of pre-eclampsia in the community. *BMJ* 2005;330:576–580.

27 Duckitt K, Harrington D. Risk factors for pre-eclampsia at antenatal booking: systematic review of controlled studies. *BMJ* 2005;330:565.

28 Mires GJ, Williams FL, Leslie J, Howie PW. Assessment of uterine arterial notching as a screening test for adverse pregnancy outcome. *Am J Obstet Gynecol* 1998;179:1317–1323.

29 Meads CA, Cnossen JS, Meher S *et al.* Methods of prediction and prevention of pre-eclampsia: systematic reviews of accuracy and effectiveness literature with economic modelling. *Health Technol Assess* 2008;12(6):iii–iv,1–270.

30 Levine RJ, Maynard SE, Qian C *et al.* Circulating angiogenic factors and the risk of preeclampsia. *N Engl J Med* 2004;350:672–683.

31 Ahmad S, Ahmed A. Elevated placental soluble vascular endothelial growth factor receptor-1 inhibits angiogenesis in preeclampsia. *Circ Res* 2004;95:884–891.

32 Kendall RL, Thomas KA. Inhibition of vascular endothelial cell growth factor activity by an endogenously encoded soluble receptor. *Proc Natl Acad Sci USA* 1993;90:10705–10709.

33 Livingston JC, Chin R, Haddad B, McKinney ET, Ahokas R, Sibai BM. Reductions of vascular endothelial growth factor and placental growth factor concentrations in severe preeclampsia. *Am J Obstet Gynecol* 2000;183:1554–1557.

34 Dugoff L, Hobbins JC, Malone FD *et al.* First-trimester maternal serum PAPP-A and free-beta subunit human chorionic gonadotropin concentrations and nuchal translucency are associated with obstetric complications: a population-based screening study (the FASTER Trial). *Am J Obstet Gynecol* 2004;191:1446–1451.

35 Gagnon A, Wilson RD, Audibert F *et al.* Obstetrical complications associated with abnormal maternal serum markers analytes. *J Obstet Gynaecol Can* 2008;30:918–949.

36 Askie LM, Duley L, Henderson-Smart DJ, Stewart LA. Antiplatelet agents for prevention of pre-eclampsia: a meta-analysis of individual patient data. *Lancet* 2007;369:1791–1798.

37 Koopmans CM, Bijlenga D, Groen H *et al.* Induction of labour versus expectant monitoring for gestational hypertension or mild pre-eclampsia after 36 weeks' gestation (HYPITAT): a multicentre, open-label randomised controlled trial. *Lancet* 2009;374:979–988.

38 Thangaratinam S, Coomarasamy A, O'Mahony F *et al.* Estimation of proteinuria as a predictor of complications of pre-eclampsia: a systematic review. *BMC Med* 2009;7:10.

39 Duley L, Gülmezoglu AM, Henderson-Smart DJ, Chou D. Magnesium sulphate and other anticonvulsants for women with pre-eclampsia. *Cochrane Database Syst Rev* 2010;(11):CD000025.

40 Matthys LA, Coppage KH, Lambers DS, Barton JR, Sibai BM. Delayed postpartum preeclampsia: an experience of 151 cases. *Am J Obstet Gynecol* 2004;190:1464–1466.

41 Bellamy L, Casas JP, Hingorani AD, Williams DJ. Pre-eclampsia and risk of cardiovascular disease and cancer in later life: systematic review and meta-analysis. *BMJ* 2007;335:974.

Chapter 12
Heart Disease in Pregnancy

Catherine Nelson-Piercy
Guy's and St Thomas' Foundation Trust and Queen Charlotte's & Chelsea Hospital, London, UK

Although pregnancies complicated by significant heart disease are rare in the UK, Europe and the developed world, cardiac disease remains the leading cause of maternal death in the UK [1]. There were indirect deaths attributed to cardiac disease in 2006–2008, giving a death rate of 2.3 per 100 000 maternities. The maternal mortality rate from cardiac disease has continued to rise since the early 1980s. The major causes of cardiac deaths over the last 10 years are cardiomyopathy (predominantly peripartum), myocardial infarction and ischaemic heart disease, and dissection of the thoracic aorta and sudden adult death syndrome. In the UK, rheumatic heart disease is now extremely rare in women of childbearing age and mostly confined to immigrants. There were no maternal deaths reported from rheumatic heart disease from 1994 until 2002, but there were two deaths in the 2003–2005 triennium [2].

Women with congenital heart disease, having undergone corrective or palliative surgery in childhood and surviving into adulthood, are encountered more frequently. These women may have complicated pregnancies. Women with metal prosthetic valves face difficult decisions regarding anticoagulation in pregnancy and have a greatly increased risk of haemorrhage.

Because of significant physiological changes in pregnancy, symptoms such as palpitations and signs such as an ejection systolic murmur are very common and innocent findings. Not all women with significant heart disease are able to meet these increased physiological demands. The care of the pregnant and parturient woman with heart disease requires a multidisciplinary approach involving obstetricians, cardiologists and anaesthetists, preferably in a dedicated antenatal cardiac clinic. This allows formulation of an agreed and documented management plan encompassing management of both planned and emergency delivery.

The most common and important cardiac conditions encountered in pregnancy are discussed below.

Physiological adaptations to pregnancy, labour and delivery

Blood volume starts to rise by the fifth week after conception secondary to oestrogen- and prostaglandin-induced relaxation of smooth muscle that increases the capacitance of the venous bed. Plasma volume increases and red cell mass rises, but to a lesser degree, thus explaining the physiological anaemia of pregnancy. Relaxation of smooth muscle on the arterial side results in a profound fall in systemic vascular resistance and together with the increase in blood volume determines the early increase in cardiac output. Blood pressure falls slightly, but by term has usually returned to the pre-pregnancy value. The increased cardiac output is achieved by an increase in stroke volume and a lesser increase in resting heart rate of 10–20 bpm. By the end of the second trimester the blood volume and stroke volume have risen by between 30 and 50%. This increase correlates with the size and weight of the products of conception and is therefore considerably greater in multiple pregnancies as is the risk of heart failure in heart disease [3].

Although there is no increase in pulmonary capillary wedge pressure, serum colloid osmotic pressure is reduced. The gradient between colloid oncotic pressure and pulmonary capillary wedge pressure is reduced by 28%, making pregnant women particularly susceptible to pulmonary oedema. Pulmonary oedema will be precipitated if there is an increase in cardiac preload (such as infusion of fluids), increased pulmonary capillary permeability (such as in pre-eclampsia), or both.

In late pregnancy in the supine position, pressure of the gravid uterus on the inferior vena cava (IVC) causes a reduction in venous return to the heart and a consequent fall in stroke volume and cardiac output. Turning from the lateral to the supine position may result in a 25% reduction in cardiac output. Pregnant women should therefore be nursed in the left or right lateral position

Dewhurst's Textbook of Obstetrics & Gynaecology, Eighth Edition. Edited by D. Keith Edmonds.
© 2012 John Wiley and Sons, Ltd. Published 2012 by John Wiley and Sons, Ltd.

wherever possible. If the mother has to be kept on her back, the pelvis should be rotated so that the uterus drops forward and cardiac output as well as utero-placental blood flow is optimized. Reduced cardiac output is associated with reduction in uterine blood flow and therefore placental perfusion; this can compromise the fetus.

Labour is associated with further increases in cardiac output (15% in the first stage and 50% in the second stage). Uterine contractions lead to autotransfusion of 300–500 mL of blood back into the circulation and the sympathetic response to pain and anxiety further elevate heart rate and blood pressure. Cardiac output is increased more during contractions but also between contractions. The rise in stroke volume with each contraction is attenuated by good pain relief and further reduced by epidural analgesia and the supine position. Epidural analgesia or anaesthesia causes arterial vasodilatation and a fall in blood pressure [4]. General anaesthesia is associated with a rise in blood pressure and heart rate during induction but cardiovascular stability thereafter. Prostaglandins given to induce labour have little effect on haemodynamics but ergometrine causes vasoconstriction and Syntocinon can cause vasodilation and fluid retention.

In the third stage up to 1 L of blood may be returned to the circulation due to the relief of IVC obstruction and contraction of the uterus. The intrathoracic and cardiac blood volume rise, cardiac output increases by 60–80% followed by a rapid decline to pre-labour values within about 1 hour of delivery. Transfer of fluid from the extravascular space increases venous return and stroke volume further. Those women with cardiovascular compromise are therefore most at risk of pulmonary oedema during the second stage of labour and the immediate postpartum period. All the changes revert quite rapidly during the first week and more slowly over the following 6 weeks, but even at 1 year significant changes still persist and are enhanced by a subsequent pregnancy [5].

Normal findings on examination of the cardiovascular system in pregnancy

These may include a loud first heart sound with exaggerated splitting of the second heart sound and a physiological third heart sound at the apex. A systolic ejection murmur at the left sternal edge is heard in nearly all women and may be remarkably loud and be audible all over the precordium. It varies with posture and if unaccompanied by any other abnormality it reflects the increased stroke output. Venous hums and mammary souffles may be heard. Because of the peripheral vasodilatation the pulse may be bounding and in addition ectopic beats are very common in pregnancy.

Cardiac investigations in pregnancy

Troponin is not affected by pregnancy and remains a valid test for myocardial ischaemia. The ECG axis shifts superiorly in late pregnancy due to a more horizontal position of the heart. Small Q waves and T-wave inversion in the right precordial leads are not uncommon. Atrial and ventricular ectopics are both common.

The amount of radiation received by the fetus during a maternal chest X-ray (CXR) is negligible and CXR should never be withheld if clinically indicated in pregnancy. Transthoracic echocardiography is the investigation of choice for excluding, confirming or monitoring structural heart disease in pregnancy. Transoesophageal echocardiography is also safe with the usual precautions to avoid aspiration. Magnetic resonance imaging (MRI) and chest computerized tomography (CT) are safe in pregnancy. Routine investigation with electrophysiological studies and angiography are normally postponed until after pregnancy but angiography should not be withheld in, for example, acute coronary syndromes.

General considerations in pregnant women with heart disease

The outcome and safety of pregnancy are related to:
- presence and severity of pulmonary hypertension;
- presence of cyanosis;
- haemodynamic significance of the lesion;
- functional NYHA (New York Heart Association) class as determined by the level of activity that leads to dyspnoea [6].

Most women with pre-existing cardiac disease tolerate pregnancy well if they are asymptomatic or only mildly symptomatic (New York Heart Association class II or less) before the pregnancy, but important exceptions are pulmonary hypertension, Marfan's syndrome with a dilated aortic root, and some women with mitral or aortic stenosis.

Cardiac events such as stroke, arrhythmia, pulmonary oedema and death complicating pregnancies in women with structural heart disease are predicted by [7]:
- a prior cardiac event or arrhythmia;
- NYHA classification above class II;
- cyanosis;
- left ventricular ejection fraction <40%;
- left heart obstruction, i.e. mitral valve area <2 cm², aortic valve area <1.5 cm², aortic valve gradient (mean – non-pregnant) >30 mmHg.

These features therefore also act as reasons to refer to specialist centres for counselling and management of the pregnancy.

Women with cyanosis (oxygen saturation below 80–85%) have an increased risk of fetal growth restriction, fetal loss, and thromboembolism secondary to the reactive polycythaemia. Their chance of a live birth in one study was less than 20% [8].

Women with the above risk factors for adverse cardiac or obstetric events should be managed and counselled by a multidisciplinary team including cardiologists with expertise in pregnancy, obstetricians with expertise in cardiac disease, fetal medicine specialists and paediatricians. There should be early involvement of obstetric anaesthetists and a carefully documented plan for delivery.

Specific cardiac conditions

Congenital heart disease

Asymptomatic acyanotic women with simple defects usually tolerate pregnancy well. Many defects will have been treated surgically or by the interventional paediatric cardiologist but others are first discovered during pregnancy. Women with congenital heart disease are at increased risk of having a baby with congenital heart disease, and should therefore be offered genetic counselling if possible before pregnancy [9] and detailed scanning for fetal cardiac anomalies with fetal echocardiography by 18–20 weeks' gestation.

Acyanotic congenital heart disease
Atrial septal defect

After bicuspid aortic valve (which is much commoner in males), secundum atrial septal defect (ASD) is the commonest congenital cardiac defect in adults. Paradoxical embolism is rare and arrhythmias do not usually develop until middle age. Mitral regurgitation caused by mitral leaflet prolapse develops in up to 15% of uncorrected ASDs. Pulmonary hypertension is rare.

No problems are anticipated during pregnancy but acute blood loss is poorly tolerated. It can cause massive increase in left-to-right shunting and a precipitous fall in left ventricular output, blood pressure and coronary blood flow and even lead to cardiac arrest.

Ventricular septal defect and patent ductus

Like regurgitant valve disease, these defects, which increase the volume load of the left ventricle, are well tolerated in pregnancy unless the defects are large and complicated by pulmonary vascular disease.

Pulmonary stenosis

Pulmonary stenosis does not usually give rise to symptoms during pregnancy. However, when severe and causing right ventricular failure, balloon pulmonary valvotomy has been successfully carried out during pregnancy. The procedure is best performed during the second trimester with uterine shielding.

Aortic stenosis

Left ventricular outflow tract obstruction at any level can cause problems during pregnancy. Pre-pregnancy assessment is the ideal. Significant obstruction results if aortic valve area is less than $1\,cm^2$ or if the non-pregnant mean gradient across the valve is above 50 mmHg. Indications that pregnancy will be high risk include failure to achieve a normal rise in blood pressure without the development of ST- or T-wave changes during exercise, impaired left ventricular function and symptoms including chest pain syncope or pre-syncope.

The ECG will normally show left ventricular hypertrophy and the Doppler transaortic valve velocity will rise during pregnancy if the stroke volume increases in a normal fashion. If left ventricular systolic function is impaired, the left ventricle may not be capable of generating a high gradient across the valve. Therefore a low gradient may be falsely reassuring.

Any patient who develops angina, dyspnoea or resting tachycardia should be admitted to hospital for rest. Administration of a β-adrenergic blocking drug will increase diastolic coronary flow time and left ventricular filling with resultant improvement in angina and left ventricular function. If despite these measures angina, pulmonary congestion and left ventricular failure persist or progress, balloon aortic valvotomy needs to be considered [10]. These valves are intrinsically not ideal and severe aortic regurgitation may be created, but if successful the procedure may buy time and allow completion of the pregnancy. The procedure can also be carried out for relief of discrete subaortic stenosis but with some risk of causing mitral regurgitation.

Coarctation of the aorta

Most cases encountered will already have been surgically corrected, although residual narrowing is not uncommon. Ideally, any narrowing or pre- or post-stenotic dilatation or aneurysm formation should be assessed with MRI prior to pregnancy. Aortic coarctation may first be diagnosed during pregnancy and should always be considered when raised blood pressure is recorded at booking, especially if investigation for secondary causes of pre-existing hypertension has not previously been undertaken.

Although the blood pressure can be lowered, adequate control cannot be maintained during exercise, which brings the risk of cerebral haemorrhage or aortic dissection [11]. The woman should therefore be advised to rest and avoid exertion. The risk of dissection is increased in patients with pre-existing aortic abnormality associated with coarctation, Marfan's syndrome or other inherited disorders of connective tissue.

Hypertension should be aggressively treated, and to minimize the risk of rupture and dissection beta-blockers are the ideal agents. Left ventricular failure is unlikely in the absence of an associated stenotic bicuspid aortic valve or endocardial fibroelastosis with impaired left ventricular function. Normal delivery is usually possible, although severe coarctation would indicate a shortened second stage.

Marfan's syndrome

A majority (80%) of patients with Marfan's syndrome have some cardiac involvement, most commonly mitral valve prolapse and regurgitation. Pregnancy increases the risk of aortic rupture or dissection usually in the third trimester or early after birth. The risk of type A aortic dissection in pregnant women with Marfan's syndrome is around 1%, even in the absence of a dilated aortic root [6]. Progressive aortic root dilatation and an aortic root dimension above 4 cm are associated with increased risk (10%) [12]. Women with aortic roots greater than 4.6 cm should be advised to delay pregnancy until after aortic root repair or root replacement with resuspension of the aortic valve [13].

Conversely, in women with minimal cardiac involvement and an aortic root of less than 4 cm pregnancy outcome is usually good, although those with a family history of aortic dissection or sudden death are also at increased risk since in some families aortic root dissection occurs in the absence of preliminary aortic dilatation [6].

Management should include counselling regarding the dominant inheritance of the condition, monthly echocardiography to assess the aortic root in those with cardiac involvement, and beta-blockers for those with hypertension or aortic root dilatation. Vaginal delivery for those with stable aortic root measurements is possible but elective Caesarean section with regional anaesthesia is recommended if there is an enlarged or dilating aortic root.

Cyanotic congenital heart disease

Cyanotic congenital heart disease in the adult is usually associated with either pulmonary hypertension (as in Eisenmenger's syndrome) or pulmonary stenosis (as in tetralogy of Fallot). Patients with single ventricle, transposition of the great arteries and complex pulmonary atresias with systemic blood supply to the lungs may all survive to adult life with or without previous palliative surgery.

Tetralogy of Fallot

The association of severe right ventricular outflow tract obstruction with a large subaortic ventricular septal defect (VSD) and overriding aorta causes right ventricular hypertrophy and right-to-left shunting with cyanosis. Pregnancy is tolerated well but fetal growth is poor with a high rate of miscarriage, prematurity and small-for-dates babies. The haematocrit tends to rise during pregnancy in cyanosed women because systemic vasodilatation leads to an increase in right-to-left shunting.

Women with a resting arterial saturation of 85% or more, a haemoglobin below 18 g/dL and a haematocrit below 55% have a reasonable chance of a successful outcome. Arterial saturation falls markedly on effort so rest is prescribed to optimize fetal growth but subcutaneous low-molecular-weight heparin (LMWH) should be given to prevent venous thrombosis and paradoxical embolism. Most women will have had previous surgical correction of the tetralogy and do well in pregnancy [14].

Postoperative congenital heart disease

Survivors of neonatal palliative surgery for complex congenital heart disease need individual assessment. Echocardiography by a paediatric or adult congenital cardiologist enables a detailed assessment to be made.

Following the Fontan operation for tricuspid atresia or transposition with pulmonary stenosis, the right ventricle is bypassed and the left ventricle provides the pump for both the systemic and pulmonary circulations. Increases in venous pressure can lead to hepatic congestion and gross oedema but pregnancy can be successful. It is important that women with a Fontan circulation are kept well filled peripartum as without optimal preload the left ventricle cannot adequately drive the pulmonary circulation. These women are usually anticoagulated with warfarin outside pregnancy and LMWH in pregnancy.

Eisenmenger's syndrome and pulmonary hypertension

Pulmonary vascular disease, whether secondary to a reversed large left-to-right shunt such as a VSD (Eisenmenger's syndrome) or to lung or connective tissue disease (e.g. scleroderma) or due to idiopathic arterial pulmonary hypertension, is extremely dangerous in pregnancy and women known to have significant pulmonary vascular disease should be advised from an early age to avoid pregnancy and be given appropriate contraceptive advice [15]. Maternal mortality is 25–40% [16].

The danger relates to fixed pulmonary vascular resistance that cannot fall in response to pregnancy, and a consequent inability to increase pulmonary blood flow with refractory hypoxaemia. Pulmonary hypertension is defined as a non-pregnant elevation of mean (not systolic) pulmonary artery pressure of 25 mmHg or more at rest or 30 mmHg on exercise in the absence of a left-to-right shunt. Pulmonary artery systolic (not mean) pressure is usually estimated using Doppler ultrasound to measure the regurgitant jet velocity across the tricuspid valve. This should be considered a screening test. There is no agreed relation between the mean pulmonary pressure and the estimated systolic pulmonary pressure. If the systolic pulmonary pressure estimated by Doppler is thought to indicate pulmonary hypertension, a specialist cardiac opinion is recommended. If there is pulmonary hypertension in the presence of a left-to-right shunt, the diagnosis of pulmonary vascular disease is particularly difficult and further investigation including cardiac catheterization to calculate pulmonary vascular resistance is likely to be necessary. Pulmonary hypertension as defined by Doppler studies may also occur in mitral stenosis and with large left-to-right shunts that have not reversed. Women with pulmonary hypertension who still have predominant left-to-right shunts are at lesser risk and may do well during pregnancy, but although such women may not have pulmonary vascular disease and a fixed pulmonary vascular resistance (or this may not have been established prior to pregnancy), they have the potential to develop it and require very careful monitoring.

Modern management of pulmonary hypertension includes drugs such as sildenafil and bosentan. With such therapies, pulmonary pressures can be reduced to within the normal range, and therefore pregnancy may be safely negotiated. Although bosentan is teratogenic in animals, the benefit of continuing therapy in pregnancy probably outweighs this risk. In the event of unplanned pregnancy a therapeutic termination should be offered. Elective termination carries a 7% risk of mortality, hence the importance of avoiding pregnancy if possible. If such advice is declined, multidisciplinary care, elective admission for bed rest, oxygen and thromboprophylaxis with LMWH are recommended [17]. Fetal growth should be carefully monitored.

Most fatalities occur during delivery or the first week after birth. There is no evidence that monitoring the pulmonary artery pressure before or during delivery improves outcome; indeed insertion of a pulmonary artery catheter increases the risk of thrombosis, which may be fatal in such women. Vasodilators given to reduce pulmonary artery pressure will (with the exception of inhaled nitric oxide and prostacyclin) inevitably result in a concomitant lowering of the systemic pressure, exacerbating hypoxaemia.

There is no evidence that abdominal or vaginal delivery or regional versus general anaesthesia improve outcome in pregnant women with pulmonary hypertension. Great care must be taken to avoid systemic vasodilatation. The patient should be nursed in an intensive care unit after delivery. Nebulized prostacyclin can be used to try to prevent pulmonary vasoconstriction. When sudden deterioration occurs (usually in the postpartum period) resuscitation is rarely successful and no additional cause is found at post-mortem, although there may be concomitant thromboembolism, hypovolaemia or pre-eclampsia. Death is usually preceded by vagal slowing, a fall in blood pressure and oxygen saturation, followed by ventricular fibrillation.

Acquired valve disease

Mitral valve prolapse

This common condition may also be called 'floppy mitral valve' and may be sporadic or inherited as a dominant condition in some families with variants of Marfan's syndrome. Pregnancy is well tolerated and for women with isolated mitral valve prolapse there are no implications for the mother or fetus in pregnancy.

Rheumatic heart disease

Mitral stenosis

Worldwide, mitral stenosis remains the most common potentially lethal pre-existing heart condition in pregnancy. There are many pitfalls because (i) an asymptomatic patient may deteriorate in pregnancy, (ii) mitral stenosis may have increased in severity since a previous uncomplicated pregnancy, (iii) stenosis can recur or worsen after valvuloplasty or valvotomy and (iv) mitral stenosis that may previously not have been recognized may be missed during routine antenatal examination because the murmur is low-pitched, usually quiet, diastolic and submammary.

Women may deteriorate secondary to tachycardia (related to pain, anxiety, exercise or intercurrent infection), arrhythmias or the increased cardiac output of pregnancy. Sinus tachycardia at rest should prompt concern. Tachycardia is the reflex response to failure to increase stroke volume and it reduces the time for left atrial emptying during diastole so that left ventricular stroke volume falls, the reflex sinus tachycardia accelerates and left atrial pressure climbs. This creates a vicious circle of increasing heart rate and left atrial pressure and can precipitate pulmonary oedema. The anxiety caused by the dyspnoea increases the tachycardia and exacerbates the problem (Fig. 12.1). Pulmonary oedema may also be precipitated by increased volume (such as occurs during the third stage of labour or following injudicious intravenous fluid therapy) [18]. The risks are increased with severe mitral stenosis (mitral valve area $<1\,cm^2$), moderate or severe symptoms prior to pregnancy, and in those diagnosed late in pregnancy.

The ECG in mitral stenosis shows left atrial P waves and right axis deviation. The CXR shows a small heart but with prominence of the left atrial appendage and left atrium and pulmonary congestion or oedema. The diagnosis is confirmed with transthoracic echocardiography.

Women with severe mitral stenosis should be advised to delay pregnancy until after balloon, open or closed mitral valvotomy, or if the valve is not amenable to valvotomy until after mitral valve replacement. Beta-blockers decrease heart rate, increase diastolic filling time and decrease the risk of pulmonary oedema [18] and should be given in pregnancy to maintain a heart rate of under 90 bpm. Diuretics should be commenced or continued if indicated. It is also important that the woman does not over-exert herself.

In the event of pulmonary oedema, the patient should be sat up, oxygen should be given and the heart rate slowed by relief of anxiety with diamorphine, and 20 mg of intravenous furosemide administered. Digoxin

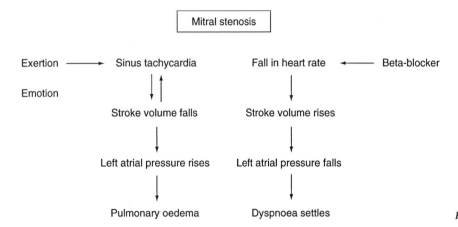

Fig. 12.1 Mitral stenosis.

should only be used if atrial fibrillation occurs as it does not slow the heart in sinus rhythm (because increased sympathetic drive easily overcomes its mild vagotonic effect).

If medical therapy fails or for those with severe mitral stenosis, balloon mitral valvotomy may be safely and successfully used in pregnancy if the valve is suitable [19], although this will require transfer to a hospital with major cardiac facilities. Percutaneous balloon valvotomy carries a risk of major complications of about 1%, whereas for surgical valvotomy the risks are as follows.
• Closed valvotomy: fetal mortality 5–15%, maternal mortality 3%.
• Open valvotomy: fetal mortality 15–33%, maternal mortality 5%.
If an open operation on the mitral valve is likely to be required, this should be deferred if possible until after delivery.

Women with mitral stenosis should avoid the supine and lithotomy positions as much as possible for labour and delivery. Fluid overload must be avoided; even in the presence of oliguria, without significant blood loss, the temptation to give intravenous colloid must be resisted. Cautious epidural analgesia or anaesthesia is suitable for the patient with mitral stenosis as is vaginal delivery but limitation of maternal effort with an instrumental delivery may be indicated.

Regurgitant valve disease
Patients with regurgitant valve disease, either mitral or aortic, tolerate pregnancy much better than patients with valvular stenosis. The systemic vasodilatation in pregnancy reduces regurgitant flow as does tachycardia in patients with aortic regurgitation. When the valve disease is of rheumatic origin the advent of sudden atrial fibrillation may precipitate pulmonary oedema. Similarly monitoring of left ventricular function is important in those with severe mitral or aortic regurgitation.

Mechanical heart valves

Most women with prosthetic heart valves have sufficient cardiovascular reserve to accomplish pregnancy safely. The optimal strategy for anticoagulation in women with metal heart valve replacements in pregnancy is controversial since the interests of the mother and the fetus are in conflict. These women require lifelong anticoagulation and this must be continued in pregnancy because of the increased risk of thrombosis. However, warfarin is associated with warfarin embryopathy (chondrodysplasia punctata) if given during the period of organogenesis (6–12 weeks' gestation) [20] and with fetal intracerebral haemorrhage in the second and third trimesters.

Despite a maternal international normalized ratio (INR) within the therapeutic range, there is a greater anticoagulant effect on the fetus than on the mother because the immature fetal liver produces only low levels of vitamin K-dependent clotting factors and maternal procoagulants do not cross the placenta due to their large molecular size. The fetal risk from warfarin is dose dependent. Women requiring more than 5 mg daily are at increased risk of teratogenesis, miscarriage and stillbirth [21,22].

Heparin and LMWH do not cross the placenta and therefore are an attractive option. However, even in full anticoagulant doses, they are associated with an increased risk of valve thrombosis and embolic events [20,21,23]. Heparins can also cause retroplacental haemorrhage so the risk of fetal loss is not eliminated. Further disadvantages of unfractionated heparin include a need for parenteral administration, powerful but short duration of action, narrow therapeutic index, a steep dose–response curve, increasing dose requirement during pregnancy, and lack of agreed optimal test or target for safe and effective activity. Overshooting with incremental dosage brings a risk of bleeding. High doses of unfractionated heparin long term may also cause osteoporosis.

LMWHs have a better safety profile in pregnancy and, provided there is close monitoring of anti-Xa levels with appropriate dose adjustments and good compliance with twice-daily injections, recent data would suggest a low risk of thrombotic events [23,24]. Most clinicians use concomitant low-dose aspirin and many women need an increase in the LMWH dose in order to maintain peak anti-Xa levels of 0.8–1.2 IU/mL [24].

There are three basic options for anticoagulation management.

1 Continue warfarin throughout pregnancy, stopping only for delivery. This is the safest option for the mother [20,21].

2 Replace warfarin with high-dose LMWH from 6 to 12 weeks' gestation to avoid warfarin embryopathy.

3 Use high-dose LMWH throughout pregnancy.

Which option is chosen will depend on several factors.

• *The type of mechanical valve.* The risk of thrombosis is less with the newer bileaflet valves (e.g. carbomedics) than with first-generation ball and cage (e.g. Starr–Edwards) or second-generation single tilting disc (e.g. Björk–Shiley) valves.

• *The position of the valve replacement.* Valves in the aortic rather than the mitral position are associated with a lower risk of thrombosis [24].

• *The size of the mechanical valve.* If a valve was replaced before the woman had finished growing, it may be relatively small and this increases the risk of thrombosis.

• *The number of mechanical valves.* Two valves give a higher risk of thrombosis.

• *The dose of warfarin* required to maintain a therapeutic INR. If this is less than 5 mg, the risk to the fetus is reduced.

• Any previous history of embolic events.

If warfarin is used in pregnancy, serial fetal scans are indicated to detect embryopathy and intracerebral haemorrhage. Warfarin should be discontinued and substituted for LMWH for 10 days prior to delivery to allow clearance of warfarin from the fetal circulation. For delivery itself, LMWH therapy is interrupted.

Conversion from LMWH back to warfarin should be delayed for at least 3–5 days after delivery to minimize the risk of obstetric haemorrhage. There is a high risk of antenatal but particularly postpartum bleeding in women with mechanical valves [24].

In the event of bleeding or the need for urgent delivery in a fully anticoagulated patient, warfarin may be reversed with recombinant human factor VIIa fresh frozen plasma and vitamin K, and heparin with protamine sulphate. High doses of vitamin K should be avoided if possible since it renders the woman extremely difficult to anticoagulate with warfarin after delivery.

Thrombolytic treatment can be used for prosthetic valve thrombosis during pregnancy, and although it may cause embolism or bleeding or placental separation, the risks are lower than those of cardiothoracic surgery.

Coronary artery disease

Myocardial infarction and ischaemic heart disease are now seen more commonly in pregnant and postpartum women and pregnancy increases the risk of myocardial infarction [25]. When myocardial infarction occurs in pregnancy it often develops without a preceding history of typical angina. Pregnant women may present with atypical epigastric pain or nausea or dizziness as well as with chest, neck and left arm pain. In pregnancy the underlying cause may be due to non-atherosclerotic conditions. Spontaneous coronary artery dissection and coronary artery thrombosis are more common in pregnancy [2,26]. Most occur during late pregnancy or around or after delivery. Coronary ischaemia may be associated with drug abuse from crack cocaine. Embolic occlusion should always be considered and an embolic source such as mitral stenosis or infective endocarditis sought.

The risk factors for ischaemic heart disease in pregnancy are the same as for the non-pregnant woman. The risk is increased in older multigravid women and in those who smoke and those with diabetes, obesity, hypertension, hypercholesterolaemia or a family history of coronary artery disease [25,27]. There should be a low threshold for investigating chest pain and other symptoms that could be due to acute coronary syndrome particularly in women with risk factors. Troponin I is not affected by pregnancy and this should be requested along with serial ECGs in women in whom acute coronary syndrome is suspected.

The management of acute myocardial infarction and acute coronary syndrome is as for the non-pregnant woman. Coronary angiography should be undertaken without hesitation in order to define the pathology and determine management. Intravenous and intracoronary thrombolysis and percutaneous transluminal coronary angioplasty and stenting have all been successfully performed in pregnancy. Both aspirin and beta-blockers are safe in pregnancy. Clopidogrel may be used following stenting but should ideally be discontinued prior to delivery. There are less data for glycoprotein IIb/IIIa inhibitors, which are normally avoided. Statins should be discontinued for the duration of pregnancy as they are associated with an increased risk of malformations [28].

Hypertrophic cardiomyopathy

Hypertrophic cardiomyopathy (HCM) is an autosomal dominant disease characterized by hypertrophy of the undilated left ventricle in the absence of an abnormal haemodynamic load and with underlying myocyte and myofibrillar disarray. Family studies, now sometimes aided by genetic identification of a responsible mutant gene, have indicated the broad spectrum of phenotypic abnormality that exists not only between individuals at different ages but within families. Patient series previously described from specialist centres represented a highly skewed population of high-risk patients referred because of disabling symptoms or a malignant family history. In the years before echocardiography only gross examples of the disorder could be identified but these patients formed the basis of many of the published natural history studies.

HCM is not infrequently first diagnosed in pregnancy when a systolic murmur leads to an ECG and echocardiographic study. Most patients are asymptomatic and do well. HCM used to be regarded as a rare disease with a high risk of sudden death but is now recognized to be relatively common, being found in 1 in 500 young adults in a recent study and in most patients the disorder is benign.

Patients with HCM respond well to pregnancy by a useful increase in their normally reduced left ventricular cavity size and stroke volume. The danger relates to left ventricular outflow tract obstruction that may be precipitated by hypotension or hypovolaemia. Symptoms of shortness of breath, chest pain, dizziness or syncope indicate the need for a beta-blocker [29]. Ventricular arrhythmias are commoner in older patients but uncommon in the young. Sudden death has only very rarely been reported during pregnancy. It is most important in all patients to avoid vasodilatation during labour and delivery and during regional anaesthesia/analgesia. Any hypovolaemia will have the same effect and should be rapidly and adequately corrected. It is most unusual to find hypertrophy in the infants of mothers with HCM.

Peripartum cardiomyopathy

This pregnancy-specific condition is defined as the development of cardiac failure between the last month of pregnancy and 5 months after delivery, in the absence of an identifiable cause or recognizable heart disease prior to the last month of pregnancy, and left ventricular systolic dysfunction demonstrated by the following echocardiographic criteria [30]:
- left ventricular ejection fraction <45%;
- fractional shortening <30%;
- left ventricular end-diastolic dimension >2.7 cm/m^2.

Echocardiography shows dilatation that usually involves all four chambers but is dominated by left ventricular hypokinesia, which may be global or most marked in a particular territory.

The condition is rare but the true incidence is unknown as mild cases undoubtedly go unrecognized. Recognized risk factors include multiple pregnancy, hypertension (pre-existing or related to pregnancy or pre-eclampsia), multiparity, increased age and Afro-Caribbean race.

Peripartum cardiomyopathy does not differ clinically from dilated cardiomyopathy except in its temporal relationship to pregnancy. The severity varies from catastrophic to subclinical, when it may be discovered only fortuitously through echocardiography. Diagnosis should be suspected in the peripartum patient with breathlessness, tachycardia or signs of heart failure. Pulmonary oedema is often a major feature and may be precipitated by the use of Syntocinon or by fluids given to maintain cardiac output during spinal anaesthesia for delivery. The CXR shows an enlarged heart with pulmonary congestion or oedema and often bilateral pleural effusions. Systemic embolism from mural thrombus may herald the onset of ventricular arrhythmias or precede the development of clinical heart failure and pulmonary embolism may further complicate the clinical picture.

The differential diagnosis includes pre-existing dilated cardiomyopathy, pulmonary thromboembolism, amniotic fluid embolism, myocardial infarction and pulmonary oedema related to pre-eclampsia or β_2-agonist therapy for preterm labour. Echocardiography immediately implicates the left ventricle and excludes pulmonary embolism as the cause. Pre-eclampsia may rarely cause transient impairment of left ventricular function but this normally recovers rapidly after delivery.

Management is as for other causes of heart failure, with oxygen, diuretics, vasodilators and angiotensin-converting enzyme (ACE) inhibitors if after delivery. Thromboprophylaxis is imperative. The cautious addition of a cardioselective β-adrenergic blocking drug may be helpful if tachycardia persists, particularly if the cardiac output is well preserved. The most gravely ill patients will need intubation, ventilation and monitoring with use of inotropes and sometimes temporary support from an intra-aortic balloon pump or ventricular assist device. Heart transplantation may be the only chance of survival in severe cases.

About 50% of women make a spontaneous and full recovery. Most case fatalities occur close to presentation and cardiomyopathy is the cause of almost one-quarter of maternal cardiac deaths [2]. Recent data show a 5-year survival of 94% [31]. Patients should remain on an ACE inhibitor for as long as left ventricular function remains abnormal. Prognosis and recurrence depend on the normalization of left ventricular size, which may continue to improve for several years after delivery [32,33]. Those women with severe myocardial dysfunction (defined as left ventricular end-diastolic dimension ≥6 cm and fractional shortening ≤21%) are unlikely to regain normal cardiac function on follow-up [34]. Those whose left ventricular function and size do not return to normal within 6 months and prior to a subsequent pregnancy are at significant risk of worsening heart failure (50%) and death (25%) or recurrent peripartum cardiomyopathy in the next pregnancy. They should therefore be advised against pregnancy [32]. Women who have recovered normal left ventricular size and function should have their functional reserve assessed using stress (exercise) echocardiography. Even if this is normal there is a risk of recurrent heart failure in subsequent pregnancies [29].

Arrhythmias

Atrial and ventricular premature complexes are common in pregnancy. Many pregnant women are symptomatic from forceful heart beats that occur following a compensatory pause after a ventricular premature complex. Most women with symptomatic episodes of dizziness, syncope and palpitations do not have arrhythmias [35].

A sinus tachycardia requires investigation for possible underlying pathology such as blood loss, infection, heart failure, thyrotoxicosis or pulmonary embolus. The commonest arrhythmia encountered in pregnancy is supraventricular tachycardia (SVT). First onset of SVT (both accessory pathway mediated and atrioventricular nodal re-entrant) is rare in pregnancy but exacerbation of symptoms is common in pregnancy [35]. Half of SVTs do not respond to vagal manoeuvres.

Propranolol, verapamil and adenosine have Food and Drug Administration approval for acute termination of SVT. Adenosine has advantages over verapamil including probable lack of placental transfer and may be safely used in pregnancy for SVTs that do not respond to vagal stimulation [35]. For prevention of SVTs, beta-blockers or verapamil may be used. Flecainide is safe and is used in the treatment of fetal tachycardias. Propafenone and amiodarone should be avoided [36], the latter because of interference with fetal thyroid function [37]. Temporary and permanent pacing, cardioversion and automatic implantable defibrillators (AICD) are also safe in pregnancy. Care is needed when bipolar diathermy is used at Caesarean section since this may also be misinterpreted by the AICD as venticular fibrillation leading to deployment of a shock. The device is therefore usually inactivated during Caesarean section.

Cardiac arrest

This should be managed according to the same protocols as used in the non-pregnant woman. Pregnant women (especially those in advanced pregnancy) should be 'wedged' to relieve any obstruction to venous return from pressure of the gravid uterus on the IVC. This can be most rapidly achieved by turning the patient into the left lateral position. If cardiopulmonary resuscitation is required, then the pelvis can be tilted while keeping the torso flat to allow external chest compressions. Emergency Caesarean section may be required to aid maternal resuscitation.

Endocarditis prophylaxis

Infective endocarditis (IE) is rare in pregnancy but threatens the life of both mother and child. Fatal cases of endocarditis in pregnancy have occurred antenatally, rather than as a consequence of infection acquired at the time of delivery [2]. Treatment is essentially the same as outside pregnancy, with emergency valve replacement if indicated. As always, the baby should be delivered if viable before the maternal operation.

The current UK recommendations from the National Institute for Health and Clinical Excellence [38] are that antibiotic prophylaxis against IE is not required for childbirth. The British Society for Antimicrobial Chemotherapy [39] and the American Heart Association have recommended cover only for patients deemed to be at high risk of developing IE (such as women with previous IE) and for those who have the poorest outcome if they develop IE (such as those with cyanotic congenital heart disease). If antibiotic prophylaxis is used it should be with amoxicillin 2 g i.v. plus gentamicin 120 mg i.v. at the onset of labour or ruptured membranes or prior to Caesarean section, followed by amoxicillin 500 mg orally (or i.m/i.v. depending on the patient's condition) 6 hours later. For women who are penicillin allergic, vancomycin 1 g i.v. or teicoplanin 400 mg i.v. may be used instead of amoxicillin.

 Summary box 12.1

- Cardiac disease is the commonest cause of death in pregnancy or the puerperium in the UK.
- Mortality of pulmonary hypertension in pregnancy is 25–40%.
- Women with Marfan's syndrome are at risk of aortic dissection in pregnancy, particularly if they have a dilated aortic root.
- Women with mitral stenosis are at risk of pulmonary oedema in mid-pregnancy and during or immediately after delivery.
- If women with mechanical valves in pregnancy are managed with therapeutic doses of low-molecular-weight heparin, this should be closely monitored and doses adjusted to maintain therapeutic levels. These women have an increased risk of bleeding, particularly after delivery.

References

1 Lewis G. Centre for Maternal and Child Enquiries (CMACE). Saving Mother's Lives: reviewing maternal deaths to make motherhood safer: 2006–2008. The Eigth Report of the Confidential Enquiries into Maternal Deaths in the UK. *BJOG* 2011; 118(Suppl 1).

2 Lewis G (ed.) *Saving Mothers' Lives: Reviewing Maternal Deaths to Make Motherhood Safer 2003–2005. The Seventh Report on Confidential Enquiries into Maternal Deaths in the United Kingdom.* London: The Confidential Enquiry into Maternal and Child Health, 2007. Available at: www.cmace.org.uk/getattachment/26dae364-1fc9-4a29-a6cb-afb3f251f8f7/Saving-Mothers'-Lives-2003-2005-(Full-report).aspx

3 Robson SC, Hunter S, Boys RJ, Dunlop W. Serial study of factors influencing changes in cardiac output during human pregnancy. *Am J Physiol* 1989;256:H1060–H1065.

4 Robson SK, Hunter S, Boys R, Dunlop W, Bryson M. Changes in cardiac output during epidural anaesthesia for Caesarean section. *Anaesthesia* 1986;44:465–479.

5 Clapp JF III, Capeless E. Cardiovascular function before, during and after the first and subsequent pregnancies. *Am J Cardiol* 1997;80:1469–1473.

6 Thorne SA. Pregnancy in heart disease. *Heart* 2004;90:450–456.

7 Siu SC, Sermer M, Colman JM et al. Prospective multicenter study of pregnancy outcomes in women with heart disease. *Circulation* 2001;104:515–521.

8 Presbitero P, Somerville J, Stone S et al. Pregnancy in cyanotic congenital heart disease. Outcome of mother and fetus. *Circulation* 1994;89:2673–2676.

9 Burn J, Brennan P, Little J et al. Recurrence risks in offspring of adults with major heart defects: results from first cohort of British Collaboration study. *Lancet* 1998;351:311–316.

10 Presbitero P, Prever SB, Brusca A. Interventional cardiology in pregnancy. *Eur Heart J* 1996;17:182–188.

11 Beauchesne LM, Connolly HM, Ammash NM, Warnes CA. Coarctation of the aorta: outcome of pregnancy. *J Am Coll Cardiol* 2001;38:1728–1733.

12 Lind J, Wallenburg HC. The Marfan syndrome and pregnancy: a retrospective study in a Dutch population. *Eur J Obstet Gynecol Reprod Biol* 2001;98:28–35.

13 Lipscomb KJ, Clayton Smith J, Clarke B, Donnai P, Harris R. Outcome of pregnancy in women with Marfan's syndrome. *Br J Obstet Gynaecol* 1997;104:201–206.

14 Singh H, Bolton PJ, Oakley CM. Outcome of pregnancy after surgical correction of tetralogy of Fallot. *BMJ* 1983;285:168.

15 Thorne SA, Nelson-Piercy C, MacGregor A. Risks of contraception and pregnancy in heart disease. *Heart* 2006;92:1520–1525.

16 Bédard E, Dimopoulos K, Gatzoulis MA. Has there been any progress made on pregnancy outcomes among women with pulmonary arterial hypertension? *Eur Heart J* 2009;30: 256–265.

17 Weiss BM, Zemp L, Seifert B, Hess OM. Outcome of pulmonary vascular disease in pregnancy: a systematic overview from 1978 through 1996. *J Am Coll Cardiol* 1998;31:1650–1657.

18 Tsiaras S, Poppas A. Mitral valve disease in pregnancy: outcomes and management.. *Obstet Med* 2009;2:6–10.

19 Horstkotte D, Fassbender D, Piper C. Balloon valvotomy during pregnancy. *J Heart Valve Dis* 2005;14:144–146.

20 Chan WS, Anand S, Ginsberg JS. Anticoagulation of pregnant women with mechanical heart valves. *Arch Intern Med* 2000;160:191–196.

21 Sadler L, McCowan L, White H, Stewart A, Bracken M, North R. Pregnancy outcomes and cardiac complications in women with mechanical, bioprosthetic and homograft valves. *BJOG* 2000;107:245–253.

22 Cotrufo M, De Feo M, De Santo L, Romano G, Della Corte A, Renzulli A. Risk of warfarin during pregnancy with mechanical valve prostheses. *Obstet Gynecol* 2002;99:35–40.

23 Oran B, Lee-Parritz A, Ansell J. Low molecular weight heparin for the prophylaxis of thromboembolism in women with prosthetic mechanical heart valves during pregnancy. *Thromb Haemost* 2004;92:747–751.

24 McClintock C. Use of therapeutic dose low molecular weight heparin during pregnancy in women with mechanical heart valves. *Obstet Med* 2010;3:40–42.

25 James AH, Jamison MG, Biswas MS, Brancazio LR, Swamy GK, Myers ER. Acute myocardial infarction in pregnancy: a United States population-based study. *Circulation* 2006;113: 1564–1571.

26 Roth A, Elkayam U. Acute myocardial infarction associated with pregnancy. *Ann Intern Med* 1996;125:751–757.

27 Ladner HE, Danielsen B, Gilbert WM. Acute myocardial infarction in pregnancy and the puerperium: a population-based study. *Obstet Gynecol* 2005;105:480–484.

28 Edison RJ, Muenke M. Central nervous system and limb anomalies in case reports of first-trimester statin exposure. *N Engl J Med* 2004;350:1579–1582.

29 Steer P, Gatzoulis M, Baker P (eds) *Cardiac Disease in Pregnancy.* London: RCOG Press, 2006.

30 Pearson GD, Veille JC, Rahimtoola S et al. Peripartum cardiomyopathy. National Heart, Lung and Blood Institute and Office of Rare Diseases (NIH). Workshop Recommendations and Review. *JAMA* 2000;283:1183–1188.

31 Felker GM, Thompson RE, Hare JM et al. Underlying causes and long-term survival in patients with initially unexplained cardiomyopathy. *N Engl J Med* 2000;342:1077–1084.

32 Elkayam U, Tummala PP, Rao K et al. Maternal and fetal outcomes of subsequent pregnancies in women with peripartum cardiomyopathy. *N Engl J Med* 2001;344:1567–1571.

33 Sliwa K, Fett J, Elkayam U. Peripartum cardiomyopathy. *Lancet* 2006;368:687–693.

34 Witlin AG, Mabie WC, Sibai BM. Peripartum cardiomyopathy: a longitudinal echocardiographic study. *Am J Obstet Gynecol* 1997;177:1129–1132.

35 Cordina R, McGuire MA. Maternal cardiac arrhythmias during pregnancy and lactation. *Obstet Med* 2010;3:8–16.

36 James PR. Drugs in pregnancy. Cardiovascular disease. *Best Pract Res Clin Obstet Gynaecol* 2001;15:903–911.

37 Magee LA, Downar E, Sermer M et al. Pregnancy outcome after gestational exposure to amiodarone. *Am J Obstet Gynecol* 1995; 172:1307–1311.

38 NICE Short Clinical Guidelines Technical Team. *Prophylaxis Against Infective Endocarditis: Antimicrobial Prophylaxis Against Infective Endocarditis in Adults and Children Undergoing Interventional Procedures.* NICE Clinical Guideline 64, 2008. Available at: www.nice.org.uk/nicemedia/pdf/CG64NICEguidance.pdf

39 Gould FK, Elliott TS, Foweraker J et al. Guidelines for the prevention of endocarditis: report of the Working Party of the British Society for Antimicrobial Chemotherapy. *J Antimicrob Chemother* 2006;57:1035–1042.

Chapter 13
Diabetes and Endocrine Disease in Pregnancy

Anne Dornhorst[1] *and Catherine Williamson*[2]

[1] Hammersmith Hospital, Imperial College Healthcare NHS Trust, London, UK
[2] Institute of Reproductive and Developmental Biology, Imperial College London, London, UK

Diabetes in pregnancy

Recent years have seen a rapid rise in the prevalence of diabetes in pregnancy. This increase reflects the increasing number of women of childbearing age with pre-gestational type 2 diabetes mellitus (type 2 DM) and the rise in women being diagnosed with gestational diabetes mellitus (GDM). Over the last two decades across Europe the antenatal population has become older, more obese and more ethnically diverse, all risk factors for type 2 DM and GDM. Today in many European urban antenatal clinics the number of women with pre-gestational type 2 DM outnumber those with type 1 DM. Not only are pregnant women with type 2 DM likely to be older, more obese and belong to an non-white ethnic minority, they are also more likely to have higher levels of social deprivation than either women with type 1 DM or the general antenatal population without diabetes [1,2]. Women with type 2 DM therefore enter pregnancy with established risk factors for a poor pregnancy outcome (Fig. 13.1).

The increasing proportion of women with type 2 DM, with their associated risk, in today's antenatal clinics helps to explain why pregnancy outcomes in women with diabetes have not appreciably improved over the last 40 years despite major advances in obstetric, neonatal and diabetic care. Despite some improvement in pregnancy outcomes reported from specialized obstetric units for women with type 1 DM, overall congenital abnormalities, stillbirths and perinatal deaths remain twofold to fourfold higher among women with pre-gestational diabetes [3]. In addition around 40–50% of all births have evidence of growth acceleration above the 90th percentile for gestational age. The rate of Caesarean births also remains unacceptably high at 67% of all births in an audit of over 3800 births in 2003 in England, Wales and Northern Ireland to women with type 1 and type 2 DM. Of these Caesarean births, 56% were performed as emergencies [2].

A small percentage of women with diabetes in pregnancy have a monogenetic or mitochondrial cause for their diabetes that would have been misclassified as type 1 or 2 DM in the past but which is now being diagnosed due to advances in genetic screening. The importance of recognizing this cohort is that pregnancy outcome is determined as much by the genetic mutation as by the diabetes.

Diabetic and obstetric management, from pre-conceptual counselling through to postnatal care, is influenced by the type of diabetes the woman is experiencing (the main categories of diabetes are shown in Table 13.1). This chapter covers the clinical management of pregnancies complicated by pre-gestational diabetes and the screening and management of GDM. The consequences of a diabetic pregnancy for neonates and their long-term health are also discussed.

General principles for the management of diabetic pregnancies

Maternal hyperglycaemia increases the risk of poor pregnancy outcomes (Table 13.2). Congenital abnormalities, miscarriage, accelerated fetal growth, late stillbirth, birth trauma and neonatal hypoglycaemia all increase with increasing maternal glycaemia. Similarly, the long-term health risks for the child of obesity and future risk of type 2 DM all increase with increasing maternal glycaemia. For these reasons the principal tenet for management, from the time of conception to the time of delivery, is to strive for maternal euglycaemia. Apart from glycaemic management, diabetic-specific complications such as retinopathy and nephropathy need to be screened for and treated when necessary.

For women with pre-gestational diabetes the association between pre-pregnancy glycaemic control and the risk of congenital malformations begins at the upper level of the normal non-diabetic range [4]. The teratogenic

Dewhurst's Textbook of Obstetrics & Gynaecology, Eighth Edition. Edited by D. Keith Edmonds.
© 2012 John Wiley and Sons, Ltd. Published 2012 by John Wiley and Sons, Ltd.

RISK FACTORS
Adverse pregnancy outcome
Obesity
Age
Ethnicity
Social deprivation

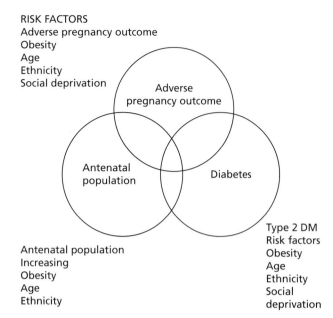

Antenatal population
Increasing
Obesity
Age
Ethnicity

Type 2 DM
Risk factors
Obesity
Age
Ethnicity
Social deprivation

Fig. 13.1 Shared risk factors for poor pregnancy outcomes and type 2 diabetes.

Table 13.1 The main categories of diabetes encountered in obstetric practice.

Type 1 diabetes
Absolute or near absolute insulin deficiency due to autoimmune destruction of pancreatic β cells. Typical presentation under 20 years old, with only 10% having a first-degree relative affected. Not associated with obesity. Accounts for approximately 5% of all diabetes outside pregnancy, but approximately 50% among women of childbearing age

Type 2 diabetes
Relative insulin deficiency and decreased insulin sensitivity. Presents typically over 20 years old, with approximately 60% having a first-degree relative affected. Strongly associated with obesity. Accounts for approximately 90% of all diabetes outside pregnancy and approximately 50% among women of childbearing age

Monogenetic diabetes
Maturity-onset diabetes of the young. Owing to a single gene mutation causing a defect in pancreatic β-cell insulin secretion. Present from birth but typically diagnosed within the second and third decade. Autosomal dominant with approximately 95% having a first-degree relative affected. Not associated with obesity. Accounts for less than 2% of all diabetes outside pregnancy

Mitochondrial diabetes
Arises from a mutation in mitochondrial DNA leading to a defect in insulin secretion; it is thus maternally inherited. Associated with a number of other medical problems including sensorineural deafness, a tendency for stroke and lactic acidosis. Diabetes usually develops in the mid thirties. Not associated with obesity. Accounts for less than 1% of all diabetes outside pregnancy

Secondary diabetes
Diabetes due to other medical conditions, i.e. pancreatitis, cystic fibrosis, glucocorticoids and other drugs. Accounts for approximately 2% of all diabetes outside pregnancy

Table 13.2 The influence of maternal hyperglycaemia on mother, fetus, neonate and young adult.

First trimester	
Implantation	Inhibits trophectoderm differentiation
Embryogenesis	Increases oxidative stress affecting expression of critical genes essential for embryogenesis
Organogenesis	Activates the diacylglycerol–protein kinase C cascade, increasing congenital defects
Miscarriage	Increases premature programmed cell death of key progenitor cells of the blastocyst
Second trimester	
Endocrine pancreas	Stimulates fetal β cells
Fetal growth	Stimulates fetal hyperinsulinaemia that results in growth acceleration seen on ultrasound by 26 weeks
Third trimester	
Fetal growth	A major fetal substrate and determinant for accelerated fetal growth
Adipose disposition	Stimulates hyperinsulinaemia that promotes fat disposition including intra-abdominal fat
Lung maturation	Stimulates hyperinsulinaemia that delays lung maturation by inhibiting surfactant proteins
Stillbirth	Is associated with defects in placental maturation that increase the risk of fetal hypoxia
Delivery	
Birth trauma	By causing accelerated fetal growth there is an increased risk of shoulder dystocia predisposing to birth trauma and asphyxia
Neonate	
Hypoglycaemia	Stimulates fetal hyperinsulinaemia that predisposes to neonatal hypoglycaemia
Hypocalcaemia	Alters the placental expression of calbindin mRNA that affects calcium status at birth
Polycythaemia	Stimulates fetal hyperinsulinaemia that enhances antepartum haemopoiesis as does fetal hypoxia
Cardiomyopathy	Stimulates fetal hyperinsulinaemia that predisposes to hypertrophic cardiomyopathy
Adolescence/adulthood	
Obesity	Intrauterine exposure predisposes to the metabolic syndrome, independent of any genetic susceptibility
Type 2 diabetes	Intrauterine exposure predisposes to type 2 diabetes, independent of any genetic susceptibility

effect of maternal hyperglycaemia occurs during blastocyst formation and continues through the period of embryogenesis and fetal organogenesis until the 12th gestational week. In order to significantly limit early fetal loss and the added risk of congenital abnormalities, women with diabetes need to optimize their glycaemic control prior to pregnancy. Hence the importance of planned pregnancies, pre-conception counselling and the continuation of contraception before glycaemic control has been optimized.

The normal physiological changes in pregnancy facilitate maternal–placental–fetal transfer of glucose, especially postprandially. In pregnancies complicated by diabetes, maternal glucose is transferred to the fetus rather than being taken up preferentially in maternal muscle or fat stores. From the 12th gestational week circulating glucose in the fetus stimulates secretion of fetal insulin, which acts as a potent intrauterine growth factor. Hence the need for exemplary maternal glycaemic control throughout the whole of pregnancy.

Gestational diabetes occurring *de novo* in the latter half of pregnancy as a consequence of the physiological metabolic changes of pregnancy is not associated with congenital malformations but is associated with accelerated fetal growth. There is a clear continuum of risk, beginning within the range of normal maternal glycaemic levels and extending up to the levels seen in type 2 DM [5].

With the rise of obesity among today's general antenatal population the impact of obesity on pregnancy outcomes is becoming clearer. Obesity is an independent risk factor for late stillbirth, birth trauma and maternal complications after delivery [6,7]. The prevention and management of obesity in women of childbearing age has become a public health issue and is not covered in this chapter.

All pregnancies complicated by diabetes should be under the care of a hospital-based multidisciplinary consultant-led team, with a named obstetrician and diabetologist working to locally agreed guidelines based on national and international guidelines [8] (Table 13.3).

 Summary box 13.1

Increasing maternal hyperglycaemia is associated with an increasing risk of:
- congenital malformations;
- stillbirth;
- accelerated fetal growth;
- neonatal hypoglycaemia.

Pre-conception counselling

Women with diabetes who attend a pre-conception clinic have better pregnancy outcomes than those who do not. In addition to giving general healthy lifestyle advice on healthy weight management, diet, exercise, alcohol and cigarette smoking, these clinics provide an opportunity for glycaemic control to be intensified, high-dose folic acid supplements (5mg) to be prescribed and medications to be reviewed so that potentially harmful drugs, such as angiotensin-converting enzyme (ACE) inhibitors,

Table 13.3 A structured approach to the management of diabetic pregnancies.

Prior to pregnancy
Pre-conception counselling

First trimester
Referral to a combined multidisciplinary diabetic obstetric antenatal clinic
Dating scan
Screening for diabetic complications
Screening for non-diabetic comorbidities
Assessment and optimization of glycaemia
Advice on hypoglycaemia prevention

Second trimester
Optimization of glycaemic control
Screening for congenital abnormalities
Surveillance for medical obstetric complications
Assessment of fetal growth

Third trimester
Optimization of glycaemic control
Assessment of fetal growth
Timing and mode of delivery

Delivery
Protocols for insulin during labour and delivery

Post partum
Adjustment of insulin dosage
Breast-feeding
Discussing contraception

---

angiotensin receptor blockers and statins (HMG-CoA reductase inhibitors), can be stopped or switched to safer alternatives.

Pre-conception clinics provide an opportunity to engage positively with women planning pregnancy and allow discussion of the diabetic care pathway, including how to rapidly access the obstetric service once pregnant. These clinics should explain the reason for increased fetal and maternal surveillance and provide reassurance that with good glycaemic control the risks associated with a diabetic pregnancy can be reduced to those approaching the background antenatal population. It is important to stress that any improvement in glycaemic control before a pregnancy reduces the risk for that pregnancy [9]. The high numbers of women who fail to engage in pre-conception counselling is often attributed to the negative and unsupportive messages that these women have received over the years. Overall, 95% of women with pregestational diabetes give birth to a healthy infant, although this figure would be higher if glycaemic control in early pregnancy could be improved.

Pre-conception clinics provide an opportunity to screen for diabetic microvascular disease, retinopathy, nephropathy and neuropathy. In addition women at risk of macrovascular disease can be identified. These complications increase with duration of diabetes and are therefore more common in women with type 1 than type 2 DM as many of these women will have had type 1 DM for over 20 years.

Retinopathy can worsen with rapid improvement in glycaemic control, as can occur during the pre-conception period and in early pregnancy. It is therefore recommended that pregnancy is postponed if significant retinopathy is present to allow laser treatment to be given. Women should be reassured that although retinopathy can deteriorate in pregnancy, it usually reverts to pre-pregnancy levels after the birth and if required laser treatment is safe in pregnancy.

As a generalization women can be reassured that any deterioration in renal function during pregnancy usually reverts to pre-pregnancy levels of function after the birth. Women who have significant diabetic nephropathy (proteinuria >2 g per 24 hours) should be informed of their high risk of pre-eclampsia and preterm birth. Women with microalbuminuria and lesser degrees of proteinuria should be made aware that they will require meticulous blood pressure monitoring during pregnancy as they are at increased of pregnancy-induced hypertension.

Diabetic neuropathy is more common in women with type 1 DM, and autonomic neuropathy is particularly problematic in pregnancy as it blunts the adrenergic and metabolic response to hypoglycaemia, potentially leading to frequent and severe episodes of hypoglycaemia. This risk is especially prevalent in early pregnancy before maternal and placental hormones have increased sufficiently to increase insulin resistance and minimize this risk. Women with autonomic neuropathy should receive dietary advice to reduce this risk of hypoglycaemia and their partners instructed on how to administer glucagon for the management of severe hypoglycaemia.

Diabetes is associated with macrovascular disease and premature coronary heart disease, and this risk increases with duration of diabetes and increasing maternal age. A previous history of cardiovascular disease or its diagnosis in pregnancy is associated with significant maternal morbidity, and therefore women with a previous history of ischaemic heart disease or considered at risk from it should be referred to a cardiologist prior to pregnancy.

To achieve the pre-pregnancy guideline glycaemic targets ($HbA_{1c} < 6.1\%$, fasting blood glucose <5.5 mmol/L, 2-hour post-meal glucose <7.8 mmol/L) requires most women to intensify their glycaemic management prior to pregnancy. This is best done with frequent home glucose monitoring and the help of a diabetic specialist nurse.

For all women with type 1 DM, four to five daily insulin injections or an insulin pump will be required. For women not on an insulin pump, insulin should be given as part of a basal-bolus regimen with a long-acting basal insulin, usually given at night, and rapid or short-acting insulin boluses taken with each meal. There is some evidence that the risk of hypoglycaemia for women with type 1 DM in early pregnancy is lessened with the use of an insulin pump and suitable patients should be considered for an insulin pump prior to pregnancy.

For women with type 2 DM, a basal-bolus regimen is also recommended as it offers the most flexibility around food timing and exercise and lessens the risk of hypoglycaemia in early pregnancy. For some women who have had type 2 DM for only a short time and have been well controlled on diet and metformin alone, adequate glycaemic control may be achievable prior to and early in pregnancy with either a twice-daily mixture (of a short- and medium-acting insulin) or with just a rapid-acting insulin with meals. However, by the second trimester most women will require a basal-bolus regimen.

Continuing with the oral agent metformin for women with type 2 DM before pregnancy is recommended by the UK clinical guidelines, although this is not endorsed by other national guidelines. While there is no evidence that the sulphonylureas are teratogenic in early pregnancy, these agents are associated with less good glycaemic control in pregnancy than insulin and less favourable pregnancy outcomes.

 Summary box 13.2

Women with pre-gestational diabetes should be informed to:
- take 5 mg folic acid prior to conception and for the following 12 weeks;
- achieve the best possible HbA_{1c} prior to conception;
- ensure that all routine medications are safe for pregnancy;
- be screened for possible diabetic eye and kidney disease.

First trimester

Referral to a combined multidisciplinary diabetic obstetric antenatal clinic

Pregnant women with diabetes should be cared for by a multidisciplinary diabetic obstetric antenatal clinic. The team should comprise a named obstetrician, diabetologist, specialized midwife, diabetic nurse and dietitian. There needs to be clear guidance for how women and their primary care team can access this clinic rapidly once pregnancy is confirmed, to enable glycaemic management to be intensified promptly. Between antenatal clinic visits regular phone contact with the diabetic nurse throughout the first trimester can help lessen clinic visits.

Dating ultrasound scan

An early ultrasound at 6–8 weeks should be performed to assess viability and for dating purposes. Relying on ultrasound scanning later in pregnancy for dating is less accurate and this is important as the majority of women will go on to have an elective birth before 40 gestational weeks.

Screening for diabetic complications

Retinal screening is usually performed annually using retinal photographs taken in primary care. All women should have dilated eye examination preferably by retinal photography in the first trimester with referral to an ophthalmologist if retinopathy is present.

Screening for diabetic nephropathy comprises measurement of the albumin/creatinine ratio and serum creatinine level. If either is elevated, meticulous attention should be paid to blood pressure control, with the early introduction of safe hypertensive agents if the blood pressure is elevated. For women with significant proteinuria or serum creatinine above 120 μmol/L, the introduction of aspirin or heparin should be considered.

Women with diabetic autonomic neuropathy are at increased risk of gastroparesis that can increase in early pregnancy, causing nausea and vomiting, poor glycaemic control and an increased risk of hypoglycaemia. Dietary advice and non-pharmacological treatment should be given prior to treatment with antiemetics such as antihistamines.

Screening for non-diabetic maternal comorbidities

Women with type 1 DM are more susceptible to other autoimmune diseases. The prevalence of autoimmune thyroid disease is sufficiently high to warrant all women with type 1 DM, not known to have thyroid disease, to be screened in early pregnancy. Other associated autoimmune diseases associated with type 1 DM should only be screened for if clinically indicated.

Women with type 2 DM are likely to have a number of related comorbidities associated with insulin resistance, such as obesity, hypertension and dyslipidaemia. Hypertriglyceridaemia associated with type 2 DM is associated with increased circulating glycerol and fatty acids that can act as fetal fuel substrates increasing the risk of accelerated growth. Women with type 2 DM who are obese should receive appropriate dietary advice that should include an appropriate weight gain target. General encouragement to increase walking especially after meals is helpful to lessen postprandial blood glucose rises as well as weight gain.

Screening for chromosomal anomalies

Chromosomal abnormalities such as Down's syndrome are not increased in women with diabetes. However, screening for Down's syndrome at the end of the first trimester (13 weeks 6 days) using the 'combined' test (nuchal translucency, β-human chorionic gonadotrophin and pregnancy-associated plasma protein A) may detect increased nuchal translucency due to diabetic-related malformations such as structural malformations of the heart.

Assessment and optimization of glycaemia

The first HbA_{1c} measurement taken in pregnancy provides an assessment of the level of glycaemic control around the time of organogenesis and is an indicator of the risk of major congenital malformations.

To optimize maternal glycaemic control in order to minimize excess maternal glucose transfer requires fasting maternal plasma glucose levels below 6 mmol/L and 1-hour postprandial levels below 7.8 mmol/L. As previously mentioned, this degree of glycaemic control requires a highly flexible insulin regimen, best provided by a basal-bolus insulin regimen or an insulin pump. The newer rapid-acting insulin analogues are well suited for targeting postprandial glycaemia and NovoRapid is licensed for use in pregnancy; the long-acting insulin analogues such as insulin glargine and insulin detemir, although providing better basal cover than the human intermediate-acting NHP insulins, have yet to be licensed for use in pregnancy.

The adjustment of insulin dose is based on frequent daily blood glucose monitoring that should include a fasting value, a 1-hour post-meal value and a bedtime reading. The skill in adjusting the insulin dose around individual patients with varying lifestyles, duration of diabetes and diabetic complications is considerable. There is no one formula that is applicable for all women with type 1 or type 2 DM, and the precise insulin regimen has to be formulated on an individual basis between the woman, who is often extremely adept in doing this herself, and the diabetic team.

Diabetic ketoacidosis is associated with high fetal loss and requires prompt hospital admission and treatment. Ketoacidosis develops more quickly in pregnancy and at lower blood glucose levels due to enhanced maternal lipolysis. It is therefore important to remind women with type 1 DM never to stop their insulin even if not eating due to nausea or vomiting. Women with type 1 DM should be able to test for ketones, preferably using blood testing strips rather than urine ketone dipsticks. Advice needs to be given on how to manage and monitor low levels of ketonaemia (<1.5 mmol/L) and when to seek hospital advice urgently if unwell or if blood ketones are higher than 1.5 mmol/L. Positive tests for urinary ketones are common before breakfast but these should clear rapidly after the breakfast insulin dose and eating; if urinary ketonuria is persistent, urgent medical advice is required. Women with type 2 DM usually have sufficient insulin to prevent ketoacidosis outside pregnancy; however, because of the profound insulin resistance associated with pregnancy and increased maternal lipolysis, ketoacidosis can occasionally occur especially in the presence of vomiting.

Advice on prevention of hypoglycaemia

Maternal hypoglycaemia is frequent during early pregnancy in insulin-treated women. Hypoglycaemia is not by itself harmful to the fetus but can occasionally be life-threatening for the woman. Maternal deaths among women with type 1 DM continue to be reported in the triennial report of the Confidential Enquiries into Maternal Deaths in the UK. Risk factors for severe hypoglycaemia are duration of type 1 DM, poor hypoglycaemic awareness, autonomic neuropathy, gastroparesis, renal impairment and sleeping alone. All women must be aware of the risk of hypoglycaemia as they intensify their insulin management and be given advice on timing of meals and snacks; in addition family members need to be aware of how to recognize and treat hypoglycaemia, including how to give glucagon. All women should carry identifications cards specifying that they are taking insulin and what to do if they become hypoglycaemic. Specific advice on driving should include the need to perform a blood test before getting into a car and not to drive if experiencing hypoglycaemic episodes without warning signs. The rapid-acting insulin analogues such as NovoRapid have been shown to reduce severe hypoglycaemic episodes, especially at night, in pregnancy.

Summary box 13.3

Women treated with insulin should be informed that:
- maternal hypoglycaemia is frequent in early pregnancy;
- the risk of hypoglycaemia is increased with increasing duration of type 1 diabetes;
- to carry sweets and a sweet drink with them at all times;
- to carry/wear some form of identification specifying that they are taking insulin;
- to instruct their partners on how and when to be able to give glucagon;
- to stop driving if they lose their awareness of hypoglycaemia.

Second trimester

Optimization of glycaemic control

By the start of the second trimester in non-diabetic pregnancies there is a fall in fasting glucose and a rise in postprandial glucose levels. By the middle of the second trimester, maternal insulin resistance starts to increase due to high concentrations of circulating maternal fatty acids and placental hormones. By term in women without diabetes insulin secretion has to increase two to three times to control blood glucose levels after meals. Before 20 weeks' gestation, women with diabetes who started pregnancy well controlled may not have needed to increase their overall insulin dosage and some may have actually reduced it due to nausea and decreased food intake. However, after 20 weeks' gestation insulin requirements begin to rise, usually doubling or trebling by term. The diabetic nurse should ensure that the woman has the knowledge and confidence to increase her own insulin in response to her glucose readings. As the basal night-time

insulin is increased, it may be necessary to give half this dose in the morning to avoid nocturnal hypoglycaemia.

Women with type 2 DM are usually insulin resistant prior to pregnancy and by the second trimester, when insulin resistance increases further, may require doses that by the end of pregnancy exceed 300 units daily. The coadministration of metformin can help to reduce the total insulin dose required and help limit overall weight gain.

Screening for congenital abnormalities

A detailed ultrasound scan should be offered to all women between 18 and 20 weeks' gestation to look for major congenital abnormalities. This scan should specifically examine those structures most commonly affected in diabetic pregnancies, namely the spine, skull, kidneys and heart. The scan should also ensure visualization of the four chambers of the heart together with the ventricular outflow tracts.

Surveillance for medical obstetric complications

Women should be rescreened for retinopathy using digital retinal photographs at 26 weeks if there was any evidence of retinopathy in the first trimester; referral to an ophthalmologist is required if the retinopathy has progressed.

Women with diabetes have an increased risk of hypertension in pregnancy, including pre-eclampsia. Serial clinic blood pressure measurements and urine dipstick for protein and laboratory analysis for albumin/creatinine ratio should be performed and any sign of hypertension treated promptly and appropriately (see Chapter 11).

Assessment of fetal growth

Ultrasound scans for assessment of fetal growth should start at the end of the second trimester and be repeated every 4 weeks until 36 weeks of gestation. Serial measurements of the fetal abdominal circumference expressed as a percentile can provide an indication of growth acceleration or restriction. Measurement of liquor volume should also be recorded serially as polyhydramnios is more common in diabetic pregnancies.

Third trimester

Optimization of glycaemic control

During the third trimester maternal insulin resistance continues to increase along with insulin requirements. Achieving good glycaemic control tends to become easier as the insulin resistance protects women from severe hypoglycaemic episodes.

If glucocorticosteroids are required for lung maturation, insulin requirements over the following 72 hours will need to increase. If two 12-mg beclomethasone or dexamethasone injections are given at 12–24-hour intervals, it is important that the insulin dose is proactively increased or the woman admitted and intravenous insulin (on a sliding scale) administered over the 72 hours, given in addition to her normal insulin dose.

Assessment of fetal growth

Evidence on serial ultrasound scans of a rising abdominal circumference percentile in relation to head circumference or biparietal diameter is indicative of accelerated fetal growth. This pattern of fetal growth is seen in association with poor maternal control and the resulting fetal hyper-insulinaemia. Fetal insulin is a potent growth factor that promotes excessive fat disposition within the abdomen and enlargement of the visceral organs, including the liver and heart. While the term 'macrosomia' is widely used clinically and in the literature to describe infants of mothers with diabetes, the precise definition of macro-somia is poorly characterized, with definitions varying from an absolute birthweight above 4, 4.5 or 5 kg to a percentile birthweight in excess of 90, 95 or 97.5%. As birthweight is dependent on gestational age, sex, ethnic origin, parental height and maternal weight, any defini-tion based on absolute weight is best avoided. With diabe-tes it is the pattern of fetal growth rather than the absolute or percentile birthweight that is important. The influence of maternal obesity alone accounts for many of the infants of mothers with type 2 DM having high birthweights.

Serial ultrasound scans also help identify infants with fetal growth restriction or asymmetrical growth restric-tion (poor increase in abdominal circumference centile growth compared with head circumference). Such growth patterns are indicative of uteroplacental insufficiency, as frequently seen in women with renal impairment, vascu-lar disease or hypertension. If detected, fetal monitoring should be intensified to assess the optimal timing of birth.

Timing and mode of delivery

Because of the approximately fourfold higher risk of late unexpected stillbirth among women with diabetes [1,10], national and international guidelines advocate that birth should occur before 39 weeks' gestation, ideally between weeks 38 and 39. The exact timing and mode of delivery is best deferred to after the fetal ultrasound at 36 weeks, when a more informed discussion can take place based on maternal and fetal well-being and the estimated fetal weight.

The high rates of emergency Caesarean section among women with diabetes (as high as 56% of all births to all mothers with pre-gestational diabetes between 2002 and 2003 in England, Wales and Northern Ireland) is partly a consequence of failed induction at 38 weeks' gestation in nulliparous women with type 1 DM. While women with type 2 DM are more likely to be multiparous and there-fore induction of labour before term should be more suc-cessful, obesity is a risk factor for poor uterine contractility and this is probably a contributing factor to the high Caesarean rates among women with type 2 DM.

The risk of birth trauma increases with increasing birth-weight. The risk of shoulder dystocia is approximately 3% when the birthweight is 4–4.5 kg, and 10–14% when the birthweight is above 4.5 kg. However, a policy based purely on estimated birthweight by ultrasound (4000 or 4500 g) would result in an unacceptable rate of Caesarean section. Planning mode of delivery of a large baby detected on ultrasound of a mother with diabetes needs to include other medical, obstetric and fetal factors.

Birth

Protocols for insulin during labour and delivery

There need to be clear written guidelines for the manage-ment of women with diabetes on the labour ward and how insulin therapy is managed during labour. Most women will be admitted electively, be it for induction or Caesarean section, and clear instructions of what diabetic medication to take the evening prior to admission should be given.

Women being admitted for a planned induction should be encouraged to take their normal insulin doses the night before. Once admitted they should continue with their short-acting bolus insulin to cover meals, only switching to an intravenous insulin sliding scale once in labour or a decision has been taken to perform a Caesarean section.

Ideally, elective Caesarean section should be planned for early morning, with the woman advised to take her normal bolus insulin with her evening meal and two-thirds of her usual basal insulin the night before admis-sion. Once on the ward an insulin sliding scale can be started, with the dose adjusted downwards straight after delivery (see below).

Although there is no absolute right or wrong way to give insulin during this period, it is usual hospital policy to start an intravenous insulin sliding scale with a 5% glucose–insulin infusion during active labour or for an operative delivery and this is continued until the mother starts taking meals. During labour and delivery hourly blood glucose monitoring should be done. Immediately following the birth the insulin dose must be halved (see below).

After birth

Insulin requirements drop to pre-pregnancy levels once the placenta is delivered. Insulin is not excreted into breast milk and is considered completely safe for use during breast-feeding. Women with type 1 DM can recom-mence their pre-pregnancy insulin regimen as soon as they are eating and drinking normally. Women with type 2 DM prior to pregnancy can also restart their pre-pregnancy doses of insulin. The post-delivery dose of insulin should be clearly written in the hospital notes as part of the delivery plan.

Women with type 2 DM previously treated with metformin can continue this while breast-feeding as only very low levels are excreted in breast milk. The oral sulphonylureas in use today are highly protein bound and, as this binding is non-ionic, they are unlikely to be displaced by other drugs and to be free to pass into breast milk. However, there are theoretical concerns that they could cause neonatal hypoglycaemia if they were to be excreted into breast milk, and for this reason metformin is favoured over the sulphonylurea drugs when oral hypoglycaemic drugs are required while breast-feeding.

During the postpartum period advice on suitable contraception should be offered and the need for preconception counselling before any future pregnancy.

Screening for and management of gestational diabetes

Gestational diabetes is glucose intolerance first recognized in pregnancy. This definition includes women with previously undiagnosed diabetes at one end of the spectrum and those with disturbances of glucose intolerance resulting form the metabolic changes in late pregnancy that abut onto the upper limit of the normal range. Glucose intolerance in pregnancy is a continuum and there has been enormous controversy over where the risk to pregnancy outcome actually occurs. There is no controversy that women with undiagnosed diabetes that is detected in pregnancy should be as vigorously managed as those women with pre-gestational diabetes. As the background prevalence of type 2 DM increases, the percentage of women identified as having GDM who have truly had undiagnosed diabetes prior to that pregnancy will increase. A much smaller percentage of women will be in the preclinical stages of type 1 DM. How best to screen for pre-existing diabetes in early pregnancy has not been resolved.

The Hyperglycemia and Adverse Pregnancy Outcome (HAPO) study published in 2008 was a 7-year international study that recruited 23 325 pregnant women with no prior diabetes from nine countries. Each woman underwent a 75-g oral glucose tolerance test (OGTT) between 24 and 32 weeks of gestation and was followed to the end of the pregnancy [5]. This study showed that increasing fasting glucose as well as the 1- and 2-hour post-OGTT level were all linearly correlated to maternal, perinatal and neonatal outcomes, defined as a birthweight above the 90th percentile for gestational age, primary Caesarean delivery, clinically diagnosed neonatal hypoglycaemia, and cord-blood serum C-peptide level above the 90th percentile. The study was also able to demonstrate that there was a strong interaction between maternal obesity, GDM and pregnancy outcome. The prevalence of macrosomia among the 17 244 non-obese women in HAPO with no GDM was 6.7% (1147),

Table 13.4 Risk factors for gestational diabetes.

Body mass index >30 kg/m^2
Gestational diabetes in a previous pregnancy
Age >25 years
Family history of diabetes
Ethnicity: belonging to a non-white ethnic group
Previous delivery of a large baby
Previous stillbirth

compared with 10.2% for non-obese women with GDM, 13.6% for obese women without GDM, and 20.2% for obese women with GDM.

Since the HAPO, the International Association of Diabetes in Pregnancy Study Groups (IADPSG) Consensus Panel has recommended cut-off thresholds for GDM after a 75-g OGTT between 24 and 32 weeks' gestation as follows: plasma glucose greater than 5.1 mmol/L fasting, 10.0 mmol/L at 1 hour or 8.5 mmol/L at 2 hours [11]. These cut-offs were based on the risk of the primary adverse outcomes being 1.75 times the estimated odds for these outcomes. These new guidelines identified approximately 16% of the entire HAPO study cohort as having GDM. While different criteria exist across Europe and the USA for its diagnosis, there has been a general recognition internationally to move towards the 75-g OGTT as a screening test for GDM. The decision to screen universally or to only target those women with recognized risk factors (Table 13.4) has not been resolved. Universal screening has cost and personnel resource implications.

The benefits of treating women who fulfil the WHO criteria for impaired glucose tolerance (IGT) between 24 and 34 weeks' gestation has been shown in an Australian randomized clinical trial involving 1000 women with GDM in which perinatal outcomes were reduced [12]. The 500 women with GDM randomized to active intervention (which included diet, glucose monitoring and insulin if required) showed better neonatal outcomes than those of women who received no intervention. This study also highlighted the 10% higher rate of induction of labour among the intervention group, although the Caesarean section rate was similar in both groups.

Once GDM is diagnosed the glycaemic targets set for GDM in pregnancy should be similar to those for all women with diabetes, namely fasting blood glucose below 6 mmol/L and 1-hour postprandial glucose below 7.8 mmol/L. The first line of treatment of GDM is with diet and modest exercise alone; however if the glycaemic targets are not met, metformin alone or metformin and insulin is required.

In the UK the use of metformin for the management of GDM has been endorsed since the publication of the MiG trial (Metformin versus Insulin for the treatment of

Gestational diabetes [13]) in 2008. This trial randomized 751 women with GDM at 20–33 weeks of gestation to open treatment with metformin (supplemented with insulin if required) or insulin alone. Of the 363 women assigned to metformin, 92.6% continued to receive metformin until delivery and 46.3% required insulin therapy to be added. No difference was seen in the primary composite outcome of neonatal hypoglycaemia, respiratory distress, need for phototherapy, birth trauma, 5-min Apgar score less than 7 or prematurity. The metformin-treated women compared with the insulin group had the added benefit of less pregnancy weight gain and less weight retention at 6 weeks after delivery. In addition, more women in the metformin-treated than the insulin-treated group stated that they would choose to receive their assigned treatment again in a further pregnancy (76.6% vs. 27.2%).

Although the newer sulphonylurea agents such as glibenclamide appear safe when given after 15 weeks' gestation, their use with or with out metformin is not widely used in those parts of the world where insulin is readily accessible [14]. However, when access to insulin is problematic, oral hypoglycaemic agents provide an alternative therapeutic option.

Among women identified as having GDM, excluding those who have diabetes after delivery, approximately 50% will progress to type 2 DM over the subsequent 20 years. Lifestyle intervention that minimizes weight gain and encourages physical activity has been shown to halve the progression rate from IGT to diabetes over a 4–5 year period among women with previous GDM, as does the administration of metformin. It is therefore important that all women diagnosed with GDM receive lifestyle counselling and have their glucose tolerance status checked annually with a fasting plasma glucose, HbA_{1c} or OGTT. These women should also be advised to seek early screening for glucose intolerance in any future pregnancy as recurrence rates are high.

> ### Summary box 13.4
>
> - The glycaemic targets for GDM are similar to those for pre-gestational diabetes.
> - The UK guidelines endorse the use of metformin during pregnancy.
> - Approximately 50% of women will progress to type 2 DM over 20 years.
> - After a GDM pregnancy annual screening for diabetes should occur.
> - Pre-conception counselling is required for future pregnancies.
> - Early screening for diabetes or GDM in future pregnancies.

Neonatal and longer-term consequences of a diabetic pregnancy

The neonate of mothers with diabetes, in addition to the increased risk of congenital abnormalities, is at increased risk of a number of transient metabolic disturbances as outlined in Table 13.2 [15]. The commonest metabolic disturbance is hypoglycaemia, a result of persistent fetal hyperinsulinaemia after birth when the maternal transfer of glucose has ceased. The other metabolic conditions are transient and can be attributed to overexposure to maternal glucose and other fuel substrates.

Recent studies on children of mothers with both type 1 and type 2 DM have shown that there is an increased risk of childhood obesity and metabolic disturbances in adolescence including an increased risk of glucose intolerance [16–18]. This risk is higher among children of mothers whose glycaemic control was poor in pregnancy. As young adults, children of mothers with diabetes have an increased risk of type 2 DM, the diabetes emerging at an earlier age than did their mother's diabetes. These follow-up studies of children of mother with diabetes are highly suggestive that maternal diabetes can influence aspects of fetal metabolic programming, and stresses the importance of achieving exemplary glycaemic control in all diabetic pregnancies.

> ### Summary box 13.5
>
> The neonate of a women with diabetes is at increased risk of:
> - neonatal hypoglycaemia;
> - childhood obesity;
> - metabolic changes in adolescents that predispose to type 2 DM.

Endocrine disease

Thyroid disease is the commonest endocrine disorder in pregnant women and this is therefore considered in more detail than other endocrinopathies. However, pituitary, adrenal and parathyroid disease may have serious consequences for the mother and fetus and these are also discussed.

Thyroid disease

Thyroid function in normal pregnancy

The thyroid hormones thyroxine (T4) and triiodothyronine (T3) are synthesized within the thyroid follicles. Thyroid-stimulating hormone (TSH) stimulates synthesis and release of T3 and T4, in addition to uptake of iodide which is essential for thyroid hormone synthesis. Although T4 is synthesized in greater quantities, it is

Table 13.5 Normal ranges for thyroid function tests in pregnancy.

	FT4 (pmol/L)	FT3 (pmol/L)	TSH (mU/L)
Non-pregnant	11–23	4–9	0–4
First trimester	11–22	4–8	0–1.6
Second trimester	11–19	4–7	0.1–1.18
Third trimester	7–15	3–5	0.7–7.3*

* Current guidance for management of thyroxine replacement in women with autoimmune hypothyroidism is to maintain TSH ≤2.5 mU/L.
Source: Parker [19], Chan & Swaminathan [20] and Kotarba *et al.* [21].

converted into the more potent T3 by deiodination in peripheral tissues.

During normal pregnancy the circulating levels of thyroid-binding globulin increase, and as a consequence total T3 and T4 levels also increase. Therefore, free hormone levels should be measured in pregnant women. TSH levels should be interpreted with caution in the first trimester as human chorionic gonadotrophin has a weak stimulatory effect on the TSH receptor. Table 13.5 summarizes the normal ranges for TSH, free T4 and free T3 in pregnancy.

The fetus cannot synthesize T4 and T3 until the 10th week of gestation, and it is therefore dependent on transplacental transfer of the maternal hormone. There is increased maternal synthesis of thyroid hormones in the first trimester as a result of transplacental passage and the high levels of thyroid-binding globulin, and this in turn results in an increased maternal requirement for iodide. In areas of relative iodide deficiency this may result in the development of maternal hypothyroxinaemia and goitre.

Hypothyroidism

Hypothyroidism affects approximately 1% of pregnant women. Providing thyroxine replacement therapy is adequate, hypothyroidism is not associated with an adverse pregnancy outcome for the mother or fetus. There is an established association between poorly controlled hypothyroidism and a variety of adverse outcomes, including congenital abnormalities, hypertension, premature delivery, fetal growth restriction and postpartum haemorrhage. Overt hypothyroidism also causes subfertility, and the presence of thyroid autoantibodies, even if the mother is euthyroid, is associated with an increased risk of miscarriage [22,23]. Furthermore, a study that compared 404 women with subclinical hypothyroidism (i.e. raised TSH with normal free T4) with 16 894 controls demonstrated an association with placental abruption and premature delivery [24].

Severe hypothyroidism affects the subsequent intelligence of the offspring of affected mothers. There is now an emerging body of research demonstrating a relationship between maternal subclinical hypothyroidism, isolated hypothyroxinaemia and even positive thyroid peroxidase antibodies and reduced intelligence and motor development in the offspring [25–27]. It is likely that larger prospective studies will clarify the relationship between maternal thyroid status and fetal neurodevelopment.

Given the concerns about the fetal effects of maternal subclinical hypothyroidism, current advice from the British Endocrine Society is that women with hypothyroidism should be given thyroxine replacement at a dose that ensures their thyroid function tests are normal, with free T4 at the upper end of the normal range and TSH at 2.5 mU/L or less [28]. The exception is for women who have had a thyroidectomy for thyroid cancer as it is necessary to suppress TSH secretion, and in whom the thyroxine dose should be increased if required. Thyroxine absorption is decreased by certain drugs including iron and calcium supplements, and therefore it is best taken on an empty stomach and 4 hours apart from any iron or other supplements.

Hyperthyroidism

Hyperthyroidism affects 1 in 500 pregnant women, 90% of whom have Graves' disease. Graves' disease is caused by TSH receptor-stimulating antibodies. Women with well-treated disease rarely have maternal complications of pregnancy. The disease may remit during the latter trimesters such that treatment may need to be reduced or stopped. In the postpartum period the disease may flare and require treatment with the same or higher doses of antithyroid medication. Poorly controlled hyperthyroidism is associated with several pregnancy complications, including maternal thyrotoxic crisis, miscarriage, gestational hypertension, pre-eclampsia and intrauterine growth restriction [29,30]. The risk of these complications is reduced if the disease is adequately controlled before delivery.

The principal drugs used to treat hyperthyroidism (propylthiouracil and carbimazole) inhibit thyroid hormone synthesis. The early reports of an association between carbimazole treatment and aplasia cutis in the fetus have not been confirmed by subsequent studies, and there is no other evidence that either drug is associated with congenital abnormalities. Both drugs may rarely cause neutropenia and agranulocytosis. Therefore patients should be aware that symptoms of infection, particularly sore throat, may be associated with this complication and they must have a neutrophil count checked immediately should they occur. Once drug treatment has been commenced thyroid function tests should be carried out and checked regularly. A recent joint publication from the Food and Drug Administration and American Thyroid

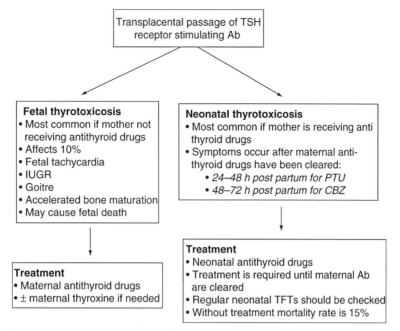

Fig. 13.2 Fetal and neonatal effects of transplacental passage of thyroid stimulating hormone (TSH) receptor-stimulating antibodies. IUGR, intrauterine growth restriction; CBZ, carbimazole; PTU, propylthiouracil; TFT, thyroid function test.

Association reported that propylthiouracil treatment is associated with acute liver failure in 1 in 10000 adults and 1 in 2000 children [31]. It was therefore advised that this drug should not be used as a first-line agent for hyperthyroidism in children or adults. However, an exception was made for the first trimester of pregnancy due to the possible rare association of carbimazole with aplasia cutis. As has been mentioned above, this association is theoretical and therefore we recommend a preference for the use of carbimazole for new cases of hyperthyroidism diagnosed in pregnancy.

Propylthiouracil and carbimazole both cross the placenta. However, fetal hypothyroidism is rarely seen. TSH receptor-stimulating antibodies also cross the placenta and may influence fetal and neonatal thyroid status. The potential consequences of transplacental passage of thyroid-stimulating antibodies (and the relevance of concurrent administration of antithyroid medication) are summarized in Fig. 13.2.

Women requiring antithyroid medication should not be discouraged from breast-feeding. However, if they are taking more than 15mg carbimazole or 150mg propylthiouracil daily, the infant should be reviewed. They should also be encouraged to feed before taking the medication and to take divided doses.

Thyrotoxic crisis, also called 'thyroid storm', is a medical emergency that can present with exaggerated features of hyperthyroidism in addition to hyperpyrexia, congestive cardiac failure, dysrhythmias and an altered mental state. It may be precipitated by infection, abrupt cessation of treatment, surgery, labour or delivery and must be treated immediately as it can be life-threatening. Treatment involves administration of intravenous fluids, hydrocortisone, propranolol, oral iodine and carbimazole or propylthiouracil.

Postpartum thyroiditis

Postpartum thyroiditis is associated with the presence of thyroid antiperoxidase antibodies. The quoted incidence varies between 2 and 16%. It is characterized by an initial hyperthyroid phase that classically occurs 1–3 months after delivery, followed by a hypothyroid phase that usually resolves by 12 months after delivery. The hypothyroidism may require treatment with thyroxine, but treatment should be stopped after 1 year as many cases resolve. However, the likelihood of developing subsequent hypothyroidism in women who have had postpartum thyroiditis is quoted at 5% per year, so affected women should have their thyroid function checked regularly.

Pituitary disease

The anterior pituitary secretes prolactin, growth hormone (GH), adrenocorticotrophic hormone (ACTH), follicle-stimulating hormone (FSH), luteinizing hormone (LH) and TSH.

Pituitary tumours

Prolactinomas

In normal pregnancy the pituitary gland increases in size by 50–70% as a consequence of normal lactotroph hyperplasia, and therefore a tumour that did not cause pressure effects in the non-pregnant state may do so during pregnancy. The most frequently seen pituitary tumours in pregnant women are prolactinomas, although ACTH- or GH-secreting tumours and non-functioning (i.e. non-hormone-secreting) tumours may also be seen. Common symptoms that occur as a consequence of enlargement of a pituitary tumour are headache and visual disturbance, in particular bitemporal field loss. Rarely a woman may develop pituitary apoplexy or diabetes insipidus.

Prolactinomas are subdivided according to their size. Tumours that measure less than 10 mm in diameter are defined as microprolactinomas and constitute the majority. In non-pregnant patients, 5% of tumours are defined as macroprolactinomas (>10 mm). Women with microprolactinomas can be reassured that these tumours rarely enlarge in pregnancy. It is not necessary to continue treatment with dopamine agonists once a woman with a microprolactinoma has conceived. Surveillance should include a clinical assessment each trimester that comprises assessment of the visual fields to confrontation and enquiry for symptoms suggestive of pituitary enlargement. Serum prolactin levels should not be checked as they increase by as much as 10-fold by week 25 of gestation. Several studies have reported the frequency of symptomatic enlargement of microprolactinomas in pregnancy, and when these data are combined only 1.4% of 363 cases have symptoms of tumour enlargement [32]. In contrast, 26.2% of 84 women with macroprolactinomas had symptomatic tumour enlargement. Symptomatic tumour enlargement is less likely in women with macroprolactinomas previously treated with surgery or irradiation before pregnancy [32].

Women with macroprolactinomas should continue to take dopamine agonists throughout pregnancy and the visual fields should be checked with formal perimetry on a regular basis, i.e. at least once each trimester and more commonly if there are any concerns. Bromocriptine was the first dopamine agonist to be used, but its use is associated with relatively common side effects, including nausea, vomiting and postural hypotension. Therefore cabergoline and quinagolide are used in increasing numbers of cases as they are better tolerated and cabergoline has the additional advantage of a longer half-life, allowing it to be given once or twice weekly. The data that are available indicate that bromocriptine and cabergoline are not associated with an increased risk of congenital abnormalities or other adverse pregnancy outcomes. The Medicines and Healthcare Products Regulatory Agency (MHRA) published new guidance on the use of ergot-derived dopamine agonists in October 2008. This is because the European Medicines Agency has published warnings and recommendations related to cardiac fibrosis associated with these medications. There is a higher risk with cabergoline and it clearly states that pregnancy should be excluded before starting cabergoline. At present it is not known whether fetal cardiac fibrosis can occur. This new advice will change the current treatment of pregnant women with macroprolactinoma. Quinagolide is a non-ergot-derived dopamine agonist and is therefore not associated with cardiac fibrosis, so it is likely that this drug will be used more in future. However, there are few published data regarding its use in pregnancy.

Women taking dopamine agonists are usually unable to lactate. However, breast-feeding is not contraindicated in women with microprolactinomas as it does not cause an increase in the size of these pituitary tumours.

ACTH-secreting tumours

Cushing's syndrome is caused by excess circulating cortisol. Cushing's syndrome in non-pregnant individuals is most commonly caused by ACTH-secreting tumours (i.e. Cushing's disease), while adrenal tumours are the commonest cause in pregnant women, and 21% of the adrenal tumours are malignant [33]. The predominance of adrenal tumours may be explained by reduced fertility in women with pituitary tumours. Cushing's syndrome caused by both pituitary and adrenal tumours is considered in this section as many of the features overlap.

Plasma levels of cortisol, ACTH and cortisol-binding globulin are raised in pregnancy, as is urinary free cortisol. Therefore it is important to refer to normal ranges for pregnancy when investigating the hypothalamic–pituitary axis in a pregnant woman. A review of case reports of maternal Cushing's syndrome reported premature delivery in 12 of 23 cases, one spontaneous abortion and two stillbirths [33]. A review of the management of Cushing's syndrome secondary to adrenal tumours demonstrated that fetal and neonatal outcome is better if the tumour is removed during pregnancy rather than at completion of pregnancy [34].

Untreated Cushing's syndrome in pregnancy is associated with increased rates of maternal and fetal morbidity and mortality, and in particular the incidence of diabetes mellitus and hypertension is high. Treatment of Cushing's syndrome is primarily surgical. There have been reports of successful use of the medical agents metyrapone, ketoconazole and aminoglutethimide, all of which inhibit biosynthesis of cortisol, and of cyproheptadine which suppresses corticotrophin-releasing hormone. However, experience is limited due to the rarity of Cushing's syndrome in pregnancy.

Other pituitary tumours

GH-secreting tumours cause acromegaly, which is associated with impaired fertility and therefore pregnancy occurs rarely. Even in treated women there have been very few reports of pregnancy. Women with acromegaly usually have macroadenomas, and therefore the normal stimulation of adjacent lactotrophs may result in symptoms consistent with tumour expansion in pregnancy. It is therefore important to monitor the visual fields using formal perimetry as for women with pituitary macroadenomas. Women have an increased risk of IGT, diabetes mellitus and hypertensive disease. Treatment options include dopamine agonists to reduce the size of adjacent lactotrophs, somatostatin analogues or surgery. The somatostatin analogue octreotide has been used in a small number of cases without adverse effects. The most effective treatment for non-functioning pituitary tumours is surgery (possibly followed by radiotherapy).

Diabetes insipidus

Diabetes insipidus is caused by deficiency of the posterior pituitary hormone vasopressin. A subgroup of affected women require an increased dose of desmopressin as a consequence of placental synthesis of vasopressinase. This may also explain why some cases present *de novo* in pregnancy. Desmopressin is more effective than vasopressin as it is more resistant to vasopressinase.

Lymphocytic hypophysitis

Lymphocytic hypophysitis is an inflammatory disease of the pituitary that occurs more commonly in women and is associated with pregnancy. Approximately 60% of cases present with hypopituitarism and 20% present with diabetes insipidus [35]. It is important to distinguish lymphocytic hypophysitis from a pituitary adenoma as surgery may exacerbate hypopituitarism associated with the former. Lymphocytic hypophysitis may resolve spontaneously and approximately 50% of cases respond to corticosteroids, although the condition commonly recurs following cessation of treatment.

Sheehan's syndrome

This term describes hypopituitarism that presents in the late postpartum period, and which is caused by haemorrhage and hypotension at the time of delivery. The hypotension results in avascular necrosis that affects the anterior pituitary more commonly than the posterior pituitary. Women most frequently present with failure of lactation and subsequent amenorrhoea, but they may have any feature of hypopituitarism including the more subtle features of hypoadrenalism and hypothyroidism.

Adrenal disease

Adrenal tumours

Adrenal tumours are rare in pregnancy. The commoner tumours secrete corticosteroids, catecholamines or aldosterone, causing Cushing's syndrome, phaeochromocytoma or Conn's syndrome, respectively. Non-functioning tumours may rarely occur. Cushing's syndrome is more commonly caused by adrenal tumours in pregnant women as discussed above.

Phaeochromocytoma is rare but important to diagnose because the maternal and fetal mortality has been quoted as 50% if it is not treated adequately. The diagnosis should be suspected in women with hypertension that occurs in association with sweating, anxiety, headache or palpitations. The clinical features may be paroxysmal and some women have IGT or diabetes. The diagnosis is made with 24-hour urinary catecholamines, which should be repeated several times if an initial test is normal. Other investigations that may be used are plasma catecholamines or a pentolinium suppression test, and there should be a low threshold for performing magnetic resonance imaging. Treatment in the first instance should be with an alpha-blocker, for example phenoxybenzamine, followed by a beta-blocker, for example propranolol. Definitive treatment is surgical removal, the timing of which is dictated by the gestational age at diagnosis, the response to medical treatment and the accessibility of the tumour. Laparoscopic surgery has been performed in pregnancy to remove phaeochromocytoma with good outcomes.

Conn's syndrome

Primary hyperaldosteronism, also called Conn's syndrome, is characterized by hypertension in association with low serum potassium, raised plasma aldosterone and suppressed renin activity. The pregnancy-specific reference ranges for these hormones should be used. Conn's syndrome usually improves in pregnancy. However, when symptomatic the hypertension may be treated with conventional antihypertensives. Spironolactone should be used with caution as this may cause feminization of the male fetus. Surgery is also a treatment option.

Hypoadrenalism

Hypoadrenalism may result from haemorrhagic destruction, for example as a consequence of severe obstetric haemorrhage, or from autoimmune destruction (Addison's disease). It may present in an insidious manner with symptoms of fatigue, hypotension, nausea, vomiting, and ultimately with sepsis or circulatory collapse. Serum biochemistry may reveal hyponatraemia and a serum cortisol should be checked (ideally with a cortisol-binding globulin and in liaison with an endocrinologist). If a diagnosis of Addison's disease is made, it should be remembered that this commonly coexists with other autoimmune diseases, and there should be a low threshold for screening for conditions such as pernicious anaemia, thyroid disease or type 1 DM. Glucocorticoid replacement is mandatory if the hypoadrenalism is suspected, although this can usually be delayed until after the serum cortisol has been checked. The glucocorticoid dose should be increased to cover the stress of labour or intercurrent infections and the woman should be advised to carry a steroid card and medicalert bracelet. Women with hypoadrenalism are at particular risk if they develop hyperemesis gravidarum and are unable to take their glucocorticoid replacement orally. They should be admitted for intramuscular or intravenous glucocorticoid replacement until they are able to take their drugs by mouth.

Congenital adrenal hyperplasia

This describes several inborn errors of metabolism that affect glucocorticoid and mineralocorticoid synthesis, the commonest of which is 21-hydroxylase deficiency. They are associated with reduced fertility, particularly if associated with mineralocorticoid deficiency. Affected women who manage to conceive have increased risks of hypertension and pre-eclampsia. The steroid requirement rarely increases during pregnancy. However, the dose of glucocorticoids should be increased to cover labour. Women should receive genetic counselling prior to conception to discuss the merits of mutation screening in the partner (for 21-hydroxylase deficiency the carrier rate is 1 in 50) and the risk of having an affected fetus.

Parathyroid disease

Hyperparathyroidism is associated with a raised parathyroid hormone and may be primary, secondary or tertiary. Primary hyperparathyroidism is most commonly caused by a parathyroid adenoma, and is associated with hypercalcaemia and hypercalciuria. Secondary hyperparathyroidism is a normal physiological consequence of chronic hypocalcaemia, for example in association with vitamin D deficiency or chronic renal failure. Tertiary hyperparathyroidism occurs when a clone of cells starts to function autonomously following long-standing secondary hyperparathyroidism. Primary hyperparathyroidism is commoner in women and 25% of cases occur in the childbearing years. Most pregnant women with the disease are asymptomatic, although they may have symptoms of hypercalcaemia including nephrolithiasis, pancreatitis or altered mental state. However, the condition does have a high perinatal complication rate, with fetal death reported as 27–31% of conservatively managed pregnancies and tetany occurring in 50% of neonates of untreated mothers [36]. The perinatal complication rate is reduced considerably if the condition is treated and for most cases the appropriate therapy is surgical removal of the tumour, ideally in the first trimester.

Vitamin D deficiency

Vitamin D deficiency may be nutritional or secondary to a metabolic disease. Nutritional deficiency of vitamin D is particularly common in women from non-white ethnic groups, and severe deficiency can present with osteomalacia and pathological fractures in pregnancy. Maternal vitamin D deficiency is associated with neonatal morbidity and impaired growth within the first year, and therefore vitamin D supplementation is recommended in at-risk groups. The WHO and the UK National Institute for Health Clinical Excellence guidelines recommend 400 IU (10 µg) of vitamin D daily during pregnancy and lactation. However, this relatively low dose is unlikely to be effective in women with severe deficiency. We believe that high-dose oral replacement (or in some cases intramuscular injections) of vitamin D are appropriate in these cases.

References

1 Confidential Enquiry into Maternal and Child Health. *Pregnancy in Women with Type 1 and Type 2 Diabetes, 2002–2003. England, Wales and Northern Ireland*. London: CEMACH, 2005. Available at: www.cemach.org.uk/getattachment/8af39ba1-1cab-476b-ad8e-b9393fd35aed/Pregnancy-in-women-with-type-1-and-type-2-diab-(1).aspx

2 Confidential Enquiry into Maternal and Child Health. *Diabetes in Pregnancy: Are We Providing the Best Care? Findings of a National Enquiry: England, Wales and Northern Ireland*. London: CEMACH, 2007. Available at: www.cemach.org.uk/getattachment/07707df7-9b29-4e2b-b1cf-5de2f9715af2/Diabetes-in-Pregnancy—Are-we-providing-the-b-(1).aspx

3 Wender-Ozegowska E, Wróblewska K, Zawiejska A, Pietryga M, Szczapa J, Biczysko R. Threshold values of maternal blood glucose in early diabetic pregnancy: prediction of fetal malformations. *Acta Obstet Gynecol Scand* 2005;84:17–25.

4 Guerin A, Nisenbaum R, Ray J. Use of maternal GHb concentration to estimate the risk of congenital anomalies in the offspring of women with prepregnancy diabetes. *Diabetes Care* 2007;30:1920–1925.

5 Metzger BE, Lowe LP, Dyer AR *et al*. Hyperglycemia and adverse pregnancy outcomes. *N Engl J Med* 2008;358:1991–2002.

6 Kristensen J, Vestergaard M, Wisborg K, Kesmodel U, Secher NJ. Pre-pregnancy weight and the risk of stillbirth and neonatal death. *BJOG* 2005;112:403–408.

7 Centre for Maternal and Child Enquiries. *Management of Women with Obesity in Pregnancy*. London: CEMACH, 2010. Available at: www.cemach.org.uk/getattachment/26cfa33c-723b-45c5-abee-4d00b0d7be4c/Joint-CMACE-RCOG-Guideline—Management-of-Obesity.aspx

8 Guideline Development Group. Management of diabetes from preconception to the postnatal period: summary of NICE guidance. *BMJ* 2008;336:714–717.

9 Macintosh MC, Fleming KM, Bailey JA *et al*. Perinatal mortality and congenital anomalies in babies of women with type 1 or type 2 diabetes in England, Wales, and Northern Ireland: population based study. *BMJ* 2006;333:177.

10 Lauenborg J, Mathiesen E, Ovesen P *et al*. Audit on stillbirths in women with pregestational type 1 diabetes. *Diabetes Care* 2003;26:1385–1389.

11 Metzger BE, Gabbe SG, Persson B *et al*. International association of diabetes and pregnancy study groups recommendations on the diagnosis and classification of hyperglycemia in pregnancy. *Diabetes Care* 2010;33:676–682.

12 Crowther CA, Hiller JE, Moss JR *et al*. Effect of treatment of gestational diabetes mellitus on pregnancy outcomes. *N Engl J Med* 2005;352:2477–2486.

13 Rowan JA, Hague WM, Gao W, Battin MR, Moore MP. Metformin versus insulin for the treatment of gestational diabetes. *N Engl J Med* 2008;358:2003–2015.

14 Langer O, Conway DL, Berkus MD, Xenakis EM, Gonzales O. A comparison of glyburide and insulin in women with gestational diabetes mellitus. *N Engl J Med* 2000;343:1134–1138.

15 Nold J, Georgieff M. Infants of diabetic mothers. *Pediatr Clin North Am* 2004;51:619–637.

16 Weiss PA, Scholz HS, Haas J, Tamussino KF, Seissler J, Borkenstein MH. Long-term follow-up of infants of mothers with type 1 diabetes: evidence for hereditary and nonhereditary transmission of diabetes and precursors. *Diabetes Care* 2000;23:905–911.

17 Clausen TD, Mathiesen ER, Hansen T *et al*. High prevalence of type 2 diabetes and pre-diabetes in adult offspring of women with gestational diabetes mellitus or type 1 diabetes: the role of intrauterine hyperglycemia. *Diabetes Care* 2008;31:340–346.

18 Mughal MZ, Eelloo J, Roberts SA *et al*. Body composition and bone status of children born to mothers with type 1 diabetes mellitus. *Arch Dis Child* 2010;95:281–285.

19 Parker JH. Amerlex free tri-iodothyronine and free thyroxine levels in normal pregnancy. *Br J Obstet Gynaecol* 1985;92:1234–1238.

20 Chan BY, Swaminathan R. Serum thyrotrophin hormone concentration measured by sensitive assays in normal pregnancy. *Br J Obstet Gynaecol* 1988;95:1332–1336.

21 Kotarba DD, Garner P, Perkins SL. Changes in serum free thyroxine, free tri-iodothyronine and thyroid stimulating hormone reference intervals in normal term pregnancy. *J Obstet Gynecol* 1995;15:5–8.

22 Prummel MF, Wiersinga WM. Thyroid autoimmunity and miscarriage. *Eur J Endocrinol* 2004;150:751–755.

23 Negro R, Formoso G, Mangieri T, Pezzarossa A, Dazzi D, Hassan H. Levothyroxine treatment in euthyroid pregnant women with autoimmune thyroid disease: effects on obstetrical complications. *J Clin Endocrinol Metab* 2006;91:2587–2591.

24 Casey BM, Dashe JS, Wells CE *et al*. Subclinical hypothyroidism and pregnancy outcomes. *Obstet Gynecol* 2005;105:239–245.

25 Haddow JE, Palomaki GE, Allan WC *et al*. Maternal thyroid deficiency during pregnancy and subsequent neuropsychological development of the child. *N Engl J Med* 1999;341:549–555.

26 Pop VJ, Brouwers EP, Vader HL, Vulsma T, van Baar AL, de Vijlder JJ. Maternal hypothyroxinaemia during early pregnancy and subsequent child development: a 3-year follow-up study. *Clin Endocrinol* 2003;59:282–288.

27 Yuanbin Li, Zhongyan Shan, Weiping Teng *et al*. Abnormalities of maternal thyroid function during pregnancy affect neuropsychological development of their children at 25–30 months. *Clin Endocrinol* 2010;72:825–829.

28 Abalovich M, Amino N, Barbour LA *et al*. Management of thyroid dysfunction during pregnancy and postpartum: an Endocrine Society Clinical Practice Guideline. *J Clin Endocrinol Metab* 2007;92(8 Suppl):S1–S47.

29 Millar LK, Wing DA, Leung AS, Koonings PP, Montoro MN, Mestman JH. Low birth weight and preeclampsia in pregnancies complicated by hyperthyroidism. *Obstet Gynecol* 1994;84:946–949.

30 Mestman JH. Hyperthyroidism in pregnancy. *Best Pract Res Clin Endocrinol Metab* 2004;18:267–288.

31 Bahn RS, Burch HS, Cooper DS *et al*. The role of propylthiouracil in the management of Graves' disease in adults: report of a meeting jointly sponsored by the American Thyroid Association and the Food and Drug Administration. *Thyroid* 2009;19:673–674.

32 Molitch ME. Pituitary tumours and pregnancy. *Growth Horm IGF Res* 2003;13(Suppl A):S38–S44.

33 Pickard J, Jochen AL, Sadur CN, Hofeldt FD. Management of Cushing's syndrome secondary to adrenal adenoma during pregnancy. *Obstet Gynecol Surv* 1990;45:87–93.

34 Pricolo VE, Monchik JM, Prinz RA, DeJong S, Chadwick DA, Lamberton RP. Management of Cushing's syndrome secondary to adrenal adenoma during pregnancy. *Surgery* 1990;108:1072–1077.

35 Thodu E, Asa SL, Kontogeorgos G, Kovacs K, Horvath E, Ezzat S. Clinical case seminar: lymphocytic hypophysitis: clinicopathological findings. *J Clin Endocrinol Metab* 1995;80:2302–2311.

36 Schnatz PF, Curry FL. Primary hyperparathyroidism in pregnancy: evidence-based management. *Obstet Gynecol Surv* 2002;57:365–376.

Further reading

Arun CS, Taylor R. Influence of pregnancy on long-term progression of retinopathy in patients with type 1 diabetes. *Diabetologia* 2008;51:1041–1045.

Barrett H, McElduff A. Vitamin D and pregnancy: an old problem revisited. *Best Pract Res Clin Endocrinol Metab* 2010;24:527–539.

Bell R, Bailey K, Cresswell T, Hawthorne G, Critchley J, Lewis-Barned N. Trends in prevalence and outcomes of pregnancy in women with pre-existing type I and type II diabetes. *BJOG* 2008;115:445–452.

Catalano PM, Huston L, Amini SB, Kalhan SC. Longitudinal changes in glucose metabolism during pregnancy in obese women with normal glucose tolerance and gestational diabetes mellitus. *Am J Obstet Gynecol* 1999;180:903–916.

Conway DL. Obstetric management in gestational diabetes. *Diabetes Care* 2007;30(Suppl 2):S175–S179.

Dabelea D, Knowler WC, Pettitt DJ. Effect of diabetes in pregnancy on offspring: follow-up research in the Pima Indians. *J Matern Fetal Med* 2000;9:83–88.

Diabetes Control and Complications Trial Research Group. Effect of pregnancy on microvascular complications in the Diabetes Control and Complications Trial. *Diabetes Care* 2000;23:1084–1091.

Gautier JF, Wilson C, Weyer C *et al*. Low acute insulin secretory responses in adult offspring of people with early onset type 2 diabetes. *Diabetes* 2001;50:1828–1833.

Guideline Development Group. Management of diabetes from preconception to the postnatal period: summary of NICE guidance. *BMJ* 2008;336:714–717.

Hawthorne G. Metformin use and diabetic pregnancy: has its time come? *Diabetic Med* 2006;23:223–227.

Holing EV, Beyer CS, Brown ZA, Connell FA. Why don't women with diabetes plan their pregnancies? *Diabetes Care* 1998;21:889–895.

Kitzmiller JL, Block JM, Brown FM *et al*. Managing preexisting diabetes for pregnancy: summary of evidence and consensus recommendations for care. *Diabetes Care* 2008;31:1060–1079.

Lakasing L, Williamson C. Obstetric complications due to autoantibodies. *Baillieres Best Pract Res Clin Endocrinol Metab* 2005;19: 149–175.

Lapillonne A. Vitamin D deficiency during pregnancy may impair maternal and fetal outcomes. *Med Hypotheses* 2010;74:71–75.

Lee AJ, Hiscock RJ, Wein P, Walker SP, Permezel M. Gestational diabetes mellitus: clinical predictors and long-term risk of developing type 2 diabetes: a retrospective cohort study using survival analysis. *Diabetes Care* 2007;30:878–883.

Matsushita E, Matsuda Y, Makino Y, Sanaka M, Ohta H. Risk factors associated with preterm delivery in women with pregestational diabetes. *J Obstet Gynaecol Res* 2008;34:851–857.

Metzger BE, Buchanan TA, Coustan DR *et al*. Summary and recommendations of the Fifth International Workshop-Conference on Gestational Diabetes Mellitus. *Diabetes Care* 2007;30(Suppl 2):S251–S260.

Nader S. Thyroid disease and pregnancy. In: Creasy RK, Resnik R, Iams JD, Lockwood CJ, Moore TR (eds) *Creasy and Resnik's Maternal–Fetal Medicine: Principles and Practice*, 6th edn. Philadelphia: Saunders Elsevier, 2009:995–1014.

Nader S. Other endocrine disorders of pregnancy. In: Creasy RK, Resnik R, Iams JD, Lockwood CJ, Moore TR (eds) *Creasy and Resnik's Maternal–Fetal Medicine: Principles and Practice*, 6th edn. Philadelphia: Saunders Elsevier, 2009:1015–1040.

Nicholson W, Bolen S, Witkop CT, Neale D, Wilson L, Bass E. Benefits and risks of oral diabetes agents compared with insulin in women with gestational diabetes: a systematic review. *Obstet Gynecol* 2009;113:193–205.

Nielsen LR, Pedersen-Bjergaard U, Thorsteinsson B, Johansen M, Damm P, Mathiesen ER. Hypoglycemia in pregnant women with type 1 diabetes: predictors and role of metabolic control. *Diabetes Care* 2008;31:9–14.

Nielsen LR, Damm P, Mathiesen ER. Improved pregnancy outcome in type 1 women with diabetes with microalbuminuria or diabetic nephropathy: effect of intensified antihypertensive therapy? *Diabetes Care* 2009;32:38–44.

Pearson DW, Kernaghan D, Lee R, Penney GC. The relationship between pre-pregnancy care and early pregnancy loss, major congenital anomaly or perinatal death in type I diabetes mellitus. *BJOG* 2007;114:104–107.

Powrie RO, Greene MF, Camann W. *De Swiet's Medical Disorders in Obstetric Practice*, 5th edn. Oxford: Wiley-Blackwell, 2010: chapters 11–14.

Ratner RE, Christophi CA, Metzger BE *et al*. Prevention of diabetes in women with a history of gestational diabetes: effects of metformin and lifestyle interventions. *J Clin Endocrinol Metab* 2008;93:4774–4779.

Rosenfeld H, Ornoy A, Shechtman S, Diav-Citrin O. Pregnancy outcome, thyroid dysfunction and fetal goitre after in utero exposure to propylthiouracil: a controlled cohort study. *Br J Clin Pharmacol* 2009;68:609–617.

Sobngwi E, Boudou P, Mauvais-Jarvis F *et al*. Effect of a diabetic environment in utero on predisposition to type 2 diabetes. *Lancet* 2003;361:1861–1865.

Webster J. A comparative review of the tolerability profiles of dopamine agonists in the treatment of hyperprolactinaemia and inhibition of lactation. *Drug Saf* 1996;14:228–238.

Chapter 14
Renal Disease

Sarah Winfield[1] and John M. Davison[2]
[1]Leeds Teaching Hospital NHS Trust, Leeds, UK
[2]Institute of Cellular Medicine, Newcastle University, Newcastle upon Tyne, UK

Providing care for women with underlying renal disease contemplating pregnancy or those already pregnant requires that the obstetrician has up-to-date knowledge about pregnancy physiology, antenatal care and the technology for fetal surveillance. It is essential to appreciate the need for multidisciplinary teamwork in a centre with all the necessary facilities for dealing with high-risk patients and their babies. The quoted rates for renal disease in pregnancy range from 3 to 15 per 10000. This chapter focuses on chronic kidney disease (CKD), women on dialysis and kidney transplant recipients, aiming to provide the busy clinician with information for counselling and judicious decision-making.

Pre-pregnancy assessment

The basic components should be analysis of risks as well as provision of health education and advice plus any interventions that might be considered helpful, all united under the banner of that much-used word 'counselling' [1]. The multidisciplinary team has to decide what is important so that active preparation for pregnancy is tailored to each woman's needs, with her being encouraged to involve her partner so that all the implications can be discussed, including potential areas of disagreement, even whether infertility treatment, if needed, would be made available.

> **Summary box 14.1**
>
> - All women of childbearing age with CKD, including those on dialysis and kidney transplant recipients should be made aware of the implications regarding reproductive health, contraception, modification of remedial risk factors and optimisation of medications.
> - Active preparation for pregnancy should be individualized to each woman's needs and should involve her partner.
> - Multidiscplinary clinics are needed for the prepregnancy assessment and antenatal care of these women.

What the patient wants to know

Aside from what the team wants to discuss and achieve for the woman and her partner, she herself usually has four straightforward questions.

1 Should I get pregnant?
2 Will my pregnancy be complicated?
3 Will I have a live and healthy baby?
4 Will I have problems after my pregnancy?

Often the first, and sometimes even the second, question is bypassed, the woman immediately wanting to know the answers to the final two questions. Therefore it is essential to ensure that all relevant information and even harsh realities are passed on, based on fact not anecdote.

What the patient needs to understand

She must understand the risks and the need to improve her own knowledge, so that she can best use the guidance and support to make any necessary changes in her behaviour, attitude and medication(s). Knowledge of, and even understanding the risks, however, may not be sufficient to ensure the patient makes the changes because many other factors influence her behaviour. Even when there is an element of self-management (perhaps best exemplified with dialysis and/or diabetes) this will also be affected by the woman's repertoire of beliefs, skills, intuition, motivation and not just her so-called knowledge, however gained. The key is a strong, unwaivering, positive, supportive relationship with the team that allows pre-pregnancy advice to be included in the overall care agenda as a goal-orientated process. Thus a planned pregnancy is one that is desired well before conception, occurs when contraception is discontinued and where the woman attempts to achieve optimal health beforehand.

Even if some of the answers are not favourable, a woman, being an autonomous adult, may still choose to plan for (or proceed with) a pregnancy in an effort to re-establish a normal life in the face of chronic illness [2]. Indeed some women may not seek advice until already pregnant. Occasionally, there may be ethical dilemmas

Dewhurst's Textbook of Obstetrics & Gynaecology, Eighth Edition. Edited by D. Keith Edmonds.
© 2012 John Wiley and Sons, Ltd. Published 2012 by John Wiley and Sons, Ltd.

regarding the clinician's duty of care for women who ignore advice; interestingly, there are studies that have differentiated 'healthy' and 'pathological' levels of assumed risk and which have tried to understand the psychology of women who pursue parenthood despite big risks to their own health and the unborn child [3].

Normal pregnancy

The renal tract undergoes marked anatomical, haemodynamic, tubular and endocrine changes as part of the systemic upheaval of maternal adaptation to pregnancy [4,5]. The kidneys enlarge because both vascular volume and interstitial space increase but there is no accelerated renal growth nor morphological alterations akin to compensatory renal hypertrophy. The calyces, renal pelves and ureters dilate markedly, invariably more prominent on the right side, seen in 90% of women.

Glomerular filtration rate (GFR), measured as 24-hour creatinine clearance (C_{cr}), increases by 6–8 weeks' gestation. Serum creatinine (S_{cr}) and serum urea (S_{urea}), which average 70 μmol/L and 5 mmol/L respectively in non-pregnant women, decrease to mean values of 50 μmol/L and 3 mmol/L during pregnancy. Values for S_{cr} of 80 μmol/L and S_{urea} of 6 mmol/L, which are acceptable in the non-pregnant state, are suspect in pregnancy. At term, a 15–20% decrement in C_{cr} occurs, which affects S_{cr} minimally. It should be remembered that S_{cr} levels may increase up to 17 μmol/L shortly after ingestion of cooked meat (because cooking converts preformed creatine into creatinine), and this has to be taken into account when timing blood sampling.

The 24-hour urinary total protein excretion (TPE) increases in normal pregnancy, and up to 300 mg (some would say 500 mg) per 24 hours can be regarded as normal [6]. So-called significant proteinuria (TPE >300 mg per 24 hours) may correlate with a protein concentration of 30 mg/dL in a 'spot' urine sample, but given the problems with dipstick testing many still prefer a 24-hour or some timed quantitative determination. However, an alternative may be the use of 'spot' urine protein/creatinine ratios that equal 30 mg/μmol or more.

Chronic kidney disease

Renal impairment and the prospects for pregnancy and afterwards

A woman may lose up to 50% of her renal function and still maintain S_{cr} below 125 μmol/L because of hyperfiltration by the remaining nephrons; however, if renal function is more severely compromised, then further small decreases in GFR will cause S_{cr} to increase markedly [4,7–9]. In women with CKD, whilst the pathology may be both biochemically and clinically silent, the internal milieu may already be disrupted. Most individuals remain symptom-free until GFR declines to less than 25% of normal, and many serum constituents are frequently normal until a late stage of disease. However, degrees of functional impairment that do not appear to disrupt homoeostasis in non-pregnant individuals can jeopardize pregnancy.

Summary box 14.2

- If pre-pregnancy renal function is normal or only mildly decreased ($S_{cr} \leq 125\,\mu$mol/L) and hypertension minimal and/or well controlled, then obstetric outcome is usually successful.
- There is an increased risk of antenatal complications such as pre-eclampsia, fetal growth restriction and preterm delivery.
- Offer low-dose aspirin as prophylaxis against pre-eclampsia, starting within first trimester.
- During pregnancy target blood pressure should be 140/90 mmHg.
- Greater degrees of renal dysfunction ($S_{cr} > 125\,\mu$mol/L (and certainly >180 μmol/L) and/or the presence of poorly controlled hypertension are more ominous, at least for maternal outcome, especially long-term renal prognosis.
- The use of eGFR from the MDRD or Epi-CKD formulae is not recommended for use in pregnancy.

The basic question for a woman with CKD must be: is pregnancy advisable? If so, then the sooner she starts to have her family the better, since in many cases renal function will decline with time. Women with suspected or known CKD, not always counselled prior to pregnancy, may present already pregnant as a *fait accompli*, and then the question must be whether pregnancy should continue (Table 14.1).

Obstetric and long-term renal prognoses differ in women with different levels of dysfunction. Counselling is based on two functional parameters: the degree of renal

Table 14.1 Pre-pregnancy considerations in chronic kidney disease.

Renal pathology under consideration
Good general health
Review and optimize pre-pregnancy drug therapy
Diastolic blood pressure ≤80 mmHg or well-controlled hypertension with 'safe' medication(s)
$S_{cr} \leq 250\,\mu$mol/L but preferably ≤180 μmol/L and better still <125 μmol/L
No or minimal proteinuria
'Well-controlled' comorbidities (e.g. diabetes mellitus, infections)
Relevance of obstetric history

Table 14.2 Pre-pregnancy kidney function (S_{cr}) in CKD patients with estimates for obstetric outcome and renal functional loss.

Renal status	S_{cr} (µmol/L)	Problems in pregnancy (%)	Successful obstetric outcome (%)	Permanent loss of kidney function (%)
Mild	≤125	26	96	<3
Moderate	≥125	47	90	25
Severe	≥250	86	71	53

Estimates are based on 2420 women/3645 pregnancies (1972–2000) which attained at least 24 weeks' gestation. This (unpublished literature review) is retrospective and publications dealing with greater degrees of dysfunction comprised fewer than 400 patients.

insufficiency and the presence or absence of hypertension (Table 14.2). Although no formal guidelines have been issued by any professional groups the pregnancy and CKD literature, almost entirely retrospective, has traditionally and arbitrarily classified renal insufficiency solely by pre-pregnancy S_{cr}: ≤125 µmol/L indicates mild insufficiency, 125–250 µmol/L moderate insufficiency, and above these levels severe insufficiency [10]. Their use has been the mainstay of pre-pregnancy counselling for over 25 years, consistently showing that normotensive women with intact or only mildly decreased but stable renal function generally do very well, experiencing more than 95% live births, about 75% of which are appropriate for gestational age. These excellent statistics also reflect a literature that has shown constantly improving perinatal outcomes from the 1980s onwards, indicative of the marked advances in both antenatal and neonatal care [11–18]. With mild insufficiency there is an increased incidence of superimposed pre-eclampsia or late pregnancy hypertension, as well as increased proteinuria, exceeding the nephrotic range (3 g per 24 hours) in 50% of women in the second half of pregnancy. Pregnancy does not appear to adversely affect the course of the CKD.

However, there are exceptions to this optimistic outlook [18–21]. Certain types of CKD appear more sensitive to pregnancy, including lupus nephropathy and perhaps membranoproliferative glomerulonephritis. In addition, women with scleroderma and periarteritis nodosa do poorly (especially when there is marked renal involvement and associated hypertension) and thus should be counselled to avoid pregnancy. Furthermore, there is some disagreement about whether pregnancy adversely influences the natural history of IgA nephropathy, focal segmental glomerulosclerosis and reflux nephropathy. It seems likely that prognosis with these renal lesions is actually similar to that of women with mild impairment in general, provided pre-pregnancy function is preserved and high blood pressure absent

(Table 14.3). Lupus nephritis is considered elsewhere in this book.

Prognosis is poorer when there are greater degrees of renal dysfunction [18,22–27]. With moderate impairment, live births still approach 90%, but the incidence of pre-eclampsia, fetal growth restriction and/or preterm delivery exceeds 50%. With severe dysfunction, outlook is more drastically curtailed. Although there is a paucity of data for analysis in both these categories, what has become obvious is that a cut-off S_{cr} of 250 µmol/L is too high for moderate impairment, with 180 µmol/L more appropriate, and thus there is a tendency to designate these patient groups 'moderate to severe' (Table 14.4). This literature is slowly increasing and the message could not be clearer: hypertension is common by term (60%) as is significant proteinuria (50%) as well as deterioration in renal function (at times rapid and substantial) and although infant survival rates are good (80–90%), rates of premature delivery (60%) and fetal growth restriction (40%) underscore the very high potential for obstetric complications in these women [22,24,28,29]. Not previously so obvious are the facts that 30–50% of women with moderate insufficiency experience functional loss more rapidly than would be expected from the natural course of their renal disease and that poorly controlled hypertension might be a harbinger of poor outcome [24]. Once S_{cr} rises above 250 µmol/L there are even bigger risks of accelerated loss of renal function, and even terminating the pregnancy may not reverse the decline (Table 14.2).

Temporary dialysis

Temporary or acute dialysis has been advocated during pregnancy in the face of overall deterioration in renal function (especially when S_{urea} exceeds 20 mmol/L and/or there is refractory hyperkalaemia), severe metabolic acidosis, pulmonary oedema responding poorly to diuretics and danger of volume overload with heart failure [5,18,29,30]. Dialysis may increase the chance of successful outcome by 'buying time' for fetal maturation but it does not arrest the inexorable decline in renal function, ultimately to end-stage failure. In trying to avoid extreme prematurity in this way, it has to be asked whether such life-threatening effects on the mother's renal prognosis can be justified. Nevertheless, the awareness by some women of progress in antenatal care and neonatal provision encourages them to anticipate good outcomes and they will say that they are prepared to take a chance and even seek assisted conception in the face of their infertility. Of importance in all the current controversies is that the literature that forms the basis of our views is primarily retrospective, with most patients only having mild dysfunction and women with severe to moderate disease being limited in number. Confirmation of guidelines and prognoses therefore requires adequate prospective trials.

Table 14.3 Chronic renal disease and pregnancy.

Renal disease	Clinical watchpoints
Chronic glomerulonephritis and focal glomerular sclerosis (FGS)	Can be high blood pressure late in pregnancy but usually no adverse effect if renal function is preserved and hypertension absent before pregnancy. Some disagree, believing coagulation changes in pregnancy exacerbate disease, especially IgA nephropathy, membranoproliferative glomerulonephritis and FGS
IgA nephropathy	Some cite risks of sudden escalating or uncontrolled hypertension and renal deterioration. Most note good outcome when renal function is preserved
Chronic pyelonephritis (infectious tubulointerstitial disease)	Bacteriuria in pregnancy and may lead to exacerbation
Reflux nephropathy	Some have emphasized risks of sudden escalating hypertension and worsening of renal function. Consensus now is that results are satisfactory when pre-pregnancy function is only mildly affected and hypertension is absent. Vigilance for urinary tract infections is necessary
Urolithiasis	Ureteral dilatation and stasis do not seem to affect natural history, but infections can be more frequent. Stents have been successfully placed and sonograpically controlled ureterostomy has been performed during gestation
Polycystic kidney disease	Functional impairment and hypertension are usually minimal in childbearing years
Diabetic nephropathy	No adverse effect on the renal lesion. Increased frequency of infections, oedema or pre-eclampsia. Advanced nephropathy can be a problem
Human immunodeficiency virus with associated nephropathy (HIVAN)	Renal component can be nephrotic syndrome or severe impairment. Scanty literature should be considered when nephrotic proteinuria occurs suddenly, especially in immunocompromised patients
Systemic lupus erythematosus	Prognosis is most favourable if disease is in remission 6 months before conception. Some increase steroid dosage immediately after delivery
Periarteritis nodosa	Fetal prognosis is poor. Maternal death can occur. Therapeutic abortion should be considered
Scleroderma	If onset during pregnancy, there can be rapid overall deterioration. Reactivation of quiescent scleroderma can occur during pregnancy and after delivery
Previous urologic surgery	Depending on original reason for surgery, there may be other malformations of the urogenital tract. Urinary tract infection is common during pregnancy and renal function may undergo reversible decrease. No significant obstructive problem, but Caesarean section might be necessary for abnormal presentation or to avoid disruption of the continence mechanism if artificial sphincters or neourethras are present
After nephrectomy, solitary and pelvic kidneys	Pregnancy is well tolerated. Might be associated with other malformations of the urogenital tract. Dystocia rarely occurs with a pelvic kidney

Table 14.4 Pre-pregnancy kidney function (S_{cr}) in CKD patients with estimates for obstetric complications and outcome and renal functional loss.

S_{cr} (µmol/L)	Fetal growth restriction (%)	Preterm delivery (%)	Pre-eclampsia (%)	Perinatal deaths (%)	Loss of >25% renal function		
					Pregnancy (%)	Persists postpartum (%)	End-stage failure in 1 year (%)
≤125	25	30	22	1	2	–	–
125–180	45	70	40	6	40	20	3
≥180	70	>90	60	12	70	55	35

Estimates are based on literature from 1985 to 2009, with all pregnancies attaining at least 24 weeks' gestation (Davison and Winfield, unpublished data). Modified and supplemented from Williams & Davison [8].

Note that from more recent analyses of women with severe CKD it is now apparent that an S_{cr} cut-off of 250 µmol/L is too high a level for 'moderate' renal impairment, a cut-off of 180 µmol/L now being recommended [1,45].

Antenatal strategy and decision-making

These patients must be seen as early as possible. Thereafter assessments should be at 2–4 week intervals until 32 weeks' gestation and then every 1–2 weeks, depending on the clinical circumstances [1,8].

1 Assessment of renal function by 24-hour C_{cr} and by protein excretion (see Chapter 11), either as 24-hour excretion or a spot protein/creatinine ratio.

2 Careful blood pressure monitoring for early detection of hypertension (and assessment of its severity) and pre-eclampsia, with consideration (in early pregnancy) of the use of prophylactic low-dose aspirin.

3 Early detection and treatment of anaemia, usually by oral/intravenous iron therapy. Some recommend use of recombinant human erythropoietin if haematocrit is 20% or less, but caution is needed as hypertension can be caused or aggravated. Blood transfusion may need to be considered.

4 Early detection of covert bacteriuria or confirmation of urinary tract infection (UTI) and prompt treatment; if there are recurrent UTIs, then antibiotic prophylaxis should be given throughout pregnancy.

5 Biophysical/ultrasound surveillance of fetal size, development and well-being.

The clinician must bear in mind the balance between maternal prognosis and fetal prognosis: the effect of pregnancy on a particular disease and the effect of that disease on pregnancy. The clinical watchpoints associated with specific renal diseases are summarized in Table 14.3. The following guidelines apply to all CKD patients.

Renal function

If renal function deteriorates significantly at any stage of pregnancy, then reversible causes, such as UTI, subtle dehydration or electrolyte imbalance (occasionally precipitated by inadvertent diuretic therapy), should be sought. Near term, as in normal pregnancy, a decrease in function of 15–20%, which affects S_{cr} minimally, is permissible. Failure to detect a reversible cause of a significant decrement is grounds to end the pregnancy by elective delivery. When proteinuria occurs and persists, but blood pressure is normal and renal function preserved, pregnancy can be allowed to continue under closer scrutiny. With nephrotic syndrome prophylactic heparin is needed and should be continued for 6 weeks after delivery. The use of acute dialysis has been mentioned earlier.

Blood pressure

The conventional dividing line for obstetric hypertension is 140/90 mmHg. Most of the specific risks of hypertension in pregnancy appear to be related to superimposed pre-eclampsia (see Chapter 11). There is confusion about the true incidence of superimposed pre-eclampsia in women with CKD. This is because the diagnosis cannot be made with certainty on clinical grounds alone; hypertension and proteinuria may be manifestations of the underlying CKD and chronic hypertension alone has an increased pre-eclampsia risk fourfold that of normotensive pregnant women. Treatment of mild hypertension (diastolic blood pressure less than 95 mmHg in the second trimester or less than 100 mmHg in the third) is not necessary during normal pregnancy, but many would treat women with CKD more aggressively, believing that this preserves kidney function. There are still debates about the so-called 'tight control', accuracy of automated devices and the role of ambulatory blood pressure measurements.

Medications such as methyldopa, calcium channel blockers, labetalol and hydralazine are safe in pregnancy. Angiotensin-converting enzyme (ACE) inhibitors and angiotensin receptor blockers should not be prescribed and even if patients were taking either of these in early pregnancy (to continue the so-called renal protection from pre-pregnancy) they should not be continued or recommended later on.

Fetal surveillance and timing of delivery

Serial assessment of fetal well-being is essential. In the absence of fetal or maternal deterioration delivery should be at or near term. If complications do arise, the judicious moment for intervention might be determined by fetal status (see Chapter 28). Regardless of gestational age, most babies weighing more than 1500 g survive better in a special care nursery than in a hostile intrauterine environment. Planned preterm delivery may be necessary if there is impending intrauterine fetal death, if renal function deteriorates substantially, if uncontrollable hypertension supervenes, or if eclampsia occurs. Obstetric considerations should be the main determinant for delivery by Caesarean section.

Role of renal biopsy in pregnancy

Experience with renal biopsy in pregnancy is sparse, mainly because clinical circumstances rarely justify the risks [5,9]. Biopsy is therefore usually deferred until after delivery. Reports of excessive bleeding and other complications in pregnant women have led some to consider pregnancy as a relative contraindication to renal biopsy. When renal biopsy is undertaken immediately after delivery in women with well-controlled blood pressure and normal coagulation indices, the morbidity is certainly similar to that reported in non-pregnant patients. The few generally agreed indications for antepartum biopsy are suspicion of rapidly progressive glomerulonephritis or when severe nephrotic syndrome develops in early pregnancy.

Long-term effects of pregnancy in women with renal disease

Pregnancy does not cause deterioration or otherwise affect rate of progression of CKD beyond what might be expected in the non-pregnant state, provided pre-pregnancy kidney dysfunction was minimal and/or hypertension is absent or very well controlled before pregnancy [11,18,31–33]. An important factor in long-term prognosis could be the sclerotic effect that prolonged gestational renal vasodilatation might have in the residual (intact) glomeruli of the kidneys of these women. The situation may be worse in a single diseased kidney, where more sclerosis has usually occurred within the fewer (intact) glomeruli. Although the evidence in healthy women and those with mild renal disease argues against hyperfiltration-induced damage in pregnancy, there is little doubt that in some women with moderate, and certainly severe, dysfunction there can be unpredicted, accelerated and irreversible renal decline in pregnancy or immediately afterwards [31].

There is also a new literature focusing on relationships between CKD, pre-eclampsia and the remote prognosis in both groups in terms of cardiovascular disorders and end-stage renal failure and whether the superimposition of pre-eclampsia on CKD hastens progression to end-stage status [34–37]. It seems that pre-eclampsia is not a risk factor ('marker' is a better term) for progression (see Chapter 11).

New system for assessment of renal impairment and its implications for CKD in pregnancy

Estimated GFR

The traditional approach, with CKD defined as mild, moderate or severe, used by most clinicians is now being questioned. There are calls for guidance based on the current CKD classification that is part of the US National Kidney Foundation (NKF) K/DOQI clinical practice guidelines, endorsed by the UK National Service Framework for Renal Services, and now widely adopted by nephrologists [38,40]. The cornerstone of the classification is the use of estimated GFR (eGFR; units mL/min/1.73 m^2), calculated from a formula based on S_{cr} adjusted for age, gender and race; nowadays most chemical pathology laboratories are encouraged to report eGFR. The so-called Modified Diet in Renal Disease (MDRD) formula was developed in the USA in a multiethnic population of women and men with moderate renal impairment and, most importantly, an eGFR below 60 mL/min/1.73 m^2. The classification recognizes five stages of CKD (Table 14.5).

In non-pregnant populations, eGFR is much less reliable in patients with CKD stages 1 and 2 because of the poor correlation with actual GFR when it exceeds 60 mL/min [41]. In fact over 95% of women with underlying CKD becoming pregnant do have an actual GFR of 60 mL/min or more.

Table 14.5 Stages of CKD classified according to the US National Kidney Foundation.

Stage		eGFR (mL/min/1.73 m^2)
1	Kidney damage with normal or even increased GFR	≥90
2	Kidney damage with mild GFR decrease	60–89
3	Moderate GFR decrease	30–59
4	Severely low GFR	15–29
5	Kidney failure	<15 or dialysis

eGFR, estimated glomerular filtration rate.
Source: Davison *et al.* [5], National Kidney Foundation [38,39], Davison & Lindheimer [45], Imbasciati *et al.* [46].

Unlike many prediction formulae, the MDRD equation is not individualized for body surface area and is therefore theoretically attractive for use in the obstetric population in whom increased surface area is not a reflection of increased muscle mass and therefore of increased S_{cr}. However, reports to date have not borne this out and during pregnancy the MDRD fomula substantially underestimates GFR compared with the gold standard of inulin clearance [42]. An important clinical concern deriving from the fact that eGFR tends to underestimate true GFR is that its use might signal to the clinician an exaggerated deterioration in GFR, perhaps promoting unnecessary delivery. Therefore, the use of the MDRD equation during pregnancy to estimate GFR in women who have known renal impairment prior to conception or who develop renal complications during pregnancy cannot be recommended. The same applies for the Epi-CKD formula [43]. Also the Cockroft–Gault formula, and many others, are inaccurate in pregnancy and there is disagreement about using cystatin C to monitor renal function [44].

eGFR versus S_{cr}

It might seem that a system based on GFR would be superior to one based on S_{cr} and perhaps the database in the literature should be converted to this new CKD classification [45]. We would argue almost certainly not, as the great majority of pregnant women are those with mild disease (CKD stages 1 and 2) and, as mentioned already, the formulae for eGFR in women whose values are anticipated to be above 60 mL/min in the non-pregnant state are unreliable. Furthermore, the traditional system has been easy to disseminate and is familiar among non-nephrology specialists. Whilst defending the use of S_{cr} it must nevertheless be mentioned that very small women may present with normal or mildly elevated S_{cr}, and especially if their total muscle mass is quite low, so a timed urinary creatinine clearance (a 12-hour collection will suffice) may reveal 'true' GFR values indicative of more severe renal dysfunction [45].

If in the future clinicians start using the CKD system rather than the traditional guidelines, it might be preferable to stratify patients into two groups: stages 1–2, mild renal impairment; stages 3–5, moderate to severe renal impairment. Although no attempt has been made to revisit earlier publications and re-analyse where possible in terms of stages 1–5, there is one landmark prospective study covering 23 years that has assessed the rate of decline of maternal renal function during pregnancy in 49 white non-diabetic women with CKD stages 3–5 before pregnancy (eGFR <60 mL/min/1.73 m² pre-pregnancy) to average 39 months after delivery [46]. This multicentre Italian network effort confirmed earlier observations that such women have complicated pregnancies with poor perinatal outcomes as well as an accelerated decline in renal function. That it took 21 years to compile this series endorses how unusual pregnancy is in women with advanced CKD. The main conclusion was encouraging because while the group as a whole lost function during pregnancy, the rate of loss was not affected by pregnancy [33]. Also, 95% of the fetuses survived, albeit many were born preterm and/or growth restricted. The best outcomes were to women whose pre-pregnancy eGFR was between 60 and 40 mL/min/1.73 m², corresponding to S_{cr} values between 125 and 141–150 μmol/L or proteinuria less than 1 g/day. On the other hand, women with eGFR below 40 mL/min/1.73 m² and proteinuria above 1 g/day had poorer outcomes, the combination resulting in worse outcomes than either factor alone. Although these women developed renal failure faster than other groups, it was not possible to determine if pregnancy was a causal factor.

Patients on dialysis

Dialysis and the prospects for pregnancy and afterwards

Despite reduced libido and relative infertility, women on long-term dialysis do conceive and must therefore use contraception if they wish to avoid pregnancy [29,47–49]. Although conception is not common (an incidence of 1 in 200 patients has been quoted), its true frequency is unknown because most pregnancies in dialysis patients probably end in early spontaneous abortion. The high therapeutic abortion rate in this group of patients (which has decreased from 40% in the 1990s to under 15% today) still suggests that those who become pregnant do so inadvertently, probably because they are unaware that pregnancy is possible.

Summary box 14.3

- Incidence of conception in chronic dialysis patients of childbearing age is quoted as 1 in 200.
- Pregnancy poses big maternal risks but successful obstetric outcome is now 80%, leading to a reconsideration of counselling for these patients.
- Frequency of dialysis must be increased as soon as pregnancy is diagnosed and management of anaemia, nutritional issues and hypertension are very important.

Many authorities still do not advise chronic dialysis patients to become pregnant or to continue a pregnancy if present. In the last decade, however, fetal survival has significantly improved from 50% to almost 80%, with 90% attaining 36 weeks' gestation, which has led to a reconsideration of counselling for these patients [50,51]. Favourable prognostics for obstetric success include time on dialysis of less than 5 years, age under 35 years, residual urine production, and absence of or well-controlled hypertension as well as the early diagnosis of pregnancy thus facilitating increases in frequency and duration of dialysis. Nevertheless, pregnancy still poses big maternal risks, including volume overload, threat of preterm labour, polyhydramnios (40–70%), major exacerbations of hypertension and/or superimposed pre-eclampsia (50–80%) and rarely, fortunately, placental abruption.

Antenatal strategy and decision-making

If women on dialysis become pregnant, they may present for care in advanced pregnancy because it was not suspected by either the patient or her doctors. Irregular menstruation is common and missed periods are usually ignored. Urine pregnancy tests are unreliable (even if there is any urine available). Thus ultrasound evaluation is needed to confirm and date pregnancy.

Dialysis policy

Some patients have gestational GFR increments despite renal function being insufficient to sustain life without dialysis [9,10,47,49,52–55]. The planning of dialysis strategy has several aims.

1 Maintain S_{urea} below 20 mmol/L (some would argue <15 mmol/L), as intrauterine fetal death is more likely if values are much in excess of 20 mmol/L. Success has occasionally been achieved despite levels of around 28 mmol/L for many weeks but lower S_{urea} is definitely associated with higher birthweight and gestational age at delivery. Weekly dialysis should be 20 hours or more per week, using a dialysate with a higher potassium, lower calcium and lower bicarbonate. There is now good evidence that nocturnal dialysis (up to 36 hours per week) is associated with much better outcomes, as it can be a

haemodialfiltration protocol too. Increased dialysis hours, however minimal, should make control of weight gain and dietary management easier. The potential disadvantage of more dialysis is electrolyte imbalance, hence the need to scrutinize serum chemistries at all times. Heparin can be used for anticoagulation.

2 Avoid hypotension and maternal volume depletion during dialysis, and a biocompatible small-surface-area dialysis to reduce ultrafiltration per treatment may be helpful in this regard. In late pregnancy the enlarging uterus and supine posture may aggravate hypotensive episodes by decreasing venous return.

3 Ensure tight control of blood pressure throughout pregnancy, with the diastolic blood pressure ideally maintained at 80–90 mmHg.

4 Avoid rapid fluctuations in intravascular volume by limiting interdialysis weight gain to about 1 kg until late pregnancy.

5 Watch serum calcium closely to avoid hypercalcaemia and remember the potential for hypophosphataemia, hypokalaemia and depletion of water-soluble vitamins as well as the hazards of magnesium sulphate infusion, if required.

6 Scrutinize carefully for preterm labour, as dialysis and uterine contractions are associated.

Anaemia

Dialysis patients are usually anaemic, invariably aggravated further in pregnancy. There is some evidence of a positive correlation between maternal haemoglobin and successful obstetric outcome; however, although haemoglobin of 10 g/dL or more is advisable, the upper limit of an optimal haemoglobin level has yet to be determined [54]. Blood transfusion may be needed (especially before delivery), with caution necessary as it could exacerbate hypertension and impair the ability to control circulatory overload, even with extra dialysis. Fluctuations in blood volume can be minimized if packed red cells are transfused during dialysis. Treatment of anaemia with recombinant human erythropoietin has been 'safely' used in pregnancy, when requirements can be higher. The theoretical risks of hypertension and thrombotic complications have not been encountered, nor have adverse neonatal effects.

Hypertension

Normotension before pregnancy is reassuring. Some patients have abnormal lipid profiles and possibly accelerated atherogenesis so theoretically may not have the cardiovascular capacity to make gestational adaptations. Patients with diabetic nephropathy who become pregnant are those in whom cardiovascular problems are the most worrisome. As a generalization, blood pressure tends to be labile and hypertension is common, although control may be possible by careful dialysis. Ideally, diastolic blood pressure should be maintained between 80 and 90 mmHg.

Nutrition

Despite more frequent dialysis, uncontrolled dietary intake should be discouraged [47]. Daily oral intakes of 1.5 g/kg protein, 1.5 g calcium, 50 mmol potassium and 80 mmol sodium are advisable, with supplements of vitamin C, riboflavin, niacin, thiamine and vitamin B_6 as well as iron and folic acid supplements. Vitamin D supplements can be difficult to judge in patients who have had parathyroidectomy. Measurement of 25-hydroxyvitamin D levels should not be neglected, with supplementation if needed. In addition, oral phosphate supplements can be used if phosphate levels are low.

Fetal surveillance and timing of delivery

The same applies as with CKD. Preterm labour is common and it may even commence during dialysis. Caesarean section should be necessary only for obstetric reasons, although it has been argued that elective Caesarean section in all cases would minimize potential problems during labour.

Peritoneal dialysis

Young women can be managed with this approach and successful pregnancies have now been reported [56]. Outcome is not dependent on mode of dialysis (haemodialysis vs. peritoneal) but there may be more infertility in women receiving continuous ambulatory peritoneal dialysis (PD).

With PD, although anticoagulation and some of the fluid balance and volume problems of haemodialysis are avoided, these women nevertheless face the same problems of hypertension, anaemia, term labour, sudden intrauterine death and placental abruption. During pregnancy the number of PD exchanges must be increased and the fill volumes of fluid may need reducing to less than 1.5 L, which might be best achieved by switching to automated PD. The size of the enlarging uterus in late pregnancy may make PD impossible and a temporary switch to haemodialysis may be necessary. It should be remembered that peritonitis can be a severe complication of chronic ambulatory PD, accounting for the majority of therapy failures but an increased incidence has not been reported in pregnancy. If Caesarean section is needed then theoretically it should be undertaken extraperitoneally with the traditional approach requiring a switch to haemodialysis.

Kidney transplant recipients

Transplantation and the prospects for pregnancy and afterwards

Renal, endocrine and sexual functions return rapidly after transplantation and assisted conception techniques are also available. About 1 in 50 women of childbearing age with a functioning transplant will become pregnant. Of the conceptions, about 25% do not go beyond the initial trimester because of spontaneous or therapeutic abortion, but of those pregnancies in well women that do, 97% end successfully [1,3,5,9]. In early pregnancy there may be increased risk of ectopic pregnancy because of pelvic adhesions following surgery, PD, intrauterine contraceptive device (IUCD) and/or pelvic inflammatory disease consequent to immunosuppression. Diagnosis of ectopic pregnancy may be delayed as irregular bleeding and pain may be wrongly attributed to deteriorating renal function and/or the presence of the pelvic allograft. A renal transplant has even been performed with surgeons unaware that the recipient was in early pregnancy. Obstetric success in such cases does not negate the importance of contraception counselling for all renal failure patients and the exclusion of pregnancy prior to the surgery.

Summary box 14.4

- About 1 in 50 women of childbearing age with a functioning transplant becomes pregnant.
- Of those pregnancies that go beyond the first trimester, 97% have successful obstetric outcome. Serial assessment of renal function is essential along with early diagnosis and treatment of rejection (5%), blood pressure control and treatment of infection.
- Some immunosuppressive drugs are contraindicated in pregnancy.
- There are no obstructive problems and/or mechanical injury to the transplant during vaginal delivery.

A woman should be counselled from the time the various treatments for renal failure and the potential for optimal rehabilitation are discussed [1,2,57,58]. As mentioned at the start of this chapter, couples who want a child should be encouraged to discuss all the implications, including the harsh realities of maternal survival prospects. Individual centres have their own guidelines. In most, a wait of at least 1 year after transplantation is advised. By then, the patient will have recovered from the surgery and any sequelae, graft function will have stabilized, and immunosuppression will be at maintenance levels. Also, if function is well maintained at 2 years, there is a high probability of allograft survival at 5 years (Table 14.6). As with CKD it is preferable if pre-pregnancy S_{cr} values are below 125 μmol/L, as above this level there can be more complications and problems (Table 14.7). Interestingly, the two significant higher S_{cr} cut-offs are 160 and 180 μmol/L [1]. In the non-pregnant patient the use of eGFR is not applicable.

Antenatal strategy and decision-making

Management requires serial assessment of renal function, early diagnosis and treatment of rejection, blood pressure control, early diagnosis or prevention of anaemia,

Table 14.6 Pre-pregnancy considerations in renal transplant recipients.

Good general health for about 1 year after transplantation
Stature compatible with good obstetric outcome
No or minimal proteinuria
No or well-controlled hypertension
No evidence of graft rejection
No pelvicalyceal distension on recent ultrasound or intravenous urography
Stable graft function: $S_{cr} \leq 160$ μmol/L, preferably ≤ 125 μmol/L
Drug therapy at maintenance levels: prednisolone, azathioprine, ciclosporin and tacrolimus are 'safe'
Mycophenolate mofetil and sirolimus are contraindicated

Source: Newcastle upon Tyne 1976, revised 1987 and 2006. See Davison [1], Winfield & Davison [3], Davison *et al.* [10], Armenti *et al.* [57].

Table 14.7 Pre-pregnancy kidney function (S_{cr}) in kidney transplant recipients with estimates for obstetric complications and outcome and loss of graft function.

S_{cr} (μmol/L)	Fetal growth restriction (%)	Preterm delivery (%)	Pre-eclampsia (%)	Perinatal deaths (%)	Loss of >25% renal function		
					Pregnancy (%)	Persists postpartum (%)	End-stage failure in 1 year (%)
≤125	30	35	24	3	15	4	–
125–160	50	70	45	7	20	7	10
≥160	60	90	60	12	45	35	70

Estimates based on literature review (1991–2007) from 1076 women in 1498 pregnancies, with all pregnancies attaining at least 24 weeks' gestation.
Source: Davison, unpublished data.

treatment of any infection, and meticulous assessment of fetal well-being (Table 14.8). As well as regular renal assessments, liver function tests, plasma protein, and calcium and phosphate should be checked at 6-weekly intervals. Cytomegalovirus and herpesvirus hominis status should be checked during each trimester and HIV should be determined at first attendance. Haematinics are needed if the various haematological indices show deficiency.

Transplant function

The sustained increase in GFR characteristic of early normal pregnancy is evident in renal transplant recipients. Immediate graft function after transplantation and the better the pre-pregnancy GFR, the greater the increment in pregnancy. Transient 20–25% reductions in GFR can occur during the third trimester and do not usually represent a deteriorating situation with permanent impairment. However, significant renal functional impairment can develop in some patients during pregnancy, and this may persist following delivery, invariably being related to pre-pregnancy S_{cr} (Table 14.7). As a gradual decline in function is common in non-pregnant patients, it is difficult to delineate the specific role of pregnancy. Most agree that pregnancy does not compromise long-term graft progression unless there was already graft dysfunction before pregnancy [57,59,60]. Proteinuria occurs near term in 40% of patients but disappears after delivery and, in the absence of hypertension, is not significant unless it exceeds 1 g in 24 hours, which by some is considered to be a marker of suboptimal obstetric outcome and/or later deterioration. Whether calcineurin inhibitors are more nephrotoxic in the pregnant compared with the non-pregnant patient is not known. Certainly the literature indicates that with the advent of these immunosuppressive agents, pre-pregnancy S_{cr} levels are higher overall than during the era of azathioprine and steroids [60].

Transplant rejection

Serious rejection episodes occur in 5% of pregnant women. While this incidence is no greater than that seen in non-pregnant individuals during a similar period, it is unexpected because it has been assumed that the privileged immunological status of pregnancy might benefit the allograft. Rejection often occurs in the puerperium and may be due to a return to normal immune status (despite immunosuppression) or possibly a rebound effect from the altered gestational immunoresponsiveness [57,61].

Chronic rejection with a progressive subclinical course may be a problem in all recipients. Whether pregnancy influences the course of subclinical rejection is unknown: no factors consistently predict which patients will develop rejection during pregnancy. There may also be a non-immune contribution to chronic graft failure due to the

Table 14.8 Management summary for a renal transplant patient.

Before pregnancy

Patients should defer pregnancy for at least 1 year after transplant, with appropriate and reliable contraception
Assessment of graft function
Recent biopsy and/or organ-specific tests
Proteinuria
S_{cr}
Hepatitis B and C, cytomegalovirus, toxoplasmosis, and herpes simplex status
Maintenance immunosuppression
Azathioprine
Ciclosporin
Tacrolimus
Corticosteroids
Mycophenolate mofetil and sirolimus contraindicated
Comorbidities (e.g. diabetes, hypertension) should be optimally managed
Vaccinations should be given if needed (e.g. hepatitis, tetanus, pneumococcus, human papillomavirus and influenza)
Discuss the aetiology of the original disease and genetic issues, if appropriate
Discuss the effect of pregnancy on graft function
Discuss the risks of fetal growth restriction, preterm delivery and low birthweight

Antenatal

Early diagnosis and dating of pregnancy
Clincial and laboratory monitoring of the graft and immunosuppressive drug levels every 2–4 weeks until 32 weeks, then every 1–2 weeks until delivery
Surveillance for rejection, with transplant biopsy considered if it is suspected
Surveillance for bacterial or viral infection (e.g. cytomegalovirus, toxoplasmosis, hepatitis in first trimester and repeat if signs of rejection or tenderness over graft site)
Monthly urine cultures
Fetal surveillance after 32 weeks (e.g. non-stress test, sonographic evaluation)
Monitoring of hypertension and management
Surveillance for pre-eclampsia
Screening for gestational diabetes
For kidney recipients: proteinuria is common
For kidney–pancreas recipients: immunosuppressive agents may augment diabetogenic effect of pregnancy. All infections must be taken very seriously

Delivery

Caesarean delivery for obstetric reasons
For kidney recipients: episiotomy on side opposite to graft. Caesarean section may not be easy

Post partum

Monitor immunosuppressive drug levels for 3–4 weeks after delivery, with adjustment as needed
Surveillance for rejection and consider biopsy if it is suspected
Breast-feeding is appropriate; monitor fetal drug levels
Contraception counselling is essential

Source: modified and supplemented from Armenti *et al.* [57].

damaging effect of hyperfiltration through remnant nephrons, perhaps even exacerbated during pregnancy. An important clinical watchpoint is that rejection is difficult to diagnose: if any of the clinical hallmarks are present (fever, oliguria, deteriorating renal function, renal enlargement, and tenderness), then the diagnosis should be considered. Ultrasound assessment may be helpful but without renal biopsy, rejection cannot be distinguished from acute pyelonephritis, recurrent glomerulopathy, possible severe pre-eclampsia, and even ciclosporin nephrotoxicity and therefore renal biopsy is indicated before embarking on anti-rejection therapy [61].

Immunosuppressive therapy

Immunosuppressive therapy is usually maintained at pre-pregnancy levels. There are many encouraging registry and single centre reports of (non-complicated) pregnancies in patients taking ciclosporin and tacrolimus (FK506 or Prograf). Numerous adverse effects are attributed to calcineurin inhibitors in non-pregnant transplant recipients, including renal toxicity, hepatic dysfunction, chronic hypertension, tremor, convulsions, diabetogenic effects, haemolytic uraemic syndrome, and neoplasia. In pregnancy, some of the maternal adaptations that normally occur may theoretically be blunted or abolished by ciclosporin, especially plasma volume expansion and renal hemodynamic augmentation. There is good evidence to suggest that patients have more hypertension and smaller babies [61,62].

From registry reports and post-marketing data, it is evident that exposure to mycophenolate mofetil (MMF) in pregnancy is associated with an increased incidence and specific type of malformation, as well as a higher incidence of spontaneous abortions in female transplant recipients. A predominance of a particular type of birth defect had not been reported with previous immunosuppressive regimens and successful pregnancies with MMF exposure have also been reported but the conclusion cannot be avoided that there is a characteristic pattern of malformation after *in utero* exposure to MMF [63]. Indeed, the existence of an MMF-associated embryopathy has been proposed with consistent main features: cleft lip and palate, microtia with atresia of the external auditory canal, micrognathia and hypertelorum [64]. Ocular anomalies, corpus callosum agenesis, heart defects, kidney malformations and diaphragmatic hernia could also be a part of the phenotypic spectrum, which is supported by experimental animal studies. To date, in the babies, psychomotor development and growth have been reported as normal.

Thus MMF poses a management dilemma, as a drug with proven efficacy but of potential harm. Alternative immunosuppression may either be less effective (e.g. azathioprine) or have limited experience in this context (e.g. sirolimus). So, in these circumstances the clinician has

Table 14.9 Pregnancy safety information for immunosuppressive drugs used in transplantation.

	Animal reproductive data	Pregnancy category
Corticosteroids (prednisolone, methylprednisolone, others)	Yes	B
Azathioprine (Imuran)	Yes	D
Ciclosporin (Sandimmun, Neoral, others)	Yes	C
Tacrolimus (FK506, Prograf)	Yes	C
Antithymocyte globulin (Atgam, ATG)	No	C
Antithymocyte globulin (Thymoglobulin)	No	C
Muromonab-CD3 (Orthoclone OKT3)	No	C
Mycophenolate mofetil (CellCept)	Yes	D
Mycophenolic acid (Myfortic)	Yes	D
Basiliximab (Simulect)	Yes	B
Daclizumab (Zenapax)	No	C
Sirolimus (Rapamune)	Yes	C

B, no fetal risk, no controlled studies; C, fetal risk cannot be ruled out; D, evidence of fetal risk.
Source: US Food and Drug Administration classification. Modified from Armenti *et al.* [57,61,62].

two choices: (i) recommend pre-pregnancy changes to immunosuppression, potentially increasing rejection risk and in the absence of data on the efficacy of such switches, or (ii) recommend continuation of an efficacious regimen with potential teratogenic risk (Table 14.9).

Hypertension and pre-eclampsia

Hypertension, particularly before 28 weeks' gestation, is associated with adverse perinatal outcome. This may be due to covert cardiovascular changes that accompany and/or are aggravated by chronic hypertension. The appearance of hypertension in the third trimester, its relationship to deteriorating renal function, and the possibility of chronic underlying pathology and pre-eclampsia is a diagnostic problem. Pre-eclampsia is actually diagnosed clinically in about 30% of pregnancies.

Infections

Throughout pregnancy patients should be monitored carefully for bacterial and viral infection. Prophylactic antibiotics must be given before any surgical procedure, however trivial.

Diabetes mellitus

As the results of renal transplantation have improved in those women whose renal failure is caused by juvenile-onset diabetes mellitus, pregnancies are now being reported in these women. Pregnancy complications occur with at least twice the frequency seen in the non-diabetic patient, and this may be due to the presence of generalized cardiovascular pathology, which is part of the metabolic risk factor syndrome. Successful pregnancies have been reported after combined pancreas–kidney allografts.

Fetal surveillance and timing of delivery

The points discussed under CKD are equally applicable to renal transplant recipients. Preterm delivery is common (45–60%) because of intervention for obstetric reasons and the common occurrence of preterm labour or preterm rupture of membranes. Preterm labour is commonly associated with poor renal function, but in some it has been postulated that long-term immunosuppression may 'weaken' connective tissues and contribute to the increased incidence of preterm rupture of membranes.

Vaginal delivery should be the aim; usually there are no obstructive problems and/or mechanical injury to the transplant [3,57]. Unless there are problems, spontaneous onset of labour can be awaited but most advise not exceeding 38–39 weeks' gestation. During labour careful monitoring of fluid balance, cardiovascular status and temperature is mandatory. Aseptic technique is essential for every procedure. Surgical induction of labour (by amniotomy) and episiotomy warrant antibiotic cover. Pain relief can be conducted as for healthy women. Augmentation of steroids should not be overlooked. Caesarean section should be undertaken for obstetric reasons only.

Post-delivery management issues

Paediatric management

Over 50% of liveborns have no neonatal problems. Preterm delivery is common (45–60%), as is fetal growth restriction (20–30%), and occasionally the two problems coexist. Lower birthweights are seen in infants born to mothers who received their transplant less than 2 years previously and the use of calcineurin inhibitors can be associated with birthweight depression [3,61].

Breast-feeding

There are substantial benefits to breast-feeding. It could be argued that because the baby has been exposed to immunosuppressive agents and their metabolites in pregnancy, breast-feeding should not be allowed. However, little is known about the quantities of these drugs and their metabolites in breast milk and whether the levels are biologically trivial or substantial. For ciclosporin, levels in breast milk are usually greater than those in a simultaneously taken blood sample. There is a view that mothers who want to breast-feed should be encouraged, so long

Table 14.10 Neonatal problems in the newborn of kidney allograft recipients.

Preterm delivery and/or small for gestational age
Respiratory distress syndrome
Adrenocortical insufficiency
Septicaemia
Cytomegalovirus infection
Depressed haematopoiesis
Lymphoid and thymic hypoplasia
Reduced T lymphocyte and immunoglobulin levels
Chromosome aberrations in leucocytes

as the baby is thriving [3,62,64] and monitoring fetal drug levels could be undertaken.

Long-term assessment

There are theoretical worries about *in utero* exposure to immunosuppressive agents, with eventual development of malignant tumours in affected offspring, autoimmune complications and/or abnormalities in reproductive performance in the next generation. Thus paediatric follow-up is needed (Table 14.10). To date, information about general progress in early childhood has been good.

Maternal follow-up after pregnancy

The ultimate measure of transplant success is the long-term survival of the patient and the graft. As it is only 40 years since this procedure became widely employed in the management of end-stage renal failure, few long-term data from sufficiently large series exist from which to draw conclusions. Furthermore, the long-term results for renal transplants relate to a period when many aspects of management would be unacceptable by present-day standards. Average survival figures of large numbers of patients worldwide indicate that about 90% of recipients of kidneys from related living donors are alive 5 years after transplantation. With cadaver kidneys, the figure is approximately 70%. If renal function was normal 2 years after transplant, survival increased to over 80%. This is why women are counselled to wait about 2 years before considering a pregnancy even though a view is now emerging that 1 year would be sufficient.

A major concern is that the mother may not survive or remain well enough to rear the child she bears. Pregnancy occasionally and sometimes unpredictably causes irreversible declines in renal function. However, the consensus is that pregnancy has no effect on graft function or survival [57,59,65]. Also, repeated pregnancies do not adversely affect graft function or fetal development, provided that pre-pregnancy renal function is well preserved and hypertension minimal and/or well controlled.

Contraception

Oral contraception can cause or aggravate hypertension, thromboembolism and/or subtle changes to the immune system. This does not necessarily contraindicate its use but careful surveillance is essential. IUCDs may aggravate menstrual problems, which in turn may obscure symptoms and signs of early pregnancy abnormalities, such as threatened miscarriage or ectopic pregnancy. The increased risk of chronic pelvic infection in immunosuppressed patients with IUCDs is a problem and, as the insertion or replacement of a coil can be associated with bacteraemia of vaginal origin, so antibiotic cover is essential at this time. Lastly, the efficacy of an IUCD is reduced in women taking immunosuppressive and anti-inflammatory agents but many still request this method.

Gynaecological problems

There is a danger that symptoms secondary to genuine pelvic pathology may be erroneously attributed to the transplant because of its location near the pelvis [5]. Transplant recipients receiving immunosuppressive therapy have a malignancy rate estimated to be 100 times greater than normal and the female genital tract is no exception. This association is probably related to factors such as loss of immune surveillance, chronic immunosuppression allowing tumour proliferation and/or prolonged antigenic stimulation of the reticuloendothelial system. Regular gynaecological assessment is therefore essential and any gynaecological management should be on conventional lines, with the outcome unlikely to be influenced by stopping or reducing immunosuppression [3,61].

References

1 Davison JM. Prepregnancy care and counselling in chronic renal patients. *Eur Clin Obstet Gynaecol* 2006;2:24–29.

2 McKay DB, Josephson MA, Armenti VT *et al.* Women's Health Committee of the American Society of Transplantation: Reproduction and transplantation: Report on the AST Consensus Conference on Reproductive Issues and Transplantation. *Am J Transplant* 2005;5:1592–1599.

3 Winfield S, Davison JM. The patient with organ transplantation. In: Macklon NS, Greer IA, Steegers EAP (eds) *Textbook of Periconceptional Medicine*. Zug, Switzerland: Informa, 2009: 57–68.

4 Lindheimer MD, Conrad KP, Karumanchi SA. Renal physiology and disease in pregnancy. In: Alpern RJ, Hebert SC (eds) *Seldin and Giebisch's The Kidney*. San Diego: Elsevier, 2007, pp 2339–2398.

5 Davison JM, Nelson-Piercy C, Kehoe S, Baker P. *Renal Disease in Pregnancy*. London: RCOG Press, 2008. Available at: www.rcog.org.uk/files/rcog-corp/uploaded-files/StudyGroup ConsensuViewsRenalDisease.pdf

6 Lindheimer MD, Kanter D. Interpreting abnormal proteinuria in pregnancy: the need for a more pathophysiological approach. *Obstet Gynecol* 2010;115:365–375.

7 Williams D. Renal disorders. In: James DK, Steer PJ, Weiner CP, Gonik B (eds) *High Risk Pregnancy. Management Options*, 3rd edn. Philadelphia: Saunders, 2006: 1098–1124.

8 Williams D, Davison JM. Chronic kidney disease in pregnancy. *BMJ* 2008;336:311–315.

9 Williams DJ, Davison JM. Renal disorders. In: Creasy RK, Resnik R, Iams JD (eds) *Maternal–Fetal Medicine: Principles and Practice*, 6th edn. Philadelphia: Saunders, 2009: 767–792.

10 Davison JM, Katz AI, Lindheimer MD. Kidney disease and pregnancy: obstetric outcome and long-term renal prognosis. *Clin Perinatol* 1985;12:497–519.

11 Katz AI, Davison JM, Hayslett JP, Simpson M. Pregnancy in women with kidney disease. *Kidney Int* 1980;18:192–206.

12 Jungers P, Forget D, Henry M, Huoillier P. Chronic kidney disease and pregnancy. *Adv Nephrol* 1986;15:103–115.

13 Surian M, Imbasciati E, Cosci P. Glomerular disease and pregnancy: a study of 123 pregnancies. *Nephron* 1984;36:101–105.

14 Abe S. An overview of pregnancy in women with underlying renal disease. *Am J Kidney Dis* 1991;17:112–115.

15 Barcelo P, Lopez-Lillo J, Del Rio G. Succesful pregnancy in primary glomerular disease. *Kidney Int* 1986;30:914–919.

16 Jungers P, Houillier P, Forget D, Henry-Amar M. Specific controversies concerning the natural history of renal disease in pregnancy. *Am J Kidney Dis* 1991;17:116–122.

17 Imbasciati E, Pouticelli C. Pregnancy and renal disease: predictors of maternal outcome. *Am J Nephrol* 1991;11:353–357.

18 Jungers P, Chauveau D. Pregnancy and renal disease. *Kidney Int* 1997;52:871–885.

19 Abe S. The influence of pregnancy on the long term renal prognosis in women with IgA nephropathy. *Clin Nephrol* 1994;41: 61–64.

20 Jungers P, Houillier P, Chauveau D, Chouksonn G, Moynot A, Stihari H. Pregnancy in women with reflux nephropathy. *Kidney Int* 1996;50:593–599.

21 Jungers P, Chauveau D, Choukroun G *et al.* Pregnancy in women with impaired renal function. *Clin Nephrol* 1997;47: 281–288.

22 Hou SH, Grossman SD, Madia N. Pregnancy in women with renal disease and moderate renal insufficiency. *Am J Med* 1985; 78:185–189.

23 Imbasciati E, Pardi G, Capetta P. Pregnancy in women with chronic renal failure. *Am J Nephrol* 1986;6:193–198.

24 Cunningham FG, Cox SM, Harstad TW, Mason RA, Prichard JA. Chronic renal disease and pregnancy outcome. *Am J Obstet Gynecol* 1990;163:453–459.

25 Jones DC, Hayslett JP. Outcome of pregnancy in women with moderate or severe renal insufficiency. *N Engl J Med* 1996;335: 226–232.

26 Bar J, Ben-Rafael Z, Padoa A, Orvieto R, Bover G, Hod M. Prediction of pregnancy outcome in subgroups of women with renal disease. *Clin Nephrol* 2000;53:437–444.

27 Hou S. Historical perspective of pregnancy in chronic renal disease. *Adv Chronic Kidney Dis* 2007;14:116–118.

28 Fischer MJ. Chronic kidney disease and pregnancy: maternal and fetal outcomes. *Adv Chronic Kidney Dis* 2007;14:132–145.

29 Bramham K, Briley AL, Seed PT *et al.* Pregnancy outcome in women with chronic kidney disease. A prospective cohort study. *Reproductive Sci* 2011;18:623–630.

30 Chopra S, Suri V, Aggarwal N, Rohilla M, Keepanasseril A, Kohli HS. Pregnancy in chronic renal insufficiency: single

centre experience from North India. *Arch Gynecol Obstet* 2009; 279:691–695.

31 Epstein FH. Pregnancy and renal disease. *N Engl J Med* 1996; 335:277–278.

32 Fischer MJ, Lehnerz SD, Herbert JR, Parikh CR. Kidney disease is an independent risk factor for adverse fetal and maternal outcome in pregnancy. *Am J Kidney Dis* 2004;43:415–423.

33 Lindheimer MD, Davison JM. Pregnancy and chronic kidney disease: any progress? *Am J Kidney Dis* 2007;49:729–731.

34 Vikse BE, Irgeus LM, Bostad L, Iversen BM. Adverse outcome and later kidney biopsy in the mother. *J Am Soc Nephrol* 2006; 17:837–845.

35 Vikse BE, Irgeus LM, Leivestad T, Skjaerven R, Ivesen BM. Preeclampsia and the risk of end-stage renal disease. *N Engl J Med* 2008;359:800–809.

36 Munkhaugen J, Vikse BE. New aspects of preeclampsia: lessons for the nephrologists. *Nephrol Dial Transpl* 2009;24:2964–2967.

37 Ness RB, Roberts JM. Epidemiology of pregnancy-related hypertension. In: Lindheimer MD, Roberts JM, Cunningham FG (eds) *Chesley's Hypertensive Disorders in Pregnancy*, 3rd edn. San Diego: Academic Press, 2009: 37–50.

38 National Kidney Foundation KDQQI Clinical Practice Guidelines for Chronic Kidney Disease: Evaluation, Classification and Stratification. *Am J Kidney Dis* 2002;39(Suppl 1):S1–S266.

39 National Kidney Foundation Practice Guidelines for Chronic Kidney Disease: Evaluation, Classification and Stratification. *Ann Intern Med* 2003;139:137–147.

40 Department of Health. Estimating glomerular filtration rate (GFR): information for laboratories. Available at: www.dh.gov. uk/prod_consum_dh/groups/dh_digitalassets/@dh/@en/ documents/digitalasset/dh_4133025.pdf

41 Lin J, Knight EL, Hogan ML, Singh AK. A comparison of prediction equations for estimating GFR in adults without kidney disease. *J Am Soc Nephrol* 2003;14:2573–2580.

42 Smith MC, Moran P, Ward MK, Davison JM. Assessment of GFR during pregnancy using the MDRD formula. *BJOG* 2008; 115:109–112.

43 Smith MC, Moran P, Davison JM. Epi-CKD is a poor predictor of GFR in pregnancy. *Arch Dis Child Fetal Neonatal Ed* 2011;96: Fa99.

44 Bubay Z, Al-Wakeen J, Addar M *et al.* Serum cystatin-C in pregnant women: reference values, reliable and superior diagnostic accuracy. *Clin Exp Obstet Gynecol* 2005;32:175–179.

45 Davison JM, Lindheimer MD. Pregnancy and chronic kidney disease (CKD). *Semin Nephrol* 2011;31:86–99.

46 Imbasciati E, Gregorinin G, Cabiddu G, Gammaro L. Pregnancy in CKD stages 3 to 5: fetal and maternal outcomes. *Am J Kidney Dis* 2007;49:753–762.

47 Luders C, Castro MC, Titan SM *et al.* Obstetric outcome in pregnant women on longterm dialysis: a case series. *Am J Kid Dis* 2010;56:77–85.

48 Okendaye I, Abrinko P, Hou S. Registry of pregnancy in dialysis patients. *Am J Kidney Dis* 1998;31:766–773.

49 Holley JL, Schmidt RJ, Bender FH. Gynecologic and reproductive issues in women on dialysis. *Am J Kidney Dis* 1997;29: 685–690.

50 Hou S. Pregnancy in women on dialysis: is success a matter of time? *Clin J Am Soc Nephrol* 2008;3:312–313.

51 Piccoli GB, Conijn A, Consiglia V *et al.* Pregnancy in dialysis patients: is the evidence strong enough to lead us to change our counselling policy? *Clin Am J Soc Nephrol* 2010;5:62–71.

52 Barau M, Hladunewich M, Kenner J *et al.* Successful pregnancies on nocturnal home hemodialysis. *Clin J Am Soc Nephrol* 2008;3:392–396.

53 Asimaiya Y, Otsubo S, Matsuda Y *et al.* The importance of low blood urea nitrogen levels in pregnancy patients undergoing hemodialysis to optimise birth weight and gestational age. *Kidney Int* 2009;75:1217–1222.

54 Reddy SS, Holley JL. The implications of using dialysis and anaemia management for infant survival in pregnant women on hemodialysis. *Kidney Int* 2009;75:1133–1134.

55 Hou S. Modification of dialysis regimens for pregnancy. *J Artif Organs* 2002;25:823–826.

56 Hou S. Pregnancy in women treated with dialysis: Lessons from a large series over 20 years. *Am J Kid Dis* 2010;56:5–6.

57 Armenti VT, Constantinescu S, Moritz MJ, Davison JM. Pregnancy after transplantation. *Transplant Rev* 2008;22: 223–240.

58 McKay DB, Josephson MA. Pregnancy in recipients of solid organs: effects on mother and child. *N Engl J Med* 2006;354: 1281–1293.

59 Sturgiss SN, Davison JM. Effect of pregnancy on the long-term function of renal allografts: an update. *Am J Kidney Dis* 1995; 26:54–56.

60 Sibanda N, Briggs JD, Davison JM *et al.* Pregnancy after organ transplantation: a report from the UK Transplant Pregnancy Registry. *Transplantation* 2007;83:1301–1307.

61 Armenti VT, Moritz MJ, Cardonick EH, Davison JM. Immunosuppression in pregnancy: choices for infant and maternal health. *Drugs* 2002;62:2361–2375.

62 Armenti VT, Moritz MJ, Davison JM. Drug safety issues in pregnancy following transplantation and immunosuppression. *Drug Saf* 1998;19:219–232.

63 Perez-Aytes A, Ledo A, Boso V *et al.* In-utero exposure to mycophenolate mofetil: a characteristic phenotype? *Am J Med Genet A* 2008;146:1–7.

64 Armenti VT, Moritz MJ, Davison JM. Parenthood posttransplantation: 50 years later. *Transplantation* 2008;85:1389–1390.

65 Sifontis NM, Coscia LA, Constantinescu S *et al.* Pregnancy outcomes in solid organ transplant recipients with exposure to mycophenolate mofetil or sirolimus. *Transplantation* 2006;82: 1608–1702.

66 Kim HW, Seok HJ, Kim TH *et al.* The experience of pregnancy after renal transplantation: Pregnancies even within postoperative 1 year may be tenable. *Transplant* 2008;85:1412–1419.

Chapter 15
Haematological Problems in Pregnancy

Peter Clark[1], Andrew J. Thomson[2] and Ian A. Greer[3]
[1] Ninewells Hospital and Medical School, Dundee, UK
[2] Royal Alexandra Hospital, Paisley, UK
[3] University of Liverpool, Liverpool, UK

Anaemia

A normochromic, normocytic 'anaemia' can occur from weeks 7–8 of gestation. This is due to the physiological increase in plasma volume that is relatively greater than the increase in red cell mass. However, the haemoglobin should not fall below 11 g/dL in the first trimester or below 10.5 g/dL in the second and third trimesters [1]. More marked anaemia may be due to iron, folate or, more rarely, vitamin B_{12} deficiency or a haemoglobinopathy.

Haematinic requirements

Pregnancy requires an iron intake of around 2.5 mg/day throughout, with perhaps 3.0–7.5 mg/day required in the third trimester. Thus iron deficiency is a very common cause of anaemia in pregnancy worldwide. An average Western diet supplies around 250 μg/day of folate; however, requirements increase to around 400 μg/day during pregnancy [2], with deficiency most commonly due to a lack of folate-rich vegetables such as broccoli and peas, often linked to social deprivation. Folate deficiency is more common in multiple pregnancy, frequent childbirth and adolescent mothers. The body stores around 3 mg of vitamin B_{12}, with a daily dietary requirement of 3 μg. The only B_{12} source is animal foodstuffs and therefore vegetarians and vegans are most at risk of dietary deficiency.

The effects of haematinic deficiency

The signs and symptoms of early deficiencies are non-specific, including tiredness and features of any underlying cause (Table 15.1). Aside from anaemia, folate and B_{12} deficiency are linked to neural tube defects [3,4]. The effect of iron deficiency (before anaemia is manifest) on maternal and fetal well-being is not fully understood. Such deficiency has been associated with increased blood loss at delivery, poor fetal iron stores, an increased placenta/fetus weight ratio [5], premature delivery and low birthweight [1], although these may also relate to the underlying cause. Most subjects with folate deficiency are identified incidentally due to a raised mean red cell volume (MCV), but folate deficiency anaemia often coexists with iron deficiency and more often presents at the end of pregnancy or in the early puerperium. Severe vitamin B_{12} deficiency can also result in a demyelinating neuropathy, although mild maternal B_{12} deficiency appears compatible with normal pregnancy [6].

Diagnosis of haematinic deficiency

As the MCV may increase with normal gestation, the reduction in MCV usually seen in iron deficiency is not a reliable marker in pregnancy. Serum iron, total iron-binding capacity (TIBC), ferritin, serum transferrin receptor levels and red cell-derived protoporphyrin can all be used to diagnose iron deficiency. However, normal pregnancy leads to a progressive fall in serum iron and ferritin and an increase in TIBC, free protoporphyrin and transferrin receptor levels [7]. Thus, a number of parameters may be required to diagnose mild deficiency, although a markedly reduced serum ferritin (<12 μg/L) remains diagnostic. For practical purposes serum ferritin is therefore the best first-line investigation for suspected iron deficiency.

Megaloblastic anaemia from B_{12} or folate deficiency is suggested by an MCV in excess of 100 fL, with right-shifted neutrophils on the blood film (Table 15.2). Serum folate is sensitive to deficiency, but may be reduced with very recent shortage of dietary folate and also reduces in normal pregnancy. Red cell folate levels are less affected by recent diet, but may rise in otherwise normal pregnancy [8,9]. If necessary, megaloblastic erythropoiesis can be demonstrated by bone marrow examination. Serum B_{12} levels may fall by 30–50% during normal pregnancy, but this is probably not a true tissue deficiency [6]. Specific tests to diagnose intrinsic factor deficiency (from pernicious anaemia) involve radioisotope exposure and are contraindicated in pregnancy, but plasma intrinsic factor antibodies, if present, can point to a diagnosis of pernicious anaemia.

Dewhurst's Textbook of Obstetrics & Gynaecology, Eighth Edition. Edited by D. Keith Edmonds.
© 2012 John Wiley and Sons, Ltd. Published 2012 by John Wiley and Sons, Ltd.

Table 15.1 Causes of iron, folate and vitamin B_{12} deficiency.

Iron
Diet: vegetarian/vegan
Blood loss
Menorrhagia
Peptic ulceration
Inflammatory bowel disease
Haemorrhoids
Varices
Aspirin
Anticoagulants
von Willebrand's disease
Malabsorption
Coeliac
Gastrectomy

Folate
Dietary
Alcoholism
Poverty
Adolescence
Malabsorption: gluten-induced enteropathy (coeliac)
Increased use:
    Chronic haemolysis
    Congenital red cell disorders
    Haemoglobinopathy
    Myeloproliferative disorders
Loss: dialysis
Miscellaneous: anticonvulsants

Vitamin B_{12}
Dietary: vegans
Malabsorption
Pernicious anaemia
Partial gastric resection, ileal resection, intestinal stagnant loop
Crohn's disease
Tapeworms
Tropical sprue
Miscellaneous: folate deficiency

Table 15.2 Differential diagnosis of a raised MCV.

B_{12} deficiency
Folate deficiency
Alcohol
Hypothyroidism
Pregnancy
Liver disease
Myelodysplasia
Haemolysis

Prophylaxis

The haemoglobin concentration is often used to screen for haematinic deficiency, with an assessment at presentation and again in the early third trimester. Whether routine iron supplementation is warranted is not resolved,

Table 15.3 Elemental iron in various oral iron preparations.

Preparation	Dose (mg)	Elemental iron (mg)
Ferrous sulphate	300	60
	325	65
Ferrous sulphate (dried)	200	65
	325	105
Ferrous gluconate	300	34–35
Ferrous fumarate	325	106
	322	100
	200	65

because although it may result in fewer women with a haemoglobin level less than 10 g/dL in late pregnancy and the puerperium [1], it is not clear whether this benefits the mother or baby. If required, supplementation can be achieved with 30–60 mg of elemental iron daily, which produces few side effects. Side effects are mainly seen with replacement therapy ($\geq$200 mg/day of elemental iron). Furthermore, supplementation with more than 200 mg/day will not produce a supranormal haemoglobin or haematocrit. The amount of elemental iron present in the common oral formulations is shown in Table 15.3. To prevent neural tube defects, folic acid supplementation (400 μg/day) is routinely given in the first trimester. It should also be taken for 3 months prior to conception in those planning pregnancy and a higher dose is needed if there is a previous child with a neural tube defect or a chronic red cell disorder. Such supplementation is also of value with regard to prophylaxis of anaemia in women with potential dietary deficiency. Folate should be continued through pregnancy in women on antiepileptic drugs that antagonize folate metabolism, in those with likely dietary deficiency or those with increased demand such as multiple pregnancy.

Treatment

The treatment of established iron deficiency is with 200 mg of elemental iron daily. Higher doses are not required. Even 200 mg/day of elemental iron may lead to gastrointestinal upset, which may be dose or product related. This is usually ameliorated by either dose reduction (100 mg/day), or a change in the preparation. Iron absorption is maximized when combined with ascorbic acid, such as taking the iron supplements with fresh orange juice or a vitamin C preparation. Therapy failure occurs in malabsorption and when loss exceeds intake, but is most commonly due to poor compliance. There are also liquid oral iron preparations and parenteral therapy. Parenteral therapy is useful in malabsorption and failed compliance, but otherwise does not produce an overall faster response than oral iron and side effects are common.

Thus in practice parenteral iron is rarely required. Proven folate deficiency anaemia should be treated with folic acid (5 mg/day). In all such cases of anaemia, B_{12} deficiency must also be excluded, as folate may improve the anaemia of B_{12} deficiency but exacerbate any associated neurological deterioration [10]. In B_{12} deficiency, a single intramuscular dose of 1000 µg of B_{12} should lead to a reticulocyte response within 3–7 days. Weekly injections should be employed until anaemia resolves and lifelong replacement is often required.

Summary box 15.1

The haemoglobin decreases in normal pregnancy, but should not fall below 11 g/dL in the first trimester or below 10.5 g/dL in the second and third trimesters.

The thalassaemias

The thalassaemias are a heterogeneous group of genetic disorders of haemoglobin synthesis, named after the haemoglobin that is deficient. The mutation may result in a reduced rate of production of the affected gene or result in no chain synthesis at all [11]. The majority of thalassaemias are inherited in a Mendelian recessive manner. Given the diversity of genetic defects and the possibility of genetic combinations, thalassaemias, irrespective of their molecular basis, are often classified by their clinical effects into thalassaemia minor, thalassaemia intermedia and thalassaemia major. In general, thalassaemia carriers are often symptomless and fall into the minor category. Those with thalassaemia intermedia are more severely affected and may often have anaemia, although this does not require regular transfusion. In its major form, thalassaemia presents with lifelong transfusion dependency.

Alpha thalassaemia

Women with one or two deletions of the four α-globin genes are usually symptom-free and have a normal pregnancy outcome. With haemoglobin (Hb) H disease, where three α-globin genes are absent, there are variable clinical features ranging from mild asymptomatic anaemia to severe transfusion-dependent anaemia, with jaundice, hepatosplenomegaly, growth restriction and bone abnormalities. Mild to moderate haemolysis is the predominant feature. This is worsened by pregnancy, so prophylactic folic acid (5 mg/day) is needed. Gallstones are not infrequent due to the high red cell turnover. Infections, drugs and fever may also worsen the anaemia. A fetus affected by Hb Barts with no α-globin production (both parents carrying two α-globin deletions on the same chromosome) will develop hydrops, polyhydramnios and placentomegaly [12]. There is a high risk of pre-eclampsia in the mother. The fetus is also at risk of congenital abnormalities. Maternal carriage of alpha thalassaemia is associated with an MCV of less than 80 fL (often less than 70 fL), a mean corpuscular haemoglobin (MCH) of less than 27 pg, with, very often, no evidence of anaemia and normal mean corpuscular haemoglobin concentration (MCHC). If iron deficiency is excluded, then carriage of thalassaemia should be suspected and the diagnosis confirmed with polymerase chain reaction and globin gene analysis.

Beta thalassaemia

This condition is due to a defect in β-chain synthesis caused by heterogeneous point mutations within the β-globin gene, with nearly 180 different mutations associated with its phenotype. It interferes with red cell maturation and increases red cell destruction within the marrow and spleen. Major forms have lifelong chronic dyserythropoietic anaemia with splenomegaly and skeletal deformity. With inadequate transfusion profound anaemia, marked skeletal deformity of the long bones and skull, recurrent infections and death occurs. With adequate transfusion anaemia is controlled but transfusion-related iron overload will result in endocrine abnormalities and pancreatic, hepatic and cardiac failure. This results in failure of pubertal growth, delayed sexual development and hypogonadotrophic hypogonadism affecting fertility. Thus only a small number of successful pregnancies are reported [13–15]. With significant left ventricular dysfunction or arrhythmias, pregnancy is best avoided. Serum ferritin reflects hepatic iron stores but does not relate well to cardiac deposition, although magnetic resonance imaging can now quantify cardiac iron deposition. When pregnancy does occur Caesarean section is common for cephalo-pelvic disproportion due to the small stature of the mother and the fact that the unaffected fetus has normal growth. Spinal abnormalities should be considered with neuraxial anaesthesia. With beta thalassaemia intermedia there is a reasonable pregnancy success rate with well-controlled disease. However, growth restriction and increasing anaemia are not uncommon [16]. Correspondingly, transfusion requirements increase with increasing gestation. Where transfusion is required, the aim should be to maintain haemoglobin over 10 g/dL to reduce the risk of fetal hypoxia. Most often, chelating agents are discontinued on diagnosis of pregnancy (as the safety of chelation in pregnancy has not been established) and restarted after delivery, but folic acid supplements are required throughout pregnancy.

Beta thalassaemia minor is usually symptom-free, but anaemia is common in pregnancy and there may be a higher rate of fetal growth restriction and oligohydramnios. However there is no overall difference in perinatal mortality or congenital malformations. [17]. Carriers have normal/low haemoglobin, low MCV and MCH but normal MCHC. More severe anaemias may be encountered in those with combined dietary deficiencies. Folic acid supplementation should be prescribed (and oral iron, but only if the ferritin is low) throughout pregnancy.

Screening for thalassaemia

Population screening for haemoglobin disorders has been practised for many years and prenatal testing for haemoglobinopathies is recommended in at-risk groups [18]. Carriers are reliably detected by screening red cell indices, traditionally an MCV of 80 fL or less, although (as red cells may swell with storage) an MCH of less than 27 pg is more reliable. Electrophoresis (and exclusion of iron deficiency where appropriate) is then used to make the diagnosis (e.g an elevated HbA$_2$ of 3.5–7% with, or without, an increased HbF concentration, is consistent with beta thalassaemia heterozygote). If the HbA$_2$ percentage is within the normal range, and the MCH is less than 27 pg, the woman should be investigated for alpha thalassaemia trait [11]. Prenatal diagnosis, with samples obtained via chorionic villous sampling (CVS), amniocentesis or fetal blood sampling, is possible using a variety of methods [18,19], including pre-implantation genetic diagnosis [20], and the diagnostic accuracy is high in specialist centres. However, examination of fetal material in the maternal circulation is not yet suitable for the determination of fetal carriage of the majority of haemoglobinopathies [20,21].

Sickle cell disease

Sickle cell disease varies in presentation from a lifelong crippling haemolytic disorder (characterized by crises caused by infection, aplasia, infarction and haemolysis) to a diagnosis only made on a routine blood film examination. This variation may be due to the co-inheritance of persistence of fetal haemoglobin. With repeated crises, bone deformity, osteomyelitis, renal failure, myocardial infarction, leg ulceration, gallstones and cardiac failure may develop. With repeated transfusions there is an increased risk of blood-borne infections and iron overload. The outcome of pregnancy in mothers with sickling disorders is heavily dependent on the adequacy of maternal healthcare [22]. In the USA, a maternal mortality rate of 0.25–0.5% has been reported, with 99% of pregnancies (which were viable after 28 weeks) resulting in a live birth. Around half of the pregnancies are complicated by at least one painful crisis and hospital admission is often required. There is likely to be an increased risk of pre-eclampsia and of fetal growth restriction, possibly through placental infarction [23]. In developing countries the outcome of pregnancy with a major sickling disorder may be substantially worse, with high maternal and perinatal mortality.

Sickle cell trait results in no change to the haematological indices. It is diagnosed by a positive sickle test and the demonstration of both an HbA and HbS band on gel electrophoresis.

Sickle cell disease is diagnosed by the presence of anaemia, the presence of sickled red cells on the blood film, blood film appearances of hyposplenism, a positive sickle test and the pattern of HbS and HbF, with no HbA, on haemoglobin electrophoresis. The presence of a microcytosis may suggest the co-inheritance of thalassaemia, or the presence of iron deficiency. Higher haemoglobin (11–13 g/dL) may indicate the presence of HbC or co-inheritance of another haemoglobin variant.

In all subjects with a major sickling disorder treatment includes the prevention of infection. This is achieved with prophylactic penicillin and the use of pneumococcal, meningococcal and *Haemophilus influenzae* vaccinations with antimalarial prophylaxis if appropriate. The management of a painful crisis involves adequate pain control, treatment of any infection, maintenance of oxygenation, hydration and thromboprophylaxis [24], although specific randomized controlled trials of management in pregnancy are lacking [25]. Regular blood transfusion is not usually required. However, if haemoglobin is falling (indicating an increase in haemolysis) and especially if there is evidence of a falling reticulocyte count (indicating an impending aplastic phase), then transfusion should be given. When transfusion is required and the haemoglobin is already less than 5 g/dL, it may be that a top-up transfusion to 12–14 g/dL will result in sufficient dilution of the sickle cells to the desired target level of less than 30% of the circulating red cells. When transfusion is required at a higher haemoglobin level (8–10 g/dL), then a partial exchange transfusion should be carried out (removing 500 mL by phlebotomy while transfusing two red cell units). The mainstay of management of a pregnancy in women with a severe sickling disorder is folic acid supplementation (5 mg/day throughout pregnancy), regular haemoglobin estimations, regular monitoring of fetal growth and consideration of the need for transfusion [19]. Prophylactic blood transfusions in pregnancy remains controverisal and although there may be a reduction in the frequency of vaso-occlusive events when prophylactic transfusion has been used [26], it seems likely that any improvement in pregnancy outcome may relate to improvements in the general management of pregnancy rather than from prophylactic transfusion itself [19]. However, transfusion should be considered when there is an acute anaemia (haemoglobin <5 g/dL), pre-eclampsia, septicaemia, acute renal failure, acute chest syndrome, recent cerebral ischaemia of arterial origin, and when preparing for surgery. Multiple pregnancy will require assessment for transfusion on a more regular basis.

Summary box 15.2

Most patients with sickle cell trait or thalassaemia minor are usually symptom-free and have a normal pregnancy outcome.

Haemolytic disease of the newborn

The Rh antigens on red cells result from the action of two genes (*RHD* and *RHCE*), leading to two haplotypes (combining c or C, D or no D, e or E). Of these, RhD is the most important in obstetrics. Around 15% of white people are RhD negative. If an RhD-negative mother carries an RhD-positive child, the transplacental passage of blood and immunoglobulin may result in the development of maternal anti-RhD antibody that passes to the fetus. Indeed, there is a one in six chance of maternal anti-RhD formation in the absence of prophylaxis. Whether the mother develops such antibodies depends on the amount of feto-maternal haemorrhage (FMH) and any feto-maternal ABO mismatch (as natural maternal anti-A or anti-B may clear fetal cells before immunization occurs). RhD haemolytic disease of the newborn (HDN) most often occurs in the second or subsequent pregnancies, but occasionally significant fetal haemolysis occurs in the first [27].

Since the introduction of routine prophylaxis with anti-RhD immunoglobulin in developed countries, there has been a dramatic reduction in the occurrence of severe neonatal jaundice related to RhD. Despite this, continuing vigilance is requried as anti-RhD continues to be the commonest red cell antibody associated with significant fetal and neonatal morbidity and mortality. However, other maternal alloantibodies, directed towards RhE, Rhc, RhC and Kell, as well as feto-maternal ABO incompatibility, should all be considered in the diagnosis of neonatal hyperbilirubinaemia [28].

Antenatal diagnosis and monitoring for RhD incompatibility

All women should have their blood group determined at pregnancy presentation and again at 28–32 weeks' gestation. A further estimation between 34 and 36 weeks is also recommended [29]. When a potential sensitizing event occurs in an RhD-negative woman (Table 15.4), whether she has circulating anti-RhD should be determined and (if more than 20 weeks' gestation or at delivery) an FMH estimation carried out [30]. At delivery, the ABO/RhD

Table 15.4 Potential RhD sensitizing events.

Antepartum haemorrhage
Abdominal trauma
Fetal external version
Ectopic pregnancy
Delivery
Invasive investigations
Amniocentesis
Chorionic villous sampling
Fetal blood sampling
Embryo reduction
Other *in utero* therapeutic interventions/surgery (e.g. shunt insertion, intrauterine transfusion)
Fetal loss
Intrauterine death
Stillbirth
Miscarriage with evacuation
Complete or incomplete miscarriage >12/40
Therapeutic termination

type of the baby should be determined from a cord sample. If the baby is RhD positive and HDN is suspected, a direct antiglobulin test should be performed on the cord blood sample [31].

Anti-RhD detected early in pregnancy is more likely to result in HDN than if detected for the first time later on. When any antibody associated with HDN is detected it should be quantified. For RhD, this should be by automated methods and reported in international units, rather than by manual titration [29]. In general, the absolute value may not be as important as a rising titre. In addition, the RhD (as well as Kell and c) status of the fetus can be determined from cell-free fetal DNA obtained from the maternal circulation [32,33]. Further, although most non-invasive methods are not sufficiently sensitive, weekly velocimetry of the fetal middle cerebral artery may predict moderate or severe anaemia and has begun to replace serial amniocentesis in determining when fetal blood sampling is required [34].

Fetal presentation

Fetal presentation varies from mild anaemia to severe anaemia with jaundice, oedema, cardiac failure, effusions and pulmonary haemorrhage, neurological deficits and kernicterus, which may result in stillbirth, neonatal death or complete resolution.

Intrauterine management

If fetal maturity permits, delivery of the fetus is indicated when there is evidence of significant disease. When fetal immaturity does not allow delivery, fetal transfusion (which has reduced perinatal mortality from 95% to 50%) should be carried out and such transfusion is indicated when the haematocrit is below 25% (18–26 weeks' gestation) or below 30% (after 34 weeks). The blood used should be cross-matched against maternal serum, with a haematocrit of 75–90% and both seronegative for cytomegalovirus and gamma irradiated (to prevent transfusion-related graft-versus-host disease). The aim is to increase the haematocrit to about 45% and further transfusions may be required every 1–3 weeks. In some circumstances repeated maternal plasma exchange or high-dose intravenous human normal immunoglobulin have been used, until fetal transfusion is possible.

Prevention

Sensitization can be prevented by suppression of the maternal immune response to the RhD antigen. This is achieved by the timely administration of a passive antibody [31,35–37]. Intramuscular anti-RhD should be administered to all RhD-negative women within 72 hours of delivery and, if not, within 10 days [37,38]. The dose required should be determined by the level of FMH. Given intramuscularly, 125 IU of anti-RhD is sufficient to protect against 1 mL of RhD-positive red cells. In the UK, 250 IU is routinely given for any potential sensitizing event before 20 weeks and 500 IU for any event after 20 weeks. If a further sensitizing event occurs more than 7 days after a prophylactic anti-RhD dose, a further dose should be given. Routine post-delivery anti-RhD immunoprophylaxis has markedly reduced fetal deaths, although cases of HDN still occur (due to other blood groups, unrecognized sensitization in a previous pregnancy, red cell or platelet transfusion, inadequate treatment, or unrecognized potential sensitization). Indeed, unrecognized events are now the most important cause of maternal sensitization in many developed countries. Those events relating to RhD may be amenable to the routine administration of anti-RhD to all RhD-negative women with no detectable anti-RhD antibodies in the third trimester [38].

Non-RhD antibodies

At least 40 red cell antigens have been associated with HDN, including Rhc, RhC, RhE, Kell, Duffy, MNS, Lutheran, Kidd and U. After anti-RhD, antibodies against c, Kell (K$_1$) or E are the most frequently encountered antibodies requiring treatment. The K$_1$ antigen is found in 9% of white people (who are virtually all heterozygous) and 8–18% of pregnancies with detectable maternal anti-K$_1$ result in a K$_1$-positive fetus, with hydrops in about 30% of such cases. Management of such antibodies requires a combination of ultrasound, paternal genotyping, fetal blood sampling and intrauterine transfusion [39].

Summary box 15.3

Although RhD remains a significant cause of haemolytic disease of the newborn, a number of other maternal alloantibodies should be routinely considered in the diagnosis of neonatal hyperbilirubinaemia.

Table 15.5 Thrombocytopenia in pregnancy.

Spurious (i.e. clumping or poor sampling)
Gestational
Immune thrombocytopenic purpura
Heparin-induced thrombocytopenia
Post-transfusion purpura
Acute fatty liver of pregnancy
Pre-eclampsia/HELLP syndrome
Thrombotic thrombocytopenic purpura/haemolytic uraemic syndrome
Disseminated intravascular coagulation
Drug-induced thrombocytopenia
Systemic lupus erythematosus/antiphospholipid syndrome
Viral (HIV/EBV/CMV)
Congenital thrombocythemias/thrombocytopenia
Hypersplenism
Type 2b von Willebrand's disease
Marrow dysfunction/haematinic deficiency

CMV, cytomegalovirus; EBV, Epstein–Barr virus.

Table 15.6 Investigation of thrombocytopenia.

Blood film to exclude platelet clumps, microangiopathic haemolytic anaemia or other haematological disorders
Coagulation screen (to include fibrinogen and D-dimer levels)
Renal and liver function tests
Antiphospholipid antibodies
Anti-DNA antibodies to exclude SLE (antinuclear antibody is sufficient as a screening test)

SLE, systemic lupus erythematosus.

Thrombocytopenia

Towards the end of pregnancy less than 5% of women have a platelet count below 150×10^9/L. This gestational thrombocytopenia carries no significance, but requires exclusion of other disorders (Table 15.5). If the platelet count is below 100×10^9/L, further investigations are required (Table 15.6).

Immune thrombocytopenic purpura

Immune thrombocytopenic purpura (ITP) results in thrombocytopenia from autoantibody-mediated destruction of platelets. Such antibodies occur idiopathically and

Table 15.7 Causes of immune thrombocytopenic purpura.

Idiopathic
Helicobacter pylori
Systemic lupus erythematosus
Lymphoma/chronic lymphocytic leukaemia
HIV
Drugs

Table 15.8 Causes of thrombotic thrombocytopenic purpura/ haemolytic uraemic syndrome.

Thrombotic thrombocytopenic purpura
Congenital
Pregnancy
Drugs (e.g. clopidogrel, ticlopidine, tacrolimus)
Combined contraceptive pill
Bone marrow transplant
Systemic lupus erythematosus
Malignancy
HIV
Escherichia coli 0157

Haemolytic uraemic syndrome
Pregnancy
Infection (cytotoxin-producing *E. coli* or *Shigella*)
Drugs (e.g. ciclosporin, quinine, chemotherapy)

also in association with other disorders (Table 15.7). ITP most commonly presents as asymptomatic maternal thrombocytopenia, but transplacental passage of antibodies can result in fetal thrombocytopenia in 9–15% and intracerebral haemorrhage in 1.5% of babies with affected mothers. The diagnosis of ITP in pregnancy is by exclusion of other disorders [40].

Treatment

Spontaneous bleeding is unlikely with platelet counts above $20 \times 10^9/L$, and monitoring of the patient and platelet count are often all that is required, with the aim of attaining an adequate platelet count for safe delivery (including neuraxial anaesthesia). A spontaneous vaginal delivery or Caesarean section is considered safe from a surgical perspective when the platelet count is above $50 \times 10^9/L$. If the woman wishes or requires epidural or spinal anaesthesia, then a platelet count above $80 \times 10^9/L$ is recommended [40].

When required, treatment with either oral corticosteroids or intravenous immunoglobulin (IgG) produces 50–70% response rates. This response usually lasts 2–3 weeks and repeated dosing may be required. Secondary treatments include high-dose methylprednisolone or azathioprine, or a combination of these therapies with intravenous IgG. Other treatments (vinca alkaloids and cyclophosphamide) are not suitable in pregnancy and splenectomy is also best avoided. If considered essential however, it is best carried out between 13 and 20 weeks' gestation. The anti-CD20 antibody rituximab has also been used in refractory cases of ITP, although its overall place in management is not yet defined [41]. Moreover, rituximab crosses the placenta and suppresses neonatal B-cell development. However, the overall long-term effect of this on the fetus is unknown at present [42].

Management of delivery

The baby's platelet count cannot be reliably predicted from any maternal features. Furthermore, fetal sampling is hazardous or prone to spuriously low results. Thus, procedures in labour and at delivery that pose an additional bleeding risk should be avoided (fetal scalp electrode, fetal blood sampling, ventouse and rotational forceps). However, there is no evidence that Caesarean section is safer for the thrombocytopenic fetus than an uncomplicated vaginal delivery, as the nadir in platelets is most often 24–48 hours after delivery. A cord blood platelet count should be determined in all babies and close monitoring is required over the next 2–5 days. The use of intravenous IgG may block the Fc-dependent placental transfer of maternal antibodies to the fetus.

Thrombotic thrombocytopenic purpura/haemolytic uraemic syndrome

Thrombotic thrombocytopenic purpura (TTP) and haemolytic uraemic syndrome (HUS) are characterized by thrombocytopenia, microangiopathic haemolytic anaemia and multiorgan failure [43]. TTP is more often associated with neurological abnormalities and non-renal organ ischaemia, while patients with HUS have predominantly renal manifestations and usually present after delivery. HUS can present with haemolysis, elevated liver enzymes and low platelets, making it difficult to distinguish from HELLP syndrome associated with pre-eclampsia [44–46]. TTP occurs most often as an idiopathic single episode, although there is a congenital form that may recur. Like HUS, it may also occur secondary to other influences (Table 15.8).

Von Willebrand factor (vWF) is, on release from the endothelium, cleaved by the metalloprotease ADAMTS-13, resulting in the correct balance of vWF multimers. TTP/HUS is characterized by a failure of this cleavage. In TTP, this can be due to a congenital deficiency of ADAMTS-13, but is more commonly due to an acquired autoantibody. The resultant excess of circulating ultra-large multimers of vWF leads to platelet aggregation and consumption, and in turn to microvascular thrombosis. However, in HUS, and in many cases of TTP, ADAMTS-13 is normal and indeed a reduction in ADAMTS-13 is not specific to TTP/HUS. Consequently, the exact mechanism is not fully understood. However, the physiological coagulation changes in pregnancy may predispose to the condition.

Diagnosis

HUS typically presents after birth with thrombocytopenia, haemolysis and renal failure, whilst TTP is a classic pentad of fever, haemolysis, thrombocytopenia, central nervous system signs and renal dysfunction. However, all five are only present in around 50% of cases. TTP, particularly recurrent TTP, usually presents before 24 weeks of pregnancy. Routine blood clotting tests are often normal in the early stages of TTP/HUS, but as the disease progresses there may be coagulation activation and disseminated intravascular coagulation. Although pregnancy is associated with alterations in ADAMTS-13 activity [47], measurement of ADAMTS-13 and autoantibodies against ADAMTS-13 may be of value in confirming the clinical diagnosis of TTP in pregnant subjects [48–50]. However, given the need for the rapid institution of treatment, such test results will often only be available after a presumptive diagnosis has been made and treatment has started.

Treatment

With the exception of endotoxin-related HUS (where supportive care is the main requirement) and congenital TTP, it is unlikely that a clear distinction between the two syndromes will be possible in the majority of pregnancy-related cases. As a consequence, both are often considered as a single syndrome when considering therapy, particularly as there may be benefit in plasma exchange in non-toxin-related (or atypical) HUS [51].

The mainstay of treatment is plasma exchange, which should be instituted within 24 hours of presentation [52]. Although the optimal regimen and fluid replacement is not certain, fresh frozen plasma (FFP) is the common standard. However, cryosupernatant or solvent detergent-treated FFP may be preferred. When exchange is not immediately available, FFP alone may be beneficial and indeed may be sufficient in congenital disease. Intravenous methylprednisolone and aspirin (when platelets $>50 \times 10^9$/L) are often added to plasma exchange therapy. However, platelet transfusions should be avoided in TTP. If the patient deteriorates or does not respond, higher volume or frequency of exchanges or different replacement fluid is recommended. As with ITP there may be a role for rituximab in those with resistant or recurrent disase, although, as noted above [42], its safety profile in pregnancy is not yet determined.

> **Summary box 15.4**
>
> - A mild thrombocytopenia (platelet count ≥100 × 10⁹/L) not uncommonly occurs with increasing gestation in normal pregnancy.
> - In ITP the baby's platelet count cannot be reliably predicted from any maternal feature and any procedure during delivery that poses an additional bleeding risk to the baby should be avoided.
> - The mainstay of treatment of TTP is plasma exchange, which should be commenced within 24 hours of presentation.

Venous thromboembolism

Venous thromboembolism (VTE) is a leading cause of maternal death in the developed world and remains the major direct cause of maternal mortality in the UK. VTE occurs throughout pregnancy, with an estimated antenatal and postnatal incidence of 6–12 and 3–7 per 10 000 maternities respectively. Over 40% of antenatal VTE occur in the first trimester of pregnancy [53] and a recent report examining maternal mortality in the UK found that two-thirds of antenatal cases of fatal pulmonary embolism (PE) occurred in the first trimester [54]. The incidence of fatal PE in pregnancy has fallen since the 1950s in the UK, largely through a reduction in the number of women dying after vaginal deliveries. There has been less impact on deaths in the antenatal and intrapartum period and after Caesarean section [55], although deaths from PE following Caesarean delivery appear to be declining, possibly due to thromboprophylaxis. The daily risk of VTE is fourfold higher in the postnatal period compared with the antenatal period [56].

Gestational deep venous thrombosis (DVT) usually occurs in the ileo-femoral veins (over 70% vs. 9% in the non-pregnant) and is therefore more likely to result in PE. Furthermore, it is also more likely to occur in the left leg (85–90% vs. 55% in the non-pregnant), perhaps related to compression of the left iliac vein by the right iliac artery [57]. Of pregnant women who experience DVT, 80% will develop post-thrombotic syndrome, characterized by chronic leg swelling, discomfort, skin discoloration and leg ulceration.

Physiological changes in pregnancy

VTE is up to 10 times more common in pregnancy than in comparable non-pregnant subjects, which may relate to the physiological changes in the maternal circulation and coagulation that occur in normal pregnancy as a preparation for delivery. Virchow's triad for VTE consists of alterations in normal blood flow (stasis), trauma or damage to the vascular endothelium and alterations in the constitution of blood (hypercoagulability), and describes the three broad categories of factors that contribute to thrombosis. During normal pregnancy, hypercoagulability results from increases in the levels of factor VIII and fibrinogen, reduction in protein S levels, a resistance to protein C in 40% of women and impaired fibrinolysis [58]. Studies assessing blood flow velocity in the lower limbs in pregnancy have shown extensive reduction in flow velocity of up to 50% by 29 weeks' gestation, reaching its nadir at 34–36 weeks. The changes in both blood flow velocity and coagulation factors may persist for up to 6 weeks after delivery. The third factor underlying most venous thrombosis is vascular damage and trauma to the pelvic veins, which may occur during normal vaginal delivery and perhaps particularly so during abdominal or instrumental delivery [59].

Risk factors for VTE in pregnancy

A number of risk factors for pregnancy VTE are known (Table 15.9), such as age over 35 years (1.216 vs. 0.615 per

Table 15.9 Risk factors for venous thromboembolism (VTE) in pregnancy.

Risk factor for VTE	Adjusted odds ratios	95% confidence interval
Previous VTE	24.8	17.1–36
Immobility	7.7	3.2–19
(If combined with BMI ≥25)	62	–
BMI >30	5.3	2.1–13.5
Smoking	2.7	1.5–4.9
Weight gain >21 kg (vs. 7–21 kg)	1.6	1.1–2.6
Parity >1	1.5	1.1–1.9
Age >35	1.3	1.0–1.7
Pre-eclampsia	3.1	1.8–5.3
Pre-eclampsia with intrauterine growth restriction	5.8	2.1–16
Assisted reproductive techniques	4.3	2.0–9.4
Twins	2.6	1.1–6.2
Antepartum haemorrhage	2.3	1.8–2.8
Postpartum haemorrhage	4.1	2.3–7.3
Caesarean section	3.6	3.0–4.3
Medical conditions: sickle cell disease, SLE, heart disease, anaemia, infection, varicose veins	2.0–8.7	
Blood transfusion	7.6	6.2–9.4

BMI, body mass index; SLE, systemic lupus erythematosus.
Source: Royal College of Obstetricians and Gynaecologists [72], Lindqvist *et al.* [106], Jacobsen *et al.* [107], James *et al.* [108], Knight [109].

Table 15.10 Prevalence rates (%) of congenital thrombophilia in Western populations.

Factor V Leiden	2–7
Protein C deficiency	0.2–0.33
Prothrombin 20210A	2
Antithrombin deficiency	0.25–0.55
Antiphospholipid antibodies (lupus anticoagulant and anticardiolipin antibodies	3

Table 15.11 Risk of pregnancy-associated venous thromboembolism in women with underlying thrombophilia.

Thrombophilic defect	Risk of thrombosis
Factor V Leiden (heterozygote)	9.32
Factor V Leiden (homozygote)	34.4
Prothrombin 20210A (heterozygote)	6.8
Prothrombin 20210A (homozygote)	26.4
Protein C deficiency	4.76
Protein S deficiency	3.19

Source: Robertson *et al.* [110].

1000 maternities) and Caesarean (particularly emergency) section [60]. It is well recognized that the presence of multiple risk factors increases the risk of VTE. For example, the combination of body mass index (BMI) 25 or more and immobility has been shown to carry a greater than 60-fold increase in risk, whereas both factors alone are associated with a less than 10-fold increase. Over 70% of women who suffer a fatal or non-fatal PE in the UK have identifiable risk factors, hence many episodes of PE are potentially preventable with the appropriate use of thromboprophylaxis [54]. Around 50% of episodes of pregnancy VTE have an identifiable underlying heritable thrombophilia (Tables 15.10 and 15.11). In addition, acquired persistent antiphospholipid antibodies also increase pregnancy VTE risk. From case–control and cohort studies the thrombotic risk is about 1 in 450 in factor V Leiden heterozygotes, about 1 in 200 in prothrombin G20210A heterozygotes and about 1 in 113 in those with protein C deficiency. Hence, the absolute VTE risk is low for most common thrombophilias. However, the absolute risk is much higher in those with antithrombin deficiency (VTE risk of 1 in 2.8 for type 1 and 1 in 42 for type 2 deficiency) and factor V Leiden homozygotes, while those with combined defects (e.g. factor V Leiden/prothrombin G20210A compound heterozygotes) have a pregnancy VTE risk of 4.6 in 100 [61].

Table 15.12 Association between heritable thrombophilias and pregnancy complications: meta-analyses of observational studies.

	Recurrent miscarriage	IUGR	Pre-eclampsia	Placental abruption	Late fetal loss
Factor V Leiden	2.0 (1.5–2.7)	2.7 (1.3–5.5)	2.19 (1.46–3.27)	6.7 (2.0–21.6)	3.26 (1.82–5.83)
Prothrombin G20210A	2.0 (1.0–4.0)	2.5 (1.3–5.0)	2.54 (1.52–4.23)	7.71 (3.01–19.76)	2.3 (1.09–4.87)
Protein C deficiency	1.57 (0.23–10.54)	–	21.5 (1.1–414.4)	–	1.41 (0.96–2.07)
Protein S deficiency	14.72 (0.99–218.01)	10.2 (1.1–91)	12.7 (4.0–39.7)	0.3 (0–70.1)	7.39 (1.28–42.83)
Antithrombin deficiency	–	–	7.1 (0.4–117.4)	4.1 (0.3–49.9)	–

Data are odds ratio with 95% confidence intervals in parentheses. IUGR, intrauterine growth restriction.
Source: Rodger *et al.* [66].

Thrombophilia and pregnancy complications

The obstetric antiphospholipid syndrome is characterized by the presence of maternal antiphospholipid antibodies (lupus anticoagulant or anticardiolipin antibodies of IgG and/or IgM isotype in blood, present in medium or high titres on at least two occasions at least 3 months apart) and an obstetric complication (including an episode of VTE, recurrent miscarriage, fetal growth restriction, severe pre-eclampsia or intrauterine fetal death) [62]. In this syndrome, adverse pregnancy outcomes may be the result of poor placental perfusion due to localized thrombosis or increased thrombin generation and placental damage. Antiphospholipid antibodies may also interfere with trophoblast invasion and, *in vitro*, heparin has been shown to ameliorate this effect. Low-dose aspirin and heparin are recommended in the management of women with recurrent miscarriage and antiphospholipid syndrome [63,64].

The heritable thrombophilias have also been associated with placental-mediated pregnancy complications, including fetal growth restriction, pre-eclampsia, placental abruption and intrauterine fetal death (Table 15.12). The putative mechanism may be related to reduced placental perfusion, fibrin deposition and thrombus formation in uterine vessels and intervillous spaces [65]. However, the association is largely based on retrospective case–control data and is inconsistent and not confirmed in prospective studies [66,67]. Thus there is no convincing evidence of causation. Furthermore, there is a lack of evidence to support the use of antithrombotic therapy in women who have a heritable thrombophilia and have experienced a pregnancy complication [68,69]. Although a small observational study has indicated a benefit of low-molecular-weight heparin (LMWH) [70], further information from large clinical trials is awaited. Meanwhile, antithrombotic intervention cannot be recommended for women with heritable thrombophilia and pregnancy complications.

Thromboprophylaxis during pregnancy and the puerperium

Women attending for their first antenatal visit should be assessed for risk factors for VTE. Specifically, they should be asked about a personal and family history of VTE and whether an objective diagnosis was made. Women with a personal history of VTE are at increased risk of recurrence during pregnancy and the puerperium. Recurrence rates of 1.4–11.1% have been reported [71]. The risk of recurrent VTE occurring during pregnancy is higher in women who have previously had an unprovoked or oestrogen-related episode compared with those whose VTE was provoked by a temporary risk factor that is no longer present. VTE risk assessment should occur throughout pregnancy (and particularly before and after delivery) since many risk factors (Table 15.9) may only become apparent as pregnancy advances and following delivery.

Current guidelines recommend that if a previous VTE was associated with a temporary risk factor that is no longer present and the event was not pregnancy or 'pill' related and there are no other risk factors, then antenatal thromboprophylaxis should not be routinely recommended [72]. In this situation, thromboprophylaxis with LMWH should be employed in the puerperium. Antenatally, graduated elastic compression stockings may be employed. In contrast, women with recurrent VTE, a previous VTE and a family history of VTE (in a first-degree relative), additional risk factors including thrombophilia, or where the previous event was idiopathic or pregnancy or 'pill' related should be offered antenatal LMWH thromboprophylaxis (Table 15.13). A once-daily regimen of LMWH is appropriate, starting from their first presentation in pregnancy throughout the antenatal period and for at least 6 weeks after delivery. The dose of LMWH is based on the woman's weight (Table 15.14).

There is a lack of evidence to guide management of asymptomatic inherited or acquired thrombophilia in

Table 15.13 Summary of antenatal thromboprophylaxis.

- Women who have had a previous provoked and non-oestrogen-related VTE do not routinely require antenatal thromboprophylaxis with LMWH
- Women with a previous unprovoked VTE, or oestrogen-related VTE (including pregnancy), or previous recurrent VTE, or other additional risk factors for VTE should be offered antenatal thromboprophylaxis with LMWH
- Women considered to be at high risk of VTE because of multiple risk factors (three or more) should be considered for thromboprophylaxis with LMWH antenatally
- Women with inherited or acquired thrombophilia and no previous history of VTE do not require pharmacological thromboprophylaxis antenatally. Exceptions include women with:
  - multiple thrombophilic defects (including homozygosity for factor V Leiden)
  - antithrombin deficiency
  - heritable thrombophilia and a strong family history of VTE, especially if pregnancy-related

LMWH, low-molecular-weight heparin; VTE, venous thromboembolism.

Table 15.14 Thromboprophylactic doses of LMWH during pregnancy and the puerperium.

Weight (kg)	Enoxaparin	Dalteparin	Tinzaparin
<50	20 mg daily	2500 units daily	3500 units daily
50–90	40 mg daily	5000 units daily	4500 units daily
91–130	60 mg daily*	7500 units daily*	7000 units daily*
131–170	80 mg daily*	10 000 units daily*	9000 units daily*
>170	0.6 mg/kg/day*	75 units/kg/day*	75 units/kg/day*

* May be given in two divided doses.
Source: Royal College of Obstetricians and Gynaecologists [72].

pregnancy. These women may qualify for antenatal or postnatal thromboprophylaxis, depending on the specific thrombophilia and the presence of other risk factors. Women with previous VTE who are receiving long-term anticoagulant therapy should change to LMWH by 6 weeks' gestation to avoid the risk of teratogenesis. These women should be considered at very high risk of VTE and should receive 'treatment' doses of LMWH (e.g. enoxaparin 40 mg 12-hourly, dalteparin 5000 units 12-hourly or tinzaparin 4500 units 12-hourly) throughout pregnancy.

Acute VTE in pregnancy

Diagnosis
The symptoms and signs associated with DVT are common in normal pregnancy (Table 15.15), reflecting the

Table 15.15 Symptoms and signs of venous thromboembolism.

Deep venous thrombosis
Leg pain or discomfort (especially the left leg)
Swelling
Tenderness
Increased temperature and oedema
Lower abdominal pain
Elevated white cell count

Pulmonary embolism
Dyspnoea
Collapse
Chest pain
Haemoptysis
Faintness
Raised jugular venous pressure
Focal signs in the chest
Associated symptoms and signs of DVT

physiological changes of pregnancy. Indeed, less than 10% of women presenting with suspected DVT in pregnancy have the diagnosis confirmed and less than 6% with suspected PE are treated after completion of diagnostic imaging. However, as mortality from untreated PE is high and clinical diagnosis of VTE unreliable, diagnostic imaging should be performed when VTE is suspected and anticoagulant treatment should be commenced (unless strongly contraindicated) until objective testing is concluded [73]. D-dimer estimation has high negative predictive value as a screening test for VTE in the nonpregnant. However, elevated levels are seen during normal pregnancy particularly at term and in the postnatal period [74] and are increased further in conditions such as pre-eclampsia, preterm labour and placental abruption. Further research and validation of diagnostic algorithms using D-dimer for diagnosis is required to determine whether gestation-specific reference ranges will improve the usefulness of D-dimer testing in pregnancy [75].

Deep vein thrombosis
Real-time/duplex ultrasound is used to diagnose DVT and has a sensitivity of 97% and a specificity of 94%. A negative ultrasound result with a low level of clinical suspicion should result in the discontinuation of anticoagulation (Table 15.16). With a negative ultrasound but a high level of clinical suspicion, anticoagulation should be continued and the ultrasound repeated in 1 week, or X-ray venography considered. If repeat testing is negative, anticoagulant treatment should be discontinued.

Where iliac vein thrombosis is suspected (which may present with back pain and/or swelling of the entire limb) and ultrasound does not demonstrate thrombus, pulsed

Table 15.16 Investigation of deep venous thrombosis (DVT) and pulmonary embolism (PE) in pregnancy.

Test results	Management
V/Q scan reports a 'medium' or 'high' probability of PE	Anticoagulant treatment should be continued
'Low' probability of PE on *V/Q* scan but positive ultrasound for DVT	Anticoagulant treatment should be continued
V/Q scan reports a low risk of PE and there are negative leg ultrasound examinations	Anticoagulant treatment can be discontinued
V/Q scan reports a low risk of PE and there are negative leg ultrasound examinations, yet there is a high level of clinical suspicion	Anticoagulant treatment should continue with repeat testing in 1 week (*V/Q* scan and leg ultrasound examination)
If the clinical probability of PE is high, even if the *V/Q* scan shows 'low' probability and leg ultrasound examination is negative	Alternative imaging techniques should be considered (see text)

Table 15.17 Estimates of fetal radiation dose during diagnostic tests for venous thromboembolism.

Chest X-ray	<0.01 mGy
Limited venography	<0.5 mGy
V/Q scan (depends on isotopes used)	5.8 mGy
Low-dose perfusion scanning (omitting ventilation scanning)	<0.12 mGy
CT pulmonary angiography	First trimester <0.02 mGy
	Second trimester (<0.08 mGy
	Third trimester <0.13 mGy

Source: after Ginsberg *et al.* [111], except data for CT pulmonary angiography from Winer-Muram *et al.* [112].

Doppler, magnetic resonance venography or conventional contrast venography should be considered.

Pulmonary embolism

If PE is suspected and the woman is haemodynamically stable, a chest X-ray (CXR) should be performed principally to exclude other disorders including pneumothorax, pneumonia or lobar collapse. The radiation dose to the fetus with CXR is negligible (Table 15.17). Whilst the CXR is normal in over half of pregnant patients with objectively proven PE, abnormal features caused by PE include atelectasis, effusion, focal opacities, regional oligaemia or pulmonary oedema. The ECG is of limited value and the interpretation of blood gases requires consideration of normal pregnancy physiology.

If the CXR is normal, bilateral Doppler ultrasound leg studies should be performed (Table 15.16). A diagnosis of DVT may indirectly confirm a diagnosis of PE and since

anticoagulant therapy is the same for both conditions, further investigation is not usually necessary. This would limit the radiation doses from further diagnostic tests to the mother and her fetus.

The choice of technique for definitive diagnosis of PE is normally between ventilation–perfusion (*V/Q*) scanning and CT pulmonary angiography (CTPA). During pregnancy the ventilation component of the *V/Q* scan can often be omitted, thereby minimizing the radiation dose to the fetus. In the UK, the British Thoracic Society recommends CTPA as first-line investigation for non-massive PE in non-pregnant patients [76]. However, *V/Q* scanning has a high negative predictive value in pregnancy and may be more reliable than CTPA [77]. When *V/Q* interpretation is difficult (e.g. if the CXR is abnormal), then CTPA is preferred. This technique delivers a lower radiation dose to the fetus (see section below), and may identify other pathology such as aortic dissection. The main disadvantage of CTPA is the high radiation dose to the maternal breasts, associated with an increased lifetime risk of developing breast cancer.

Radiation exposure associated with diagnostic tests

CTPA delivers less radiation to the fetus than *V/Q* scanning during all trimesters of pregnancy (Table 15.17). It has been estimated that the risk of fatal cancer to the age of 15 years is less than 1 in 1 million after *in utero* exposure to CTPA and 1 in 280 000 following a perfusion scan. While CTPA is associated with a lower risk of radiation for the fetus, this must be offset by the relatively high radiation dose (20 mGy) to the mother's thorax and in particular breast tissue. The delivery of 10 mGy of radiation to a woman's breast increases her lifetime risk of developing breast cancer. It has been estimated that the increased risk is 13.6% (background risk 1 in 200), a figure that has been cited widely [73,78]. Whilst this level of risk may be an overestimate, breast tissue is especially sensitive to radiation exposure during pregnancy. It therefore seems sensible to recommend that lung *V/Q* scans should be considered the investigation of first choice for young women, especially if there is a family history of breast cancer or the patient has had a previous chest CT scan. Radiation exposure from pulmonary angiography is approximately 0.5 mSv to fetus and 5–30 mSv to mother.

Treatment

Blood should be taken for a full blood count and coagulation screen before anticoagulant therapy is commenced. Renal or hepatic dysfunction, which are cautions for anticoagulant therapy, should also be assessed through urea, electrolytes and liver function tests.

The treatment of VTE in pregnancy is heparin, with LMWH having largely replaced unfractionated heparin (UFH). Vitamin K antagonists are rarely employed in the antenatal period for the treatment of VTE since they cross the placenta and can have adverse effects on the fetus (see below). Meta-analyses of randomized controlled trials in non-pregnant patients indicate that LMWH is more effective and is associated with a lower risk of haemorrhagic complications and lower mortality than UFH in the initial treatment of DVT. A meta-analysis of randomized controlled trials has shown equivalent efficacy of LMWH and UFH in the initial treatment of PE. A systematic review of LMWH in pregnancy has confirmed its efficacy and safety in the management of acute thrombosis and in the provision of thromboprophylaxis.

Whilst several LMWH preparations are available, most experience currently exists with enoxaparin, dalteparin and tinzaparin. In non-pregnant patients with acute VTE, LMWH is usually administered in a once-daily dose. In view of recognized alterations in the pharmacokinetics of dalteparin and enoxaparin during pregnancy, a twice-daily dosage regimen is recommended for these heparins in the initial treatment of VTE in pregnancy (enoxaparin 1 mg/kg twice daily; dalteparin 100 units/kg twice daily). Preliminary biochemical data suggest that once-daily administration of tinzaparin (175 units/kg) may be appropriate in the treatment of VTE in pregnancy. Whichever preparation of LMWH is employed, the woman should be taught to self-administer the drug by subcutaneous injection, allowing her to be managed on an outpatient basis until delivery.

Treatment with LMWH can be monitored by measuring peak anti-Xa activity (3 hours after injection) with a therapeutic range of approximately 0.5–1.2 units/mL. However, for most patients such monitoring is considered unnecessary, as reliable results are found using a dose based on weight [79]. Monitoring may be indicated at extremes of body weight (<50 and ≥90 kg) and in women with recurrent VTE or renal disease. Platelet monitoring is considered unneccessary in women treated exclusively with LMWH (see below).

Risks of anticoagulant therapy in pregnancy

Both UFH and LMWH do not cross the placenta and are not associated with teratogenicity or fetal bleeding. In contrast, vitamin K antagonists such as warfarin, cross the placenta and, with exposure between 6 and 12 weeks of gestation, are associated with a characteristic embryopathy (Table 15.18), which can be avoided by heparin

Table 15.18 The features of warfarin embryopathy.

Mid-facial, particularly nasal, hypoplasia
Stippled chondral calcification
Short proximal limbs
Short phalanges
Scoliosis

---

substitution. The risk of warfarin embryopathy was 6.4% in one systematic review of warfarin use during pregnancy in women with mechanical heart valves [80], although other reviews have found lower levels (0.6–4%) [81]. The risk of embryopathy may be higher with doses of warfarin over 5 mg/day. Warfarin is also associated with fetal and neonatal haemorrhage. With fetal liver immaturity, maternal therapeutic warfarin (INR 2–3) is likely to result in excessive anticoagulation in the fetus. Warfarin during the second and third trimesters may also result in neurodevelopmental problems.

The maternal complications of anticoagulant therapy include haemorrhage, osteoporosis, thrombocytopenia and allergy. With UFH, the rate of major bleeding in pregnant patients is 2%, which is similar to heparin and warfarin when used for the treatment of DVT in the non-pregnant. One of the potential advantages of LMWH over UFH is an enhanced anti-Xa (antithrombotic)/anti-IIa (anticoagulant) ratio, resulting in a theoretically reduced bleeding risk. UFH causes a dose-dependent loss of cancellous bone and, if administered for more than 1 month, symptomatic vertebral fractures occur in 2–3%, with significant density reduction evident in more than 30% with long-term therapy. LMWH carries a much lower risk of symptomatic osteoporosis than UFH [82]. Around 3% of non-pregnant patients receiving UFH develop an idiosyncratic immune, IgG-mediated heparin-induced thrombocytopenia (HIT), which is frequently complicated by extension of pre-existing VTE or new arterial thrombosis. The HIT risk is substantially lower with LMWH and considered negligible if LMWH is used exclusively. This condition should be suspected if the platelet count falls to below 100×10^9/L (or to less than 50% of baseline) 5–15 days after commencing heparin (or sooner with recent heparin exposure). If ongoing anticoagulation is needed in such patients, then the heparinoid danaparoid sodium is recommended. Danaparoid inhibits thrombin production and has a low rate of cross-reactivity with HIT antibodies. A review of 91 pregnancies in 83 women concluded that danaparoid is an effective and safe antithrombotic in pregnancies for women who are intolerant of heparin [83]. Guidelines from North America recommend that routine platelet count monitoring is not required in obstetric patients who have received only LMWH as heparin-induced thrombocytopenic thrombosis is not a feature in pregnancies managed exclusively with LMWH [68]. If UFH is employed or if the obstetric patient is receiving LMWH after first receiving UFH, or if she has received UFH in the past, the platelet count should ideally be monitored every 2–3 days from day 4 to day 14, or until heparin is stopped, whichever occurs first [84].

Labour and delivery

Heparin treatment should be discontinued 24 hours prior to elective induction of labour or delivery by Caesarean

Table 15.19 Heparin and neuraxial instrumentation.

Wait 12 hours after prophylactic dose LMWH before epidural
instrumentation
Wait 24 hours after the last therapeutic dose (e.g. enoxaparin
1 mg/kg/12 hours) before epidural instrumentation
Wait 10–12 hours from most recent LMWH injection before cannula
removal
No LMWH for at least 4 hours after epidural catheter removal

section. If spontaneous labour occurs, the woman should not inject any further heparin until she has been assessed. If heparin is required and there is a high risk of haemorrhage, intravenous UFH should be employed (as prompt reversal occurs on discontinuation or with protamine). Similarly, if the woman has a very high risk of recurrent VTE (e.g. a VTE diagnosed near term), then therapeutic intravenous UFH can be initiated and discontinued 4–6 hours prior to the expected time of delivery. The risk of epidural or spinal haematoma during neuraxial instrumentation in pregnant patients receiving LMWH has not been clearly quantified, but precautions are indicated (Table 15.19).

In the UK, in non-pregnant patients it is recommended that anticoagulant therapy should be continued for 6 weeks for calf vein thrombosis and 3 months for proximal DVT or PE when VTE has occurred in relation to a temporary risk factor, and 6 months for a first episode of idiopathic VTE. The presence of ongoing risk factors and the safety of LWMH have led authorities to propose that anticoagulant therapy should be continued for the duration of the pregnancy and until at least 6 weeks after delivery and to allow a total duration of treatment of at least 3 months. Both heparin and warfarin are satisfactory for use after birth and neither is contraindicated in breast-feeding.

Management of massive life-threatening PE
Massive life-threatening PE is an obstetric and medical emergency. It is defined as an embolus associated with haemodynamic compromise (systolic blood pressure <90 mmHg or a drop in systolic blood pressure of 40 mmHg or more from baseline for a period over 15 min), not otherwise explained by hypovolaemia, sepsis or new arrhythmia. Hospitals should have guidelines for the management of non-haemorrhagic obstetric shock. The collapsed shocked pregnant woman needs to be assessed by a multidisciplinary resuscitation team of experienced clinicians including senior obstetricians, physicians and radiologists, who should decide on an individual basis whether a woman receives intravenous UFH, thrombolytic therapy or thoracotomy and surgical embolectomy.

Oxygen should be administered and the circulation supported using intravenous fluids and inotropic agents if required. Intravenous UFH is the traditional method of heparin administration in acute VTE and remains the preferred treatment in massive PE because of its rapid effect and extensive experience of its use in this situation. The diagnosis should be established using either portable echocardiography or CTPA.

In massive life-threatening PE with haemodynamic compromise there is a case for considering thrombolytic therapy, as anticoagulant therapy will not reduce the obstruction of the pulmonary circulation. After thrombolytic therapy has been administered, an intravenous infusion of UFH can be given. There are now a large number of published case reports on the use of thrombolytic therapy in pregnancy, streptokinase being the agent most frequently employed. Streptokinase, and probably other thrombolytic agents, do not cross the placenta. No maternal deaths associated with thrombolytic therapy have been reported, and the maternal bleeding complication rate is approximately 6%, which is consistent with that in non-pregnant patients receiving thrombolytic therapy. Most bleeding events occur around catheter and puncture sites and, in pregnant women, from the genital tract. If the patient is not suitable for thrombolysis or is moribund, cardiothoracic surgeons should be consulted to consider urgent thoracotomy.

Summary box 15.5

- Although venous thrombosis is often associated with the post-partum period, a significant number of cases of fatal pulmonary embolus occur in the first trimester.
- Gestational venous thrombosis usually occurs in the ileo-femoral veins, particularly on the left side.
- Risk assessments for VTE should be performed throughout pregnancy and the puerperium.
- The clinical diagnosis of VTE is unreliable. Consequently, objective imaging should be performed and anticoagulant treatment used until objective testing is concluded.
- Neither unfractionated nor low-molecular-weight heparins cross the placenta.

Inherited bleeding disorders

A number of inherited bleeding disorders may be encountered by those providing pregnancy care. Of these, vWF deficiency is the most common. For some of these disorders pregnancy management also includes the diagnosis, or exclusion, of fetal carriage of these inherited defects. However, many cases of fetal carriage remain unsuspected during pregnancy. Depending on the defect, a number of pregnant haemophilia carriers may require more active management during the pregnancy, delivery and the puerperium. An outline of the issues surrounding von Willebrand's disease (vWD) and the commoner haemophilias (i.e. A, B and C) are detailed below. The particular challenges surrounding other rarer disorders such as dysfibrinogenaemia or factor (F)XIII deficiency have been the subject of a recent comprehensive review [85].

Haemophilia A and B

Heritable deficiencies of FVIII (haemophilia A) and FIX (haemophilia B) occur as X-linked recessive disorders. Consequently, most females carrying an affected gene are asymptomatic. Moreover, in the vast majority of haemophilia A carriers, FVIIIc levels will normalize during pregnancy. Women can be mildly symptomatic if (amongst other mechanisms) they are homozygous for a mutation or have significant lyonization (where the random inactivation of the X chromosome that occurs in all cells, by chance, inactivates more of the normal X chromosome in the factor-producing cells). For both haemophilias, daughters of an affected male are obligate carriers of the disease and a female carrier of haemophilia has a 50/50 chance of passing the disorder to her son and a 50/50 chance of passing the carrier state to her daughter.

Haemophlia A results from a variety of genetic mutations, although 40% of severely affected individuals have an inversion involving intron 22 of the gene, whereas the majority of mild disease results from point mutations. Haemophilia A also tends to follow a similar pattern in affected family members, reflecting the particular familial mutation, although in 60% of cases there may be no known family history. Haemophilia B is considerably less common, but is more often associated with a family history. It is also associated with a wide variety of mutations, with many of these being peculiar to an individual family. Both haemophilia A and B result in a lifelong tendency to bleed. However, it is unusual to see bleeding problems in the neonate and symptoms are often first seen when the infant begins to crawl or walk. For both haemophilias symptoms are directly related to the level of remaining factor activity: a level below 1 IU/dL leads to severe spontaneous bleeding (often haemarthrosis); a level of 1–5 IU/dL leads to moderate bleeding only after minor trauma; and a level of 6–40 IU/dL leads to mild bleeding only after major trauma. In both haemophilia and vWD (see below) the diagnosis may be suspected if there is prolongation of the activated partial thromboplastin time (APTT), although a normal time does not exclude mild disease. The diagnosis of haemophilia can be confirmed by determining FVIIIc, FIXc and FXIc levels. In milder cases, vWD may also have to be excluded.

In mild haemophilia A and vWD, there should be an assessment of the effect of the vasopressin analogue desmopressin (DDAVP), which may increase plasma FVIIIc and vWF by two to five times. DDAVP has no significant oxytocic effects [86], is not associated with teratogenicity in animal studies and has been used in early pregnancy to permit CVS or amniocentesis [87]. Theoretically, if used at delivery it could carry an increased risk of fetal hyponatraemia. However, restricting its use until after clamping of the placental cord should avoid this. Replacement with factor products in haemophilia A and B should be achieved with recombinant or high purity factor preparations where possible, with dosage based on the plasma concentration of factor required and on the body weight or plasma volume. In general, treatment should be initiated under the supervision of a physician experienced in the management of haemophilia and in the UK there is a system of regional haemophilia centres. In all cases, if a patient presents for care, the centre responsible for the patient's haemophilia care should be contacted to determine which treatment product is usually used and to ascertain if the patient is known to have any inhibitor to FVIII or FIX which might affect treatment.

Carrier detection of haemophilia

A mother is an obligate carrier of haemophilia if she has an affected father. She is also considered a carrier if she has had two affected sons, or if she has a family history and one affected son. It is also likely if she has no family history but has had an affected son. In general, the phenotype of haemophilia A remains constant in families and carriage of a mild defect should result in a mildly affected son. A reduced level of FVIIIc is consistent with carriage of haemophilia A, although a normal level does not exclude it, especially if an individual is pregnant. In suspected cases with normal FVIIIc, it has been shown that the ratio of plasma FVIIIc to vWF levels may help distinguish between carriers and non-carriers, but this is unlikely to give useful information in pregnant subjects because of the marked physiological changes in both factors. Female carriage of haemophilia B is likely if there is reduced FIX activity (which often results in a more clear-cut distinction from non-carriers than FVIII carriage in haemophilia A), but assessment of FIX antigen levels is more problematic as there may be a considerable overlap with non-haemophilic subjects. Unlike FVIII, FIX activity does not change substantially with increasing gestation, and in those carriers with a low level this level tends to persist during pregnancy.

For haemophilia A there are two types of genetic diagnosis that can be achieved: direct and indirect evidence of a mutation. In severe haemophiliacs, direct detection of the intron 22 inversion, or a further common inversion in part of the intron 22 sequence, should be carried out. In mildly affected individuals, the indirect methods using linkage analysis of polymorphisms can be carried out. This requires information from several family members, one of whom needs to carry the disease, and relies on normally occurring variations in the genetic nucleotide sequence that can be used to track the mutant gene. Alternatively, direct sequencing will give diagnostic information in the majority of subjects. For haemophilia B, confirmation of female carriage requires knowledge of the mutation within the family. In general, to be certain that an identified mutation causes haemophilia B, it is recommended that the mutation is already included in one of the international databases of haemophilia mutations, as some mutations do not affect function.

Prenatal diagnosis

In those many cases which are sporadic, elimination of fetal haemophilia cannot be achieved by prenatal diagnosis. However, when haemophilia is suspected, prenatal diagnosis can be achieved by a number of techniques. Of these, CVS is the method of choice. However, as it is carried out prior to the possibility of fetal sexing by ultrasound, CVS may result in an unnecessary risk to a female fetus. CVS is used to determine the fetal sex in the first instance and, where appropriate, a known mutation can then be detected by sequencing or, if possible, by linkage analysis. A number of polymorphisms are informative in about 90% of cases of haemophilia B in white people. However, genetic diagnosis by CVS is not infallible. In the second trimester, it is usual to offer fetal sexing by ultrasound. Amniocentesis can also be used to acquire fetal genetic material, and can be carried out after the fetal sex determination by ultrasound. However, this may lead to the possibility of termination beyond 15 weeks' gestation. Cordocentesis to determine fetal levels of FVIII or FIX can be used between 18 and 20 weeks, but is often seen as a last resort as it may lead to the stress of an even later termination. Isolation of free fetal DNA in the maternal circulation is possible in the first trimester, and may be increasingly used, in combination with ultrasound [88], to determine fetal sex prior to 11 weeks' gestation. In the future the diagnosis of haemophilia itself may be achieved by isolation of fetal cells or free fetal DNA from the maternal circulation.

Antepartum carrier management

In mild haemophilia A and vWD the levels of vWF and FVIIIc increase with gestation and thus replacement products are rarely required in carriers before birth. However, when early complications such as miscarriage or ectopic pregnancy occurs, or a procedure such as amniocentesis or CVS is required in a carrier, then problems are occasionally seen. FIXc levels do not increase during pregnancy and in more markedly affected haemophilia B carriers, haemostatic support is more likely to be required during pregnancy than with equivalent haemophilia A carriers. Such support should be with recombinant factor products, as DDAVP is usually ineffective in FIX deficiency. If there is the potential for use of blood products

(even recombinant products) during the pregnancy, then the woman should have her immunity to hepatitis A and B checked and appropriate immunization considered. FVIIIc or FIX levels should be checked in all carriers at the first antenatal visit and again in the third trimester (at 28 and 34 weeks). A level of 50 IU/dL of FVIII or FIX, as appropriate, is usually sufficient to avoid haemorrhagic problems in early pregnancy, for vaginal delivery, diagnostic procedures (such as amniocentesis) and Caesarean section, and (if the level is above 50 IU/dL and the coagulation screen is normal) epidural anaesthesia [89].

Management of delivery and puerperium

On admission to the labour suite, a full blood count, coagulation screen, appropriate factor level assessment (unless these have previously been normal) and a cross-match sample for group and save should be performed. Intramuscular analgesia should be avoided if the mother has a FVIIIc level of less than 50 IU/dL, but such therapy can be given intravenously. The management of delivery must consider the possibility of fetal haemophilia. Even if the fetus is a female it is important to remember that she may still be at risk of bleeding because of the combination of lyonization and the reduced coagulation factor production associated with liver immaturity. The mode of delivery remains controversial [90], but generally delivery should be by the least traumatic method and vaginal delivery is often preferred for known haemophilia carriers, with few obstetricians recommending Caesarean section purely on the basis of suspected (or known) fetal haemophilia. However, the main concern is fetal intracerebral bleeding in the course of delivery. Thus, where the fetus may be a carrier female or affected male, it is prudent to avoid procedures that would place the fetus at increased risk of bleeding, such as complicated forceps deliveries, rotational forceps, ventouse extraction, scalp electrodes or fetal scalp blood sampling. A straightforward mid or low cavity forceps delivery is usually considered to carry a reasonable risk. However, if there is a delay in labour and an easy vaginal delivery seems less likely, then the mother should be delivered by Caesarean section.

In haemophilia A, as pregnancy FVIIIc levels fall quickly to pre-pregnancy levels after delivery, haemorrhage is possible and FVIII levels should be maintained above 50 IU/dL for at least 3 days after vaginal delivery and for 5 days following Caesarean section [89]. DDAVP can be used, if required, in breast-feeding mothers as it does not enter breast milk. For the newborn, cord determination of appropriate factor levels, on blood aspirated by clean venepuncture from the umbilical vein, should be obtained in all suspected or known cases if possible. Vaccines should be given by the subcutaneous route and intramuscular injections and heel stabs avoided until the level of clotting factors is known. In such cases vitamin K prophylaxis is routinely given by the oral rather than intramuscular route. Follow-up for determination and, if required, treatment must be organized with the appropriate paediatric haemophilia centre.

Difficulties arise when a sporadic case of haemophilia unexpectedly presents with an intracerebral haemorrhage following vaginal delivery. In this context it is important to remember that approximately one-third of cases of haemophilia are due to new mutations. In sporadic cases, haemophilia in the child may not be immediately considered and mild prolongation of the APTT (which occurs in moderately affected individuals) may be interpreted as being within normal limits for the newborn. In all suspected cases, specific factor assays should be performed. Screening for congenital dislocation of the hip should be carried out with caution, or postponed until the results of factor levels are known. The place of early prophylaxis after birth remains controversial and in some areas serial brain ultrasound scans are used to screen for intracerebral haemorrhage. Recent advice does recommend that cranial ultrasound/computed tomography should be performed in neonates where the diagnosis of haemophilia has been made and there has been a traumatic delivery or bleeding is suspected [89].

Haemophilia C

Haemophilia C is inherited as an autosomal recessive trait and results in reduced FXIc levels. The disorder has a prevalence in the general population of about 1 in 1 million, but occurs at a higher frequency in the Ashkenazi and Iraqi Jew populations. At least 28 known mutations are known but, unlike haemophilia A and B, bleeding is more difficult to predict. Generally, bleeding does not correlate well with residual FXI activity. Haemarthrosis is uncommon and spontaneous bleeding is rare. Indeed, in many affected individuals bleeding only occurs following surgery or trauma. Although deficiency may prolong the APTT, this is only likely to detect homozygous subjects. Thus in all suspected cases a FXIc assay should be performed. Prenatal diagnosis is often difficult because of the large number of mutations associated with FXI deficiency, although two mutations predominate in Askenazi jews, making prenatal diganosis more straightforward [89].

Management in pregnancy

There are a variety of studies that show no change in FXIc levels with gestation in normal individuals [91,92], although many show a gradual reduction [93]. It has been recommended that factor levels should be checked at booking, 28 weeks, 34 weeks and prior to invasive procedures [89]. However, as there is no good correlation between FXIc levels and bleeding, close monitoring of FXIc levels may be of limited value. Postpartum haemorrhage occurs in 20% of homozygotes, but excessive

bleeding may also occur in heterozygotes. In general, subjects with a FXIc level below 15 IU/dL have a 16–30% chance of excessive bleeding during delivery [92,94] and should receive prophylactic factor concentrate at the beginning of labour or prior to a planned delivery, unless there is a history of uneventful major surgery without prophylaxis [89]. Even if specific haemostatic support is thought not to be required, products should be available. When therapy is needed, daily use of a FXI concentrate is probably justified, with the aim of achieving a target FXIc level of no greater than 70 IU/dL (as levels greater than 100 IU/dL have been associated with thrombosis [95,96]). In those with a history of thrombosis or atherosclerosis, FXI concentrate may not be advisable and support with virally inactivated FFP is an alternative. If there has been no history of bleeding, tranexamic acid could also be used to cover delivery [91], but fibrinolysis is impaired in pregnancy and this should be used with caution in view of the potential for thrombosis. The use of regional anaesthesia remains controversial, and should be avoided in severe cases or those with a history of significant haemorrhage [89]. As with any other haemophilia, the possibility of fetal carriage should be considered when planning fetal monitoring, forceps and ventouse extraction at delivery, although neonatal bleeding is uncommon. As FXI levels may be low in the neonatal period, exclusion of disease in offspring may not be possible immediately after delivery.

von Willebrand's disease

vWF binds platelets to the subendothelium at the site of vessel injury, whilst the binding of FVIII to vWF in the plasma protects FVIII from degradation. vWD results in a quantitative or qualitative defect in vWF and is the most common heritable bleeding disorder, with a frequency that has been estimated at about 1% of many populations [97,98]. There are three main types of vWD: type 1 is the most common and results in partial deficiency of vWF and is usually mild; type 2 results in a functional defect of vWF (of which four variants are recognized); and type 3 is more severe as it results in a virtual absence of vWF, with an accompanying significant effect on FVIIIc levels [99].

A reduction in vWF results in a defect of primary haemostasis leading to menorrhagia, bruising, epistaxis, postpartum haemorrhage and bleeding after dental extraction. In severe vWD, the accompanying reduction in circulating FVIII also results in a mild to moderate haemophilia A phenotype. In all suspected cases, APTT, vWF antigen and activity, and FVIIIc levels should be assessed. However, vWF/FVIII may rise in association with the acute-phase response and in pregnancy [93], so the diagnosis of mild disease can be difficult. In the mildest and commonest form of vWD, blood levels of vWF will respond to an infusion of the vasopressin analogue DDAVP [86,100]. In subjects who do not respond to DDAVP, treatment with plasma-derived factor concentrates (which contain both FVIII and vWF) is required. Although antifibrinolytic agents are often avoided in pregnancy, tranexamic acid may also be a useful adjunct to other therapy, particularly in postpartum haemorrhage and it has also been used to control or prevent bleeding at/around delivery without apparent maternal or fetal effects [87].

Management

All women with vWD who are contemplating pregnancy should be advised of the risk of bleeding and offered access to a genetic counsellor regarding the inheritance of vWD and given information on the planned evaluation of her offspring after delivery [99]. During pregnancy all affected women should have rapid access to specialized haemophilia care. If the fetus is at risk of severe (usually type 3) vWD, prenatal diagnosis may be required, achieved either by identifying a mutation or by analysing restriction fragment length polymorphisms that are known to be informative. Although vWF levels increase with gestation, it is important to assess vWF (activity and antigen) and FVIIIc levels between 34 and 36 weeks' gestation in all women with vWD to confirm that the levels have increased sufficiently to allow labour and delivery without the need for DDAVP or blood products [99].

In subjects with mild to moderate vWD, vWF levels usually increase from weeks 6–10 of gestation, increasing threefold to fourfold by the third trimester [92,101]. This makes antenatal therapy unnecessary in most cases. However, as with haemophilia A, early pregnancy complications (particularly when vWF activity is below 50 IU/dL) may require specific treatment to improve vWF levels. DDAVP has been used during pregnancy, but repeated administration and use where there is evidence of pre-eclampsia should be avoided [89]. In more severe vWD there is unlikely to be a rise in vWF with gestation [101,102] and factor therapy may be required to cover interventional procedures or spontaneous bleeding. In type 2b vWD, thrombocytopenia may develop or worsen during pregnancy as a result of increasing platelet aggregation [103]. Consequently, monitoring of the platelet count in this group may be advisable, although treatment is not usually required [104]. A vWF/FVIII activity level above 50 IU/dL is considered safe for vaginal delivery and Caesarean section [89].

After delivery, the levels of vWF rapidly return to pre-pregnancy levels. Consequently, vWD is associated with a twofold to fourfold higher risk of primary and secondary postpartum haemorrhage [87,105]. However, in most mild vWD, prophylactic therapy for vaginal delivery is not needed, although treatment may be required (particularly in type 2 vWD) for episiotomy or perineal tears. Even in mild disease, epidural analgesia should not be undertaken lightly but with due regard to the risks of spinal haematoma, and in all cases vWF acivity above 50 IU/dL is recommended before epidural analgesia is considered [89]. As with mild haemophilia A, in those who are known to respond to DDAVP, this can be used to cover Caesarean section. Overall, delayed secondary postpartum haemorrhage may be 15–20 times more common in those with vWD than in normal women [99] and even in mild vWD there will be a fall in vWF after delivery and discharge planning in women with symptomatic disease should take account of the possibility of delayed secondary postpartum haemorrhage. In particular, vWF and FVIIIc levels should be monitored in the first days after delivery and maintained above 50 IU/dL for 3–5 days. After delivery all women should be advised of the potential for postpartum haemorrhage and close contact should be maintained between affected women and healthcare providers throughout the puerperium [99]. Severe vWD is more often associated with intrapartum and postpartum haemorrhage, which may occur despite prophylaxis.

Epidural anaesthesia is not recommended for more severe disease, but if the vWF ristocetin cofactor level (vWF activity) and factor VIIIc level are above 50 IU/dL and the coagulation screen is normal, regional anaesthesia is not absolutely contraindicated [99]. As with all bleeding disorders, where a fetus is at risk of inheriting vWD, delivery should managed to minimize the risk of trauma to the fetus. In all suspected cases, the umbilical cord venous vWF level should be assessed with a sample obtained by clean venepuncture. It should be noted that this is not reliable for the exclusion of milder disease.

 Summary box 15.6

- Most mild or non-affected haemophilia carriers and patients with vWD have a normal pregnancy outcome. However, vigilance and planning are required when complications occur, or invasive investigations are required, particularly in early pregnancy.
- Given the possibility of fetal carriage of inherited bleeding disorders, the delivery of affected or carrier mothers should be by the least traumatic method.

References

1 Pena-Rosas J, Viteri F. Effects and safety of preventive oral iron or iron+folic acid supplementation for women during pregnancy. *Cochrane Database Syst Rev* 2009;(4):CD004736.

2 Ali S, Economides D. Folic acid supplementation. *Curr Opin Obstet Gynecol* 2000;12:507–512.

3 Hibbard E, Smithells R. Folic acid metabolism and human embryopathy. *Lancet* 1965;i:1254–1256.

4 Ray J, Blom H. Vitamin B12 insufficiency and the risk of fetal neural tube defects. *Q J Med* 2003;96:289–295.

5 Hindmarsh PC, Geary MP, Rodeck CH, Jackson MR, Kingdom JC. Effects of early maternal iron stores on placental weight and structure. *Lancet* 2000;356:719–723.

6 Pardo J, Peled Y, Bar J *et al.* Evaluation of low serum vitamin B(12) in the non-anaemic pregnant patient. *Hum Reprod* 2000;15:224–226.

7 van den Broek NR, Letsky EA, White SA, Shenkin A. Iron status in pregnant women: which measurements are valid. *Br J Haematol* 1998;103:817–824.

8 Andersson A, Hultberg B, Brattström L, Isaksson A. Decreased serum homocysteine in pregnancy. *Eur J Clin Chem Clin Biochem* 1992;30:377–379.

9 Qvist I, Abdulla M, Jägerstad M, Svensson S. Iron, zinc and folate status during pregnancy and two months after delivery. *Acta Obstet Gynecol Scand* 1986;65:15–22.

10 Commentary. Does folic acid harm people with vitamin B12 deficiency. *Q J Med* 1995;88:357–364.

11 Old J. Screening and genetic diagnosis of haemoglobinopathies. *Scand J Clin Lab Invest* 2007;67:71–86.

12 Chui D, Waye J. Hydrops fetalis caused by alpha-thalassaemia: an emerging health care problem. *Blood* 1998;91:2213–2222.

13 Aessopos A, Karabatsos F, Farmakis D *et al.* Pregnancy in patients with well-treated beta-thalassaemia: outcome for mothers and newborn infants. *Am J Obstet Gynecol* 1999;180: 360–365.

14 Jensen C, Tuck S, Wonke B. Fertility in beta-thalassaemia major: a report of 16 pregnancies, preconceptual evaluation and a review of the literature. *Br J Obstet Gynaecol* 1995;102: 625–629.

15 Mordel N, Birkenfeld A, Goldfarb AN, Rachmilewitz EA. Successful full-term pregnancy in homozygous beta-thalassaemia major: case report and review of the literature. *Obstet Gynecol* 1989;73:837–839.

16 Nassar AH, Usta IM, Rechdan JB, Koussa S, Inati A, Taher AT. Pregnancy in patients with beta thalassemia intermedia: outcomes of mothers and newborns. *Am J Hematol* 2006;81: 499–502.

17 Sheiner E, Levy A, Yerushalmi R, Katz M. Beta-thalassaemia minor during pregnancy. *Obstet Gynecol* 2004;103:1273–1277.

18 Ryan K, Bain BJ, Worthington D *et al.* Significant haemoglobinopathies: guidelines for screening and diagnosis. *Br J Haematol* 2010;149:35–49.

19 American College of Obstetricians and Gynecologists. Haemoglobinopathies in pregnancy. ACOG Practice Bulletin No. 78. *Obstet Gynecol* 2007;109:229–237.

20 Leung WC, Leung KY, Lau ET, Tang MH, Chan V. Alpha-thalassaemia. *Semin Fetal Neonatal Med* 2008;13:215–222.

21 Hahn S, Zhong X, Holzgreve W. Recent progress in non-invasive prenatal diagnosis. *Semin Fetal Neonatal Med* 2008;13: 57–62.

22 Rahimy MC, Gangbo A, Adjou R, Deguenon C, Goussanou S, Alihonou E. Effect of active prenatal management on pregnancy outcome in sickle cell disease in an African setting. *Blood* 2000;96:1685–1689.

23 Koshy M. Sickle cell disease and pregnancy. *Blood Rev* 1995;9:157–164.

24 Rees DC, Olujohungbe AD, Parker NE, Stephens AD, Telfer P, Wright J. Guidelines for the management of the acute painful crisis in sickle cell disease. *Br J Haematol* 2003;120:744–752.

25 Martí-Carvajal AJ, Peña-Martí GE, Comunián-Carrasco G, Martí-Peña AJ. Interventions for treating painful sickle cell crisis during pregnancy. *Cochrane Database Syst Rev* 2009;(1): CD006786.

26 Mahomed K. Prophylactic versus selective blood transfusion for sickle cell anaemia during pregnancy. *Cochrane Database Syst Rev* 2006;(3):CD000040.

27 Urbaniak S, Greiss M. RhD haemolytic disease of the fetus and the newborn. *Blood Rev* 2000;14:44–61.

28 Roberts IA. The changing face of haemolytic disease of the newborn. *Early Hum Dev* 2008;84:515–523.

29 British Committee for Standards in Haematology, Blood Transfusion Task Force. Guidelines for blood grouping and red cell antibody testing during pregnancy. *Transfus Med* 1996;6:71–74.

30 Working Party of the British Committee for Standards in Haematology, Transfusion Taskforce. *Guidelines for the Estimation of Fetomaternal Haemorrhage.* London: British Society for Haematology, 2009. Available at: www.bcshguidelines.com/documents/BCSH_FMH_bcsh_sept2009.pdf

31 British Committee for Standards in Haematology. *Guidelines for the Use of Prophylactic Anti-D Immunoglobulin.* London: British Society for Haematology, 2006. Available at: www.bcshguidelines.com/documents/Anti-D_bcsh_07062006.pdf

32 Lo Y, Bowell PJ, Selinger M *et al.* Prenatal determination of fetal rhesus D status by DNA amplification of peripheral blood of rhesus-negative mothers. *Ann NY Acad Sci* 1994;731: 229–236.

33 van der Schoot C, Hahn S, Chitty LS. Non-invasive prenatal diagnosis and determination of fetal Rh status. *Semin Fetal Neonatal Med* 2008;13:63–68.

34 Moise KJ Jr. The usefulness of middle cerebral artery Doppler assessment in the treatment of the fetus at risk for anemia. *Am J Obstet Gynecol* 2008;198:161.e1–4.

35 National Institute for Health and Clinical Excellence. *Pregnancy (Rhesus-negative Women): Routine Anti-D.* Technology appraisal TA156. London: NICE, 2008. Available at: http://guidance.nice.org.uk/TA156

36 Royal College of Obstetricians and Gynaecologists. *The Use of Anti-D Immunoglobulin for Rhesus D Prophylaxis.* Green-top Guideline No. 22, 2011. Available at: www.rcog.org.uk/files/rcog-corp/GTG22AntiD.pdf

37 Bowman J. Thirty-five years of Rh prophylaxis. *Transfusion* 2003;43:1661–1666.

38 MacKenzie IZ, Bowell P, Gregory H, Pratt G, Guest C, Entwistle CC. Routine antenatal Rhesus D immunoglobulin prophylaxis: the results of a prospective 10 year study. *Br J Obstet Gynaecol* 1999;106:492–497.

39 Daniels G, Poole J, de Silva M, Callaghan T, MacLennan S, Smith N. The clinical significance of blood group antibodies. *Transfus Med* 2002;12:287–295.

40 British Committee for Standards in Haematology General Haematology Task Force. Guidelines for the investigation and management of idiopathic thrombocytopenic purpura in adults, children and in pregnancy. *Br J Haematol* 2003;120: 574–596.

41 Arnold D, Dentali F, Crowther MA *et al.* Systematic review: efficacy and safety of rituximab for adults with idiopathic

thrombocytopenic purpura. *Ann Intern Med* 2007;146: 25–33.

42 Klink DT, van Elburg RM, Schreurs MW, van Well GT. Rituximab administration in third trimester of pregnancy suppresses neonatal B-cell development. *Clin Dev Immunol* 2008;2008:271363.

43 Franchini M, Zaffanello M, Veneri D. Advances in the pathogenesis, diagnosis and treatment of thrombotic thrombocytopenic purpura and hemolytic uremic syndrome. *Thromb Res* 2006;118:177–184.

44 George JN. The association of pregnancy with thrombotic thrombocytopenic purpura/hemolytic uremic syndrome. *Curr Opin Hematol* 2003;10:339–344.

45 Esplin M, Branch D. Diagnosis and management of thrombotic microangiopathies during pregnancy. *Clin Obstet Gynecol* 1999;42:360–367.

46 Veyradier A, Meyer D. Thrombotic thrombocytopenic purpura and its diagnosis. *J Thromb Haemost* 2005;3:2420–2427.

47 Stella CL, Dacus J, Guzman E *et al.* The diagnostic dilemma of thrombotic thrombocytopenic purpura/hemolytic uremic syndrome in the obstetric triage and emergency department: lessons from 4 tertiary hospitals. *Am J Obstet Gynecol* 2009;200:381–384.

48 Martin JN Jr, Bailey AP, Rehberg JF, Owens MT, Keiser SD, May WL. Thrombotic thrombocytopenic purpura in 166 pregnancies: 1955–2006. *Am J Obstet Gynecol* 2008;199:98–104.

49 Gerth J, Schleussner E, Kentouche K, Busch M, Seifert M, Wolf G. Pregnancy-associated thrombotic thrombocytopenic purpura. *Thromb Haemost* 2009;101:248–251.

50 Scully M, Starke R, Lee R, Mackie I, Machin S, Cohen H. Successful management of pregnancy in women with a history of thrombotic thrombocytopaenic purpura. *Blood Coagul Fibrinolysis* 2006;17:459–463.

51 Taylor CM, Machin S, Wigmore SJ, Goodship TH. Clinical practice guidelines for the management of atypical haemolytic uraemic syndrome in the United Kingdom. *Br J Haematol* 2009;148:37–47.

52 Scully MA, Machin SJ. Berend Houwen Memorial Lecture: ISLH Las Vegas May 2009: the pathogenesis and management of thrombotic microangiopathies. *Int J Lab Hematol* 2009;31: 268–276.

53 Blanco-Molina A, Trujillo-Santos J, Criado J *et al.* Venous thromboembolism during pregnancy or postpartum: findings from the RIETE Registry. *Thromb Haemost* 2007;97:186–190.

54 Centre for Maternal and Child Enquiries. *Saving Mothers' Lives: Reviewing Maternal Deaths to Make Motherhood Safer, 2003–2005. The Seventh Report of the Confidential Enquiries into Maternal Deaths in the United Kingdom.* London: CMACE, 2007. Available at: www.cmace.org.uk/getattachment/26dae364-1fc9-4a29-a6cb-afb3f251f8f7/Saving-Mothers'-Lives-2003-2005-(Full-report).aspx

55 Confidential Enquiry into Maternal and Child Health. *Stillbirth, Neonatal and Post-neonatal Mortality 2000–2003. England, Wales and Northern Ireland.* London: CEMACH, 2005. Available at: www.cmace.org.uk/getattachment/f0dc4ef6-71e9-4ec2-8221-f118522b5f3c/Stillbirth,-Neonatal-and-Perinatal-Mortality-2000-.aspx

56 Ray J, Chan W. Deep vein thrombosis during pregnancy and the puerperium: a meta-analysis of the period of risk and the leg of presentation. *Obstet Gynecol Surv* 1999;54: 265–271.

57 Chan W, Spencer F, Ginsberg J. Anatomical distribution of deep vein thrombosis in pregnancy. *Can Med Assoc J* 2010;182:641.

58 Clark P, Brennand J, Conkie JA, McCall F, Greer IA, Walker ID. Activated protein C sensitivity, protein C, protein S and coagulation in normal pregnancy. *Thromb Haemost* 1998;79: 1166–1170.

59 Greer I, Thomson A. Management of venous thromboembolism in pregnancy. *Best Pract Res Clin Obstet Gynaecol* 2001;15: 583–603.

60 McColl M, Ramsay J, Tait R. Risk factors for pregnancy-associated venous thromboembolism. *Thromb Haemost* 1997;78: 1183–1188.

61 Bates SM, Greer IA, Hirsh J, Ginsberg JS. Use of antithrombotic agents during pregnancy: the Seventh ACCP Conference on Antithrombotic and Thrombolytic Therapy. *Chest* 2004; 163:627S–644S.

62 Cohen D, Berger SP, Steup-Beekman GM, Bloemenkamp KW, Bajema IM. Diagnosis and management of the antiphospholipid syndrome. *BMJ* 2010;340:c2541.

63 Rai R, Cohen H, Dave M, Regan L. Randomised controlled trial of aspirin and aspirin plus heparin in pregnant women with recurrent miscarriage associated with phospholipid antibodies (or antiphospholipid antibodies). *BMJ* 1997;314:253–257.

64 Royal College of Obstetricians and Gynaecologists. *The Investigation and Treatment of Women with Recurrent Miscarriage.* Green-top Guideline No. 17, 2003. Available at: www.rcog.org.uk/files/rcog-corp/uploaded-files/GT17Recurrent Miscarriage2003.pdf

65 Kujovich J. Thrombophilia and pregnancy complications. *Am J Obstet Gynecol* 2004;191:412–424.

66 Rodger M, Paidas M, McLintock C *et al.* Inherited thrombophilia and pregnancy complications revisited. *Obstet Gynecol* 2008;112:320–324.

67 Rodger M, Betancourt MT, Clark P *et al.* The association of factor V Leiden and prothrombin gene mutation and placenta-mediated pregnancy complications: a systematic review and meta-analysis of prospective cohort studies. *PLoS Med* 2010;7:e1000292.

68 Bates SM, Greer IA, Pabinger I, Sofaer S, Hirsh J. Venous thromboembolism, thrombophilia, antithrombotic therapy, and pregnancy: American College of Chest Physicians Evidence-Based Clinical Practice Guidelines (8th Edition). *Chest* 2008;133(6 Suppl):844S–886S.

69 Walker M, Ferguson S, Allen V. Heparin for pregnant women with acquired or inherited thrombophilias. *Cochrane Database Syst Rev* 2003;(2):CD003580.

70 Younis JS, Ohel G, Brenner B, Haddad S, Lanir N, Ben-Ami M. The effect of thromboprophylaxis on pregnancy outcome in patients with recurrent pregnancy loss associated with factor V Leiden mutation. *BJOG* 2000;107:415–419.

71 De Stefano V, Martinelli I, Rossi E *et al.* The risk of recurrent venous thromboembolism in pregnancy and puerperium without antithrombotic prophylaxis. *Br J Haematol* 2006;135: 386–391.

72 Royal College of Obstetricians and Gynaecologists. *Reducing the Risk of Thrombosis and Embolism During Pregnancy and the*

Puerperium. Green-top Guideline No. 37a, 2009. Available at: www.rcog.org.uk/files/rcog-corp/GTG37aReducingRisk Thrombosis.pdf

73 Royal College of Obstetricians and Gynaecologists. *The Acute Management of Thrombosis and Embolism During Pregnancy and the Puerperium*. Green-top Guideline No. 37b, 2007. Available at: www.rcog.org.uk/files/rcog-corp/GTG37b1022011.pdf

74 Francalanci I, Comeglio P, Alessandrello Liotta A *et al*. D-dimer plasma levels during normal pregnancy measured by specific ELISA. *Int J Clin Lab Res* 1997;27:65–67.

75 Kovac M, Mikovic Z, Rakicevic L *et al*. The use of D-dimer with new cutoff can be useful in diagnosis of venous thromboembolism in pregnancy. *Eur J Obstet Gynecol Reprod Biol* 2010;148:27–30.

76 British Thoracic Society Standards of Care Committee Pulmonary Embolism Guideline Development Group. British Thoracic Society guidelines for the management of suspected acute pulmonary embolism. *Thorax* 2003;58:470–484.

77 Ridge CA, McDermott S, Freyne BJ, Brennan DJ, Collins CD, Skehan SJ. Pulmonary embolism in pregnancy: comparison of pulmonary CT angiography and lung scintigraphy. *AJR Am J Roentgenol* 2009;193:1223–1227.

78 Cook J, Kyriou J. Radiation from CT and perfusion scanning in pregnancy. *BMJ* 2005;331:350.

79 Rodie VA, Thomson AJ, Stewart FM, Quinn AJ, Walker ID, Greer IA. Low molecular weight heparin for the treatment of venous thromboembolism in pregnancy: case series. *BJOG* 2002;109:1020–1024.

80 Chan W, Anand S, Ginsberg J. Anticoagulation of pregnant women with mechanical heart valves: a systematic review of the literature. *Arch Intern Med* 2000;160:191–196.

81 Schaefer C, Hannemann D, Meister R *et al*. Vitamin K antagonists and pregnancy outcome. A multi-centre prospective study. *Thromb Haemost* 2006;95:949–957.

82 Greer I, Nelson-Piercy C. Low-molecular weight heparins for thromboprophylaxis and treatment of venous thromboembolism in pregnancy: a systematic review of safety and efficacy. *Blood* 2005;106:401–407.

83 Magnani H. An analysis of clinical outcomes of 91 pregnancies in 83 women treated with danaparoid. *Thromb Res* 2010;125:297–302.

84 Warkentin TE, Greinacher A, Koster A, Lincoff AM. Treatment and prevention of heparin induced thrombocytopenia: American College of Chest Physicians Evidence-Based Clinical Practice Guidelines (8th Edition). *Chest* 2008;133(6 Suppl):340S–380S.

85 Kadir R, Chi C, Bolton-Maggs P. Pregnancy and rare bleeding disorders. *Haemophilia* 2009;15:990–1005.

86 Mannucci P. Desmopressin: a nontransfusional form of treatment for congenital and acquired bleeding disorders. *Blood* 1998;72:1449–1455.

87 Kujovich J. von Willebrand disease and pregnancy. *J Thromb Haemost* 2005;3:246–253.

88 Chi C, Hyett JA, Finning KM, Lee CA, Kadir RA. Non-invasive first trimester determination of fetal gender: a new approach for prenatal diagnosis of haemophilia. *BJOG* 2006;113:239–242.

89 Lee CA, Chi C, Pavord SR *et al*. The obstetric and gynaecological management of women with inherited bleeding disorders:

review with guidelines produced by a taskforce of UK Haemophilia Centre Doctors' Organization. *Haemophilia* 2006;12:301–306.

90 Madan B, Street A. What is the optimal mode of delivery for the haemophilia carrier expecting an affected infant: vaginal delivery or caesarean delivery? *Haemophilia* 2010;16:425–426.

91 Chi C, Kulkarni A, Lee CA, Kadir RA. The obstetric experience of women with factor XI deficiency. *Acta Obstet Gynecol Scand* 2009;88:1095–1100.

92 Kadir RA, Lee CA, Sabin CA, Pollard D, Economides DL. Pregnancy in women with von Willebrand's disease or factor XI deficiency. *Br J Obstet Gynaecol* 1998;105:314–321.

93 Clark P. Changes in haemostasis variables in pregnancy. *Semin Vasc Med* 2003;3:13–24.

94 Salomon O, Steinberg DM, Tamarin I, Zivelin A, Seligsohn U. Plasma replacement therapy during labor is not mandatory for women with severe factor XI deficiency. *Blood Coagul Fibrinolysis* 2005;16:37–41.

95 Bolton-Maggs PH, Colvin BT, Satchi BT, Lee CA, Lucas GS. Thrombogenic potential of factor XI concentrate. *Lancet* 1994;344:748–749.

96 Collins PW, Goldman E, Lilley K, Pasi KJ, Lee CA. Clinical experience of factor XI deficiency: the role of fresh frozen plasma and factor XI concentrate. *Haemophilia* 1995;1:227–231.

97 Rodeghiero F, Castaman G, Dini E. Epidemiological investigation of the prevalence of von Willebrand's disease. *Blood* 1997;69:454–459.

98 Werner EJ, Broxson EH, Tucker EL, Giroux DS, Shults J, Abshire TC. Prevalence of von Willebrand disease in children: a multiethnic study. *J Pediatr* 1993;123:893–898.

99 Nichols W, Hultin MB, James AH *et al*. von Willebrand disease (VWD): evidence-based diagnosis and management guidelines, the National Heart, Lung, and Blood Institute (NHLBI) Expert Panel report (USA). *Haemophilia* 2008;14:171–232.

100 Castaman G, Tosetto A, Rodeghiero F. Pregnancy and delivery in women with von Willebrand's disease and different von Willebrand factor mutations. *Haematologica* 2010;95:963–969.

101 Conti M, Mari D, Conti E, Muggiasca ML, Mannucci PM. Pregnancy in women with different types of von Willebrand disease. *Obstet Gynecol* 1986;68:282–285.

102 Greer IA, Lowe GD, Walker JJ, Forbes CD. Haemorrhagic problems in obstetrics and gynaecology in patients with congenital coagulopathies. *Br J Obstet Gynaecol* 1991;98:909–918.

103 Rick ME, Williams SB, Sacher RA, McKeown LP. Thrombocytopenia associated with pregnancy in a patient with type IIB von Willebrand's disease. *Blood* 1987;69:786–789.

104 Pasi K, Collins PW, Keeling DM *et al*. Management of von Willebrand disease: a guideline from the UK Haemophilia Centre Doctors' Organization. *Haemophilia* 2004;10:218–231.

105 Kouides P. Current understanding of von Willebrand's disease in women: some answers, more questions. *Haemophilia* 2006;12(Suppl 3):43–51.

106 Lindqvist P, Dahlback B, Marsal K. Thrombotic risk during pregnancy: a population study. *Obstet Gynecol* 1999;94:595–599.

107 Jacobsen A, Skjeldestad F, Sandset P. Ante- and postnatal risk factors of venous thrombosis: a hospital-based case-control study. *J Thromb Haemost* 2008;6:905–912.

108 James AH, Jamison MG, Brancazio LR, Myers ER. Venous thromboembolism during pregnancy and the postpartum period: incidence, risk factors, and mortality. *Am J Obstet Gynecol* 2006;194:1311–1315.

109 Knight M. Antenatal pulmonary embolism: risk factors, management and outcomes. *BJOG* 2008;115:453–461.

110 Robertson L, Wu O, Langhorne P *et al*. Thrombophilia in pregnancy: a systematic review. *Br J Haematol* 2006;132:171–196.

111 Ginsberg JS, Hirsh J, Rainbow AJ, Coates G. Risks to the fetus of radiological procedures used in the diagnosis of maternal venous thromboembolic disease. *Thromb Haemost* 1989;61: 189–196.

112 Winer-Muram HT, Boone JM, Brown HL, Jennings SG, Mabie WC, Lombardo GT. Pulmonary embolism in pregnant patients: fetal radiation dose with helical CT. *Radiology* 2002;224: 487–492.

Chapter 16
Miscellaneous Medical Disorders

Andrew McCarthy
Imperial College Healthcare, London, UK

The Confidential Enquiry into Maternal and Child Health [1] is referred to in Chapter 32. In the latest enquiry, covering the years 2003–2005, the rate of death from indirect causes remained stable in comparison to previous years. There were a number of deaths where vulnerable women had not accessed care, and emphasis is placed on ensuring that there are no barriers to deter vulnerable members of society from seeking appropriate care.

Most medical conditions in this age group do not result in serious morbidity, though many have the potential to do so (e.g. epilepsy, asthma and migraine). It is important that women receive good advice before pregnancy about the potential impact of their medical condition, and enter pregnancy with appropriate confidence about routine medication or specific management plans to alter treatment in the first trimester. This necessitates that they have ready access to specialist help once they become pregnant. Some compromise in effectiveness of medical treatment for long-term conditions is potentially involved, and it is clearly appropriate that these issues will have been addressed prior to pregnancy, for example anticoagulation in high-risk patients or renal protection with angiotensin-converting enzyme (ACE) inhibitors. The importance of pre-conception counselling is emphasized in the latest Confidential Enquiry.

There are a variety of medical disorders which may impact on a mother's health during pregnancy and the puerperium. These may be classified as those that are incidental to the pregnancy and where no exacerbation is expected as a result of pregnancy, and those that are clearly prone to exacerbation due to pregnancy. The latter are of greatest concern to obstetricians, but incidental problems leading to serious morbidity also require careful coordinated care, and care pathways are generally much less robust for these conditions.

General considerations

Mean age of childbearing has increased steadily in recent years. This has the effect of increasing the chance of a pregnancy being complicated by coincidental medical conditions, and increases the risk that such conditions can impact on women's health. In the UK the latest figures collected over the triennium 2003–2005 reveals that 3.2% of deliveries are to women 40 years of age and over, while 2.9% of women have a body mass index (BMI) over 40. In some units 6% of women are 40 years and older. This reflects a major shift, increasing risk of morbidity from medical disorders, and may be a contributory factor towards indirect deaths in the triennial maternal mortality enquiry. The number of women delivering who were born outside the UK also continues to rise, contributing to this burden.

Management of women with medical disorders is often best coordinated within clinics with both obstetric and medical opinions and midwifery input available. When problems arise such clinics make outpatient management much more convenient for the patient, and facilitate good communication between the relevant medical teams. They also serve as a focal point with which the woman may make contact in early pregnancy when treatment changes may need to take place without delay or in later pregnancy if there are problems. Integrated care plans for women with medical disorders should be made. Good communication between the different specialties involved in a woman's care is necessary, and good communication between maternity units is necessary so that women with complications are managed in centres with all relevant expertise. Within units, consideration needs to be given to how such cross-specialty communication occurs if there is no formal multidisciplinary meeting where

Dewhurst's Textbook of Obstetrics & Gynaecology, Eighth Edition. Edited by D. Keith Edmonds.
© 2012 John Wiley and Sons, Ltd. Published 2012 by John Wiley and Sons, Ltd.

high-risk cases are discussed. The role of the midwife and support workers cannot be emphasized enough in ensuring that women feel comfortable contacting services, and in ensuring that issues such as domestic abuse are picked up (see Chapter 61).

Respiratory disorders

Women with respiratory disorders require careful assessment when they present for antenatal care. For many this will mean a specialist opinion from an obstetric physician, for others an agreed care pathway with the relevant specialist. For those with a risk of respiratory compromise during pregnancy or delivery, investigation with pulmonary functions tests may be necessary. Exclusion of associated pulmonary vascular disease by echocardiography is essential if there is any risk (see Chapter 12 for further discussion). An anaesthetic opinion prior to the third trimester is valuable, including for those with possible respiratory compromise due to musculoskeletal problems. Such musculoskeletal conditions can also hinder regional anaesthesia, and referral should occur early enough to allow imaging of the spine if necessary to allow the anaesthetist time to plan.

Breathlessness can be one of the most difficult symptoms to interpret in pregnancy. Some increase in breathlessness arises during the course of a normal pregnancy, and yet the same complaint can be a manifestation of serious and life-threatening complications such as thromboembolism, cardiac disease, or deterioration of background respiratory disease. Patients should have a careful clinical assessment by history and examination. Oxygen saturation, arterial blood gases and chest X-ray may all help in differentiating physiological breathlessness from serious disease. Experienced medical opinion should be sought if there is concern about underlying pathology, and if faced with recurrent admissions.

 Summary box 16.1

Women with recurrent admissions have been identified in the maternal mortality enquiry as a high-risk group. Readmission with the same complaint should always result in a re-evaluation of the primary diagnosis, appropriateness of treatment and of the need for more senior or specialist review.

Management of acute respiratory compromise may require delivery. While the physiological adaptation to pregnancy is not critically dependent on any respiratory change, in the presence of pathology the negative impact of pregnancy including splinting of the diaphragm may mean that delivery is an important part of the treatment plan to ensure recovery. This may mandate Caesarean delivery in difficult circumstances and in such situations experienced obstetric, medical and anaesthetic input is required. Such patients may require general anaesthesia and intensive care after delivery.

Asthma

The most common respiratory disorder is asthma, affecting approximately 4% of all pregnant women, and maternal death from asthma still occasionally occurs [1]. Most women with asthma will not suffer any adverse affect on their pregnancy as a result of their condition. It is important that women with asthma receive good advice about using medication in pregnancy and reassurance that all commonly used medications to control asthma are safe. They must be reassured that flares must not be ignored and that treatment of flares with medication such as steroids is safe for their baby. Generally, a short course of oral steroid therapy will achieve control of symptoms where conventional inhalers are failing. As these women may present directly to delivery suites, it is important that protocols for the treatment of acute asthmatic attacks are available in such units [2] and that medical back-up is available. It is clearly ideal that consultation should ensure that women presenting in the third trimester have optimal control of their asthma prior to childbirth, and this will mean serial visits for those with brittle control to ensure stepwise increases in treatment. Acute exacerbations in labour are rare.

Pneumonia

Pneumonia can be a life-threatening illness in a woman of childbearing age [1], although the incidence in pregnancy is thought to be similar to that in the non-pregnant state [3]. Productive cough and pleuritic chest pain are the most common complaints in addition to breathlessness. Acute pneumonia should be managed by experienced physicians; imaging is important in patient care and should not be withheld. In one series, 24% of patients also had asthma, and background respiratory disease must always be sought. Most antibiotics are safe for the pregnant mother (tetracyclines are contraindicated), and it is important to treat infection vigorously rather than exercise restraint due to inappropriate fear of medication. An aminoglycoside should be considered in the more severe cases in addition to first-line treatment [3]. The management objectives include preventing the respiratory compromise developing to the stage where there is a need for delivery as this will then be a very high risk delivery. It is also important to prevent the underlying infection developing into sepsis syndrome with associated haemodynamic instability. Anaesthetic input is required from an early stage where delivery may need to be considered. Adverse outcome on pregnancy has been reported, particularly a high risk of preterm delivery and possibly abruption [3].

Varicella pneumonia is a particular cause for concern for the pregnant woman. It typically arises some days after the onset of the rash [3] and is most likely to arise in the third trimester. Women with respiratory symptoms in the presence of primary varicella infection should be managed aggressively. It can occur in association with encephalitis and hepatitis, and will require prompt admission for intravenous aciclovir therapy. Aciclovir does not appear to have adverse sequelae for the fetus, and case fatality rates have reduced markedly with aciclovir treatment.

Tuberculosis

Tuberculosis can present for the first time during pregnancy. A high index of suspicion must be maintained when presented with symptoms of cough, malaise or weight loss in high-risk groups. Pregnancy poses a diagnostic difficulty as it is more difficult to interpret non-specific symptoms such as malaise. In the UK, the immigrant population is most at risk, with Somali and Asian women representing nearly all cases [4]. In the UKOSS study the mean duration of stay in the UK was between 4 and 5 years at time of diagnosis, and the median gestational age at diagnosis was 27 weeks. It is associated with increased obstetric complications, particularly a high risk of preterm delivery and intrauterine growth retardation (IUGR). Delay in diagnosis was greatest for those with extrapulmonary disease. Most treatment options appear to be safe, including ethambutol, rifampicin, isoniazid with pyridoxine and also pyrazinamide. Streptomycin carries risks of eighth nerve damage and should be avoided. Extrapulmonary disease is as common as pulmonary disease in the UK [4]. In the UKOSS study co-infection with HIV was present in a significant minority, and most had extrapulmonary disease.

Cystic fibrosis

While men with this condition are often infertile, women may be fertile and wish to conceive. Prenatal diagnosis of this autosomal recessive condition should be discussed before pregnancy and a plan made. It is also important that such women have a management plan made preconceptually that allows for the specific risks to the mother. Pulmonary disease with hypoxaemia, poor nutritional status and pulmonary hypertension will prompt the greatest concern, and may make pregnancy inadvisable. Added concerns will be liver disease, diabetes, and the ability of the woman to cope following delivery with the demands of a newborn baby in the context of limited life expectancy (late thirties). Pulmonary functions tests, echocardiography to exclude pulmonary hypertension, and arterial gases may all guide the decision about whether pregnancy is advisable. Chest infections require prompt and expert treatment antenatally, and associated problems such as diabetes also require attention. Early involvement of the anaesthetic staff is advisable, and analgesia in labour is preferably by regional anaesthesia. Most women with cystic fibrosis will have a good outcome to their pregnancy [5,6], although the most recent Confidential Enquiry emphasizes that maternal death may occur despite optimal care [1]. There are a significant number of reports of successful outcome to pregnancy following lung transplantation for cystic fibrosis patients, although risk of subsequent rejection of the transplant is a concern [7].

Respiratory failure after delivery

Respiratory failure can arise for the first time in the postpartum period. The differential diagnosis includes adult respiratory distress syndrome, pulmonary oedema secondary to pre-eclampsia or nephrotic syndrome, amniotic fluid embolism, pulmonary embolism, infection and collapse, and side effects of tocolysis. Often a single diagnosis is not reached, and care is supportive. Care must be taken to exclude undiagnosed cardiac disease or peripartum cardiomyopathy, and protect the patient from thromboembolic complications.

Neurological conditions

Serious manifestations of neurological disease are fortunately rare in pregnancy, although cerebral haemorrhage remains a significant cause of maternal death. Epilepsy and migraine are common causes of morbidity, and epilepsy remains a significant contributor to maternal mortality [1]. Deaths from epilepsy arise directly from seizures as well as from a phenomenon known as 'sudden unexpected death in epilepsy'. This condition is ill-defined, usually not witnessed and may occur remote from a seizure.

Epilepsy

Women of childbearing age who suffer from epilepsy must have their treatment designed to maximize safety and compliance in pregnancy. Antiepileptic drugs can cause congenital malformation, and the risk increases depending on the drug used, the dose, and the number of drugs used [8]. The greatest concern arises with sodium valproate, with regard to both congenital malformation risk and subsequent neurological development [9]. Ultrasound assessment for anomalies needs to exclude specific abnormalities associated with medication, but will not achieve 100% detection. Folic acid 5 mg daily is generally prescribed in view of the relative folate deficiency of many mothers on antiepileptic treatment. Serum levels of antiepileptic drugs are subject to many influences and in general fall modestly during pregnancy. Potential influences include increased plasma volume, altered protein binding and excretion. It is important that control of seizures is achieved to minimize maternal morbidity, and patients must be followed up to ensure dose adjustments are made as appropriate. Women should be maintained on as few drugs as possible. Sodium valproate is the major cause for concern in the second and third trimester, in light of data suggesting increased educational needs in children exposed *in utero* [9]. Drug doses may need to be adjusted after delivery if there are alterations during the antenatal period. Specific advice must be given to epileptic women about childcare, such as not bathing the baby on their own, and patient organizations often issue information leaflets which are very helpful.

Summary box 16.2

Antiepileptic medication must be reviewed prior to pregnancy to ensure that the patient is on as few drugs as possible, with the lowest risk of congenital malformation but with adequate control of seizures.

Migraine

Migraine is a common problem in pregnancy. Pregnant women often suffer from headaches which may resolve spontaneously in the second trimester, and the natural history of migraine in pregnancy suggests a reduction in incidence through the trimesters [10]. Strategies employed for migraine during pregnancy include low-dose aspirin as prophylaxis, paracetamol and codeine as pain relief during the acute attack, and propranolol if attacks are still troublesome despite these measures. Focal migraine can arise in pregnancy and requires an experienced opinion to exclude serious underlying causes. The available evidence suggests that the triptans are safe in pregnancy and a reasonable option for those with troublesome migraine [11].

Focal transient neurological symptoms can arise in pregnancy and usually have a benign course. One study that assessed women presenting with a first attack of dysphasia, hemisensory and hemimotor syndromes found a very low incidence of cerebral ischaemia [12]. In most cases, it was concluded that these were migraine attacks, despite the lack of prior history. Subsequently only 29% demonstrated recurrent migraine on follow-up suggesting that pregnancy can lower the threshold for a migraine attack resulting in a single episode.

Cerebral vascular disease

Cerebral haemorrhage is a major cause of maternal morbidity and mortality [1]. It can arise where there is inadequate blood pressure control or an underlying vulnerable circulation. Neurological complaints during pregnancy must be investigated just as in the non-pregnant state. Ischaemic strokes also arise in pregnancy, and it is difficult to determine whether there is an increased incidence reflecting the coagulation changes of pregnancy. Investigation of any underlying thrombophilic state can be important, and further thromboprophylaxis instigated.

In the latest maternal mortality triennial report [1], 11 of 22 cases of intracranial haemorrhage were due to subarachnoid haemorrhage. Most occurred antenatally in the second half of pregnancy, and some postnatally. One of the cases occurred during labour, raising the spectre that labour is a potential risk factor. This has not always been clear, and in this case it arose from a large middle cerebral artery aneurysm. Defining any increased risk of rupture during labour is not possible from the literature, and decisions on mode of delivery must be individualized and reflect the patient's wishes and parity. Experience based on this report suggests that neurological examination must be carried out, and neuroimaging should be offered in the presence of severe and incapacitating headaches. Of the 22 women who died from cerebral haemorrhage in this report, nine had some degree of uncontrolled hypertension. Blood pressure can often be most difficult to control postnatally.

An analysis of risk factors and timing of intracranial haemorrhage has been conducted in the USA [13]. Analysis in this population revealed advanced maternal age, African American race, hypertensive disorders, coagulopathy and drug abuse to be associated with increased risk of cerebral haemorrhage. The same study suggests that the postpartum period is the time of greatest risk, and this is exacerbated with increasing maternal age. In this study 20% of the women with intracranial haemorrhage died, although the authors accept this may be an underestimate due to their study design. When cerebral aneurysms are detected in the antenatal period, management decisions should be made jointly between the obstetricians and neurosurgeons with consideration given to issues of radiation exposure and possible embolization [14].

Summary box 16.3

Failure to control hypertension may result in cerebral haemorrhage. Severe and incapacitating headaches must be investigated.

Cerebral vein thrombosis

Cerebral vein thrombosis may be more common in pregnancy [15]. It tends to present with a very severe headache, and experienced opinion should be sought to determine if magnetic resonance imaging is warranted.

This is the investigation of choice for such a diagnosis. The treatment involves anticoagulation, in most cases with low-molecular-weight heparin until stability is achieved after delivery when conversion to warfarin can be considered.

Rheumatology

Antiphospholipid syndrome and systemic lupus erythematosus

Pregnancy outcome may be impaired in systemic lupus erythematosus (SLE), but will generally be good. Outcome is significantly better for those who conceive when the background disease is quiescent and worse for those with unstable disease or flares in the first trimester or during pregnancy. Much of the impaired outcome can be explained as a result of secondary antiphospholipid syndrome (APS), with increased risks of IUGR, placental abruption and pre-eclampsia. Lupus nephritis, with associated hypertension and proteinuria, also impacts adversely on outcome. Renal failure secondary to nephritis increases risk further. Ro and La antibodies occasionally result in morbidity or mortality from congenital heart block (2%) and congenital lupus (5%). As most immunosuppressive treatment is safe in pregnancy, generally the best approach is to maintain treatment and ensure disease quiescence. Careful monitoring of immunosuppressive treatment is required, and associated infection and flares must be treated promptly.

APS is an acquired condition characterized by an increased tendency to thrombosis, recurrent miscarriage, impaired pregnancy outcome and thrombocytopenia (see Chapter 7). Laboratory tests to confirm the diagnosis include those for anticardiolipin antibody and lupus anticoagulant. These tests must be positive on two consecutive occasions at least 6 weeks apart as transient positivity can be found in association with viral illness. The outlook is worse for APS associated with a thrombotic history than for APS associated with prior recurrent miscarriage or poor obstetric history [16]. Treatment in pregnancy involves antiplatelet therapy with low-dose aspirin and sometimes heparin. The argument for heparin treatment is greatest for those with a thrombotic history (mandatory) or prior late pregnancy complications as opposed to recurrent miscarriage.

Rheumatoid arthritis

Rheumatoid arthritis can complicate pregnancy. In the presence of mild disease a temporary improvement in the symptoms of arthritis can arise, and this is presumed to be due to the steroidal properties of placental hormones or other immune effect of pregnancy. In such cases a flare may arise after delivery. Many case series to date are heavily weighted by experience of women with mild disease, but more women with moderate or severe disease are now willing to contemplate pregnancy. This is a result, at least to some extent, of the increasing success of disease-modifying drugs such as methotrexate, leflunomide and tumour necrosis factor (TNF)-α antagonists, which then must be withdrawn prior to or early in pregnancy. Pregnancy can prove more challenging in such cases and will require careful supervision by a rheumatologist or obstetric physician, and the involvement of an anaesthetist prior to delivery. For those on long-term steroid therapy, increased surveillance for gestational diabetes is necessary. Recent evidence suggests that infliximab may be safely used for those with severe symptoms. Some consideration needs to be given to the extent of handicap which can arise from moderate or severe rheumatoid arthritis. This can seriously impair the ability of a mother to properly care for her newborn child. Early referral to an occupational therapist can ensure that the family is best prepared for any problems that may arise.

Scleroderma and mixed connective tissue disease can also complicate pregnancy. Scleroderma/systemic sclerosis is a high-risk condition in pregnancy and should be managed in very specialized units. Decisions on therapy (or withdrawal of therapy) must be made in joint consultation with rheumatologists as there is specific concern about withdrawal of ACE inhibitors and prescription of steroids. Caution is required in assessing the cardiopulmonary status of such women when pregnancy is being planned. Echocardiography must be performed to exclude pulmonary hypertension. Hypertension and renal involvement are also common and require careful management. Mixed connective tissue disorders can also present problems, akin to those with lupus or other arthritic diseases.

Liver disorders

Liver disorders frequently complicate pregnancy, but fortunately rarely result in long-term morbidity. Cholestasis of pregnancy is the most common [17] and is thought to affect about 4500 pregnancies per year in the UK. It classically presents with an itch and sleeplessness in the third trimester. It is associated with an increased risk of intrauterine death, classically from 37 weeks' gestation, an increased risk of meconium passage, and increased risk of preterm labour. The mechanism of intrauterine death is uncertain, but is likely to be related to a toxic effect on the fetus. A recent study suggests that the risk of fetal complications increases as bile acid levels rise, and that a threshold bile acid level of 40 µmol/L exists for such complications [18]. Laboratory investigation includes liver function tests and assay of serum bile acids. It is currently uncertain whether the bile acids themselves may be directly responsible for fetal demise. Treatment strategies include timely delivery, cool aqueous menthol cream to relieve itch and ursodeoxycholic acid. Ursodeoxycholic acid is currently the mainstay of treatment and is prescribed at doses commencing at 500 mg twice daily and may be increased to a maximum of 2 g daily. The value of the main treatment strategies of ursodeoxycholic acid and delivery at 37–38 weeks is uncertain [19]. There is a high likelihood of recurrence (approximately 80%). Some women who present with this condition will have underlying liver disease and this is most likely to be noted with early-onset disease, or failure of liver function to return to normal after delivery.

Acute fatty liver of pregnancy (AFLP) is a serious but rare liver condition arising in pregnancy that can be very non-specific at time of presentation. It is associated with nausea, vomiting, abdominal pain and jaundice. Diagnosis is normally made when faced with this clinical picture in association with significantly elevated aspartate aminotransferase (AST) and alanine aminotransferase (ALT) and no direct evidence of pre-eclampsia. The diagnosis may be supported by imaging suggestive of fatty change. Manifestations of liver failure include coagulopathy, haemodynamic instability and hypoglycaemia and such patients must be managed in an intensive care or high-dependency setting. Hypoglycaemia may be profound and requires immediate correction. It is a common omission in maternity units for the blood sugar level not to be checked. Serial assessment of blood clotting is important. Delivery must be achieved prior to the development of coagulation failure if possible, where necessary at the expense of fetal maturity. It is often not possible to clearly distinguish AFLP from HELLP syndrome (haemolysis, elevated liver enzymes, low platelets) or pre-eclampsia.

Liver dysfunction in pregnancy can also be caused by incidental viral or autoimmune hepatitis. Where it is unexplained, serology for acute hepatitis must be investigated and medical help requested. It is often difficult to determine whether liver dysfunction is due to a pregnancy-related complication or incidental liver disease, and consideration must be given to delivery when there is uncertainty. Liver failure is rare in or after pregnancy. The more common causes include paracetamol overdose, viral hepatitis, HELLP syndrome and AFLP. Correct diagnosis is important as early referral to a liver unit with a view to transplantation may be appropriate. Delivery will not affect the natural course of a viral hepatitis, but is likely to be beneficial in HELLP syndrome and AFLP. The issue of referral to specialist liver units most commonly arises after delivery if liver function continues to deteriorate rather than improve. Such decisions should be made in consultation with a specialist unit and will require senior input.

Hyperemesis

Hyperemesis gravidarum is defined as vomiting in early pregnancy sufficient to warrant hospital admission. Vomiting is clearly very common in early pregnancy, but some women suffer disproportionately, occasionally resulting in serious sequelae including severe dehydration and increased risk of thromboembolism. Pregnancy outcome is generally unaffected, though there may be an increased incidence of IUGR where sustained vomiting results in maternal weight loss. Treatment options include small light snacks, intravenous rehydration and sometimes antiemetic treatment. Promethazine and metoclopramide are commonly used for this indication. There is uncertainty regarding the effectiveness of antiemetics. It is important that B vitamins are replenished as Wernicke's encephalopathy can occur. Corticosteroids may have a role in exceptional cases. When all else fails total parenteral nutrition may be required, but this is very rare. It is difficult to predict recurrence risks in a subsequent pregnancy, but some women undoubtedly experience severe nausea and vomiting with every pregnancy.

It is very important that hyperemesis is regarded as a diagnosis of exclusion. Serious underlying causes for ongoing vomiting must be sought such as central nervous system pathology, gastrointestinal disease or surgical problems. Peptic ulceration is rare in pregnancy but can arise. It is sometimes appropriate to consider endoscopy for women with persistent vomiting or a trial of treatment. Gastro-oesophageal reflux is a much more common problem. The diagnosis is not usually in doubt and the condition can be treated with antacids, metoclopramide, histamine H_2 antagonists and proton pump inhibitors.

Abdominal complications and inflammatory bowel disease

Problems such as appendicitis, pancreatitis and cholecystitis can arise in pregnancy, and it is estimated that 0.2–1.0% of all pregnant women will require general surgery [20]. These problems must be managed aggressively to minimize any risk of associated peritonitis, which can result in premature labour and associated sepsis. The estimated risk of fetal loss is 20% with a perforated appendix as opposed to 5% if uncomplicated [20]. Diagnosis of such complications can be difficult and requires an experienced opinion.

Inflammatory bowel disease can also complicate pregnancy. Pregnancy outcome is generally satisfactory, although there may be some increased risk of preterm birth and IUGR, particularly if there is active disease. It is usually treated in the same way in pregnancy as in the non-pregnant state, with steroids and sulfasalazine the mainstays of therapy. Supplementation of haematinics and vitamin D may be required. There is increasing evidence that infliximab may be used safely in the more severe and difficult cases [21]. Possible sequelae, such as perineal and perianal disease and intra-abdominal adhesions, need to be considered when discussing mode of delivery. In the presence of ileal pouch anal anastomosis, limited evidence suggests that vaginal delivery can be safely considered [22], although the possibility of deterioration in function with time is not excluded given the duration of follow-up in the current studies.

 Summary box 16.4

In the presence of severe or uncontrolled inflammatory bowel disease, the patient should be booked into a unit that can provide multidisciplinary care and counselling, and provide care for the neonate in the event of prematurity.

Dermatoses of pregnancy

There are a number of specific dermatological conditions that arise only in pregnancy. The most common is termed 'polymorphic eruption of pregnancy' and affects approximately 0.5% of pregnancies. This maculopapular rash presents on the abdomen and thighs with umbilical sparing. It causes irritation and can be treated with steroid cream if localized, or systemic steroids. Skin biopsy is sometimes necessary in pregnancy, typically when there is a relatively early presentation and significant maternal symptoms. Polymorphic eruption tends to arise in the late third trimester, and not to recur in subsequent pregnancies. It does not affect fetal outcome.

Pemphigoid gestationis is much more rare (1 in 60 000 incidence) and commences around the umbilicus. It starts as pruritic papules and plaques that develop into vesicles and bullae after a lag of a few weeks. It is thought to be immunological in origin and is associated with other autoimmune disorders. Severe cases should be treated with systemic steroids. This rash can be slow to resolve after delivery and has a high risk of recurrence in subsequent pregnancies, often at earlier gestations. This condition appears to be associated with some fetal risk and IUGR, and therefore fetal surveillance must be instituted.

Prurigo of pregnancy is another papular eruption affecting extensor surfaces and the abdomen. It may be associated with atopy, and can be treated with antihistamines and topical steroids. There are other dermatoses that can arise specifically in pregnancy. Dermatological opinion and biopsy tend to be reserved for those that are particularly disabling or which have failed to respond to topical steroids.

Human immunodeficiency virus

If a mother has HIV, in the absence of intervention her baby has a one in four chance of infection. This is reduced to around 1% with the main treatment strategies, including antiretroviral treatment, elective Caesarean and avoidance of breast-feeding. Routine antenatal testing for HIV is now the norm in most developed countries in view of this, and appears to be most effective if an opt-out approach is taken. Rapid testing for unbooked patients is increasingly achievable. In the UK, 95% of women are diagnosed by the time of delivery. Infection with HIV poses specific problems in pregnancy, and antiretroviral treatment must be supervised by experienced physicians. Infected women will be offered such treatment with the aim of reducing vertical transmission and minimizing disease progression. Choice of antiretroviral treatment will depend on clinical status, viral load and CD4 counts. There is no evidence of reproducible congenital abnormality with different antiretroviral agents, but clearly some caution is required with newer agents and treatment regimens until long-term follow-up data become available. Risks of perinatal transmission are reduced by Caesarean delivery, appropriate intrapartum antiretroviral treatment, avoidance of breast-feeding and treatment for the neonate. If a woman labours, invasive monitoring and artificial rupture of the membranes should be avoided, and a plan made for antiretroviral treatment for the mother and neonate.

Psychiatric disorders in the antenatal period

It is increasingly clear that psychiatric problems can lead to maternal mortality and very significant morbidity [1]. Reference to the latest maternal mortality report confirms the major contribution psychiatric disease makes. Antenatal assessment must include an evaluation of risk of psychiatric morbidity. This will involve review of any previous episodes of psychiatric care or social vulnerability. Patients at risk of such problems are often poor attendees for antenatal care, and are disproportionately represented in refugee or ethnic minority subgroups. Language and culture are too often barriers to appropriate care. It is clear that healthcare workers need to be aware of these factors, that systems need to be in place to ensure that such patients can access appropriate antenatal care, and that plans are made to ensure provision of support in the puerperium.

Depressive symptoms are as common in the antepartum as postpartum period, though major depressive illness is a greater problem after delivery. Symptoms include sleeplessness, lack of energy, anxiety and an inability to take pleasure from the pregnancy. Women will often have a history of a previous depressive episode, but up to one-third will not. In those with a prior diagnosis, a judgement needs to be made about continuing any previous medication. Strategies to minimize medication are reasonable provided they are supported by the mental health team. Often the woman is best served by continuing her previous treatment despite an instinctive desire to stop for fear of harming her child.

Most psychotropic medication is relatively safe in pregnancy, with few overt congenital abnormalities described in association. The exceptions include lithium, which appears to be associated with an increased incidence of Ebstein's anomaly. This is a serious consideration for those patients with bipolar disorders, where a balanced judgement must be made reflecting psychiatric stability versus a 5% risk of a potentially surgically correctable anomaly. There is some concern about an association between selective serotonin reuptake inhibitors and risk of cardiovascular defects in the fetus [23]. There is also some concern that these agents may increase the risk of pulmonary hypertension in the neonate. For many women suffering from anxiety disorders and mild depression, psychotherapy and counselling may be a better option than medication. Tricyclic antidepressants such as imipramine or amitriptyline appear to be safe in pregnancy but some of the evidence is conflicting, There are arguments for reducing the dose or stopping treatment completely prior to delivery in view of the potential for anticholinergic side effects in the neonate. Benzodiazepines may carry some teratogenic risk and are best avoided. It is reasonable for many women on antidepressant medication at conception to have a trial off treatment provided this is supported by their psychiatrist.

Manic depressive illness and schizophrenia both carry substantial risks of relapse following delivery and care in the initial postpartum phase, including reintroduction of medication, must be planned in advance. Antipsychotic medication in pregnancy may carry some risk to the fetus, but this will often be outweighed by the need for stability. It is important that decisions on long-term therapy during pregnancy are made in consultation with a psychiatrist. The incidence of severe depressive illness increases markedly in the months following delivery, while 10% of women will suffer from a milder form of depressive illness after delivery. Puerperal psychosis occurs following 1 in 500 deliveries, and about half will have presented by 7 days after delivery. Admissions following delivery should be to specialized mother and baby units [1].

Malignant disease

In the Confidential Enquiry, the major categories of tumour resulting in death were breast, brain, haemato-logical, melanoma, lung and gastrointestinal. As with other categories of death, women with social and domestic problems who could not present for care were over-represented. Delayed diagnosis can be a problem in pregnancy as symptoms may be explained as being due to a pregnancy, or signs may be masked by the abdominal and breast changes of pregnancy. Treatment options may be more limited in view of greater vascularity with pregnancy, more difficult surgical access, and greater thromboembolic risk. Chemotherapy [24] and radiotherapy [25] can be considered in pregnancy, with the greater volume of reassuring evidence for chemotherapy.

Pregnancy may exacerbate the growth of hormone-dependent tumours such as breast. The incidence of a pregnancy-related breast cancer is approximately 1 in 3000 [24]. This is likely to increase modestly with increases in maternal age. The median gestational age at diagnosis is 21 weeks. Breast cancer is more likely to present with later-stage disease in pregnancy, and prognosis is similar to the non-pregnant state when allowance is made for this. Termination of pregnancy is most likely to be considered if breast cancer is diagnosed in the first trimester. Treatment can involve surgery as in the non-pregnant. Radiotherapy has been used but requires careful counselling and is dependent on the gestational age, the dose required and the potential to shield the fetus. Chemotherapeutic protocols can be used that do not pose a significant risk to the fetus, but are generally avoided in the weeks preceding delivery to minimize the risk of coincident neutropenia or thrombocytopenia. Tamoxifen is not recommended in pregnancy. Current advice is that women should defer pregnancy for at least 2 years after a diagnosis of breast cancer, and longer with later staging of disease. Similar principles will apply to other tumours. A pragmatic approach has to be taken following a diagnosis of cancer in pregnancy that allows for the individual's wishes, the gestational age, and the feasibility of treating most forms of cancer in pregnancy with reasonable success rates.

Summary box 16.5

Stage the tumour and determine the correct treatment protocol prior to discussion about outcome of pregnancy or need to terminate.

Conclusion

This chapter has involved discussion of many medical disorders that may affect pregnancy, with emphasis on those contributing to indirect deaths in the triennial enquiry into maternal death. It is worth emphasizing that appropriate management of these conditions can lead to a woman having far greater confidence during her pregnancy and the avoidance of unnecessary morbidity, for example pregnancy blighted by migraine or arthritis and avoidance of stillbirth associated with medical conditions such as obstetric cholestasis. Good-quality antenatal care can also facilitate preparation for a difficult puerperium, and avoidance of long-term morbidity associated with flares in the postpartum period, when it is difficult for women to attend for medical appointments and routine patterns of referral often break down.

References

1 Lewis G (ed.) *Saving Mothers' Lives: Reviewing Maternal Deaths to Make Motherhood Safer 2003–2005. The Seventh Report on Confidential Enquiries into Maternal Deaths in the United Kingdom.* London: The Confidential Enquiry into Maternal and Child Health, 2007. Available at: www.cmace.org.uk/getattachment/26dae364-1fc9-4a29-a6cb-afb3f251f8f7/Saving-Mothers'-Lives-2003-2005-(Full-report).aspx

2 British Thoracic Society Scottish Intercollegiate Guidelines Network. British guideline on the management of asthma. *Thorax* 2008;63(Suppl 4):1–121.

3 Graves CR. Pneumonia in pregnancy. *Clin Obstet Gynecol* 2010;53:329–336.

4 Knight M, Kurinczuk JJ, Nelson-Piercy C et al. Tuberculosis in pregnancy in the UK. *BJOG* 2009;116:584–588.

5 Whitty JE. Cystic fibrosis in pregnancy. *Clin Obstet Gynecol* 2010;53:369–376.

6 Boyd J, Mehta A, Murphy D. Fertility and pregnancy outcomes in men and women with cystic fibrosis in the United Kingdom. *Hum Reprod* 2004;19:2238–2243.

7 Gyi KM, Hodson ME, Yacoub MY. Pregnancy in cystic fibrosis lung transplant recipients: case series and review. *J Cyst Fibros* 2006;171:175.

8 Morrow J, Russell A, Guthrie E et al. Malformation risks of antiepileptic drugs in pregnancy: a prospective study from the UK Epilepsy and Pregnancy Register. *J Neurol Neurosurg Psychiatry* 2006;77:193–198.

9 Adab N, Kini U, Vinten J. The longer term outcome of children born to mothers with epilepsy. *J Neurol Neurosug Psychiatry* 2004;76:1575–1583.

10 Goadsby PJ, Goldberg J, Silberstein SD. Migraine in pregnancy. *BMJ* 2008;336:1502–1504.

11 Duong S, Bozzo P, Nordeng H et al. Safety of triptans for migraine headaches during pregnancy and breastfeeding. *Can Fam Physician* 2010;56:537–539.

12 Liberman A, Karussis D, Ben-Hur T et al. Natural course and pathogenesis of transient focal neurological symptoms during pregnancy. *Arch Neurol* 2008;65:218–220.

13 Bateman BT, Schumacher HC, Bushnell J et al. Intracerebral haemorrhage in pregnancy: frequency, risk factors, and outcome. *Neurology* 2006;67:424–429.

14 Laurence AG, Marshman A, Aspoas R et al. The implications of ISAT and ISUIA for the management of cerebral aneurysms during pregnancy. *Neurosurg Rev* 2007;30:177–180.

15 Jeng J, Tang S, Yip P. Stroke in women of reproductive age: comparison between stroke related and unrelated to pregnancy. *J Neurol Sci* 2004;221:25–29.

16 Bramham K, Hunt BJ, Germain S et al. Pregnancy outcome in different clinical phenotypes of antiphospholipid syndrome. *Lupus* 2010;19:58–64.

17 Geenes V, Williamson C. Intrahepatic cholestasis of pregnancy. *World J Gastroenterol* 2009;15:2049–2066.

18 Glantz A, Marschall H, Mattsson L. Intrahepatic cholestasis of pregnancy: relationships between bile acid levels and fetal complication rates. *Hepatology* 2004;40:467–474.

19 Gurung V, Williamson C, Chappell L et al. Pilot study for a trial of ursodeoxycholic acid and/or early delivery for obstetric cholestasis. *BMC Pregnancy Childbirth* 2009;9:19.

20 Parangi S, Levine D, Henry A et al. Surgical gastrointestinal disorders during pregnancy. *Am J Surg* 2007;193:223–232.

21 O'Donnell S, O'Morain C. Review article: use of antitumour necrosis factor therapy in inflammatory bowel disease during pregnancy and conception. *Aliment Pharmacol Ther* 2008;27:885–894.

22 Hahnloser D, Pemberton JH, Wolff BG et al. Pregnancy and delivery before and after ileal pouch-anal anastomosis for inflammatory bowel disease: immediate and long-term consequences and outcomes. *Dis Colon Rectum* 2004;47:1127–1135.

23 Pedersen LH, Henriksen TB, Vestergaard M, Olsen J, Bech BH. Selective serotonin reuptake inhibitors in pregnancy and congenital malformations: population based cohort study. *BMJ* 2009;339:b3569.

24 Vinatier E, Merlot B, Poncelet E et al. Breast cancer during pregnancy. *Eur J Obstet Gynecol Reprod Biol* 2009;147:9–14.

25 Luis SA, Christie DR, Kaminski A, Kenny L, Peres MH. Pregnancy and radiotherapy: management options for minimising risk, case series and comprehensive literature review. *J Med Imaging Radiat Oncol* 2009;53:559–568.

Part 5
Fetal Medicine

Chapter 17
Antenatal Screening

Ruwan C. Wimalasundera
Queen Charlotte's & Chelsea Hospital, London, UK

There are several definitions of screening, but the one used by the National Screening Committee (NSC) in the UK [1] is as follows:

Screening is a public health service in which members of a defined population who do not necessarily perceive they are at risk of, or already affected by, a disease or complications of a disease, are asked a question or offered a test to identify those who are more likely to be helped than harmed by further tests or treatments to reduce the risks of a disease or its complications.

Antenatal screening is the screening of a low-risk pregnant population to identify individuals at risk of a disease or condition which may affect either the mother or the fetus. The aims of antenatal screening are several. Firstly, to allow women at high risk of a condition to have a further diagnostic test, which may itself have a risk of miscarriage, to confirm the diagnosis. Secondly, to allow counselling of the parents about the impact of the diagnosed condition on the mother or fetus as well as enabling timely medical or surgical treatment of the condition before or after birth. If the condition carries a significant risk to the mother or fetus and is not treatable, it gives the parents the chance to decide on termination if appropriate. Finally, it allows the parents and family a chance to prepare emotionally, financially and socially for a child if born with the condition.

In terms of deciding which maternal or fetal conditions should be screened, it is important to understand the fundamental principles of screening for disease initially described by Wilson and Jungner in 1968 [2].
- The condition must have a high enough prevalence in the population screened and be a significant health problem in terms of morbidity or mortality.
- The natural history of the disease and its stages of progression need to be understood.
- The screening test for the condition should have high sensitivity and specificity and be acceptable to the population.

- There must be further diagnostic testing available for screen-positive individuals.
- There must be mechanisms for counselling, prevention, treating and/or managing screen-positive patients.
- The screening policy must be cost-effective, i.e. the cost of case finding (including diagnosis and treatment) should be economically balanced in relation to possible expenditure on medical care as a whole.

Screening programmes need to be managed on a population level, and must be effective and accountable in terms of disseminating information to clinicians as well as the public. In the UK this supervising function is carried out by the NSC, which was established in 1996. Using these criteria, the NSC programme for antenatal screening includes fetal anomaly screening for Down's syndrome and fetal structural anomalies, screening for sickle cell anaemia and thalassaemia, and screening for infectious diseases (HIV, hepatitis B, rubella and syphilis).

Other screening tests are offered routinely in pregnancy following national guidelines but are not governed on a national basis, such as screening for maternal anaemia and blood group antibodies. These are managed at a regional level or within individual hospitals. There are also conditions that do not fit the criteria for population screening, but which may be offered on an individual basis because of specific risk factors such as gestational diabetes, cystic fibrosis, Tay–Sachs disease, cervical length screening for preterm labour, group B streptococcal infection or uterine artery Doppler. However, these are outside the remit of this chapter. Finally, there are screening tests still in the research phase but which may be applicable in the future, such as non-invasive fetal genotyping.

All these screening tests have the potential for harm as well as good. It is therefore essential that information is available to pregnant women explaining the benefits as well as the risks involved in screening for a particular condition including the implications of a positive screen result in terms of the pathway of further investigations, treatments and potential miscarriage as well as psychological trauma. Parents need this information early in pregnancy and they need to know they have a choice to accept or decline a test and that their decision will be respected and supported by the health professionals.

Diagnosis of fetal anomaly

The National Institute of Health and Clinical Excellence (NICE) guidance on antenatal care in the UK stipulates that all women should be offered a minimum of two scans in pregnancy [3]: a first-trimester scan between 10 and 14 weeks as part of the screening programme for Down's syndrome or, if this is declined, for dating the pregnancy; a further scan is offered between 18 and 22 weeks to screen for any structural anomalies in the fetus.

Down's syndrome screening

There are several tests that can be offered for screening for Down's syndrome. Each consists of a risk assessment based on maternal age and a scan performed in the first trimester or a blood test in the first or second trimester or a combination of scans and blood tests. The current tests offered in the UK include the following.

- *Nuchal translucency.* A first-trimester (11 to 13+6 weeks) test based on measurement of the fold of skin on the back of the fetal neck (nuchal translucency) together with maternal age.
- *Quadruple test.* Early second-trimester (14 to 20 weeks) test based on measurement of α-fetoprotein (AFP), unconjugated oestriol, free β-human chorionic gonadotrophin (hCG) or total hCG, and inhibin-A together with maternal age.
- *Combined test.* Late first-trimester (10 to 14+1 weeks) test based on combining nuchal translucency measurement with free β-hCG, pregnancy-associated plasma protein A (PAPP-A) and maternal age.
- *Integrated test.* The integration of different screening markers measured at different stages of pregnancy into a single test result. Unless otherwise qualified, 'integrated test' refers to the integration of nuchal translucency meas-

urement and PAPP-A in the first trimester with serum AFP, hCG, inhibin-A and unconjugated oestriol from 14+2 to 20 weeks' gestation.

The NSC has been given the responsibility for implementing a national strategy for Down's syndrome and fetal anomaly screening in the UK. In 2003 the Committee produced a screening policy known as the Model of Best Practice [4] which stated that all pregnant women should be offered screening for Down's syndrome with a test that provides a detection rate above 75% and a false-positive rate of less than 3% using a cut-off of 1 in 250 at term. These guidelines were based on the SURUSS report [5], a multicentre study of nearly 50000 singleton pregnancies that analysed the most effective, safe and cost-effective methods of screening for Down's syndrome using nuchal translucency, maternal serum and urine markers in the first and second trimester and maternal age in various combinations. The authors concluded that the integrated test was the best-performing with the highest detection and lowest false-positive rates at any given risk cut-off (Table 17.1). The Model of Best Practice also concluded that the integrated test resulted in the lowest loss rate of unaffected fetuses (Table 17.2).

However, in 2008 [6] and again in 2010 [7] the Model of Best Practice was reviewed, the report concluding that all trusts in the UK should offer a screening test that

Table 17.1 SURUSS study of screening performance with a constant early second-trimester risk cut-off of 1 in 250.

Screening test	Detection rate (%)	False-positive rate (%)
Triple test	81	6.9
Quadruple test	84	5.7
Combined test	83	5
Integrated test	90	2.8

Source: data from Wald *et al.* [5].

Table 17.2 Outcome in 100000 women screened with a constant detection rate of 75%.

Test	Unaffected women referred for CVS or amniocentesis	No. of Down's syndrome diagnosed	No. of unaffected fetuses lost	No. of Down's syndrome diagnosed per unaffected fetuses lost
Triple	4200	152	30	5.1
Quadruple	2500	152	18	8.5
Combined	2300	152	17	9
Integrated	300	152	2	76.3

Assumes an 80% acceptance rate of amniocentesis/CVS and 0.9% loss rate from the procedure.
Source: derived from Wald *et al.* [5].

detected 90% of Down's syndrome with a 2% false-positive rate using a cut-off of 1 in 150. The current screening test supported by the NSC is the combined test. The Committee concluded that as the combined test is a single-stage procedure, it was the most cost-effective and simplest to implement nationally and at the same time deliver the standard required (current detection rate for this test is 85% with a 2.2% false-positive rate). It is anticipated that 15% of women will be too late for combined testing at booking and should be offered the quadruple test from 14 to 20 weeks' gestation [7]. Although the integrated test had the slightly better detection rate, the fact that it needed two serum tests on different occasions increased the risk of women missing the second test, which affected the accuracy as well as increased the workload on healthcare staff in coordinating the test and tracing defaulters.

However, there are some clinical situations which may have implications in terms of interpreting any Down's syndrome screening programme.

1 *Twin pregnancy.* Since 2009 twin pregnancies can access combined testing. However, it is essential that the 'chorionicity' of the pregnancy is diagnosed on scan and reported to the laboratory as the adjustment factor for the serum biochemistry would vary depending on whether it is a dichorionic or monochorionic pregnancy [8]. Although single-centre data suggest a 75% detection rate with a 6.9% false-positive rate [9], there are as yet no population data in twin pregnancies. With triplets or higher-order pregnancy, there are no data available regarding the biochemistry adjustments. Therefore, the risk of Down's syndrome can only be calculated using maternal age and nuchal translucency measurement.

2 *Nuchal translucency measurement of 3.5 mm or more.* When measurement of nuchal translucency in the first trimester is 3.5 mm or more, it is associated with an increased risk of fetal cardiac anomalies (2.5%) and aneuploidy. Therefore referral should be made for specialist scanning and counselling even if Down's syndrome screening has been declined. There is no indication for completing the serum biochemistry under these circumstances.

3 *Maternal vaginal bleeding in first trimester.* If there is a history of significant maternal vaginal bleeding at the time of first-trimester screening for Down's syndrome, this may affect maternal blood levels of the biochemical markers used in the combined test, perhaps secondary to placental disruption. However the NSC suggest that the combined test is performed, because current data suggest that the biochemical marker levels are not significantly different in women with this history.

4 *'Vanished' twin.* When a first-trimester ultrasound shows that there is an empty second pregnancy sac, the biochemical markers appear no different to those in a singleton pregnancy and the combined test can be used to calculate the risk. If ultrasound shows that there is a second sac containing a dead fetus (sometimes called 'vanished' twin), it is possible that there could be a contribution to the maternal biochemical markers for many weeks. Under these circumstances the risk calculation should be based on the maternal age and nuchal translucency only (i.e. without biochemistry).

Screen-positive result

All women who have a screen-positive result should be referred for possible confirmatory testing. This involves initial counselling regarding the implications of the screen-positive result and the possible confirmatory tests available. The confirmatory tests would be either chorionic villous sampling (CVS) or amniocentesis. This counselling should be based on the risk of aneuploidy, the voluntary nature of the test, the option of no testing, the technique of the proposed test, the procedure-related loss rate and other common complications associated with the test, the timing of the result and the possible management options depending on the result of the test. This decision to balance the potential risk of the loss of an unaffected fetus against that of having an affected child is a very difficult and traumatic one and it is important that the parents are not rushed into a decision.

Amniocentesis

Amniocentesis can only be performed after 15 weeks when the uterus is an abdominal organ and the proportion of fluid needed to be removed (15–20 mL) is relatively small compared with the overall liquor volume at this gestation (150–250 mL). The procedure is performed under aseptic conditions, under continuous ultrasound guidance using a gauge 20–22 needle introduced transabdominally. The miscarriage rate for amniocentesis is generally quoted as 1 in 100 (1%) and is based on the single randomized controlled trial of second-trimester amniocentesis by Tabor *et al.* [10] in Denmark in 1986. They demonstrated that the women randomized to the group not undergoing amniocentesis had a miscarriage rate of 0.7% compared with 1.7% in the group who had amniocentesis and therefore suggested that amniocentesis increased the background miscarriage rate by 1%.

Amniotic fluid will contain fetal skin, urogenital and pulmonary epithelial cells and cells from the extraembryonic membranes. The cells are first concentrated by centrifuging and then cultured for 7–10 days, with the result of the karyotype being available in 14–15 days. However, over the last decade, chromosome-specific probes and fluorescence *in situ* hybridization (FISH) techniques have been developed to detect numerical aberrations in interphase non-dividing cells, eliminating the need for prolonged cell culture. Therefore, rapid prenatal diagnosis of amniotic fluid using fluorescence-based probes for short tandem repeat (STR) markers on chromosomes 21, 13 and 18 and polymerase chain reaction (PCR) amplification of these STRs [11] can be performed to give a result within three working days.

It is now routine practice that all amniocentesis and CVS performed purely for a high-risk combined test result are only sent for PCR analysis of chromosomes 21, 18 and 13 and not for a full karyotype. A full karyotype is only performed if there are structural anomalies on scan or there is a previous history of other chromosome anomalies. If the PCR confirms trisomy 21, 18 or 13, then the same sample will be cultured for a confirmatory full karyotype. This has led to situations where an initial PCR result is normal with no ultrasound anomalies seen at the time of amniocentesis, but detailed anomaly scans several weeks later detect a structural anomaly that may be consistent with other chromosomal anomalies. This is rare but may necessitate a further amniocentesis for a full karyotype.

Chorionic villous sampling

This involves sampling of placental tissue rather than amniotic fluid and can be performed soon after the screen-positive result of the combined test becomes available between 11 and 14 weeks. There are two routes used for CVS: transabdominal, which is now the preferred option, or transcervical if the former is not possible. CVS should not performed before 10 weeks because of the reported association of early CVS and isolated fetal limb disruption and oromandibular hypoplasia [12]. Cytogenetic analysis of the CVS sample is similar to that of amniocentesis. However, placental karyotype may not be exactly the same as the fetus, known as confined placental mosaicism, and occurs in around 1% of chorionic villous samples. This may require reanalysis with a second-trimester amniocentesis. Mosaicism is only confirmed in the fetus in about 10% of cases.

Multiple pregnancies

Invasive prenatal diagnosis should only be performed in multiple pregnancies by a specialist in tertiary-level fetal medicine units who have experience of performing selective termination of pregnancy if required. The uterine contents need to be mapped thoroughly before the procedure is undertaken to ensure that separate samples are taken from each fetus and that each twin can be identified accurately at a later stage. Amniocentesis is the preferred option in most units because of the relatively high risk of cross-contamination of chorionic tissue with CVS in dichorionic twins (2–6%), leading to false-positive or false-negative results. Recent series suggest that total fetal loss rates in twins after amniocentesis (3.5–4.0%) or CVS (2–4%) may not be much higher than background rates.

Non-invasive genetic testing

Given the procedure-related pregnancy loss rates associated with invasive prenatal diagnosis, many research groups have tried to investigate non-invasive methods for determining fetal genetic and chromosomal anomalies. The initial focus of research was to try to isolate fetal cells in the maternal circulation [13], but the frequency of fetal cells in the maternal blood is very low and they are difficult to isolate. Furthermore, fetal cells appear to remain in the maternal circulation for many years after a delivery and so any fetal cells isolated from an index pregnancy may be from previous pregnancies and so of little use [14]. Hence it has been difficult to isolate fetal whole cells for reliable non-invasive prenatal genetic testing [15].

However, in 1997 Lo *et al.* [15] reported the presence of cell-free fetal (CFF) DNA in the maternal circulation, which contributed to 10% of overall free DNA in the maternal circulation and could be readily detected using basic molecular techniques [16,17]. Significantly, this CFF DNA was detectable in the maternal circulation within a few weeks of pregnancy [18] and completely cleared from the maternal circulation within 2 hours of delivery [19]. CFF DNA consists of short fragments of DNA rather than whole chromosomes and originates from the placenta [20,21]. These properties make CFF DNA an ideal source of fetal material for non-invasive genetic prenatal diagnosis. Furthermore, free fetal RNA derived from genes active in the placenta and therefore fetal in origin has also been isolated in the maternal circulation [22]. Although it is still difficult to extract pure fetal DNA or RNA from the maternal serum, using the intrinsic difference between maternal and fetal DNA [21], the relative proportion of fetal DNA can be increased.

Most research has focused on DNA sequences that are paternally derived or which occur *de novo* and are therefore not present in the mother. The best-developed example of this is non-invasive testing for fetal sex determination in fetuses at risk of X-linked diseases such as congenital adrenal hyperplasia (CAH) [23]. This searches for CFF DNA for the Y chromosome in the maternal circulation, with the presence of the Y-chromosome DNA denoting a male fetus and absence a female fetus. Various studies have shown sensitivities of 87–100% with 98–100% specificity and, more significantly, a 45% reduction in the need for invasive testing in pregnancies with a history of CAH [24]. The technique has also been developed for use in single gene disorders not found in the mother, such as Huntington's disease, achondroplasia or cystic fibrosis.

However, the clinical situation where CFF DNA has had the greatest impact on routine clinical management is in fetal RhD genotyping in RhD-negative women. It is now routine practice to perform non-invasive fetal genotyping in all alloimmunized RhD-negative women who have had a previously affected child or increasing antibody titres, with a false-negative rate of only 0.2% [25].

The most significant recent advance has been the use of CFF DNA for detecting trisomy 21. In 2011 Chiu *et al.*

[26] reported the use of 'massively parallel genomic sequencing' to measure the small increase in fetal chromosome 21 DNA concentration in pregnancies affected by Down's syndrome. Using this technique in 753 pregnancies, they detected trisomy 21 fetuses with 100% sensitivity and 97.9% specificity, which resulted in a positive predictive value of 96.6% and negative predictive value of 100%. The authors concluded that multiplexed maternal plasma DNA sequencing analysis could be used to rule out fetal trisomy 21 among high-risk pregnancies and that, if referrals for amniocentesis or CVS were based on the sequencing test results, about 98% of invasive diagnostic procedures could be avoided. Currently this test is still in the research phase and is too expensive and time-consuming for population screening. However, with further development is likely to completely alter screening for Down's syndrome in the next decade.

Positive confirmatory result

Once a positive diagnosis of trisomy 21 is made on amniocentesis or CVS, the parents need to be referred for specialist counselling, usually with a genetic counsellor or a screening coordinator. The parents need to be counselled regarding the findings and the implications of a baby with trisomy 21, including the risks of physical and neurological handicap. They also need counselling as to the options for continuation of the pregnancy or termination.

Summary box 17.1

- NSC has recommended combined testing for Down's syndrome screening in all women. This involves nuchal translucency scan and maternal serum measurement for PAPP-A and hCG between 10+6 and 14+1 weeks. Using risk cut-off of 1 in 150 there is an 85% detection rate for a 2.2% false-positive rate.
- Combined testing should be offered for twins, but need to define chorionicity. Higher-order multiple pregnancies would need to rely on nuchal translucency measurement alone.
- Diagnostic testing with CVS or amniocentesis involves risk of miscarriage of approximately 1:100.
- Non-invasive diagnostic testing for trisomy 21 using free fetal DNA is technically possible but not economically practical as yet.

Ultrasound screening for fetal anomalies

In the UK there is a policy of routine second-trimester ultrasound screening for fetal anomalies [3]. However, detection of fetal anomalies varies considerably depending on the anomaly being screened for as well as the gestation at screening, the skill of the operator and the quality of the equipment used. A systematic review of routine ultrasound screening for fetal anomalies [27]

Table 17.3 Percentage of fetal anomalies detected by routine second-trimester ultrasound screening according to anatomical systems.

Condition	Detection rate (%) expected 2010
Anencephaly	98
Open spina bifida	90
Cleft lip	75
Diaphragmatic hernia	60
Gastroschisis	98
Exomphalos	80
Serious cardiac abnormalities	50
Bilateral renal agenesis	84
Lethal skeletal dysplasia	60
Edwards' syndrome (trisomy 18)	95
Patau's syndrome (trisomy 13)	95

Source: National Institute for Health and Clinical Excellence [3].

in 96 633 babies between 1996 and 1998 found an overall detection rate of 44.7%, with detection being considerably higher after 24 weeks (41.3%) than before 24 weeks (18.6%) (Table 17.3). In the UK although detection rates appear to be higher, there is considerable geographic variation. Chitty *et al.* [28] reported an overall detection rate of 74% in an inner London unit, whereas Boyd *et al.* [29] reported a detection rate of 50% in Oxford.

Although an anomaly scan has been routine in the UK for the last three decades, the NSC has only recently (2010) produced guidance on minimum standards for fetal anomaly screening to improve the detection rates of specific anomalies, particularly cardiac [30]. The structures that need to be viewed as standard and the specific views to be obtained are detailed in Table 17.4.

Fetal cardiac protocol

The detection of cardiac anomalies is of particular interest. Early prenatal detection of congenital heart disease (CHD) has increased due to advances in ultrasound resolution and the incorporation of at least a four-chamber cardiac view in the routine anomaly scan, which is now accepted as standard care in the UK. However, there is regional variation in antenatal detection of CHD, with those obstetric centres close to cardiac units performing better than those situated in more remote areas. The risk of aneuploidy varies with the structural anomaly detected and it would be outside the scope of this chapter to detail the risk for each structural anomaly. However, cardiac anomalies are the commonest type of structural anomaly detected in fetal life and at birth, with a frequency of 8 per 1000. Table 17.5 illustrates the variation in risk of aneuploidy with the various cardiac defects [31].

Fetal echocardiography involving the four-chamber view of the heart and the outflow tracts forms part of the

Table 17.4 Fetal anomaly ultrasound base menu: 18+0 to 20+6 weeks.

Area	Structure	View

Head and neck	Skull
	Neck:skin fold (NF)
	Brain
	Cavum septum
	   pellucidum
	Ventricular atrium
	Cerebellum
		Shape
		Subjective: measure NF
		   if it looks increased

Face	Lips	Coronal view
Chest	Heart Four-chamber view Outflow tracts Lungs	Refer to fetal cardiac protocol (see text)

Abdomen	Stomach: stomach and
	   short intrahepatic
	   section of umbilical vein
	Abdominal wall
	Bowel
	Renal pelvis
	Bladder
		Transverse, sagittal
		Transverse
		Transverse:
		   measure AP
		Sagittal and transverse

Spine	Vertebrae Skin covering	Sagittal and transverse Sagittal and transverse
Limbs (a)	Femur	Length (one leg only)

Limbs (b)	Hands: metacarpals (left
	   and right)
	Feet: metatarsals (left and
	   right)
		Visible (not counted)
		Visible (not counted)

Uterine cavity	Amniotic fluid Placenta	Subjective volume Visible and position noted

Source: Kirwan [30].

ultrasound scan base menu (see Table 17.4) [30]. As a minimum, four basic intracardiac views are required: laterality, the four-chamber view, the left ventricular outflow tract and the right ventricular outflow tract. A description of all the structures that require assessment is outlined in Table 17.4. The use of colour flow Doppler is not a requirement, but it should be encouraged as it may help provide additional information and improve detection of CHD. It is likely that the use of colour flow Doppler will be incorporated into the assessment of fetal echocardiography in 2013.

Mid-trimester ultrasound markers
Soft-tissue markers are signs detected on a second-trimester anomaly scan that in themselves are not structural defects but which have an association with aneuploidy, and therefore their presence increases the risk of aneuploidy. Markers include nuchal skin oedema, short femoral or humeral length measurements, choroid plexus cysts, bilateral renal pelvic dilatation, echogenic fetal bowel and hyperechogenic foci ('golf balls') in the fetal heart. Early publications reporting increased prevalence of these markers in Down's syndrome fetuses compared with euploid fetuses were used to derive increased risks for trisomy 21. However, a meta-analysis of 56 studies by Smith-Bindmen *et al.* [32] found sensitivities for individual markers in isolation of only 1–16% (Table 17.5), whereas the sensitivity of multiple markers in association with structural anomalies was 69%. Most of the markers in isolation had low relative risks (positive predictive values or likelihood ratios of 3–7 only). In 2010 the NSC clarified soft-tissue markers in its statement on normal variant screening in pregnancy [30]:

The introduction of a national Down syndrome screening programme in early pregnancy has changed the way in which the 18+0 to 20+6 fetal anomaly scan findings should be interpreted. The Programme Centre has recommended that an established Down syndrome screening test result should not be recalculated at this time. Women who are found to be 'low risk' through testing in either first or second trimesters, or who have declined screening for Down syndrome should not be referred for further assessment of chromosomal abnormality even if normal variants such as the examples below (whether single or multiple) are seen at the 18+0 to 20+6 weeks fetal anomaly screening scan. Indeed we encourage that the term ultrasound 'Down's soft marker' is no longer used.
1 Choroid plexus cyst(s).
2 Dilated cisterna magna.
3 Echogenic foci in the heart.
4 Two vessel cord.

However, the appearances listed below are examples of findings which should be reported and the woman referred for further assessment and treated as for any other suspected fetal anomaly.
1 Nuchal fold (greater than 6 mm).
2 Ventriculomegaly (atrium greater than 10 mm).
3 Echogenic bowel (with density equivalent to bone).
4 Renal pelvic dilatation (AP measurement greater than 7 mm).
5 Small measurements compared to dating scan (significantly less than 5th centile on national charts).

Management options
Following a diagnosis of fetal abnormality, women should be referred for appropriate counselling regarding the nature of the abnormality, the possibility of therapy, and the probable outcome for the child. Further consultation with the relevant paediatric specialist may be indicated, especially where postnatal interventions are contemplated or where there is a major risk of serious handicap. Counselling should address the certainty of the diagnosis, the possible association with other anomalies and the

Table 17.5 Meta-analysis performed by Wimalasundera and Gardiner [31].

Cardiac anomaly	Overall aneuploid rate (%)	Trisomy 21 (%)	Trisomy 18 (%)	Trisomy 13 (%)	45XO (%)	Other (%)	22q11 deletion
AVSD	46	79	13			8	
VSD	46	43	45	2	4	6	10–17
TOF	31	43	29	7		21	6–30
CoA	33	18	24	24	12	22	
CAT	19				25	75	10
IAAb							17–50
APVS	20						
HLHS	7		56	22	11	11	
DORV	21	10	40	20	30		1
Mitral atresia	18						
UVH	15						
PS/PA + IVS	5						
Tricuspid atresia	7				50	50	
TVD	4						
Aortic stenosis	5						
ASD	17						
TGA	0						
cTGA	0						
Tumours	0						
Cardiomyopathy	0						
Cardiosplenic syndromes	0						
DIV	0						

Data expressed as overall rate of aneuploidy (%) for individual congenital cardiac defects.
APVS, absent pulmonary valve syndrome; ASD, atrial septal defect; AVSD, atrioventricular septal defect; CAT, common arterial trunk; CoA, Coarctation of the aorta; DIV, double inlet ventricle; DORV, double outlet right ventricle; HLHS, hypoplastic left heart syndrome; IAAb, interrupted aortic arch type B; PS/PA + IVS, pulmonary stenosis/pulmonary atresia with intact ventricular septum; TGA, transposition of the great arteries; cTGA, corrected transposition of the great arteries; TOF, Tetralogy of Fallot; TVD, tricuspid valve dysplasia; UVH, univentricular heart; VSD, ventricular septal defect.

associated risk of aneuploidy or other serious undiagnosed genetic syndromes. Women also need to be advised of the prognosis for the fetus, including perinatal morbidity and the risk of intrauterine death, the postnatal morbidity associated with the findings and the life expectancy of the child. Finally, they need to be counselled about whether any curative or ameliorating procedures can be offered in the neonatal period, whether early delivery and what mode of delivery may be required, and if any procedures could be offered whilst the fetus is *in utero*.

There are no treatments for chromosomal anomalies and some structural abnormalities, and the management issues are essentially limited to termination versus continuation of pregnancy. Unless the abnormality is trivial, termination of pregnancy is a management option that should be discussed in parental counselling. The Royal College of Obstetricians and Gynaecologist (RCOG) report on termination of pregnancy for fetal abnormality [33] advises that where abortion falls within the grounds specified in the Abortion Act of 1967, doctors must advise the woman that she has this option. They must ensure she understands the nature of the fetal abnormality, and the probable outcome of the pregnancy, whether it continues to term or is aborted. The woman is then able to decide whether she wishes to have an abortion and to give her informed consent.

Parents who decide to continue with a pregnancy where the prognosis is universally fatal, such as anencephaly or trisomy 18, need to be supported in their decision by all staff concerned in their care. However, women need to be counselled regarding the high risk of intrauterine death and if they should reach term, management of the labour needs to be discussed. The parents should be given the option of no monitoring in labour to avoid deliver by Caesarean section, which would not improve neonatal survival and would significantly increase maternal morbidity. Neonatal resuscitation with an option of no active resuscitation also needs to be discussed by the neonatologist and carefully detailed in the notes.

Summary box 17.2

- Detailed anomaly scan should be offered to all women between 18+0 and 20+6 weeks.
- Choroid plexus cysts, intracardiac echogenic foci, single umbilical artery and enlarged cisterna magna, if they occur in isolation, should no longer be considered as markers for aneuploidy and should not be reported on.
- If an anomaly is detected, the parents need to be certian of their decision to continue the pregnancy or have a termination of pregnancy if it is offered.

Haemoglobinopathy screening

Sickle cell disorders and thalassaemia are the most common inherited haemoglobinopathies. They are caused by single gene defects, with 5% of the world's population being carriers and about 300 000 births worldwide affected by severe forms of the disease each year. The options for antenatal screening are based on early diagnosis to allow informed reproductive choice about whether to continue the pregnancy as there are as yet no measures to improve outcome antenatally.

Screening policy in the UK has been complicated by the variation in ethnic minorities in different regions and therefore the prevalence, particularly of sickle cell disease. Policy options in the UK were evaluated in two systematic reviews [34,35] that led to the introduction in 2004 of a screening policy in areas of high prevalence, based on an estimate of the fetal prevalence of sickle cell disease of greater than 1.5 per 10 000 live births. The key standard of antenatal screening for sickle cell disease and thalassaemia is for 50% of at-risk couples to be identified by 10 weeks' gestation to enable the completion of prenatal diagnostic testing by 13 weeks for those who want it [36]. The screen involved universal maternal blood screening in high prevalence areas without specific reference to family origin questionnaires. This estimated that 40% of the high-risk antenatal population would be within the high prevalence trusts [37].

In the low prevalence areas, which covered the remaining 60% of the antenatal population, the programme suggested the use of a family origin questionnaire (FOQ) to target screening. The currently used FOQ was adapted from an original pilot study by Dyson *et al.* [38], who looked at two questionnaires and evaluated their value in the detection of high-risk groups. This was later adapted from further trials in low prevalence areas and involves questions on the ethnic origins of the mother and the father of the baby [39].

The current policy in the UK for low prevalence populations (<1.5 per 10 000 live births) is to perform thalassaemia screening in all women on routine blood analysis and target high-risk women for sickle cell screening based on the answers to the FOQ. This has been shown to be an effective screening tool in low prevalence populations [40].

Haemoglobin variants

Haemoglobin (Hb) is composed of tetraglobin chains, two α-chains and two non-α-chains. The α-chains are encoded by the two closely related genes, *HBA1* and *HBA2*, on chromosome 16. The non-α-chains (β, γ and δ) are encoded by a cluster of genes on chromosome 11 [41]. In normal adults, HbA is the main type of haemoglobin (96–98%) while HbA_2 and HbF are only present in 2–3% and less than 1%, respectively [42].

Haemoglobin variants are characterized by gene mutation of the globin chains. In normal haemoglobin, glutamic acid is in position 6 on the β-chain, while in sickle cell disease this glutamic acid is replaced by valine leading to the formation of sickle cells. The sickling process can be activated by infections, hypoxia, acidosis, physical exercise, vaso-occlusion due to cold as well as dehydration [43]. Many types of haemoglobin variant have been found, depending on racial background. Normally, carriers of haemoglobin variants, especially heterozygous, have no symptoms. However, combination of haemoglobin variants and thalassaemia gene on the same globin chain may result in severe symptoms. For example, combination of HbE with thalassaemia gene becomes a double heterozygote that shows symptoms similar to homozygous thalassaemia.

Thalassaemia, which is slightly different from haemoglobin variants, involves gene mutations that cause production of an insufficient amount of normal globin chains. All types of thalassaemia are considered quantitative haemoglobin disease. Thalassaemia can be categorized into three classes, major, intermediate and minor, according to the severity of the symptoms. The two main thalassaemia syndromes (thalassaemia major) are α and β thalassaemia, which involve homozygous genetic defects in the α-globin and β-globin chain production respectively [41].

Screening tests

Screening for thalassaemia and haemoglobin variants are based on full blood count and haemoglobin electrophoresis. If mean corpuscular volume (MCV) is less than 80 fL and mean corpuscular haemoglobin (MCH) less than 27 pg, this would suggest a microcytic anaemia and the possibility of thalassaemia or iron deficiency anaemia. This would then be analysed further using techniques such as high-performance liquid chromatography [44]. Electrophoresis is one of the widely used techniques for analysing haemoglobin variants based on the movement of different haemoglobins or different globin chains, containing different charges, in an electric field [41].

Screen-positive result

Once a woman has been detected as a carrier in a high-risk or low-risk population, the father of the baby would be offered screening to determine the risk status of the baby. If both parents are carriers or the carrier status of the father cannot be identified, then the couple/woman needs to be referred for further counselling regarding the findings and the potential effects of an affected baby as well as the reproductive options available. Depending on the outcome of this counselling, if they have decided that they wish to proceed to diagnostic testing, they should then be referred to a fetal medicine centre for fetal geno-typing. This would involve either CVS or amniocentesis and genotyping of the fetus for thalassaemia or sickle cell variants depending on the parental genotype. Results are usually available in three to five working days. Further counselling following these results is usually warranted. This may involve referral to a paediatric haematologist to discuss further what the parents may expect for an affected child, including the current treatments available, before the parents make a decision on continuation of the pregnancy or a termination.

 Summary box 17.3

- In high-risk areas, thalassaemia and sickle cell screening should be offered to all women based on a full blood count and haemoglobin electrophoresis. If the mother is affected or a carrier, then the partner needs screening before considering offering diagnostic fetal testing.
- In low-risk areas, thalassaemia screening is offered to all and sickle cell screening targeted to high-risk women based on a family origin questionaire.

Red cell antibodies

The rhesus (Rh) system of red cell proteins is one of the most complex blood group systems. There are several different antigens, of which D, C, c, E and e are the most important. The function of the Rh complex is thought to be critical to the structure of the membrane [45]. More than 50 different red cell antigens have been reported to be associated with haemolytic disease of the fetus and newborn (HDN). However, only three antibodies seem to be associated with severe fetal disease: anti-RhD, anti-Rhc and anti-Kell (K_1). HDN is most commonly caused by maternal sensitization to Rh, specifically to the D antigen. HDN due to D incompatibility was prevalent in white people, who have the highest incidence of the D-negative phenotype (15–17%), but was rare in other ethnic groups. However, the incidence has dramatically decreased with the use of anti-D immunoglobulin as prophylaxis in Rh-negative women, which has been shown to effectively prevent isoimmunization against RhD [46].

Screening for blood group antibodies in the UK should be performed at booking (8–12 weeks' gestation) [3]. This initial testing should include ABO and RhD typing as well as a screening test to detect any irregular red cell antibodies. Testing should be undertaken again at 28 weeks' gestation for all women with no antibodies on initial testing to ensure that no additional antibodies have developed. Antibody screening should be undertaken using an indirect antiglobulin test and a red cell panel conforming to current UK guidelines [47].

Guidance on the routine administration of antenatal anti-D prophylaxis recommends that anti-D is offered to all pregnant women who are RhD-negative [48]. Routine anti-D prophylaxis can be given as two doses of 500 units anti-D immunoglobulin (one at 28 weeks and one at 34 weeks), as two doses of 1000–1650 units (one at 28 weeks and one at 34 weeks), or as a single dose of 1500 units between 28 and 30 weeks' gestation [48].

However, as anti-D is a blood product and can be associated with a small risk of allergic reaction, in the case where a woman is RD-negative, consideration should also be given to offering partner testing because if the biological father of the fetus is negative as well, anti-D prophylaxis need not be administered. Other situations where antenatal anti-D prophylaxis may not be necessary include where a woman has opted to be sterilized after the birth of the baby or when a woman is otherwise certain that she will not have another child after the current pregnancy [3].

Screen-positive result

When a red cell antibody is detected on maternal screening, the clinician responsible for the woman's antenatal care must be informed of its likely significance, with respect to both the risk of HDN and transfusion problems. Management of pregnancies in which red cell antibodies are detected varies depending on the clinical significance and titre of the antibody detected. If an Rh antibody such as D, E or c or Kell is detected, fetal Rh or Kell genotyping is now routinely performed using CFF DNA in the maternal sera, as described previously. If the fetus is found to be antigen positive for the Rh or Kell antigen, then maternal titres should be repeated every month until approximately 28 weeks' gestation, when the testing interval should be increased to every 2 weeks. If the titres go above 4 IU/mL, the woman needs to be referred to a tertiary fetal medicine centre for further monitoring and the possibility of *in utero* therapy for fetal anaemia.

Intrauterine therapy for fetal anaemia by intravascular fetal transfusion was probably the first major success story in fetal medicine. There have been two recent advances that have revolutionized the management of fetal anaemia. Firstly, the development of PCR techniques to identify fetal Rh genotype from free fetal DNA in the maternal serum, as described previously [49]. The second major advance is the abandonment of invasive amniocentesis for detecting ΔOD450 of amniotic fluid as a surrogate for fetal haemolysis in favour of non-invasive monitoring for fetal anaemia using fetal middle cerebral artery Doppler velocimetry. Mari *et al.* [50] demonstrated that by using a cut-off of 1.5 multiples of the median (MOM) that the middle cerebral artery Doppler peak systolic velocity (MCA PSV) could be used with a sensitivity of 100% and false-positive rate of 12% to detect fetal anaemia (Plate 17.1).

Once an isoimmunized woman has been detected to have an antigen-positive fetus with rising antibody titres over 4 IU/mL, the women will then be monitored with weekly MCA PSV monitoring using ultrasound. If the MCA PSV is above 1.5 MOM [50], fetal blood sampling under continuous ultrasound guidance is performed with immediate access to fetal blood analysis. If the fetus is anaemic, it is transfused using maternally cross-matched O, Rh-negative, cytomegalovirus-negative, irradiated, concentrated (haematocrit 70–90%) blood. Weekly MCA PSV monitoring is continued and further fetal blood sampling is performed if indicated on MCA PSV. Women who have been transfused are usually delivered electively at 37–38 weeks and the neonate should undergo double phototherapy postnatally. *In utero* therapy has dramatically improved the outcome of pregnancies with alloimmunization to red cell antibodies, with over 92% survival rates if transfusions occur prior to the development of fetal hydrops [51].

 Summary box 17.4

- All women should be screened for red cell antibodies at booking (8–14 weeks) and again at 28 weeks' gestation.
- Prophylactic use of anti-D at 28 and 34 weeks' gestation in Rh-negative women has dramatically reduced the incidence of RhD alloimmunization.
- Women with rising RhD, Rhc or RhE antibodies or any detectable anti-Kell antibodies need to be referred to an appropriate fetal medicine unit for monitoring and possible fetal blood transfusion.

Infection screening

The UK screening programme for infectious disease in pregnancy advocates routine screening for HIV, hepatitis B, rubella and syphilis. The policy and standards are agreed by the NSC and published in the NICE antenatal care guidelines [3]. The prevalence of all four of these

Table 17.6 Prevalence of infections in London (data based on annual reports).

Infection	London prevalence (%) 2007/2008	London prevalence (%) 2008/2009	London prevalence (%) 2009/2010
Syphilis	0.36	0.41	0.38
Hepatitis B	10.4	1.02	1.02
HIV	0.39	0.39	0.46
Rubella	4.15	5.0	4.6

infections is still significant in the UK and particularly in inner cities such as London [52] (Table 17.6) and therefore routine antenatal screening is essential to prevent mother-to-child transmission of hepatitis B, HIV and syphilis. The screening programme also identifies women for whom postnatal MMR (measles, mumps, rubella) vaccination could protect future pregnancies.

The programme stipulates the following.

1 All pregnant women are offered screening at the booking visit for rubella antibody, syphilis, HIV and hepatitis B as an integral part of their antenatal care during their first and all subsequent pregnancies regardless of immunization history.

2 Although every woman has a right to decline screening, if screening has been declined at booking, they should be re-offered screening at 28 weeks' gestation.

3 Pregnant women arriving in labour who have not received antenatal care elsewhere are offered screening for infectious diseases. Priority is given to hepatitis B and HIV screening and presumptive action is taken on a preliminary positive result until the result is confirmed. If an HIV test result is not available, appropriate preventive measures should be offered. In cases where consent is withheld for screening during labour, screening is offered again after delivery.

4 If there is a screen-positive result, the current national standards state a second sample should be taken for syphilis, hepatitis B and HIV to confirm the screening result. Following this result the women should be referred for specialist counselling and appropriate follow-up and management [53].

Hepatitis B

Hepatitis B is an infectious disease caused by hepatitis B virus (HBV). It is transmitted through infected blood and other body fluids. Transmission can occur through sexual contact or perinatal vertical transmission from mother to baby. The risk of perinatal transmission is dependent on the status of the maternal infection. Approximately 70–90% of mothers who are positive for HBV e antigen (HBeAg) will transmit the infection to the baby. The rate of transmission is approximately 10% in women with antibody to e antigen (anti-HBe). Infection can result in acute or chronic infection. A chronic infection with HBV may result in cirrhosis of the liver and liver cancer. The earlier in life the infection occurs, the greater the risk that it will lead to chronic infection, liver disease and early death.

Vaccination of the baby within 24 hours of delivery and at 1, 2 and 12 months is effective in preventing transmission of infection from mother to baby. In babies born to women with a higher risk of transmission, the addition of hepatitis B-specific immunoglobulin can reduce the risk further. With this strategy, transmission can be prevented in over 90% of infants exposed to maternal infection [54].

Screen-positive result

If a woman is screen-positive for HBV, she should be referred to an appropriate specialist (hepatologist, gastroenterologist or infectious disease specialist) within 6 weeks of a positive result. There, she should be fully evaluated in terms of any acute management and arrangements made for appropriate postnatal vaccination of the baby. There should also be discussion about testing of other family members.

Notification and contact tracing

Notification of hepatitis B, HIV and syphilis are a legal requirement under the Public Health (Control of Disease) Act and the Public Health (Infectious Diseases) Regulations. Notification is particularly important as it ensures correct contact tracing and treatment of family and close contacts, in accordance with the recommendations of the Joint Committee on Vaccination and Immunisation [55] and the Department of Health [56].

Summary box 17.5

- Women who are HBV surface-antigen positive but e-antigen negative should be offered postnatal vaccination of the baby to prevent vertical transmission.
- Women who are e-antigen positive are offered both vaccination and hepatitis B immunoglobulin.

Human immunodeficiency virus

HIV is a retrovirus that infects and damages T lymphocytes, resulting in immunosuppression and eventually leading to AIDS. Two forms of the virus have been identified, HIV-1 and HIV-2. The commonest and most virulent form is HIV-1, with HIV-2 being relatively uncommon in Western countries. HIV can be transmitted through sexual contact or via contaminated blood, for example needle sharing or vertical transmission from mother to child, which can occur *in utero*, during delivery or through breast-feeding [57].

Vertical transmission is a gobal problem and most HIV-infected children in the UK have acquired the infection from their mothers. Pregnant women should be offered screening for HIV infection at their booking appointment because appropriate antenatal interventions can reduce mother-to-child transmission of HIV infection.

Antiretroviral therapy has been shown to significantly reduce the rate of vertical transmission. Zidovudine chemoprophylaxis given in the prenatal and intrapartum period and to the newborn reduces vertical transmission from 27.7% to 7.9% [58]. However, zidovudine monotherapy is considered inappropriate in mothers with high viral load or low CD4 counts because it fails to suppress viral replication and increases the risk of development of viral resistance [59]. The British HIV Association [57,60] recommend the use of combination antiretroviral therapy in order to achieve prolonged viral suppression when treatment is indicated, with the aim of reducing the viral load to below detectable levels, and recommend that HIV infection in pregnant women should be treated as infection in non-pregnant patients. It is therefore recommended that advanced HIV infection in pregnant women should be treated with combination antiretroviral therapy, which through more complete suppression of viral replication allows greater and prolonged recovery of immune function [61].

Screen-positive result

If there is a primary laboratory screen-positive result, the samples are referred for testing by a specialist laboratory to confirm the reactivity is specific for HIV (involving at least two further independent assays). All women who have confirmed positive test results should be counselled in person and offered specialist counselling and support, which is also available for their partners and family if requested.

Women found to be positive are referred for specialist HIV treatment within a multidisciplinary framework. This would involve advice about management of their infection and interventions to reduce the risk of vertical and sexual transmission, including discussions on the use of antiretrovirals and Caesarean section, early treatment and care for the child, and decisions about breast-feeding. It also provides an opportunity to reinforce health promotion advice and to discuss arrangements for partner notification and testing of previous children [53].

HIV-positive results also need to be accessible to members of staff, at all times, to inform appropriate clinical care particularly in the delivery suite when the woman arrives in labour. It is also important to ensure that a paediatric care plan is determined prior to the birth to ensure the mother understands and has consented to testing and potential treatment regimens after delivery.

Rubella

Rubella acquired in pregnancy, particularly in the first 12 weeks, may result in fetal loss or serious congenital abnormalities. It is therefore essential that all susceptible women in pregnancy are identified and advice given on avoidance of exposure to rubella and offered the first dose of MMR vaccine by the maternity service on the completion of the pregnancy [3].

Established childhood rubella immunization programmes mean that coverage in the UK is generally high and that, for most pregnant women, the detection of rubella-specific IgG implies immunity following immunization or infection before pregnancy. Detection of rubella IgG in women who have recently arrived from countries where rubella is endemic (or where rubella immunization is not available or not effectively implemented) may rarely indicate rubella infection acquired in early pregnancy [62]. However, recent data from Health Protection Agency national surveillance systems in the UK have reported a national increase in the number of women susceptible to rubella [63].

Rubella antibody testing should be offered at least in a first pregnancy irrespective of a single previous report of rubella-specific IgG and immunization history. A history of exposure to, or possible recent infection with, rubella in early pregnancy is actively sought, particularly in recent immigrants, and the laboratory is informed of a suspicious history so that the appropriate tests for primary rubella infection (IgM and IgG avidity) are performed [64]. Testing is considered unnecessary if there is documented evidence of two tests on different blood samples both confirming the presence of rubella-specific IgG [65].

Screen-positive result

Tests such as enzyme-linked immunosorbent assay (ELISA) and radial haemolysis are suitable for rubella antibody screening; latex agglutination is a suitable second-line assay [53].

If a low level (<10 IU/mL) of rubella-specific IgG is detected yet the woman has received two or more documented doses of rubella vaccine, further doses of vaccine are unlikely to be of value and protection against rubella is assumed. Such women are advised to report any rash, illness or contact with a rubella-like rash for further investigation.

Screening results are reported as rubella-specific IgG detected/not detected rather than immune/susceptible. The laboratory advises on any further follow-up required (e.g. 'immunization advised, postpartum if pregnant' for results reported as rubella-specific IgG not detected). As detection of rubella-specific IgG does not exclude the possibility of recent infection, evidence of rash in early pregnancy is sought and communicated to the laboratory to allow interpretation of results [64]. Immunization of pregnant women is avoided where feasible [53].

Syphilis

Syphilis is an infectious disease caused by *Treponema pallidum*. It is transmitted primarily through sexual contact but can be transmitted from mother to baby during pregnancy. Acquired and congenital syphilis infection is staged according to the time from acquisition of the primary infection. The risk of transmission from mother to baby declines as maternal syphilis infection progresses. Risk ranges from 70 to 100% in primary syphilis, 40% in early latent syphilis and 10% in late latent syphilis. Maternal syphilis infection can result in a range of adverse pregnancy and neonatal outcomes, including late miscarriage, stillbirth, hydrops and low birthweight [54].

The aim of antenatal screening for syphilis is to detect pregnant women with congenitally transmissible syphilis so that they can be treated with antibiotics to prevent transmission of infection. This can significantly reduce the risk of congenital syphilis, stillbirths, premature births, neonatal deaths, and severe illness in infancy and beyond. The pregnant woman can also be treated to prevent progression of disease, as well as giving the opportunity of treatment for their sexual partners [66].

Despite its low prevalence in the UK, economic analyses carried out in Norway, England and Thailand have consistently found that the benefits of antenatal syphilis screening outweigh its costs, even where the prevalence of maternal infection is as low as 1–11 per 100 000 [67,68].

Screen-positive result

The false-negative rate of single blood samples tested for syphilis serology will depend on the stage of infection. In primary syphilis it may be up to 20–30% and a high index of clinical suspicion is therefore critical when there is a significant risk of primary infection. However, later in infectious syphilis (i.e. in secondary and early latent infection) the false-negative rate should effectively be below 0.1% (sensitivity of 99.9%) [69].

A screen-positive test is then followed by confirmation of the reactive result by a second test employing independent methodology. The false reactivity rate of single blood samples tested in this way should effectively be zero (specificity of 100%) [69]. Once a screen-positive result is confirmed, the woman and her family should be referred to a specialist in genitourinary medicine for assessment, counselling and possible treatment [53].

Group B streptococcus

Group B streptococcus (*Streptococcus agalactiae*) is a major cause of early-onset infection in newborn infants. Although screening is offered routinely in North America [70], there is still controversy about its benefits. The incidence of early-onset group B streptococcal disease in the UK in the absence of systematic screening or widespread intrapartum antibiotic prophylaxis is 0.5 per 1000 births, which is similar to that seen in the USA after universal screening and intrapartum antibiotic prophylaxis, despite comparable vaginal carriage rates [71].

There have been no randomizsed controlled trials (RCTs) on antenatal screening or comparing the different screening strategies. Estimates of the efficacy of the screening strategies are based on observational studies. Therefore, currently the RCOG have produced guidance suggesting that pregnant women should not be offered routine antenatal screening for group B streptococcus because evidence of its clinical and cost effectiveness remains uncertain [71].

Hepatitis C virus

Pregnant women should not be offered routine screening for hepatitis C virus because there is insufficient evidence to support its clinical and cost effectiveness.

Toxoplasmosis

Routine antenatal serological screening for toxoplasmosis should not be offered because the risks of screening may outweigh the potential benefits. Pregnant women should be informed of primary prevention measures to avoid toxoplasmosis infection, such as:
- washing hands before handling food;
- thoroughly washing all fruit and vegetables, including ready-prepared salads, before eating;
- thoroughly cooking raw meats and ready-prepared chilled meals;
- wearing gloves and thoroughly washing hands after handling soil and gardening;
- avoiding cat faeces in cat litter or in soil.

Conclusions

Antenatal screening is the testing of apparently healthy pregnant women to identify undiagnosed diseases or pregnancies at high risk of developing a disease. There are clear economic arguments in favour of some forms of antenatal screening, such as that for Down's syndrome, structural anomalies, blood group antibodies, certain infections and haemoglobinopathies. However, population screening for other conditions such as group B streptococcal infection do not have the same economic, epidemiological or clinical values. Nevertheless, there are continuous advances in current screening techniques that will alter the detection rate and false-positive rates, warranting a change in the risk cut-off levels as in the case of Down's syndrome screening. More significantly, there are recent advances in techniques such as non-invasive fetal genotyping and aneuploidy screening using CFF DNA in maternal sera, which may allow more accurate and safer screening programmes in the future.

It is important to remember that screening programmes have the potential for harm as well as good. Therefore, it is essential that clear and comprehensive information is available to the parents as early as possible in pregnancy to allow them to make an informed decision on undertaking the screening test and the implications of a screen-positive or screen-negative result.

References

1 National Screening Committee. Definition of screening. Available at: www.screening.nhs.uk/screening.

2 Wilson JM, Jungner YG. [Principles and practice of mass screening for disease.] *Bol Oficina Sanit Panam* 1968;65:281–393.

3 National Institute for Health and Clinical Excellence. *Antenatal Care: Routine Care for the Healthy Pregnant Women*. Clinical Guideline 62, 2008. Available at: http://guidance.nice.org.uk/CG62.

4 Department of Health. *Model of Best Practice for Providing Down's Syndrome Screening*, 2003. Available at: www.dh.gov.uk/publications.

5 Wald NJ, Rodeck C, Hackshaw AK, Walters J, Chitty L, Mackinson AM. First and second trimester antenatal screening for Down's syndrome: the results of the Serum, Urine and Ultrasound Screening Study (SURUSS). *Health Technol Assess* 2003;7(11):1–77.

6 Department of Health. *Fetal Anomaly Screening Programme. Screening for Down's Syndrome: UK NSC Policy Recommendations 2007–2010: Model of Best Practice*. Available at: www.dh.gov.uk/prod_consum_dh/groups/dh_digitalassets/@dh/@en/documents/digitalasset/dh_084731.pdf

7 NHS Fetal Anomaly Screening Programme. Review of the Model of Best Practice 2008: Down's syndrome screening for England. Gateway reference 9674. Available at: www.screening.nhs.uk.

8 Spencer K, Kagan KO, Nicolaides KH. Screening for trisomy 21 in twin pregnancies in the first trimester: an update of the impact of chorionicity on maternal serum markers. *Prenat Diagn* 2008;28:49–52.

9 Spencer K, Nicolaides KH. Screening for trisomy 21 in twins using first trimester ultrasound and maternal serum biochemistry in a one-stop clinic: a review of three years experience. *BJOG* 2003;110:276–280.

10 Tabor A, Philip J, Madsen M, Bang J, Obel EB, Norgaard-Pedersen B. Randomised controlled trial of genetic amniocentesis in 4606 low-risk women. *Lancet* 1986;i:1287–1293.

11 Verma L, Macdonald F, Leedham P, McConachie M, Dhanjal S, Hulten M. Rapid and simple prenatal DNA diagnosis of Down's syndrome. *Lancet* 1998;352:9–12.

12 Froster UG, Jackson L. Limb defects and chorionic villus sampling: results from an international registry, 1992–94. *Lancet* 1996;347:489–494.

13 Cheung MC, Goldberg JD, Kan YW. Prenatal diagnosis of sickle cell anaemia and thalassaemia by analysis of fetal cells in maternal blood. *Nat Genet* 1996;14:264–268.

14 Bianchi DW, Simpson JL, Jackson LG *et al.* Fetal gender and aneuploidy detection using fetal cells in maternal blood: analysis of NIFTY I data. National Institute of Child Health and

Development Fetal Cell Isolation Study. *Prenat Diagn* 2002;22: 609–615.

15 Lo YM, Corbetta N, Chamberlain PF *et al.* Presence of fetal DNA in maternal plasma and serum. *Lancet* 1997;350:485–487.

16 Lun FM, Chiu RW, len Chan KC, Yeung LT, Kin LT, nis Lo YM. Microfluidics digital PCR reveals a higher than expected fraction of fetal DNA in maternal plasma. *Clin Chem* 2008;54: 1664–1672.

17 Lo YM, Tein MS, Lau TK *et al.* Quantitative analysis of fetal DNA in maternal plasma and serum: implications for noninvasive prenatal diagnosis. *Am J Hum Genet* 1998;62:768–775.

18 Galbiati S, Smid M, Gambini D *et al.* Fetal DNA detection in maternal plasma throughout gestation. *Hum Genet* 2005;117: 243–248.

19 Lo YM, Zhang J, Leung TN, Lau TK, Chang AM, Hjelm NM. Rapid clearance of fetal DNA from maternal plasma. *Am J Hum Genet* 1999;64:218–224.

20 Alberry M, Maddocks D, Jones M *et al.* Free fetal DNA in maternal plasma in anembryonic pregnancies: confirmation that the origin is the trophoblast. *Prenat Diagn* 2007;27:415–418.

21 Chan KC, Zhang J, Hui AB *et al.* Size distributions of maternal and fetal DNA in maternal plasma. *Clin Chem* 2004;50:88–92.

22 Poon LL, Leung TN, Lau TK, Lo YM. Presence of fetal RNA in maternal plasma. *Clin Chem* 2000;46:1832–1834.

23 Rijnders RJ, van der Schoot CE, Bossers B, de Vroede MA, Christiaens GC. Fetal sex determination from maternal plasma in pregnancies at risk for congenital adrenal hyperplasia. *Obstet Gynecol* 2001;98:374–378.

24 Wright CF, Chitty LS. Cell-free fetal DNA and RNA in maternal blood: implications for safer antenatal testing. *BMJ* 2009;339: b2451.

25 van der Schoot CE, Hahn S, Chitty LS. Non-invasive prenatal diagnosis and determination of fetal Rh status. *Semin Fetal Neonatal Med* 2008;13:63–68.

26 Chiu RW, Akolekar R, Zheng YW *et al.* Non-invasive prenatal assessment of trisomy 21 by multiplexed maternal plasma DNA sequencing: large scale validity study. *BMJ* 2011;342:c7401.

27 Bricker L, Garcia J, Henderson J *et al.* Ultrasound screening in pregnancy: a systematic review of the clinical effectiveness, cost-effectiveness and women's views. *Health Technol Assess* 2000; 4(16):i–193.

28 Chitty LS, Hunt GH, Moore J, Lobb MO. Effectiveness of routine ultrasonography in detecting fetal structural abnormalities in a low risk population. *BMJ* 1991;303:1165–1169.

29 Boyd PA, Chamberlain P, Hicks NR. 6-year experience of prenatal diagnosis in an unselected population in Oxford, UK. *Lancet* 1998;352:1577–1581.

30 NHS Fetal Anomaly Screening Programme. *18+0 to 20+6 Weeks Fetal Anomaly Scan: National Standards and Guidance for England.* Royal College of Obstetricians and Gynaecologists, 2010. Available at: http://fetalanomaly.screening.nhs.uk/getdata.php?id=11218

31 Wimalasundera RC, Gardiner HM. Congenital heart disease and aneuploidy. *Prenat Diagn* 2004;24:1116–1122.

32 Smith-Bindman R, Hosmer W, Feldstein VA, Deeks JJ, Goldberg JD. Second-trimester ultrasound to detect fetuses with Down syndrome: a meta-analysis. *JAMA* 2001;285:1044–1055.

33 Royal College of Obstetricians and Gynaecologists. *Termination of Pregnancy for Fetal Abnormality in England, Wales and Scotland.*

May 2010. Available at: www.rcog.org.uk/files/rcog-corp/TerminationPregnancyReport18May2010.pdf

34 Davies SC, Cronin E, Gill M, Greengross P, Hickman M, Normand C. Screening for sickle cell disease and thalassaemia: a systematic review with supplementary research. *Health Technol Assess* 2000;4(3):i–99.

35 Zeuner D, Ades AE, Karnon J, Brown J, Dezateux C, Anionwu EN. Antenatal and neonatal haemoglobinopathy screening in the UK: review and economic analysis. *Health Technol Assess* 1999;3(11):i–186.

36 NHS Sickle Cell and Thalassaemia Screening Programme. *Standards for the Linked Antenatal and Newborn Screening Programme.* Available at: http://sct.screening.nhs.uk/cms.php?folder=2493.

37 Streetly A, Claske M, Downing M *et al.* Implementation of the newborn screening programme for sickle cell disease in England: results for 2003–2005. *J Med Screen* 2008;15:9–13.

38 Dyson SM, Culley L, Gill C *et al.* Ethnicity questions and antenatal screening for sickle cell/thalassaemia (EQUANS) in England: a randomised controlled trial of two questionnaires. *Ethn Health* 2006;11:169–189.

39 Family Origin Questionnaire. Available at: http://sct.screening.nhs.uk/cms.php?folder=2506.

40 Anglin A, Gill C, Latinovic R, Henthorn J, Streetly A. *Review of Antenatal Screening Implementation in Low Prevalence Trusts.* Available at: http://sct.screening.nhs.uk/getdata.php?id=11051

41 Hartwell SK, Srisawang B, Kongtawelert P, Christian GD, Grudpan K. Review on screening and analysis techniques for haemoglobin variants and thalassemia. *Talanta* 2005;65: 1149–1161.

42 Clarke GM, Higgins TN. Laboratory investigation of hemoglobinopathies and thalassemias: review and update. *Clin Chem* 2000;46:1284–1290.

43 Little RR, Roberts WL. A review of variant hemoglobins interfering with hemoglobin A1c measurement. *J Diabetes Sci Technol* 2009;3:446–451.

44 Colah RB, Surve R, Sawant P *et al.* HPLC studies in hemoglobinopathies. *Indian J Pediatr* 2007;74:657–662.

45 Ballas SK, Clark MR, Mohandas N *et al.* Red cell membrane and cation deficiency in Rh null syndrome 7. *Blood* 1984;63: 1046–1055.

46 Freda VJ, Gorman JG, Pollack W. Rh factor: prevention of isoimmunization and clinical trial on mothers. *Science* 1966;151: 828–830.

47 UK Blood Transfusion and Tissue Transplantation Service. *Guidelines for the Blood Transfusion Services in the UK*, 7th edn. Available at: www.transfusionguidelines.org.uk/index.aspx?Publication=RB&Section=25

48 National Institute for Health and Clinical Excellence. *Pregnancy (Rhesus Negative Women): Routine Anti-D (Review).* Technology Appraisal 156. Available at: http://guidance.nice.org.uk/TA156

49 Lo YM, Bowell PJ, Selinger M *et al.* Prenatal determination of fetal rhesus D status by DNA amplification of peripheral blood of rhesus-negative mothers. *Ann NY Acad Sci* 1994;731: 229–236.

50 Mari G, Deter RL, Carpenter RL *et al.* Noninvasive diagnosis by Doppler ultrasonography of fetal anaemia due to maternal red-cell alloimmunization. Collaborative Group for Doppler

Assessment of the Blood Velocity in Anaemic Fetuses. *N Engl J Med* 2000;342:9–14.

51 van Kamp IL, Klumper FJ, Meerman RH, Oepkes D, Scherjon SA, Kanhai HH. Treatment of fetal anemia due to red-cell alloimmunization with intrauterine transfusions in the Netherlands, 1988–1999. *Acta Obstet Gynecol Scand* 2004;83: 731–737.

52 Permalloo N, Chapple J. NHS antenatal and newborn screening programmes London region report 2009–2010. Available at: www.screening.nhs.uk/getdata.php?id=10098.

53 Department of Health. *Screening for Infectious Diseases in Pregnancy. Standards to Support the UK Antenatal Screening Programme*. Available at: www.dh.gov.uk/assetRoot/04/06/61/91/04066191.pdf.

54 National Screening Committee. *Infectious Diseases in Pregnancy Screening Programme. Programme Standards*. Available at: http://infectiousdiseases.screening.nhs.uk/getdata.php?id=10640

55 Department of Health. Joint Committee on Vaccination and Immunisation. Available at: www.dh.gov.uk/ab/JCVI/index.htm?ssSourceSiteId=en.

56 Department of Health. *Immunisation Against Infectious Disease: The 'Green Book'*. Available at: www.dh.gov.uk/en/Publicationsandstatistics/Publications/PublicationsPolicyAndGuidance/DH_079917

57 de Ruiter A., Mercey D, Anderson J *et al*. British HIV Association and Children's HIV Association guidelines for the management of HIV infection in pregnant women 2008. *HIV Med* 2008; 9:452–502.

58 Connor EM, Sperling RS, Gelber R *et al*. Reduction of maternal–infant transmission of human immunodeficiency virus type 1 with zidovudine treatment. Pediatric AIDS Clinical Trials Group Protocol 076 Study Group. *N Engl J Med* 1994;331: 1173–1180.

59 Carpenter CC, Fischl MA, Hammer SM *et al*. Antiretroviral therapy for HIV infection in 1998: updated recommendations of the International AIDS Society-USA Panel. *JAMA* 1998;280: 78–86.

60 Taylor GP, Lyall EG, Mercey D *et al*. British HIV Association guidelines for prescribing antiretroviral therapy in pregnancy (1998). *Sex Transm Infect* 1999;75:90–97.

61 Lyall EG, Blott M, de Ruiter A *et al*. Guidelines for the management of HIV infection in pregnant women and the prevention of mother-to-child transmission. *HIV Med* 2001;2:314–334.

62 Tookey PA, Cortina-Borja M, Peckham CS. Rubella susceptibility among pregnant women in North London, 1996–1999. *J Public Health Med* 2002;24:211–216.

63 Health Protection Agency and UK National Screening Committee. Infectious Diseases in Pregnancy Screening Programme: 2005–2007 data. Available at: http://infectiousdiseases.screening.nhs.uk/publications.

64 Mehta NM, Thomas RM. Antenatal screening for rubella: infection or immunity? *BMJ* 2002;325:90–91.

65 Morgan-Capner P, Crowcroft NS. Guidelines on the management of, and exposure to, rash illness in pregnancy (including consideration of relevant antibody screening programmes in pregnancy). *Commun Dis Public Health* 2002;5:59–71.

66 Greenwood AM, D'Alessandro U, Sisay F, Greenwood BM. Treponemal infection and the outcome of pregnancy in a rural area of The Gambia, west Africa. *J Infect Dis* 1992;166:842–846.

67 Williams K. Screening for syphilis in pregnancy: an assessment of the costs and benefits. *Community Med* 1985;7:37–42.

68 Connor N, Roberts J, Nicoll A. Strategic options for antenatal screening for syphilis in the United Kingdom: a cost effectiveness analysis. *J Med Screen* 2000;7:7–13.

69 Egglestone S, Turner AJ. The PHLS Syphilis Serology Working Group. Serological diagnosis of syphilis. *Commun Dis Public Health* 2000;3:158–162.

70 Centers for Disease Control and Prevention. Prevention of perinatal group B streptococcal disease: a public health perspective. *MMWR* 1996;45:1–24.

71 Royal College of Obstetricians and Gynaecologists. *Prevention of Early-onset Neonatal Group B Streptococcal Disease*. Green-top Guideline No. 36, 2003. Available at: www.rcog.org.uk/files/rcog-corp/uploaded-files/GT36GroupBStrep2003.pdf

Chapter 18
Disorders of Fetal Growth and Assessment of Fetal Well-being

Gordon C.S. Smith and Christoph C. Lees
The Rosie Hospital, Cambridge, UK

Defining disorders of growth requires relating a given achieved growth to an expected growth. In the case of fetal growth, three further levels of complexity arise. First, growth is determined in part by gestational age and an apparent growth disorder may reflect inaccurate assessment of gestational age. Second, even if gestational age is known accurately, the size of the fetus can only be assessed indirectly by ultrasound. Third, even accepting these limitations, fetal measurements are typically related to a population-based norm. Deviation from normal may arise from parental determinants of growth, such as race and stature. The primary interest in assessing fetal growth is to avoid the complications associated with a fetus that is poorly grown due to uteroplacental insufficiency. The most important consequence of fetal compromise is perinatal death, principally antepartum stillbirth.

Endocrine regulation of fetal growth

Fetal growth is critically regulated by the insulin-like growth factors (IGFs). There are two IGFs, numbered I and II. There are two main receptors for the IGFs, numbered 1 and 2. The type 1 IGF receptor mediates most of the major biological effects of IGF-I and IGF-II and it binds the two growth factors with similar affinity. The type 2 IGF receptor appears to be mainly involved in clearance of IGF-II. Mice lacking IGF-I, IGF-II or the type 1 IGF receptor are growth restricted at birth. Mice lacking the type 2 receptor are large at birth. Following birth, IGF levels are stimulated by growth hormone (GH). However, in fetal life, levels of the IGFs appear largely independent of GH and are stimulated by human placental lactogen. The effects of IGFs are influenced by six distinct IGF-binding proteins (IGFBP). Binding of IGF to an IGFBP may decrease or enhance its physiological effect. A number of IGFBP proteases exist, such as pregnancy-associated plasma protein A (PAPP-A), a protease for IGFBP-4 and IGFBP-5. Many associations have been described between cord blood, amniotic fluid and maternal serum levels of components of the IGF system and fetal growth.

Placental regulation of fetal growth

The placenta is clearly crucial for fetal growth as it provides all the substrates for fetal growth and performs gaseous exchange in fetal life. Some of the associations between IGF system proteins and eventual birthweight involve placentally derived components, such as PAPP-A, as IGFs are also important in controlling placentation. A number of tests of placental function demonstrate associations with eventual fetal growth (see below). A view emerged that many complications of pregnancy associated with poor placental function may be due to failure of the so-called 'second wave' of trophoblast invasion in the second trimester. However, more recent studies have suggested that trophoblast invasion takes place as a continuous process during the first half of pregnancy. The process of implantation and early placentation may be crucial in determining fetal growth disorder and there are associations between both the size of the fetus in the first trimester of pregnancy and maternal levels of PAPP-A and the eventual birthweight of the baby (Fig. 18.1).

Genomic imprinting and fetal growth

Key genes of the IGF system are imprinted. Genomic imprinting is the selective inactivation of a gene in the conceptus in relation to whether it is the maternal or paternal copy. This is an epigenetic process, i.e. it is an inheritable alteration in gene expression that is not due to

Dewhurst's Textbook of Obstetrics & Gynaecology, Eighth Edition. Edited by D. Keith Edmonds.
© 2012 John Wiley and Sons, Ltd. Published 2012 by John Wiley and Sons, Ltd.

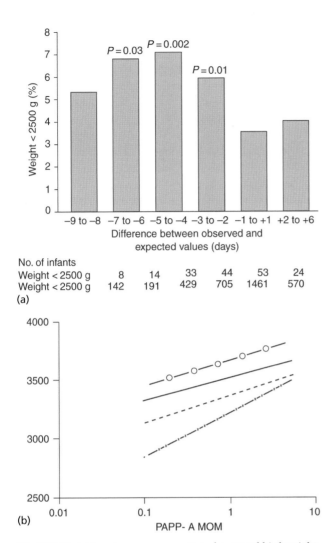

No. of infants						
Weight < 2500 g	8	14	33	44	53	24
Weight < 2500 g	142	191	429	705	1461	570

Fig. 18.1 First-trimester measurements and eventual birthweight. (a) Relationship between observed and expected crown–rump length and the incidence of low birthweight. (b) Relationship between first-trimester levels of PAPP-A and eventual birthweight at term. Red line, 41 weeks; black line, 40 weeks; blue line, 39 weeks; green line, 38 weeks.

a change in DNA sequence. Genomic imprinting is primarily a feature of placental mammals and is thought to be important in controlling the conflict of the paternal interest in fathering large offspring and the maternal interest of dividing resources equally among all her offspring. Imprinted genes may act in balancing these conflicting interests at all stages of development. In fetal life, this is primarily manifested in the control of fetal growth. The key role of the placental IGF system is underlined by the fact that IGF-II, a stimulator of placental invasion, is paternally imprinted and the type 2 IGF receptor, which degrades IGF-II, is maternally imprinted. The importance of imprinting in the regulation of human fetal growth is illustrated by a number of genetic conditions that are

manifestations of aberrant expression of imprinted genes. These can result in fetal overgrowth (e.g. Beckwith–Wiedemann syndrome) or intrauterine growth restriction (e.g. Silver–Russell syndrome).

Definition of fetal growth disorder

Fetal growth disorder is strictly defined as the failure of a fetus to grow according to its genetic potential. In practice this is never known and fetal growth is defined on the basis of the expected dimensions of the infant in relation to its gestational age. At birth, these measurements can be made directly. In fetal life, ultrasound is employed (see below). Defining whether a given value of a continuous variable is normal, whether weight or an ultrasonic measurement, involves identifying a value which is thought to be the limit of the normal range. Often, measurements which are within two standard deviations of the mean are regarded as normal: this includes approximately 95% of the population. It follows that approximately 2.5% of the population will be regarded as small and 2.5% large, assuming a normal distribution. In practice, due to error in estimating gestational age, inaccuracy in weight estimation and variation in true genetic potential, there will be no cut-off that correctly separates normal and abnormal. In practice, if the threshold is set at an extreme low value, most of the fetuses less than that level will be growth restricted. As the threshold increases, the proportion which are truly growth restricted will decrease. The converse follows for identifying large infants. In practice, three percentile thresholds are commonly employed: less than the 3rd, less than the 5th, and less than the 10th percentile and the equivalent upper limits used for large infants. Fetuses outside the given threshold are called small for gestational age (SGA) or large for gestational age (LGA), as appropriate, and those within the range are called appropriate for gestational age (AGA). The terms SGA and intrauterine growth restriction (IUGR) are often used interchangeably although they are clearly not synonymous.

Epidemiology of fetal growth disorder

The epidemiological associations with delivering an SGA infant are shown in Table 18.1. These can be classified as primarily genetic, primarily environmental or mixed genetic and environmental, although clearly the distinctions are not absolute. Similar factors will be involved in determining a large fetus, although the associations will clearly be reversed. Fetal growth may also be affected by pathological processes. These in turn can be classified as maternal disease, abnormalities of the placenta and fetal disease. Maternal cardiovascular and connective tissue

Table 18.1 Epidemiological associations with intrauterine growth restriction.

Risk factor	Risk
Previous affected pregnancy	About 20% recurrence risk, depending on persistence of risk factors
Smoking	Reduction in average birthweight of 458 g in smokers of 20 cigarettes/day
	Odds ratio (OR) 2.28 (2.29–2.76) for SGA
Alcohol	At <1 unit/day, OR 1.1 (95% CI 1.00–1.13) for SGA
	1–2 units a day, OR 1.62 (1.26–2.09)
	3–5 units a day, OR 1.96 (1.16–3.31)
Caffeine	No significant effect on risk of 10th centile birthweight when smoking controlled for
Diabetes	20% incidence in women with tight control vs. 10% in less-tight control for birthweight <10th centile
Hypertension	Risk of SGA (in mild chronic hypertension) from 8.0 to 15.5% depending on series
Renal disease	Incidence of SGA ~23% with chronic proteinuria during pregnancy
	37% risk of SGA with moderate to severe renal insufficiency
Bowel disease	OR 2.4 (1.6–3.7) of low birthweight in Crohn's disease
	No evidence of increased risk of IUGR in ulcerative colitis
	OR 3.4 (95% CI 1.6–7.2) of 'IUGR' in untreated coeliac disease
Cardiac disease	No increase in risk of SGA (<10th centile)
Thrombophilia	Factor V Leiden heterozygote: pooled OR 0.8 (0.3, 2.3)
	Prothrombin gene G20210A heterozygote: pooled OR 5.7 (1.2, 27.4)
	MTFHR heterozygote: pooled OR 5 (1.8, 13.8)
	Protein S deficiency: pooled OR 10.2 (1.1–91.0)
	Anticardiolipin antibodies: OR 33.9 (1.6–735.8)
Assisted conception	Relationship between IVF pregnancy and IUGR remains controversial but OR for SGA (<10th centile) of 1.6 (95% CI 1.3–2.0) in recent meta-analysis
Systemic lupus erythematosus	28.5% incidence of IUGR in pregnancies with active lupus, but only 7.6% in inactive lupus patients
Maternal age	No evidence of increased risk of low maternal age, but OR of 1.28 of <5th centile birth weight for >35 years and 1.49 >40 years
Weight/BMI	No evidence of increased risk of SGA with maternal obesity
	BMI <20 OR 1.37 (1.29–1.45) for birthweight <5th centile
Low socioeconomic status	OR 2.91 (95% CI 2.14–7.51) for IUGR

BMI, body mass index; CI, confidence interval; IUGR, intrauterine growth restriction; IVF, *in vitro* fertilization; MTFHR, methylene tetrahydrofolate reductase; SGA, small for gestational age.

disease are particularly associated with poor growth. Conversely, maternal diabetes and obesity are common causes of a large infant. Placental causes of growth restriction include confined placental mosaicism but more commonly poor growth is associated with biochemical and ultrasonic tests that suggest poor placental function but which do not establish the cause of the dysfunction. Intrinsic fetal causes of poor growth include chromosomal abnormalities (in particular aneuploidy), nonchromosomal syndromes (such as Cornelia de Lange syndrome) and congenital infection. Careful elucidation of history, structural and Doppler assessment of the placenta and fetus and other appropriate investigations will help clarify whether a growth abnormality is pathological.

Physiological fetal response to adverse intrauterine environment

In cases where a fetus is poorly grown due to an adverse intrauterine environment, it adapts in order to survive the challenge. The primary purpose of these adaptations is to maintain oxygen supply to the key organs, namely the brain, heart and adrenal. These reflexes are stimulated by the peripheral arterial chemoreceptors. Unlike the child or adult, chemoreceptor stimulation inhibits breathing movements in the fetus. These adaptive responses underlie many of the biophysical assessments of fetal wellbeing. The responses and the biophysical measurements are listed in Table 18.2.

Consequences of fetal growth disorder

The most common single cause of perinatal death is unexplained antepartum stillbirth. Analysis of these events suggests that poor fetal growth is the major single determinant of these deaths. Moreover, antepartum stillbirth of structurally normal fetuses is also associated with abruption and pre-eclampsia. Both of these outcomes are associated with IUGR. Poor growth is also associated with perinatal death due to prematurity. It has been

Table 18.2 Physiological basis for biophysical assessment of the poorly grown fetus.

Organ	Normal state	Association with adverse environment	Biophysical measurement
Fetal placenta	Low-resistance circulation	Poor placental development results in high resistance	Doppler velocimetry of umbilical arteries demonstrates increased resistance
Fetal body	Moderately high-resistance circulation	Peripheral arterial chemoreceptors stimulate vasoconstriction in non-vital organs	Doppler velocimetry of descending aorta demonstrates high resistance. The descending aorta also supplies the umbilical arteries and increased resistance in the fetal side of the placenta also contributes
Maternal placenta	Low-resistance circulation	Poor placental development results in high resistance	Doppler velocimetry of the uterine artery demonstrates high-resistance flow and notching: predictive of IUGR, abruption and stillbirth
Cerebrovascular circulation	High resistance	Peripheral arterial chemoreceptors stimulate vasodilation to maintain brain oxygen supply	Doppler velocimetry of middle cerebral artery demonstrates reduced resistance
Kidney	Adequate blood flow and urine output	Increased vasopressin and reduced blood flow reduces urine output	Decreased liquor volume
Thorax	Breathing movements prepare for birth	Peripheral arterial chemoreceptors inhibit breathing movements	Decreased fetal breathing movements
Heart	Low central venous pressure	Central venous pressure rises as heart fails when fetus fails to compensate for adverse intrauterine environment	High-resistance flow in the ductus venosus, absent or reversed flow during atrial systole, pulsatile flow in umbilical vein
Central nervous system	Stimulation of fetal movement in cycles of activity	Fetal movements inhibited to reduce oxygen consumption by non-vital organs	Decreased or absent fetal movements

shown that growth restriction in early pregnancy is associated with an increased risk of spontaneous preterm birth. Labour appears to be initiated by activation of the fetal hypothalamic–pituitary–adrenal axis. In sheep, the effector hormone from the adrenal is cortisol, whereas in primates and – it is assumed – in the human it is likely to be androgenic precursors of oestrogen. The effect in both species is stimulation of labour. Therefore, spontaneous preterm delivery may be a physiologically indicated response to a poor environment. Poor growth is also directly related to prematurity in the context of elective delivery for suspected fetal compromise. Poor fetal growth is also associated with increased morbidity and mortality in infancy. For example, the risk of sudden infant death syndrome varies inversely with the birthweight percentile (Fig. 18.2). It is thought that the susceptibility of the adult to a range of diseases may also be affected by IUGR (the Barker hypothesis). The basis for this is associations between birthweight and birth proportions and the rates of disease in later life. These associations are not particularly strong, however, with a relative risk of death from ischaemic heart disease

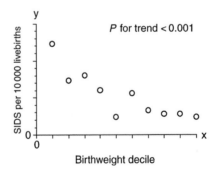

Fig. 18.2 Association between birthweight percentile and the risk of sudden infant death syndrome.

(IHD) of approximately 1.7 across the range of birthweights. Interestingly, the mother who delivers a low birthweight infant has a much higher relative risk of IHD, suggesting a genetic component. Nevertheless, animal models appear to confirm associations between intrauterine stress and later cardiovascular and metabolic function.

Investigation and management of fetal growth disorder

The challenge of perinatal care is to distinguish those fetuses that are small but healthy ('constitutionally small') from those with pathologically reduced growth. In practice, fetal growth disorders are rare as an isolated finding before 24 weeks and routine assessment of fetal growth is therefore normally performed only after 24 weeks. While fetal size may be assessed both clinically and by ultrasound, fetal growth may only be ascertained by serial assessments.

The concept of symmetric and asymmetric IUGR has been taken to describe early-onset (chromosomal/genetic) and later-onset (uteroplacental) IUGR respectively. Thus poor fetal growth before 24 weeks is more commonly associated with genetic and chromosomal abnormalities or fetal infection, whereas after 24 weeks fetal growth is determined to a far greater extent by maternal influences and uteroplacental function. As ultrasound techniques have advanced, it has become clear that the symmetric/asymmetric IUGR dichotomy is somewhat of an oversimplification. The growth restriction thought to be inherent to chromosomal and genetic conditions may in fact be mediated by uteroplacental insufficiency; hence severely growth restricted trisomy 18 babies in the third trimester frequently exhibit asymmetrical growth restriction with abnormal uteroplacental and fetal Doppler. Conversely, ultrasound assessment of fetuses with severe early-onset uteroplacental insufficiency often reveals symmetrically reduced abdominal and head measurements.

Prediction of fetal growth restriction

The epidemiological factors described above might be used to identify fetuses that are likely to have growth abnormalities allowing an increased level of surveillance. However, although many statistical associations are described, few of these are particularly strong. Therefore, although a study may show that a woman with a body mass index of 17 has an increased risk of delivering an SGA infant, the majority of these women would deliver an AGA infant. Most adverse pregnancy outcomes occur to women with no identified risk factors. These statements can be expressed in terms of screening: maternal history has low sensitivity and low positive predictive value in detecting fetal growth disorder. Biochemical prediction of IUGR has been investigated primarily using analytes measured in the first or second trimesters in the context of Down's syndrome screening programmes. While low first-trimester PAPP-A levels are associated with low birthweight, studies of first and second trimester α-fetoprotein, human chorionic gonadotrophin and inhibin-A have shown a less consistent picture. None of these biochemical analytes has sufficient predictive value to be useful in a clinical context.

Uterine artery Doppler allows indirect assessment of downstream resistance in the arteries, arterioles and capillaries of the maternal side of the placenta. It is a quick, simple and non-invasive technique that involves the placement, using colour Doppler ultrasound, of a sample gate over the uterine artery just distal to its origin from the internal iliac artery. Pulsed wave Doppler is then applied, and a flow–velocity waveform is obtained from which resistance indices such as resistance index, pulsatility index (PI) and A/B or S/D ratios can be derived. Low-resistance waveforms indicate good trophoblast invasion to the spiral arterioles (Plate 18.1a), whereas high-resistance waveforms (characterized by low levels of end-diastolic flow and notches) indicate abnormal placentation (Plate 18.1b). The higher the uterine artery PI, the higher the risk of severe adverse outcome due to abnormal placentation (Fig. 18.3). Large studies with good reproducibility reported in the last decade have suggested its potential utility as a screening tool in predicting both pre-eclampsia and fetal growth restriction.

Although the sensitivity of uterine Doppler is poor for growth restriction at any gestation, it is good for severe and early-onset forms, particularly if performed at 22–24 weeks. For example, its sensitivity in predicting IUGR below the 10th centile requiring delivery before 34 weeks is around 80%, for a 5% screen-positive rate in an unselected population. However, it is less reliable at predicting IUGR in twins and if performed earlier in gestation. It has not become a feature of routine antenatal care as

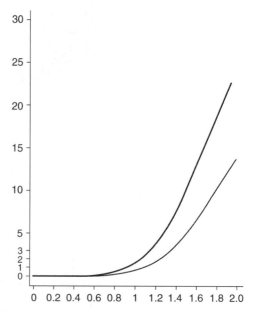

Fig. 18.3 Likelihood ratio for severe adverse outcome (vertical axis) relating to mean pulsatility index (horizontal axis). Smokers are represented by a thick black line (left), non-smokers by a thin line.

controversy still exists over its utility in screening low-risk populations, although concerns over reproducibility have now been largely overcome.

First-trimester screening models incorporating uterine artery impedance, maternal history and maternal serum measurements of, for example, PAPP-A generally do not perform as well as 22–24 week uterine artery Doppler in screening for SGA or growth restriction, having a relatively high false-positive rate. The models do tend to be more effective for pre-eclampsia screening, and for SGA with pre-eclampsia, than for SGA/IUGR alone. The prospect of enhancing these risk prediction models with assessment of maternal cardiac and vascular function in the first trimester is alluring, though the techniques presently are time-intensive and relatively poorly reproducible, rendering them not useful in population screening.

Clinical assessment of fetal growth

Clinical examination is most commonly by symphysis–fundal height (SFH) measurement. SFH assessment has traditionally been performed from 24 weeks' gestation onwards by measuring the distance from the mother's pubic symphysis to the uterine fundus, and successive measurements recorded in the woman's notes or on a chart. The SFH measurement after 24 weeks has been taken to be equal in centimetres to the week of gestation, ±2 cm to 36 weeks and ±3 cm from 36–42 weeks. The problems associated with SFH measurement are poor intra- and inter-observer reproducibility and those inherent to the technique. As it relies on assessment of the height of the uterine fundus as a proxy measure of fetal growth, it can therefore take no account of confounding maternal factors such as height, weight and physical build, and uterine/fetal factors such as fibroids, polyhydramnios or oligohydramnios, multiple pregnancy and fetal lie. Two large retrospective studies in the 1980s suggested that reduced SFH measurements correctly identified only 25–50% of fetuses whose birthweight was below the 10th centile.

One approach to improving the predictive ability of SFH measurement for SGA infants has been to adjust the measurement for maternal characteristics, such as maternal height, weight, parity and ethnicity. A non-randomized controlled trial of customised SFH measurement demonstrated increased antenatal detection of SGA infants (48% with customized SFH vs. 29% with standard measurements). However, no differences in clinical outcome were apparent between the two groups. Customization has also been applied to other obstetric measurements, such as fetal biometry and birthweight. Although in increasingly widespread use, the role of customization of obstetric measurements remains to be defined fully. This relates in part to distinguishing between physiological and pathological determinants of variability in fetal growth. For example, nulliparity is associated with both a lower birthweight and an increased risk of stillbirth. It is plausible

therefore that poor growth is on the causal pathway between nulliparity and stillbirth. If this were the case, it is questionable whether obstetric measurements should be automatically adjusted for nulliparity.

Ultrasound biometry

Ultrasound is the most sensitive method of assessing fetal growth. It is important to note that while a single ultrasound measurement may give an indication of whether the fetal abdominal circumference or estimated fetal weight is above or below a predefined centile, this does not in itself diagnose a fetal growth abnormality. Abnormal fetal growth can only be ascertained by successive measurements, usually of the abdominal circumference, plotted either manually or by specialized software on a centile chart.

Growth parameters, primarily biparietal diameter, head circumference, femur length and abdominal circumference, are plotted on charts which delineate the normal range of growth within a population. In an attempt to refine identification of true IUGR, ultrasound growth charts that adjust for baseline maternal and fetal characteristics have been devised. They also allow differentiation between fetuses that are small but which have normal growth rate (hence might have been mislabelled 'growth restricted' using normal population centile charts) and those whose growth was originally within the normal range but has fallen below a given centile.

Fetal arterial and venous Doppler

The decision to deliver an SGA infant is based on a combination of investigations. Fetal arterial and venous Doppler assessment has shown itself to be useful and reproducible in tracking the cardiovascular responses to hypoxia and acidaemia in fetuses compromised through uteroplacental insufficiency. Fetal vessels most commonly assessed are the umbilical and middle cerebral arteries, thoracic aorta and the ductus venosus. Meta-analysis of randomized controlled trials has shown that in high-risk pregnancies umbilical artery Doppler improves perinatal outcome. It remains unclear why this should be, as no consistent management plan was followed.

As the fetoplacental unit becomes more hypoxic, the normal umbilical artery Doppler impedance (Plate 18.2a) increases, eventually leading to reduction and absence of end-diastolic flow (Plate 18.2b,c respectively). In extreme circumstances, there might be reversed umbilical end-diastolic flow; this is rarely seen after 3 weeks however. Throughout this process, there is a concomitant fall in middle cerebral artery resistance, known as centralization or 'brain sparing'. Later venous changes can be observed with pulsed wave Doppler of the ductus venosus: as acidaemia and impaired contractility of the heart supervene, the biphasic waveform (Fig. 18.4a) becomes abnormal with an exaggerated *a* wave, sometimes reaching or falling below the baseline, indicating 'back pressure'

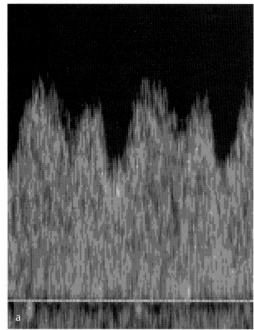

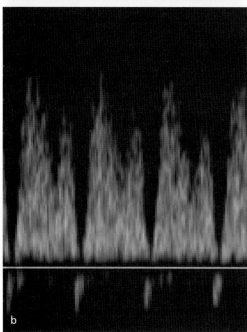

Fig. 18.4 Assessment of ductus venosus Doppler: (a) normal waveform; (b) reversed *a* wave.

during atrial contraction (diastole) (Fig. 18.4b). This finding in the ductus venosus, often mirrored by increased pulsatility in the umbilical vein, is an ominous and usually pre-terminal event.

Cardiotocography and biophysical assessment

The most reproducible method of assessing the fetal heart rate is by computerized analysis; several software packages allow storage, comparison and print-out of successive

traces. Chronic uteroplacental insufficiency may lead to hypoxia and in severe cases to acidaemia. The short-term variation (STV) in fetal heart rate, assessed by computerized analysis, is the best indicator of fetal compromise in this context. STV increases with gestational age: the 2.5th centile is approximately 4.4 ms at 26 weeks and 6 ms at 34 weeks. It is very rare for there to be fetal acidaemia at values above these, whereas reduced STV correlates well with fetal hypoxia and metabolic acidaemia.

Successive recordings of an at-risk growth-restricted fetus over days or weeks will often show a gradual reduction in STV in parallel with other findings such as reduced amniotic fluid, reduced fetal movements and raised umbilical artery resistance with centralization of blood flow. Spontaneous decelerations seen on cardiotocography (CTG) are a relatively late finding and usually coincide with reduced STV on computerized recordings. Unprovoked decelerations on CTG are related to the occurrence of fetal hypoxaemia and acidaemia.

Other elements of the biophysical profile, such as fetal tone, movements and amniotic fluid, should be reported alongside fetal growth, Doppler findings, maternal condition and CTG at every ultrasound scan of a potentially compromised fetus. However, in UK and European practice, a formal biophysical score is rarely used to dictate management and timing of delivery.

Timing of delivery

The optimal timing of delivery in hypoxic growth-restricted fetuses is simply not known. There have been no randomized studies that give an indication as to which method of fetal assessment to use and when to deliver. The Growth Restriction Intervention Trial (GRIT) reported on over 500 compromised babies where the timing of delivery was in doubt. This demonstrated a non-significant trend towards better long-term outcome when delivery was delayed among infants recruited between 24 and 30 weeks, but not at later gestations. The risk of fetal hypoxaemia and acidaemia (hence possible intrauterine death) must be weighed against the complications arising from prematurity. There is considerable geographical variation in practice: in North America the biophysical profile usually determines timing of delivery whereas in Europe this decision is usually made on a combination of CTG and Doppler findings. The inconsistency reflects the lack of very strong evidence favouring one method over another.

There is a consensus that reversed umbilical artery Doppler end-diastolic flow after 32 weeks' gestation, and absent end-diastolic flow after 34 weeks is an indication for immediate delivery. However, reversed umbilical end-diastolic flow at 26 or even 28 weeks is not necessarily an indication for delivery as in earlier gestation these Doppler findings may follow a more chronic course. There is compelling evidence from observational studies that in severe fetal growth restriction, delaying delivery to after 29 weeks confers a 'step change' improvement in both neonatal mortality and morbidity. However, an assessment of all Doppler and biophysical parameters is most informative before making a decision for delivery.

Summary box 18.1

- Fetal growth in the second half of pregnancy is associated with a number of measurements in the first trimester (smaller than expected crown rump length and low PAPP-A), indicating that late placental dysfunction may have its origins in the immediate weeks post conception.
- Placental effects of insulin-like growth factors (IGFs), acting through the type 1 IGF receptor, are critical determinants of fetal growth.
- Maternal characteristics, biochemical measurements and uterine artery Doppler are all associated with the risk of poor fetal growth but the main clinical approach to detecting small babies in the low risk population is measurement of the symphysis-fundal height.
- The primary form of assessment of fetuses with suspected growth restriction is umbilical artery Doppler flow velocimetry, but serial monitoring is performed using biometry, arterial Dopplers, venous Dopplers and computerized cardiotocography.

Further reading

Baschat AA, Cosmi E, Bilardo CM *et al.* Predictors of neonatal outcome in early-onset placental dysfunction. *Obstet Gynecol* 2007;109:253–261.

Breeze AC, Lees CC. Prediction and perinatal outcomes of fetal growth restriction. *Semin Fetal Neonatal Med* 2007;12:383–397.

Das UG, Sysyn G. Abnormal fetal growth: intrauterine growth retardation, small for gestational age, large for gestational age. *Pediatr Clin N Am* 2004;51:639–654.

Smith GCS. First trimester origins of fetal growth impairment. *Semin Perinatol* 2004;28:41–50. This whole issue of the journal was a series of reviews on disorders of fetal growth and contains eight recent relevant reviews.

Zhong Y, Tuuli M, Odibo AO. First-trimester assessment of placenta function and the prediction of pre-eclampsia and intrauterine growth restriction. *Prenat Diagn* 2010;30:293–308.

Chapter 19
Fetal Medical Conditions

Janet Brennand
Southern General Hospital, Glasgow, UK

Fetal thyroid function

The advent of fetal blood sampling has allowed direct and accurate quantification of fetal thyroid function. Fetal thyroid hormone synthesis commences at 10–12 weeks' gestation. Prior to this the fetus relies on placental transfer of maternal thyroid hormones. Fetal serum thyroid-stimulating hormone (TSH), thyroxine-binding globulin (TBG), free and total thyroxine (T4) and triiodothyronine (T3) increase with advancing gestation, from 14–16 weeks onwards [1,2]. The concentrations of total and free T4 (FT4) reach adult levels by 36 weeks' gestation. In contrast T3 concentrations are lower than adult levels throughout pregnancy. There is no relationship between maternal and fetal thyroid hormone levels, confirming that development of the fetal pituitary–thyroid axis is independent of the mother. Fetal TSH concentrations are low until 15–18 weeks' gestation, and the lack of correlation between it and thyroid hormone concentrations indicates that thyroid maturation is independent of TSH. Fetal TSH receptors become responsive to TSH at 20 weeks' gestation.

Thyroid hormones promote normal growth, development and neurological function. Disruption of normal thyroid function, if unrecognized and untreated, can therefore have significant long-term sequelae. Thyroid dysfunction in the fetus can result from a primary problem affecting the fetus. More commonly it occurs secondary to maternal thyroid disease and/or its treatment.

The presence of fetal goitre indicates thyroid dysfunction, provided other differential diagnoses of a fetal neck mass, such as cystic hygroma, cervical teratoma and haemangioma, have been excluded. The goitre may represent fetal hyperthyroidism or hypothyroidism. The serious adverse consequences of fetal hyperthyroidism are miscarriage and intrauterine death, and of hypothyroidism neonatal cretinism.

Fetal hyperthyroidism

Fetal hyperthyroidism is most likely to occur secondary to maternal Graves' disease as a result of placental transfer of autoantibodies. TSH receptor-stimulating antibodies (TRAbs) are of the IgG class and therefore readily able to cross the placenta and stimulate the fetal thyroid gland. TRAbs can stimulate the fetal thyroid from 20 weeks' gestation. TRAbs are increased in at least 80% of women with Graves' disease. It has been estimated that neonatal thyrotoxicosis occurs in 2–10% of babies born to women with Graves' disease [3]. The risk of fetal hyperthyroidism is related to TRAb concentrations. The placenta is more permeable to IgG in the second half of pregnancy and fetal concentrations of TRAbs reach maternal levels at around 30 weeks' gestation. As a result, fetal hyperthyroidism usually develops in the second half of pregnancy

Pregnancies at risk

A pregnant woman with Graves' disease can be categorized as follows [3].

1 Euthyroid, not on medication, but who has previously received antithyroid drugs: the risk of fetal/neonatal hyperthyroidism is negligible and measurement of TRAbs is not necessary.

2 Euthyroid, previously treated with radioactive iodine or surgery: TRAbs should be measured in early pregnancy to detect presence and, if present, their concentration. High concentrations of antibodies identify a pregnancy at risk of fetal hyperthyroidism. TRAbs should be measured again in the third trimester to identify risk of neonatal hyperthyroidism.

3 Requiring antithyroid drugs to achieve normal thyroid function: TRAbs should be measured in the last trimester.

Features

Fetal tachycardia (>160bpm) is the most common feature of fetal hyperthyroidism. Other findings include

---

intrauterine growth restriction (IUGR), accelerated bone maturation, cardiomegaly, cardiac failure and hydrops. A large fetal goitre can cause hyperextension of the fetal neck resulting in malpresentation. Oesophageal compression may result in polyhydramnios with its associated risk of preterm labour.

Management

Ultrasound can detect fetal goitre, which is the earliest ultrasound feature of fetal thyroid dysfunction and appears before fetal tachycardia. Fetal goitre is defined as a thyroid circumference equal to or greater than the 95th centile for gestational age and normative fetal thyroid measurements have been defined [4]. Colour flow Doppler may help differentiate between a hyperthyroid and hypothyroid goitre. Hyperthyroidism is associated with a signal throughout the gland, whereas a signal confined to the periphery of the gland is suggestive of hypothyroidism [5,6]. In at-risk pregnancies monthly ultrasound should be carried out from around 20 weeks' gestation to assess thyroid size.

Amniotic fluid thyroid concentrations do not reflect fetal thyroid status [7] and therefore amniocentesis is not indicated in the assessment of fetal thyroid function. Cordocentesis is the only direct method of assessing this. This is an invasive procedure, with a risk of miscarriage, and should be reserved for cases in which it is impossible to distinguish fetal hyperthyroidism from fetal hypothyroidism on clinical grounds, or for cases where the response to fetal therapy is not as anticipated (i.e. deterioration despite treatment).

Treatment

Treatment by maternal administration of antithyroid drugs is both safe and effective in the management of fetal hyperthyroidism. Propylthiouracil is the drug of choice because of the reduced risk of side effects. If the mother is euthyroid she may require thyroxine supplementation. This may also be necessary for women already on antithyroid medication who need to increase the dose.

Fetal hypothyroidism

Causes of fetal hypothyroidism are shown in Table 19.1 [8]. Worldwide, iodine deficiency is the leading cause. Maternal thyroid disease associated with thyroid autoantibodies can cause fetal hypothyroidism. Antithyroperoxidase antibodies cross the placenta in the third trimester but have little effect on fetal thyroid function. However, although TRAbs are generally stimulatory, they can be inhibitory, resulting in fetal hypothyroidism.

Features

Ultrasound features include IUGR, goitre and decreased fetal movements. There may be tachycardia or bradycardia and in severe cases complete heart block. Cardiomegaly

Table 19.1 Causes of fetal/neonatal hypothyroidism.

Disorder	Transmission
Thyroid dysgenesis (aplasia, hypoplasia, ectopy)	Sporadic
Thyroid dyshormonogenesis	Familial, autosomal recessive
Hypothalamic–pituitary dysfunction	Sporadic, autosomal recessive
TSH receptor mutations	Autosomal recessive, dominant
TSH receptor blocking IgG	Maternal thyroid disease with transplacental transmission
Iatrogenic	
Antithyroid drugs	
Radioactive iodine after 10–12 weeks' gestation	
Excess iodine/iodide	
Endemic iodine deficiency	

Source: adapted from Fisher [8].

and delayed skeletal maturation may occur. Fetal hypothyroidism is often unrecognized and should be considered in all women with a history of thyroid disease and/or antithyroid medication.

Management

If fetal hypothyroidism is secondary to maternal antithyroid therapy, the dose of the drug should be reduced with the aim of keeping maternal FT4 levels at the upper end of the normal range for gestational age. Ultrasound of the fetal thyroid should be carried out at no greater than fortnightly intervals to ensure reduction in size, which is usually noted within 2 weeks of reducing therapy [9].

Transplacental transfer of T4 is inadequate to treat hypothyroid goitre. The intra-amniotic route is used and 250–500 µg of T4 at 7–10 day intervals is a proposed regimen [10]. The success of treatment can be monitored by ultrasound assessment as above. If the fetal condition deteriorates despite treatment, cordocentesis is needed to measure fetal TSH and FT4 levels.

 Summary box 19.1

- There is a risk of fetal thyroid dysfunction in women who are thyroid receptor antibody positive or who are taking antithyroid medication.
- Fetal goitre, present on ultrasound, indicates fetal thyroid dysfunction if other differential diagnoses have been excluded.
- It should be possible to distinguish fetal hyperthyroidism from hypothyroidism on clinical grounds in most cases.
- Cordocentesis is reserved for those cases in which this distinction on clinical grounds is not possible.
- Fetal thyroid dysfunction can be treated successfully *in utero*.

Congenital adrenal hyperplasia

Congenital adrenal hyperplasia (CAH) occurs when abnormal adrenal steroidogenesis results in androgen excess. Five hormones are responsible for the conversion of cholesterol to cortisol, and a defect in any one of these will cause precursors to be diverted to the production of androgens. CAH is an autosomal recessive condition and in 90–95% of cases is due to a deficiency of 21-hydroxylase. Androgen excess *in utero* leads to virilization of a female fetus and in the severe form is associated with salt loss secondary to aldosterone deficiency. Androgen excess does not affect development of fetal male genitalia. Virilized females may be assigned the wrong gender at birth and are likely to require corrective genital surgery.

The aim of therapy is therefore to prevent virilization of a female fetus. The fetal adrenal gland can be suppressed by maternal administration of dexamethasone. A minimum dose of 20 µg per kilogram pre-pregnancy weight in two divided doses is the recommended regimen and therapy must be commenced at 6–7 weeks' gestation when the external genitalia begin to differentiate [11].

Approach to management

• A family with an index case should be offered pre-pregnancy counselling and identification of the genetic mutation.
• The risk of an affected fetus in a subsequent pregnancy is 1 in 4, and of a virilized female fetus 1 in 8.
• Commence dexamethasone treatment at 6–7 weeks' gestation.
• Perform chorionic villous sampling (CVS) at 10–11 weeks' gestation to identify an affected fetus.
• Discontinue dexamethasone in all male fetuses and all unaffected female fetuses.
• If the fetus is an affected female, continue treatment for the remainder of the pregnancy.

The above regimen means that seven of eight pregnancies are exposed to unnecessary steroid therapy. Non-invasive analysis of cell-free fetal DNA from maternal blood can identify the Y chromosome from 7 weeks' gestation and therapy could be discontinued in the pregnancies with a male fetus without waiting for CVS results. If the fetus is female, treatment will have to continue until genetic results from CVS are available, still exposing three of eight fetuses to potentially unnecessary treatment. Future detection of the genetic defect by non-invasive means will be the only way to eliminate this blind approach to early therapy. There are no reported teratogenic effects of antenatal dexamethasone treatment. Information regarding longer-term effects is limited and parents must be made aware of this when discussing the pros and cons of therapy.

Fetal dysrhythmias

These comprise irregular fetal heart rhythm, fetal tachycardias and fetal bradycardias. Rhythm disturbances are encountered in approximately 2% of pregnancies during routine ultrasound [12]. M-mode and pulsed-wave Doppler echocardiography are the main diagnostic techniques. The common dysrhythmias are discussed here. The reader is referred to other literature for a more comprehensive discussion of all dysrhythmias and their diagnosis [13,14].

Irregular fetal heart rate

This is typically described as a 'missed beat' and is usually due to atrial extrasystoles. These extrasystoles are more common in the third trimester and are detected in 1.7% of fetuses after 36 weeks' gestation. Ventricular extrasystoles are much rarer. The extrasystoles are benign and usually resolve prior to delivery. Occasionally (2–3% of cases) a sustained tachycardia develops and it is wise to auscultate the heart regularly to ensure this does not occur.

Tachycardia

A fetal tachycardia is defined as a sustained heart rate above 180 bpm. Fetal tachycardia occurs in 0.5% of pregnancies and is therefore relatively common. Supraventricular tachycardia (SVT) is the most common type (66–90% of cases), followed by atrial flutter (10–30%). Atrial fibrillation and chaotic atrial tachycardia are much less common and ventricular tachycardia is extremely rare during fetal life [15].

Supraventricular tachycardia

The most common type of SVT is a re-entry phenomenon where an accessory conducting pathway allows rapid retrograde passage of the electrical impulse from ventricle to atrium, establishing a re-entry circuit. This is defined as atrioventricular (AV) re-entrant tachycardia. In this type of SVT the time interval between ventricular and atrial contraction (VA interval) is short. In SVT caused by atrial ectopic tachycardia or permanent junctional reciprocating tachycardia, the VA interval is long. Establishing the length of the VA interval is important when deciding on therapy. In SVT the fetal heart rate is often in the region of 240 bpm with reduced variability. The ratio of atrial to ventricular contractions (AV ratio) is 1:1.

Atrial flutter

The atrial rate is very fast at 350–500 bpm. At such a fast rate 1:1 AV conduction is not possible. More commonly there is a degree of AV block, usually 2:1, but it can be greater.

Table 19.2 Antiarrhythmic drugs for treatment of fetal tachycardia.

Drug	Loading dose	Maintenance dose	Plasma levels	Notes
Digoxin	0.5–1.0 mg i.v.	0.25–0.5 mg t.d.s.	1–2.5 ng/mL	A first-line antiarrhythmic drug
				Maternal administration ineffective if fetal hydrops present
Flecainide		100 mg t.d.s.	0.4–0.8 µg/mL	Pro-arrhythmic
				Regular maternal ECG monitoring
				Good placental transfer: first-line therapy if hydrops present
				Should see an effect (sinus rhythm) in 72 hours
Sotalol		80–160 mg b.d.		Pro-arrhythmic
				Regular maternal ECG monitoring
				Good placental transfer: fetal levels almost the same as maternal
				First-line therapy if fetal hydrops
Amiodarone	800–1600 mg/day oral or i.v.	400–800 mg/day		Poor placental transfer (10–40%)
				Long half-life facilitates accumulation in the fetal compartment

Source: adapted from Simpson and Silverman [14].

Management options

The fetus with a sustained fetal tachycardia is at risk of developing cardiac failure, hydrops and ultimately fetal death. Fetal mortality is 27% if hydrops develops, compared with 0–4% if it is absent [16]. The aim of management is to reduce this risk. If the fetus is managed conservatively, close fetal monitoring is necessary to detect early signs of cardiac failure. Delivery, followed by postnatal therapy, is an option if close to term, but it is recognized that pharmacological control of the heart rate in the neonatal period is not always straightforward. *In utero* therapy is effective in restoring sinus rhythm and is the preferred option for treating preterm infants, reserving delivery for those cases that fail to respond to indirect or direct fetal therapy.

The transplacental route is the route of choice for fetal therapy. The drugs used in the management of fetal tachycardia are illustrated in Table 19.2. If there is no response to maternal drug administration or there is severe hydrops, direct fetal therapy via cordocentesis is required. The risks associated with cordocentesis are greater in the presence of hydrops. Maternal administration of drugs should take place in a hospital setting owing to potential pro-arrhythmic effects (flecainide, sotalol, amiodarone). A baseline ECG should be performed prior to medication, and repeated after starting therapy or increasing drug dosage, looking for prolongation of the QT interval.

Bradycardia

This is defined as a fetal heart rate persistently below 100 bpm.

Atrioventricular block

In AV block there is disturbance of electrical conduction between the atria and ventricles. Three types are described.

In first-degree block there is a prolonged AV interval and this cannot be detected on routine ultrasound. Second-degree block is of two types. In type I there is progressive lengthening of AV conduction time until an impulse is blocked; this results in an irregular rhythm but the fetal heart rate may be normal. In type II second-degree block there is conduction of some beats and not others, without lengthening of the AV conduction time. On M-mode the atrial rate may be twice that of the ventricular rate (2:1 block) and occasionally 3:1 block is seen.

In complete AV block (CAVB) there is complete dissociation of atrial and ventricular contractions. This rare condition (1 in 15000–22000 live births) has two important causes: congenital heart disease (CHD) and immune-mediated disease. CHD accounts for 50% of cases of CAVB, the most common defects being left atrial isomerism and congenitally corrected transposition of the great vessels. Immune-mediated disease has been the subject of fetal therapy. Transplacental transfer of maternal anti-Ro and anti-La antibodies results in inflammation and damage of the fetal myocardium and conduction tissue. These antibodies may be present in women with a history of Sjögren's syndrome or systemic lupus erythematosus. The risk of CAVB in a woman with antibodies is approximately 2%, with a recurrence risk of 16%. The risk to the fetus is maximal between 16 and 26 weeks' gestation. Poor prognostic features for CAVB include hydrops, heart rate below 55 bpm and premature delivery. The mortality ranges from 18 to 43% [13].

There are no treatment options that are clearly effective. Steroids, either dexamethasone or betamethasone, have been administered with variable results. The same is true for β sympathomimetics, which are given with the aim of increasing the fetal heart rate. The current lack of evidence confirming efficacy of therapy, and the potential maternal and fetal side effects of medication, must be borne in mind in the evaluation of whether or not to treat.

Summary box 19.2

- Fetal cardiac arrhythmias are common, affecting 1–2% of pregnancies.
- Ectopic beats usually resolve spontaneously.
- Fetal therapy for tachycardias is preferred to premature delivery.
- Detailed fetal echocardiography and testing for maternal anti-Ro and anti-La antibodies should be performed in cases of complete heart block.
- There is currently no therapy of proven benefit for complete heart block.

Fetal and neonatal alloimmune thrombocytopenia

The incidence of fetal and neonatal alloimmune thrombocytopenia (FNAIT) is estimated to be 1 in 1000–2000 pregnancies [17]. It occurs when maternal platelets lack antigens that are present on the fetal platelets. An alloimmune response develops whereby maternal antibodies (IgG) are produced that cross the placenta, cause fetal platelet destruction and thrombocytopenia. Fetal platelets express specific antigens from the first trimester. FNAIT is the platelet equivalent of red cell alloimmunization. However, in contrast to red cell alloimmunization, FNAIT can complicate 50% of first pregnancies.

The following human platelet antigen (HPA) systems are described: HPA-1, HPA-2, HPA-3, HPA-4, HPA-5 and HPA-15 [18]. The distribution of HPA systems is affected by race, with 2% of white women being HPA-1a negative. HPA-1a antibodies account for 85% of cases of FNAIT. The other antibodies most frequently encountered in white people are HPA-5b and HPA-3a [19]. HPA-5b is associated with milder FNAIT than that induced by HPA-1a. In some cases a responsible antibody cannot be identified, despite a clear clinical diagnosis of FNAIT.

FNAIT is rare, but platelet incompatibility is not infrequent: 1 in 50 pregnancies will be incompatible for HPA-1a. The observed frequency of alloimmunization is much less than this. The development of HPA-1a alloantibodies is related to HLA phenotype. Major histocompatibility class II antigen DR3 is found in 60–80% of people who develop antibodies and HLA DRw52 antigen is found in 100% of responders. Therefore platelet incompatibility does not equal alloimmunization, which in turn does not equal fetal thrombocytopenia [20].

Most affected infants are asymptomatic or present with signs of minor haemorrhage such as petechiae. In more severe cases there will be internal haemorrhage, and intracranial haemorrhage (ICH) is most frequent. The

sequelae of ICH can be severe, and include perinatal mortality, hydrocephalus and long-term neurological handicap. The risk of perinatal ICH is approximately 11% (15% if fetal deaths are included) [21]. The severity of FNAIT is not correlated to maternal antibody titre, and therefore this cannot be used to guide management in subsequent pregnancies. There is at least a similar or increased risk of thrombocytopenia in a subsequent pregnancy when the father is homozygous for the responsible antigen. Obstetric history is relevant. If there was no ICH in the index pregnancy, the risk of ICH in a subsequent affected pregnancy is 7%. If a previous sibling was affected by ICH, the recurrence risk is 75% [21]. Most cases of ICH occur in the third trimester, with maximal risk at 30 weeks' gestation, but there are documented cases as early as 20 weeks' gestation [22]. The risk is related to the length of time the fetus is exposed to thrombocytopenia and therefore the rationale is that therapy should start at 18–20 weeks.

Management

The aim of treatment is to reduce the risk of *in utero* and perinatal ICH. The only method of assessing the fetal platelet count is cordocentesis. If the fetus is thrombocytopenic, the risk of exsanguination as a result of cordocentesis is greater. Direct transfusion of platelets at the time of cordocentesis will increase the fetal platelet count, but the lifespan of platelets is only 4–5 days, necessitating repeat transfusions at 7–10 day intervals if a normal platelet count is to be maintained. The mean fetal loss rate is 1.6% per procedure in FNAIT and the incidence of emergency delivery estimated at 2.4% per procedure [21]. Degranulation of transfused platelets may augment the risk of fetal bradycardia. The cumulative fetal loss rate per pregnancy is 6% if cordocentesis and platelet transfusion is the chosen option [17]. An alternative approach is to defer cordocentesis until prior to delivery at which point a single platelet transfusion can be given, if indicated, and the baby delivered a couple of days later. This obviously reduces the risks associated with multiple procedures. However, the fetus may have already been exposed to prolonged thrombocytopenia and suffered an ICH.

Because of the risks associated with invasive therapy, a more conservative approach has been developed. The use of intravenous immunoglobulin (IVIG) in the management of FNAIT was first reported by Bussel *et al.* [23]. A dose of 1 g/kg/week resulted in a significant increase in fetal platelet count. The mechanism of action of IVIG remains unclear but a number of possible explanations are described [17]. Firstly, anti-HPA antibodies in the maternal circulation will be diluted by the presence of immunoglobulin and therefore less will be transferred across the placenta. Secondly, IVIG may block placental Fc receptors, thus preventing transmission of maternal antibodies. Finally, IVIG may block Fc receptors on fetal macrophages, preventing destruction of antigen–antibody complex-coated cells. IVIG reduces the risk of ICH even in those fetuses that do not show an increase in platelet count. There must therefore be some additional protective effect of this therapy. The addition of corticosteroids to the IVIG regimen does not improve efficacy [24].

IVIG is the treatment of choice for FNAIT in many centres. Although invasive management gives direct information about the fetal platelet count, it must be shown to as good as, or indeed superior to, conservative management in order to justify the complication rates, which may exceed the risks associated with untreated disease. Recent evidence shows that this is not the case, IVIG having a 100% success rate compared with 94–96% success rates for cordocentesis and platelet transfusion [17].

Delivery is a time of high risk of ICH in the thrombocytopenic fetus. Elective Caesarean section is not free from risk of ICH, and cases of vaginal delivery are reported without adverse effects. Ideally, the fetal platelet count should be in excess of 50×10^9/L if vaginal delivery is contemplated. If invasive testing is avoided, and hence the fetal platelet count unknown, elective section should be chosen.

Fetal anaemia

This can result from red cell alloimmunization or parvovirus infection. The mechanism of fetal anaemia, its management and treatment are discussed for both aetiologies.

Red cell alloimmunization

If a pregnant woman is exposed to fetal red cells that possess different antigens to her own red cells (i.e. the antigens have been inherited from the father), she will mount an immune response. The initial response is production of IgM antibodies, which do not cross the placenta and therefore the pregnancy in which antibodies are first detected is unlikely to be affected. However, on further exposure to the foreign red cell antigen IgG antibodies are produced, which do cross the placenta and cause fetal haemolytic anaemia. The antibodies most commonly associated with haemolytic disease of the fetus and newborn (HDN) are the rhesus system antibodies RhD, Rhc and RhE, and Kell.

Some aspects of the assessment and management of pregnancies at risk of HDN are discussed in Chapter 15. Fig. 19.1 outlines a proposed management strategy for

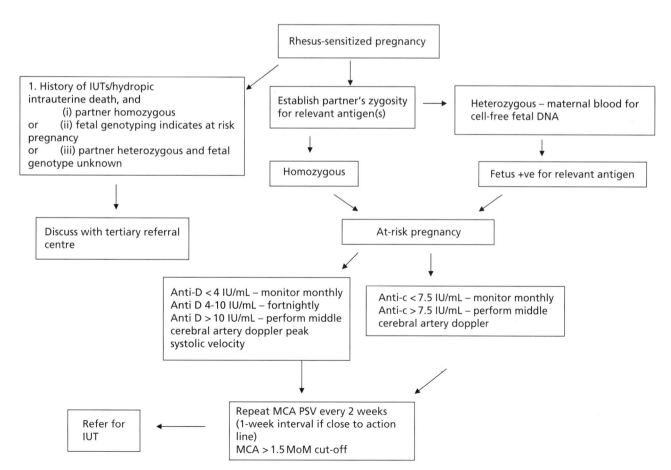

Fig. 19.1 Algorithm for the management of rhesus-sensitized pregnancies. IU, international units; MCA PSV middle cerebral artery peak systolic velocity; IUT, intrauterine transfusion; MoM, multiples of the median.

rhesus-sensitized pregnancies. Important points to recognize include the following.

• If the father is heterozygous for the relevant antigen, fetal blood group should be established using the non-invasive technique of assessing cell-free fetal DNA in maternal blood.

• Anti-D and anti-c concentrations can be quantified; this is not possible for anti-E or Kell antibodies.

• The trend of rise in antibody concentration is as important as a particular cut-off level.

Monitoring: middle cerebral artery Doppler

Having established that a pregnancy is at risk of fetal anaemia secondary to red cell alloimmunization, the aim of monitoring is to determine the point at which fetal therapy is indicated, before the fetus becomes severely anaemic. Fetal hydrops indicates the presence of severe anaemia. The early ultrasound features of hydrops are ascites and cardiomegaly, followed by progressive skin oedema, pericardial and pleural effusions and placental oedema. The entire purpose of the monitoring described below is to intervene before hydrops develops.

Doppler is informative in fetal anaemia because of some basic principles of blood flow. If the cross-sectional area of a vessel remains constant, blood velocity is directly proportional to blood flow. In addition, decreased blood viscosity will increase blood flow [25]. The anaemic fetus has a reduced blood viscosity and a hyperdynamic circulation, both of which will increase blood flow and hence blood velocity. In the middle cerebral artery (MCA) this is reflected by an increase in peak systolic velocity (PSV). MCA PSV measurements that are above a cut-off of 1.5 multiples of the median for gestational age identify moderate to severely anaemic fetuses with a sensitivity of 100% and a false-positive rate of 12% [26]. MCA PSV is not a good predictor of mild anaemia, but this is not a concern since this group of fetuses does not require *in utero* therapy. MCA PSV measurement is shown in Fig. 19.2 and the technique is described by Mari *et al.* [26].

Non-invasive monitoring using MCA Doppler has replaced serial amniocentesis in the management of at-risk pregnancies. Amniocentesis is an invasive procedure with a procedure-related loss rate of up to 1%. Repeated procedures are usually necessary in the same pregnancy and each procedure carries a risk of feto-maternal haemorrhage and of exacerbating the degree of fetal anaemia. A multicentre study comparing MCA Doppler with amniocentesis for monitoring at-risk pregnancies has demonstrated that MCA Doppler has a significantly greater accuracy and sensitivity [27]. In addition, 51% of women would have avoided an invasive procedure if MCA Doppler had been solely relied on. It is therefore the monitoring modality of choice in the majority of centres.

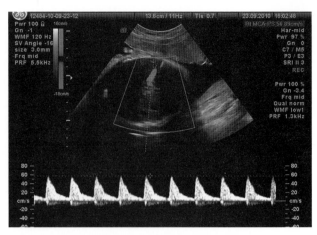

Fig. 19.2 Middle cerebral artery peak systolic velocity measurement.

> ## Summary box 19.3
>
> • The main antibodies causing fetal anaemia are anti-RhD, anti-Kell and anti-Rhc.
> • Parvovirus infection is an important cause of fetal anaemia, and should be considered in all cases of non-immune hydrops.
> • Non-invasive testing has replaced invasive testing for the management of fetal anaemia.
> • Fetal blood group should be determined on cell-free fetal DNA in maternal blood.
> • Middle cerebral artery Doppler has replaced amniocentesis for timing intrauterine transfusion in the majority of centres.
> • The need for intrauterine transfusion should be predicted before hydrops develops.

Treatment: intrauterine transfusion

The first intrauterine transfusion (IUT) was performed by Liley in 1963 [28] via the intraperitoneal route. Donor red blood cells are absorbed into the circulation via the diaphragmatic lymphatics. This results in slower restoration of fetal haemoglobin than if blood is given directly into the circulation, and as a result is no longer the route of choice for fetal therapy. It does still have a place in those cases requiring transfusion before 18–20 weeks' gestation, when intravascular access may not be possible. Intraperitoneal transfusion from 16 weeks' gestation has been employed successfully in a small cohort of severe cases of rhesus alloimmunization, until a gestation at which intravascular access could be achieved [29].

The introduction of real-time ultrasound facilitated needle-guided intraperitoneal transfusion in 1977 [30]. The first intravascular transfusion was performed fetoscopically by Rodeck *et al.* in 1981 [31]. A variety of techniques for IUT have been employed. Direct intravascular transfusion is the preferred technique in which the

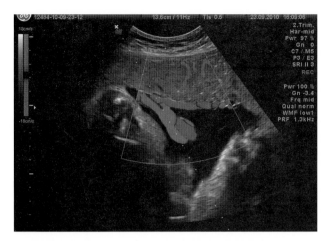

Fig. 19.3 Anterior placental cord insertion, with needle guideline.

additional volume is absorbed by the fetoplacental circulation, thus 'protecting' the fetus from fluid overload. The fetal circulation is accessed via the umbilical cord at its placental insertion (Fig. 19.3) or the intrahepatic portion of the umbilical vein. Intracardiac transfusion has also been described [32]. The choice of route will be influenced by placental site and fetal position. Access to the cord insertion is easiest if the placenta is anterior. When accessing the cord insertion the vein is targeted rather than an artery, as the latter is prone to spasm and there is an increased risk of complications.

Technical aspects of the procedure are listed below.
• Maternal sedation, antibiotics, single course of steroids at 26 weeks' gestation and above.
• Aseptic technique.
• Needle guide and free-hand approach; 20 gauge needle.
• Cord insertion/intrahepatic vein.
• Cross-matched, O, Rh-negative, cytomegalovirus-irradiated blood.
• Repeat at 2-week intervals.
• Aim for delivery at 34–35 weeks' gestation.
Once the chosen vessel is punctured, a sample of fetal blood is analysed immediately by on-site laboratory staff to obtain the fetal haematocrit. The volume of blood to be transfused is calculated by a formula incorporating fetal haematocrit, donor haematocrit and fetoplacental blood volume. It is important that the donor haematocrit is as high as possible (≥75%) to reduce the risk of volume overload. The aim is for a post-transfusion haematocrit of 40–45%. The estimated post-procedure decline in haematocrit is 1–2% per day [33], and in general a transfusion interval of 14 days is used, although cases vary individually, as will the policies of different centres. If the fetus is severely anaemic and/or hydropic, a stepwise transfusion is given, aiming for a haematocrit of 30%, with repeat transfusion 1 week later.

Complications of IUT
There are a number of procedure-related complications of IUT. The perinatal mortality rate is 1.6–2% [34]. Complications include vasospasm and fetal bradycardia, chorioamnionitis and preterm labour/delivery, emergency delivery and augmentation of the alloimmunization with implications for future pregnancies.

Outcomes
A review of 19 studies using IUT shows an overall survival rate of 84% [34]. The survival rate is higher for non-hydropic fetuses (94%) compared with hydropic fetuses (74%). There is evidence that infants severely affected by rhesus disease have lower birthweights than matched controls [35]. Infants treated with IUT show evidence of catch-up growth *in utero* and birthweights comparable to controls [36]. Existing data for short-term neurodevelopmental outcome following IUT suggest that this can be expected to be normal in more than 90% of cases, irrespective of a history of hydrops [37,38].

Kell alloimmunization
This can result in profound fetal anaemia, hydrops and intrauterine death. It differs from rhesus alloimmunization for a number of reasons. Past obstetric history is not reliable in predicting outcome in a subsequent pregnancy [39]. Maternal antibody titres do not correlate well with the severity of fetal anaemia; poor outcomes have been reported with low titres [40]. The type of anaemia is not solely haemolytic, but is also due to erythroid suppression [41]. For these reasons management of a Kell immunized pregnancy is challenging. Fortunately, the incidence of HDN due to Kell is low; only 9% of the white population is Kell positive and 0.2% are homozygous [42]. MCA PSV monitoring has been shown to be reliable in the management of Kell alloimmunization. Fortnightly MCA PSV measurements once the antibody titre is 1:32 is a reasonable approach to management.

> ### 💡 Summary box 19.4
>
> • Ultrasound-guided cordocentesis has revolutionized fetal investigation and therapy.
> • Intrauterine transfusion can treat anaemia secondary to alloimmunization or parvovirus infection.
> • Intravascular access is obtained at the placental cord insertion or the intrahepatic portion of the umbilical vein.
> • The procedure-related loss rate of intrauterine transfusion is 1–2%.
> • This risk is higher if fetal hydrops is present.

Parvovirus
Parvovirus infection should be considered in any fetus presenting with non-immune hydrops. Alternatively, a woman contracting parvovirus infection during

pregnancy requires appropriate monitoring to detect developing fetal anaemia. The topic has been reviewed extensively by other authors [43–45].

Parvovirus B19 is thought to exclusively infect humans, and it binds to the blood group P antigen cellular receptor that is present on haematopoietic precursors, endothelial cells, fetal myocytes and placental trophoblast. Its effect on the haematopoietic system results in profound anaemia and non-immune hydrops fetalis (NIHF). In addition, viral particles have been identified in fetal myocardial tissue, and cardiac dysfunction due to myocarditis may also contribute to the development of cardiac failure.

Approximately 50% of pregnant women are susceptible to infection, and outbreaks occur every 3–4 years, most commonly in late winter and spring. The peak incidence of hydrops occurs with infection between 17 and 24 weeks' gestation [45]. Quoted risks for hydrops developing if infection occurs at 9–20 weeks' or 13–20 weeks' gestation are 2.9% [46] and 7.1% [45] respectively. The virus infects the fetal liver, which in the second trimester is the main source of haematopoietic activity. Haematopoiesis is augmented at this gestation to meet the demands of the growing fetus, and the lifespan of red blood cells is decreased, rendering the fetus particularly susceptible to any arrest in haematopoietic production.

Levels of the P-antigen are negligible in the third trimester, and hence the risk of anaemia and hydrops appears to be low. The risk of vertical transmission during pregnancy is 30%, and the mean interval from maternal infection to development of NIHF is 2–6 weeks [47], although longer intervals have been reported [46].

Maternal serology will confirm recent infection. If IgM titres exceed IgG titres, the infection took place within the previous month and the fetus remains at risk of complications, even if none are present at initial presentation [48]. Maternal serology can be misleading if checked earlier than 7 days after contact as IgG and IgM could both be negative at this stage. Similarly, by the time of clinically established hydrops, IgM levels may already be low or, rarely, undetectable [43]. Fetal serology is of no help diagnostically as the fetal immune system is too immature to mount a detectable IgG/IgM immune response. Polymerase chain reaction techniques to detect viral DNA are required.

Management

MCA PSV is reliable in predicting fetal anaemia secondary to parvovirus infection [49]. The anaemia can be successfully treated by IUT, which reduces the mortality rate of severe hydrops [45]. Generally a single transfusion is

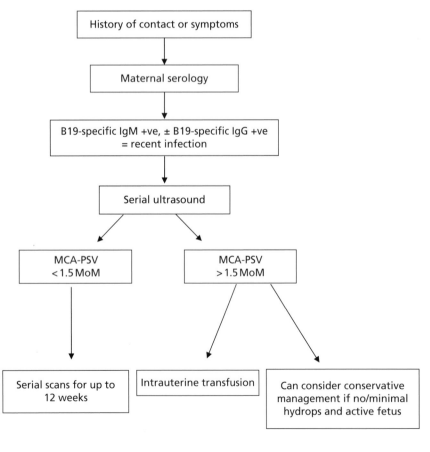

Fig. 19.4 Algorithm for the management of parvovirus infection. MoM, multiples of the median.

required. Cordocentesis and IUT are obviously not without risk, and the risks are higher when the fetus is hydropic. Thrombocytopenia is often a feature of parvovirus infection and this will potentially increase the procedure-related risk of exsanguination. In addition to red cell transfusion, consideration should be given to transfusion of platelets in those fetuses with severe thrombocytopenia.

Close fetal surveillance is required following maternal seroconversion prior to 24 weeks' gestation. Weekly MCA PSV should be carried out and IUT considered for results above the cut-off of 1.5 multiples of the median. Serial surveillance for 8–12 weeks after conversion is indicated. Anaemia due to parvovirus has the potential to resolve as the fetus mounts its own immune response. As a result, MCA Doppler monitoring may identify some fetuses that are anaemic at presentation but which are actually in the recovery phase of the infection. If other signs of fetal well-being are present, such as good fetal movements and normal liquor volume, it may be possible to continue conservative management and avoid IUT in these particular cases. A proposed management plan is summarized in Fig. 19.4.

References

1 Ballabio M, Nicolini U, Jowett T *et al*. Maturation of thyroid function in normal human foetuses. *Clin Endocrinol* 1989;31: 565–571.

2 Thorpe-Beeston JG, Nicolaides KH, Felton C *et al*. Maturation of the secretion of thyroid hormone and thyroid stimulating hormone in the fetus. *New Engl J Med* 1991;324:532–536.

3 Laurberg P, Nygaard B, Glinoer D *et al*. Guidelines for TSH-receptor antibody measurement in pregnancy: results of an evidence-based symposium organised by the European Thyroid Association. *Eur J Endocrinol* 1998;139:584–586.

4 Ranzini AC, Ananth CV, Smulian JC *et al*. Ultrasonography of the fetal thyroid: normograms based on biparietal diameter and gestational age. *J Ultrasound Med* 2001;20:613–617.

5 Polak M, Leger J, Luton D *et al*. Fetal cord blood sampling in the diagnosis and the treatment of fetal hyperthyroidism in the offsprings of a euthyroid mother producing thyroid stimulating immunoglobulins. *Ann Endocrinol* 1997;4:348–352.

6 Luton D, Fried D, Sibony O *et al*. Assessment of fetal thyroid function by colored Doppler echography. *Fetal Diagn Ther* 1997;12:24–27.

7 Hollingsworth DR, Alexander NM. Amniotic fluid concentrations of iodothyronines and thyrotropin do not reliably predict fetal thyroid status in pregnancies complicated by maternal thyroid disorders of anencephaly. *J Clin Endocrinol Metab* 1983;57:349–355.

8 Fisher DA. Fetal thyroid function: diagnosis and management of fetal thyroid disorders. *Clin Obstet Gynecol* 1997;40:16–31.

9 Thorpe-Beeston JG. Goitre. In: Fisk NM, Moise KJ Jr (eds) *Fetal Therapy*. Cambridge: University Press, 1997: 252–260.

10 Polak M, Le Gac I, Vuillard E *et al*. Fetal and neonatal thyroid function in relation to maternal Graves' disease. *Best Pract Res Clin Endocrinol Metab* 2004;18:289–302.

11 Van Vliet G, Polak M, Ritzen EM. Treating fetal thyroid and adrenal disorders through the mother. *Nat Clin Pract Endocrinol Metab* 2008;4:675–682.

12 Southall DP, Richards J, Hardwick RA *et al*. Prospective study of fetal heart rate and rhythm patterns. *Arch Dis Child* 1980;55:506–511.

13 Api O, Carvalho JS. Fetal dysrhythmias. *Best Pract Res Clin Obstet Gynaecol* 2008;22:31–48.

14 Simpson JM, Silverman NH. Diagnosis of cardiac arrhythmias during fetal life. In: Yagel S, Silverman NH, Gembruch U (eds) *Fetal Cardiology*. London: Taylor & Francis, 2005: 333–343.

15 Simpson JM. Fetal arrhythmias. *Ultrasound Obstet Gynecol* 2006;27:599–606.

16 Simpson JM, Sharland GK. Fetal tachycardias: management and outcome of 127 consecutive cases. *Heart* 1998;79:576–581.

17 Van den Akker ESA, Oepkes D. Fetal and neonatal alloimmune thrombocytopenia. *Best Pract Res Clin Obstet Gynaecol* 2008;22: 3–14.

18 Metcalfe P, Watkins NA, Ouwehand WH *et al*. Nomenclature of human platelet antigens. *Vox Sang* 2003;85:240–245.

19 Porcelijn L, Kanhai HHH. Diagnosis and management of fetal platelet disorders. In: Rodeck CH, Whittle MJ (eds) *Fetal Medicine: Basic Science and Clinical Practice*. London: Churchill Livingstone, 1999:805–815.

20 Kelsey H, Rodeck CH. Fetal thrombocytopenia. In: Fisk NM, Moise KJ Jr (eds) *Fetal Therapy*. Cambridge: University Press, 1997: 164–183.

21 Radder CM, Brand A, Kanhai HHH. Will it ever be possible to balance the risk of intracranial haemorrhage in fetal or neonatal alloimmune thrombocytopenia against the risk of treatment strategies to prevent it? *Vox Sang* 2003;84:318–325.

22 Giovangrandi Y, Daffos F, Kaplan C *et al*. Very early intracranial haemorrhage in alloimmune fetal thrombocytopenia. *Lancet* 1990;336:310.

23 Bussel JB, Richard MD, Berkowitz L *et al*. Antenatal treatment of neonatal alloimmune thrombocytopenia. *N Engl J Med* 1988;319:1374–1378.

24 Bussel JB, Berkowitz RL, Lynch L *et al*. Antenatal management of alloimmune thrombocytopenia with intravenous gamma-globulin: a randomised trial of the addition of low-dose steroid to intravenous gamma-globulin. *Am J Obstet Gynecol* 1996;174:1414–1423.

25 Giles WB, Trudinger BJ. Umbilical cord whole blood viscosity and the umbilical artery flow velocity time waveforms: a correlation. *Br J Obstet Gynaecol* 1986;93:466–470.

26 Mari G, Deter RL, Carpenter RL *et al*. Noninvasive diagnosis by Doppler ultrasonography of fetal anemia due to maternal red-cell alloimmunization. Collaborative group for Doppler assessment of the blood velocity in anemic fetuses. *N Engl J Med* 2000;342:9–14.

27 Oepkes D, Seaward G, Vandenbussche FPHA *et al*. Doppler ultrasonography versus amniocentesis to predict fetal anemia. *N Engl J Med* 2006;355:156–164.

28 Liley AW. Intrauterine transfusion of foetus in haemolytic disease. *BMJ* 1963;2:1107–1109.

29 Fox C, Martin W, Somerset DA *et al*. Early intraperitoneal transfusion and adjuvant maternal immunoglobulin therapy in the

treatment of severe red cell alloimmunisation, prior to fetal intravascular transfusion. *Fetal Diagn Ther* 2008;23:159–163.

30 Cooperberg PL, Carpenter CW. Ultrasound as an aid in intrauterine transfusion. *Am J Obstet Gynecol* 1977;128:239–241.

31 Rodeck CH, Kemp JR, Holman CA *et al*. Intravascular fetal blood transfusion by fetoscopy in severe rhesus isoimmunisation. *Lancet* 1981;i:625–627.

32 Westgren M, Selbing A, Stangenberg M. Fetal intracardiac transfusions in patients with severe rhesus isoimmunisation. *BMJ* 1988;296:885–886.

33 MacGregor SN, Socol ML, Pielet BW *et al*. Prediction of hematocrit decline after intravascular transfusion. *Am J Obstet Gynecol* 1989;161:1491–1493.

34 Schumacher B, Moise KJ. Fetal transfusion for red blood cell alloimmunization in pregnancy. *Obstet Gynecol* 1996;88:137–150.

35 Binks AS, Lind T, McNay RA. Effects of rhesus haemolytic disease upon birthweight. *J Obstet Gynaecol Br Commonw* 1973;80:301–304.

36 Roberts A, Grannum P, Belanger K *et al*. Fetal growth and birthweight in isoimmunized pregnancies after intravenous intrauterine transfusion. *Fetal Diagn Ther* 1993;8:407–411.

37 Janssens HM, de Haan MJ, van Kamp IL *et al*. Outcome for children treated with fetal intravascular transfusions because of severe blood group antagonism. *J Pediatr* 1997;131:373–380.

38 Hudon L, Moise KJ Jr, Hegemier SE *et al*. Long-term neurodevelopmental outcome after intrauterine transfusion for the treatment of fetal hemolytic disease. *Am J Obstet Gynecol* 1998;179:858–863.

39 Caine ME, Mueller-Heubach E. Kell sensitzation in pregnancy. *Am J Obstet Gynecol* 1986;154:85–90.

40 Leggat HM, Gibson JM, Barron SL *et al*. Anti-Kell in pregnancy. *Br J Obstet Gynaecol* 1991;98:162–165.

41 Weiner CP, Widness JA. Decreased fetal erythropoiesis and hemolysis in Kell haemolytic anemia. *Am J Obstet Gynecol* 1996;174:547–551.

42 Weinstein L. Irregular antibodies causing haemolytic disease of the newborn. *Obstet Gynecol Surv* 1976;31:581–591.

43 de Jong EP, de Haan TR, Kroes AC *et al*. Parvovirus B19 infection in pregnancy. *J Clin Virol* 2006;36:1–7.

44 Heegaard ED, Brown KE. Human parvovirus B19. *Clin Microbiol Rev* 2002;15:485–505.

45 Enders M, Weidner A, Zoellner I *et al*. Fetal morbidity and mortality after acute human parvovirus B19 infection in pregnancy: prospective evaluation of 1018 cases. *Prenat Diagn* 2004;24:513–518.

46 Miller E, Fairley CK, Cohen BJ *et al*. Immediate and long term outcome of human parvovirus B19 infection in pregnancy. *Br J Obstet Gynaecol* 1998;105:174–178.

47 Yaegashi N, Niinuma T, Chisaka H *et al*. The incidence of, and factors leading to, parvovirus B19-related hydrops fetalis following maternal infection: report of 10 cases and meta-analysis. *J Infect* 1998;37:28–35.

48 Beersma MFC, Claas ECJ, Sopaheluakan T *et al*. Parvovirus B19 viral loads in relation to VP1 and VP2 antibody responses in diagnostic blood samples. *J Clin Virol* 2005;34:71–75.

49 Delle Chiaie L, Buck G, Grab D *et al*. Prediction of fetal anemia with doppler measurement of the middle cerebral artery peak systolic velocity in pregnancies complicated by maternal blood group alloimmunization or parvovirus B19 infection. *Ultrasound Obstet Gynecol* 2001;18:232–236.

Chapter 20
Fetal Anomalies

Sailesh Kumar
Queen Charlotte's & Chelsea Hospital, London, UK

Almost 5% of newborns have a congenital malformation. In many cases these malformations are minor and do not impact on either the short- or long-term outcome for the individual. However, major congenital malformations are a significant contributor to both perinatal morbidity and mortality and indeed the detection of such anomalies has been the goal of antenatal screening programmes worldwide. In many countries the antenatal detection of fetal anomalies and the subsequent termination of these fetuses have been responsible for the decline in perinatal mortality rate seen over the last three decades. The detection of fetal structural abnormalities is generally made by ultrasound with additional more sophisticated techniques, such as three/four-dimensional ultrasound, fetal magnetic resonance imaging (MRI) or fetoscopy, reserved for complex cases where standard two-dimensional ultrasound fails to clarify the diagnosis.

The objectives of an antenatal screening programme should be (i) to provide appropriate information for women so that they are able to make an informed choice about their screening options and pregnancy management, (ii) to identify serious fetal abnormalities, either incompatible with life or associated with morbidity, allowing women to make timely decisions about pregnancy outcome, (iii) to identify abnormalities that may benefit from antenatal intervention and (iv) to identify abnormalities that may require early intervention following delivery. Clearly the successful implementation of an antenatal fetal anomaly screening programme depends on many factors, including the provision of adequate patient information, the availability of trained sonographers and good ultrasound equipment and clear management pathways for patients once an anomaly has been detected.

The European Surveillance of Congenital Anomalies (EUROCAT) recorded a total prevalence of major congenital anomalies of 23.9 per 1000 births for 2003–2007. Congenital heart defects were the most common non-chromosomal anomalies (6.5 per 1000 births), followed by limb defects (3.8 per 1000), anomalies of urinary system (3.1 per 1000) and nervous system malformations (2.3 per 1000). It has been estimated that the perinatal mortality rate associated with congenital anomalies is in the region of 0.9–1 per 1000 births.

Although first- and second-trimester aneuploidy screening is widely available in the UK, Europe, North America and many parts of Australasia, for many women the first antenatal ultrasound scan will be the mid-trimester fetal anomaly scan which is generally done at 18–22 weeks' gestation. The majority of fetal structural anomalies will be detected during this examination. With better high resolution machines and trained sonographers, many structural anomalies are now diagnosed during the late first and early second trimester, which is clearly preferable for women.

Timing and development of fetal malformations

The crucial morphogenetic window during which the fetus is particularly susceptible is the period of blastogenesis, which extends throughout the first 4 weeks of development (from fertilization until the end of the gastrulation stage, days 27 to 28 after conception). Any insult during this period can result in structural malformations, including patterns of multiple congenital anomalies arising from developmental field defects. Severe damage may cause demise of the fetus or, because of the pluripotent nature of the embryo and early fetus in general, compensatory changes may occur allowing development to continue in a normal or near-normal fashion. Because the fetus is less susceptible to damage when the development of the majority of organs has been completed, the most common anomalies associated with teratogenic exposures during the fetal period are fetal growth restriction (intrauterine growth retardation) and mild abnormalities of phenotype (e.g. epicanthic folds, clinodactyly). However, teratogenic drugs can result in a wide variety of effects that range from infertility, prenatal onset growth

Dewhurst's Textbook of Obstetrics & Gynaecology, Eighth Edition. Edited by D. Keith Edmonds.
© 2012 John Wiley and Sons, Ltd. Published 2012 by John Wiley and Sons, Ltd.

restriction, structural defects and functional central nervous system (CNS) abnormalities to miscarriage or fetal death. Similarly various perinatal infections (particularly viruses) can have significant teratogenic effects on the developing fetus with an extremely wide spectrum of resulting malformations.

 Summary box 20.1

- The fetus is most vulnerable in the first 4 weeks of life.
- Many maternal conditions, drugs and infections can cause structural malformations in specific organ systems.
- Ultrasound is the usual modality of imaging in pregnancy and detects the vast majority of anomalies.

Selected fetal anomalies in specific organ systems

Cardiovascular system anomalies

The fetal heart develops from the splanchnic mesoderm and in its earliest and most rudimentary form is represented by two tubes which subsequently fuse and then canalize. Repeated rotations and septations then occur that ultimately results in a four-chamber organ.

Congenital heart disease affects 6–8 per 1000 live births, at least half of which should be detectable before birth. Cardiac malformations are also associated with a wide variety of fetal and maternal conditions and medications. Fetal echocardiography should be considered for the following.

- First-degree relative with congenital heart disease: one previous sibling affected, 2–4% risk; two or more previous siblings affected, 10% risk; mother affected, 5–12% risk; father affected, 1–3% risk.
- Maternal insulin-dependent diabetes: 3–4% risk.
- Autoimmune antibodies (anti-Ro and anti-La).
- Drug therapy: lithium 10% risk.
- Epilepsy: 4–7% risk with monotherapy, 15% risk with polytherapy.
- Monochorionic twins: 4% risk.
- Increased nuchal translucency ≥3.5 mm: 3% risk, rising to 23% risk if >5.5 mm.
- High-risk structural anomalies: tracheo-oesophageal fistula, 15–40% risk; duodenal atresia, 17% risk; omphalocele, 20–30% risk; diaphragmatic hernia, 10–20% risk.

Detection of any cardiac abnormality should prompt a detailed evaluation for extracardiac anomalies. Karyotyping should be offered (risk 1–50%) depending on the type of lesion. Concomitant 22q deletion testing should be performed for outflow tract abnormalities (1% risk overall but 10% with outflow tract lesions). Delivery should generally take place in a tertiary unit. The mode and timing of delivery is usually decided on standard obstetric criteria.

Aortic stenosis

Aortic stenosis accounts for 4–6% of all cardiovascular abnormalities and is four times more common in males. It has an incidence of 3–4 per 10 000 live births. It may be either subvalvular, valvular or supravalvular. Stenosis secondary to valve abnormalities is usually due to cusp malformations seen in unicuspid or bicuspid aortic valves. The incidence of bicuspid aortic valves is approximately 1 in 100 newborns. Critical aortic stenosis causes reduced left ventricular output and increased diastolic filling pressure, which then causes hypertrophy followed by dilatation of the left ventricle.

Critical aortic stenosis can cause coronary hypoperfusion, subendocardial ischaemia and significant metabolic acidosis. The development of hydrops fetalis carries a very poor prognosis. Differential diagnoses include hypoplastic left heart syndrome (HLHS), coarctation of the aorta and cardiomyopathy. HLHS is frequently associated with both aortic and mitral valve atresia.

In many congenital heart centres, transcatheter balloon valvuloplasty is the initial procedure of choice in newborns with congenital aortic stenosis who are either duct dependent or have low cardiac output. Post-delivery patency of the ductus arteriosus should be maintained with prostaglandin (PG)E$_2$ and any associated metabolic acidosis corrected. Early neonatal echocardiography should be performed to confirm the cardiac abnormality and treatment then planned.

Pulmonary stenosis

This is a fairly common abnormality with the diagnosis often made after delivery. It has an incidence of approximately 1 in 1500 live births. Pulmonary stenosis may be isolated, occur in association with other abnormalities (Fallot's tetralogy) or occur in association with genetic syndromes (William's syndrome, Noonan's syndrome) or secondary to congenital rubella infection. Narrowing of the pulmonary valve can lead to hypertrophy of the right ventricle and, in severe cases, hypoplasia of the right ventricle. Pulmonary stenosis may progress *in utero*, resulting in tricuspid regurgitation, heart failure and hydrops.

Delivery of the baby should take place in a tertiary unit. The ductus arteriosus should be kept patent with a PGE$_2$ infusion. Early echocardiography to confirm the diagnosis and to exclude other cardiac malformations should be performed. Cardiac catheterization and balloon valvuloplasty is the treatment of choice although some cases may require open heart surgery.

Hypoplastic left heart syndrome

HLHS is a major congenital heart anomaly accounting for 1% of congenital cardiac abnormalities (Fig. 20.1). Without treatment, newborn babies with HLHS usually die and it is responsible for 25% of all cardiac deaths in the first

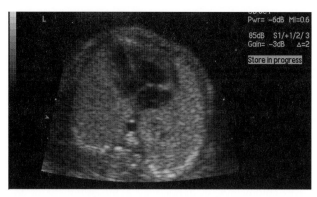

Fig. 20.1 Hypoplastic left heart.

week of life. HLHS is the end result of a spectrum of conditions that includes aortic valve stenosis/atresia, mitral valve stenosis/atresia, proximal aortic hypoplasia and left ventricular hypoplasia. Important associated anomalies include pulmonary venous return abnormalities. CNS anomalies including agenesis of the corpus callosum, microcephaly and holoprosencephaly have been reported. HLHS is associated with aneuploidy, genetic syndromes (Holt–Oram, Noonan's) and extracardiac abnormalities.

The patient should be referred to a tertiary centre and jointly managed by a fetal medicine specialist and paediatric cardiologist. Karyotyping should be performed and termination of pregnancy should be discussed with parents as the outcome for the majority of cases is very poor.

Hypoplastic right heart syndrome

This anomaly is due to pulmonary valve atresia with an intact interventricular septum. Occasionally the tricuspid valve is also atretic. The left ventricle supplies both the systemic as well as the pulmonary circulation (by retrograde flow through the ductus arteriosus). The malformation is suspected if there is obvious discrepancy in size between the two ventricles. Karyotyping may be indicated if additional anomalies are present. However, the overall risk for aneuploidy is low. Termination of pregnancy should be discussed, particularly if hydrops is present.

Atrioventricular septal defect

This anomaly covers a spectrum of congenital heart malformations characterized by a common atrioventricular junction coexisting with deficient atrioventricular septation. In ostium primum atrial septal defect there are separate atrioventricular valvular orifices despite a common junction, while in complete atrioventricular septal defect there is a common valve. There is a strong association (30–50%) with Down's syndrome. Additional cardiac malformations are present in more than 70% of cases.

The key diagnostic feature on the four-chamber view of the heart is the presence of a common atrioventricular valve. Once the abnormality is detected referral to a tertiary centre and paediatric cardiologist is advisable. Karyotyping is essential and careful assessment of the fetus for additional anomalies is important. Termination of pregnancy should be offered for large lesions with fetal hydrops, if aneuploidy is detected or if there are other major associated anomalies.

Tetralogy of Fallot

Tetralogy of Fallot occurs in approximately 1 in 3600 live births and accounts for 3.5% of infants born with congenital heart disease. It comprises a ventricular septal defect, right ventricular outflow tract obstruction, aorta overriding the interventricular septum, and right ventricular hypertrophy. The spectrum of severity is wide, ranging from right outflow tract obstruction to pulmonary atresia; 15% of cases may be associated with DiGeorge's syndrome caused by a deletion on the long arm of chromosome 22 (22q11.2). Once the diagnosis is suspected, referral to a paediatric cardiologist is essential. Karyotyping should be offered (including 22q deletion studies). The development of hydrops is a poor prognostic sign and termination of pregnancy should be discussed.

Central nervous system anomalies

Development of the human CNS involves several complex steps, including neural proliferation, neuroblast migration and neuronal differentiation. This is an extremely complex process influenced by both genetic and environmental factors and continues *ex utero* for several years.

Agenesis of the corpus callosum

Agenesis of the corpus callosum (ACC) is a failure to develop the large bundle of fibres that connect the two cerebral hemispheres. It occurs in 1 in 4000 individuals and has been estimated to have an incidence of 4 per 1000 live births. ACC can be either complete or partial. It may occur in isolation, associated with aneuploidy, part of a genetic syndrome or in association with other brain malformations. Various teratogens (alcohol, antiepileptic medication and cocaine), environmental factors and viral infections (rubella) have also been associated with ACC. If ACC is suspected a careful search for both intracranial and extracranial anomalies is required. Karyotyping should be offered and fetal MRI to assess the brain in greater detail should also be performed.

Counselling by a paediatric neurologist is essential as the spectrum of potential problems is wide. Termination of pregnancy should be offered if the diagnosis is made prior to 24 weeks (in the UK) or after this gestation if there is evidence of progressive ventriculomegaly or the presence of additional abnormalities. The outcome for complete and partial ACC is conflicting, with the majority of studies showing no difference in behavioural and medical outcomes between the two. Most children with isolated ACC will have mild behavioural problems.

Dandy–Walker malformation

Dandy–Walker malformation is the most common congenital malformation of the cerebellum, with an incidence of 1 in 5000 births. Classic Dandy–Walker malformation is characterized by absence of the cerebellar vermis accompanied by dilatation of the fourth ventricle and a posterior fossa cyst. The cerebellum itself may be hypoplastic. In the Dandy–Walker variant, the posterior fossa is minimally enlarged; there is partial agenesis of the vermis, the fourth ventricle communicates with the arachnoid space, and no hydrocephalus is present. There is an association with a variety of genetic syndromes, chromosomal abnormalities, infections and environmental teratogens. Associated CNS malformations are present in up to 68% of cases, the most common of which is agenesis or hypoplasia of the corpus callosum. Karyotyping should be offered. In selected cases, particularly if Dandy–Walker variant is suspected, fetal MRI is extremely helpful. Termination of pregnancy is an option regardless of gestation if a classic Dandy–Walker malformation is detected because of the very poor long-term prognosis. The situation is more difficult with isolated Dandy–Walker variant as many of these children may have good long-term outcome. Counselling by a paediatric neurologist is essential.

Holoprosencephaly

Holoprosencephaly (HPE) is a spectrum of congenital malformations involving the brain and face and is characterized by impaired or incomplete midline division of the embryonic forebrain (prosencephalon). HPE has an incidence of 1 in 16000 live births. Only 3% of fetuses with HPE survive to birth. Facial anomalies associated with HPE include cyclopia, ethmocephaly, cebocephaly, median cleft lip, and less severe facial manifestations. Midline facial defects occur in the majority (>80%) of cases. Approximately 40% of live births with HPE have a chromosomal anomaly and trisomy 13 accounts for over half of these cases.

Alobar HPE is the most severe form. There is incomplete division of the cerebral hemispheres with a single midline forebrain ventricle (monoventricle), which often communicates with a dorsal cyst. The interhemispheric fissure and corpus callosum are completely absent. In semi-lobar HPE, there is a failure of separation of the anterior hemispheres, with some separation of the posterior hemispheres. The frontal horns of the lateral ventricle are absent, but posterior horns are present. The corpus callosum is absent anteriorly. In lobar HPE (the mildest form), the cerebral hemispheres are fairly well divided, with fusion of only the most rostral/ventral aspects.

Karyotyping must be offered. Termination of pregnancy should be discussed and offered. Alobar and most cases of semi-lobar HPE are not compatible with prolonged *ex utero* survival. Lobar HPE can be associated with long-term survival and will need evaluation for endocrine abnormalities and/or craniofacial surgery. Genetic counselling is essential and prenatal diagnosis may be an option in selected cases. HPE due to euploid non-syndromic causes have an empiric recurrence risk of 6%.

Ventriculomegaly

Ventriculomegaly is defined as a measurement of the atrium of the posterior or anterior horns of the lateral ventricles of more than 10 mm at any gestation. A measurement above 15 mm is considered severe. Once detected it is important to obtain a detailed history, especially of recent viral illness or significant maternal trauma, family genetic history, previous congenital abnormality or fetal/neonatal thrombocytopenia. Karyotyping should be offered (7–15% risk of aneuploidy). Amniotic fluid should also be sent for viral polymerase chain reaction (PCR) analysis. Maternal blood for infection screening, particularly *Toxoplasma*/cytomegalovirus (CMV) and rubella should be performed. If the ventriculomegaly is associated with intracerebral haemorrhage, evidence of fetal alloimmune thrombocytopenia should be sought (antiplatelet antibodies/HPA typing).

Fetal MRI should be arranged and further review with a paediatric neurologist is essential, particularly if the prognosis is in doubt. Neurodevelopmental outcome for mild isolated ventriculomegaly is variable and in general more than 85% will have normal outcome or minimal delay. However, asymmetric bilateral ventriculomegaly may carry a worse prognosis, with these children at significant risk for behavioural abnormalities. Poor prognostic factors include coexistent cerebral anomalies and progression of the ventriculomegaly. In severe ventriculomegaly, the outcome may still be variable but less than 30% of children will develop normally. Termination of pregnancy should be offered for severe ventriculomegaly (>15 mm), aneuploidy, spina bifida or other associated major malformations. The mode of delivery is on standard obstetric criteria. In the presence of severe macrocephaly, Caesarean section or cephalocentesis may be required. Cephalocentesis is associated with a high incidence of procedural/intrapartum demise.

Neural tube defects

Most neural tube defects are multifactorial in origin, with a genetic component that interacts with a number of environmental risk factors. The ccommonest forms of neural tube defects are referred to as 'open', where the involved neural tissues are exposed to the body surface. They include anencephaly, craniorachischisis and myelomeningocele. Between 2% and 16% of isolated open neural tube defects occur in association with aneuploidy or a single gene defect. If additional structural anomalies are present the risk may be as high as 24%. Anticonvulsant use, mutations in the MTHFR (methylene tetrahydrofolate reductase) gene, maternal hyperthermia, obesity, diabetes mellitus and a previous family history are all risk factors. Recurrence in any subsequent pregnancy can be significantly reduced by taking high-dose (4–5 mg) folic acid periconceptually. Some neural tube defects are lethal (anencephaly, craniorachischisis) whereas others are compatible with long-term survival. However, there is risk of significant morbidity including mobility issues and bladder and bowel dysfunction and counselling by a neurologist is essential.

Gastrointestinal tract anomalies

Duodenal atresia

Duodenal atresia has an incidence of 1 in 5000–10 000 live births. The diagnosis is suspected when ultrasound shows polyhydramnios and a double bubble appearance (due to a dilated stomach and proximal duodenum). Although occasionally seen earlier in gestation, the diagnosis is usually only made after 24 weeks. Approximately 50% of cases of duodenal atresia have associated structural anomalies. Almost 30% are associated with Down's syndrome and other anomalies are usually related to the VACTERL group (*V*ertebral, *A*norectal, *C*ardiac, *T*racheo*E*sohageal, *R*enal and *L*imb). If the diagnosis is suspected on antenatal ultrasound, karyotyping must be offered because of the high risk of Down's syndrome. If aneuploidy is confirmed, termination of pregnancy is an option. Because of the significant risk of polyhydramnios (50%), frequent scans are required and amnioreduction offered if the amniotic fluid index is 40 cm or more or if the patient is symptomatic. Preterm labour occurs in approximately 40% of cases. Delivery should take place in a tertiary centre with neonatal and paediatric surgical facilities.

Meconium ileus/peritonitis

Meconium ileus is impaction of abnormally thick meconium in the distal ileum. Meconium peritonitis occurs when there is *in utero* perforation of bowel resulting in a sterile chemical peritonitis. Ultrasound features of meconium peritonitis include intra-abdominal calcifications, hyperechogenic bowel, ascites and bowel dilatation. Polyhydramnios may also be present. Serial ultrasound scans should be performed to assess progression of bowel dilatation, development of ascites or intra-abdominal cysts and polyhydramnios, which might indicate complicated meconium peritonitis with a 50% chance of requiring neonatal surgery. If these are present, consideration should be given to delivering the baby in a tertiary centre with neonatal surgical facilities.

Parental cystic fibrosis carrier testing and/or invasive fetal testing should be offered. If cystic fibrosis is diagnosed, appropriate genetic counselling should be offered and termination of pregnancy discussed if the diagnosis is made early in pregnancy. Long-term outcome depends on the underlying cause for the meconium peritonitis. In simple isolated meconium peritonitis the prognosis is usually excellent. In infants with cystic fibrosis the long-term outlook is guarded because of other extra-abdominal complications that can develop.

Abdominal wall defects

Omphalocele (exomphalos)

This is a midline anterior abdominal wall defect of variable size characterized by the absence of abdominal muscles, fascia and skin. It can occur in the upper, mid or lower abdomen. A defect in cranial folding results in a high or epigastric omphalocele classically seen in pentalogy of Cantrell (epigastric omphalocele, anterior diaphragmatic defect, sternal cleft and pericardial/cardiac defects). Lateral folding defects result in a mid-abdominal omphalocele and caudal defects cause a hypogastric omphalocele seen in bladder or cloacal exstrophy. The herniated viscera are covered by a membrane consisting of peritoneum on the inner surface, amnion on the outer surface and Wharton's jelly between the two layers. The umbilical cord inserts into the sac and not the body wall. It has an incidence of 1.5–3 per 10 000 births. Most cases are sporadic and are associated with advanced maternal age. It may occur in isolation or associated with aneuploidy (40%) or as part of a genetic syndrome. Smaller defects are more likely to be associated with chromosome abnormalities. Associated abnormalities are common (50–70%), with cardiac lesions predominating (30–40% of cases). Fetal mortality is strongly associated with the presence of additional structural malformations. The diagnosis can be made in the first trimester, although most are detected at mid-trimester anomaly scan. Maternal serum α-fetoprotein is usually raised by an average of 4 multiples of the median.

Once the abnormality has been detected the patient should be referred to a tertiary centre where there are facilities for detailed evaluation of the fetus. Karyotyping and fetal echocardiography should be performed. If macroglossia and other organomegaly are detected, Beckwith–Wiedemann syndrome should be suspected and the cytogenetics laboratory alerted to specifically look for abnormalities in the 11p15 region. Multidisciplinary counselling with paediatric surgeons, neonatologists, paediatric cardiologists and fetal medicine specialists should take place. The parents should be advised about increased incidence of fetal growth restriction, preterm labour and intrauterine death. Delivery should take place in a tertiary centre. Although vaginal delivery is reasonable and does not appear to influence outcome, elective Caesarean section may be preferable in order that delivery takes place in a more controlled environment and timing of neonatal surgery can be better planned. Large omphaloceles are probably best delivered by Caesarean section because of the possibility of trauma or soft tissue dystocia during a vaginal delivery.

The aim of surgery is to reduce the herniated viscera into the abdomen and to close the fascia and skin to create a solid abdominal wall with a relatively normal umbilicus. However, treatment can vary depending on the size and type of defect, the size of the baby, and any associated neonatal problems. Most surgeons prefer primary closure whenever possible. Nevertheless, large defects with significant visceral herniation may require a more gradual or phased approach using silos to achieve reduction over a period of time before the abdominal wall is finally closed.

Gastroschisis

This anomaly is believed to result secondary to an ischaemic insult to the developing abdominal wall. There is a full-thickness defect that occurs secondary to incomplete closure of the lateral folds during the sixth week of gestation. The right paraumbilical area is usually affected. The incidence of gastroschisis is 0.4–3 per 10 000 births and appears to be increasing. It has a strong association with young maternal age (<20 years), cigarette smoking, illicit drugs (cocaine), vasoactive over-the-counter drugs (such as pseudoephedrine) and environmental toxins. The diagnosis is usually obvious on ultrasound, with free floating bowel or rarely the liver floating in the amniotic fluid without a covering membrane. Differential diagnoses include ruptured omphalocele sac or limb–body wall complex.

Associated anomalies occur in 10–20% of cases and most of these are in the gastrointestinal tract. Chromosomal abnormalities or genetic syndromes are very rare. There is a slight increase in the incidence of cardiac abnormalities but this is not as high as seen in omphalocele. There is an increased incidence of preterm labour (30%), fetal growth restriction (70%), oligohydramnios (25%) and fetal death. The cause of fetal growth failure is unclear but could be partially due to increased protein loss from the exposed viscera. The herniated bowel is at risk from volvulus and long segment necrosis and/or more localized atretic and stenotic segments. Increasing bowel dilatation, progressive oligohydramnios or decreased growth velocity may all be indicative of a fetus that is at increased risk of intrauterine death or greater neonatal complications. Early referral to a tertiary centre with multidisciplinary management is essential. Fetal echocardiography should be performed because of the increased association with cardiac anomalies. Serial scans should be performed to assess fetal growth and liquor volume, degree of bowel dilatation and bowel wall thickness. There is no contraindication for vaginal delivery but, as for omphalocele, elective Caesarean section may also be an option to facilitate neonatal care. Overall survival is good (90–95%), with most deaths occurring in babies who have significant bowel loss, sepsis or long-term complications of short bowel syndrome. There is a 10% risk of hypoperistalsis syndrome, which may require longer hospitalization and hyperalimentation. Gastrointestinal reflux occurs in 10% of cases and there is a 5–10% risk of obstruction due to adhesions in the longer term. A significant number of cases will also develop inguinal hernias due to increased intra-abdominal pressure after surgery. The risk of recurrence is small but exposure to vasoactive substances should be avoided in any subsequent pregnancy.

Genitourinary tract anomalies

Congenital anomalies of the kidney and urinary tract account for one-third of all anomalies detected by routine fetal ultrasonography. In humans, fetal glomeruli develop by 8–9 weeks, tubular function commences after week 14 and nephrogenesis is largely complete by birth. After 20 weeks, the kidneys provide over 90% of the amniotic fluid. Any bilateral renal malformation can be associated with oligohydramnios/anhydramnios, lung hypoplasia, joint contractures and facial abnormalities collectively termed the Potter sequence.

Renal agenesis

Unilateral renal agenesis has an incidence of 1 in 500–1000 births compared with bilateral renal agenesis which occurs in 1 in 5000–10 000 births. Bilateral renal agenesis is not compatible with extrauterine life. It occurs more commonly in males and there is also an increased incidence in twins. Poorly controlled maternal diabetes or ingestion of renotoxic drugs are other aetiologic factors. The diagnosis is usually made at the mid-trimester fetal anomaly scan. Although earlier diagnosis is sometimes possible, it is often difficult in the first trimester as the amniotic fluid volume is not significantly reduced at that stage. Anhydramnios is usually present by mid-trimester in bilateral renal agenesis. The liquor volume is usually normal in unilateral agenesis and the normal kidney can be larger due to compensatory hypertrophy.

There is an increased incidence of additional anomalies particularly in the genital (blind vagina, uterine malformations, seminal vesicle cysts), cardiovascular and gastrointestinal systems in up to 44% of fetuses with renal agenesis. If the diagnosis of bilateral renal agenesis is made antenatally, the parents must be counselled about the dismal outcome and offered termination of pregnancy. Karyotyping and post-mortem is essential to help diagnose aneuploidy or a specific syndrome. Ultrasound of parental kidneys should be considered and genetic counselling offered. The risk of recurrence is low in unilateral renal agenesis (2–4%) but can be as high as 6–10% in bilateral cases.

Multicystic dysplastic kidney

Unilateral multicystic dysplastic kidney (MCDK) has an incidence of 1 in 3000–5000 live births compared with 1 in 10 000 for bilateral dysplasia. It is one of the commonest causes of an abdominal mass in the neonatal period. The abnormal kidneys contain undifferentiated cells and metaplastic elements such as cartilage. On ultrasound, large hyperechogenic kidneys containing multiple cysts of varying sizes are present. Contralateral renal abnormalities can occur in 30–50% of cases. The prognosis for the fetus depends on whether there is unilateral or bilateral dysplasia. Bilateral MCDK is often lethal, with fetuses dying from pulmonary hypoplasia after birth. Termination of pregnancy should be offered in these cases.

No specific fetal intervention is required in cases of isolated unilateral MCDK. Serial ultrasound scans to monitor size of the abnormal kidney and liquor volume should be performed. Occasionally gradual resorption (autonephrectomy) of the abnormal kidney can occur. Karyotyping should be offered to exclude aneuploidy. The mode of delivery is based on standard obstetric criteria. The prognosis is usually good. There is a small risk of long-term hypertension and malignant transformation in the dysplastic kidney.

Lower urinary tract obstruction

In male fetuses, posterior urethral valves are the most common cause (90%) of bladder outlet obstruction. In female fetuses, urethral atresia accounts for the majority of cases. Oligohydramnios and a large thick-walled bladder with a keyhole sign and bilateral hydroureters and hydronephrosis are usually evident on ultrasound. Other causes of lower urinary tract obstruction are prune belly syndrome and urethral atresia. The prognosis is worse (95% mortality) in those diagnosed antenatally when mid-trimester oligohydramnios is present. Features that suggest poor prognosis include dilatation of the upper tract, increased bladder wall thickness, oligohydramnios and evidence of renal dysplasia (echogenic renal cortex and cystic renal change), especially before 24 weeks. Obstruction can be complete or partial and the amount of liquor volume usually gives some idea as to the severity of the obstruction. In complete obstruction anhydramnios rapidly develops. In addition, renal dysplasia can occur from an early gestation if the obstruction is severe. Karyotyping is important as aneuploidy is present in up to 10% of cases. Termination of pregnancy is an option, particularly if there is severe oligohydramnios/anhydramnios, the diagnosis is made early in pregnancy or if there is evidence of renal dysplasia on ultrasound.

Fetal therapy is possible, although there are no randomized trials as to the efficacy of any particular option. Treatment can include serial vesicocentesis, percutaneous vesico-amniotic shunting or cystoscopy (experimental). The rationale for vesico-amniotic shunting is to decompress the urinary tract and therefore relieve the back-pressure on the fetal kidneys and to hopefully prevent the development of renal dysplasia. Shunting also allows restoration of flow of fetal urine into the amniotic cavity and thus prevents pulmonary hypoplasia. The risk of requiring dialysis and subsequent renal failure is approximately 30–50% is several series. Additional long-term problems include reflux, recurrent infections, bladder compliance and voiding issues, and sexual function.

Head and neck anomalies

Cleft lip and palate

The incidence of cleft lip and palate varies with ethnicity and geographical region but in a white population it is approximately 1 in 800–1000 for cleft lip and palate and 1 in 100 for cleft palate alone. Orofacial clefts can be classified as non-syndromic (isolated) or syndromic based on the presence of other congenital anomalies. Approximately 20–50% of all orofacial clefts are believed to be syndromic. The aetiology of cleft lip/cleft palate is complex and multifactorial, involving both genetic and environmental factors. Many environmental factors are associated with orofacial clefting, including maternal alcohol consumption and cigarette smoking. Folate deficiency is also associated with cleft lip/cleft palate and prenatal folic acid supplementation has been shown to decrease this risk. Maternal corticosteroid use causes a threefold to fourfold increase in orofacial clefting. Anticonvulsants, including phenytoin and valproic acid, also cause cleft lip and palate. Phenytoin causes a nearly 10-fold increase in the incidence of facial clefting.

Associated anomalies include brain, cardiac and limb/spine deformities. There is a high risk of cerebral anomaly with midline clefts. Karyotyping should be offered in all cases. All patients should be promptly referred to a multidisciplinary craniofacial team following fetal diagnosis, where all aspects of the baby's management including feeding, surgery and cosmetic results can be discussed with parents. It is important to exclude any underlying syndrome after birth and genetic counselling for the risk of recurrence should be offered.

Cystic hygroma/lymphangioma

Cystic hygroma is a rare congenital malformation of the lymphatic system and has an incidence of 1 in 6000–16 000 births. Among aborted fetuses the incidence may be as high as 1 in 300. Approximately 75% occur in the neck, usually in the posterior triangle more commonly on the left side and 20% occur in the axillary region. Chromosome abnormalities are present in almost 70% of cases, with Turner's syndrome and Down's syndrome particularly common. There is also an association with non-chromosomal conditions (Noonan's syndrome, multiple pterygium syndrome). Once detected a careful search for additional abnormalities is vital. Karyotyping should always be offered. The presence of hydrops is a poor prognostic feature, with a perinatal mortality rate above 80%. Fetal echocardiography should be performed. There is an increased incidence of preterm labour and polyhydramnios particularly if the cystic hygroma impairs fetal swallowing. In very large lesions obstruction of the pharynx and larynx may develop making intubation very difficult. The EXIT procedure (*ex utero* intrapartum treatment) may be required before the umbilical cord is divided.

Skeletal system anomalies

Skeletal dysplasias are a heterogeneous group of genetic disorders characterized by differences in the size, shape and mineralization of the skeletal system that frequently result in disproportionate short stature. The diagnosis is usually made by clinical features, radiological criteria, family history and, increasingly, by genetic testing. It is estimated that 30–45 per 100 000 newborns have a skeletal dysplasia. Antenatal management depends on identifying the presence of a skeletal dysplasia and making an assessment of the lethality of the condition. Karyotyping should be offered, particularly in the presence of other abnormalities. DNA should be stored for future genetic testing. A precise diagnosis often needs to await postnatal or post-abortal radiology or molecular testing. Most cases of skeletal dysplasias are autosomal recessive, for which genetic counselling is important. Others may be due to a new dominant mutation. Family history of skeletal dysplasia, malformations and short stature should be obtained. Termination of pregnancy is an option for most cases of skeletal dysplasia as many have a poor outcome. A narrow thorax in particular indicates a high chance of lethal pulmonary hypoplasia. Specific genetic mutations are known for some skeletal dysplasias (achondroplasia and thanatophoric dysplasia, *FGFR3* mutation; campomelic dysplasia, *SOX9* mutation; diastrophic dysplasia, *DTDST* mutation; osteogenesis imperfecta, *COL1A* or *COL2A* mutation) and therefore prenatal diagnosis may be possible in selected cases.

Thoracic anomalies

Pulmonary development requires normal fetal breathing movements, an adequate intrathoracic space, sufficient amniotic fluid, normal intra-lung fluid volume and pulmonary blood flow. Maternal health, including nutrition, endocrine factors, smoking and disease, can also adversely influence fetal lung development. There are five stages of lung development: embryonic (0–7 weeks *in utero*), pseudoglandular (7–17 weeks *in utero*), canalicular (17–27 weeks *in utero*), saccular (28–36 weeks *in utero*) and alveolar (36 weeks *in utero* to 2 years postnatal).

Diaphragmatic hernia

Congenital diaphragmatic hernia has an incidence of 1 in 3000–5000 births. The combination of lung hypoplasia, lung immaturity and pulmonary hypertension can result in high mortality for this condition. The degree of pulmonary hypoplasia depends entirely on the length of time and extent the herniated organs have compressed the fetal lungs. Associated abnormalities may be present in 30–60% of cases and can involve any organ system. Aneuploidy is present in 10–20% of cases and it may also be associated with some genetic syndromes (Fryn's syndrome, Beckwith–Wiedemann syndrome). Congenital diaphragmatic hernia should be suspected if the fetal stomach is not in its usual intra-abdominal position. Liver, mesentery and bowel and spleen may be present in the chest. Differential diagnoses include congenital cystic adenomatoid malformations, bronchogenic cysts, pulmonary sequestration or thoracic teratomas. Polyhydramnios and/or hydrops may sometimes be present. Increased liquor is usually due to impaired swallowing and hydrops may occur if there is significant cardiac compression. Liver herniation is a poor predictive factor for the development of pulmonary hypoplasia.

Management includes detailed assessment of the fetus for additional anomalies, karyotyping and fetal echocardiography. Fetal MRI or three-dimensional ultrasound can sometimes be considered to evaluate lung volume. Parents should be counselled by a paediatric surgeon regarding neonatal management. Termination of pregnancy is an option if significant visceral herniation (particularly liver) is present. The aim is to deliver at term. The mode of delivery is made on standard obstetric criteria. However, it is essential that delivery takes place in a tertiary centre where the baby can be closely monitored to assess the degree of pulmonary compromise (hypoplasia and vascular hypertension) before surgery is undertaken.

Cystic congenital adenomatoid malformation

Cystic congenital adenomatoid malformation (CCAM) is characterized by lack of normal alveoli and excessive proliferation and cystic dilatation of terminal respiratory bronchioles. The incidence of CCAM is 1 in 11 000–35 000 live births and the condition is slightly more common in males. CCAMs are usually unilateral (>85%) and usually involve only one lobe of the lung; 60% are left-sided lesions. The diagnosis is usually made on antenatal ultrasound by the detection of enlarged hyperechogenic lungs sometimes containing cysts of varying sizes. Mediastinal shift, cardiac compression, polyhydramnios and hydrops may also be present. Between 45 and 85% of prenatally identified CCAMs will spontaneously regress. However, large macrocystic or solid lesions can cause hydrops, pulmonary hypoplasia, cardiac dysfunction and perinatal death. The majority of fetal CCAMs follow a characteristic growth pattern that is highly dependent on gestational age. There is usually an increase in size between 17 and 26 weeks before possible regression after 30 weeks. Large lesions can cause pulmonary hypoplasia, impairment of fetal swallowing and polyhydramnios, cardiac compression and hydrops. Serial scans are essential to monitor the size of the lesion (particularly macrocystic CCAM), the development of cardiac compression and/or hydrops. In selected cases fetal therapy (either aspiration of the cyst or insertion of a shunt to drain the cyst) may be an option. The mode and timing of delivery is on standard obstetric criteria. Postnatally the baby will require careful monitoring and a chest X-ray. Surgery may be deferred for up to 24 months.

Pleural effusions

Fetal pleural effusions have an incidence of 1 in 10000–15000 pregnancies. Effusions may be primary (due to leak of chyle into the pleural cavity) or secondary (seen in hydrops). Complications include mediastinal shift, cardiac compression, hydrops and pulmonary hypoplasia (Plate 20.1). Affected fetuses are at significant risk for respiratory distress at birth. Once detected the patient should be referred to a fetal medicine unit for further investigations. The presence of other anomalies should be excluded. Fetal echocardiography should be performed as cardiac abnormalities are present in 5% of cases. Karyotyping should be offered as there is a significant association (10%) with aneuploidy. Maternal serology for infection should be performed. Serial scans should be arranged to assess the size of the effusion. The development of hydrops or polyhydramnios is a poor prognostic feature. There are several treatment options. Firstly, a period of expectant observation is reasonable if the fetus is not hydropic and the effusion is small or moderate in size. Thoracocentesis or pleuro-amniotic shunting are other options. The risks associated with pleuro-amniotic shunting include miscarriage or preterm labour, rupture of membranes, blockage of the shunt and shunt migration. Survival after pleuro-amniotic shunting is approximately 80%.

Fetal tumours

Teratomas

Teratomas are tumours that contain tissue from all three germinal layers (ectoderm, mesoderm and endoderm). Most prenatally diagnosed teratomas are situated in the brain, oropharynx, sacrococcygeal region, mediastinum, abdomen and gonad. Teratomas are the most common perinatal tumour, comprising 37–52% of congenital neoplasms and having a yearly incidence of approximately 1 in 40000 live births. The majority of teratomas occur in the sacrococcygeal region (60%), followed by the gonads (20%) and thoraco-abdominal lesions (15%).

Sacrococcygeal teratomas are the most common neoplasm in the fetus and newborn, with an estimated prevalence of 1 in 30000–40000. There is a 3:1 female preponderance. The diagnosis is often made when a complex mass is detected at the base of the spine. It can be either predominantly solid and vascular or predominantly cystic with relatively little vascularity, or mixed with equal amounts of solid and cystic structures. Associated anomalies are present in 10–40% of cases. Arteriovenous shunting through the vascular component of the tumour can result in hydrops, polyhydramnios and high-output cardiac failure. Poor prognostic factors include large solid tumours (>10 cm), hydrops and polyhydramnios. Other complications include gastrointestinal or bladder outlet obstruction. Most sacrococcygeal teratomas are histologically benign, with malignancy more common in solid tumours and in males.

Tumour dystocia, rupture and haemorrhage during delivery are the main causes of perinatal morbidity and mortality. Additionally, polyhydramnios can precipitate preterm delivery. Maternal complications including pre-eclampsia (mirror syndrome) can occur if there is significant placentomegaly and hydrops. Delivery should take place in a tertiary centre with facilities for immediate surgery. Elective Caesarean section should be the mode of delivery, with particular care taken during delivery to avoid trauma to the tumour. Blood should be available in the delivery room in case of tumour haemorrhage.

Fetal hydrops

Hydrops is an end-stage process for a number of fetal diseases resulting in tissue oedema and/or fluid collection (ascites, pleural effusion, pericardial effusion) in various sites (Fig. 20.2). Its aetiology may be either immune or non-immune depending on the presence or absence of red cell alloimmunization. Non-immune causes now account for more than 90% of all cases of hydrops. Congenital heart abnormalities, cardiac arrhythmias (supraventricular tachycardia, complete heart block), twin–twin transfusion syndrome, congenital anomalies, aneuploidy, infections, congenital anaemia and congenital chylothorax are all possible causes for hydrops. Regardless of the aetiology, hydrops has a very poor outcome (>80% mortality). Early development of hydrops has a particularly poor prognosis. The

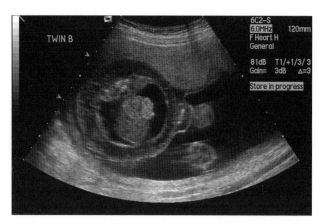

Fig. 20.2 Severe hydrops with skin oedema and ascites.

mortality rate is highest among neonates with congenital anomalies (60%) and lowest among neonates with congenital chylothorax (6%). Mortality is significantly higher in premature infants and those delivered in poor condition.

It is important to obtain a detailed family, medical, obstetric and genetic history. A history of prior exposure to possible viral infections (maternal rash, arthralgia/myalgia) is especially important. Detailed ultrasound to detect structural abnormalities, particularly cardiac and thoracic abnormalities, should be performed. The umbilical cord and placenta should be carefully examined to exclude vascular malformations. The fetal heart rate and rhythm should be examined to exclude fetal tachyarrhythmias or bradyarrhythmias. Maternal blood should be taken for full viral screen (CMV, parvovirus, rubella, herpes), *Toxoplasma* serology, blood group and antibody screen and haemoglobin electrophoresis. Fetal anaemia should be excluded by middle cerebral artery peak systolic velocity monitoring. Fetal echocardiography should be performed in all cases. If anaemia is suspected the most likely cause is parvovirus infection. This is a treatable condition usually requiring a single fetal transfusion. Karyotyping is mandatory in all cases. Samples should be sent for cytogenetics and infection screen using PCR. If hydrops is secondary to fetal arrhythmia, maternal antiarrhythmic therapy may be of benefit. There is usually a delay in response because of the slow transplacental transfer into the fetal circulation. Occasionally, direct fetal treatment may be required in cases of fetal supraventricular tachycardia unresponsive to maternal treatment. If the hydrops is secondary to a structural anomaly (e.g. pleural effusion), *in utero* therapy (pleuroamniotic shunting) may be necessary. Termination of pregnancy should be offered if hydrops is severe or if major malformations or aneuploidy is present. Parents should be counselled that untreated hydrops carries a very high perinatal mortality rate and that outcome is likely to be poor.

Conclusions

When a fetal structural anomaly is identified, regardless of gestation, there are several key issues that must be considered. Firstly, it is crucial to remember that to the pregnant woman the detection of any anomaly is a source of great anxiety and stress. Women should receive information regarding the abnormal ultrasound findings in a clear, sympathetic and timely fashion, and in a supportive environment that ensures privacy. Whenever appropriate, referral to a tertiary fetal medicine unit should be made. A full and frank discussion with a senior obstetrician or fetal medicine specialist is important to explain the diagnosis and further management of the pregnancy. Further testing (amniocentesis, chorionic villous sampling or fetal blood sampling) may be required. More complex imaging with fetal MRI may sometimes help delineate anatomy (particularly for CNS anomalies). Additional counselling by a genetic counsellor or geneticist may be necessary. Counselling should always be unbiased and respectful of the patient's choice, culture, religion and beliefs.

In many cases serial scans will be necessary to assess evolution of the abnormality and to attempt to detect other anomalies not previously identified, as this may influence counselling as well as the obstetric or neonatal management. In some cases parental imaging and testing may be required. Referral to an appropriate paediatric or surgical specialist should be considered to enable the woman to receive the most accurate information possible concerning the anomaly and the associated prognosis. It may be important to stress that, not infrequently, both major and minor structural anomalies, whether isolated or multiple, may sometimes be part of a genetic syndrome (despite a normal fetal karyotype) and that long-term prognosis will depend on the final diagnosis. Critically, it is important to stress that antenatal ultrasound is geared towards evaluating anatomy rather than function and that sometimes normal anatomy does not always correlate with normal function and vice versa.

Although fetal therapy is possible for some conditions, it is generally not an option for the majority of fetal structural anomalies. If early or urgent postnatal management is required, delivery at a centre that can provide the appropriate neonatal care should be considered. In cases of termination of pregnancy, stillbirth or neonatal death, the health professional should encourage the performance of a complete post-mortem by a perinatal pathologist to provide maximum information about the fetal anomaly. If this is refused, at least a partial or external post-mortem (including X-rays and photographs) should be considered.

Summary box 20.2

- When an abnormality is detected consider further investigations, including karyotyping, parental testing, fetal MRI and fetal echocardiography.
- Counselling should be non-directive, sympathetic and wherever possible should include a paediatric specialist.
- For some conditions termination of pregnancy is an option but it must be broached sensitively.
- The importance of a post-mortem should be explained to parents.
- When appropriate, genetic input should be arranged.
- Pre-pregnancy counselling may be helpful for some parents.

Further reading

NHS Fetal Anomaly Screening Programme. *18+0 to 20+6 Weeks Fetal Anomaly Scan: National Standards and Guidance for England*. Royal College of Obstetricians and Gynaecologists, 2010. Available at: http://fetalanomaly.screening.nhs.uk/getdata.php?id=11218

Chapter 21
Multiple Pregnancy

Mark D. Kilby[1,2] *and Dick Oepkes*[3]

[1]School of Clinical and Experimental Medicine, College of Medical and Dental Sciences, University of Birmingham, Birmingham, UK

[2]Fetal Medicine Centre, Birmingham Women's Foundation Trust, Birmingham, UK

[3]Department of Obstetrics, Leiden University Medical Centre, Leiden, Netherlands

Multiple pregnancy has a global impact on both maternal and perinatal risk in any pregnancy and impacts on society in terms of both social and economic effects. Improvements in the health of the population, and in particular perinatal care, have led to a reduction in overall total pregnancy complications (both maternal and perinatal). However, the proportion of these attributed to twins and higher-order pregnancies is increasing and of significant importance. Almost every maternal and obstetric problem occurs more frequently in a multiple pregnancy and there are, in addition, a number of potential intrapartum considerations that complicate routine management. The modern management of a multiple pregnancy initially concentrates on the recognition of fetal risk, as mediated primarily by chorionicity, and then the monitoring of fetal growth and well-being using ultrasound. Attempts to reduce the risks of preterm delivery and pre-eclampsia in the mother are equally important and equally as frustrating (as in singleton pregnancy care), with little improvement in overall management of these conditions in the last 20 years. Recognizing the specialized nature of multiple pregnancy management has led to the publication of recommendations by two scientific study groups of the Royal College of Obstetricians and Gynaecologists (RCOG) [1,2] and the commissioning of recommendations of care for multiple pregnancies by the National Institute of Health and Clinical Excellence (NICE) in 2009 [3]. At the heart of care is the recommendation that such pregnancies are managed within specialist multidisciplinary teams and in designated multiple pregnancy clinics so as to organize antenatal, intrapartum and indeed postnatal care.

Incidence

The considerable geographical and temporal variation in multiple pregnancy incidence reflects factors including dizygotic twinning as the result of multiple ovulation [4]. The incidence of twinning ranges from 4 per 1000 births in Japan to as frequent as 54 per 1000 in some regions of Nigeria. In addition, this 'complication' is more prevalent in pregnancies with advancing maternal age (presumed to be secondary to the rise in follicle-stimulating hormone concentrations). Familial predisposition to multiple ovulations (dizygous twining) may occur and is presently best explained by an autosomal dominant inheritance pattern. In contrast, monozygous twinning, the result of early cleavage division of a single blastocyst, occurs with a relatively constant incidence of approximately 3.9 per 1000.

Time trends of multiple pregnancy demonstrate a remarkable change in reproductive behaviour and consequence. Some of the first documented records from Scandinavia in the eighteenth century indicate that multiple pregnancy rates may have been higher then than they are today, reaching a zenith of 17 per 1000 maternities [5]. However, during the twentieth century, twin pregnancy rates appeared to be in decline until the early 1970s, since when there has been a clear rise in prevalence [6]. Since the early 1980s, the twinning rate in the UK has risen from 9.8 to 13.6 and the triplet rate from 0.14 to 0.44 per 1000 maternities. Such an increase is reflected internationally, with the greatest rise being noted in the USA (Fig. 21.1). Multiple pregnancies accounted for 1.6% of all births in the UK during 2007, with approximately 98% of these being twin births [7]. A considerable proportion of the increase is due to assisted reproductive technologies, such as super-ovulation (using antioestrogens or gonadotrophins) and *in vitro* fertilization (IVF) with embryo transfer. There is evidence that the number of multiple pregnancies is influenced by the number of embryo transfers and, as such, the number of multiple pregnancies associated with IVF has reduced since the recommendation that embryo transfer numbers be reduced (in the UK, at least). In addition, epidemiological evidence suggests that both types of assisted reproduction techniques increase the incidence of monozygous twinning by up to eightfold [8]. This is particularly associated with the techniques of 'blastocyst hatching'. Monochorionic twins

Dewhurst's Textbook of Obstetrics & Gynaecology, Eighth Edition. Edited by D. Keith Edmonds.
© 2012 John Wiley and Sons, Ltd. Published 2012 by John Wiley and Sons, Ltd.

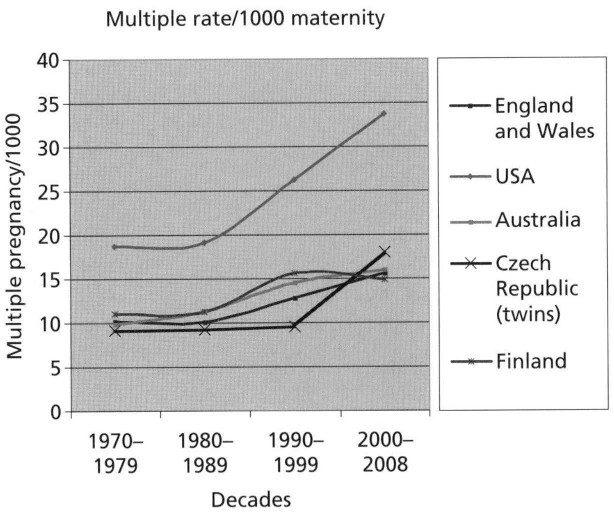

Multiple rate/1000 maternity

Fig. 21.1 Changes in multiple birth rates (all modes of conception) internationally. (From the Office of National Statistics, 2010, with permission.)

comprise 20% of spontaneous and 5% of iatrogenic twin gestations. This is important as monochorionic twins have the greatest pregnancy-related complication rates.

However, it is also important to recognize other influences. The association between increasing maternal age (strongest at 30–39 years) and spontaneous dizygous twinning is worthy of note. The combined effects of delayed childbearing and high uptakes of assisted reproductive technologies at advanced maternal age have been responsible for this rise [9].

Perinatal wastage

Cumulative fetal loss rate in twins is up to five times higher (and in triplets 10 times higher) than in corresponding singleton pregnancies. Rates of stillbirth and neonatal mortality for a multiple pregnancy are 14.9 and 19.8 per 1000 live births, respectively. This high perinatal wastage and morbidity is largely attributed to the increased risk of prematurity and also intrauterine growth restriction (IUGR) with associated iatrogenic prematurity (irrespective of chorionicity, see below).

Cerebral palsy is approximately three times more common in twins and 10 times more common in triplets compared with singletons. These figures are per fetus, whereas the more relevant figure when counselling parents is the chance of their multiple pregnancies producing any one baby with these complications.

Chorionicity and zygosity

Approximately two-thirds of twins are dizygous and one-third monozygous. However, it is chorionicity rather than zygosity that mediates the degree of perinatal risk in any individual multiple pregnancy. This is most important as it is clinically identifiable. Cumulative fetal loss rates and perinatal mortality are up to five times higher in monochorionic twins compared with dichorionic twins [10]. This study, and a more contemporary one (during a period when modern management was possible including more widespread recognition of feto-fetal transfusion syndrome and its fetoscopically directed treatment [11]), noted that in monochorionic diamniotic twin pregnancies, 85% resulted in double survivors, 7.5% in a single survivor and 7.5% in no surviving baby. These deaths occurred spontaneously or iatrogenically. Perinatal morbidity appears similarly related, with prenatal acquired cerebral lesions evident in the early neonatal period on ultrasound in up to one-third of monochorionic twins compared with 3% of dichorionic twins delivered preterm [12]. Such excess morbidity and mortality is mediated predominantly (but not exclusively) through the inter-twin placental vascular anastomoses that connect the two fetal circulations.

The relationship between zygosity and chorionicity is demonstrated in Fig. 21.2. Monozygotic pregnancies assume one of three placental configurations. Division within 3 days of fertilization results in separate dichorionic placentae, which in up to 50% of cases may have the appearance on ultrasound of being adjacent to each other and 'fused'. Splitting after formation of the inner cell mass at 4 days after fertilization results in a single monochorionic diamniotic placenta, whereas splitting after 7 days results in monochorionic monoamniotic twins. Approximately one in five of all twins are monochorionic.

Ultrasonic determination of chorionicity

Chorionicity may be clinically determined during pregnancy using ultrasound, with up to 90–100% accuracy in the first trimester. Ultrasound allows the following features to be ascertained.

• Determination of the number of constituent layers of the dividing membranes (and therefore of membrane thickness).
• Qualitative interpretation of the membrane as 'thick' (dichorionic) or 'thin' (monochorionic) appears as accurate as inter-twin membrane/septal measurement.
• Demonstration of a tongue of placental tissue within the base of the inter-twin membrane, known as the 'twin peak' sign, is diagnostic of a dichorionic pregnancy. In contrast, a thin septum with a single placental mass is suggestive of monochorionicity.
• Presence (or not) of a single placental mass.

Chorionicity should be determined on ultrasound in all multiple pregnancies, as a screening test, ideally within the first trimester between 11 and 14 weeks of gestation (when specificity and sensitivity are greatest). A digital or hardcopy image(s) should be stored demonstrating the

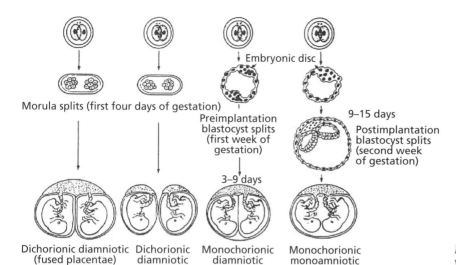

Dichorionic diamniotic (fused placentae)   Dichorionic diamniotic   Monochorionic diamniotic   Monochorionic monoamniotic

Fig. 21.2 Zygosity and chorionicity. (From Ward and Whittle [1] with permission.)

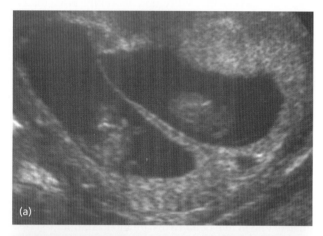

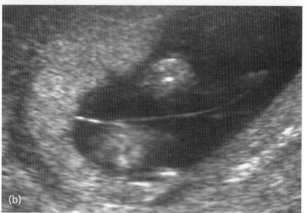

Fig. 21.3 (a, b) First-trimester ultrasound determination of chorionicity. (From Ward and Whittle [1] with permission.)

signs of chorionicity (Fig. 21.3). This is because chorionicity is relevant to:
- counselling parents in relation to the risk of perinatal morbidity and mortality;
- counselling parents in relation to their risk of genetic and structural abnormalities;
- invasive testing and the management of discordant congenital anomaly;
- feasibility of multiple fetal pregnancy reduction;
- risk of complications that may occur in a multiple pregnancy and potential sequelae that may ensue;
- early detection and management of feto-fetal transfusion syndrome.

Such an examination should be routine and allow the stratification of prospective pregnancy care. In addition, ultrasonic visualization of the inter-twin membrane/septum and genitalia may be difficult later on in pregnancy or when there is significant oligohydramnios complicating the pregnancy. The first ultrasound allocation of chorionicity should be performed in the first trimester between 11 and 14 weeks at a time when increasing numbers of pregnancies are undergoing nuchal translucency screening [13]. Ultrasonic sexing is performed for medical rather than social reasons in multiple pregnancies and, as such, achieves a high degree of accuracy, usually between 16 and 20 weeks.

Zygosity determination

Monochorionic twins by definition are monozygotic, while discordant sex twins are dizygous. In the remaining 50%, zygosity cannot be determined without DNA fingerprinting, such as the polymerase chain reaction technique that compares parental inheritance patterns of a number of dinucleotide and trinucleotide short tandem repeats which are highly polymorphic in copy number. Such determination is rarely performed prospectively in clinical practice. Just as placental chorionicity is rechecked at birth (usually by clinical or histopathological examination), cord blood zygosity studies may be offered to parents of twins where there is indeterminate zygosity. Not only are parents curious but knowledge of zygosity influences the twins' rearing, their sense of identity, their genetic risks and their transplantation compatibility.

However, it is not routine to offer this in current practice within the NHS in the UK. Rarely there may be indications for zygosity testing *in utero* on invasive collection of fetal tissue, such as excluding contamination, deducing genetic risk or demonstrating dichorionicity in the presence of fetal compromise.

Miscarriage

Twins have a high incidence of spontaneous early pregnancy loss. Estimates suggest that approximately 12% of human conceptions start as twins [14]. Studies of ultrasound or miscarriage pathology indicate that twins are found at least twice as commonly in the first trimester as at birth. First-trimester early pregnancy loss and resorption of one previously indefinable twin on ultrasound is known as the 'vanishing twin' phenomenon and is estimated to occur in up to 20% of twin pregnancies [15]. Spontaneous first-trimester loss of one or more fetuses in high-order pregnancies is estimated to occur approximately 50% of the time. When one twin dies *in utero* in mid-trimester, a papyraceous fetus (the squashed paper-like remains of the baby) may be found alongside the placenta after delivery. In some cases, this is only identifiable histopathologically.

Prenatal diagnosis

The widespread use of ultrasound in the first trimester and for routine mid-trimester anomaly scanning to detect structural congenital malformations and Down's syndrome is relevant to all multiple pregnancies. Zygosity determines the risk of congenital abnormality and chorionicity what can be done if it is found to be present.

Zygosity may be deduced definitively in cases of monochorionicity or discordant external genitalia (dizygous), while in dichorionic concordant-sex twins the chance of dizygosity is 75–80%. Monozygous twins have a 50% increase in structural abnormalities per baby. In particular, they have twice the frequency of congenital heart disease (a fourfold increase per pregnancy). Women with dizygous twins can be counselled that the chance of their pregnancy producing a child with Down's syndrome is theoretically double their age-related risk, whereas women with monozygous twins simply have their age-related risk that both twins will be aneuploid. Serum screening is, in general, inapplicable to multiple pregnancies. In contrast, nuchal translucency and first-trimester ultrasound scanning as a fetal-specific screening test is readily applicable and recommended by the National Screening Committee in the UK. At 18–24 weeks, women with multiple pregnancies should be offered a mid-trimester fetal anomaly scan (which includes visu-alization of the four chambers of the heart and the great vessel outflow tracts) irrespective of chorionicity (as in singleton pregnancies). In addition, in the first trimester between 11 and 13 + 6 weeks, all women with multiple pregnancies should be offered nuchal translucency screening for the detection of chromosome anomalies (as well as the formal documentation of chorionicity). In dichorionic twins, the risk of aneuploidy is that of each of the individual fetuses. In monochorionic twin pregnancies, the risk of aneuploidy is the average between the twins. The use of first-trimester serum screening as an adjunct to nuchal translucency, taking chorionicity into account, may slightly improve detection rates for Down's syndrome in twins, but the results of large prospective studies are awaited [16].

Invasive procedures

Invasive procedures in twins and other higher-order multiple pregnancies are potentially complex procedures and should only be performed in fetal medicine referral centres [17]. The *in utero* topography (placental and membranes) is mapped using ultrasound. The location of fetuses, the placental site(s) and the plane of the dividing septum in three dimensions should be noted and recorded. Such is a prerequisite for interpretation of discordant results and for selective termination of pregnancy. The operator performing the diagnostic procedure should also undertake any selective termination so as to minimize uncertainty and obviate any need for confirmatory invasive testing.

In monochorionic twins, it is acceptable practice to sample only one fetus by either amniocentesis or chorionic villous sampling (CVS). However, rare cases of heterokaryotypic monochorionic twins may be missed (occurring in <1%). For this reason, amniocentesis on both amniotic sacs is worthy of consideration if monochorionic twins are discordant for structural anomalies, nuchal translucencies or growth.

In dichorionic twins, there has been controversy about whether CVS is less desirable than amniocentesis for performing karyotyping. Because of problems with contamination, some investigators suggest restricting CVS to high-risk cases such as monogenic disease or where there is an aneuploidy risk of greater than 1 in 50. The risk of contamination is likely to be higher than the published figures (2%) since the literature is confined to discordant-sex twins. Any benefits of CVS are outweighed by the potentially disastrous consequences of misdiagnosis due to contamination, with subsequent termination of a diploid fetus or the wrongful birth of a fetus with a chromosome abnormality. For these reasons, the RCOG guidelines [17] discuss potential advantages to amniocentesis as the preferred option for karyotyping in dichorionic twins. Such a decision has to be weighed against the increased risks of selective reduction at increased gestational ages.

When performing fetal blood sampling, the intrahepatic vein may be sampled to avoid confusing the cord origins in twins.

There are no randomized controlled trials to indicate procedure-related loss rates in twins. However, background loss rates are appreciably higher. Recent data suggest that total fetal loss rate in twins is up to 4% after amniocentesis and between 2 and 4% for CVS. A case–control study of 220 twins undergoing mid-trimester amniocentesis reported a loss rate of only 0.3% higher than in control twins [18].

In dichorionic twins discordant for fetal anomaly, selective termination of pregnancy by the induction of asystole using an abortifacient is associated with an 8% loss rate in the international registry, with lower rates if the procedure is performed before 16 weeks' gestation [19]. Selective termination of monochorionic twins cannot be performed using injection of an abortifacient as this would lead to death of the healthy twin due to sharing of the circulation along vascular anastomoses. However, a variety of cord occlusion techniques has been developed to render selective termination feasible. However, there is evidence that there is an associated increased risk of co-twin demise and co-twin morbidity when these procedures are performed [20]. Survival rates of the co-twin vary between 70 and 80% in reported single-centre series.

Maternal homeostatic responses

All the normal physiological adaptations such as increased cardiac output, glomerular filtration rate and renal blood flow are further increased in a multiple pregnancy. Women with twins increase their plasma volume by one-third more than women with singletons. Red cell mass increases approximately 300 mL more than in singleton pregnancies but because this is disproportionately less than the increase in plasma volume, haemoglobin and haematocrit values fall. Maternal iron stores are diminished in 40% of women with twins so routine haematinic supplementation is recommended (usually as combined iron sulphate and folic acid supplementation).

Hyperemesis gravidarum is more common in multiple pregnancies and is managed as in singleton pregnancies. Severe cases may respond to maternal steroid therapy and require pyroxidine (B_6) supplementation. The majority of minor pregnancy complications such as backache, symphysis pubis dysfunction, oedema, varicose veins, haemorrhoids and stria are all increased as a result of both the physical effects of greater uterine size and greater placental hormone production [21].

Hypertensive disease of pregnancy and pre-eclampsia are up to 10 times more common in multiple compared with singleton pregnancies but are managed once diagnosed on standard principles (as in singletons). Consideration should be given to low-dose aspirin prophylaxis but there are no national/international recommendations to this effect. Maternal pregnancy-related hypertension remains a significant cause of maternal morbidity (and mortality) in multiple pregnancies and a significant cause of iatrogenic preterm delivery, increasing perinatal morbidity and mortality. This occurs in 15–20% of twin pregnancies, 25% of triplets and up to 60% of higher-order multiple pregnancies [22].

Postnatally, the physical difficulties and socioeconomic impact of coping with the demands of two or more babies are considerable. Postnatal depression is more common in women nursing twins than singletons [23]. With the high perinatal loss rates there are often associated problems of postnatal grieving and bereavement. Families of women who give birth to babies after a multiple pregnancy may require addition social support.

Intrauterine growth restriction

Ultrasound is the primary tool for monitoring growth in multiple pregnancies for several reasons. The risk of IUGR (~25%) is higher than in singleton pregnancy, and in two-thirds of cases growth will be discordant (affecting one twin only). In addition, abdominal palpation and symphysis–fundal height measurement are unreliable as indices of growth in individual fetuses as they reflect total intrauterine growth.

There is no proven agreement on the ideal frequency of ultrasound examination. However, it is common policy to scan dichorionic twins at up to 4-weekly intervals from 24 weeks' gestation with or without Doppler measurements as indicated. Monochorionic twins are often scanned more frequently, at 2–3 weekly intervals, usually from 16–18 weeks onwards. At this gestational age, there is significant overlap in diagnosis between early twin–twin transfusion syndrome and selective IUGR. The evidence informing scan interval (for either chorionicity) is minimal.

There is controversy as to whether singleton or twin biometric charts should be used. The former appears more sensible, as twins have a higher risk of IUGR with potential morbidity and the use of twin charts thus seems akin to using separate charts for other high-risk groups. Furthermore, increasing emphasis is placed on growth profile and fetal condition (i.e. liquor volume estimation and umbilical artery Doppler velocimetry). Many centres use the measurement of discordancy in estimated fetal weight (EFW) as an index of discordant IUGR:

$$EFW = 100 \times (EFW_{larger} - EFW_{smaller}) / EFW_{larger}$$

This parameter has some predictive value in monochorionic twins for bad outcome in feto-fetal transfusion syndrome and stillbirth [24], but in dichorionic twins it is a relatively poor predictor of perinatal death [25].

The standard principle of management of IUGR (i.e. delivery when the risks of continued intrauterine life outweigh those of extrauterine existence) needs modification in twin pregnancy to account for the risks to both twins. The latency between absent end-diastolic flow velocity in IUGR in twins is longer before 'pre-terminal' factors precipitate delivery than in singleton pregnancies. In addition, this latency is longest in monochorionic twins. However, careful and specialist surveillance of such pregnancies using cerebral, peripheral and intracardiac arterial and venous Doppler velocimetry is required. For example, cessation of fetal growth with pre-terminal arterial and venous Doppler studies may warrant delivery at 26 weeks in a singleton fetus. However, discordant IUGR at such an early gestation in dichorionic twins might better be managed by allowing the severely affected IUGR fetus to die *in utero*, sparing the healthy fetus the risks of iatrogenic prematurity. Such risks and the balancing of decision-making are always difficult and should be individualized. Decisions should be made in concert with parents and multidisciplinary teams (including neonatologists).

In monochorionic twins, such decisions are even more complex. There is some evidence that the presence or absence of umbilical artery Doppler flow during diastole is indicative of prognosis. Positive end-diastolic velocities indicate the best prognostic group when there is significant discordancy between monochorionic twins in terms of growth. Absent end-diastolic velocity indicates an intermediate risk group and so-called intermittent absent end-diastolic velocity indicates the worst prognostic group and, in particular, the worst outcomes in terms of perinatal morbidity [26]. Indeed, in monochorionic twin pregnancies complicated by IUGR in one fetus, there is evidence that the 'larger' twin may have the highest morbidity in terms of neurodevelopmental sequelae. In some cases (of early onset) it may be necessary to consider selective cord occlusion rather than delivery of the whole pregnancy (depending on the gestational age of diagnosis). However, these again are difficult decisions evoking clinical complexity and parental anxieties. Management in a tertiary centre is therefore vital and individual discussions relating to procedure-related morbidity and mortality are essential.

Preterm labour

Multiple pregnancies contribute disproportionately to preterm deliveries. Recent data indicate that, overall, 52.2% of multiple births deliver before 37 weeks and 10.7% prior to 32 weeks [27]. This is the major cause of neonatal death in multiple pregnancies: mortality rates are up to seven times higher in twins than singleton pregnancies; in triplets and higher-order pregnancies, rates of nearly 40 per 1000 live births have been recorded [28]. The median gestational ages at delivery in twins and triplets is 37 and 34 weeks respectively. However, the proportion of these pregnancies delivering before 30 weeks (twins 7%, triplets 15%) is much more concerning because of the associated long-term morbidity. Parents should be informed of the symptoms and signs of threatened preterm labour and the advisability of early presentation. The stimulus to this increased risk is not clearly defined. Certainly (as in polyhydramnios) there is increased uterine distension (i.e. stretch), which may influence autocrine and paracrine intramyometrial processes. There is also focus on the potential materno–fetal endocrine interaction, which may predispose to this increased risk (Fig. 21.4).

There is little evidence that the screening techniques available are highly predictive of preterm delivery (although some demonstrate promise); however, more reliable identification of twin pregnancies at risk of preterm birth may improve outcome if effective interventions are used. Management of preterm labour in multiple pregnancies differs little from that of singletons, except that the consequences of prematurity affect a greater number of babies. The following discussion concentrates on those aspects which appertain especially to multiple pregnancies.

Prediction

The prediction of preterm labour in twins and multiple pregnancies is as problematic as it is in singletons. One of the most promising methods of prediction of spontaneous labour in twins is the measurement of maternal cervical length using transvaginal ultrasound. A systematic review of 11 studies in the published literature (1436 pregnancies) has indicated the potential efficacy of cervical length in predicting risk of spontaneous preterm delivery in twins. Between 23 and 24 weeks' gestation, the mean maternal cervical length is similar to that of singleton pregnancies (38mm). At this gestation, a cervical length of 25mm or less will have a positive summary likelihood ratio of 5.02 (95% CI 3.21–7.61) and a negative summary likelihood ratio of 0.75 (95% CI 0.54–106) for delivery prior to 34 weeks. This correlates with a change from pre-test probability of preterm birth of 18.5% to a post-test probability of 14.2% (12.9–15.9) with a negative test and 47.6% (38.9–56.4) with a positive test [29].

The use of home uterine activity monitoring or fetal fibronectin estimation [30] has not been demonstrated conclusively to be useful in prediction and therefore cannot be advocated.

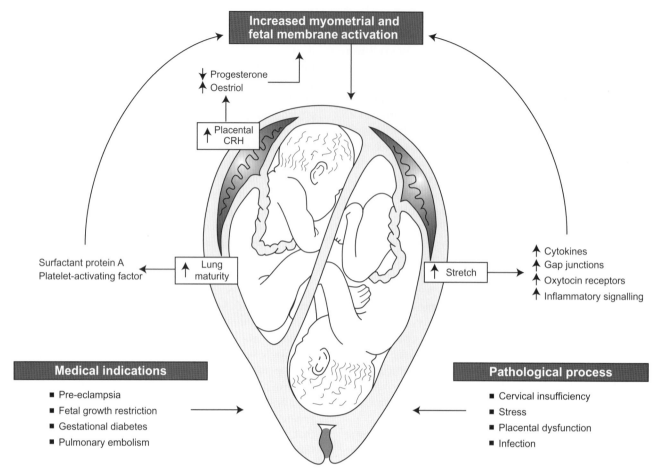

Fig. 21.4 Factors affecting risk of preterm delivery in twins. (a) Dichorionic twins. (b) Monochorionic twins. (With permission from Elsevier.)

Prevention

Preterm labour in a multiple pregnancy (as in polyhydramnios) is attributed to over-distension ('stretch') of the uterus. Accordingly, there is no specific preventive measure (aside from fetal reduction in higher-order multiple pregnancies as discussed below).

Although hospitalization for bed rest has been widely practised in the past, there is little evidence to support its use. Critical appraisal of the literature and meta-analysis of four randomized controlled trials indicates that bed rest in twins significantly increases the chances of preterm delivery, with a trend to greater perinatal mortality [31]. In contrast, a single randomized controlled trial in triplets demonstrated a non-significant trend to less premature delivery and fewer neonatal deaths but was based on a very small number of cases [32].

Meta-analysis of seven randomized controlled trials demonstrated that prophylactic β_2-sympathomimetic therapy was of no benefit in preventing preterm labour in twin pregnancies [33]. This was not surprising given its lack of efficacy in singleton pregnancies and is presumably due to tachyphylaxis. As in singleton pregnancies, this therapy is no longer used. In addition, cervical cer-

clage, and most recently vaginal progesterone therapy, has not been shown to be helpful and indeed may actually be harmful [34]. Indeed, an individual patient-level meta-analysis of randomized trials of cervical cerclage in women with a 'short' cervix (on ultrasound at 20–23 weeks) indicated an increased risk of preterm delivery prior to 35 weeks [35].

Most contemporary focus has fallen on the role of maternal administration of progesterone in potentially reducing the risk of preterm delivery. The Study Of Progesterone for the Prevention of Preterm Birth In Twins (STOPPIT) was a randomized, double-blind, controlled trial to assess the role of daily vaginal progesterone (90 mg) for 10 weeks from 24 weeks' gestation [34]. This study indicated that progesterone did not reduce the composite outcome risk of delivery or intrauterine death before 34 weeks in women with twin pregnancy. These effect was independent of chorionicity (although there was a trend towards worsening of outcome in monochorionic twins). Such findings are in concordance with another study demonstrating no efficacy [36], in which progesterone was administered as intramuscular 17-hydroxyprogesterone caproate (250 mg).

As such there is no evidence that prophylactic measures, either physical or pharmacological, prevent spontaneous preterm labour in multiple pregnancies.

Management

The use of β_2-sympathomimetic infusions in multiple pregnancy, along with steroids and fluid overload, are known risk factors for the rare but potentially fatal complication of pulmonary oedema. As in singleton pregnancies, such active tocolysis has all but been abandoned. Equally, tocolysis with maternally administered oral nifedipine or intravenous atosiban (an oxytocin receptor antagonist) only leads to a relatively modest prolongation of gestation and studies informing efficacy of use in multiple pregnancies are sparse. Certainly, as in singleton pregnancies, the use of such therapy is usually only advocated to allow prophylaxis with corticosteroids. This is exemplified in a retrospective cohort study of 432 twin pregnancies (1982–1986), which noted that 54% of twins were born after spontaneous preterm delivery; of these, 23% were associated with preterm premature rupture of membranes and a further 23% were iatrogenic [37]. In these iatrogenic indications, 44% were secondary to maternal hypertension, 33% secondary to fetal compromise and/or IUGR, 9% secondary to antepartum haemorrhage and 7% associated with one or more fetal death.

Maternal glucocorticoids have been clearly demonstrated to reduce the incidence of respiratory distress syndrome and its perinatal consequences in numerous randomized controlled trials [38]. However, only one uncontrolled study with separate data from multiple pregnancies suggested reduced benefits from antenatal corticosteroid administration in multiple pregnancies compared with singleton pregnancies [39]. The relative 'resistance' of multiple pregnancies to pulmonary surfactant maturation compared with singleton pregnancies has been postulated and has raised the possibility that a larger dose is required in multiple pregnancies but this remains to be objectively tested [40].

A report by Holmes *et al.* [41] has indicated that among 18% of 325 twin pregnancies delivering before 34 weeks' gestation, 70% did so within 24 hours of presentation, the usual interval required for maximal corticosteroid efficacy. It has therefore been proposed that corticosteroids be administered prophylactically. Such a proposal is controversial. It is certainly theoretically possible that this could do more harm than good, as such therapy would potentially need to be administered on a weekly basis and there is no evidence that repeat doses of steroids are of increased value. Furthermore, and not withstanding the safety of steroids in follow-up studies, there remain concerns about the potential adverse fetal effects of repeated steroid courses on glial formation and hippocampal development in children exposed *in utero*.

Complications of monochorionic twinning

Monochorionic twinning, which complicates 20% of all twin pregnancies, may be said to be a congenital anomaly of the placenta where the inter-twin circulations communicate through placental vascular anastomoses. These occur in almost all monochorionic twin pregnancies. Bidirectional superficial arterial–arterial or venous–venous anastomoses may potentially compensate for any haemodynamic imbalance created by deep unidirectional arterial–venous anastomoses. Relatively small inter-twin 'transfusions' are thus likely to be a normal physiological event in monochorionic twins. However, the imbalance of flow between twins may well be pathological and is always a potential risk in such pregnancies (increasing perinatal mortality considerably).

Acute feto-fetal transfusion

When one of a monochorionic twin dies *in utero*, there is a significant risk of ischaemic damage predominantly to the fetal brain (18% in monochorionic twins), although there are reports of damage to pulmonary and hepatic systems, intestinal atresia, limb reduction and renal necrosis. For twin pregnancies overall, a recent systematic review derived a risk of 9% (95% CI 6–13) for neurological abnormality [42]. Death of one of a monochorionic twin substantially increases the risk of co-twin demise *in utero*. Again, a recent systematic review has reported that surviving monochorionic twin fetuses have a six times greater risk of intrauterine fetal death (12%) following single fetal demise after 20 weeks' gestation than initially surviving dichorionic twins (4%; OR 6, 95% CI 1.8–19.8) [42]. Gestational age at the time of intrauterine fetal death influences the extent and type of fetal brain injury. Single intrauterine fetal death after the second trimester can lead to periventricular leucomalacia, multicystic encephalomalacia or germinal matrix haemorrhage. In the third trimester of pregnancy, subcortical leucomalacia, basal ganglion damage or lenticulostriate vasculopathy may develop. There is debate about whether development of such central nervous system (CNS) anomalies are gestationally dependent. However, the long-term morbidity of such an event prior to 14 weeks is controversial and the association less pronounced.

Unlike dichorionic twins, discordant fetal compromise with risks of intrauterine demise in one twin have to be balanced against the potentially adverse effects of iatrogenic prematurity in the co-twin if delivery needs to be expedited in monochorionic twins. A balanced and sometimes complex discussion may ensue, not only to prevent intrauterine death in the potentially compromised twin but also to prevent sequelae in the co-twin. However, once single intrauterine fetal death has occurred in a monochorionic twin, delivery should not be immediate. The pregnancy should be evaluated for secondary sequelae, initially by the use of ultrasound. Such assessment should be within a tertiary fetal medicine centre. The assessment often includes the use of sequential ultrasound scanning (with increasingly the adjuvant investigation of fetal magnetic resonance imaging) to prospectively evaluate the presence of CNS neuropathology that may develop up to 4 weeks after the sentinel event.

Chronic feto-fetal transfusion

Chronic feto-fetal transfusion syndrome (FFTS) occurs in approximately 15% of monochorionic pregnancies (twins and triplets). It is responsible for up to 40% of deaths in monochorionic twins, where it is more commonly known as twin–twin transfusion syndrome (TTTS). The underlying pathophysiology involves chronic shunting of blood from the donor twin to the recipient twin, leading to an inter-twin haemodynamic imbalance. Such a vicious circle of events leads to the 'donor' twin becoming hypoperfused, growth restricted and with associated oliguria and the development of anhydramnios. The co-twin, the 'recipient', becomes polyuric with often severe polyhydramnios and a hyperdynamic circulation that may cause both diastolic and systolic cardiac dysfunction, ending in the development of hydrops fetalis and death (if no treatment ensues). FFTS/TTTS is diagnosed when there is gross discordancy in amniotic fluid volume in monochorionic twins with polyhydramnios in the recipient and anhydramnios in the donor sac. It constitutes severe disease if the onset is prior to 26 weeks. A staging system has been described and is useful in annotating the condition in a consistent manner but does not always denote a logical order of disease progression (Table 21.1). In general

terms, the prognosis is better in early stage disease (stage I and II) and worse in more advanced disease (stages III and IV). However, cardiac dysfunction may be present in up to 20% of fetuses with stage I disease (by Quintero staging) and as a consequence complicated monochorionic twin pregnancies may progress to the most adverse stages without warning.

Untreated, perinatal loss rates in the mid-trimester approach 95%. The principal clinical problem is severe polyhydramnios, which may be associated with premature rupture of membranes or preterm labour (or a combination of these) usually before 26 weeks' gestation. In addition, differences in inter-twin haemodynamics may be associated with single or double twin demise (with antecedent CNS morbidity). Fetoscopic laser ablation/coagulation of the inter-twin communicating vessels (Fig. 21.5) has been demonstrated by critical appraisal of the literature to be the optimal treatment in FFTS/TTTS [43]. This is therefore the treatment of choice in monochorionic twin pregnancies presenting with this complication prior to 26 weeks' gestation.

Table 21.1 Staging system for FFTS/TTTS.

Stage I	Polyhydramnios /oligohydramnios with bladder of the donor still visible
Stage II	Bladder of the donor not visible
Stage III	Presence of absent end-diastolic flow velocity in the umbilical artery, reverse flow in the ductus venosus or pulsatile umbilical venous flow in either twin
Stage IV	Hydrops in either twin
Stage V	Demise of one or both twins

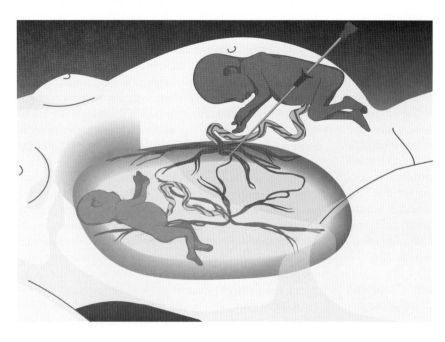

Fig. 21.5 Fetoscopic laser ablation. (With permission from Elsevier.)

Twin reversed arterial perfusion sequence

This rare condition (complicating 1 in 35 000 pregnancies) arises in monochorionic twins with two umbilical cords often linked by large arterio-arterial anastomoses. Flow from one, the 'pump' twin, supplies the other, the 'perfused' twin, in a retrograde fashion. The perfused twin almost always has associated significant congenital malformations, often including a rudimentary heart and aorta. The term 'twin reversed arterial perfusion (TRAP) sequence' is preferred, so named because reversed deoxygenated arterial supply is associated with only rudimentary development of the upper body structures within the fetus. Thus the acardiac twin is perfused by its co-twin (the pump twin) via the inter-twin placental anastomoses (Fig. 21.6). Perinatal mortality in the pump twin in untreated cases is approximately 50% due to associated polyhydramnios and cardiac failure that may ensue [44]. Although polyhydramnios may be elevated by amnioreduction, definitive treatments that cause occlusion of the perfused (acardiac) twin's cord or rudimentary aorta may be achieved by a variety of fetoscopic or ultrasound-guided techniques (intrafetal laser ablation, radiofrequency thermal ablation and fetoscopic cord occlusion). With careful case selection improved outcome for the pump twin is described in up to 85% [45,46]. Most significant complications include co-twin demise or hypoperfusion (with cerebral morbidity) and/or preterm ruptured membranes.

Monoamniotic twins

Of monozygotic twins, 1% lie in the same sac (monoamniotic) exposing them to the risks of cord entanglement. This may prove problematic most commonly (but not exclusively) in the intrapartum period. For this reason most cases are delivered by elective Caesarean section. These twins also have higher reported overall perinatal mortality rates of approximately 30%. This appears largely related to the risk of sudden unexplained intrauterine death (often before 34 weeks' gestation). Therefore the timing of delivery of these twins is controversial. Anecdotal and cohort studies have suggested that use of prophylactic maternal sulindac (cyclooxygenase-2

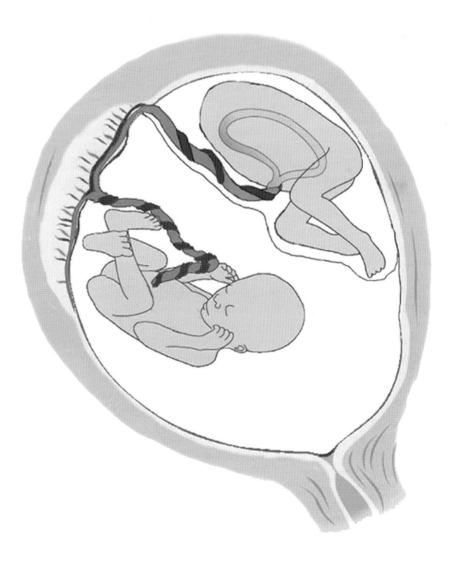

Fig. 21.6 Twin reversed arterial perfusion sequence. (Image reproduced with permission from Professor Neil Sebire.)

inhibitor) to reduce fetal urine output and thus amniotic fluid volume reduces the risk of cord entanglement [47]. In combination with this, others have advocated hospitalization from 26–28 weeks onwards and elective premature delivery of these twins between 32 and 34 weeks' gestation. The most recent evidence indicates that the risk of these events are relatively low, with close outpatient surveillance being recommended rather than very early elective delivery [48–50]. However, the consensus view suggests a course of prophylactic corticosteroids followed by elective delivery by 34 completed weeks in these rare twin pregnancies.

Labour and delivery of twins and multiple pregnancies

Whatever the chorionicity of the twin pregnancy it is best practice for intrapartum care to be discussed and a multidisplinary plan set out in the early third trimester of pregnancy. The indications for elective Caesarean section are relatively few. Congenital anomalies associated with significant risk of cephalopelvic disproportion (including conjoined twins) would be an obvious indication and potentially monoamniotic twins would be another (see below). In addition, monochorionic pregnancies, complicated by placental anomalies associated with increased perinatal mortality (i.e. TTTS or TRAP), are generally delivered at 34–36 weeks and usually by Caesarean section [2].

Perinatal mortality increases slightly after 38 weeks' gestation in twins and there are therefore many obstetricians who elect for delivery then. However, there are no data to indicate whether or not this rise in mortality applies to twins whose growth and well-being are known to be normal on ultrasound. Induction of labour is not contraindicated in twin pregnancies. Mode of delivery is decided on standard principles based on presentation of the first twin (cephalic in 70%, breech in 30%) and the documentation of optimal fetal growth and well-being. Those with previous Caesarean section scars are probably best delivered by repeat Caesarean section because of the greater risk of scar dehiscence/rupture due to both uterine distension and intrauterine manipulation of the second twin. Recent data have indicated that a planned elective Caesarean section may achieve an up to 75% reduction in the risk of perinatal death compared with vaginal delivery by reducing risks of acidosis and anoxia (especially to the second twin) [51–54].

Caesarean section has been advised when the first twin is breech, which would obviate the rare risk of interlocking twins and entrapment of the head of a presenting breech above the second cephalic twin. The use of intrapartum ultrasound may allow detection of such problems with early recourse to emergency Caesarean section. However, there is no evidence that vaginal delivery of a presenting breech that would otherwise satisfy criteria for vaginal delivery (estimated fetal weight less than 3.5–4 kg, flexed head and not footling) is inappropriate in selected cases. The presentation of the second twin is of no importance until after birth of the first.

Even in twins where the first twin is cephalic presentation (at term), there may be the need for obstetric delivery of the second twin with potentially an increased risk of perinatal morbidity. However, a Cochrane Review (on delivery of the second twin not presenting cephalically) indicates that Caesarean section increases maternal febrile morbidity without improving neonatal outcome [55]. This awaits critical appraisal.

For vaginal delivery, continuous cardiotocography of both twins is best achieved by a combination of internal and external monitoring on a dual-channel recorder. An intravenous line is sited and maternal blood drawn for group and save, in view of the increased incidence of Caesarean section and postpartum haemorrhage. Augmentation of labour with oxytocin may be used as in singletons. An epidural anaesthetic is strongly advised in case of the unexpected need for internal manipulation of the second twin. If one is not sited, an anaesthetist will be required at delivery with early recourse to spinal or even general anaesthesia. The place of delivery is debatable but there is an increasing trend for twins to be delivered in operating theatres so that there is immediate redress to emergency Caesarean section if necessary.

Delivery of the first twin proceeds as for a singleton. Its cord is clamped to prevent fetal haemorrhage (from the second twin along any placental anastomoses). An experienced obstetrician discerns the presentation of the second twin, either by abdominal or vaginal examination or, increasingly, by the use of transabdominal ultrasound. Oblique or transverse lies are then converted to a longitudinal lie by external version and held in place by an assistant. Uterine contractions should be monitored and if necessary augmented using oxytocin. The membranes should be left intact to facilitate version. External cephalic version may be used to manipulate the fetal head over the pelvic inlet. Internal cephalic version is preferred as a primary procedure by many experienced obstetricians, as it seems to be associated with a higher success and lower complication rate than external cephalic version. One or preferably both feet are grasped and brought down into the vagina followed by an assisted breech delivery with contractions and maternal effort.

Historical series suggest that the risk to the second twin is increased the greater the delay until delivery. Classically, intervals of greater than 30 min are acceptable providing the cardiotocograph is satisfactory and the presenting part is descending. Uterine inertia with a longitudinal lying second twin is corrected by oxytocin infusion. This is a not uncommon occurrence in the intrapartum management of twins.

Fetal distress may be managed by ventouse delivery, even if the head is high or breech extraction. The already stretched vaginal tissues after the birth of the first twin allow these procedures in circumstances where they would normally be contraindicated. Caesarean section for second twin is rarely indicated for disproportion, usually where the second twin is much bigger than the first. An oxytocin infusion is given prophylactically in the third stage of labour to minimize the risks of postpartum haemorrhage.

There is some evidence that the risk of perinatal loss is greater at the end of the third trimester in monochorionic twins compared with dichorionic twins. Therefore, a recent recommendation was that monochorionic twin pregnancies should be induced by 37 completed weeks of gestation. However, this is a consensus opinion rather than driven by critical appraisal of the published literature.

Higher-order multiples

Perinatal and maternal risk increases exponentially with increasing fetal number. Most higher-order multiple pregnancies are the result of assisted reproductive technologies and thus should be preventable with closer monitoring of follicular response and single (or, at most, two) embryo transfers in IVF therapy. Indeed, there are proven arguments for restricting the number of embryos transferred to one in order to minimize twin and triplet risk, and this course of action appears to have limited adverse effect on live birth rates when more cycles are allowed [56,57].

Every woman/couple with a higher-order multiple pregnancy should have a discussion with a senior obstetrician relating to increased maternal and perinatal risks. This should involve the discussion and option of multiple fetal pregnancy reduction. In addition to perinatal mortality rates, parents should be counselled as to the mean gestational age at delivery (33 weeks for triplets, 31 weeks for quadruplets). In addition, 10% of triplets and 25% of quadruplets deliver before 28 weeks' gestation, with severe neurological sequelae rates of 12% and 25% (respectively) in survivors [58]. The chief perceived disadvantage of multiple fetal pregnancy reduction, usually accomplished by administration of a percutaneous fetal intrathoracic injection of abortifacient (commonly potassium chloride), is complete miscarriage. International registry data demonstrate that this is lowest with reduction to twins, with rates for starting triplets and quadruplets of 7% and 15% respectively [59]. There is now a consensus that multifetal pregnancy reduction between 10 and 12 weeks should be recommended for quadruplets and higher multiples so as to lower both maternal and fetal risks.

The situation with triplets has been more controversial, with many considering this a social issue for parents. However, recent data indicate that in a fetal reduction group (N = 482) compared with an expectantly managed group (N = 411), the rate of miscarriage was significantly higher (8.1% vs. 4.4%, RR 1.83, 95% CI 1.08–3.16; P = 0.036) and the rate of preterm delivery lower (10.4% vs. 26.7%, RR 0.37, 95% CI 0.27–0.51; P < 0.0001) [60].

Higher-order multiple pregnancies should be managed in tertiary perinatal centres with a fetal medicine service. Management is along standard lines for twins but with greater emphasis on preventing preterm delivery and on monitoring fetal growth and well-being. Although there have been successful reports of triplets and even quadruplets being delivered vaginally, most higher-order pregnancies are now delivered by Caesarean section. This alleviates difficulties with electronic fetal monitoring, avoids unrecognized hypoxaemia (especially given the high incidence of IUGR) and prevents birth trauma from manipulative delivery of non-cephalic presenting fetuses. Given the higher incidence of preterm labour in the mid-trimester, the option after delivery of the presenting fetus of conservative management with passive retention of residual fetus to prolong gestational age should be considered [61].

The concept of a multiple pregnancy clinic
Increasingly, there is consensus opinion that the management of multiple pregnancies should be concentrated in a designated 'multiple pregnancy clinic' with experienced midwifery and obstetric discussion and decision-making and with access to immediate diagnostic ultrasound and multidisciplinary opinions (i.e. anaesthetic, neonatal paediatric and psychological services). This care should be holistic in approach (in the widest sense) and could be organized regionally or in subregional centres depending on local population needs and numbers. Such clinics would allow the timely diagnosis of complications of multiple pregnancy along with an individualized plan of care for the prenatal, intrapartum and postnatal periods in women with multiple pregnancies.

Conclusion

The rate of multiple pregnancies appears to be rising, a phenomenon elevated by increased maternal age and the use of assisted reproduction technologies. Even so, the greatest proportion of multiple pregnancies are twins. Obstetric care should be undertaken with specialist teams in a multiples clinic so that prenatal care (influenced by chorionicity), intrapartum care and postnatal well-being may be discussed and planned prospectively. Such developments will hopefully minimize the increased maternal and perinatal risks that exist in such complex pregnancies.

Summary box 21.1

- The prevalence of twin and triplet pregnancies is increasing worldwide. This is associated with a significantly increased risk of maternal and perinatal adverse outcomes in such pregnancies.
- The modification of artificial reproduction techniques with transfer of single embryos reduces significantly (but not completely) the risk of multiple pregnancy.
- Chorionicity is an important factor to determine using ultrasound in the first trimester. Monochorionic twin pregnancies are associated with an increased risk of perinatal mortality and morbidity.
- Multiple pregnancies should be managed in designated multidisciplinary clinics where a holistic approach to pregnancy management can be adopted. This includes the discussion and planning of intrapartum care.
- In the postnatal period, women who have children from multiple pregnancies require increased support as they are at increased risk of emotional/psychological morbidity and this may also lead to socioeconomic stress.

References

1 Ward RH, Whittle MJ (eds) *Multiple Pregnancy*. London: RCOG Press, 1995.

2 Royal College of Obstetricians and Gynaecologists. *Multiple Pregnancy: Study Group Statement*. Available at: www.rcog.org.uk/womens-health/clinical-guidance/multiple-pregnancy-study-group-statement.

3 National Institute for Health and Clinical Excellence. *Multiple Pregnancy: the Management of Twin and Triplet Pregnancies in the Antenatal Period*. Available at: http://guidance.nice.org.uk/CG/Wave16/8.

4 Martin NG, Robertson DM, Chenevix-Trench G, de Kretser DM, Osborne J, Burger HG. Elevation of follicular phase inhibin and luteinising hormone levels in mothers of dizygotic twins suggests non-ovarian control of human multiple ovulation. *Fertil Steril* 1991;56:469–474.

5 Eriksson AW, Fellman J. Demographic analysis of the variation in the rates of multiple maternities in Sweden since 1751. *Hum Biol* 2004;76:343–359.

6 Office for National Statistics. *Birth Statistics. Review of the National Statistician on births and patterns of family building in England and Wales, 2006*. Series FM1 No. 35. Births, maternities and multiple births. Available at: www.statistics.gov.uk/downloads/theme_population/FM1_35/FM1_No35.pdf.

7 Office for National Statistics. *Birth Statistics. Review of the National Statistician on births and patterns of family building in England and Wales, 2008*. Series FM1 No. 37. Births 1938–2004. Maternities with multiple birth. Available at: www.statistics.gov.uk/downloads/theme_population/FM1-37/FM1_37_2008.pdf.

8 Derom C, Derom R, Vlietinck R, Maes H, Van den Berghe H. Iatrogenic multiple pregnancies in East Flanders, Belgium. *Fertil Steril* 1993;60:493–496.

9 Office for National Statistics Report. Series FM1 No. 30–33. Birth Statistics 2008. Available at: www.statistics.gov.uk/downloads/theme_population/FM1_33/FM1_33.pdf.

10 Sebire NJ, Snijders RJ, Hughes K, Sepulveda W, Nicolaides KH. The hidden mortality of monochorionic twin pregnancies. *Br J Obstet Gynaecol* 1997;104:1203–1207.

11 Lewi L, Jani J, Blickstein I *et al*. The outcome of monochorionic diamniotic twin gestations in the era of invasive fetal therapy: a prospective cohort study. *Am J Obstet Gynecol* 2008;199:514.e1–e8.

12 Bejar R, Vigliocco G, Gramajo H *et al*. Antenatal origin of neurological damage in newborn infants. II. Multiple gestations. *Am J Obstet Gynecol* 1990;162:1230–1236.

13 Royal College of Obstetricians and Gynaecologists. *Management of Monochorionic Twin Pregnancy*. Green-top Guideline No. 51, 2008. Available at: www.rcog.org.uk/files/rcog-corp/uploaded-files/T51ManagementMonochorionicTwinPregnancy2008a.pdf.

14 Boklage CE. Survival probability of human conceptions from fertilisation to term. *Int J Fertil* 1990;35:75, 79–80, 81–94.

15 Landy HJ, Keith LG. The vanishing twin: a review. *Hum Reprod Update* 1998;4:177–183.

16 Spencer K, Kagan KO, Nicolaides KH. Screening for trisomy 21 in twin pregnancies in the first trimester: an update of the impact of chorionicity on maternal serum markers. *Prenat Diagn* 2008;28:49–52.

17 Royal College of Obstetricians and Gynaecologists. *Amniocentesis and Chorionic Villus Sampling*. Green-top Guideline No. 8, 2010. Available at: www.rcog.org.uk/files/rcog-corp/GT8Amniocentesis0111.pdf.

18 Ghidini A, Lynch L, Hicks C, Alvarez M, Lockwood CJ. The risk of second-trimester amniocentesis in twin gestations: a case-control study. *Am J Obstet Gynecol* 1993;169:1013–1016.

19 Evans MI, Ciorica D, Britt DW, Fletcher JC. Update on selective reduction. *Prenat Diagn* 2005;25:807–813.

20 O'Donoghue K, Rutherford MA, Engineer N, Wimalasundera RC, Cowan FM, Fisk NM. Transfusional fetal complications after single intrauterine death in monochorionic multiple pregnancy are reduced but not prevented by vascular occlusion. *BJOG* 2009;116:804–812.

21 Malone FD, D'Alton ME. Multiple gestation: clinical characteristics and management. In: Creasy RK, Resnik R (eds) *Creasy and Resnik's Maternal–Fetal Medicine*, 6th edn. Philadelphia: Saunders Elsevier, 2009: 453–476.

22 Malone FD, Kauffman GE, Chelmow D, Athanassiou A, Nores JA, D'Alton ME. Maternal morbidity in twin and triplet pregnancies. *Am J Perinatol* 1998;15:73–76.

23 Thorpe K, Golding J, MacGillivray I, Greenwood R. Comparison of prevalence of depression in mothers of twins and mothers of singletons. *BMJ* 1991;302:875–878.

24 Blickstein I, Goldman RD, Smith-Levitin M, Greenberg M, Sherman D, Rydhstroem H. The relation between inter-twin birth weight discordance and total twin birth weight. *Obstet Gynecol* 1999;93:113–116.

25 Bronsteen R, Goyert G, Bottoms S. Classification of twins and neonatal morbidity. *Obstet Gynecol* 1989;74:98–10.

26 Gratacós E, Lewi L, Muñoz B *et al*. A classification system for selective intrauterine growth restriction in monochorionic pregnancies according to umbilical artery Doppler flow in the smaller twin. *Ultrasound Obstet Gynecol* 2007;30:28–34.

27 Information Services Division, NHS Scotland. Scottish Perinatal and Infant Mortality and Morbidity Report, 2008. Available at: www.isdscotland.org/Health-Topics/Maternity-and-Births/Publications/index.asp#742.

28 Confidential Enquiry into Maternal and Child Health. *Perinatal Mortality 2007*. London: CEMACH, 2009. Available at: www.cemach.org.uk/getattachment/bc6ad9f0-5274-486d-b61a-8770a0ab43e7/Perinatal-Mortality-2007.aspx.

29 Honest H, Bachmann LM, Coomarasamy A, Gupta JK, Kleijnen J, Khan KS. Accuracy of cervical transvaginal sonography in predicting preterm birth: a systematic review. *Ultrasound Obstet Gynecol* 2003;22:305–322.

30 Goldenberg RL, Iams JD, Miodovnik M *et al.* The preterm prediction study: risk factors in twin gestations. National Institute of Child Health and Human Development Maternal–Fetal Medicine Units Network. *Am J Obstet Gynecol* 1996;175:1047–1053.

31 Crowther C, Han S. Hospitalisation for bed rest in twin pregnancy. *Cochrane Database Syst Rev* 2010;(7):CD000110.

32 Dodd JM, Crowther CA. Hospitalisation for bed rest for women with a triplet pregnancy: an abandoned randomised controlled trial and meta-analysis. *BMC Pregnancy Childbirth* 2005;5:8.

33 Keirse MJ. New perspectives for the effective treatment of preterm labour. *Am J Obstet Gynecol* 1995;173:618–628.

34 Norman JE, Mackenzie F, Owen P *et al.* Progesterone for the prevention of preterm birth in twin pregnancy (STOPPIT): a randomised, double-blind, placebo-controlled study and meta-analysis. *Lancet* 2009;373:2034–2040.

35 Berghella V, Odibo AO, To MS, Rust OA, Althuisius SM. Cerclage for short cervix on ultrasonography: meta-analysis of trials using individual patient-level data. *Obstet Gynecol* 2005;106:181–189.

36 Rouse DJ, Caritis SN, Peaceman AM *et al.* A trial of 17 alpha-hydroxyprogesterone caproate to prevent prematurity in twins. *N Engl J Med* 2007;357:454–461.

37 Gaardner MO, Goldenberg RL, Cliver SP, Tucker JM, Nelson KG, Copper RL. The origin and outcome of preterm twin pregnancies. *Obstet Gynecol* 1995;85:553–557.

38 Brownfoot FC, Crowther CA, Middleton P. Different corticosteroids and regimens for accelerating fetal lung maturation for women at risk of preterm birth. *Cochrane Database Syst Rev* 2008;(4):CD006764.

39 Burkett G, Bauer C, Morrison J, Curet L. Effects of prenatal dexamethasone administration on prevention of respiratory distress syndrome in twin pregnancies. *J Perinatol* 1986;6:304–308.

40 Choi SJ, Song SE, Seo ES, Kim JH, Roh CR. The effects of single or multiple courses of antenatal corticosteroids therapy on neonatal respiratory distress syndrome in singleton vs. multiple pregnancies. *Aust NZ J Obstet Gynaecol* 2009;29:173–179.

41 Holmes R, Wardle P. Tuohy J. Antenatal steroids administration in twin pregnancy. *Contemp Rev Obstet Gynaecol* 1996;8:181–184.

42 Ong SS, Zamora J, Khan KS, Kilby MD. Prognosis for the co-twin following single-twin death: a systematic review. *BJOG* 2006;113:992–998.

43 Roberts D, Neilson JP, Kilby MD, Gates S. Interventions for the treatment of twin–twin transfusion syndrome. *Cochrane Database Syst Rev* 2008;(1):CD002073.

44 Moore TR, Gale S, Benirschke K. Perinatal outcome of forty-nine pregnancies complicated by acardiac twinning. *Am J Obstet Gynecol* 1990;163:907–912.

45 Lee H, Wagner AJ, Sy E, Ball R, Feldstein VA, Goldstein RB. Effacacy of radioferequency ablation in management of TRAP. *Am J Obstet Gynecol* 2007;196:459e1–e4.

46 O'Donoghue K, Barigye O, Pasquini L, Chappell L, Wimalasundera RC, Fisk NM. Interstitial laser therapy for fetal reduction in monochorionic multiple pregnancy: loss rate and association with aplasia cutis congenita. *Prenat Diagn* 2008;28:535–543.

47 Peek MJ, McCarthy A, Kyle P, Sepulveda W, Fisk NM. Medical amnioreduction with sulindac to reduce cord complications in monoamniotic twins. *Am J Obstet Gynecol* 1997;176:334–336.

48 Dias T, Mahsud–Dornan S, Bhide A, Papageorghiou AT, Thilaganathan B. Cord entanglement and perinatal outcome in monoamnionic twin pregnancies. *Ultrasound Obstet Gynecol* 2010;35:201–204.

49 Hack KE, Derks JB, Schaap AH *et al.* Perinatal outcome of monoamniotic twin pregnancies. *Obstet Gynecol* 2009;113:353–360.

50 Baxi LV, Walsh CA. Monoamniotic twins in contemporary practice: a single-center study of perinatal outcomes. *J Matern Fetal Neonatal Med* 2010;23:506–510.

51 Smith GCS, Shah I, White IR, Pell JP, Dobbie R. Mode of delivery and the risk of perinatal death amongst twins at term. *BJOG* 2005;112:1139–1144.

52 Smith GCS, Fleming KM, White IR. Birth order in twins and the risk of perinatal death related to delivery in England, Northern Ireland and Wales, 1994–2003. *BMJ* 2007;334:576.

53 Armson BA, O'Connell C, Persad V, Joseph KS, Young DC, Baskett TF. Determinants of perinatal mortality and serious neonatal morbidity in the second twin. *Obstet Gynecol* 2006;108:556–564.

54 Herbst A, Kallen K. Influence of mode of delivery on neonatal mortality in the second twin, at and before term. *BJOG* 2008;115:1512–1517.

55 Crowther CA. Caesarean delivery for the second twin. *Cochrane Database Syst Rev* 2000;(2):CD000047.

56 Templeton A, Morris JK. Reducing the risk of multiple births by transfer of two embryos after in vitro fertilisation. *N Engl J Med* 1998;339:573–577.

57 Gelbaya TA, Tsoumpou I, Nardo LG. The likelihood of live birth and multiple birth after single versus double embryo transfer at the cleavage stage: a systematic review and meta-analysis. *Fertil Steril* 2010;94:936–945.

58 Lipitz S, Reichman B, Uval J *et al.* A prospective comparison of the outcome of triplet pregnancies managed expectantly or by multifetal reduction to twins. *Am J Obstet Gynecol* 1994;170:874–879.

59 Evans MI, Berkowitz RL, Wapner RJ *et al.* Improvement in outcomes of multifetal pregnancy reduction with increased experience. *Am J Obstet Gynecol* 2001;184:97–103.

60 Papageorghiou AT, Avgidou K, Bakoulas V, Sebire NJ, Nicolaides KH. Risks of miscarriage and early preterm birth in trichorionic triplet pregnancies with embryo reduction versus expectant management: new data and systematic review. *Hum Reprod* 2006;21:1912–1917.

61 Antsaklis A, Daskalakis G, Papageorgiou I, Aravantinos D. Conservative treatment after miscarriage of one fetus in multifetal pregnancies. Report of three cases and review of the literature. *Fetal Diagn Ther* 1996;11:366–372.

Part 6
Birth

Chapter 22
The Normal Mechanisms of Labour

Andrés López Bernal[1] and Errol R. Norwitz[2]

[1]School of Clinical Sciences, University of Bristol, and St Michael's Hospital, Bristol, UK

[2]Department of Obstetrics, Gynecology and Reproductive Sciences Yale, New Haven Hospital, New Haven, Connecticut, USA

Labour is the physiological process by which the products of conception are passed from the uterus to the outside world, and is common to all mammalian viviparous species. The mean duration of a human singleton pregnancy is 40 weeks (280 days) from the first day of the last normal menstrual period. 'Term' is defined as the period from 37 to 42 weeks of gestation. Both preterm birth (defined as delivery prior to 37 weeks) and post-term pregnancy (continuation beyond 42 weeks' gestation) are associated with increased neonatal morbidity and mortality. Considerable evidence suggests that the fetus is in control of the timing of labour, although maternal factors are also involved. This chapter summarizes the current state of knowledge on the mechanisms responsible for the onset of labour and for the safe and timely delivery of the fetus.

Morphological changes in the uterus during pregnancy

The uterus provides a safe environment for the embryo to implant and develop. The nutritious endometrial layer becomes 'receptive' during a specific window of time in the luteal phase of the menstrual cycle, thereby facilitating implantation of the blastocyst and development of a viable fetoplacental unit. Over a period of 40 weeks, the fetus, placenta and amniotic fluid increase their mass considerably, posing remarkable haemodynamic, metabolic and mechanical demands on the mother. The uterus alone increases in both weight (from 40–70 g in the non-pregnant state to 1100–1200 g at term) and volume (from 10 mL to 5 L). At the same time as it expands, the uterus must remain relaxed with a closed cervix to allow for growth and differentiation of the fetus to a stage when it is ready to cope with extrauterine life. At the onset of labour, the uterus is responsible for driving the process of birth through a complex set of structural, biochemical and electrophysiological changes that result in the establishment of synchronized myometrial contractions and cervical ripening and dilatation. The process of cervical ripening involves localized changes in the connective tissue content and attributes, with an increase in collagen solubility and alterations in the proteoglycan composition of the ground substance. This remodelling results from a proinflammatory reaction within the cervix, with elevated levels of cytokines and other proinflammatory molecules signalling through Toll-like receptors [1,2]. The process ends with the delivery of the newborn and the placenta, followed by an intense period of uterine remodelling and involution.

Diagnosis of labour

Summary box 22.1

Labour is a clinical diagnosis characterized by regular phasic uterine contractions increasing in frequency and intensity resulting in effacement and dilatation of the uterine cervix.

Labour is a clinical diagnosis characterized by an increase in myometrial activity or, more precisely, a switch in the myometrial contractility pattern from 'contractures' (long-lasting, low-frequency activity) to 'contractions' (frequent, high-intensity, high-frequency activity) [3] resulting in effacement and dilatation of the uterine cervix. In normal labour, there appears to be a time-dependent relationship between these various factors. The biochemical connective tissue changes in the cervix usually precede uterine contractions and cervical dilatation which, in turn, occur before spontaneous rupture of the fetal membranes. Cervical dilatation in the absence of uterine contractions is seen most commonly in the second trimester and is suggestive of cervical incompetence. Similarly, the presence of uterine contractions in the absence of cervical change does not meet criteria for the diagnosis of labour, and should be referred to as 'preterm' or 'prelabour' contractions.

Dewhurst's Textbook of Obstetrics & Gynaecology, Eighth Edition. Edited by D. Keith Edmonds.
© 2012 John Wiley and Sons, Ltd. Published 2012 by John Wiley and Sons, Ltd.

Timing of labour and birth

> **Summary box 22.2**
>
> The ability of obstetric care providers to predict and prevent preterm labour and birth is poor, resulting in potentially severe complications for the newborn, distress to the parents and high medical costs.

The timely onset of labour and birth is a critical determinant of perinatal outcome. Considerable evidence suggests that, in most viviparous animals, the fetus is in control of the timing of labour [4–9]. The slow progress in our understanding of the molecular and cellular mechanisms responsible for the onset of labour is due primarily to the lack of an adequate animal model and to the autocrine/paracrine nature of the parturition cascade in humans, which precludes direct investigation. As noted above, alterations in the timing of birth are the leading cause of neonatal mortality and morbidity. The ability of obstetric care providers to predict and prevent preterm labour and birth is poor, resulting in potentially severe complications for the newborn, distress to the parents and high medical costs. Despite the routine use of antenatal corticosteroids and considerable improvements in special care baby units, the perinatal mortality rates for preterm birth remain steady, and there is a wide range of both short-term and long-term complications and handicap in surviving preterm infants [10]. Thus, there is an urgent need to investigate the mechanisms of spontaneous preterm labour, which may or may not result from the same endocrine and intracellular pathways as the physiological onset of labour at term. The genetic, endocrine and biochemical factors implicated in the onset of normal labour at term are discussed in detail below.

Genetic influences on the timing of labour

Horse–donkey cross-breeding experiments performed in the 1950s resulted in a gestational length intermediate between that of horses (340 days) and that of donkeys (365 days), suggesting an important role for the fetal genotype in the initiation of labour [4,11]. In contrast, familial clustering [12,13], racial disparities [14–18] and the high incidence of recurrent preterm birth [19,20] suggest an important role for maternal genetic factors in the timing of labour. For example, black (including African American,

African and Afro-Caribbean) women have a preterm birth rate that is twofold higher than that observed in white women [14–18]. Even after adjusting for potential confounding demographic and behavioural variables, the rate of premature deliveries in black women remains higher than that for white women [16,17]. Interestingly, the risk of preterm birth in interracial (black–white) couples is significantly different and intermediate between that of white–white (8.6%) and black–black couples (14.8%) [21]. Taken together, these data suggest that genetic influences of both the mother and fetus may be involved in the timing of labour. Recent studies estimate that genetic factors – or, more correctly, gene–environment interactions – may account for up to 20% of preterm births [22–24]. For example, maternal carriage of the $-308(G \rightarrow A)$ polymorphism in the promoter region of the tumour necrosis factor (TNF)-α gene is associated with an increased risk of spontaneous preterm birth (odds ratio [OR] 2.7, 95% CI 1.7–4.5) [25,26], which is further increased in the presence of bacterial vaginosis (OR 6.1, 95% CI 1.9–21.0) [25–27]. Interestingly, the risk of spontaneous preterm birth is increased even further if the woman with the TNF-α gene promoter polymorphism and bacterial vaginosis also happens to be black (OR 17) [27].

Endocrine control of labour

It is likely that a 'parturition cascade' exists at term in the human (Fig. 22.1) that is responsible for the removal of mechanisms maintaining uterine quiescence and for the recruitment of factors acting to promote uterine activity [7,28]. Given its teleological importance, such a cascade would probably have multiple redundant loops to ensure a fail-safe system of securing pregnancy success and ultimately the preservation of the species. In such a model, each element is connected to the next in a sequential fashion, and many of the elements demonstrate positive feed-forward characteristics typical of a cascade mechanism. The sequential recruitment of signals that serve to augment the labour process suggest that it may not be possible to identify any one signalling mechanism as being uniquely responsible for the initiation of labour. It may therefore be prudent to describe such mechanisms as being responsible for *promoting*, rather than *initiating*, the process of labour [29].

A comprehensive analysis of each of the individual paracrine/autocrine pathways implicated in the process

Fig. 22.1 Proposed 'parturition cascade' for the onset of labour at term. The spontaneous onset of labour at term is regulated by a series of paracrine/autocrine hormones acting in an integrated parturition cascade. The factors responsible for maintaining uterine quiescence throughout gestation (a) and for the onset of labour at term (b) are shown. This includes the withdrawal of the inhibitory effects of progesterone on uterine contractility and the

recruitment of cascades that promote oestrogen (oestriol) production and lead to upregulation of the contraction-associated proteins within the uterus. ACTH, adrenocorticotrophic hormone (corticotrophin); CAPs, contraction-associated proteins; CRH, corticotrophin-releasing hormone; DHEAS, dehydroepiandrosterone sulphate; 11β-HSD, 11β-hydroxysteroid dehydrogenase; SROM, spontaneous rupture of membranes.

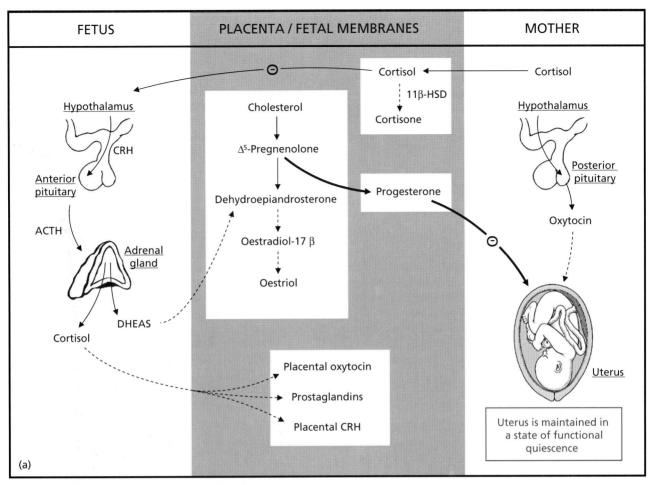

(a)

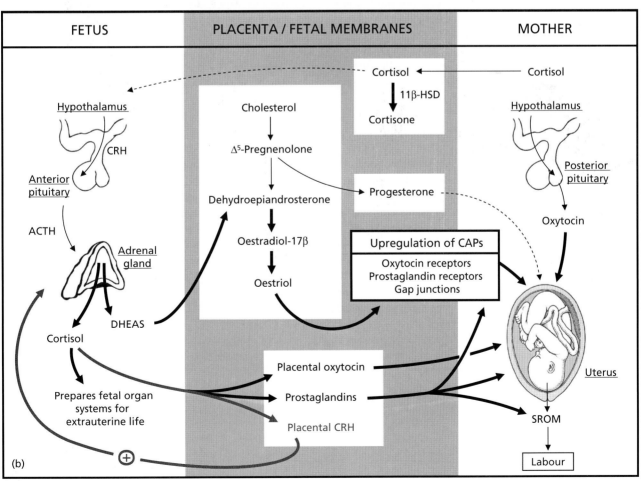

(b)

of labour have been reviewed in detail elsewhere [4–9,29,30]. In brief, human labour is a multifactorial physiological event involving an integrated set of changes within the maternal tissues of the uterus (myometrium, decidua and uterine cervix) and fetal membranes which occur gradually over a period of days to weeks. Such changes include, but are not limited to, an increase in prostaglandin synthesis and release within the uterus, an increase in myometrial gap junction formation, and upregulation of myometrial oxytocin receptors ('uterine activation'). Once the myometrium and cervix are prepared, endocrine and/or paracrine/autocrine factors from the fetal membranes and placenta bring about a switch in the pattern of myometrial activity from irregular contractures to regular contractions ('uterine stimulation'). The fetus may coordinate this switch in myometrial activity through its influence on placental steroid hormone production, through mechanical distension of the uterus, and through secretion of neurohypophyseal hormones and other stimulators of prostaglandin synthesis.

Fetal hypothalamic–pituitary–adrenal axis

The final common pathway towards the onset of labour appears to activation of the fetal hypothalamic–pituitary–adrenal axis, and is probably common to all species. In the human, the fetal adrenal provides abundant C_{19} oestrogen precursor (dehydroepiandrosterone) directly from its intermediate (fetal) zone. This is because the human placenta is an incomplete steroidogenic organ and oestrogen synthesis by the human placenta has an obligate need for C_{19} steroid precursor (see Fig. 22.1) [6,31]. In the rhesus monkey, infusion of the C_{19} precursor androstenedione leads to preterm delivery [32,33]. This effect is blocked by concurrent infusion of an aromatase inhibitor [34], demonstrating that conversion to oestrogen is important. However, systemic infusion of oestrogen failed to induce delivery [32,33], suggesting that the action of oestrogen is likely paracrine/autocrine. Just as important to the onset of labour as the local surge in oestrogen production is the functional withdrawal of progesterone activity at the level of the uterus, which appears to be common to all species [35]. In most laboratory animals (except for the guinea pig and armadillo), progesterone withdrawal occurs by decreasing progesterone concentrations in the maternal circulation (i.e. systemic progesterone withdrawal) [36,37]. In women, however, parturition occurs without a systemic progesterone withdrawal. Progesterone levels in the maternal and fetal circulations are relatively high in pregnancy (10- to 100-fold higher than in the luteal phase of the menstrual cycle), and remain elevated throughout pregnancy as well as during labour and delivery, decreasing only after delivery of the placenta [38,39]. Building on the earlier pioneering work by George Corner and colleagues [40], Arpad Csapo writing in the 1950s proposed the 'progesterone block' hypothesis [41]. This hypothesis proposes that progesterone maintains pregnancy by actively blocking myometrial contractions, and that labour is initiated by withdrawal of the progesterone blockade which transforms the muscle to the labouring state. This paradigm is supported by a considerable body of research in multiple species [35–37]. For example, administration of a progesterone receptor antagonist (such as RU486) increases myometrial contractility and excitability at all stages of pregnancy and, in most cases, induces labour and delivery [42,43]. It is now generally accepted that progesterone is essential for the maintenance of human pregnancy, and interruption of its synthesis or action in the latter half of pregnancy initiates labour. In support of this argument, recent clinical studies have shown that progesterone supplementation may decrease the incidence of recurrent preterm birth in women at high risk by virtue of one or more prior spontaneous preterm births [44,45] or cervical shortening [46].

Fetal pulmonary surfactant

Recent studies in mice suggests that surfactant protein-A (SP-A) secreted from the lungs of near-term pups may provide an additional trigger for parturition in that species [47]. Whether SP-A or any of the other multimeric surfactant-associated proteins (SP-B, SP-C or SP-D) have a comparable role in human labour remains to be determined. Interestingly, concentrations of SP-A and SP-D increase sharply in amniotic fluid from 26 weeks of gestation to term [48], and have been localized to fetal membranes and decidua [48] where they appear to exert potent innate immune functions acting in part through the Toll-like receptors TLR-2 and TLR-4 [48,49]. The concept that fetal surfactant (a mixture of lipids and apoproteins) may provide a signal for parturition is appealing, because it provides a link between fetal lung maturation, which is essential for extrauterine life, and the onset of labour. In addition to its protein component, amniotic fluid surfactant is also an important intrauterine source of the bioactive lipid arachidonic acid, which is required for prostaglandin synthesis [50].

'Decidual activation' and the onset of labour

Activation of decidual cells, especially resident macrophages, have long been implicated in the mechanism of labour by promoting the synthesis and release of prostaglandins and proinflammatory cytokines [51,52]. Prostaglandins are the final common pathway for parturition in many species, and act as local hormones to synchronize uterine activation and cervical ripening through specific receptor signalling pathways in decidua and myometrium [53,54]. It has been proposed that a delicate balance exists within the decidua between 'classically activated' (M1 or proinflammatory) and 'alternatively activated' (M2 or anti-inflammatory) macrophages, and that this balance changes in a predictable pattern throughout pregnancy [55]. Although the M1/M2 terminology is outdated and macrophages rarely fit a particular classification due to their functional plasticity, it remains useful for descriptive purposes. It is proposed that, in early pregnancy, a specific subpopulation of M2 decidual macrophages provides critical immunosuppressive function through the secretion of the cytokines interleukin (IL)-10 and transforming growth factor (TGF)-β to facilitate immunological tolerance of the semi-allogeneic conceptus [56]. This is accompanied by simultaneous downregulation of classically activated M1 macrophages within the decidua, characterized by reduced production of proinflammatory cytokines (IL-1β, TNF-α) in response to interferon (IFN)-γ or bacterial lipopolysaccharide (LPS). Uterine natural killer (NK) cells are the dominant source of IFN-γ, and decidual macrophages express IFN-γ receptors. Decidual macrophages fail to respond to IFN-γ (as measured by the induction of indoleamine 2,3-dioxygenase) in early pregnancy [57], but do respond at term [58]. Thus, decidual macrophages appear to have an immunosuppressive and angiogenic role in early pregnancy due in large part to their high levels of IL-10. It is thought that progesterone provides the stimulus for the inhibition of the proinflammatory phenotype of decidual macrophages [59], either directly or through cross-stimulation of glucocorticoid receptors [57]. As gestation progresses, uterine NK cells decline and are virtually absent at term; in contrast, the number of decidual macrophages remains high throughout gestation [60,61]. In term decidua, nearly 50% of cells are of bone marrow origin, comprising up to 20% macrophages [60]. Moreover, decidual macrophages prepared from women delivered at term are the major decidual source of PGF [62] and produce superoxide radicals and TNF-α when challenged with LPS [63]. In addition, TNF-α and IL-1β have a strong paracrine effect on decidual macrophages and stromal cells at term, stimulating the release of large amounts of PGF [64,65]. Taken together, these data suggest that labour at term is characterized by 'decidual activation' and a localized upregulation of prostaglandins and proinflammatory cytokines.

Local biochemical factors involved in the onset of labour

Regardless of whether the trigger for labour begins in the mother or the fetus, the final common pathway ends in the maternal tissues of the uterus. At the level of the uterus, labour results from a cascade of intrauterine biochemical events that culminates in the development of regular phasic uterine contractions as well as cervical dilatation and effacement. As in other smooth muscles, myometrial contractions are mediated through the adenosine triphosphate (ATP)-dependent binding of myosin to actin. In contrast to vascular smooth muscle, however, myometrial cells have a sparse innervation which is further reduced during pregnancy [66]. The regulation of the contractile mechanism of the uterus is therefore dependent not on systemic factors but on intrinsic biochemical and endocrine factors within myometrial cells. The molecular basis of uterine contractions and the local factors affecting myometrial contractility are discussed in detail below.

Myometrial contractility

Physiological basis of uterine contractility

The uterus contracts because the myometrial layer contains specialized smooth muscle cells arranged in bundles embedded in a matrix of collagenous connective tissue. The collagen fibres facilitate the transmission of force generated by myometrial bundles. Myometrial smooth muscle cells contain actin (thin filaments) and myosin (thick filaments) in a less organized fashion than in striated muscle, but nevertheless forming efficient contractile units due to their intricate cytoskeletal organization [67]. Mammalian smooth muscle myosin belong to the class II myosins, which are characterized by a hexameric protein structure composed of two heavy chains (~200 kDa) and two pairs of light chains: the 20-kDa regulatory myosin light chain (MYL_{20}) and the 17-kDa essential light chain. Functionally, myosin consists of three domains: the motor domain (which interacts with actin and binds ATP), the neck domain (which binds the light chains and is the site of calmodulin interaction), and the tail or anchoring domain (which helps position the motor domain so that it interacts with actin) [68]. Myosin generates contractile force by pulling actin filaments of opposite polarity towards one another (Fig. 22.2).

Myosin is both a structural protein and an enzyme (Mg-ATPase) capable of hydrolysing ATP to generate mechanical energy. The ATPase region of myosin is located in the head and is activated by actin. Its level of activity is low when MYL_{20} is unphosphorylated, but increases enormously on phosphorylation of the regulatory chains. The enzyme responsible for MYL_{20} phosphorylation is the calcium/calmodulin-dependent myosin light chain kinase (MLCK). There are three isoforms of MLCK: skeletal, cardiac and smooth muscle. All three isoforms have a common conserved serine threonine kinase domain, but smooth muscle MLCK has unique immunoglobulin and fibronectin domains [69]. Despite its name, smooth muscle MLCK is expressed in almost all tissues and is involved not only in contractions but also in many other cellular activities. Although kinases are often portrayed as promiscuous enzymes with multiple substrates, the only known substrate of MLCK is myosin. In addition to a myosin-binding domain, smooth muscle MLCK also has binding domains for actin at the N-terminus and

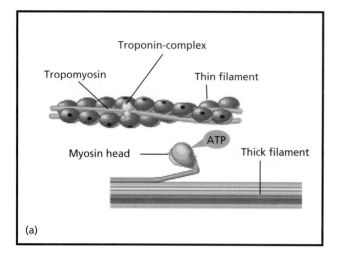

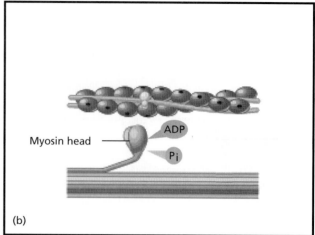

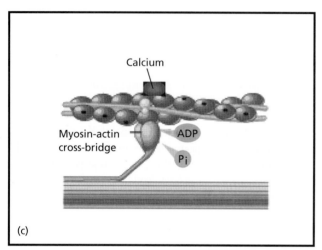

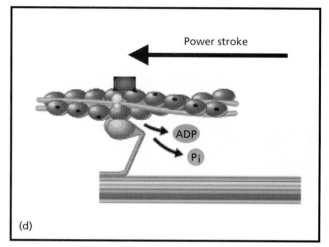

Fig. 22.2 Mechanics of muscle contraction. (a) Appearance of the contractile unit in the resting state. The thick filament refers to myosin; the thin filament is actin. Myosin-binding sites on the actin filaments are covered with by a thin filament known as tropomyosin that obscures the myosin-binding sites, therefore preventing the myosin heads from attaching to actin and forming cross-bridges. Adenosine triphosphate (ATP) is hydrolysed into adenosine diphosphate (ADP) and inorganic phosphate (Pi). The troponin complex is attached to the tropomyosin filament. (b) As intracellular calcium concentrations increase, calcium binds to the troponin complex resulting in a conformational change that allows binding sites between actin and myosin to be exposed with the formation of actin–myosin cross-bridges. (c) Formation of actin–myosin cross-bridges results in release of Pi and ADP, causing the myosin heads to bend and slide past the myosin fibres. This 'power stroke' results in shortening of the contractile unit and generation of force within the muscle. (d) At the end of the power stroke, the myosin head releases the actin-binding site, is cocked back to its furthest position, and binds to a new molecule of ATP in preparation for another contraction. The binding of myosin heads occurs asynchronously (i.e. some myosin heads are binding while other heads are releasing the actin filaments), which allows the muscle to generate a continuous smooth force. Cross-bridges must therefore form repeatedly during a single muscle contraction.

calmodulin. Purified MLCK can only bind to calmodulin in the presence of calcium. The protein structure of MLCK suggests that it is a long and flexible molecule capable of attaching itself to actin through its N-terminus and to the neck region of myosin through the C-terminal domain. In this position, the catalytic core of the enzyme is able to phosphorylate MYL_{20} in the thick filaments while being tightly anchored to the thin filaments.

Human myometrium expresses the 137-kDa and 218-kDa isoforms of MLCK in both the pregnant and non-pregnant state [70,71]. Interestingly, a small 19-kDa non-catalytic C-terminal fragment of MLCK called telokin is highly expressed in pregnant compared with non-pregnant myometrium, suggesting it may have a regulatory role in gestation [71]. Telokin belongs to a group of kinase-related proteins, but its expression appears to be restricted to smooth muscle, especially phasic smooth muscle. Despite its sequence homology with the C-terminal domain, telokin is not simply a proteolytic fragment of MLCK but is expressed independently, especially in myometrium [71]. Since telokin binds to myosin at the same site as MLCK but has no catalytic activity, an increase in telokin concentrations may compete with MLCK and reduce actin–myosin interactions [72]. In some tissues, telokin acts to enhance myosin phosphatase activity and induce calcium desensitization, thereby promoting smooth muscle relaxation [73], but these mechanisms have not been investigated in human myometrium.

Generation of uterine contractions

Myometrial smooth muscle is myogenic; that is to say, it can generate contractions spontaneously without the need for external stimulation. Myometrial cell contractions are initiated by action potentials that depolarize the cell membrane allowing the rapid entry of calcium through voltage-operated channels. The rise in intracellular calcium concentration ($[Ca^{2+}]_i$) is picked up by the Ca^{2+} sensor, calmodulin, which activates MLCK and provokes the phosphorylation of MYL_{20}. Phosphorylation of MYL_{20} stimulates the formation of cross-bridges between actin and myosin filaments and the generation of force [70,74]. The phasic nature of myometrial contractions (recurrent episodes of force separated by intervals of relaxation) is necessary to allow blood flow through the placenta and exchange of oxygen and waste products with the fetus during the several hours of labour. In order to promote relaxation between contractions, myometrial cells have efficient Ca^{2+} extrusion mechanisms including Ca^{2+} pumps and Na^+/Ca^{2+} exchangers in the cell membrane as well as in the sarcoplasmic reticulum to promote Ca^{2+} entry into intracellular stores [75,76] (Fig. 22.3).

The increase in steroid hormones and placental-derived growth factors in pregnancy has important effects on the structure of the uterus. Myometrial tissue becomes more vascularized during pregnancy, and there is hyperplasia and hypertrophy of myometrial cells. The cellular content of actin and myosin and of the actin-binding proteins caldesmon and calponin increases several fold compared with non-pregnant cells [70]. Comparisons between strips of myometrial tissue from pregnant and non-pregnant women show that the relationship between the level of MLCK phosphorylation and the amount of force is more favourable in pregnant tissue [70].

Calcium homeostasis

The phasic nature of uterine contractions is an intrinsic property of uterine smooth muscle, and is related to the capacity of myometrial cells to modify $[Ca^{2+}]_i$ through complex activation/inhibition of membrane receptors, ion channels and Ca^{2+} pumps. The main source of Ca^{2+} is the extracellular fluid, but intracellular stores such as the sarcoplasmic reticulum have important regulatory functions [77].

Myometrial cells are depolarized by action potentials which provoke the influx of Ca^{2+} through voltage-operated channels [78,79]. Spontaneous action potentials in pregnant human myometrial cells are inhibited in sodium-deficient or calcium-free solutions [80–82], thereby demonstrating the essential role of extracellular Ca^{2+} and of membrane Na^+/Ca^{2+} exchangers in the generation of action potentials and myogenic contractility. L-type calcium channels appear to be particularly important in this regard. Use of L-type calcium channel inhibitors (nifedipine, magnesium) abolish both spontaneous and oxytocin-induced contractions in myometrial strips from term pregnant women, confirming the essential role of external Ca^{2+} in the development of phasic uterine contractions in late pregnancy.

The role of intracellular calcium stores in smooth muscle physiology has been the subject of intense investigation for at least two decades [83]. In human myometrium, sporadic increases in $[Ca^{2+}]_i$ occur primarily as a consequence of Ca^{2+} release from intracellular stores (such as the sarcoplasmic reticulum) rather than from Ca^{2+} entry through the plasma membrane. These increases are transient and are followed by Ca^{2+} entry into the cells through voltage-dependent channels. Without this Ca^{2+} influx from extracellular sources, the intracellular stores are rapidly depleted. Two types of intracellular stores can be distinguished based on the nature of their regulatory mechanisms: (i) those containing ryanodine receptors (RYR), which are activated by ryanodine or caffeine, and (ii) the inositol 1,4,5-trisphosphate receptor (IP_3R)-containing stores. The latter are associated with activation of G protein-coupled receptors (GPCR) in the cell membrane resulting in activation of phospholipase C. Several isoforms of RYR and IP_3R have been described in human myometrium [84,85].

Electrophysiological coupling

A model for the activation of human myometrium has been proposed based on electrophysiological and receptor mechanisms [76,86–88]. In this model, activation of uterine contractility during labour is driven by action potentials initiated by slow depolarization of clusters of pacemaker myometrial cells. The action potentials trigger Ca^{2+} entry into the cells through L-type voltage-operated channels, and the rise in $[Ca^{2+}]_i$ provokes contractions, thus linking the electrical signal with force (excitation–contraction coupling). This model envisages that the balance of depolarization and hyperpolarization in the cell membrane is controlled by multiple pumps and channels, including a Na^+/Ca^{2+} exchanger, a Na^+/K^+ pump and a Ca^{2+}-activated K^+ channel (see Fig. 22.3), all of which contribute to relaxation (hyperpolarization). On the other hand, Ca^{2+}-sensitive chloride channels, T-type channels and a putative channel that senses whether the

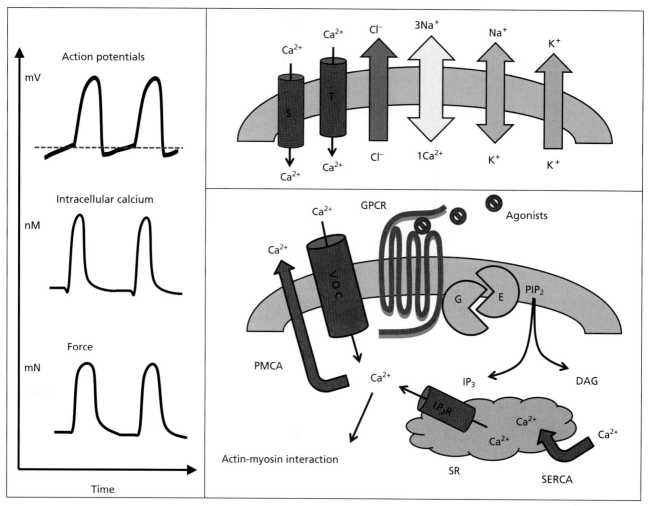

Fig. 22.3 The physiological basis of myometrial contractility. Action potentials are generated by pacemaker depolarization of the cell membrane (top) which is regulated by a complex interaction of several channels and ion pumps. These include store-operated (S) and T-type calcium channels (T) as well as calcium (Ca^{2+})-sensitive chloride (Cl^-) channels, all of which contribute to membrane depolarization. This is balanced by the Na^+/Ca^{2+} exchanger, and the strong hyperpolarizing effect of the Na^+/K^+ pump and the Ca^{2+}-sensitive potassium (K^+) channels. Action potentials (measured in mV) provoke rapid entry of Ca^{2+} into the cell by opening voltage-operated L-type channels (VOC). The resultant increase in intracellular Ca^{2+} concentrations (typically from 100 to 500 nmol/L) provokes tension (measured in mN) by enhancing actin–myosin interaction. Stimulatory agonists such as oxytocin operate through G protein-coupled receptors (GPCR) which activate G protein effector complexes (G/E). A common G/E interaction involves G_q/phospholipase C which generates two second messengers from membrane phosphatidylinositol 4,5-bisphosphate (PIP_2), namely inositol 1,4,5-trisphosphate (IP_3) and diacylglycerol (DAG). IP_3 stimulates contractility by releasing Ca^{2+} from intracellular stores in the sarcoplasmic reticulum (SR) through IP_3 receptor (IP_3R) channels. DAG stimulates protein kinase C. The phasic nature of myometrial contraction requires the activation of Ca^{2+} extrusion mechanisms to rapidly lower intracellular Ca^{2+} concentrations. These mechanisms include plasma membrane Ca^{2+}-ATPases (PMCA), which transports Ca^{2+} out of the cell, and smooth endoplasmic reticulum Ca^{2+}-ATPases (SERCA), which encourages Ca^{2+} uptake into the SR.

level of Ca^{2+} in the sarcoplasmic reticulum store is low (so called 'store operated channel') appear to tip the balance of the 'pacemaker' towards depolarization [86]. GPCR agonists like oxytocin can initiate depolarization by generating IP_3 and emptying the sarcoplasmic reticulum store through IP_3R channels, whereas RYR channels contribute to myometrial contractions by directly increasing $[Ca^{2+}]_i$ [89].

Regulation of myometrial contractility

The exact mechanisms responsible for the transition of the pregnant uterus from a long period of relative relaxation to a short period of active contractions in labour remain unknown. Greater understanding of the factors involved in the loss of uterine quiescence may assist in the anticipation and prevention of preterm labour. Therapeutic approaches to inhibit uterine contractility in women in preterm labour are still largely rudimentary, and rely on the use of drugs that are not effective or which have potentially serious side effects. We need to increase our research efforts into the endocrine control of parturition and to improve our understanding of myometrial physiology. This research is essential so that we can devise better techniques for the prediction and early diagnosis of labour, and better pharmacological strategies to control uterine contractility when indicated. A number of specific factors involved in the regulation of myometrial contractility are discussed in detail below.

Role of cell surface receptors

In addition to the spontaneous uterine activity driven by action potentials, there is strong evidence that cell surface receptors and their cell signalling pathways have a physiological influence on the regulation of uterine contractility. The uterus is richly endowed with cell surface receptors, many of which are upregulated in pregnancy and respond to classical hormones and transmitters (such as oxytocin and 5-hydroxytryptamine) as well as local modulators (prostaglandins, thromboxanes). The link between the myometrial cell membrane receptor and the initiation of a signalling cascade is mediated, in most cases, through a regulatory GTP-binding protein (G protein) (summarized in Table 22.1). G proteins can activate effector enzymes such as phospholipase Cβ (PLCβ), adenylyl cyclase or phosphoinositide 3-kinase. The PLCβ pathway is activated by receptors usually coupled to G_q, which stimulate myometrial contractility. Endogenous agonists include peptide hormones (oxytocin, endothelin),

Table 22.1 G protein-coupled receptors in myometrium and their signalling pathways.

Endogenous ligands	Receptors	G protein class	Signalling pathway	Effect on myometrial contractility
Amines				
Catecholamines	ADRA1	$G_{q/11}$	$\uparrow$PLCβ/IP$_3$–Ca^{2+}/DAG–PKCβ	Stimulation
			$\uparrow$PLCD/IP$_3$–Ca^{2+}	
	ADRA2	$G_{i/0}$	$\downarrow$ADCY/cAMP/PKA	Stimulation
	ADRB2	G_s	$\uparrow$ADCY/cAMP/PKA	Inhibition
	ADRB3	G_s	$\uparrow$ADCY/cAMP/PKA	Inhibition
		$G_{i/0}$	$\downarrow$ADCY/cAMP/PKA	
Histamine	HRH1	$G_{q/11}$	$\uparrow$PLCβ/IP$_3$–Ca^{2+}/DAG–PKCβ	Stimulation
	HRH2	G_s	$\uparrow$ADCY/cAMP/PKA	Inhibition
Serotonin	HTR1,2	$G_{i/0}$	$\downarrow$ADCY/cAMP/PKA	Stimulation
		$G_{q/11}$	$\uparrow$PLCβ/IP$_3$–Ca^{2+}/DAG–PKCβ	
	HTR4,7	G_s	$\uparrow$ADCY/cAMP/PKA	Inhibition
Eicosanoids				
PGD$_2$	PTGDR	G_s	$\uparrow$ADCY/cAMP/PKA	Inhibition
PGE$_2$	PTGER1	$G_{q/11}$	$\uparrow$PLCβ/IP$_3$–Ca^{2+}/DAG–PKCβ	Stimulation
	PTGER2,4	G_s	$\uparrow$ADCY/cAMP/PKA	Inhibition
	PTGER3	$G_{i/0}$	$\downarrow$ADCY/cAMP/PKA	Stimulation
		G_s	$\uparrow$ADCY/cAMP/PKA	Inhibition
		$G_{q/11}$	$\uparrow$PLCβ/IP$_3$–Ca^{2+}/DAG–PKCβ	
PGF$_{2\alpha}$	PTGFR	$G_{q/11}$	$\uparrow$PLCβ/IP$_3$–Ca^{2+}/DAG–PKCβ	Stimulation
Prostacyclin	PTGIR	G_s	$\uparrow$ADCY/cAMP/PKA	Inhibition
Thromboxane A$_2$	TBXA1R	$G_{q/11}$	$\uparrow$PLCβ/IP$_3$–Ca^{2+}/DAG–PKCβ	Stimulation
		$G_{12/13}$	$\uparrow$ARHGEF/RHOA/ARF6/PLD	
Peptides				
Angiotensin	AGTR2	$G_{12/13}$	$\uparrow$ARHGEF/RHOA/ARF6/PLD	Stimulation
Calcitonin-related	CL-RAMP	G_s	$\uparrow$ADCY/cAMP/PKA	Inhibition
Chorionic gonadotrophin	LHCGR	G_s	$\uparrow$ADCY/cAMP/PKA	Inhibition
Endothelin	EDNRA	$G_{q/11}$	$\uparrow$PLCβ/IP$_3$–Ca^{2+}/DAG–PKCβ	Stimulation
		G_i	$\downarrow$ADCY/cAMP/PKA	
Oxytocin/vasopressin	OXTR/AVPR1A	$G_{q/11}$	$\uparrow$PLCβ/IP$_3$–Ca^{2+}/DAG–PKCβ	Stimulation
		G_i	$\downarrow$ADCY/cAMP/PKA	

ADCY, adenylyl cyclase; ARF6, ADP-ribosylation factor 6; ARHGEF, RHO guanine nucleotide exchange factor; DAG, 1,2-diacylglycerol; GRK, G protein-coupled receptor kinase; IP$_3$, inositol 1,4,5-trisphosphate; PLCβ, phospholipase C beta; PLD, phospholipase D; PKA, protein kinase A; PKCβ, protein kinase C beta.

prostanoids (PGF$_{2\alpha}$, thromboxane A$_2$), catecholamines, muscarinic agents and inflammatory mediators (bradykinin, serotonin). The response is initiated by the hydrolysis of a receptor-sensitive pool of phosphatidylinositol 4,5-bisphosphate (PIP$_2$) in the cell membrane. The breakdown of PIP$_2$ generates two molecules with potent signalling effects: IP$_3$ which releases calcium from the sarcoplasmic reticulum, and 1,2-diacylglycerol (DAG) which activates protein kinase C (PKC) and stimulates the phosphorylation of many target proteins, including ion channels, Ca^{2+} pumps, proteins involved in GPCR function and coupling to PLC, and proteins involved in IP$_3$R regulation [90]. DAG also has PKC-independent effects. For example, in human myometrial cells, DAG analogues directly facilitate Ca^{2+} entry through the cell membrane via L-type channels and Na$^+$/Ca^{2+} exchangers [91].

Some ligands can activate more than one type of myometrial receptor, thereby creating complex responses depending on the relative abundance and affinity of each receptor subtype and the presence of other agonists competing for, or interacting with, related receptors. Moreover, G proteins are heterotrimers ($\alpha\beta\gamma$ subunits) and the effects of G$_\alpha$ subunits on PLCβ, adenylyl cyclase and other effectors are modulated by the interaction of the various G$_{\beta\gamma}$ subunits, especially those liberated from G$_i$/G$_0$ or G$_{12}$, with the same or with other effector proteins including phosphoinositide 3-kinase and ion channels. For each receptor, the effect on myometrial contractility will depend on the integration of these signals and on the physiological state of the organ under different endocrine influences. Changes in myometrial sensitivity to agonists are likely to be an important mechanism for maintaining the balance between uterine quiescence and contractility.

Oxytocin receptors

There are many genes potentially involved in the regulation of uterine contractility whose expression is modulated by oestrogens, progesterone and other pregnancy hormones. Oxytocin (OT) is a potent stimulatory peptide. Levels of OT in the maternal and fetal circulations do not change significantly during pregnancy or the first stage of labour, but the uterus becomes increasingly sensitive to circulating levels of OT at term through an increase in oxytocin receptor (OTR) concentrations in myometrial cells [92]. Indeed, it has been proposed that an increase in the concentration of OTR in the uterus may be a trigger for parturition [93]. Concentrations of OTR in the myometrium increase progressively throughout gestation reaching maximal levels in late pregnancy, and appear to remain stable during labour and delivery [85,94,95]. Uncoupling or blocking of the OTR may provide a mechanism to maintain uterine quiescence until parturition. However, the precise role of OT–OTR signalling in the

onset of labour is still uncertain. For example, both OT- and OTR-deficient mice have normal pregnancies and deliveries [96,97]. The accumulated evidence in mice suggests that inhibition of OTR function is not responsible for uterine relaxation in pregnancy, although OT retains a critical role in luteal function [98], nursing response [97] and social behaviour [96,99]. Nevertheless, the design of OTR antagonists is seen as a good approach for the management of preterm labour in women, because these drugs have relatively high uterine selectivity and few side effects [100].

Chorionic gonadotrophin receptors

In addition to its role in maintaining the corpus luteum and thereby progesterone production in early pregnancy, human chorionic gonadotrophin (hCG) also appears to have a direct effect on myometrial smooth muscle contractility. Receptors for hCG (hCGR) have been identified in human pregnant and non-pregnant myometrium, and binding of hCG to myometrial tissue decreases with the onset of labour at both term and preterm [101]. The application of hCG to human myometrial strips obtained from late pregnant women inhibits contractility [102], raising the possibility that placental gonadotrophins may serve as endogenous tocolytic agents. The action of hCG involves coupling to adenylyl cyclase through hCGR–G$_{\alpha s}$ and inhibition of intracellular Ca^{2+} fluxes through a cAMP/protein kinase A (PKA) mechanism [103]. It is not clear what PKA targets are phosphorylated on stimulation of the hCGR, but the available evidence suggest that hCG antagonizes proteins involved in OT signalling [103]. Moreover, activation of hCGR in human myometrial cells leads to loss of gap junction formation and downregulation of GJA1 (connexin 43) protein through a PKA-mediated effect [104]. Another mechanism by which the hCGR can promote uterine quiescence is through inhibition of the phosphodiesterase 5 gene in myometrial cells, thus potentiating the effect of cyclic nucleotides (such as cGMP and cAMP) [105].

β$_2$-Adrenergic receptors

The β$_2$-adrenergic receptor (ADRB2) has been a pharmacological target to relax the uterus for many years through the use of so-called beta-mimetic drugs. Exposure of human pregnant myometrial strips to the β$_2$-agonists isoproterenol and ritodrine results in a significant decrease in contractile force and in the frequency of spontaneous contractions [106–108]. Inhibitory receptors such as ADRB2 and the PGE receptor (PGER2) couple through G$_{\alpha s}$ to increase intracellular adenylyl cyclase activity and cAMP production, thereby suppressing myometrial contractility. In contrast, receptors coupled to G$_i$/G$_0$ (e.g. α$_2$-adrenoceptor, ADRA2) inhibit adenylyl cyclase and decrease cAMP production, which favours uterine contractions. Changes in the sensitivity of the uterus to endogenous agonists (catecholamines, prostaglandins) operating through these receptors may be responsible for the transition from uterine quiescence to the onset of labour. Although attractive, this hypothesis remains to be verified. Beta-mimetics (ritodrine, terbutaline, salbutamol) were among the earliest agents used clinically to inhibit uterine contractions in the setting of preterm labour, but their efficacy remains questionable [109]. Moreover, since ADRB2 receptors are widely expressed in many organ systems, the use of beta-mimetics in pregnancy is associated with potentially serious cardiovascular, neuromuscular and metabolic side effects.

Role of gap junction proteins

Uterine relaxation during pregnancy is due in part to a lack of electrical and metabolic coordination between adjacent myometrial smooth muscle cells. Gap junctions are specialized protein channels that facilitate the propagation of electrical activity and the exchange of small molecules between adjacent cells. Thus, the appearance of gap junctions in myometrium is thought to herald the onset of labour [110–112]. GJA1 (connexin 43) is one of the main structural proteins in myometrial gap junctions. Its expression is stimulated by oestradiol and retinoic acid, and inhibited by progesterone [113–115]. The function of gap junctions is tightly regulated through phosphorylation of specific serine residues at the C-terminal of GJA1. Conditional deletion of the *GJA1* gene in a murine model was associated with a dramatic delay in parturition [116].

Uterine stimulants and relaxants

The list of uterine stimulants and relaxants implicated in the onset of labour at term are summarized in Table 22.2. Some of these are discussed in further detail below.

Uterine stimulants

Oxytocin

Oxytocin is a potent endogenous uterotonic agent. The uterus is very sensitive to OT and it is capable of stimulating uterine contractions if given exogenously at intravenous infusion rates of 1–2 mU/min at term. However, many uncertainties remain about its mechanism of action. For instance, analysis of the Ca^{2+}–tension relationship in pregnant myometrial strips reveals a strong component of 'Ca^{2+} sensitization' during OT-induced contractions [117,118] probably involving inhibition of myosin phosphatase. The pathways involved are under investigation, but likely involve small GTP-binding proteins of the RHO family and activation of RHO-dependent kinases [119].

Table 22.2 Endogenous and exogenous factors affecting myometrial contractility during labour.

Uterine stimulants

Endogenous
Oxytocin
Prostaglandins
Endothelin
Epidermal growth factor

Exogenous
Oxytocin
Prostaglandins

Uterine relaxants

Endogenous
Relaxin
Nitric oxide
L-Arginine
Magnesium
Corticotrophin releasing hormone

Exogenous
β-Adrenergic agonists (ritodrine hydrochloride, terbutaline sulphate, salbutamol, fenoterol)
Oxytocin receptor antagonist (atosiban)
Magnesium sulphate
Calcium channel blockers (nifedipine, diltiazem, verapamil)
Prostaglandin inhibitors (indometacin)
Phosphodiesterase inhibitor (aminophylline)
Nitric oxide donor (nitroglycerine, sodium nitroprusside)

Prostaglandins

Summary box 22.3

Prostaglandins are the final common pathway of the parturition cascade. Prostaglandins given by any route to any species at any stage of gestation will result in pregnancy termination.

Prostaglandins cause uterine contractions and cervical effacement and dilatation, and can be used clinically for induction of labour. A detailed discussion of the central role that prostaglandins play in the onset of labour is beyond the scope of this chapter and has been reviewed elsewhere [4–9,29,30].

Endothelin

Endothelin is a 21-amino-acid peptide with potent vasoconstrictor properties that binds to specific receptors on vascular endothelial cells to regulate vascular haemostasis. Endothelin receptors have also been isolated in amnion, chorion, endometrium and myometrium [120,121], and increase in the myometrium during labour [121,122]. Endothelin promotes uterine contractility directly by increasing $[Ca^{2+}]_i$ [120,123] and indirectly by stimulating prostaglandin production by the decidua and fetal membranes [121].

Epidermal growth factor

Epidermal growth factor (EGF) is a ubiquitous growth factor that plays an important role in the regulation of cell growth, proliferation and differentiation. It acts by binding to specific cell-surface tyrosine kinase receptors that have been identified also in decidua and myometrium, and appear to be upregulated by oestrogen [120]. EGF appears to promote uterine contractility directly by increasing $[Ca^{2+}]_i$ [124] and indirectly by mobilizing arachidonic acid and increasing the synthesis and release of prostaglandins by the decidua and fetal membranes [121].

Uterine relaxants

Relaxin

Relaxin is secreted by the corpus luteum, placenta and myometrium, and relaxin binding sites have been identified on myometrial cells [125]. Relaxin inhibits myometrial contractility by promoting calcium efflux thereby decreasing $[Ca^{2+}]_i$ and inhibiting agonist-mediated activation of Ca^{2+} channels; it also directly inhibits MLCK phosphorylation [81,125,126]. Unfortunately, exogenous administration of relaxin has not been shown to consistently inhibit uterine contractile activity [127].

Parathyroid hormone-related protein

Parathyroid hormone-related protein (PTHrP) is produced by many tissues and has several functions in both developing and adult tissues including regulation of vascular tone, bone remodelling, placental calcium transport and myometrial relaxation. In rat myometrium, levels of PTHrP mRNA increase during late gestation and are higher in gravid compared with non-gravid myometrium [128]. In pregnant rats, administration of PTHrP(1–34) inhibits spontaneous contractions in the longitudinal layer of the myometrium; in non-pregnant rats, PTHrP(1–34) inhibits both OT- and acetylcholine-stimulated uterine contractions [129,130] and delays but does not completely abrogate the increase in connexin 43 and OTR gene expression [131]. PTHrP(1–34) has been shown to exert a significant relaxant effect on human myometrium collected from late gestation tissues obtained before but not after the onset of labour [132]. Taken together, these data suggest that the onset of labour is associated with a removal of the ability of PTHrP to exert its myometrial relaxant effect.

Calcitonin gene-related peptide and adrenomedullin

Circulating levels of calcitonin gene-related peptide (CGRP) and adrenomedullin are increased in pregnancy, and have been implicated in the maintenance of myometrial quiescence throughout gestation [133–135]. CGRP has been shown to inhibit myometrial contractility in rats [133], humans [136] and mice [137]. However, this effect disappears after the onset of labour, suggesting that progesterone may be required to mediate GCRP activity [133]. Adrenomedullin has been shown to inhibit spontaneous as well as bradykinin- and galanin-induced uterine contractions in rats [134,138], but its role in human pregnancy is not well established.

Magnesium

Magnesium is present in high concentrations in the myometrium. Here, it inhibits Ca^{2+} entry into myometrial cells via L- and T-type voltage-operated calcium channels and enhances the sensitivity of Ca^{2+}-activated K^+ channels [126,139], which leads to hyperpolarization and myometrial cell relaxation. Moreover, since they are both cations, magnesium competes with calcium within the cell for calmodulin binding resulting in decreased affinity of calmodulin complexes for MLCK, which further favours myometrial relaxation [140].

Nitric oxide

In the early 1980s, Furchgott and colleagues described a factor released by the endothelium of blood vessels that relaxed vascular smooth muscle cells. It was upregulated by acetylcholine, bradykinin, histamine and 5-hydroxytryptamine, and inhibited by haemoglobin. This so-called 'endothelium-derived relaxing factor' was subsequently shown to be nitric oxide (NO) [141,142]. NO activates the guanylate cyclase pathway leading to the production of cGMP, which decreases $[Ca^{2+}]_i$ and interferes with myosin light chain phosphorylation [143,144]. NO and its substrate L-arginine, as well as NO donors (such as sodium nitroprusside), have been shown to cause relaxation of myometrial contractile activity both *in vitro* and *in vivo* [145]. Under physiological conditions, L-arginine is converted to L-citrulline and NO by the enzyme nitric oxide synthase (NOS). There are three distinct NOS isoforms: neuronal NOS (nNOS or NOS1), inducible NOS (iNOS or NOS2) and endothelial NOS (eNOS or NOS3). nNOS and eNOS are calcium-dependent constitutive isoforms, whereas iNOS is a calcium-independent inducible enzyme that is highly expressed in macrophages and other tissues especially in the setting of inflammation. The role of NO in the cardiovascular, nervous and immune systems has been extensively studied and confirmed, but its involvement in uterine relaxation remains more controversial. iNOS is expressed in human myometrium, and some studies have suggested that its expression decreases before the onset of labour at both term and preterm [146]. However, other studies have been unable to confirm these observations [147–149]. Moreover, the addition of L-arginine or the NOS inhibitor

L-nitro-arginine methyl ester (L-NAME) does not affect myometrial contractility *in vitro* [145,150]. Taken together, these studies suggest that the NO pathway is not directly involved in the regulation of uterine contractility in human pregnancy.

Phosphodiesterase

The phosphodiesterase (PDE) multigene family of enzymes attenuate the effects of cAMP and cGMP by catalysing their hydrolysis and inactivation, and so occupy a key position in modulating intracellular cyclic nucleotide levels. Twelve distinct but related families of PDE have been established according to sequence homology, substrate specificity, inhibitor sensitivity, and function. Several isoforms of PDE have been identified in the human uterus [151–153]. All PDE1 subtypes are activated by Ca^{2+}/calmodulin [154,155] and are therefore uniquely placed to integrate Ca^{2+} and cyclic nucleotide signalling pathways. The activity of the PDE enzymes responsible for cAMP degradation was found to be significantly inhibited in myometrial tissue during pregnancy [156], likely as a consequence of high progesterone levels [157], suggesting that PDE inhibition may be part of the mechanism responsible for myometrial relaxation and pregnancy maintenance. Several non-selective and selective PDE inhibitors have been studied in an effort to develop an effective tocolytic agent to treat preterm labour, including 3-isobutyl-1-methylxanthine (a non-specific PDE inhibitor), rolipram (a PDE4-specific inhibitor), vinpocetin (a PDE1-specific inhibitor) and sildenafil (a PDE5-specific inhibitor) [151,158]. Despite their ability to exert potent relaxant [151,159–162] and anti-inflammatory effects [160] on strips of myometrial tissues collected from pregnant women, the therapeutic value of these agents appears to be limited by their lack of specificity, low potency and maternal side effects.

Exogenous uterine relaxants

A number of uterine relaxants have been developed in an attempt to prevent and stop preterm labour (see Table 22.2). Unfortunately, the ability of these tocolytic agents to prevent preterm birth has been largely disappointing.

β₂-Adrenergic receptor agonists

ADRB2 agonists act through specific receptors on myometrial cells to activate cAMP-dependent PKA, which in turn inhibits myosin light chain phosphorylation [163] and decreases $[Ca^{2+}]_i$ [126,139], thereby leading to myometrial relaxation.

Oxytocin receptor antagonists

Synthetic competitive OTR antagonists such as atosiban (which has mixed vasopressin/oxytocin receptor specificity) inhibit uterine contractility both *in vitro* and *in vivo* [164–166]. The relative absence of OTR in other organ systems (with the exception of the kidney) suggests that such agents should have few side effects, and this has been borne out by a number of clinical trials [167–169].

Calcium channel blockers

Calcium channel blockers function primarily by inhibiting the entry of Ca^{2+} via voltage-dependent L-type calcium channels. This causes uterine relaxation, but may also have adverse effects on the atrioventricular conduction pathway in the heart.

Prostaglandin synthesis inhibitors

Prostaglandin synthesis inhibitors inactivate the cyclooxygenase enzyme responsible for the conversion of arachidonic acid to the intermediate metabolite PGH_2, which is subsequently converted to PGE_2 and $PGF_{2\alpha}$. Aspirin causes irreversible acetylation of the cyclooxygenase (COX) enzyme, whereas indometacin is a competitive (reversible) inhibitor. Although relatively effective in suppressing uterine contractions, the adverse effects of these agents on the developing fetus (including premature closure of the ductus arteriosus and persistent pulmonary hypertension) have significantly limited their use. Moreover, these adverse effects can be seen with both non-selective COX inhibitors (such as indometacin) and those that are selective for the inducible isoform COX-2 (meloxicam, celecoxib).

Mechanics of normal labour at term

Labour and delivery is not a passive process in which uterine contractions push a rigid object through a fixed aperture. The ability of the fetus to successfully negotiate the pelvis is dependent on the complex interaction of three variables: the powers, the passenger and the passage.

The powers

The powers refers to the forces generated by the uterine musculature. Uterine activity is characterized by the frequency, amplitude (intensity) and duration of contractions. It can be assessed by observation, palpation, external monitors (such as external tocodynamometry, which measures changes in shape of the abdominal wall as a function of uterine contractions and is therefore more qualitative than quantitative), and direct measurement of intrauterine pressure (which requires insertion of a pressure transducer directly into the uterine cavity usually through the cervix after rupture of the fetal membranes). It is generally believed that the more optimal the powers, the more likely a woman is to have a successful vaginal delivery; however, there are few data to support this statement. Classically, three to five contractions in 10 min has been used to define 'adequate' uterine activity in labour, and is seen in around 95% of women in spontaneous labour at term. Various units have been devised to objectively measure uterine activity using an intrauterine pressure transducer, the most common of which are *Montevideo units* (the average strength of contractions in mmHg multiplied by the number of contractions per 10 min), which is a measure of average frequency and amplitude above basal tone; 200–250 Montevideo units defines adequate labour [170,171]. The ultimate measure of uterine activity is a clinical one. If uterine contractions are 'adequate', one of two events will occur: either the cervix will efface and dilate and the fetal head will descend, or there will be worsening caput succedaneum (scalp oedema) and/or moulding (overlapping) of the skull bones. The latter situation suggests a diagnosis of cephalopelvic disproportion.

The passenger

The passenger is the fetus. There are several fetal variables that may influence the course of labour and delivery.

1 Fetal size: can be estimated clinically through the use of the four Leopold's manoeuvres or by ultrasound.

2 Fetal lie: refers to the longitudinal axis of the fetus relative to the longitudinal axis of the uterus.

3 Fetal presentation: refers to the fetal part that directly overlies the pelvic inlet.

4 Attitude: refers to the position of the head with regard to the fetal spine (i.e. the degree of flexion and/or extension of the fetal head).

5 Position of the fetus: refers to the orientation of the fetal presenting part relative to the maternal pelvis.

6 Station: a measure of descent of the presenting part of the fetus through the birth canal.

The presence of a multifetal pregnancy increases the probability of abnormal lie and malpresentation in labour.

The passage

The passage consists of the bony pelvis (sacrum, ilium, ischium and pubis) and the resistance provided by the pelvic soft tissues (cervix and muscles of the pelvic floor). Measurements of the various parameters of the female bony pelvis have been made with great precision, both directly in cadavers and through the use of imaging (computed tomography and magnetic resonance imaging) in living women, and four distinct shapes have been defined (gynecoid, anthropoid, android and platypelloid). In practice, however, the use of clinical pelvimetry to assess the pelvic shape and capacity is of limited value. The only way to determine whether a given fetus will be able to pass safely through a given pelvis is for a woman to undergo a trial of labour.

Stages of labour

Although labour is a continuous process, for reasons of study and to assist in clinical management, it has been

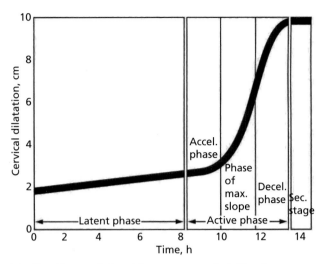

Fig. 22.4 Characteristics of the average cervical dilatation curve for nulliparous labour. The 2-hour 'action line' is shown as a stippled line. (Modified from Friedman EA. *Labour: Clinical Evaluation and Management*, 2nd edn. New York: Appleton-Century-Crofts, 1978 with permission.)

 Summary box 22.4

Labour and delivery is not a passive process in which uterine contractions push a rigid object through a fixed aperture. The ability of the fetus to successfully negotiate the pelvis is dependent on the complex interaction of three variables: the powers, the passenger and the passage.

divided into three stages as described by Friedman (Fig. 22.4) [172,173]. The first stage refers to the interval between the onset of labour and full cervical dilatation (10 cm). It has been subdivided into several phases according to the rate of cervical dilatation. The duration and rate of cervical change during the second stage of labour varies between nulliparous and multiparous women (Table 22.3). The second stage refers to the interval between full cervical dilatation and delivery of the infant. The third stage refers to delivery of the placenta and fetal membranes and usually lasts less than 10 min, but up to 30 min may be allowed in the absence of excessive bleeding before active intervention is considered.

Cardinal movements in labour

The mechanisms of labour, also known as the cardinal movements, refer to the changes in position of the fetal head during its passage through the birth canal. Because of the asymmetry of the shape of both the fetal head and the maternal bony pelvis, such rotations are required for the fetus to successfully negotiate the birth canal. Although labour and birth is a continuous process, seven discrete cardinal movements of the fetus are described: engagement (passage of the widest diameter of the pre-

Table 22.3 Progression of spontaneous labour at term.

Parameter	Mean	Fifth percentile
Nulliparas		
Total duration of labour	10.1 hours	25.8 hours
Duration of first stage of labour	9.7 hours	24.7 hours
Duration of second stage of labour	33.0 min	117.5 min
Duration of latent phase	6.4 hours	20.6 hours
Rate of cervical dilatation during active phase	3.0 cm/hour	1.2 cm/hour
Duration of third stage of labour	5.0 min	30.0 min
Multiparas		
Total duration of labour	6.2 hours	19.5 hours
Duration of first stage of labour	8.0 hours	18.8 hours
Duration of second stage of labour	8.5 min	46.5 min
Duration of latent phase	4.8 hours	13.6 hours
Rate of cervical dilatation during active phase	5.7 cm/hour	1.5 cm/hour
Duration of third stage of labour	5.0 min	30.0 min

Source: data from Friedman EA. *Labour: Clinical Evaluation and Management*, 2nd edn. New York: Appleton-Century-Crofts, 1978 with permission.

senting part to a level below the plane of the pelvic inlet), descent, flexion, internal rotation, extension, external rotation (also known as restitution) and expulsion (Fig. 22.5).

Management of uncomplicated labour and delivery

Intrapartum management

Initial assessment in labour should include a focused history (time of onset of contractions, status of the fetal membranes, presence or absence of vaginal bleeding, perception of fetal movement), physical examination and routine necessary laboratory testing (full blood count, blood type). Physical examination should include documentation of the patient's vital signs, notation of fetal position and presentation, an assessment of fetal well-being, and an estimation of the frequency, duration and quality of uterine contractions. The size, lie, presentation and engagement of the fetus should be assessed by abdominal palpation. If there are no contraindications to pelvic examination, the degree of cervical dilatation, effacement, status of the fetal membranes, and the position and station of the presenting part should be noted. If the practitioner is still uncertain about fetal presentation or if the clinical examination suggests an abnormality (such as a multifetal pregnancy, low amniotic fluid volume or intrauterine growth restriction), an ultrasound examination is indicated. Assessment of the quality of

uterine contractions and degree of cervical dilatation should be performed at appropriate intervals in order to follow the progress of labour. Vaginal examinations should be kept to a minimum to avoid promoting intra-amniotic infection. Pain management should be discussed and implemented when desired. The fetal heart rate should be recorded before, during and after a uterine contraction at least every 30 min in the first stage of labour and every 15 min in the second stage.

Clinical assistance at delivery

Preparation for delivery should take into account the patient's parity, presentation of the fetus and the progression of labour. The goals of clinical assistance at delivery are the reduction of maternal trauma, prevention of fetal injury and initial support of the newborn if required. When the fetal head crowns and delivery is imminent, pressure from the practitioner's hand is used to hold the head flexed and to control delivery, thereby preventing precipitous expulsion, which has been associated with perineal tears as well as intracranial trauma. Once the fetal head is delivered, external rotation (restitution) is allowed to occur. If the cord is around the neck, it should be looped over the head or, if not reducible, doubly clamped and transected. Use of suction to clear secretions from the fetal mouth, oropharynx and nares has not been shown to reduce the incidence of meconium aspiration syndrome [174] and, as such, is not routinely recommended. Thereafter, a hand is placed on each parietal eminence and the anterior shoulder of the fetus is delivered with the next contraction by downwards traction towards the mother's sacrum in concert with maternal expulsive efforts. The posterior shoulder is then delivered by upwards traction. The infant should be held securely and wiped dry with a sterile towel. The timing of cord clamping is dictated by convenience and is usually performed immediately after delivery.

Delivery of the placenta and fetal membranes

The third stage of labour can be managed either passively or actively. *Passive management* involves waiting for the three classic signs of placental separation (lengthening of the umbilical cord, a gush of blood from the vagina signifying separation of the placenta from the uterine wall, and a change in the shape of the uterine fundus from discoid to globular with elevation of the fundal height) before applying traction to the umbilical cord. *Active management* of the third stage has been shown to reduce total blood loss and the incidence of postpartum haemorrhage [175], but can complicate management in cases involving an undiagnosed second twin or placenta accreta. In active management, uterotonic agents such as oxytocin are administered at birth to hasten delivery of the placenta. Two techniques of controlled cord traction are described

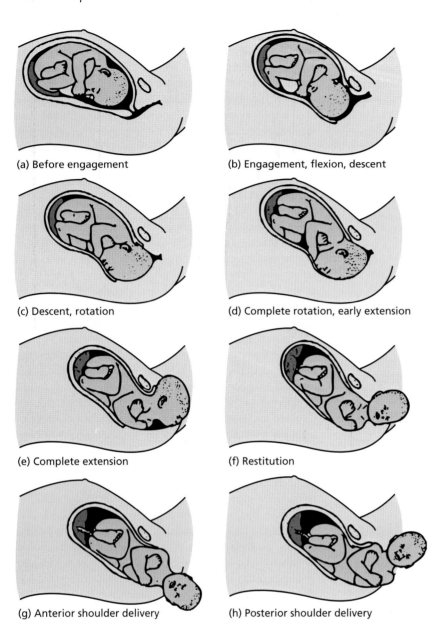

(a) Before engagement

(b) Engagement, flexion, descent

(c) Descent, rotation

(d) Complete rotation, early extension

(e) Complete extension

(f) Restitution

(g) Anterior shoulder delivery

(h) Posterior shoulder delivery

Fig. 22.5 Cardinal movements of the fetus during labour and birth.

to facilitate separation and delivery of the placenta: (i) the Brandt–Andrews manoeuvre, in which an abdominal hand secures the uterine fundus to prevent uterine inversion while the other hand exerts sustained downwards traction on the umbilical cord; or (ii) the Créde manoeuvre, in which the cord is fixed with the lower hand while the uterine fundus is secured and sustained upwards traction applied using the abdominal hand. Care should be taken to avoid avulsion of the cord.

After delivery, the placenta, umbilical cord and fetal membranes should be examined. A missing placental cotyledon or a membrane defect may suggest retention of a portion of the placenta, which can lead to postpartum haemorrhage or infection. In this setting, manual and/or surgical exploration of the uterus may be required to remove the offending tissue. The cervix, vagina and peri-

neum should also be carefully examined for evidence of birth injury. If a laceration is seen, its length and position should be noted and repair initiated. Adequate analgesia (either regional or local) is essential for repair. Special attention should be paid to repair of the perineal body, the external rectal sphincter, and the rectal mucosa. Failure to recognize and repair rectal injury can lead to serious long-term morbidity, most notably faecal incontinence.

Conclusions

The timely onset of labour and birth is an important determinant of perinatal outcome. Labour is a physiological and continuous process. The factors responsible for the onset and maintenance of labour at term are not completely understood, and continue to be under active investigation. A better understanding of the mechanisms responsible for the onset of labour will further our knowledge about disorders of parturition, such as preterm and prolonged (post-term) labour, and will improve our ability to secure a successful pregnancy outcome.

Acknowledgements

Work described here has been supported by Wellbeing of Women, the SAFE network of Excellence, the Wellcome Trust (A.L.B.) and the March of Dimes (E.R.N.).

References

1 Sennstrom MB, Ekman G, Westergren-Thorsson G *et al.* Human cervical ripening, an inflammatory process mediated by cytokines. *Mol Hum Reprod* 2000;6:375–381.

2 Dubicke A, Andersson P, Fransson E *et al.* High-mobility group box protein 1 and its signalling receptors in human preterm and term cervix. *J Reprod Immunol* 2010;84:86–94.

3 Nathanielsz PW, Giussani DA, Wu WX. Stimulation of the switch in myometrial activity from contractures to contractions in the pregnant sheep and nonhuman primate. *Equine Vet J* 1997;24:83–88.

4 Liggins GC. Initiation of labour. *Biol Neonate* 1989;55: 366–394.

5 Challis JRG, Gibb W. Control of parturition. *Prenat Neonat Med* 1996;1:283–291.

6 Nathanielsz PW. Comparative studies on the initiation of labour. *Eur J Obstet Gynecol Reprod Biol* 1998;78:127–132.

7 Norwitz ER, Robinson JN, Challis JRG. The control of labour. *N Engl J Med* 1999;341:660–667.

8 Challis JRG, Matthews SG, Gibb W, Lye SJ. Endocrine and paracrine regulation of birth at term and preterm. *Endocr Rev* 2000;21:514–550.

9 Mendelson CR. Fetal–maternal hormonal signalling in pregnancy and labour. *Mol Endocrinol* 2009;23:947–954.

10 Wen SW, Smith G, Yang Q, Walker M. Epidemiology of preterm birth and neonatal outcome. *Semin Fetal Neonatal Med* 2004;9:429–435.

11 Liggins GC. The onset of labour: an overview. In: McNellis D, Challis JRG, MacDonald PC, Nathanielsz PW, Roberts JM (eds) *The Onset of Labour: Cellular and Integrative Mechanisms.* A National Institute of Child Health and Human Development Research Planning Workshop (29 November to 1 December, 1987). Ithaca, NY: Perinatology Press, 1988: 1–3.

12 Iams JD, Goldenberg RL, Mercer BM *et al.* The Preterm Prediction Study: recurrence risk of spontaneous preterm birth. National Institute of Child Health and Human Development Maternal–Fetal Medicine Units Network. *Am J Obstet Gynecol* 1998;178:1035–1040.

13 Winkvist A, Mogren I, Hogberg U. Familial patterns in birth characteristics: impact on individual and population risks. *Int J Epidemiol* 1998;27:248–254.

14 Carmichael SL, Iyasu S, Hatfield-Timajchy K. Cause-specific trends in neonatal mortality among black and white infants, United States, 1980–1995. *Matern Child Health J* 1998;2: 67–76.

15 Ventura SJ, Bachrach CA. Nonmarital childbearing in the United States, 1940–99. *Natl Vital Stat Rep* 2000;48:1–10.

16 Blackmore CA, Ferre CD, Rowley DL, Hogue CJ, Gaiter J, Atrash H. Is race a risk factor or a risk marker for preterm delivery? *Ethn Dis* 1993;3:372–377.

17 Blackmore-Prince C, Kieke B Jr, Kugaraj KA *et al.* Racial differences in the patterns of singleton preterm delivery in the 1988 National Maternal and Infant Health Survey. *Matern Child Health J* 1999;3:189–197.

18 Ekwo E, Moawad A. The risk for recurrence of premature births to African-American and white women. *J Assoc Acad Minor Phys* 1998;9:16–21.

19 Mercer BM, Goldenberg RL, Moawad AH *et al.* The Preterm Prediction Study: effect of gestational age and cause of preterm birth on subsequent obstetric outcome. National Institute of Child Health and Human Development Maternal–Fetal Medicine Units Network. *Am J Obstet Gynecol* 1999;181:1216–1221.

20 Ananth CV, Getahun D, Peltier MR, Salihu HM, Vintzileos AM. Recurrence of spontaneous versus medically indicated preterm birth. *Am J Obstet Gynecol* 2006;195:643–650.

21 Getahun D, Ananth CV, Selvam N, Demissie K. Adverse perinatal outcomes among interracial couples in the United States. *Obstet Gynecol* 2005;106:81–88.

22 Esplin MS. Preterm birth: a review of genetic factors and future directions for genetic study. *Obstet Gynecol Surv* 2006; 61:800–806.

23 Gibson CS, MacLennan AH, Dekker GA *et al.* Genetic polymorphisms and spontaneous preterm birth. *Obstet Gynecol* 2007;109:384–391.

24 Menon R, Forunato SJ, Thorsen P, Williams S. Genetic associations in preterm birth: a primer of marker selection, study design, and data analysis. *J Soc Gynecol Investig* 2006;13: 531–541.

25 Genç MR, Vardhana S, Delaney ML, Witkin SS, Onderdonk A for the MAP Study Group. TNFA –308 G → A polymorphism influences the TNF-alpha response to altered vaginal flora. *Eur J Obstet Gynecol Reprod Biol* 2007;134:188–191.

26 Macones GA, Parry S, Elkousy M, Clothier B, Ural SH, Strauss JF III. A polymorphism in the promoter region of TNF and bacterial vaginosis: preliminary evidence of gene–environment interaction in the aetiology of spontaneous preterm birth. *Am J Obstet Gynecol* 2004;190:1504–1508.

27 Nguyen DP, Genç MR, Vardhana S, Babula O, Onderdonk A, Witkin SS. Ethnic differences of polymorphisms in cytokine and innate immune system genes in pregnant women. *Obstet Gynecol* 2004;104:293–300.

28 Norwitz ER, Lye SJ. Biology of parturition. In: Creasy RK, Resnick R, Iams JD, Lockwood CJ, Moore T (eds) *Creasy and Resnick's Maternal–Fetal Medicine*, 6th edn. Philadelphia: Elsevier, 2009: 69–85.

29 Myers DA, Nathanielsz PW. Biologic basis of term and preterm labour. *Clin Perinatol* 1993;20:9–28.

30 Honnebier MB, Nathanielsz PW. Primate parturition and the role of the maternal circadian system. *Eur J Obstet Gynecol Reprod Biol* 1994;55:193–203.

31 Madden JD, Gant NF, MacDonald PC. Study of the kinetics of conversion of maternal plasma dehydroisoandrosterone sulfate to 16 alpha-hydroxydehydroisoandrosterone sulfate, estradiol, and estriol. *Am J Obstet Gynecol* 1978;132:392–395.

32 Mecenas CA, Giussani DA, Owiny JR *et al*. Production of premature delivery in pregnant rhesus monkeys by androstenedione infusion. *Nat Med* 1996;2:443–448.

33 Figueroa JP, Honnebier MBOM, Binienda Z, Wimsatt J, Nathanielsz PW. Effect of 48 hour intravenous Δ^4 androstenedione infusion on pregnant rhesus monkeys in the last third of gestation: changes in maternal plasma estradiol concentrations and myometrial contractility. *Am J Obstet Gynecol* 1989; 161:481–486.

34 Nathanielsz PW, Jenkins SL, Tame JD, Winter JA, Guller S, Giussani DA. Local paracrine effects of estradiol are central to parturition in the rhesus monkey. *Nat Med* 1998;4: 456–459.

35 Mesiano S, Wang Y, Norwitz ER. Progesterone receptors in the human pregnancy uterus: do they hold the key to birth timing? *Reprod Sci* 2011;18:6–19.

36 Young IR, Renfree MB, Mesiano S, Shaw G, Jenkin G, Smith R. The comparative physiology of parturition in mammals: hormones and parturition in mammals. In: Norris D, Lopez K (eds) *Hormones and Reproduction in Vertebrates*. London: Academic Press, 2010.

37 Young IR. The comparative physiology of parturition in mammals. *Front Horm Res* 2001;27:10–30.

38 Tulchinsky D, Hobel CJ, Yeager E, Marshall JR. Plasma estrone, estradiol, estriol, progesterone, and 17-hydroxyprogesterone in human pregnancy. I. Normal pregnancy. *Am J Obstet Gynecol* 1972;112:1095–1100.

39 Boroditsky RS, Reyes FI, Winter JS, Faiman C. Maternal serum oestrogen and progesterone concentrations preceding normal labour. *Obstet Gynecol* 1978;51:686–691.

40 Corner GW. *The Hormones in Human Reproduction*. London: Princeton University Press, 1946.

41 Csapo A. Progesterone block. *Am J Anat* 1956;98:273–291.

42 Avrech OM, Golan A, Weinraub Z, Bukovsky I, Caspi E. Mifepristone (RU486) alone or in combination with a prostaglandin analogue for termination of early pregnancy: a review. *Fertil Steril* 1991;56:385–393.

43 Chwalisz K, Stockemann K, Fuhrmann U, Fritzemeier KH, Einspanier A, Garfield RE. Mechanism of action of antiprogestins in the pregnant uterus. *Ann NY Acad Sci* 1995;761: 202–223.

44 Meis PJ, Klebanoff M, Thom E *et al*. Prevention of recurrent preterm delivery by 17 alpha-hydroxyprogesterone caproate. *N Engl J Med* 2003;348:2379–2385.

45 da Fonseca EB, Bittar RE, Carvalho MH, Zugaib M. Prophylactic administration of progesterone by vaginal suppository to reduce the incidence of spontaneous preterm birth in women at increased risk: a randomised placebo-controlled double-blind study. *Am J Obstet Gynecol* 2003;188:419–424.

46 Fonseca EB, Celik E, Parra M, Singh M, Nicolaides KH. Progesterone and the risk of preterm birth among women with a short cervix. *N Engl J Med* 2007;357:462–469.

47 Condon JC, Jeyasuria P, Faust JM, Mendelson CR. Surfactant protein secreted by the maturing mouse fetal lung acts as a hormone that signals the initiation of parturition. *Proc Natl Acad Sci USA* 2004;101:4978–4983.

48 Miyamura K, Malhotra R, Hoppe HJ *et al*. Surfactant proteins A (SP-A) and D (SP-D): levels in human amniotic fluid and localization in the fetal membranes. *Biochim Biophys Acta* 1994; 1210:303–307.

49 Crouch E, Wright JR. Surfactant proteins A and D and pulmonary host defence. *Annu Rev Physiol* 2001;63:521–554.

50 López Bernal A, Phizackerley PJ. Fetal surfactant as a source of arachidonate in human amniotic fluid. *Prostaglandins Other Lipid Mediat* 2000;60:59–70.

51 Casey ML, MacDonald PC. Biomolecular processes in the initiation of parturition: decidual activation. *Clin Obstet Gynecol* 1988;31:533–552.

52 Nagamatsu T, Schust DJ. The immunomodulatory roles of macrophages at the maternal–fetal interface. *Reprod Sci* 2010;17:209–218.

53 Kang J, Chapdelaine P, Laberge PY, Fortier MA. Functional characterisation of prostaglandin transporter and terminal prostaglandin synthases during decidualization of human endometrial stromal cells. *Hum Reprod* 2006;21:592–599.

54 Olson DM. The role of prostaglandins in the initiation of parturition. *Best Pract Res Clin Obstet Gynaecol* 2003;17: 717–730.

55 Gordon S. Alternative activation of macrophages. *Nat Rev Immunol* 2003;3:23–35.

56 Lidstrom C, Matthiesen L, Berg G, Sharma S, Ernerudh J, Ekerfelt C. Cytokine secretion patterns of NK cells and macrophages in early human pregnancy decidua and blood: implications for suppressor macrophages in decidua. *Am J Reprod Immunol* 2003;50:444–452.

57 Cupurdija K, Azzola D, Hainz U *et al*. Macrophages of human first trimester decidua express markers associated to alternative activation. *Am J Reprod Immunol* 2004;51:117–122.

58 Heikkinen J, Mottonen M, Komi J, Alanen A, Lassila O. Phenotypic characterisation of human decidual macrophages. *Clin Exp Immunol* 2003;131:498–505.

59 Kudo Y, Hara T, Katsuki T *et al*. Mechanisms regulating the expression of indoleamine 2,3-dioxygenase during decidualization of human endometrium. *Hum Reprod* 2004;19: 1222–1230.

60 Vince GS, Starkey PM, Jackson MC, Sargent IL, Redman CW. Flow cytometric characterisation of cell populations in human pregnancy decidua and isolation of decidual macrophages. *J Immunol Methods* 1990;132:181–189.

61 Abrahams VM, Kim YM, Straszewski SL, Romero R, Mor G. Macrophages and apoptotic cell clearance during pregnancy. *Am J Reprod Immunol* 2004;51:275–282.

62 Norwitz ER, Starkey PM, López Bernal A, Turnbull AC. Identification by flow cytometry of the prostaglandin-producing cell populations of term human decidua. *J Endocrinol* 1991;131:327–334.

63 Singh U, Nicholson G, Urban BC, Sargent IL, Kishore U, Bernal AL. Immunological properties of human decidual macrophages: a possible role in intrauterine immunity. *Reproduction* 2005;129:631–637.

64 Mitchell MD, Chang MC, Chaiworapongsa T *et al*. Identification of 9alpha,11beta-prostaglandin F2 in human amniotic fluid and characterisation of its production by human gestational tissues. *J Clin Endocrinol Metab* 2005;90:4244–4248.

65 Norwitz ER, López Bernal A, Starkey PM. Tumour necrosis factor-alpha selectively stimulates prostaglandin F2 alpha

production by macrophages in human term decidua. *Am J Obstet Gynecol* 1992;167:815–820.

66 Pauerstein CJ, Zauder HL. Autonomic innervation, sex steroids and uterine contractility. *Obstet Gynecol Surv* 1970;25: S617–S630.

67 Yu JT, López Bernal A. The cytoskeleton of human myometrial cells. *J Reprod Fertil* 1998;112:185–198.

68 Sellers JR. Myosins: a diverse superfamily. *Biochim Biophys Acta* 2000;1496:3–22.

69 Takashima S. Phosphorylation of myosin regulatory light chain by myosin light chain kinase, and muscle contraction. *Circ J* 2009;73:208–213.

70 Word RA, Stull JT, Casey ML, Kamm KE. Contractile elements and myosin light chain phosphorylation in myometrial tissue from nonpregnant and pregnant women. *J Clin Invest* 1993; 92:29–37.

71 Moore F, López Bernal A. Myosin light chain kinase and the onset of labour in humans. *Exp Physiol* 2001;86:313–318.

72 Hong F, Haldeman BD, John OA *et al.* Characterisation of tightly associated smooth muscle myosin–myosin light-chain kinase–calmodulin complexes. *J Mol Biol* 2009;390:879–892.

73 Choudhury N, Khromov AS, Somlyo AP, Somlyo AV. Telokin mediates Ca²⁺-desensitization through activation of myosin phosphatase in phasic and tonic smooth muscle. *J Muscle Res Cell Motil* 2004;25:657–665.

74 Mackenzie LW, Word RA, Casey ML, Stull JT. Myosin light chain phosphorylation in human myometrial smooth muscle cells. *Am J Physiol* 1990;258:C92–C98.

75 Szal SE, Repke JT, Seely EW, Graves SW, Parker CA, Morgan KG. [Ca²⁺]ᵢ signalling in pregnant human myometrium. *Am J Physiol* 1994;267:77–87.

76 Wray S, Shmygol A. Role of the calcium store in uterine contractility. *Semin Cell Develop Biol* 2007;18:315–320.

77 Kupittayanant S, Luckas MJ, Wray S. Effect of inhibiting the sarcoplasmic reticulum on spontaneous and oxytocin-induced contractions of human myometrium. *BJOG* 2002;109: 289–296.

78 Shmygol A, Blanks AM, Bru-Mercier G, Gullam JE, Thornton S. Control of uterine Ca²⁺ by membrane voltage: towards understanding the excitation–contraction coupling in human myometrium. *Ann NY Acad Sci* 2007;1101:97–109.

79 Young RC, Schumann R, Zhang P. Nifedipine block of capacitative calcium entry in cultured human uterine smooth-muscle cells. *J Soc Gynecol Investig* 2001;8:210–215.

80 Inoue Y, Nakao K, Okabe K *et al.* Some electrical properties of human pregnant myometrium. *Am J Obstet Gynecol* 1990;162: 1090–1098.

81 Sanborn BM. Relationship of ion channel activity to control of myometrial calcium. *J Soc Gynecol Investig* 2000;7:4–11.

82 Sanborn BM, Ku CY, Shlykov S, Babich L. Molecular signalling through G-protein-coupled receptors and the control of intracellular calcium in myometrium. *J Soc Gynecol Investig* 2005;12: 479–487.

83 Bolton TB. Calcium events in smooth muscles and their interstitial cells: physiological roles of sparks. *J Physiol* 2006;570: 5–11.

84 Awad SS, Lamb HK, Morgan JM, Dunlop W, Gillespie JI. Differential expression of ryanodine receptor RyR2 mRNA in the non-pregnant and pregnant human myometrium. *Biochem J* 1997;322:777–783.

85 Rivera J, Lopez Bernal A, Varney M, Watson SP. Inositol 1,4,5-trisphosphate and oxytocin binding in human myometrium. *Endocrinology* 1990;127:155–162.

86 Berridge MJ. Smooth muscle cell calcium activation mechanisms. *J Physiol* 2008;586:5047–5061.

87 Young RC. Myocytes, myometrium, and uterine contractions. *Ann NY Acad Sci* 2007;1101:72–84.

88 Nakao K, Inoue Y, Okabe K, Kawarabayashi T, Kitamura K. Oxytocin enhances action potentials in pregnant human myometrium: a study with microelectrodes. *Am J Obstet Gynecol* 1997;177:222–228.

89 López Bernal A. Mechanisms of labour: biochemical aspects. *BJOG* 2003;110:S39–S45.

90 Sanborn BM. Hormonal signalling and signal pathway crosstalk in the control of myometrial calcium dynamics. *Semin Cell Develop Biol* 2007;18:305–314.

91 Chung D, Kim YS, Phillips JN *et al.* Attenuation of canonical transient receptor potential-like channel 6 expression specifically reduces the diacylglycerol-mediated increase in intracellular calcium in human myometrial cells. *Endocrinology* 2010; 151:406–416.

92 Turnbull AC, Anderson AB. Uterine contractility and oxytocin sensitivity during human pregnancy in relation to the onset of labour. *J Obstet Gynaecol Br Commonw* 1968;75:278–288.

93 Fuchs AR, Fuchs F, Husslein P, Soloff MS. Oxytocin receptors in the human uterus during pregnancy and parturition. *Am J Obstet Gynecol* 1984;150:734–741.

94 Bossmar T, Akerlund M, Fantoni G, Szamatowicz J, Melin P, Maggi M. Receptors for and myometrial responses to oxytocin and vasopressin in preterm and term human pregnancy: effects of the oxytocin antagonist atosiban. *Am J Obstet Gynecol* 1994;171:1634–1642.

95 Phaneuf S, Rodriguez Linares B, TambyRaja RL, MacKenzie IZ, López Bernal A. Loss of myometrial oxytocin receptors during oxytocin-induced and oxytocin-augmented labour. *J Reprod Fertil* 2000;120:91–97.

96 Takayanagi Y, Yoshida M, Bielsky IF *et al.* Pervasive social deficits, but normal parturition, in oxytocin receptor-deficient mice. *Proc Natl Acad Sci USA* 2005;102:16096–16101.

97 Nishimori K, Young LJ, Guo Q, Wang Z, Insel TR, Matzuk MM. Oxytocin is required for nursing but is not essential for parturition or reproductive behavior. *Proc Natl Acad Sci USA* 1996;93:11699–11704.

98 Imamura T, Luedke CE, Vogt SK, Muglia LJ. Oxytocin modulates the onset of murine parturition by competing ovarian and uterine effects. *Am J Physiol* 2000;279:R1061–R1067.

99 Kavaliers M, Choleris E, Agmo A *et al.* Inadvertent social information and the avoidance of parasitised male mice: a role for oxytocin. *Proc Natl Acad Sci USA* 2006;103:4293–4298.

100 Melin P. Oxytocin antagonists in preterm labour and delivery. *Baillieres Clin Obstet Gynaecol* 1993;7:577–600.

101 Zuo J, Lei ZM, Rao CV. Human myometrial chorionic gonadotropin/luteinising hormone receptors in preterm and term deliveries. *J Clin Endocrinol Metab* 1994;79:907–911.

102 Slattery MM, Brennan C, O'Leary MJ, Morrison JJ. Human chorionic gonadotrophin inhibition of pregnant human myometrial contractility. *BJOG* 2001;108:704–708.

103 Eta E, Ambrus G, Rao CV. Direct regulation of human myometrial contractions by human chorionic gonadotropin. *J Clin Endocrinol Metab* 1994;79:1582–1586.

104 Ambrus G, Rao CV. Novel regulation of pregnant human myometrial smooth muscle cell gap junctions by human chorionic gonadotropin. *Endocrinology* 1994;135:2772–2779.

105 Belmonte A, Ticconi C, Dolci S *et al*. Regulation of phosphodiesterase 5 expression and activity in human pregnant and non-pregnant myometrial cells by human chorionic gonadotropin. *J Soc Gynecol Investig* 2005;12:570–577.

106 Word RA, Casey ML, Kamm KE, Stull JT. Effects of cGMP on $[Ca^{2+}]_i$, myosin light chain phosphorylation, and contraction in human myometrium. *Am J Physiol* 1991;260:C861–867.

107 Saade GR, Taskin O, Belfort MA, Erturan B, Moise KJ Jr. *In vitro* comparison of four tocolytic agents, alone and in combination. *Obstet Gynecol* 1994;84:374–378.

108 Chanrachakul B, Pipkin FB, Warren AY, Arulkumaran S, Khan RN. Progesterone enhances the tocolytic effect of ritodrine in isolated pregnant human myometrium. *Am J Obstet Gynecol* 2005;192:458–463.

109 Moutquin J. Treatment of preterm labor with the beta-adrenergic agonist ritodrine. The Canadian Preterm Labour Investigators Group. *N Engl J Med* 1992;327:308–312.

110 Garfield RE, Hayashi RH. Appearance of gap junctions in the myometrium of women during labor. *Am J Obstet Gynecol* 1981;140:254–260.

111 Cluff AH, Bystrom B, Klimaviciute A *et al*. Prolonged labour associated with lower expression of syndecan 3 and connexin 43 in human uterine tissue. *Reprod Biol Endocrinol* 2006;4:24.

112 Chow L, Lye SJ. Expression of the gap junction protein connexin-43 is increased in the human myometrium towards term and with the onset of labour. *Am J Obstet Gynecol* 1994; 170:788–795.

113 Petrocelli T, Lye SJ. Regulation of transcripts encoding the myometrial gap junction protein, connexin-43, by oestrogen and progesterone. *Endocrinology* 1993;133:284–290.

114 Tanmahasamut P, Sidell N. Up-regulation of gap junctional intercellular communication and connexin43 expression by retinoic acid in human endometrial stromal cells. *J Clin Endocrinol Metab* 2005;90:4151–4156.

115 Tyson-Capper AJ, Cork DM, Wesley E, Shiells EA, Loughney AD. Characterisation of cellular retinoid-binding proteins in human myometrium during pregnancy. *Mol Hum Reprod* 2006;12:695–701.

116 Doring B, Shynlova O, Tsui P *et al*. Ablation of connexin43 in uterine smooth muscle cells of the mouse causes delayed parturition. *J Cell Sci* 2006;119:1715–1722.

117 McKillen K, Thornton S, Taylor CW. Oxytocin increases the $[Ca^{2+}]_i$ sensitivity of human myometrium during the falling phase of phasic contractions. *Am J Physiol* 1999;276:E345–E351.

118 Woodcock NA, Taylor CW, Thornton S. Effect of an oxytocin receptor antagonist and rho kinase inhibitor on the $[Ca^{++}]_i$ sensitivity of human myometrium. *Am J Obstet Gynecol* 2004;190:222–228.

119 Lartey J, López Bernal A. RHO protein regulation of contraction in the human uterus. *Reproduction* 2009;138:407–424.

120 Fuchs AR. Plasma membrane receptors regulating myometrial contractility and their hormonal modulation. *Semin Perinatol* 1995;19:15–30.

121 Yallampalli C. Role of growth factors and cytokines in the control of uterine contractility. In: Garfield RE, Tabb TN (eds) *Control of Uterine Contractility*. Boca Raton, FL: CRC Press, 1994: 285–294.

122 Honore JC, Robert B, Vacher-Lavenu MC, Chapron C, Breuiller-Fouche M, Ferre F. Expression of endothelin receptors in human myometrium during pregnancy and in uterine leiomyomas. *J Cardiovasc Pharmacol* 2000;36:386–389.

123 Kaya T, Cetin A, Cetin M, Sarioglu Y. Effects of endothelin-1 and calcium channel blockers on contractions in human myometrium. *J Reprod Med* 1999;44:115–121.

124 Anwer K, Monga M, Sanborn BM. Epidermal growth factor increases phosphoinositide turnover and intracellular free calcium in an immortalised human myometrial cell line independent of the arachidonic acid metabolic pathway. *Am J Obstet Gynecol* 1996;174:676–681.

125 Hollingsworth M, Downing SJ, Cheuk JMS *et al*. Pharmacological strategies for uterine relaxation. In: Garfield RE, Tabb TN (eds) *Control of Uterine Contractility*. Boca Raton, FL: CRC Press, 1994: 401.

126 Sanborn BM. Hormones and calcium: mechanisms controlling uterine smooth muscle contractile activity. *Exp Physiol* 2001; 86:223–237.

127 Kelly AJ, Kavanagh J, Thomas J. Relaxin for cervical ripening and induction of labour. *Cochrane Database Syst Rev* 2001;(2): CD03103.

128 Thiede MA, Daifotis AG, Weir EC *et al*. Intrauterine occupancy controls expression of the parathyroid hormone-related peptide gene in preterm rat myometrium. *Proc Natl Acad Sci USA* 1990;87:6969–6973.

129 Williams ED, Leaver DD, Danks JA, Moseley JM, Martin TJ. Effect of parathyroid hormone-related protein (PTHrP) on the contractility of the myometrium and localisation of PTHrP in the uterus of pregnant rats. *J Reprod Fertil* 1994;102:209–214.

130 Barri ME, Abbas SK, Care AD. The effects in the rat of two fragments of parathyroid hormone-related protein on uterine contractions in situ. *Exp Physiol* 1992;77:481–490.

131 Mitchell JA, Ting TC, Wong S, Mitchell BF, Lye SJ. Parathyroid hormone-related protein treatment of pregnant rats delays the increase in connexin 43 and oxytocin receptor expression in the myometrium. *Biol Reprod* 2003;69:556–562.

132 Slattery MM, O'Leary MJ, Morrison JJ. Effect of parathyroid hormone-related peptide on human and rat myometrial contractility *in vitro*. *Am J Obstet Gynecol* 2001;184:625–629.

133 Dong YL, Gangula PRR, Fang L, Wimalawansa SJ, Yallampalli C. Uterine relaxation responses to calcitonin gene-related peptide and calcitonin gene-related peptide receptors decreased during labor in rats. *Am J Obstet Gynecol* 1998;179:497–506.

134 Upton PD, Austin C, Taylor GM *et al*. Expression of adrenomedullin (ADM) and its binding sites in the rat uterus: increased number of binding sites and ADM messenger ribonucleic acid in 20-day pregnant rats compared with nonpregnant rats. *Endocrinology* 1997;138:2508–2514.

135 Gangula PRR, Wimalawansa SJ, Yallampalli C. Pregnancy and sex steroid hormones enhance circulating calcitonin gene-related peptide levels in rats. *Hum Reprod* 2000;15:949–953.

136 Dong YL, Fang L, Kondapaka S, Gangula PRR, Wimalawansa SJ, Yallampalli C. Involvement of calcitonin gene-related peptide in the modulation of human myometrial contractility during pregnancy. *J Clin Invest* 1999;104:559–565.

137 Naghashpour M, Dahl G. Relaxation of myometrium by calcitonin gene-related peptide is independent of nitric oxide synthase activity in mouse uterus. *Biol Reprod* 2000;63: 1421–1427.

138 Yanagita T, Yamamoto R, Sugano T *et al.* Adrenomedullin inhibits spontaneous and bradykinin-induced but not oxytocin- or prostaglandin F(2alpha)-induced periodic contraction of rat uterus. *Br J Pharmacol* 2000;130:1727–1730.

139 Sanborn BM. Ion channels and the control of myometrial electrical activity. *Semin Perinatol* 1995;19:31–40.

140 Ohki S, Ikura M, Zhang M. Identification of magnesium binding sites and the role of magnesium on target recognition by calmodulin. *Biochemistry* 1997;36:4309–4316.

141 Furchgott RF. Endothelium-derived relaxing factor: discovery, early studies, and identification as nitric oxide. *Biosci Rep* 1999;19:235–251.

142 Ignarro LJ, Buga GM, Byrns RE, Wood KS, Chaudhuri G. Endothelium-derived relaxing factor and nitric oxide possess identical pharmacologic properties as relaxants of bovine arterial and venous smooth muscle. *J Pharmacol Exp Ther* 1988;246:218–226.

143 Wu X, Somlyo AV, Somlyo AP. Cyclic GMP-dependent stimulation reverses G-protein-coupled inhibition of smooth muscle myosin-light chain phosphatase. *Biochem Biophys Res Commun* 1996;220:658–663.

144 Van Riper DA, McDaniel NL, Rembold CM. Myosin light chain kinase phosphorylation in nitrovasodilator-induced swine carotid artery relaxation. *Biochim Biophys Acta* 1997;1355:323–330.

145 Garfield RE, Ali M, Yallampalli C, Izumi H. Role of gap junctions and nitric oxide in control of myometrial contractility. *Semin Perinatol* 1995;19:41–51.

146 Bansal RK, Goldsmith PC, He Y, Zaloudek CJ, Ecker JL, Riemer RK. A decline in myometrial nitric oxide synthase expression is associated with labor and delivery. *J Clin Invest* 1997;99:2502–2508.

147 Thomson AJ, Telfer JF, Kohnen G *et al.* Nitric oxide synthase activity and localisation do not change in uterus and placenta during human parturition. *Hum Reprod* 1997;12:2546–2552.

148 Norman JE, Thompson AJ, Telfer JF, Young A, Greer IA, Cameron IT. Myometrial constitutive nitric oxide synthase expression is increased during human pregnancy. *Mol Hum Reprod* 1999;5:175–181.

149 Bartlett SR, Bennett PR, Campa JS *et al.* Expression of nitric oxide synthase isoforms in pregnant human myometrium. *J Physiol* 1999;521:705–716.

150 Jones GD, Poston L. The role of endogenous nitric oxide synthesis in contractility of term or preterm human myometrium. *Br J Obstet Gynaecol* 1997;104:241–245.

151 Leroy MJ, Cedrin I, Breuiller M, Giovagrandi Y, Ferre F. Correlation between selective inhibition of the cyclic nucleotide phosphodiesterases and the contractile activity in human pregnant myometrium near term. *Biochem Pharmacol* 1989;38:9–15.

152 Leroy MJ, Pichard AL, Cabrol D, Ferre F. Cyclic 3'5'-nucleotide phosphodiesterase in human myometrium at the end of pregnancy: partial purification and characterisation of the different soluble isoenzymes. *Gynecol Obstet Invest* 1985;20:27–36.

153 Robinson MF, Levin J, Savage N. Characterisation of soluble cyclic AMP phosphodiesterases and partial purification of a major form in human leiomyoma of the uterus. *Clin Physiol Biochem* 1987;5:249–260.

154 Sonnenburg WK, Seger D, Kwak KS, Huang J, Charbonneau H, Beavo JA. Identification of inhibitory and calmodulin-binding domains of the PDE1A1 and PDE1A2 calmodulin-stimulated cyclic nucleotide phosphodiesterases. *J Biol Chem* 1995;270:30989–31000.

155 Hoeflich KP, Ikura M. Calmodulin in action: diversity in target recognition and activation mechanisms. *Cell* 2002;108:739–742.

156 Kofinas AD, Rose JC, Meis PJ. Changes in cyclic adenosine monophosphate-phosphodiesterase activity in nonpregnant and pregnant human myometrium. *Am J Obstet Gynecol* 1987;157:733–738.

157 Kofinas AD, Rose JC, Koritnik DR, Meis PJ. Progesterone and estradiol concentrations in nonpregnant and pregnant human myometrium. Effect of progesterone and estradiol on cyclic adenosine monophosphate-phosphodiesterase activity. *J Reprod Med* 1990;35:1045–1050.

158 Berg G, Andersson RG, Ryden G. Effects of different phosphodiesterase-inhibiting drugs on human pregnant myometrium: an *in vitro* study. *Arch Int Pharmacodyn Ther* 1987;290:288–292.

159 Leroy MJ, Lugnier C, Merezak J *et al.* Isolation and characterisation of the rolipram-sensitive cyclic AMP-specific phosphodiesterase (type IV PDE) in human term myometrium. *Cell Signal* 1994;6:405–412.

160 Oger S, Mehats C, Barnette MS, Ferre F, Cabrol D, Leroy MJ. Anti-inflammatory and utero-relaxant effects in human myometrium of new generation phosphodiesterase 4 inhibitors. *Biol Reprod* 2004;70:458–464.

161 Khan RN, Hamoud H, Warren A, Wong LF, Arulkumaran S. Relaxant action of sildenafil citrate (Viagra) on human myometrium of pregnancy. *Am J Obstet Gynecol* 2004;191:315–321.

162 Mehats C, Schmitz T, Breuiller-Fouche M, Leroy MJ, Cabrol D. Should phosphodiesterase 5 selective inhibitors be used for uterine relaxation? *Am J Obstet Gynecol* 2006;195:184–185.

163 Wen Y, Anwer K, Singh SP, Sanborn BM. Protein kinase-A inhibits phospholipase-C activity and alters protein phosphorylation in rat myometrial plasma membranes. *Endocrinology* 1992;131:1377–1382.

164 Goodwin TM, Valenzuela G, Silver H, Creasy G. Dose ranging study of the oxytocin antagonist atosiban in the treatment of preterm labor. *Obstet Gynecol* 1996;88:331–336.

165 Buscher U, Chen FC, Riesenkampff E, von Dehn D, David M, Dudenhausen JW. Effects of oxytocin receptor antagonist atosiban on pregnant myometrium *in vitro*. *Obstet Gynecol* 2001;98:117–121.

166 Wilson RJ, Allen MJ, Nandi M, Giles H, Thornton S. Spontaneous contractions of myometrium from humans, non-human primate and rodents are sensitive to selective oxytocin receptor antagonism *in vitro*. *BJOG* 2001;108:960–966.

167 European Atosiban Study Group. The oxytocin antagonist atosiban versus the beta-agonist terbutaline in the treatment of preterm labor. A randomized, double-blind, controlled study. *Acta Obstet Gynecol Scand* 2001;80:413–422.

168 French/Australian Atosiban Investigators Group. Treatment of preterm labor with the oxytocin antagonist atosiban: a double-blind, randomized, controlled comparison with salbutamol. *J Obstet Gynecol Reprod Biol* 2001;98:177–185.

169 Worldwide Atosiban versus Beta-agonists Study Group. Effectiveness and safety of the oxytocin antagonist atosiban versus beta-adrenergic agonists in the treatment of preterm labour. *BJOG* 2001;108:133–142.

170 Caldeyro-Barcia R, Sica-Blanco Y, Poseiro JJ *et al.* A quantitative study of the action of synthetic oxytocin on the pregnant human uterus. *J Pharmacol Exp Ther* 1957;121:18–31.

171 Miller FC. Uterine activity, labor management, and perinatal outcome. *Semin Perinatol* 1978;2:181–186.

172 Friedman EA. The graphic analysis of labor. *Am J Obstet Gynecol* 1954;68:1568.

173 Friedman EA. Primigravid labor: a graphicostatistical analysis. *Obstet Gynecol* 1955;6:567–589.

174 Vain NE, Szyld EG, Prudent LM, Wiswell TE, Aguilar AM, Vivas NI. Oropharyngeal and nasopharyngeal suctioning of meconium-stained neonates before delivery of their shoulders: multicentre, randomised controlled trial. *Lancet* 2004; 364:597–602.

175 Rogers J, Wood J, McCandlish R, Ayers S, Truesdale A, Elbourne D. Active versus expectant management of third stage of labour: The Hinchingbrooke randomised controlled trial. *Lancet* 1998;351:693–699.

Chapter 23
Post-term Pregnancy

Aaron B. Caughey
Oregon Health & Science University, Portland, Oregon, USA

Gestational age is an important determinant of perinatal outcomes. Most attention to this issue has been focused on predicting and preventing preterm births, defined as delivery prior to 37 weeks of gestation. This seems entirely appropriate as preterm birth is the greatest cause of perinatal morbidity, mortality and costs [1,2]. However, post-term births are also associated with increased perinatal morbidity and mortality [3]. Furthermore, post-term pregnancy is easily preventable by inducing delivery. Thus, this potentially problematic condition of pregnancy deserves further attention, research and careful consideration. This chapter discusses what is known about the existing epidemiology of post-term birth and associated outcomes, the methodological issues related to studying post-term pregnancy, that complications associated with post-term pregnancy rise in a continuous manner as opposed to suddenly at any specific threshold, and the management and prevention of post-term births and future directions for research and clinical care.

Definitions

Post-term pregnancy is currently defined as a pregnancy progressing to 42 weeks (294 days) of gestation or beyond [4]. Other terms such as 'prolonged' or 'post-dates' have also been used but for the sake of nomenclature 'post-term' should be used [5]. Further, although 42 weeks is the current threshold designation for post-term pregnancy, up until the 1980s 43 weeks was the threshold while many clinicians currently use the term to describe pregnancies of 41 weeks' gestation and beyond.

To make things even more confusing, 'prolonged' has been proposed as a term to describe pregnancies of 41 to 41 + 6/7 weeks of gestation, but this has not become common usage. It is sensible that there should be a term to describe either the range of 41 to 41 + 6/7 weeks of gestation or 40 to 41 + 6/7 weeks of gestation, the designation 'late term' having been suggested for the latter, in contrast to 'early term' to describe pregnancies from 37 + 0/7 to 38 + 6/7 weeks of gestation.

Given the wide range of terminology, it is best to always include the gestational age along with the descriptor for clarity, for example 'post-term pregnancy at 42 + 1/7 weeks gestation' or 'prolonged pregnancy at 41 + 2/7 weeks gestation'.

Incidence

In order to accurately determine the 'natural' incidence of post-term pregnancy, there must be meticulous early pregnancy dating, universal follow-up of all pregnancies, and absence of obstetric intervention.

The 14% post-term pregnancy rate quoted for the Hawaiian island Kauai [6] may be regarded as informative because of low rates of obstetric intervention and full follow-up, but lacks correction for potential gestational age dating error. In the UK, the fall in incidence of post-term pregnancy from 11.5% in 1958 [7] to 4.4% in 1970 [8] illustrates the effect of the rise in rates of induction of labour from 13 to 26% over the same period. More recently, in the USA in 2005, 14% of all pregnancies progressed beyond 41 weeks of gestation and just under 6% progressed beyond 42 weeks of gestation [9]. This is lower than the approximately 18% of pregnancies beyond 41 weeks and 10% beyond 42 weeks in 1998, with these changes attributed to increases in the use of induction of labour [10,11]. An analysis of 171 527 births in residents of the North-east Thames region in 1989–1991 gave an incidence of 6.2% for post-term pregnancy [12]. In a study of 1514 healthy pregnant women in whom the discrepancy between date of last menstrual period (LMP) and dating based on first-trimester crown–rump length (CRL) was less than −1 to +1 days, the duration of pregnancy was estimated using time-to-event analysis: non-elective delivery was taken to be the event while elective delivery was taken to be censoring [13]. The median time

Dewhurst's Textbook of Obstetrics & Gynaecology, Eighth Edition. Edited by D. Keith Edmonds.
© 2012 John Wiley and Sons, Ltd. Published 2012 by John Wiley and Sons, Ltd.

to non-elective delivery was 283 days from LMP. The life-table graph published in this study gives an incidence of post-term pregnancy of about 6%. This study likely underscores the importance of accurate dating in the actual incidence of post-term pregnancy.

As noted earlier, accuracy of gestational age is an important component of determining whether a pregnancy is post-term. This has been demonstrated in several studies of pregnancy dating. For example, one study found that reliance on menstrual dates gave an incidence of post-term pregnancy of 10.7%, whereas the use of basal body temperature (BBT) charts gave a much lower rate of 4.7% [14]. In another study, the routine use of ultrasound to confirm pregnancy dating decreased the overall incidence of post-term pregnancy from 12 to 3% [15]. The impact of BBT or ultrasound dating is likely because women are far more likely to be oligo-ovulatory and have delayed ovulation than polyovulatory with earlier ovulation. Delayed ovulation in any given menstrual cycle would place a pregnancy at an earlier gestational age than that predicted by the first day of the LMP.

Other studies have demonstrated that the use of ultrasound to establish gestational age lowers the incidence of post-term pregnancy. Eik-Nes *et al.* [16] showed that adjustment of dates following measurement of the biparietal diameter at 17 weeks' gestation led to an incidence of post-term pregnancy of 3.9%. Three other studies of routine ultrasound examination for dating have demonstrated a reduction in the rate of false-positive diagnoses of post-term pregnancy, and thereby the overall rate of post-term pregnancy, from 10–15% to approximately 2–5% [17–19]. In a Cochrane review of randomized trials of routine versus selective second-trimester ultrasound, routine second-trimester biometry was found to reduce the number of pregnancies classified as post-term [20].

Moreover, early ultrasound for pregnancy dating may be superior to mid-trimester ultrasound in this regard. In a small prospective randomized trial, Bennett *et al.* [21] demonstrated that routine first-trimester ultrasound for pregnancy dating reduced the incidence of post-term pregnancy from 13% to 5% compared with second-trimester ultrasound dating. In another recent study, it was demonstrated that not only did first-trimester ultrasound dating lead to lower rates of post-term pregnancy beyond 42 weeks' gestation, but the same was true for diagnosis of pregnancy beyond 41 weeks' gestation [22]. Improved dating also reveals a greater difference in the rate of perinatal complications between term and post-term pregnancies. This is due to the misclassification bias that usually occurs with misdating. Such misclassification of women who are term as post-term and women who are post-term as term both lead to a smaller difference in the rate of complications between term and post-term pregnancies. Thus, older studies of women whose pregnancies did not have dating confirmation by ultrasound

underestimate the rates of complications seen in post-term pregnancies. The multicentre First and Second Trimester Evaluation for Aneuploidy Trial (FASTER) studied 3588 women undergoing first-trimester ultrasound [23]. Gestational age determination using CRL as opposed to LMP reduced the apparent incidence of pregnancies greater than 41 weeks' gestation from 22.1 to 8.2% ($P < 0.001$). Of note, ultrasound at 12–14 weeks' gestation, while considered early, can often lead to worse estimates of gestational age than ultrasound at 18–22 weeks. Thus, reliance on standard nuchal translucency ultrasound over an earlier first-trimester ultrasound may be problematic and requires further research.

 Summary box 23.1

- Post-term gestation is defined as 42 weeks of gestation and beyond.
- Many other terms, such as 'post-dates' and 'prolonged pregnancy', are used interchangeably with 'post-term'.
- It is likely that many so-called post-term pregnancies are due to misdating.
- Pregnancies with dating confirmed by ultrasound are less likely to become post-term.
- First-trimester ultrasound is even better than second-trimester ultrasound with respect to the prevention of misdiagnosed post-term pregnancy.

Aetiology

It is likely that the majority of post-term pregnancies represent the upper range of a normal distribution. Further, as noted above, the most common 'cause' of post-term pregnancy is inaccurate pregnancy dating. However, it does appear that there are specific associations with a range of predictors that may help point to potential aetiologies of post-term pregnancy.

Rare but classically described causes of post-term pregnancy include placental sulphatase deficiency (an X-linked recessive disorder characterized by low circulating oestriol levels), fetal adrenal insufficiency or hypoplasia, and fetal anencephaly (in the absence of polyhydramnios) [24,25].

Genetic factors may also play a role in prolonging pregnancy. In one study, women who were the product of a pregnancy beyond 41 weeks' gestation were more likely themselves to have a pregnancy progress beyond 41 weeks' gestation (RR 1.3) [26]. Similarly, women who have had a prior post-term pregnancy are more likely to have another such pregnancy [26,27]. For example, after one pregnancy beyond 41 + 0/7 weeks of gestation, the risk of a second such pregnancy in the subsequent birth is increased 2.7-fold (from 10 to 27%). If there have been two successive prolonged pregnancies, the incidence rises to 39% [28]. Paternal genes expressed in the feto-placental unit also appear to influence length of gestation. In a recent Danish case–control study [29] of women with two consecutive births, the risk of a second post-term pregnancy among 21 746 women whose first delivery was post-term was 20% as compared with 7.7% among 7009 women whose first delivery was at term. However, the risk of recurrent post-term delivery was reduced to 15% when the first and second child had different fathers (OR 0.73, 95% CI 0.63–0.84).

Low vaginal levels of fetal fibronectin at 39 weeks are predictive of an increased likelihood of post-term pregnancy [30]. Ramanathan *et al.* [31] showed how transvaginal measurement of cervical length at 37 weeks predicts both post-term pregnancy and failed induction. These observations suggest that a defect or delay in the remodelling of the cervix that takes place prior to successful initiation of labour may cause post-term pregnancy and may also be associated with some of the apparent increase in dystocia associated with post-term pregnancy.

Post-term pregnancy could result from variations in the corticotrophin-releasing hormone (CRH) system during pregnancy, such as alteration in the number or expression of myometrial receptor subtypes, altered signal transduction mechanisms or increase in the capacity of CRH-binding protein to bind and inactivate CRH. Prospective longitudinal studies have shown that women destined to deliver before term tend to have a more rapid exponential rise in CRH in mid-pregnancy while women who go on to deliver post-term babies have a slower rate of rise [32]. Efforts currently directed towards researching the initiation of labour before term may lead to greater understanding of the aetiology of post-term pregnancy.

Epidemiology

There are a number of risk factors associated with post-term pregnancy which may have biological causal association. First among these is nulliparity, with a greater proportion of nulliparas reaching 40, 41 or 42 weeks' gestation and the median duration of pregnancy being 2 days longer in nulliparas compared with multiparas. Recent data have also shown an association with male fetuses [33]. Additionally, it has been described that African American women have higher rates of preterm delivery [34], raising the possibility that race/ethnicity may be associated with overall gestational age and prolonged pregnancy in particular. One recent study found a decreased risk of post-term pregnancy among African Americans, Asians and Latinas compared with white women [35]. Further, some effects of race/ethnicity have been described to vary between obese and non-obese patients [36]. Obesity has been found to be associated with post-term pregnancy in several studies [37,38]. The association may have actual causality: studies have demonstrated this finding consistently and have shown a dose–response effect, with greater response among women who are obese than those who are overweight.

The theoretical mechanisms for the association between obesity and post-term pregnancy remain unclear. Since adipose tissue is hormonally active [39] and since obese women may have an altered metabolic status, it is possible that endocrine factors involved in the initiation of labour are altered in obese women. The long-noted associations between lower pre-pregnancy body mass index (BMI) and increased spontaneous preterm birth [40,41] are consistent with our findings and may be explained by a common, as yet unknown, mechanism regarding parturition, potentially related to circulating levels of oestrogen or progesterone. Since, evolutionarily, as a species we have evolved to face the environmental pressures of food scarcity, it is likely that the outcomes of a post-term pregnancy rarely served as an evolutionary pressure related to obesity 10 000 years ago when we existed primarily as nomadic tribes with a lower median BMI than today. Thus there is likely little benefit to the fetus for the pregnancy to proceed beyond 42 weeks' gestation, and such post-term pregnancies may be a product of current intrinsic and environmental factors.

Summary box 23.2

Post-term gestation is seen more commonly with:
- anencephaly;
- placental sulphatase deficiency;
- fetal adrenal hypoplasia;
- male fetuses;
- previous post-term pregnancy;
- maternal obesity;
- nulliparity;
- white race.

The aetiology of post-term pregnancy appears to have both a maternal and fetal component. It seems likely that there is some genetic predilection towards post-term pregnancy.

Risks associated with post-term pregnancy

Perinatal mortality

Post-term pregnancy is associated with an increased risk of perinatal mortality, both antepartum stillbirth as well as infant death. There is an important methodological distinction to make when measuring complications by gestational age. Some complications can only happen to women and infants who are delivered at that week of gestation. Other complications can occur to all women

Table 23.1 Perinatal mortality rates term versus post-term pregnancies.

Reference	Source	Outcome	37–41 weeks	42 weeks and over
Campbell *et al.* [56]	444 241 births Norway 1978–1987	Relative risk of perinatal death	1	1.30 (1.13–1.50)
Fabre *et al.* [130]	547 923 births Spain 1980–1992	Stillbirth rate Early neonatal mortality rate Perinatal mortality rate	3.3 1.7 4.9	3.6 2.8 6.4
Olesen *et al.* [131]	78 033 post-term pregnancies Danish birth register 1978–1993 5% sample of deliveries at term	Adjusted odds ratio: stillbirth Adjusted odds ratio: neonatal death Adjusted odds ratio: perinatal death	1 1 1	1.24 (0.93–1.66) 1.60 (1.07–2.37) 1.36 (1.08–1.72)

who are pregnant at that week of gestation, both those delivering as well as those who remain pregnant. For example, an antepartum stillbirth can occur in anyone who is pregnant at a given gestational age, i.e. in ongoing pregnancies. Alternatively, a neonatal death can only occur to the group that actually delivers at that week of gestation [42]. When considering the outcomes related to post-term pregnancy, we see the association with antepartum stillbirth regardless of how the effect is measured, but when the appropriate denominator of ongoing pregnancies is used, we see the risk of antepartum stillbirth begin to increase earlier at 39 and 40 weeks' gestation. Yudkin *et al.* [43] questioned the validity of using perinatal mortality rates as a means of relating outcome to gestational age, arguing that the population at risk of intrauterine fetal death at a given gestational age is the population of fetuses *in utero* at that gestational week and not those delivered at that week. However, the population at risk of intrapartum and neonatal complications such as cord prolapse or meconium aspiration syndrome is clearly the population of babies delivered at that week of pregnancy [44]. These issues are clearly explained by Smith [44], who related the perinatal risks at each gestational week to the appropriate denominators. Antepartum deaths were related to the number of ongoing pregnancies, intrapartum deaths to all births at that gestational age, excluding antepartum stillbirths, and neonatal deaths were related to the number of live births. Yudkin *et al.* [43] expressed the prospective risk of stillbirth for the next 2 weeks of the pregnancy; Hilder *et al.* [12] expressed the risk as a rate over the next week; Cotzias *et al.* [3] generated considerable controversy [45,46] by expressing the risk of prospective stillbirth for the remainder of the pregnancy. This is a counter-intuitive concept for most obstetricians, whereas many find the concept of the prospective risk of stillbirth over the coming week an accessible concept, particularly in pregnancies of 40–42 weeks' gestation ('If this woman remains undelivered in the next 7 days, what is the chance of a fetal death occurring *in utero*?').

In the broad range of literature, studies which dichotomize gestational age at 42 weeks demonstrate increased perinatal mortality (Table 23.1). The outcomes presented in this table compare pregnancies fulfilling the epidemiological definition of post-term pregnancy with those delivered at 'term'. In modern obstetric practice, women with epidemiological and obstetric risk factors are more likely to be delivered before 42 weeks. Thus women with twin pregnancies, pre-eclampsia, diagnosed intrauterine growth restriction, antepartum haemorrhage or previous perinatal death are likely to be over-represented in the 37–41 week population and under-represented among those delivered at 42 weeks and later, potentially underestimating the increased risks from progressing to the post-term period.

Studies have also examined these outcomes by week of gestation across all term pregnancies by week and demonstrate similar findings (Table 23.2). Specifically, this table addresses the argument that the duration of pregnancy is a continuum and that perinatal risks are unlikely to alter abruptly on day 294 of a pregnancy. Outcomes are presented by week of gestational age from 37 weeks up to and including 43 weeks' gestation. Outcome statistics are presented in a variety of forms as discussed above.

At first sight, it might seem that whether studies have used thresholds like 42 and 43 weeks of gestation or examined complications by week was only a matter of whether the strata required increased subgroup sample size due to needs for increased statistical power. However, examining these outcomes by threshold or in a continuous fashion is an important methodological issue. If complication rates increase as gestational age increases, then one would see an increase regardless of what threshold was chosen. And it is true, if one examines stillbirth rates before and after 39, 40, 41, 42 or 43 weeks, there is always a higher rate beyond the threshold. More importantly is how such information can be utilized to inform clinical management. Thus, a comparison of one week to the next is truly what needs to be examined. Are the

Table **23.2** Perinatal outcomes by week of gestation, 37–43 weeks.

Reference	Source	Outcome	38–39	39–40	40–41	41–42	42–43	43 and more
Bakketeig & Bergsjo [26]	157 577 births Sweden 1977–1978	Perinatal mortality rate	7.2	3.1	2.3	2.4	3	4
Ingemarsson & Kallen [49]	914 702 births Sweden 1982–1991	Stillbirth rate in nulliparas	2.72	1.53	1.23	1.86	2.26	
		Neonatal mortality rate nulliparas	0.62	0.54	0.54	0.9	1.03	
		Stillbirth rate in multiparas	2.1	1.42	1.35	1.4	1.51	
		Neonatal mortality rate multiparas	0.55	0.45	0.53	0.5	0.86	
Divon et al. [132]	181 524 singleton pregnancies Reliable dates, ≥40 weeks Sweden 1987–1992	Odds ratio for fetal death			1	1.5	1.8	2.9
Hilder et al. [11]	171 527 births London 1989–1991	Stillbirth rate	3.8	2.2	1.5	1.7	1.9	2.1
		Infant mortality rate	4.7	3.2	2.7	2	4.1	3.7
		Stillbirth rate per 1000 OP*	0.56	0.57	0.86	1.27	1.55	2.12
		Infant mortality rate per 1000 OP	0.7	0.83	1.57	1.48	3.29	3.71
Caughey & Musci [52]	Hospital based California 1992–2002 45673 births after 37 weeks	Fetal death rate per 1000 OP	0.36	0.4	0.26	0.92	3.47	
Smith [43]	700878 births in Scotland 1985–1996 Multiple births and congenital anomalies excluded	Cumulative probability of antepartum stillbirth	0.0008	0.0013	0.0022	0.0034	0.0053	0.0115
		Estimated probability of intrapartum and neonatal death	0.0006	0.0005	0.0006	0.0006	0.0006	0.0008

* Ongoing pregnancies.

risks higher of delivering at a given gestational age or of waiting an additional week of gestation? For such comparisons, examining complications week by week is of more use than simply comparing before and after a given threshold.

There are other methodological problems with this literature. Of course, there may be errors or biases in recording of information relating to gestational age. Women with uncertain dates have been repeatedly shown to be at increased risk of perinatal mortality [47,48]. Their inclusion may inflate the apparent perinatal risks of post-term pregnancy. Older studies of perinatal outcome in post-term pregnancy showed that about 25% of the excess mortality risk in post-term pregnancy relates to congenital malformations [24]. Of the studies quoted in Tables 23.1 and 23.2, only that by Smith [44] specifies that cases of lethal congenital malformation have been excluded from the analysis. Hilder *et al.* [45] reanalysed the data presented in their 1998 study [12] after correcting for congenital malformation, showing that the outcomes presented were not biased by fetuses with congenital malformation being preferentially represented among post-term pregnancies. Another potential bias is the interval between intrauterine death and delivery. A fetus that dies *in utero* at 41 weeks and is delivered at 42 weeks will be counted as a perinatal death at 42 weeks' gestation. If this happened regularly, this would suggest that perinatal mortality risks actually increase half a week to a week earlier.

Both tables show that post-term pregnancy is associated with an increased risk of perinatal death. However, there is no consistency between studies as to the timing of that increased risk from fetal death before labour, to antepartum death to early neonatal death or even infant mortality. The studies summarized in Table 23.1 suggest that an increased risk of neonatal death is the main source of the increased perinatal risk. This has been further substantiated by a recent study from California which finds higher rates of infant death in births at 41 weeks and beyond even in a low-risk population [49]. However, Table 23.2 shows that when pregnancies ending at 42 weeks are compared with those delivered at 41 weeks, every adverse outcome is increased with the exception of the 'estimated probability of intrapartum and neonatal death' from the Smith study [44]. When pregnancies ending at 41 weeks are compared with those ending at 40 weeks, this outcome is again unchanged, as is the neonatal mortality rate in multiparas in the Ingemarsson and Kallen series [50] and the infant mortality rate in the Hilder series [12]. All other outcomes deteriorate from 40 weeks to 41 weeks and again from 41 weeks to 42 weeks.

Perinatal morbidity

Epidemiological studies identify birth after 41 weeks or after 42 weeks as a risk factor for a variety of adverse neonatal outcomes. One retrospective cohort study of all low-risk, term, cephalic and singleton births delivered at the University of California, San Francisco, between 1976 and 2001 examined the incidence of adverse neonatal morbidity outcomes at 40, 41 and 42 weeks' gestation and compared these with the rates in pregnancies delivered at 39 weeks' gestation, after controlling for maternal demographics, length of labour, induction, mode of delivery and birthweight (except macrosomia) [51]. Compared with the outcome at 39 weeks' gestation, the relative risk of meconium aspiration increased significantly from 2.18 at 40 weeks to 3.35 at 41 weeks and 4.09 (95% CI 2.07–8.08) at 42 weeks. A composite outcome of 'severe neonatal complications', including skull fracture and brachial plexus injuries, neonatal seizures, intracranial haemorrhage, neonatal sepsis, meconium aspiration syndrome and respiratory distress syndrome, increased from a relative risk of 1.47 at 40 weeks to 2.04 at 41 weeks to 2.37 (95% CI 1.63–3.49) at 42 weeks. Similar findings have been demonstrated in multiple other studies that examined perinatal morbidity including pre-eclampsia, meconium, meconium aspiration syndrome, macrosomia, neonatal acidaemia, need for neonatal mechanical ventilation, Caesarean delivery and perinatal infectious morbidity [52–56].

For example, dystocia, shoulder dystocia and obstetric trauma are all increased in post-term pregnancy [57]. Here, the risks increase with increasing fetal weight, but gestational age remains a risk factor independent of birthweight. In a case-matched study of 285 women with uncomplicated singleton post-term pregnancy and spontaneous onset of labour and 855 women with uncomplicated singleton term pregnancy, Luckas *et al.* [58] showed that Caesarean delivery was significantly more common in women with post-term pregnancy (RR 1.90, 95% CI 1.29–2.85). The increase was equally distributed between Caesarean deliveries performed for failure to progress in labour (RR 0.74, 95% CI 1.02–3.04) and fetal distress (RR 2.00, 95% CI 1.14–3.61). This finding is consistent with the hypothesis that some cases of post-term pregnancy are associated with a defect in the physiology of labour, in addition to any increase in risk of fetal hypoxia. However, the possibility of bias in management arising out of the knowledge that a pregnancy is post-term cannot be excluded as a factor in the increase in Caesarean delivery rates.

A strong association between neonatal seizures and delivery at 41 weeks' gestation or more has also been identified in previous case–control studies. Minchom *et al.* [59] found that delivery after 41 weeks' gestation was associated with an odds ratio of 2.7 (95% CI 1.6–4.8). Curtis *et al.* [60] studied 89 babies with early neonatal seizures delivered after 42 weeks' gestation in Dublin; 27 were delivered after 42 weeks' gestation compared with 6 of 89 controls (OR 4.73, 95% CI 2.22–10.05).

Cerebral palsy

Neonatal encephalopathy may be followed by the development of cerebral palsy, while other cases of cerebral palsy may occur following a clinically normal neonatal period. It is accepted that the presence of neonatal encephalopathy indicates that a neurological insult has taken place during labour or the early neonatal period, while its absence is thought to indicate an insult at some earlier time in pregnancy [61]. Gaffney *et al.* [62] examined the obstetric background of 141 children from the Oxford Cerebral Palsy Register; 41 children whose cerebral palsy was preceded by neonatal encephalopathy were compared with 100 who had not suffered from neonatal encephalopathy. The babies with neonatal encephalopathy were more likely to have been delivered at 42 weeks' gestation or more (OR 3.5, 95% CI 1–12.1). Babies born at 42 weeks or more to nulliparous women were at particular risk of this sequence of events (OR 11.0, 95% CI 1.2–102.5).

Effect of parity and birthweight

Whether these outcomes, their rates, peaks and nadirs are affected by other demographics such as maternal age, race/ethnicity, socioeconomic status and medical complications of pregnancy has been minimally studied. However, it has been examined by parity. One series [50] shows that the increasing risks of adverse outcome associated with advancing age of gestation are more marked in nulliparas than in multiparas (Table 23.2). The aetiology for the modification of these outcomes by parity is unclear and could be due to true biological differences or perhaps differences in dating accuracy between the two groups. Birthweight has also been examined as a modifier of outcomes by gestational age. In an analysis of 181 524 singleton pregnancies with reliable dates delivered at 40 weeks or later in Sweden between 1987 and1992, birthweight of two standard deviations or more below the mean for gestational age was associated with a significantly increased odds ratios for both fetal (OR 7.1–10.0) and neonatal death (OR 3.4–9.4) [50]. A Norwegian cohort [57] also showed that small-for-gestational age babies were more vulnerable to the risks of post-term pregnancy. In this study, babies weighing less than the 10th centile had a relative risk of 5.68 (95% CI 4.37–7.38) of perinatal death at 42 weeks' gestation or later compared with babies between the 10th and 90th centile at the same gestational age. In this series, birthweight above the 90th centile was associated with the lowest relative risk of perinatal death (RR 0.51, 95% CI 0.26–1.0). These findings make biological sense in that one might suspect that there would be a subgroup of fetuses whose growth is affected due to intrauterine factors that increase the risk for fetal or neonatal demise. The practice pattern of delivering such fetuses at an earlier gestational age is thus supported by such findings.

Summary box 23.3

Post-term gestation is associated with:
- stillbirth;
- Caesarean delivery;
- fetal macrosomia;
- meconium-stained amniontic fluid;
- birth trauma;
- neonatal acidaemia;
- cerebral palsy;
- neonatal mortality.

A key methodological point when examining outcomes by gestational age in term and post-term pregnancies is properly determining the population at risk, i.e. *ongoing pregnancies* (all women pregnant at a particular gestational age) or *pregnancies delivered* (just the women who deliver at a particular gestational age).

   While the outcomes listed above are all more frequent in pregnancies at 42 weeks' gestation and beyond, they are also increased (though not as high) in pregnancies at 41 weeks' gestation.

Management

Management of post-term pregnancies actually starts before a pregnancy becomes post-term. The goals of managing such otherwise low-risk pregnancies is to prevent the complications of post-term pregnancy and to prevent post-term pregnancy itself. Thus, the mainstay of management involves the use of antepartum testing to reduce risks of complications from expectantly managing these pregnancies. It also includes reducing the risk of post-term pregnancy through good pregnancy dating, outpatient cervical ripening and induction of labour, all before a pregnancy becomes post-term. These broad topics are discussed below.

Antenatal testing

The evidence of increased perinatal mortality and morbidity in late term and post-term pregnancy compared with delivery at 39 or 40 weeks' gestation inevitably leads to the conclusion that some cases of post-term pregnancy could be prevented by earlier delivery. It would seem logical to use screening tests to identify pregnancies destined to have an adverse outcome and to intervene selectively in these cases.

   The ideal test of fetal well-being in post-term pregnancy would allow identification of all fetuses at risk of adverse outcome, at a stage where delivery would result in a universally good outcome. Thus a 'negative' test would indicate that the fetus is safe *in utero* for an interval of a few days until either delivery or a repeat test is performed and that the women would eventually deliver with a good outcome. At present, no method of monitoring post-term pregnancy is backed up by strong evidence

Table 23.3 Randomized trials of routine versus selective induction at 41–42 weeks' gestation.

Reference	No.	Gestation at trial entry (days)	Method of induction	Method of fetal surveillance	Perinatal deaths
Augensen et al. [133]	409	290	Oxytocin and amniotomy	CTG	0
Bergsjo et al. [119]	188	284	Membrane sweep, oxytocin, amniotomy	Fetal movement, ultrasound, urinary oestriol	1 in induction arm 2 in selective arm
Cardozo et al. [120]	363	290	PGE$_2$, oxytocin, amniotomy	Fetal movement, CTG	1 in selective arm 1 in induction arm
Chanrachakul & Herabutya [134]	249	290	Amniotomy and oxytocin	CTG, AFI	0
Dyson et al. [117]	302	287	PGE$_2$, oxytocin, amniotomy	CTG, AFI	1 in selective arm
Hannah et al. [109]	3407	287	PGE$_2$, oxytocin, amniotomy	Fetal movement, CTG, AFI	2 in selective arm
Heden et al. [135]	238	295	Amniotomy, oxytocin	CTG, AFI	0
Henry [118]	112	290	Amniotomy and oxytocin	Amnioscopy	2 in selective arm
Herabutya et al. [136]	108	294	PGE$_2$, oxytocin	CTG	1 in selective arm
James et al. [137]	74	287	Extra-amniotic saline if Bishop score <5; membrane sweep, amniotomy and oxytocin	Fetal movement, BPS	0
Katz et al. [116]	156	294	Amniotomy, oxytocin	Fetal movement, amnioscopy, oxytocin challenge	1 in each arm
Martin et al. [138]	22	287	Laminaria, oxytocin	CTG, AFI	0
NICHD [139]	440	287	CTG, oxytocin, amniotomy	CTG, AFI	0
Roach & Rogers [140]	201	294	PGE$_2$	CTG, AFI	0
Suikkari et al. [141]	119	290	Amniotomy, oxytocin	CTG, human placental lactogen, oestriol, AFI	0
Witter & Weitz [142]	200	287	Oxytocin, amniotomy	Oestriol, oxytocin challenge	0

AFI, amniotic fluid index; BPS, biophysical profile scoring; CTG, cardiotocography.

of effectiveness. There is some observational evidence that some pregnancies at risk of adverse outcome can be identified, but less evidence that prediction of the adverse outcome confers prevention.

Fetal movement counting

The least invasive monitoring is maternal assessment of fetal movements, also known as fetal kick counts. This test is used commonly in the supervision of term and post-term pregnancies (Table 23.3) but is not supported by firm evidence of efficacy. Generally, women are asked to count fetal movements once or twice per day and are expected to experience four to six such movements in 20–30 min. Two randomized trials have addressed the question of whether clinical actions taken on the basis of fetal movement improve fetal outcome [63,64]. The larger of these trials involved over 68 000 women [64]. These

trials collectively provide evidence that routine formal fetal movement counting does not reduce the incidence of intrauterine fetal death in late pregnancy. Routine counting results in more frequent reports of diminished fetal activity, with a greater use of other techniques of fetal assessment, more frequent admission to hospital and an increased rate of elective delivery. It may be that fetal movement counting in post-term pregnancy will perform more effectively than it does in low-risk pregnancies. However, in the end, if this test did demonstrate reduction in perinatal morbidity or mortality, it is likely that such a protocol also leads to maternal anxiety and high rates of false positives.

Ultrasound assessment of amniotic fluid

Ultrasound monitoring of amniotic fluid volume was first described in 1980 when a subjective classification of 'normal', 'reduced' or 'absent' amniotic fluid was described, based on the presence or absence of echo-free space between the fetal limbs and the fetal trunk or the uterine wall [65]. To test the value of the classification, 150 patients with pregnancies of 42 weeks or more underwent ultrasound examination in the 48 hours prior to delivery. The patients classified as having reduced or absent amniotic fluid had a statistically significant excess incidence of meconium-stained liquor, fetal acidosis, and birth asphyxia and meconium aspiration. Manning *et al.* [66] described a semi-quantitative method based on the largest vertical pool of amniotic fluid and used a 1-cm pool depth as the cut-off for intervention in a population of babies with suspected growth restriction. This was subsequently modified to 2 cm to improve detection of the growth-retarded infant [67]. Crowley *et al.* [68] found an increase in adverse outcomes in post-term pregnancies where the maximum pool depth was less than 3 cm. Fischer *et al.* [69] found that a maximum vertical pool of less than 2.7 cm was the best predictor of abnormal perinatal outcome.

Phelan *et al.* [70] described the amniotic fluid index (AFI), the sum of the maximum pool depth in four quadrants. Fischer *et al.* [69] found that maximum pool depth performed better than AFI in predicting adverse outcomes in post-term pregnancies. Alfirevic and Walkinshaw [71] randomly allocated women with post-term pregnancy to monitoring using either maximum pool depth or AFI. Both groups underwent computerized fetal heart rate monitoring every 3 days in addition to amniotic fluid measurements. The threshold for intervention was a maximum pool depth of less than 1.8 cm or an AFI of less than 7.3 cm. These figures had been identified as the third centiles for the local population. The number of women found to have an abnormal AFI was significantly higher than the number found to have an abnormal maximum pool depth and more women underwent induction of labour in the AFI arm of the trial. There were no perinatal deaths and no statistically significant differences in perinatal outcome between the two groups.

Morris *et al.* [72] performed an observational study of 1584 pregnant women at or beyond 40 weeks' gestation in Oxford. Women underwent measurement of amniotic fluid, using both the single deepest pool and AFI. The results of these ultrasound measurements were concealed from caregivers. These authors agreed with Alfirevic and Walkinshaw [71] that more women 'test positive' using AFI than with single deepest pool; 125 women (7.9%) had an AFI of less than 5 cm in contrast to 22 women (1.4%) who had single deepest pool less than 2 cm. There were no perinatal deaths. There were seven cases of severe perinatal morbidity, an incidence of 0.44%. Two of these had an AFI below 5 cm and four had an AFI of less than 6 cm. None of the seven cases had a deepest pool measurement of less than 2 cm, thus emphasizing the trade-off between specificity and sensitivity.

Locatelli *et al.* [73] conducted a similar study, but measured AFI twice weekly from 40 weeks until delivery. A composite adverse outcome of fetal death, 5-min Apgar score less than 7, umbilical artery pH less than 7 and Caesarean delivery for fetal distress occurred in 19.8% of those with an AFI below 5 compared with 10.7% of those with an AFI above 5 ($P = 0.001$).

These studies of amniotic fluid after 40 weeks suggest some association between reduction in volume and adverse outcome, but overall it performs with poor sensitivity and specificity. There is no evidence to suggest that it can be relied on as a means of monitoring pregnancies after 41 weeks' gestation. In a meta-analysis of studies on the relationship of amniotic fluid with adverse fetal outcome, Chauhan *et al.* [74] concluded that there was some association between oligohydramnios and an increased risk of Caesarean delivery for non-reassuring fetal heart rate patterns and low Apgar scores; however, the data relating to neonatal acidosis were insufficient. Fundamentally, while there is biological plausibility that decreases in amniotic fluid volume may predate complications in the term and post-term pregnancy, there are inadequate data to definitively state that such assessment followed by intervention will necessarily affect perinatal outcomes, by how much and with what timing. Furthermore, confidence in ultrasound assessment of amniotic fluid volume is undermined by studies which show a poor correlation between ultrasound AFI and actual amniotic fluid volumes measured by dye-dilution studies [75,76]. Development of a better test to identify the senescent placenta or changing fetal–placental–maternal physiology at term and post-term that will prevent perinatal complications is paramount.

Biophysical profile

Observational studies indicate that low biophysical scores identify babies at higher risk of adverse outcome [77]. However, evidence of ability to predict adverse outcome must not be interpreted as proof of the ability to prevent these outcomes.

A systematic review of four trials, comparing biophysical profile scoring with other forms of antepartum fetal monitoring, yields insufficient data to show that the biophysical profile is better than any other form of fetal monitoring [78]. Only one of these randomized controlled trials deals specifically with post-term pregnancy [71]. This trial compares monitoring of post-term pregnancy using a modified biophysical profile score (consisting of computerized cardiotocography, AFI and the rest of the components of the conventional biophysical profile) with simple monitoring using cardiotocography and measurement of amniotic fluid depth. The more complex method of monitoring post-term pregnancy is more likely to yield an abnormal result, but does not improve pregnancy outcome as evidenced by umbilical cord pH.

An observational study of biophysical profile scoring in the management of post-term pregnancy showed that 32 of 293 women who had abnormal biophysical profiles had significantly higher rates of neonatal morbidity, Caesarean delivery for fetal distress and meconium aspiration than the women with reassuring biophysical profiles [79]. A further observational study of 131 post-term pregnancies showed that a normal biophysical profile score was highly predictive of normal outcome, but an abnormal test had only a 14% predictive value of poor neonatal outcome [80].

Cardiotocography

Antenatal cardiotocography (CTG), also known as a contraction stress test, has been widely used for more than 20 years to monitor moderate- to high-risk pregnancies. Observational studies have reported very low rates of perinatal loss in high-risk pregnancies monitored in this way [81,82]. Four randomized controlled trials comparing CTG with other methods of antepartum fetal monitoring have been the subject of a Cochrane review [83]. Women with post-term pregnancies were included in these trials. On the basis of the information presented in this review, the antenatal CTG has no significant effect on perinatal outcome or on interventions such as elective delivery. Miyazaki and Miyazaki [84] reported a series of 125 women with post-term pregnancies where a reactive CTG was recorded within 1 week of delivery. Ten adverse outcomes were reported from this group: four antepartum deaths, one neonatal death, one case of neonatal encephalopathy and four cases of fetal distress on admission in early labour. The poor performance of antenatal CTG in this series and in the randomized trials may relate to errors in interpretation or excessive intervals between tests. Numerical analysis using computerized calculations of the baseline rate and variability may reduce the potential for human error [85]. Weiner *et al.* [86] compared the value of antenatal testing with computerized CTG, conventional CTG, biophysical profile scores and umbilical artery Doppler; 337 pregnant women who were delivered after 41 weeks' gestation and who had 610 antenatal tests were included in this study. Of 12 fetuses with reduced fetal heart rate variation on computerized CTG, 10 had a trial of labour. Of these 10 fetuses, nine had fetal distress during labour. Of the 12 fetuses with reduced fetal heart rate variation, seven were acidotic at delivery (umbilical artery pH <7.2). Overall, there were 10 acidotic fetuses at delivery in the study group. Only two of them had an umbilical systolic/diastolic ratio above the 95th percentile, three had an amniotic fluid index greater than 5, and five had fetal heart rate decelerations before labour. Fetuses who demonstrated an abnormal intrapartum fetal heart rate tracing or who were acidotic at delivery had a significantly higher rate of reduced fetal heart rate variation or decelerations before labour. The authors conclude that computerized CTG may improve fetal surveillance in post-term pregnancy. The obvious criticism of this study is the circular argument of using an antepartum CTG abnormality to predict an intrapartum CTG abnormality.

Doppler velocimetry

Two studies of umbilical artery Doppler velocimetry [87,88] in post-term pregnancy indicate that it is of no benefit. In a small observational study comparing the predictive values of CTG, AFI, biophysical profile scoring and the ratio of middle cerebral artery (MCA) Doppler to umbilical artery Doppler, Devine *et al.* [88] found that the ratio of MCA Doppler to umbilical artery Doppler was the best predictor of 'adverse outcome' in this study, defined by meconium aspiration syndrome or Caesarean delivery for fetal distress or fetal acidosis.

Prevention of post-term pregnancy

The prevention of post-term pregnancy centres around efforts to ensure that a misdiagnosis is not made from improper pregnancy dating and encouraging the onset of labour prior to post-term pregnancy developing. While the first demands public health action to ensure that all patients have the option to obtain first-trimester ultrasound dating confirmation, widespread adoption of this practice seems limited at this point. However, most women undergo second-trimester ultrasound, which also reduces the risk of being misdiagnosed with a post-term pregnancy, though not as much as first-trimester ultrasound.

Post-term pregnancy can absolutely be prevented by simply inducing all patients before they reach 42 weeks of gestation. This appears to be a reasonable approach, but does carry some costs due to the prolonged admissions to labour and delivery units for induction of labour. A better way of preventing such post-term pregnancies would use techniques to encourage spontaneous labour. Several minimally invasive interventions have been recommended to encourage the onset of labour at term and prevent post-term pregnancy, including membrane stripping, unprotected coitus and acupuncture. *Stripping or sweeping of the fetal membranes* refers to digital separation of the membranes from the wall of the cervix and lower uterine segment. This technique, which likely acts by releasing endogenous prostaglandins from the cervix, requires the cervix to be sufficiently dilated to admit the practitioner's finger. Although stripping of the membranes may be able to reduce the interval to spontaneous onset of labour, there is no consistent evidence of a reduction in operative vaginal delivery, Caesarean delivery rates, or maternal or neonatal morbidity [90–92]. *Unprotected sexual intercourse* causes uterine contractions through the action of prostaglandins in semen and potential release of endogenous prostaglandins similar to stripping of the membranes. Indeed, prostaglandins were originally isolated from extracts of prostate and seminal vesicle glands, hence their name. Despite some conflicting data, it appears that unprotected coitus may lead to the earlier onset of labour, reduction in post-term pregnancy rates, and less induction of labour [93–95]. In one small randomized trial which attempted to address this question, women were randomized to a group advised to have coitus versus a control group which was not. In this study, the women advised to have coitus did so more often (60% vs. 40%), but there was no measurable difference in the rate of spontaneous labour in this underpowered study [96]. Similarly, the efficacy of *acupuncture* for induction of labour cannot be definitively assessed because of the paucity of trial data and requires further examination [97,98].

Ultrasound to establish accurate gestational age

The first step towards managing post-term pregnancy is to reduce the number of cases of post-term pregnancy by providing ultrasound verification of gestational age for all pregnancies. A systematic review shows that routine second-trimester ultrasound reduces the number of cases of post-term pregnancy [20]. A recent randomized controlled trial of first- versus second-trimester ultrasound showed a lower rate of post-term pregnancy in pregnancies dated by first-trimester ultrasound [21]. A secondary analysis of data from the FASTER trial showed that first-trimester ultrasound determination of gestational age by CRL as opposed to LMP reduces the apparent incidence of pregnancies greater than 41 weeks from 22.1 to 8.2% [23]. It does seem that obtaining a first-trimester ultrasound to assess viability and gestational age at the first visit is a good idea and may impact the overall number of diagnosed post-term pregnancies.

Induction of labour for post-term pregnancy

Given that a patient cannot have a stillbirth at 42 weeks if she is induced at 41 weeks, induction of labour has been identified as the principal intervention to reduce perinatal morbidity from post-term pregnancy. However, there is a concern that such inductions of labour are in turn driving up the Caesarean delivery rate. Thus, obstetric providers have responded in various ways to the apparently increased perinatal mortality and morbidity associated with post-term pregnancy. Such potential clinical options include induction at term to prevent pregnancies reaching 42 weeks, routine induction at 41 or 42 weeks or shortly before, and selective induction at 41 or 42 weeks in cases identified by tests as being at risk of adverse outcome. Fortunately, the benefits and hazards of some of these strategies have been evaluated in randomized controlled trials. Randomized or quasi-random trials comparing elective induction at term versus expectant management, and elective induction after 41 weeks versus moni-

toring of post-term pregnancies were identified using the search strategy described by the Cochrane Pregnancy and Childbirth Group and formed the basis of a systematic review of management options in post-term pregnancy [99]. The main outcomes of interest are those already identified in the analysis of post-term pregnancy risks: perinatal mortality, neonatal encephalopathy, meconium-stained amniotic fluid, Caesarean delivery. In addition, evidence was sought relating to the effect of the various management options on maternal satisfaction. Subsequently, there have been other systematic reviews of randomized trials comparing induction of labour with expectant management in pregnancies of 41 weeks' gestation and more [100] or 41 weeks' gestation or less [101].

One major concern regarding induction of labour has been that of increased risk of Caesarean delivery. However, this conclusion has not been universally accepted [102]. One component of the concern regarding induction of labour is the large number of retrospective studies which demonstrate higher rates of Caesarean delivery in the induced patients [103,104]. The methodological problem with these studies is that they generally compare women who are induced to those in spontaneous labour [105]. A recent study which compared women who were induced to those who underwent expectant management actually found lower rates of Caesarean delivery in the women who were induced [106]. Further, in a recent meta-analysis of three small studies of elective induction of labour prior to 41 weeks' gestation, induction of labour led to lower rates of Caesarean delivery [107].

An alternative approach to the prevention of post-term pregnancy is selective or preventive rather than routine induction of labour at an earlier gestational age. In a small preliminary study of active management of risk in pregnancy at term (AMOR-IPAT) in which induction of labour at 41 weeks was recommended for all women with risk factors for cephalopelvic disproportion or intrapartum non-reassuring fetal testing, Nicholson *et al.* [108] were able to decrease the Caesarean delivery rate from 17% in the expectantly managed group (induction rate, 26%) to 4% in the risk-factor managed group (induction rate, 63%).In a recent, prospective, randomized controlled trial, there was a trend towards lower Caesarean rates in the risk-factor managed group, but the study was underpowered for this outcome [109]. However, it did find lower rates of admission to neonatal intensive care and an improved adverse outcome index in the risk-factor managed group, which was induced in the majority of cases.

Induction of labour at 41 weeks

Sixteen randomized trials comparing 'routine' induction of labour at a specified gestational age with a policy of selective induction of labour in response to an abnormal antepartum test are summarized in Table 23.3. These trials form the basis of a systematic review by Sanchez-Ramos *et al.* [100]. Twelve of them had been previously included in the Cochrane Review by Crowley [99]. One trial is larger than all others and contributes considerable weight to both meta-analyses [110].

Both meta-analyses adopt an inclusive approach and include trials of variable size and quality. The gestational age at trial entry varies from 287 to 294 days' gestation. A variety of methods of antepartum fetal testing are used to supervise pregnancies in the expectant arm of the trials.

Induction at or before 40 weeks

Pre-emptive induction of labour, where women with uncomplicated pregnancies were routinely offered induction at or before 40 weeks, was practised in some obstetric units in some countries in the 1970s. Six randomized trials compare a policy of 'routine' induction at 39 weeks [111,112] or 40 weeks [113–116], with either 'expectant' management of an indefinite duration or expectant management until 42 weeks' gestation. These trials reveal no evidence of any major benefit or risk to 'routine' induction at 40 weeks. Two perinatal deaths of normally formed babies occurred in the expectant arm of these trials and none in the induction arm. Obviously, this is not a significant difference. There was no effect on rate of Caesarean delivery (OR 0.60, 95% CI 0.35–1.03), instrumental delivery or use of analgesia in labour. Not surprisingly, given the relationship between gestational age and meconium staining of the amniotic fluid in labour, induction around 40 weeks reduces the incidence of meconium staining in labour (OR 0.50, 95% CI 0.31–0.86). Unfortunately, the authors of these trials did not address the important question of women's views of induction of labour at this stage of pregnancy. The authors therefore missed a golden opportunity in failing to measure women's satisfaction with their care. 'Routine' induction of labour at 40 weeks would no longer be considered a realistic option for the prevention of post-term pregnancy. The number of inductions at 40 weeks required to prevent an adverse outcome at 41 or 42 weeks would be excessive and intervention at this level would be unlikely to be welcomed by women, obstetricians or midwives.

Induction of labour and perinatal morbidity and mortality

Even the largest trial [110] has insufficient statistical power to detect a significant reduction in the perinatal mortality rate. To have an 80% chance of detecting a 50% reduction in a perinatal mortality rate of 3 per 1000, a sample size of 16 000 is required. Table 23.3 records the 13 perinatal deaths that occurred in the randomized trials, three among 3159 women allocated to induction and 10 among 3067 women allocated to selective induction. One normally formed baby, among those allocated to induction [117], died from asphyxia following emergency Caesarean delivery for meconium-stained amniotic fluid and bradycardia 2 hours after induction of labour. The other two deaths among those allocated to routine induction occurred in babies with lethal congenital anomalies. Three further deaths occurred in babies with anomalies among those allocated to selective induction. The other seven deaths occurred in normally formed babies. Two deaths in the Canadian Post-term Pregnancy Trial [110] occurred despite adherence to the monitoring protocol of daily movement counting and three times weekly CTG and ultrasound assessment of amniotic fluid volume. These babies were both small, weighing 2600 g and 3175 g. In the trial by Dyson *et al.* [118], a neonatal death from meconium aspiration occurred in a 43-week baby delivered for acute fetal bradycardia following spontaneous labour. Fetal heart rate monitoring and ultrasound assessment of amniotic fluid had been reassuring 48 hours before the spontaneous onset of labour. One of the deaths in the trial by Henry [119] was attributed to gestational diabetes. The second occurred due to meconium aspiration in a woman who refused induction following detection of meconium at amnioscopy. The deaths in the trials by Bergsjo *et al.* [120] and Cardozo *et al.* [121] were due to pneumonia and abruptio placentae, respectively.

The authors of systematic reviews adopt a different approach to the inclusion of perinatal deaths in babies with fetal abnormalities. These are excluded in the Cochrane review [99] and included by Sanchez-Ramos *et al.* [100]. Thus, the Cochrane systematic review shows that induction of labour is associated with a significant reduction in perinatal mortality in normally formed babies (OR 0.23, 95% CI 0.06–0.90), while Sanchez-Ramos *et al.* confirm the reduction in risk of perinatal death (0.9 vs. 0.33%) but with the 95% confidence intervals for the odds ratio of 0.41 crossing unity (95% CI 0.14–1.28).

Both systematic reviews report a significant reduction in the incidence of meconium-stained amniotic fluid but this does not affect the rate of meconium aspiration (0.82, 95% CI 0.49–1.37) [99]. There is no effect on fetal heart rate abnormalities during labour. The odds ratio for neonatal jaundice (3.39, 95% CI 1.42–8.09), based on the small number of trials that reported this outcome, indicate that it is increased by induction. The systematic reviews do not show any beneficial or hazardous effects on Apgar scores, neonatal intensive care admission or neonatal encephalopathy.

Effect of induction of labour on risk of Caesarean delivery

Sanchez-Ramos *et al.* [100] report that induction of labour is associated with a reduction in the rate of Caesarean delivery (OR 0.88, 95% CI 0.78–0.99). Crowley [99] reported a similar outcome, but interpreted it as evidence that a policy of 'routine' induction of labour does not increase the likelihood of Caesarean delivery. She believed that a post-randomization bias in the Hannah trial [110] may have weighted the results towards a spurious reduction in risk of Caesarean delivery. Women in the expectant arm of the Hannah trial who required induction because of abnormal antenatal tests were denied vaginal prostaglandins whereas those allocated to 'routine' induction were treated with prostaglandin E$_2$. This could potentially lead to an increase in dystocia or failed induction in those denied prostaglandins. However, this does not account for the 8.3% rate of Caesarean delivery for fetal distress in the selective induction arm of the Hannah trial compared with 5.7% in the routine induction arm. The effect of a policy of induction of labour on reducing the rate of Caesarean delivery for fetal distress is consistent across the trials reviewed. No significant heterogeneity was detected by Sanchez-Ramos *et al.* [100]. These authors also performed funnel plots, which were symmetric, indicating no evidence of publications bias.

Because the reduced rate of Caesarean delivery associated with induction of labour is contrary to a traditionally held view among obstetricians that induction of labour increases the likelihood of delivery by Caesarean section, a number of secondary analyses were carried out by Crowley [99]. These showed that induction of labour for post-term pregnancy does not increase the Caesarean delivery rate, irrespective of parity, cervical ripeness, method of induction or ambient Caesarean delivery rates.

Women's views of induction for post-term pregnancy

Regrettably, randomized trials give little information on women's views of induction versus conservative management. Only one trial assessed maternal satisfaction with induction of labour [121]. These authors showed that satisfaction was related to the eventual outcome of labour and delivery, rather than to the mode of onset of labour. Women's views are likely to be influenced by the local culture, by the attitude of their caregivers and by practical considerations such as the duration of paid maternity leave. Few obstetricians, midwives or childbirth educators are capable of giving women unbiased information about the risks of post-term pregnancy and the benefits and hazards of induction of labour. In a prospective questionnaire study of women's attitudes towards induction of labour for post-term pregnancy, Roberts and Young [122] found that despite a stated obstetric preference for conservative management, only 45% of women at 37 weeks' gestation were agreeable to conservative management if undelivered by 41 weeks. Of those undelivered by 41 weeks' gestation, 31% still desired conservative management. This significant decrease was unaffected by parity or certainty of gestational age. In a subsequent study, Roberts *et al.* [123] offered women a choice between

induction and conservative management at 42 weeks; 45% of women opted for conservative management. Certainly, an intervention that is common practice in more than 20–25% of pregnancies in most developed countries deserves more study with respect to its impact on women as well as the neonates who are the product of these pregnancies.

Post-term pregnancy and home birth

There is a lack of good-quality epidemiological evidence on the outcome of post-term pregnancy when delivery occurs at home. Bastian *et al.* [124] used multiple methods of case identification and follow-up to assemble a population-based cohort of 7002 home births in Australia; 50 perinatal deaths occurred, giving a perinatal mortality rate of 7.1 per 1000. Of 44 perinatal deaths in women of known gestational age, seven (15.9%) occurred post-term (≥42 weeks). A study conducted among Native Americans examined an increase in perinatal mortality in home births attended by midwives compared with those attended by doctors and identified post-dates pregnancies, breech deliveries and twins as the source of the difference in mortality rates between the two groups [125]. Given these relatively weak findings combined with the overall evidence regarding post-term pregnancy and intrapartum complications and perinatal morbidity and mortality, many home birth providers will refer such patients to an in-hospital practice.

Summary box 23.4

Antenatal testing

The following tests are often started at 40–41 weeks of gestation.

- Fetal movement or 'kick' counts.
- Non-stress test.
- Assessment of amniotic fluid volume.
- Biophysical profile.
- CTG or contraction stress test.

Post-term pregnancy

Post-term pregnancy may be prevented by:

- induction of labour;
- stripping/sweeping the membranes;
- vaginal intercourse;
- accupuncture.

While induction of labour has been asociated with Caesarean deliveries in previous retrospective literature, current prospective literature finds and supports the premise the Caesarean delivery is lower among those induced at 41 or 42 weeks' gestation compared with those managed expectantly beyond these thresholds.

Clinical guidelines for management of post-term pregnancy

Following the publication of the Canadian Post-term Pregnancy Trial [110] and the Cochrane review on post-term pregnancy management [111], the Society of Obstetricians and Gynaecologists of Canada (SOGC) issued a clinical practice guideline [126] that recommended the following.

1 After 41 weeks' gestation, if the dates are certain, women should be offered elective delivery.
2 If the cervix is unfavourable, cervical ripening should be undertaken.
3 If expectant management is chosen, assessment of fetal health should be initiated.

The Royal College of Obstetricians and Gynaecologists (RCOG) issued a clinical guideline on induction of labour in 2001 that included recommendations on management of post-term pregnancy [127].

1 An ultrasound to confirm gestation should be offered prior to 20 weeks, as this reduces the need for induction for perceived post-term pregnancy.
2 Women with uncomplicated pregnancies should be offered induction of labour beyond 41 weeks.
3 From 42 weeks, women who decline induction of labour should be offered increased antenatal monitoring, consisting of twice-weekly CTG and ultrasound estimation of maximum amniotic pool depth.

The American College of Obstetricians and Gynecologists Practice Guidelines [5] are somewhat similar, but specifically include the following.

1 The definition of post-term pregnancy should remain at 42 weeks of gestation and beyond.
2 Women with post-term pregnancies who have unfavourable cervices can either undergo labour induction or be managed expectantly.
3 Prostaglandin can be used in post-term pregnancies to promote cervical ripening and induce labour.
4 Delivery should be effected if there is evidence of fetal compromise or oligohydramnios.
5 Despite a lack of evidence that monitoring improves perinatal outcome, it is reasonable to initiate antenatal surveillance of post-term pregnancies between 41 weeks and 42 weeks' gestation because of evidence that perinatal morbidity and mortality increase as gestational age advances.

The SOGC guidelines provoked an impassioned response [102]. These authors challenged the evidence of increased morbidity and mortality as pregnancy advances and the evidence from randomized trials that induction of labour post-term does not increase Caesarean delivery rates and may reduce perinatal mortality rates. In particular, they were concerned that the recommendation from SOGC and RCOG that induction should be 'offered' at 41 weeks' gestation would be interpreted as a policy of mandatory induction at 41 weeks' gestation.

Thus, these three professional organizations, each with presumably capable and thoughtful members, arrived at a range of varied conclusions. Certainly this suggests, at the very least, there is a need for further research in this area, both on the effects of induction of labour, but also in ways to screen and prevent complications in late term and post-term pregnancies.

Practical management of post-term pregnancy

The RCOG recommendations are an excellent guide to practice. Every effort should be made to ensure that dates are as accurate as possible. When a woman reaches 41 weeks she should meet with a consultant obstetrician. Women have a right to be informed of the small increase in risk associated with continuing the pregnancy after 41 weeks. Thornton and Lilford [128] showed that pregnant women are much more risk averse than their caregivers. Following a vaginal examination, induction of labour should be offered on a date after 41 weeks that is acceptable to both the woman's wishes and the hospital resources. The vaginal examination could be accompanied by sweeping of the membranes, provided women are warned about the discomfort associated with this and are agreeable to proceed. Membrane sweeping reduces the need for 'formal' induction of labour [92]. The vaginal examination allows the obstetrician to inform the woman of the likely ease and success of induction of labour. For women who have previously delivered vaginally and for women with a favourable cervix, induction of labour is unlikely to be a difficult process. Women who wish to avoid induction of labour should be supported but should be made aware of the lack of reliability of antenatal tests and the lack of evidence that avoiding induction of labour reduces the risk of Caesarean delivery. As induction of labour with prostaglandins is associated with an increased risk of uterine scar dehiscence compared with spontaneous onset of labour [129], women who have had a previous Caesarean delivery, especially those with no vaginal deliveries, require carefully individualized management at 41 weeks' gestation.

References

1 Schmitt SK, Sneed L, Phibbs CS. Costs of newborn care in California: a population-based study. *Pediatrics* 2006;117: 154–160.
2 Saigal S, Doyle LW. An overview of mortality and sequelae of preterm birth from infancy to adulthood. *Lancet* 2008;371: 261–269.
3 Cotzias CS, Paterson-Brown S, Fisk NM. Prospective risk of unexplained stillbirth in singleton pregnancies at term: population based analysis. *BMJ* 1999;319:287–288.

4 World Health Organisation. *International Classification of Disease*, 10th edn. Geneva: WHO, 2003: chapter XV, 048.

5 ACOG Committee on Practice Bulletins. ACOG Practice Bulletin. Clinical management guidelines for obstetricians-gynecologists. Number 55, September 2004. Management of Postterm Pregnancy. *Obstet Gynecol* 2004;104:639–646.

6 Bierman J, Siegel E, French F, Simonian K. Analysis of the outcome of all pregnancies in a community. *Am J Obstet Gynecol* 1965;91:37–45.

7 Butler NR, Bonham DG. *Perinatal Mortality*. Edinburgh: Churchill Livingstone, 1963.

8 Chamberlain R, Chamberlain G, Howlett B, Masters K. *British Births 1970, Vol. 2. Obstetric Care*. London: Heinemann Medical, 1978.

9 Martin JA, Hamilton BE, Sutton PD *et al*. Births: final data for 2005. *Natl Vital Stat Rep* 2007;56(6):1–103.

10 Ventura SJ, Martin JA, Curtin SC, Mathews TJ, Park MM. Births: final data for 1998. *Natl Vital Stat Rep* 2000;48(3):1–100.

11 Sue A, Quan AK, Hannah ME, Cohen MM, Foster GA, Liston RM. Effect of labour induction on rates of stillbirth and caesarean delivery in post-term pregnancies. *Can Med Assoc J* 1999; 160:1145–1149.

12 Hilder L, Costeole K, Thilaganathan B. Prolonged pregnancy: evaluating gestation-specific risks of fetal and infant mortality. *Br J Obstet Gynaecol* 1998;105:169–173.

13 Smith GC. Use of time to event analysis to estimate the normal duration of human pregnancy. *Hum Reprod* 2001;16: 1497–1500.

14 Boyce A, Mayaux MJ, Schwartz D. Classical and true gestational postmaturity. *Am J Obstet Gynecol* 1976;125:911–913.

15 Savitz DA, Terry JW Jr, Dole N, Thorp JM Jr, Siega-Riz AM, Herring AH. Comparison of pregnancy dating by last menstrual period, ultrasound scanning, and their combination. *Am J Obstet Gynecol* 2002;187:1660–1666.

16 Eik-Nes SH, Okland O, Aure JC, Ulstein M. Ultrasound screening in pregnancy: a randomised controlled trial. *Lancet* 1984;i:1347.

17 Waldenstrom U, Axelsson O, Nilsson S *et al*. Effects of routine one-stage ultrasound screening in pregnancy: a randomised controlled trial. *Lancet* 1988;ii:585–588.

18 Saari-Kemppainen A, Karjalainen O, Ylostalo P, Heinonen OP. Ultrasound screening and perinatal mortality: controlled trial of systematic one-stage screening in pregnancy. The Helsinki Ultrasound Trial. *Lancet* 1990;336:387–391.

19 Ewigman BG, Crane JP, Frigoletto FD, LeFevre ML, Bain RP, McNellis D. Effect of prenatal ultrasound screening on perinatal outcome. RADIUS Study Group. *N Engl J Med* 1993;329: 821–827.

20 Neilson JP. Ultrasound for fetal assessment in early pregnancy. *Cochrane Database Syst Rev* 1998;(4):CD000182.

21 Bennett KA, Crane JM, O'Shea P, Lacelle J, Hutchens D, Copel JA. First trimester ultrasound screening is effective in reducing postterm labor induction rates: a randomized controlled trial. *Am J Obstet Gynecol* 2004;190:1077–1081.

22 Caughey AB, Nicholson JM, Washington AE. First- versus second-trimester ultrasound: the effect on pregnancy dating and perinatal outcomes. *Am J Obstet Gynecol* 2008;198:703.e1–5.

23 Bukowski R, Saade G, Malone F, Hankins G, D'Alton M. A decrease in postdate pregnancies is an additional benefit of first trimester screening for aneuploidy. *Am J Obstet Gynecol* 2001;185(Suppl):S148.

24 Naeye RL. Causes of perinatal mortality excess in prolonged gestations. *Am J Epidemiol* 1978;108:429–433.

25 Shea KM, Wilcox AJ, Little RE. Postterm delivery: a challenge for epidemiologic research. *Epidemiology* 1998;9:199–204.

26 Mogren I, Stenlund H, Hogberg U. Recurrence of prolonged pregnancy. *Int J Epidemiol* 1999;28:253–257.

27 Olesen AW, Basso O, Olsen J. Recurrence of prolonged pregnancy. *Int J Epidemiol* 1999;10:468–469.

28 Boyd ME, Usher RH, McLean FH *et al*. Obstetric consequences of postmaturity. *Am J Obstet Gynecol* 1988;158:334–338.

29 Laursen M, Bille C, Olesen AW, Hjelmborg J, Skytthe A, Christensen K. Genetic influence on prolonged gestation: a population-based Danish twin study. *Am J Obstet Gynecol* 2004;190:489–494.

30 Lockwood CJ, Moscarelli RD, Lynch L, Lapinski RH, Ghidini A. Low concentrations of vaginal fetal fibronectin as a predictor of deliveries occurring after 41 weeks. *Am J Obstet Gynecol* 1994;171:1–4.

31 Ramanathan G, Yu C, Osei E, Nicolaides KH. Ultrasound examination at 37 weeks' gestation in the prediction of pregnancy outcome: the value of cervical assessment. *Ultrasound Obstet Gynecol* 2003;22:598–603.

32 McLean M, Bisits A, Davies J, Woods R, Lowry P, Smith R. A placental clock controlling the length of human pregnancy. *Nat Med* 1995;1:460–463.

33 Divon MY, Ferber A, Nisell H, Westgren M. Male gender predisposes to prolongation of pregnancy. *Am J Obstet Gynecol* 2002;187:1081–1083.

34 Stotland NE, Caughey AB, Lahiff M, Abrams B. Weight gain and spontaneous preterm birth: the role of race or ethnicity and previous preterm birth. *Obstet Gynecol* 2006;108:1448–1455.

35 Caughey AB, Stotland NE, Washington AE, Escobar GJ. Who is at risk for prolonged and postterm pregnancy? *Am J Obstet Gynecol* 2009;200:683.e1–5.

36 Ramos GA, Caughey AB. Interrelationship between ethnicity and obesity on obstetrical outcomes. *Am J Obstet Gynecol* 2005;193:1089–1093.

37 Usha Kiran TS, Hemmadi S, Bethel J, Evans J. Outcome of pregnancy in a woman with an increased body mass index. *BJOG* 2005;112:768–772.

38 Stotland NE, Washington AE, Caughey AB. Pre-pregnancy body mass index and length of gestation at term. *Am J Obstet Gynecol* 2007;197:378.e1–5.

39 Baranova A, Gowder SJ, Schlauch K *et al*. Gene expression of leptin, resistin, and adiponectin in the white adipose tissue of obese patients with non-alcoholic fatty liver disease and insulin resistance. *Obes Surg* 2006;16:1118–1125.

40 Dietz PM, Callaghan WM, Cogswell ME, Morrow B, Ferre C, Schieve LA. Combined effects of prepregnancy body mass index and weight gain during pregnancy on the risk of preterm delivery. *Epidemiology* 2006;17:170–177.

41 Hickey CA, Cliver SP, McNeal SF, Goldenberg RL. Low pregravid body mass index as a risk factor for preterm birth: variation by ethnic group. *Obstet Gynecol* 1997;89:206–212.

42 Caughey AB, Stotland NE, Escobar G. What is the best measure of maternal complications of term pregnancy: ongoing pregnancies or pregnancies delivered? *Am J Obstet Gynecol* 2003;189:1047–1052.

43 Yudkin PL, Wood L, Redman CW. Risk of unexplained stillbirth at different gestational ages. *Lancet* 1987;i:1192–1194.

44 Smith GC. Life-table analysis of the risk of perinatal death at term and post term in singleton pregnancies. *Am J Obstet Gynecol* 2001;184:489–496.

45 Hilder L, Costeloe K, Thilaganathan B. Prospective risk of stillbirth. Study's results are flawed by reliance on cumulative prospective risk. *BMJ* 2000;320:444–445.

46 Yudkin P, Redman CW. Impending fetal death must be identified and pre-empted. *BMJ* 2000;320:444.

47 Buekens P, Delvoie P, Woolast E, Robyn C. Epidemiology of pregnancies with unknown last menstrual period. *J Epidemiol Commun Health* 1984;38:79–80.

48 Hall MH, Carr-Hill RA. The significance of uncertain gestation for obstetric outcome. *Br J Obstet Gynaecol* 1985;92:452–460.

49 Bruckner TA, Cheng YW, Caughey AB. Increased neonatal mortality among normal-weight births beyond 41 weeks of gestation in California. *Am J Obstet Gynecol* 2008;199:421.e1–7.

50 Ingemarsson I, Kallen K. Stillbirths and rate of neonatal deaths in 76,761 postterm pregnancies in Sweden, 1982–91: a register study. *Acta Obstet Gynecol Scand* 1997;76:658–662.

51 Caughey AB, Washington AE, Laros RK. Neonatal complications of term pregnancy: rates by gestational age increase in a continuous, not threshold, fashion. *Am J Obstet Gynecol* 2005;192:185–190.

52 Cheng YW, Nicholson J, Nakagawa S, Bruckner TA, Washington AE, Caughey AB. Perinatal outcomes in term pregnancies: do they differ by week of gestation? *Am J Obstet Gynecol* 2008;199:370.e1–7.

53 Caughey AB, Musci TJ. Complications of term pregnancies beyond 37 weeks of gestation. *Obstet Gynecol* 2004;103:57–62.

54 Caughey AB, Bishop J. Maternal complications of pregnancy increase beyond 40 weeks of gestation in low risk women. *J Perinatol* 2006;26:540–545.

55 Heimstad R, Romundstad PR, Eik-Nes SH, Salvesen KA. Outcomes of pregnancy beyond 37 weeks of gestation. *Obstet Gynecol* 2006;108:500–508.

56 Caughey AB, Stotland NE, Washington AE, Escobar GJ. Maternal obstetric complications of pregnancy are associated with increasing gestational age at term. *Am J Obstet Gynecol* 2007;196:155.e1–6.

57 Campbell MK, Ostbye T, Irgens LM. Post-term birth, risk factors and outcomes in a 10-year cohort of Norwegian births. *Obstet Gynecol* 1997;89:543–548.

58 Luckas M, Buckett W, Alfirevic Z. Comparison of outcomes in uncomplicated term and post-term pregnancy following spontaneous labor. *J Perinat Med* 1998;26:475–479.

59 Minchom P, Niswander K, Chalmers I *et al.* Antecedents and outcome of very early neonatal seizures in infants born at or after term. *Br J Obstet Gynaecol* 1987;94:431–439.

60 Curtis P, Matthews T, Clarke TA *et al.* The Dublin Collaborative Seizure Study. *Arch Dis Child* 1988;63:1065–1068.

61 MacLennan A. A template for defining a causal relation between acute intrapartum events and cerebral palsy: international consensus statement. *BMJ* 1999;319:1054–1059.

62 Gaffney G, Flavell V, Johnson A, Squier M, Sellers S. Cerebral palsy and neonatal encephalopathy. *Arch Dis Child* 1994;70:F195–F200.

63 Neldam S. Fetal movement as an indication of fetal wellbeing. *Lancet* 1980;i:1222–1224.

64 Grant A, Elbourne D, Valentin L, Alexander S. Routine formal fetal movement counting and risk of antepartum late death in normally formed singletons. *Lancet* 1989;ii:345–349.

65 Crowley P. Non-quantitative estimation of amniotic fluid volume in suspected prolonged pregnancy. *J Perinat Med* 1980;8:249–251.

66 Manning FA, Hill LM, Platt LD. Qualitative amniotic fluid volume determination by ultrasound: antepartum detection of intrauterine growth retardation. *Am J Obstet Gynecol* 1981;151:304–308.

67 Chamberlain PF, Manning FA, Morrison I, Harman CR, Lange IR. Ultrasound evaluation of amniotic fluid. 1. The relationship of marginal and decreased amniotic fluid volumes to perinatal outcome. *Am J Obstet Gynecol* 1984;150:245–249.

68 Crowley P, O'Herlihy C, Boylan P. The value of ultrasound measurement of amniotic fluid volume in the management of prolonged pregnancies. *Br J Obstet Gynaecol* 1980;91:444–448.

69 Fischer RL, McDonnell M, Bianculli RN, Perry RL, Hediger ML, Scholl TO. Amniotic fluid volume estimation in the post-date pregnancy: a comparison of techniques. *Obstet Gynecol* 1993;81:698–704.

70 Phelan JP, Smith CV, Broussard P, Small M. Amniotic fluid volume assessment with the four quadrant technique at 36–42 weeks' gestation. *J Reprod Med* 1987;32:540–542.

71 Alfirevic Z, Walkinshaw SA. A randomised controlled trial of simple compared with complex antenatal fetal monitoring after 42 weeks of gestation. *Br J Obstet Gynaecol* 1995;102:638–643.

72 Morris JM, Thompson K, Smithey J *et al.* The usefulness of ultrasound assessment of amniotic fluid in predicting adverse outcome in prolonged pregnancy: a prospective blinded observational study. *Br J Obstet Gynaecol* 2003;110:989–994.

73 Locatelli A, Zagarell A, Toso L, Assi F, Ghidini A, Biffi A. Serial assessment of amniotic fluid index in uncomplicated term pregnancies: prognostic value of amniotic fluid reduction. *J Matern Fetal Neonatal Med* 2004;15:233–236.

74 Chauhan SP, Sanderson M, Hendrix NW, Magann EF, Devoe LD. Perinatal outcome and amniotic fluid index in the antepartum and intrapartum periods: a meta-analysis. *Am J Obstet Gynecol* 1999;181:1473–1478.

75 Chauhan SP, Magann EF, Morrison JC, Whitowrth NS, Hendrix NW, Devoe LD. Ultrasonographic assessment of amniotic fluid does not reflect actual amniotic fluid volume. *Obstet Gynecol* 1994;84:856–860.

76 Magann EF, Chauhan SP, Barrilleaux PS, Whitworth NS, Martin JN. Amniotic fluid index and single deepest pocket: weak indicators of abnormal amniotic volumes. *Obstet Gynecol* 2000;96:737–740.

77 Manning F, Morrison J, Lange IR, Harmann CR, Chamberlain PF. Fetal assessment based on fetal biophysical profile: experience in 12,620 referred high-risk pregnancies. 1. Perinatal mortality by frequency and etiology. *Am J Obstet Gynecol* 1985;151:343–350.

78 Alfirevic Z, Neilson JP. Biophysical profile for fetal assessment in high risk pregnancies. *Cochrane Database Syst Rev* 1996;(1):CD000038.

79 Johnson JM, Harman CR, Lange IR, Manning F. Biophysical scoring in the management of the postterm pregnancy. An analysis of 307 patients. *Am J Obstet Gynecol* 1986;154:269–273.

80 Hann L, McArdle C, Sachs B. Sonographic biophysical profile in the postdate pregnancy. *J Ultrasound Med* 1987;6:191–195.

81 Keegan KA, Paul RH. Antepartum fetal heart rate testing. IV. The non-stress test as the primary approach. *Am J Obstet Gynecol* 1980;136:75–80.

82 Mendenhall HW, O'Leary J, Phillips KO. The nonstress test: the value of a single acceleration in evaluating the fetus at risk. *Am J Obstet Gynecol* 1980;136:87–91.

83 Pattison N, McCowan L. Cardiotocography for antepartum fetal assessment. *Cochrane Database Syst Rev* 1999;(1):CD001068.

84 Miyazaki FS, Miyazaki BA. False reactive nonstress tests in postterm pregnancies. *Am J Obstet Gynecol* 1981;140:269–276.

85 Dawes GS, Moullden M, Redman CWG. System 8000: computerised antenatal FHR analysis. *J Perinat Med* 1991;19:47–51.

86 Weiner Z, Farmakides G, Schulman H, Kellner L, Plancher S, Maulik D. Computerised analysis of fetal heart rate variation in post-term pregnancy: prediction of intrapartum fetal distress and fetal acidosis. *Am J Obstet Gynecol* 1994;171: 1132–1138.

87 Guidetti DA, Divon MY, Cavalieri RL, Langer O, Merkatz IR. Fetal umbilical artery flow velocimetry in postdate pregnancies. *Am J Obstet Gynecol* 1987;157:1521–1523.

88 Stokes HJ, Roberts RV, Newnham JP. Doppler flow velocity analysis in postdate pregnancies. *Aust NZ J Obstet Gynaecol* 1991;31:27–30.

89 Devine PA, Bracero LA, Lysikiewicz A, Evans R, Womack S, Byrne DW. Middle cerebral to umbilical artery Doppler ratio in post-date pregnancies. *Obstet Gynecol* 1994;84:856–860.

90 Kashanian M, Akbarian A, Baradaran H, Samiee MM. Effect of membrane sweeping at term pregnancy on duration of pregnancy and labor induction: a randomized trial. *Gynecol Obstet Invest* 2006;62:41–44.

91 de Miranda E, can der Bom JG, Bonsel GJ, Bleker OP, Rosendaal FR. Membrane sweeping and prevention of post-term pregnancy in low-risk pregnancies: a randomised controlled trial. *BJOG* 2006;113:402–408.

92 Boulvain M, Stan C, Irion O. Membrane sweeping for induction of labour. *Cochrane Database Syst Rev* 2005;(1):CD000451.

93 Tan PC, Andi A, Azmi N, Noraihan MN. Effect of coitus at term on length of gestation, induction of labor, and mode of delivery. *Obstet Gynecol* 2006;108:134–140.

94 Schaffir J. Sexual intercourse at term and onset of labor. *Obstet Gynecol* 2006;107:1310–1314.

95 Kavanagh J, Kelly AJ, Thomas J. Sexual intercourse for cervical ripening and induction of labour. *Cochrane Database Syst Rev* 2001;(2):CD003093.

96 Tan PC, Yow CM, Omar SZ. Effect of coital activity on onset of labor in women scheduled for labor induction. *Obstet Gynecol* 2007;110:820–826.

97 Rabl M, Ahner R, Bitschnau M, Zeisler H, Husslein P. Acupuncture for cervical ripening and induction of labor at term: a randomized controlled trial. *Wien Klin Wochenschr* 2001;113:942–946.

98 Smith CA, Crowther CA. Acupuncture for induction of labour. *Cochrane Database Syst Rev* 2004;(1):CD002962.

99 Crowley P. Interventions for preventing or improving the outcome of delivery at or beyond term. *Cochrane Database Syst Rev* 2000;(1):CD000170.

100 Sanchez-Ramos L, Olivier F, Delke I, Kaunitz AM. Labor induction versus expectant management for postterm pregnancies: a systematic review with meta-analysis. *Obstet Gynecol* 2003;101:1312–1318.

101 Caughey AB, Sundaram V, Kaimal A *et al.* Elective induction of labor vs. expectant management of pregnancy: a systematic review. *Ann Intern Med* 2009;151:252–263.

102 Menticoglou SM, Hall PF. Routine induction of labour at 41 weeks gestation: nonsensus consensus. *BJOG* 2002;109: 485–491.

103 Vahratian A, Zhang J, Troendle JF, Sciscione AC, Hoffman MK. Labor progression and risk of cesarean delivery in electively induced nulliparas. *Obstet Gynecol* 2005;105:698–704.

104 Seyb ST, Berka RJ, Socol ML, Dooley SL. Risk of cesarean delivery with elective induction of labor at term in nulliparous women. *Obstet Gynecol* 1999;94:600–607.

105 Caughey AB. Measuring perinatal complications: methodologic issues related to gestational age. *BMC Pregnancy Childbirth* 2007;7:18.

106 Caughey AB, Nicholson JM, Cheng YW, Lyell DJ, Washington AE. Induction of labor and cesarean delivery by gestational age. *Am J Obstet Gynecol* 2006;195:700–705.

107 Gülmezoglu AM, Crowther CA, Middleton P. Induction of labour for improving birth outcomes for women at or beyond term. *Cochrane Database Syst Rev* 2006;(4):CD004945.

108 Nicholson JM, Kellar LC, Cronholm PF, Macones GA. Active management of risk in pregnancy at term in an urban population: an association between a higher induction of labor rate and a lower cesarean delivery rate. *Am J Obstet Gynecol* 2004;191:1516–1528.

109 Nicholson JM, Parry S, Caughey AB, Rosen S, Keen A, Macones GA. The impact of the active management of risk in pregnancy at term on birth outcomes: a randomized clinical trial. *Am J Obstet Gynecol* 2008;198:511.e1–15.

110 Hannah ME, Hannah WJ, Hellman J *et al.* Induction of labour as compared with serial antenatal monitoring in post-term pregnancy. A randomised controlled trial. Canadian Multicenter Post-Term Pregnancy Trial Group. *N Engl J Med* 1992; 326:1587–1592.

111 Cole RA, Howie PW, MacNaughton MC. Elective induction of labour. A randomised prospective trial. *Lancet* 1975;i:767–770.

112 Martin DH, Thompson W, Pinkerton JHM, Watson JD. Randomised controlled trial of selective planned delivery. *Br J Obstet Gynaecol* 1978;85:109–113.

113 Breart G, Goujard J, Maillard F, Chavigny C, Rumeau-Rouquette C, Sureau C. Comparison of two obstetrical policies with regard to artificial induction of labour at term. A randomised trial. *J Obstet Biol Reprod (Paris)* 1982;11:107–112.

114 Egarter CH, Kofler E, Fitz R, Husselein PI. Is induction of labour indicated in prolonged pregnancy? Results of a prospective randomised trial. *Gynecol Obstet Invest* 1989;27:6–9.

115 Tylleskar J, Finnstrom O, Leijon I, Hedenskog S, Ryden G. Spontaneous labor and elective induction: a prospective randomised study. Effects on mother and fetus. *Acta Obstet Gynecol Scand* 1979;58:513–518.

116 Sande HA, Tuveng J, Fonstelien T. A prospective randomised study of induction of labor. *Int J Gynaecol Obstet* 1983;21: 333–336.

117 Katz Z, Yemini M, Lancet M, Mogilner BM, Ben-Hur H, Caspi B. Non-aggressive management of post-date pregnancies. *Eur J Obstet Gynecol Reprod Biol* 1983;15:71–79.

118 Dyson D, Miller PD, Armstrong MA. Management of prolonged pregnancy: induction of labour versus antepartum testing. *Am J Obstet Gynecol* 1987;156:928–934.

119 Henry GR. A controlled trial of surgical induction of labour and amnioscopy in the management of prolonged pregnancy. *J Obstet Gynaecol Br Commonw* 1969;76:795–798.

120 Bergsjo P, Gui-dan H, Su-qin Y, Zhi-zeng G, Bakketeig LS. Comparison of induced vs non-induced labor in post-term pregnancy. *Acta Obstet Gynecol Scand* 1989;68:683–687.

121 Cardozo L, Fysh J, Pearce JM. Prolonged pregnancy: the management debate. *BMJ* 1986;293:1059–1063.

122 Roberts LJ, Young KR. The management of prolonged pregnancy: an analysis of women's attitudes before and after term. *Br J Obstet Gynaecol* 1991;98:1102–1106.

123 Roberts L, Cook E, Beardsworth SA, Trew G. Prolonged pregnancy: two years experience of offering women conservative management. *J Royal Army Med Corps* 1994;140:32–36.

124 Bastian H, Keirse MJ, Lancaster PA. Perinatal death associated with planned home birth in Australia: a population based study. *BMJ* 1998;317:384–388.

125 Mehl-Madrona L, Madrona MM. Physician- and midwife-attended home births. Effects of breech, twin, and post-dates outcome data on mortality rates. *J Nurse Midwifery* 1997;42:91–98.

126 Society of Obstetricians and Gynaecologists of Canada. Post-term pregnancy. SOGC Clinical Practice Guidelines, No. 15, 1997. Available at www.sogc.org/guidelines/index_e.asp

127 Royal College of Obstetricians and Gynaecologists. *Induction of Labour*. Evidence-based Clinical Guideline No. 7, 2001. Updated July 2008 by National Institute for Health and Clinical Excellence, Clinical Guidelines CG70. Available at http://guidance.nice.org.uk/CG70/Guidance/pdf/English

128 Thornton J, Lilford R. The caesarean delivery decision: patients' choices are not determined by immediate emotional reactions. *J Obstet Gynaecol* 1989;9:283–288.

129 Lydon-Rochelle M, Holt VL, Easterling TR, Martin DP. Risk of uterine rupture during labor among women with a prior caesarean delivery. *N Engl J Med* 2001;345:3–8.

130 Fabre E, Gonzalez de Aguero R, de Agustin JL, Tajada M, Repolles S, Sanz A. Perinatal mortality in term and post-term births. *J Perinat Med* 1996;24:163–169.

131 Olesen AW, Basso O, Olsen J. Risk of recurrence of prolonged pregnancy. *BMJ* 2003;326:476.

132 Divon MY, Haglund B, Nisell H, Otterblad PO, Westgren M. Fetal and neonatal mortality in the post-term pregnancy: the impact of gestational age and fetal growth restriction. *Am J Obstet Gynecol* 1998;178:726–731.

133 Augensen K, Bergsjo P, Eikeland T, Ashvik K, Carlsen J. Randomised comparison of early versus late induction of labour in post-term pregnancy. *BMJ* 1987;294:1192–1195.

134 Chanrachakul B, Herabutya Y. Postterm with favorable cervix: is induction necessary? *Eur J Obstet Gynecol Reprod Biol* 2003;106:154–157.

135 Heden L, Ingemarsson I, Ahlstrom H, Solum T. Induction of labor vs conservative management in prolonged pregnancy: controlled study. *Int J Fetomaternal Med* 1991;4:148–152.

136 Herabutya Y, Prasertsawat PO, Tongyai T, Isarangura Na Ayudthya N. Prolonged pregnancy: the management dilemma. *Int J Gynaecol Obstet* 1992;37:253–258.

137 James C, George SS, Gaunekar N, Seshadri L. Management of prolonged pregnancy: a randomised trial of induction of labour and antepartum foetal monitoring. *Natl Med J India* 2001;14:270–273.

138 Martin JN, Sessums JK, Howard P, Martin RW, Morrison JC. Alternative approaches to the management of gravidas with prolonged post-term postdate pregnancies. *J Miss State Med Assoc* 1989;30:105–111.

139 National Institute of Child Health and Human Development Network of Maternal-Fetal Medicine Units. A clinical trial of induction of labor versus expectant management in postterm pregnancy. *Am J Obstet Gynecol* 1994;170:716–723.

140 Roach VJ, Rogers MS. Pregnancy outcome beyond 41 weeks gestation. *Int J Gynaecol Obstet* 1997;59:19–24.

141 Suikkari AM, Jalkanen M, Heiskala H, Koskela O. Prolonged pregnancy: induction or observation. *Acta Obstet Gynecol Scand Suppl* 1983;116:58.

142 Witter FR, Weitz CM. A randomised trial of induction at 42 weeks of gestation vs expectant management for postdates pregnancies. *Am J Perinatol* 1987;4:206–211.

Chapter 24
Induction and Augmentation of Labour

Jane E. Norman
MRC Centre for Reproductive Health, University of Edinburgh, Queen's Medical Research Centre, Edinburgh, UK

Definition

Induction of labour is defined as the artificial initiation of labour [1]. It is performed when it is considered that there are benefits to the baby and/or mother if the baby is delivered, compared with the alternative of the baby remaining *in utero*. Rates of induction of labour have increased significantly over the last 15 years in the USA [2] but have remained relatively stable in the UK over this period (Fig. 24.1). Current rates of induction of labour are around 20.2% in the UK (2005–2008) and 22% in the USA [2].

Indications for induction of labour

Both the UK and the USA have produced guidelines on the indications and methods for this common clinical procedure [1,3]. Suggested indications for induction of labour include a range of conditions associated with maternal or fetal compromise (Table 24.1), although the risks and benefits of induction in the majority of these particular scenarios (with the exception of post-term pregnancy) have not been subjected to randomized trials. In practice, the timing of induction requires careful clinical judgement, and it is not always obvious at which point in these disease or physiological processes that the interests of the mother or baby, or both, will be better served by ending the pregnancy by induction of labour.

Given the lack of randomized trials for the majority of these indications, it is perhaps not surprising that clinical conditions are not the only factor in affecting induction rates, with one recent study suggesting that over 25% of the variation in induction rates is unexplained by such factors [4]. This variation may reflect differences in physicians' willingness to induce labour for maternal or caregiver convenience, greater or lesser demand from women for induction of labour in different areas, or uncertainties about the benefits and risks of induction across a range of scenarios.

Contraindications to induction of labour

There is greater consensus about the contraindications to induction of labour. Contraindications relate either to factors which make labour or vaginal delivery unsuitable or to indications for immediate delivery (these latter include complete placenta praevia, vasa praevia, transverse fetal lie, umbilical cord prolapse and previous classical Caesarean section). The American College of Obstetrics and Gynecology also includes 'previous myomectomy entering the endometrial cavity' as a contraindication to labour induction [3]. These contraindications are absolute and are fairly uncontroversial. In clinical practice, however, a frequent but challenging scenario is the woman with a previous Caesarean section; such women commonly present with recognized indications for induction but are increased risk of uterine rupture. Their management is discussed further below.

Predicting success of induction of labour

Induction of labour is most successful when the cervix is 'ripe' at the time of labour induction [5,6]. Ripening is the process by which the cervix changes in consistency prior to the onset of labour: collagen content and cross-linking decline and water content increases [7]. Physiologically, this facilitates the cervix being progressively dilated by contractions of the myometrium once labour starts. Prior to the onset of labour, ripeness can be measured by using a strain gauge to determine the force required to dilate the cervix. In clinical practice, however, the most commonly used assessment of cervical ripening is the Calder modification of the Bishop score [6] (Table 24.2). This score comprises five components of the cervix, all assessed on vaginal examination: cervical length, dilation, position, consistency and its station relative to the ischial spines. Labour induction with an unripe cervix will

Dewhurst's Textbook of Obstetrics & Gynaecology, Eighth Edition. Edited by D. Keith Edmonds.
© 2012 John Wiley and Sons, Ltd. Published 2012 by John Wiley and Sons, Ltd.

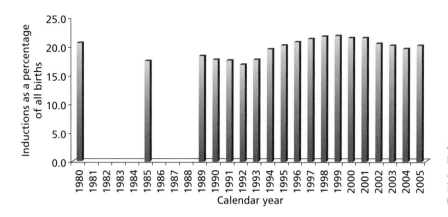

Fig. 24.1 Rates of induction of labour in England and Wales, 1980–2005. Available from www.hesonline.nhs.uk/Ease/servlet/ContentServer?siteID=1937&categoryID=1022

Table 24.1 Indications for induction of labour.

Abruptio placentae
Chorioamnionitis
Fetal demise
Gestational hypertension
Pre-eclampsia, eclampsia
Pre-labour rupture of membranes
Post-term pregnancy
Maternal medical conditions
Fetal compromise
Logistical

Source: adapted from American College of Obstetricians and Gynecologists [3].

Table 24.2 Calder modification of Bishop score.

Score	0	1	2	3
Dilation (cm)	<1	1–2	2–4	>4
Length of cervix (cm)	>4	2–4	1–2	<1
Station (relative to ischial spines)	−3	−2	−1/0	+1/+2
Consistency	Firm	Average	Soft	–
Position	Posterior	Mid/anterior		

require more uterine activity to effect cervical dilation, potentially causing a longer labour, more pain and stress for both mother and baby, a higher risk of uterine rupture and evidence of an increased odds ratio (OR) of delivery by Caesarean section (2.29, 95% CI 1.53–3.41) [8].

Digital assessment of the cervix at vaginal examination is subjective and is not surprisingly subject to considerable bias. Ultrasound measurement of cervical length is therefore a superficially more attractive option to predict success of induction of labour. Several studies have evaluated this approach, and a recent systematic review reports a meta-analysis of these data [9]. A variety of cervical lengths ranging from 16 to 32 mm have been used to indicate cervical ripeness. When these varying cervical lengths are assessed together, a 'short' cervical length predicts success and a 'long' cervical length predicts failure of labour induction, with likelihood ratios (LR) of success after a positive test of 1.66 (95% CI 1.20–2.31) and after a negative test of 0.51 (95% CI 0.39–0.67). These data are based on results from 19 trials and 3065 women, with 'success' in labour induction being defined variously as achieving vaginal delivery, achieving delivery with 24 hours of labour induction, or achieving the active stage of labour. Although there is a statistically significant association between an ultrasound measurement of short cervical length and the success of induction, the predictive value of these measurements do not support the clinical use of this test in practice. It is widely considered that a diagnostic test should have a positive LR of 5 or greater or a negative LR of 0.2 or less to be clinically useful; ultrasound measurement of cervical length for predicting success of induction of labour is clearly suboptimal when measured against this standard [10].

Although there has been no systematic assessment of the efficacy of the Bishop score in determining success of labour induction, comparison of Bishop score and ultrasound measurement of cervical length ($N = 454$ and 677, respectively) indicates similar efficacy of each [9]. It could be concluded therefore that the Bishop score is also ineffective as a tool to predict success of induction of labour. This does not mean that the Bishop score should be abandoned, as it may be useful in determining whether the cervix is ripe or whether further doses of prostaglandins are required to achieve ripeness. However, when used alone to determine the likely outcome of induction of labour, the Bishop score does not achieve current standards required of an effective diagnostic test.

Pharmacological and mechanical methods of induction of labour

In order to reduce the risk of adverse events associated with labour induction with an unripe cervix, induction is

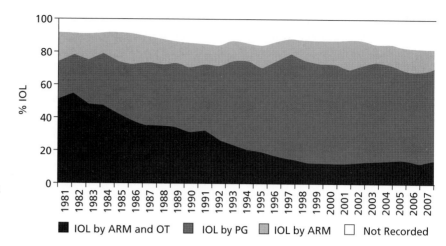

Fig. 24.2 Methods of induction of labour in Scotland, 1981–2007. ARM, artificial rupture of membranes; IOL, induction of labour; OT, oxytocin; PG, prostaglandin.

Table 24.3 Pharmacological agents for cervical ripening.

Agent	Route of administration	Dose	Maximum dose
PGE$_2$ tablets	Intravaginal	3 mg every 6 hours	6 mg
PGE$_2$ gel (dinoprostone)	Intravaginal	1 mg every 6 hours	3 mg (4 mg in unfavourable primigravidae)
PGE$_2$ controlled-release pessary (dinoprostone)	Intravaginal	Pessary releases 10 mg in 24 hours	One
PGE$_1$ (misoprostol) tablets*	Intravaginal	25 µg every 3–5 hours	None stated
PGE$_2$ (dinoprostone)*	Intracervical	0.5 mg every 6–12 hours	1.5 mg

*US practice.

often preceded by strategies to induce cervical ripening. In the UK, this is most commonly achieved with prostaglandins, normally intravaginal prostaglandin (PG)E$_2$. The increasing use of prostaglandins in association with induction of labour in Scotland over the last three decades is shown in Fig. 24.2.

In the USA, a wider variety and routes of administration of prostaglandins are endorsed, including intracervical and intravaginal PGE$_2$ and intravaginal misoprostol; intrauterine administration of a Foley catheter followed by extra-amniotic saline is also used to induce cervical ripening. Oral administration of prostaglandins is not recommended because it is associated with gastrointestinal side effects. Commonly used dose regimens in the UK and USA are shown in Table 24.3.

Prostaglandins for cervical ripening and induction of labour

The efficacy of prostaglandins for cervical ripening was shown in a seminal paper by Calder *et al.* [11]. Although highly effective in this regard, the cervical ripening effects of prostaglandins cannot easily be separated from their stimulatory effect on uterine contractions and it is largely this that causes the potential adverse effects of induction of labour with prostaglandins. Excessive uterine contrac-

tions are termed 'hyperstimulation' and can be associated with abnormalities of the fetal heart rate (FHR). In some women, an abnormal FHR may require immediate delivery by Caesarean section.

There are now extensive trial data on the use of prostaglandins for induction of labour. Demonstrated benefits of PGE$_2$ for cervical ripening compared with placebo or no treatment include reduced risk of vaginal delivery not being achieved within 24 hours (18.1% vs. 98.9%, risk ratio [RR] 0.19, 95% CI 0.14–0.25) and a reduced risk of requiring oxytocin administration (35.1% vs. 43.8%, RR 0.83, 95% CI 0.73–0.94) [12]. Although prostaglandins are associated with a greater risk of uterine hyperstimulation with FHR changes (4.4% vs. 0.49%, RR 4.14, 95% CI 1.93–8.90), this does not lead to an increased risk of Caesarean section [12].

 Summary box 24.1

Prostaglandins for induction of labour reduce the risk of the woman not being delivered within 24 hours of the start of induction and reduce the requirement for oxytocic agents, but increase the risk of uterine hyperstimulation with FHR changes.

When formulations of vaginal PGE_2 are compared, the sustained-release pessary appears to reduce operative vaginal delivery rates (9.9% vs. 19.5%, RR 0.51, 95% CI 0.35–0.76) [12], although it is a somewhat more expensive option than vaginal tablets.

The effects of vaginal PGE_1 (commonly administered as misoprostol) are similar to those of PGE_2 when placebo is used as the direct comparator of each; in other words PGE_1 also reduces the risk of vaginal delivery not occurring and the requirement for oxytocin compared with placebo [13]. However, direct comparison between vaginal PGE_2 and misoprostol shows that labour induction with vaginal misoprostol is associated with a greater likelihood of vaginal birth within 24 hours (RR 1.19, 95% CI 1.11–1.26) and a reduced need for oxytocin augmentation (RR 0.64, 95% CI 0.56–0.73) but a greater risk of uterine hyperstimulation both with FHR changes (RR 2.32, 95% CI 1.62–3.32) and without FHR changes (RR 2.93, 95% CI 2.04–4.20) [13]. Authorities in the UK and USA have come to different conclusions about the benefits of misoprostol over and above those of PGE_2. A 25-μg dose of misoprostol is not routinely available in either the UK or the USA, so that to administer the correct dose of misoprostol involves either cutting a 100-μg tablet into four or dissolving the tablet in suspension, with consequent risk of an incorrect dose. In light of the risks of both the uncertainty of dosing and the increased risk of uterine hyperstimulation with FHR abnormality, the National Institute for Health and Clinical Excellence (NICE) in the UK recommends that misoprostol not be used routinely except in the situation of intrauterine fetal death. In contrast, the American College of Obstetricians and Gynecologists endorses the use of misoprostol for induction of labour in a woman with an unfavourable cervix (assuming there has been no previous uterine surgery) [3].

Intracervical PGE_2 has been shown to be superior to placebo for cervical ripening, but inferior to vaginal prostaglandin in terms of the risk of not achieving vaginal delivery within 24 hours (RR 1.26, 95% CI 1.12–1.41) [14], leading NICE to conclude that 'intracervical PGE2 should not be used for induction of labour'.

Other methods of cervical ripening and induction of labour

Various alternative induction strategies have been investigated in order to avoid the stimulatory effects of prostaglandins on uterine contractions and hence avoid the adverse effects of prostaglandins in labour induction. Mechanical methods commonly involve extra-amniotic saline solution infusion and laminaria, or the hygroscopic dilator. Although extra-amniotic Foley catheter placement is endorsed in the USA, the use of any of the above methods increases the risk of maternal infection [15] and none are therefore endorsed for use in the UK. Membrane sweeping is recommended on routine antenatal visits post term as an adjunct to labour induction as it reduces the risk of pregnancy prolongation beyond 41 weeks [16]. Of the pharmacological methods, nitric oxide donors [17] and intracervical hyaluronidase [18] both appear to ripen the cervix without inducing myometrial contractility, but there is insufficient evidence as yet to recommend their use in clinical practice. Mifepristone, a progesterone antagonist, has less stimulatory effects on myometrial contractions than prostaglandins but concerns about safety currently preclude use with a live baby [1].

Once the cervix is ripe, continuation of labour induction may involve forewater amniotomy (artificial rupture of the membranes) with or without augmentation of labour with the oxytocic agent Syntocinon. Forewater amniotomy for induction of labour (without PGE_2 but sometimes with oxytocin) is commonly used as a primary method of induction in women with a ripe cervix, but is not routinely advised because of the increased requirement for oxytocin augmentation [19] if used alone, and because of lower acceptability compared with prostaglandin if used in combination with oxytocin [1]. It is probably for these reasons that use of artificial rupture of membranes with or without oxytocin is now much less commonly used as the primary method of induction of labour in the UK.

Augmentation of labour

Augmentation of labour is the process of speeding up the first stage of labour. For decades, amniotomy with or without oxytocin has been the standard intervention in this scenario, but recent systematic reviews suggest that these practices may not be evidence based.

Amniotomy

A meta-analysis of 14 trials in nearly 5000 women indicated that routine amniotomy had no effect on the duration of the first stage of labour, maternal satisfaction or Apgar scores at delivery, but that there was a trend to increased risk of Caesarean section (RR 1.26, 95% CI 0.98–1.62) [20]. These facts support the authors' conclusion that 'we cannot recommend that amniotomy should be introduced routinely as part of standard labour management and care'.

There is a little more evidence in support of the use of amniotomy with oxytocin (Syntocinon) for augmentation of labour. As with prostaglandins, Syntocinon has to be used carefully because the myometrial contractions it induces cause a reduction in blood flow to the uterus. This reduction in blood flow can lead to fetal distress, especially if the fetus is already compromised. A meta-analysis of 12 trials in 7792 women showed that early amniotomy and oxytocin augmentation has a modest (non-significant) benefit in reducing the risk of Caesarean section (RR 0.89,

95% CI 0.79–1.01) [21]. A significant (but again modest) reduction in the duration of the first stage of labour was observed with a mean difference of –1.43 hours (95% CI –2.01 to –0.84). There were no differences in any neonatal outcomes or in maternal satisfaction rates.

Summary box 24.2

The use of oxytocin for augmentation of labour reduces the total duration of the first stage of labour by about 90 min.

There is great variability in uterine response to oxytocin, both between different women and, during the course of labour, within individual women. Thus, if oxytocin is used, it should be started in a low dose initially, with increasing doses titrated against the clinical response, and the dose reduced in the presence of frequent contractions. Possible benefits of higher doses of oxytocin more rapidly escalated (compared with lower doses) include a faster labour and a reduced risk of Caesarean section, at the expense of increased rates of hyperstimulation but the evidence for this is considered to be weak [1]. Commonly suggested starting doses range from 0.0005 to 0.006 units/min to a maximum of 0.004–0.042 units/min. The British National Formulary (BNF) suggests a starting regimen of oxytocin of 0.001–0.002 units/min and notes that although the maximum licensed dose in the UK is 0.02 units/min, in clinical practice it is reasonable to administer oxytocin in doses up to a maximum of 0.032 units/min. Both the BNF and the NICE intrapartum care guideline [22] indicate that oxytocin should be increased at intervals not less than every 30 min. Regardless of the regimen used, the target frequency of uterine contractions is three to five every 10 min.

Complications of induction of labour

The most common complication of induction of labour is the risk that the procedure is not successful and that labour does not ensue, which occurs in around 15% of primigravidae with an unfavourable cervix, but less commonly in multiparous women or those with a higher Bishop score at the start of the induction process [23].

Caesarean section is widely considered a complication of induction of labour, although again the evidence for this is sparse. Indeed, in the clinical scenario for which there is most evidence, that of post-term pregnancy, meta-analyses indicate that induction either modestly reduces the risk [24] or has no effect on rates of Caesarean section compared with expectant management [25]. Whilst a large cohort study of primigravidae undergoing induction of labour showed an absolute rate of Caesarean section of 18–27% [26], a recent systematic review suggests that the risk of Caesarean section is no higher following induction of labour when an appropriate comparator group of women who are not induced are used [27]. These data are in agreement with our own, evaluating the effect of 'elective' induction of labour in Scotland during the period 1981–2007 (S.J. Stock *et al.*, unpublished data, see below). Thus current evidence suggests that Caesarean section is not a risk of induction of labour.

Hyperstimulation

The contractile response to prostaglandins varies from woman to woman and is not easily predictable. Thus it is not surprising that some women contract excessively after administration of standard doses of prostaglandins. Uterine hyperstimulation is defined as a contraction frequency of more than five in 10 min or contractions exceeding 2 min in duration; tachysystole occurs when uterine hyperstimulation is accompanied by an abnormal FHR pattern. NICE quotes a rate of hyperstimulation across a range of induction agents of 1–5% [1], although this may be less common with the low-dose PGE_2 regimens in use in the UK.

Profound alterations in FHR pattern may require immediate delivery by Caesarean section. In the presence of less severe FHR alterations, tocolysis (e.g. with terbutaline 250 μg i.v. or s.c.) may be sufficient to treat hyperstimulation in the majority of women.

Monitoring and setting during induction of labour

Monitoring

The evidence base for monitoring of maternal and fetal well-being during induction of labour is sparse. Most authorities suggest that a cardiotocograph should be performed to confirm that the FHR is normal prior to prostaglandin insertion. Thereafter, the onset of labour can be identified by the presence of uterine contractions. If contractions do not ensue spontaneously, digital cervical assessment should be performed at intervals no more frequently than every 6 hours to determine if there has been any change in the Bishop score. The cardiotocographic assessment should be repeated when contractions begin, normally 2–6 hours after prostaglandin administration.

Setting

There is increasing interest in carrying out induction on an outpatient basis, with the induction agent being administered at home or being administered in hospital and the woman then going home to await the onset of labour. Although there is some evidence that this approach increases maternal satisfaction, there is currently insufficient evidence to determine whether it is safe to recommend widespread use [28].

Table 24.4 Effect of induction of labour after 41+ weeks' gestation.

Outcome	RR	95% CI	Amount of evidence
Perinatal death	0.30	0.09–0.99	12 trials, 5939 women
Meconium aspiration syndrome	0.29	0.12–0.68	4 trials, 1325 women
Caesarean section	0.92	0.76–1.12	18 trials, 7865 women

Source: data from Gulmezoglu *et al.* [25].

Induction of labour at term (>37 weeks' gestation): risks and benefits

Post-term pregnancy

The highest-quality evidence on the risks and benefits of induction of labour relates to the scenario of post-term pregnancy. The cumulative risk of perinatal death rises progressively after 38 weeks of gestation [29] and many authorities have suggested that induction of labour might reduce perinatal death. A recent meta-analysis for the Cochrane collaboration, reporting on 19 randomized trials incorporating 7984 women at 41 weeks' gestation or beyond, compared a policy of labour induction to a policy of awaiting spontaneous onset of labour [25]. The babies of women in the induction arm were significantly less likely to have either perinatal death or meconium aspiration syndrome, but induction had no effect on Caesarean section rates (Table 24.4). Translating the above data into numbers needed to treat (NNT), 469 women would have to be induced at 41 weeks' gestation to prevent one perinatal death. However, these data should perhaps be interpreted with caution, as the total number of fetal or neonatal deaths was small: one in the induction group and nine in the actively managed group in this most recent meta-analysis [25].

A previous systematic review showed a significant reduction in Caesarean section rates (OR 0.88, 95% CI 0.78–0.99) but no significant difference in perinatal death (OR 0.41, 95% CI 0.14–1.18) [24], and these findings are consistent with those in the largest single randomized trial [30].

Taken together, these data suggests that induction of labour at or beyond 41 weeks probably reduces perinatal death without increasing the risk of Caesarean section. For these reasons, many authorities (including NICE) suggest that induction of labour should be routinely offered at 41 weeks' gestation and beyond in order to improve neonatal outcome. Additionally, there is some evidence that the majority of women at this gestation prefer induction of labour to conservative management [31].

Summary box 24.3

Post-term induction of labour reduces perinatal death (estimated NNT 469) without an increase in Caesarean section.

Pre-labour membrane rupture at term

Another common indication for induction of labour is when the fetal membranes rupture at term prior to the onset of labour, but labour fails to start. If the pregnancy continues without the baby being delivered, there is a risk of ascending infection which could lead to chorioamnionitis and attendant fetal and maternal compromise. However, 95% of women will labour spontaneously within 24 hours of membrane rupture, and thus early recourse to induction of labour might involve the adverse consequences of induction of labour in a woman who would have laboured spontaneously with conservative management. Again, this issue has been subject to randomized trials. At 37 weeks of gestation or more, compared with expectant management (no active management for at least 24 hours), induction within 24 hours reduces the risk of chorioamnionitis (RR 0.74, 95% CI 0.56–0.97), endometritis (RR 0.30, 95% CI 0.12–0.74) and (for the baby) neonatal intensive care admission (RR 0.72, 95% CI 0.57–0.92) without increasing rates of Caesarean section (RR 0.94, 95% CI 0.82–1.08) [32]. Importantly, women undergoing induction of labour were happier with their treatment than those managed expectantly. However, a conservative approach in order to await the onset of labour is justifiable if the woman wishes, given that induction does not significantly reduce rates of neonatal infection (RR 0.83, 95% CI 0.61–1.12). Current advice from NICE is that women with pre-labour rupture of the membranes at term (≥37 weeks' gestation) should be offered a choice of induction of labour or expectant management, and that if labour has not commenced approximately 24 hours after rupture of membranes, then induction of labour is appropriate [22]. In practice, management decisions are likely to be based on local organization of care and the individual woman's request.

Maternal request

The most controversial area, and the issue for which there is little evidence from randomized trials, relates to induction of labour in the absence of any medical indications, i.e. induction of labour on maternal request. Women and their partners are increasingly able to control many aspects of their lives, and this wish to plan their life extends (for many women) into where, when and how they have their baby. Although maternal choice is promoted in the UK, at least in regard to place of delivery and more 'natural' childbirth (such as delivery under water), there is less support for women who opt for delivery by elective Caesarean section or who wish to have their labour induced before 41 weeks' gestation unless there are 'medical' indications to do this. Elective Caesarean section on request can increase the rate of some maternal complications and may also have resource implications for the health service: the issues around this have been comprehensively debated elsewhere.

Induction of labour on request (elective induction) might be a suitable compromise for women who wish to choose the date of delivery of their baby but who hope for a vaginal delivery. Popular mythology is that elective induction is associated with an increased risk of Caesarean section. However, only three randomized trials, none of optimal quality, have assessed the effects of induction of labour prior to 41 weeks' gestation for this indication. Although the relative risk of Caesarean section was 1.73 when data from these trials was combined, the confidence intervals cross unity and thus this apparent increase in Caesarean section rate is not statistically significant (95% CI 0.67–4.50) [27]. Caughey reviewed the observational data around elective induction of labour and found no significant increase in Caesarean section rates from observational data when women having elective induction were compared with women undergoing expectant management. We subsequently completed a retrospective cohort study of over 300 000 women undergoing induction in Scotland between 1981 and 2007 and showed either no increase or a very modest increase in Caesarean section rates in association with elective induction of labour after adjustment for confounding variables of age at delivery, parity, period of birth, deprivation quintile and birthweight (S.J. Stock *et al.*, unpublished data). Additionally, we showed a reduction in perinatal mortality, with NNT at 40 weeks' gestation of 1040 inductions for every one perinatal death prevented. This beneficial effect on perinatal death reduction was achieved at the expense of one extra admission to the neonatal intensive care unit for every 131 women induced. We believe that these data provide support for a policy of agreeing to individual women's requests for elective induction of labour, and for extending choice to the timing of delivery.

Summary box 24.4

There is little evidence that induction of labour 'on request' for women with an uncomplicated pregnancy and without a previous Caesarean section increases the risk of Caesarean section compared with a policy of expectant management.

Prevention of shoulder dystocia

In the scenario where birthweight is expected to be high (e.g. babies already diagnosed with macrosomia or babies of diabetic mothers), a strategy of induction has been hypothesized to prevent further intrauterine growth, thus reducing the risk of both fetal macrosomia and shoulder dystocia and increasing the chance of vaginal delivery. However, neither randomized trials nor observational data support this hypothesis [33,34] and thus induction of labour cannot be recommended for this indication.

Intrauterine fetal death

In the absence of induction of labour, 90% of women will spontaneously deliver within 3 weeks of intrauterine fetal death. The risks of conservative management include disseminated intravascular coagulation and (particularly in the presence of ruptured membranes) ascending infection. Additionally, many women with a diagnosis of intrauterine fetal death will wish to deliver the baby as soon as possible. There are no randomized trials comparing a policy of induction with conservative management in this situation, and NICE recommends that conservative management is reasonable if 'the woman appears to be physically well, her membranes are intact and there is no evidence of infection or bleeding' [1].

In the presence of intrauterine fetal death, mifepristone 200 mg three times daily significantly reduces the induction to delivery interval [35]. In practice, a single dose of mifepristone (200 mg) followed by either low-dose vaginal misoprostol (e.g. 25–50 µg 4-hourly up to six doses) or vaginal PGE_2 is commonly used for induction of labour with intrauterine fetal death at 24 weeks or greater; higher doses of prostaglandin may be needed at earlier gestations and lower doses should be used if the woman has had a previous Caesarean section.

Induction of labour in the presence of previous Caesarean section

Women with a previous Caesarean section who undergo induction of labour are considered to have an increased risk of repeat Caesarean section and uterine rupture compared with those who labour spontaneously. There is some evidence for this: one systematic review showed that women with a previous Caesarean have a risk of Caesarean delivery of 24% (range 18–51%) during a spontaneous labour but a risk of 48% (range 28–51%) following induction of labour with PGE_2 [36]. There are no randomized trials of sufficient size to inform the risks of repeat Caesarean section or uterine rupture, but a large cohort study indicated increased odds of uterine rupture when labour was induced with prostaglandins compared with spontaneous labour (OR 2.9, 95% CI 2.0–4.3) [37]. In 14% of women with uterine rupture the baby suffered a perinatal death.

In view of the above data, induction of labour in women with a previous Caesarean section should be undertaken with caution and in an environment where uterine rupture can be rapidly diagnosed and treated if necessary. Some clinicians may feel that the possible risks of induction of labour in the presence of a previous Caesarean section are too great, and that such women are best delivered by elective Caesarean section if immediate delivery is indicated. Whilst this approach is reasonable on an empirical basis, there are no trials comparing induction of labour with elective repeat lower segment Caesarean section [38].

Pre-eclampsia

The final indication for induction of labour is the scenario of mild pre-eclampsia. Severe pre-eclampsia at term is an absolute indication for delivery, either by Caesarean section or attempting to expedite vaginal delivery by induction of labour. Mild pre-eclampsia is often managed conservatively, but there is evidence from a recent paper that liberal induction of labour in women with mild pre-eclampsia or gestational hypertension improves maternal outcomes expressed as a composite of maternal mortality, maternal morbidity, progression to severe hypertension or proteinuria, and major postpartum haemorrhage (RR 0.71, 95% CI 0.59–0.86) [39].

Summary

Induction of labour is one of the most commonly undertaken procedures in obstetric practice, but the evidence regarding risks and benefits is sparse, with the exception of the indications of post-term pregnancy and pre-labour membrane rupture. Prostaglandins are the agents most commonly used, with good evidence that they speed up the process of induction of labour. Further randomized trials are required to determine the effects of induction in a variety of clinical scenarios. Meanwhile, clinicians should discuss the current literature and its implications with pregnant women prior to making decisions about their management.

References

1 National Collaborating Centre for Women's and Children's Health on behalf of the National Institute for Health and Clinical Evidence (NICE). *Induction of Labour*. Clinical Guideline CG70, 2008. Available at: http://guidance.nice.org.uk/CG70/Guidance/pdf/English.

2 Martin JA, Hamilton BE, Sutton PD, Ventura SJ, Menacker F, Kirmeyer S. Births: final data for 2004. *Natl Vital Stat Rep* 2006; 55(1):1–101.

3 American College of Obstetricians and Gynecologists. ACOG Practice Bulletin No. 107. Induction of labor. *Obstet Gynecol* 2009;114:386–397.

4 Humphrey T, Tucker JS. Rising rates of obstetric interventions: exploring the determinants of induction of labour. *J Public Health (Oxf)* 2009;31:88–94.

5 Bishop EH. Pelvic scoring for elective induction. *Obstet Gynecol* 1964;24:266–268.

6 Calder A, Embrey M, Tait T. Ripening of the cervix with extra-amniotic prostaglandin E2 in viscous gel before induction of labour. *Br J Obstet Gynaecol* 1977;84:264–268.

7 Norman JE. Preterm labour. Cervical function and prematurity. *Best Pract Res Clin Obstet Gynaecol* 2007;21:791–806.

8 Vrouenraets FP, Roumen FJ, Dehing CJ, van den Akker ES, Aarts MJ, Scheve EJ. Bishop score and risk of cesarean delivery after induction of labor in nulliparous women. *Obstet Gynecol* 2005;105:690–697.

9 Hatfield AS, Sanchez-Ramos L, Kaunitz AM. Sonographic cervical assessment to predict the success of labour induction: a systematic review with metaanalysis. *Am J Obstet Gynecol* 2007; 197:186–192.

10 Honest H, Forbes CA, Durée KH *et al.* Screening to prevent spontaneous preterm birth: systematic reviews of accuracy and effectiveness literature with economic modelling. *Health Technol Assess* 2009;13(43):1–627.

11 Calder AA, Embrey MP, Hillier K. Extra-amniotic prostaglandin E2 for the induction of labour at term. *J Obstet Gynaecol Br Commonw* 1974;81:39–46.

12 Kelly AJ, Malik S, Smith L, Kavanagh J, Thomas J. Vaginal prostaglandin (PGE2 and PGF2a) for induction of labour at term. *Cochrane Database Syst Rev* 2009;(4):CD003101.

13 Hofmeyr GJ, Gulmezoglu AM. Vaginal misoprostol for cervical ripening and induction of labour. *Cochrane Database Syst Rev* 2003;(1):CD000941.

14 Boulvain M, Kelly A, Irion O. Intracervical prostaglandins for induction of labour. *Cochrane Database Syst Rev* 2008;(1):CD006971.

15 Heinemann J, Gillen G, Sanchez-Ramos L, Kaunitz AM. Do mechanical methods of cervical ripening increase infectious morbidity? A systematic review. *Am J Obstet Gynecol* 2008;199: 177–187; discussion 187–188.

16 Boulvain M, Stan C, Irion O. Membrane sweeping for induction of labour. *Cochrane Database Syst Rev* 2005;(1):CD000451.

17 Ledingham MA, Thomson AJ, Lunan CB, Greer IA, Norman JE. A comparison of isosorbide mononitrate, misoprostol and combination therapy for first trimester pre-operative cervical ripening: a randomised controlled trial. *BJOG* 2001;108:276–280.

18 Kavanagh J, Kelly AJ, Thomas J. Hyaluronidase for cervical ripening and induction of labour. *Cochrane Database Syst Rev* 2006;(2):CD003097.

19 Bricker L, Luckas M. Amniotomy alone for induction of labour. *Cochrane Database Syst Rev* 2000;(4):CD002862.

20 Smyth RM, Alldred SK, Markham C. Amniotomy for shortening spontaneous labour. *Cochrane Database Syst Rev* 2007;(4): CD006167.

21 Wei S, Wo BL, Xu H, Luo ZC, Roy C, Fraser WD. Early amniotomy and early oxytocin for prevention of, or therapy for, delay in first stage spontaneous labour compared with routine care. *Cochrane Database Syst Rev* 2009;(2):CD006794.

22 National Collaborating Centre for Women's and Children's Health on behalf of National Institute for Clinical Excellence (NICE). *Intrapartum Care: Management and Delivery of Care to Women in Labour*. Clinical Guidelines CG55, 2007. Available at: http://guidance.nice.org.uk/CG55.

23 Rayburn WF. Prostaglandin E2 gel for cervical ripening and induction of labour: a critical analysis. *Am J Obstet Gynecol* 1989; 160:529–534.

24 Sanchez-Ramos L, Olivier F, Delke I, Kaunitz AM. Labor induction versus expectant management for postterm pregnancies: a systematic review with meta-analysis. *Obstet Gynecol* 2003;101: 1312–1318.

25 Gulmezoglu AM, Crowther CA, Middleton P. Induction of labour for improving birth outcomes for women at or beyond term. *Cochrane Database Syst Rev* 2006;(4):CD004945.

26 Smith GC, Dellens M, White IR, Pell JP. Combined logistic and Bayesian modelling of cesarean section risk. *Am J Obstet Gynecol* 2004;191:2029–2034.

27 Caughey AB, Sundaram V, Kaimal AJ *et al.* Systematic review: elective induction of labor versus expectant management of pregnancy. *Ann Intern Med* 2009;151:252–263.

28 Kelly AJ, Alfirevic Z, Dowswell T. Outpatient versus inpatient induction of labour for improving birth outcomes. *Cochrane Database Syst Rev* 2009;(2):CD007372.

29 Smith GC. Life-table analysis of the risk of perinatal death at term and post term in singleton pregnancies. *Am J Obstet Gynecol* 2001;184:489–496.

30 Hannah ME, Hannah WJ, Hellman J *et al.* Induction of labour as compared with serial antenatal monitoring in post-term pregnancy. A randomised controlled trial. Canadian Multi-center Post-Term Pregnancy Trial Group. *N Engl J Med* 1992;326: 1587–1592.

31 Heimstad R, Romundstad PR, Hyett J, Mattsson LA, Salvesen KA. Women's experiences and attitudes towards expectant management and induction of labor for post-term pregnancy. *Acta Obstet Gynecol Scand* 2007;86:950–956.

32 Dare MR, Middleton P, Crowther CA, Flenady VJ, Varatharaju B. Planned early birth versus expectant management (waiting) for prelabour rupture of membranes at term (37 weeks or more). *Cochrane Database Syst Rev* 2006;(1):CD005302.

33 Witkop CT, Neale D, Wilson LM, Bass EB, Nicholson WK. Active compared with expectant delivery management in women with gestational diabetes: a systematic review. *Obstet Gynecol* 2009;113:206–217.

34 Sanchez-Ramos L, Bernstein S, Kaunitz AM. Expectant management versus labor induction for suspected fetal macrosomia: a systematic review. *Obstet Gynecol* 2002;100:997–1002.

35 Cabrol D, Dubois C, Cronje H *et al.* Induction of labor with mifepristone (RU 486) in intrauterine fetal death. *Am J Obstet Gynecol* 1990;163:540–542.

36 McDonagh MS, Osterweil P, Guise JM. The benefits and risks of inducing labour in patients with prior caesarean delivery: a systematic review. *BJOG* 2005;112:1007–1015.

37 Smith GC, Pell JP, Pasupathy D, Dobbie R. Factors predisposing to perinatal death related to uterine rupture during attempted vaginal birth after caesarean section: retrospective cohort study. *BMJ* 2004;329:375.

38 Dodd J, Crowther C. Induction of labour for women with a previous Caesarean birth: a systematic review of the literature. *Aust NZ J Obstet Gynaecol* 2004;44:392–395.

39 Koopmans CM, Bijlenga D, Groen H *et al.* Induction of labour versus expectant monitoring for gestational hypertension or mild pre-eclampsia after 36 weeks' gestation (HYPITAT): a multicentre, open-label randomised controlled trial. *Lancet* 2009;374:979–988.

Chapter 25
Obstetric Emergencies

Sara Paterson-Brown
Queen Charlotte's & Chelsea Hospital, London, UK

General principles for minimizing the risk of an emergency occurring

Promote good antenatal health

Good general health and a supportive home environment promote good health during pregnancy. The Confidential Enquiry into Maternal and Child Health [1] reminds us of the increased risks not only of those with pre-existing disease, but also of socially excluded immigrant women, the obese and those abusing substances. Good antenatal care is paramount in promoting health: women should be screened for a variety of risk factors and any problems that are identified should be acted on [2]. We know from the confidential enquiries over the years that we sometimes fail to recognize, communicate or act on risk factors which are apparent in the antenatal period. This makes it even more important, when considering intrapartum care, to make every effort to review a woman's antenatal health to identify any such risks, and pay heed to any instructions made in the antenatal period.

Organized intrapartum care

The senior sister in charge and the senior obstetrician on the delivery suite should work together as a team to coordinate clinical activity. It is worthy of mention that when some people are in charge of a delivery suite, no matter how busy it is things are calm and in control, while at other times even a quiet day can feel hectic. The skills required to coordinate workload and staffing are multiple and often acquired over years, but if you recognize either of the above characteristics in those you work with take a moment or two to try to define what they are doing differently and try to emulate the one and avoid features of the other.

Triage

The principles behind effective triage have hinged on the ABC approach to prioritizing casualties according to whether they have an airway (A) problem (which can lead to death within minutes if left untreated) through difficulties with breathing (B) to circulatory disorders (C).

Although this can also be useful in obstetrics, it does not address the fact that obstetricians have to prioritize between two patients: the mother and the baby. Indeed there is little written about obstetric triage [3,4] and how to fit the fetus (F) into the equation. Clearly it is not as easy as ABCF and emergency care to save a baby may take priority over a less than life-threatening maternal condition. However, it is true to say that in most societies the life of the mother is given priority over that of an unborn baby and, most importantly, the fetus is best treated by adequate, rapid and effective resuscitation or stabilization of the mother anyway [3].

> **Summary box 25.1**
>
> Hints for keeping the workload under control:
> - Keep your mind open to all the activity going on.
> - Try to coordinate activity so that things happen in sequence and not all at the same time.
> - Listen to your midwives' and doctors' concerns and address them.
> - Prioritize according to risk (triage).
> - Get simple things done quickly, as once resolved they relieve staff.
> - Do not defer decisions unnecessarily (work just builds up).
> - Give each woman a carer with the appropriate skills to match the complexity of the clinical problem.
> - Recognize if doctor or midwife is out of their depth: support them and encourage them to call for help.
> - Regularly revisit women with risk factors to check the situation is not deteriorating (do not assume you will be called).

General principles for minimizing adverse consequences resulting from an emergency

If risk factors have been identified, preparations can be made to deal with the anticipated problem and staff should be informed, briefed and their roles defined. It is

---

Dewhurst's Textbook of Obstetrics & Gynaecology, Eighth Edition. Edited by D. Keith Edmonds.
© 2012 John Wiley and Sons, Ltd. Published 2012 by John Wiley and Sons, Ltd.

not uncommon that when such problems are prepared for, everything goes smoothly: this does not mean that staff are over-cautious; it means they did their job well. Sadly, things do not always go smoothly, or an unexpected emergency occurs, and in such situations there are some features of general care which are important:

Communication and team working

In any emergency multiple workers will become involved, which can produce problems in itself:

- some staff may not know each other;
- no-one knows what anyone else is doing;
- activity can become disordered and inefficient;
- basic important treatment can be forgotten.

Although the most senior obstetrician present is likely to become the team leader, this is not always either necessary or appropriate and an anaesthetist or senior midwife may take the lead in some emergencies. Senior personnel need to talk to each other and interchange roles as dictated by the needs of the clinical scenario. In all situations the team leader should keep a cool head and deal with problems logically and efficiently as this will help keep others calm and promote a cohesive team.

 Summary box 25.2

Aids to good communication:

- Someone needs to take the lead role and coordinate activity in a systematic way such that staff work together as a team.
- The skills of any unknown staff need to be clarified.
- Roles need to be allocated which match the skills of the staff concerned.
- Specific jobs need to be given to specific people to avoid duplications and omissions.
- When someone is asked to do something, it is worth checking that they understand and are happy with what is being asked of them.
- Someone needs to document timings and actions.
- Someone needs to talk to the patient (and her partner) even if only briefly to keep them calm and informed and help them feel confident and supported.

Documentation

This has been mentioned briefly above, but in all emergencies it helps to have someone looking at the clock, holding pen and paper, who is responsible for documenting the important facts as they happen. Remember that if, as is often the case, this person is fairly junior, he or she may not understand exactly what is going on and may fail to document key activity, and therefore it is imperative that senior members of the team ensure that all essential information is communicated. Once the emergency is over, notes should be written carefully and comprehensively and signed legibly. This is the best time to account

for what has happened and any relevant diagnosis, follow-up care plan and prognosis for future pregnancies should be spelt out clearly whenever possible at this stage.

Risk management

After the emergency is over, reviewing the event with staff is hugely appreciated and very important: this is usually multidisciplinary but will sometimes be in small groups. Healthcare assistants and porters may need this support too and should not be forgotten. If everything went well, everyone should be congratulated; if some things were less than perfect, discussing why the difficulties were encountered and what might make things easier/work better another time is often helpful. This is a time for positive critical reflection; any negative feedback can wait and be dealt with privately.

Emergency training

With the reduced duration of junior doctors' training, combined with the dramatic cuts in their working hours, it is unsurprising that their clinical experience of obstetric emergencies is much less than that of their predecessors. They rely increasingly on formal training, which can be gained locally to an extent but tends to be supplemented by regional or national courses, a few of which are listed below.

- ALSO (Advanced Life Support in Obstetrics). This course is geared to midwives, obstetric senior house officers and junior specialist registrars and deals with the main obstetric emergencies in a structured systematic fashion. Candidates should gain a sound understanding of the problems and the structured approaches in how to manage them (www.also.org.uk).
- MOET (Managing Obstetric Emergencies and Trauma). This course is geared to a more senior and multidisciplinary group: obstetric consultant and senior specialist registrars (post MRCOG and at least specialty training year 5), anaesthetic consultant and senior specialist registrars, and senior accident and emergency doctors. These courses also include midwives (as 'observers' because they are not formally assessed) who receive the same training during the course and their presence emphasizes and promotes the team approach that is so important in the obstetric emergency. This course deals with more advanced and complex aspects of emergency obstetrics (www.moet.org.uk).
- MOSES (Multidisciplinary Obstetric Simulated Emergency Scenarios). This course focuses on emergency behaviour and team-working dynamics as they apply to the obstetric patient, rather than training on knowledge or techniques. It involves midwives, anaesthetists and obstetricians who often attend together from the same department. This course is very different from, and complements, MOET or ALSO (blsimcentre@bartsandthelondon.nhs.uk).

These acute obstetric emergency training courses are now well established, but they are no substitute for local multidisciplinary training. Indeed the latter has been shown to be as effective in improving knowledge [5,6] and has also been shown to improve clinical outcomes [7,8]. The recipe for successful local training appears to be a local commitment with incentives to train, multi-professional training of all staff, teamwork training combined with clinical teaching, and use of high fidelity models [9]. These optimistic reports, together with the fact that multidisciplinary emergency drills and scenarios are a requirement for CNST (Clinical Negligence Scheme for Trusts) ratings, mean that this form of training is becoming established within UK maternity departments. The other advantage of local training is that it can also be an invaluable aid to identifying problems within the system [10].

Collapse

Collapse as it presents to the obstetrician can be due to a variety of causes, from the sometimes innocent vasovagal faint through to cardiac arrest, but the initial assessment and management of the patient is remarkably similar and requires a systematic disciplined ABC approach combined with lateral tilting of the pregnant patient to minimize aortocaval compression. The essential steps of how to approach the apparently lifeless patient are summarized in Fig. 25.1, and aim to make the crucial diagnosis of cardiac arrest (as opposed to reduced consciousness due to another cause) so that cardiopulmonary resuscitation (CPR) can be commenced early. Most other conditions require basic resuscitation with attention to airway and breathing combined with intravenous access and circulatory support while the cause of the problem is diagnosed and then treated (Table 25.1).

Cardiac arrest (Fig. 25.1)

CPR is not only difficult to administer but is particularly inefficient in the pregnant patient due to:
- difficulties in performing CPR on a tilted patient;
- increased oxygen requirement in pregnancy (20% increase in resting oxygen consumption);
- decreased chest compliance due to splinting of the diaphragm (20% decrease in functional residual capacity);
- reduced venous return due to caval compression limiting cardiac output from chest compressions (stroke volume 30% at term compared with non-pregnant state);
- risk of gastric regurgitation and aspiration (relaxation of cardiac sphincter).

For these reasons it is considered appropriate to empty the uterus to aid maternal survival by performing a peri-mortem Caesarean section if CPR performed with lateral tilt is ineffective after 5 min [3,11]. To achieve this the obstetrician at such an arrest should be preparing for Caesarean section almost immediately. It is reiterated that the point of emptying the uterus is to aid in the resuscitation of the

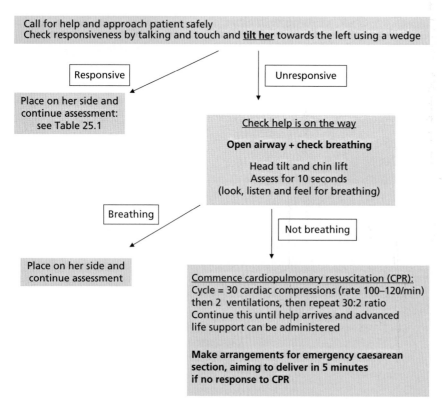

Fig. 25.1 Basic life support: approaching and treating the apparently lifeless patient.

Table 25.1 Causes, features and initial treatment of collapse in the obstetric patient (distinguishing features in bold).

	Cause/risk factors	Specific clinical Features	Specific treatment points: all need ABC + lateral tilt if undelivered
Adrenal insufficiency	Inadequate or absent steroid cover in someone previously taking steroids	Drug history can be sought Hypotensive collapse Metabolic imbalance	Supportive with intravenous fluids (check electrolytes especially sodium may be low) Hydrocortisone (200 mg i.v. stat) Check BM: may need glucose
Amniotic fluid embolism	Uterine tachysystole Syntocinon hyperstimulation Previous uterine surgery Multiparity Polyhydramnios	Restless, shortness of breath and cyanosis **Vaginal bleeding follows within 30 min due to disseminated intravascular coagulation [11]**	Oxygen + ventilate Deliver the baby as soon as possible Hydrocortisone (200 mg i.v. stat) (Aminophylline, diuretics, adrenaline, morphine)*
Anaphylaxis	Drug administration, e.g. antibiotics, Voltarol, anaesthetic agents, Haemaccel, latex	History of drugs/latex Rash Stridor Oedema	Adrenaline (1 mL of 1 in 1000 i.m. or 1 mL of 1 in 10 000 i.v. repeated as needed) with intravenous fluids Hydrocortisone (200 mg i.v. stat) Chlorpheniramine (20 mg i.v.)
Aspiration (Mendelson's syndrome)	Inhalation after vomiting/passive regurgitation (reduced consciousness with unprotected airway)	Shortness of breath, restlessness, cyanosis **Bronchospasm**	Oxygen + ventilate (Aminophylline, steroids, diuretics, and antibiotics)*
Bacteraemic shock	Overwhelming sepsis due to especially Gram-negative rods or streptococci	Hypotensive **Warm/fever/blotchy**	Replenish circulation, systems support Antibiotics intravenously (e.g. imipenem)
Cardiogenic shock	Congenital or acquired disease Cardiomyopathy	History Restless, **shortness of breath, chest pain**	**Sit up** Oxygen + frusemide
Eclampsia	Associated with cerebrovascular events or pulmonary oedema or magnesium toxicity	Hypertensive Proteinuria	Magnesium sulphate (antidote is calcium gluconate) Control blood pressure with hypotensives
Hyperglycaemia	Diabetes	Hyperventilation and **ketosis**	Intravenous fluids, insulin (and potassium)
Hypoglycaemia	Diabetes, Addison's disease, hypopituitary, hypothyroid	**Sweating/clammy** Loss of consciousness	Intravenous glucose
Intracerebral bleed	Arteriovenous malformation	Fits, CNS signs and **neck stiffness**	Supportive
Massive pulmonary embolism	Usually deep pelvic thrombosis	Restless, cyanosis, **elevated jugular venous pressure**	**Lie down** + oxygen Intravenous fluids + anticoagulation
Neurogenic	Vasovagal (uterine inversion)	**Vaginal examination**	Intravenous fluids ± atropine Reduce uterine inversion
Oligaemic	Haemorrhage (can be concealed)	**Tachycardia, pale and cold**	Restore circulation and treat
Pneumothorax Pneumomediastinum	Previous history of labour/pushing	Chest pain, shortness of breath	Aspirate/drain

*These treatments should be undertaken under anaesthetic supervision in a high-dependency or intensive care unit.

mother and is not for fetal reasons. Fetal viability issues should not delay this procedure, which is worthwhile when the pregnancy is of sufficient size to compromise resuscitation; as a guide, if the uterus has reached the level of the umbilicus it should be considered.

To perform a peri-mortem Caesarean section rapidly, the skin incision should be that with which the operator is most familiar, and the uterine incision will be influenced by the gestation of pregnancy. These details matter little compared with the pressing need to evacuate the uterus and render the mother more receptive to life-saving resuscitation techniques. A large Caesarean section pack is unnecessary and *in extremis* all the obstetrician needs is a scalpel to commence the procedure whilst other instruments are being collected.

It is stressed again that this is not done for fetal reasons but there is no doubt that fetal viability is more likely the more quickly the baby is delivered: 70% survive intact if delivered within 5 min, falling to 13% after 10 min [12].

To detail the management of each possible condition that can cause maternal collapse is beyond the scope of this chapter, but Table 25.1 summarizes the different possibilities and those features specific to them in terms of risk factors, clinically distinguishing features, and specific points of treatment. More detailed accounts can be found with references in the MOET manual [3] but a few summary points are highlighted below.

Airway problems

The airway of an obstetric patient is more vulnerable than in the non-pregnant state. Not only is there more likely to be swelling and oedema, but the progestogenic effects that reduce gastric emptying and relax the cardiac sphincter increase the chance of regurgitation and subsequent aspiration of gastric contents. For these reasons the management of any obstetric patient with reduced consciousness requires careful attention to maintaining and protecting the airway, and this should involve an anaesthetist. In simple circumstances, the patient should at the very least be nursed on her side, and a jaw thrust and chin lift can aid in bringing the tongue forward to open the airway. Severe laryngeal oedema due to pre-eclampsia or anaphylaxis are examples of situations that can critically compromise the airway in the obstetric patient, and in these circumstances an anaesthetist is needed extremely urgently to establish and maintain the airway (usually by a cuffed endotracheal tube).

Breathing problems

If the airway is patent but breathing is laboured or consciousness impaired, then supplementary oxygen is vital. This should be given by face-mask with a reservoir bag, and the oxygen should be turned up to maximum at the wall in the emergency situation. Restlessness and confu-sion are signs of hypoxaemia, can precede collapse and should be taken extremely seriously. Oxygen saturation should be measured in air by a pulse oximeter, and arterial blood taken for gas analysis if there is any concern, and results of these should be reviewed with the anaesthetist on duty.

Circulatory problems

Circulatory problems can be due to cardiac disease (where the resulting pathology is usually pulmonary oedema and low-output failure), inadequate venous return with resultant low-output failure (massive pulmonary embolus) or an underfilled circulation (hypovolaemia, due to haemorrhage or sepsis). Early intravenous access with large-bore cannulae is vital, but treatment needs to be specific to the cause. Cardiac failure patients do not require (and indeed may be killed by) volume expansion, but are helped by being sat up and given diuretics. On the other hand, a woman with a pulmonary embolus or who is hypovolaemic needs volume expansion and to be lain down flat. Distinguishing between these conditions is vital as the management of each would clearly be dangerous to the other. Hypovolaemia, which can be due to loss from the intravascular compartment (e.g. haemorrhage) or due to relative underfilling caused by vasodilatation (e.g. sepsis), is managed by volume expansion. Fluid replacement strategies with crystalloid or colloid remain controversial but the use of crystalloids in critically ill patients is supported by a Cochrane review [13] and Hartmann's solution is preferable to dextrose [14].

Haemorrhage

Obstetric haemorrhage is one of the most common causes of major maternal morbidity and mortality [1,15] and recent triennial reports raised the unhappy truth that these deaths were increasing (7 in 1997–1999, 17 in 2000–2002 and 17 in 2003–2005); fortunately, this trend has reversed in the recent report, where there were 9 deaths [1]. Over the years the confidential enquiries into maternal deaths in the UK have highlighted a variety of substandard care issues and once again emphasis is placed on the importance of clear local procedures and policies to trigger rapid and appropriate responses which should be rehearsed regularly. Furthermore, there should be senior input in high-risk cases and women at high risk of bleeding should be delivered in centres equipped for blood transfusion [1]. Particular mention is made of women with a previous Caesarean section and a low-lying placenta, as their risk of a morbidly adherent placenta is increased. In such cases antenatal and intrapartum multidisciplinary consultant input is advocated with clear plans for surgery and with conservative options for treatment considered in advance [16].

Summary box 25.3

Care bundle components for women with suspected placenta accreta:

- Consultant obstetrician involved in antenatal plan and present at delivery.
- Consultant anaesthetist involved in antenatal plan and present at delivery.
- Blood and blood products available on site.
- Multidisciplinary involvement in preoperative planning.
- Consent to include possible interventions.
- Level 2 critical care bed available.

Clinical care should concentrate on identifying risk factors for haemorrhage to enable preparations and avoiding action to be taken. However, once massive haemorrhage occurs management should follow a logical sequence of diagnostic and therapeutic options as illustrated in Figs 25.2 and 25.3.

Summary box 25.4

Hints to minimize morbidity from haemorrhage:

- Antepartum haemorrhage: if it is due to severe abruption with an accompanying bradycardia, the urgency of delivery is clear and an interval from decision to delivery of 20 min or less is associated with reduced neonatal adverse outcome [17].
- The descriptions 'heavy lochia' or 'she's trickling' are dangerous and should not be accepted: the woman should be reviewed and the problem resolved before it develops into a bigger problem.
- Continued vaginal bleeding with a contracted uterus is either due to retained placenta/membrane/clot or due to trauma and needs to be managed actively and not ignored. The problem will only get worse, so the woman should undergo examination under anaesthesia while she is well.
- Hypotension is a very late sign: blood pressure is maintained until very late in the obstetric patient who is bleeding, and tachycardia, peripheral perfusion, skin colour and urine output should be heeded early.
- If the lower segment of the uterus or the cervix fills up with blood or clot, it can cause vagal stimulation producing a bradycardia that can mislead. Vaginal examination should be done if in doubt.
- Bleeding can be concealed:
  - A uterus filling up is suggested by a rising fundus.
  - Intra-abdominal bleeding: massive volumes of blood can be accommodated within the peritoneal cavity without affecting girth measurements, which are unhelpful and can be falsely reassuring.
  - The uterus that is not central but shifted to one side should raise alarm bells. It suggests a broad ligament haematoma.
- Petechiae suggest disseminated intravascular coagulation [18].

Life-saving measures and advanced techniques for massive postpartum haemorrhage

Aortic compression

If bleeding is out of control and the anaesthetist needs to stabilize the patient, it is worth trying aortic compression while waiting for senior or specialist help to arrive. In the woman who has been delivered vaginally tilt the uterus forward and press a closed fist down onto the abdomen just below the umbilicus. If the abdomen is already open, sweep the small bowel mesentery up towards the liver and with a swab on a stick or with finger and thumb squeeze the aorta. The effect is dramatic and can be life-saving.

Uterine packing

This is useful for placental bed bleeding but can also be used with uterine atony when there is an element of uterine tone present. The technique is not new, but rather than using a gauze pack an inflatable balloon has the advantage of being quick and expandable. Various balloon catheters have been reported for this technique including the Sengstaken–Blakemore and specifically designed ones, but the urological Rusch balloon catheter is cheaper and effective [19]. Some have used a condom attached to the end of a urinary catheter, but the balloon of a normal urinary catheter itself is not suitable as its capacity is far too small. The volume needed is very dependent on the individual and the key is to insert the balloon catheter and gently fill it up whilst keeping the uterus as contracted as possible. As a rough guide approximately 200–400 mL or so is usually required, and as the balloon is blown up resistance is met and bleeding is seen to reduce. Once bleeding is controlled the balloon is usually left in for approximately 24 hours and then, again an advantage over the traditional uterine pack, it can be deflated in stages. Whatever is used to pack the uterus, antibiotic cover should be given for the procedure and until the pack/balloon is removed; similarly the bladder should be catheterized until the pack is removed.

Brace suture

The B-Lynch brace suture, first described in 1997 [20], can avoid hysterectomy in cases of bleeding from uterine atony. It aims to exert longitudinal lateral compression to the uterus combined with a tamponade effect and is performed by means of one long suture placed as illustrated in Fig. 25.4. The key to this technique is to check the hypothesis that it works by exteriorizing the uterus and compressing it (bleeding should be controlled) before continuing. Since its first description there have been many reports of its successful use but there have been modifications suggested that have confused the understanding of the principles behind it, and some of these have been

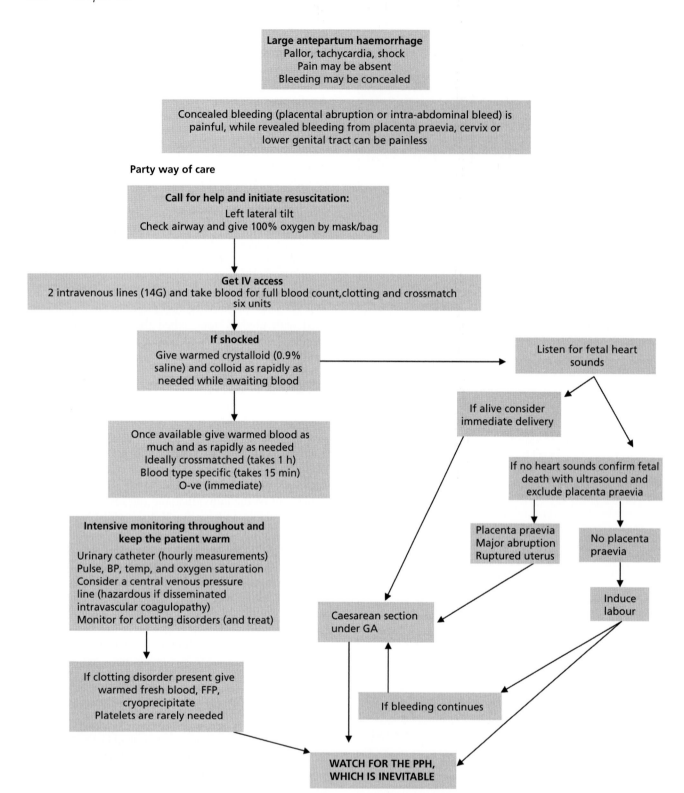

Fig. 25.2 Large antepartum haemorrhage. BP, blood pressure; CVP, central venous pressure; DIC, disseminated intravascular coagulation; FBC, full blood count; FFP, fresh frozen plasma; GA, general anaesthesia; PPH, postpartum haemorrhage.

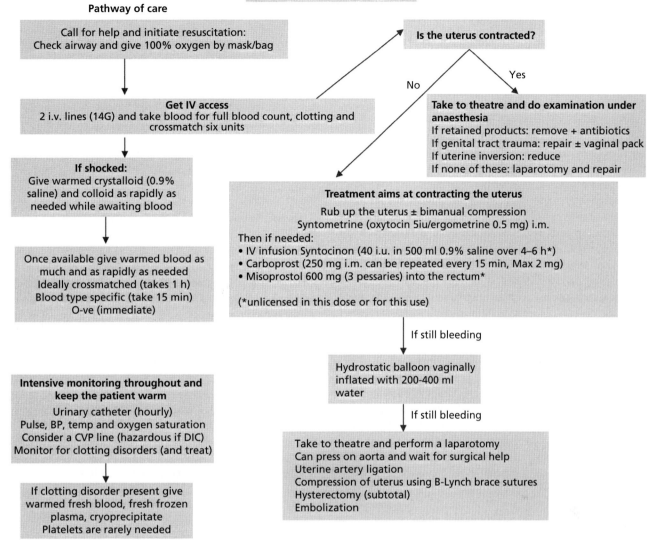

Large postpartun haemorrhage
Pallor, tachycardia, shock
bleeding can be concealed
bradycardia can be present

Pathway of care

Is the uterus contracted?

Call for help and initiate resuscitation:
Check airway and give 100% oxygen by mask/bag

No   Yes

Get IV access
2 i.v. lines (14G) and take blood for full blood count, clotting and crossmatch six units

Take to theatre and do examination under anaesthesia
If retained products: remove + antibiotics
If genital tract trauma: repair ± vaginal pack
If uterine inversion: reduce
If none of these: laparotomy and repair

If shocked:
Give warmed crystalloid (0.9% saline) and colloid as rapidly as needed while awaiting blood

Treatment aims at contracting the uterus
Rub up the uterus ± bimanual compression
Syntometrine (oxytocin 5iu/ergometrine 0.5 mg) i.m.
Then if needed:
• IV infusion Syntocinon (40 i.u. in 500 ml 0.9% saline over 4–6 h*)
• Carboprost (250 mg i.m. can be repeated every 15 min, Max 2 mg)
• Misoprostol 600 mg (3 pessaries) into the rectum*

(*unlicensed in this dose or for this use)

Once available give warmed blood as much and as rapidly as needed
Ideally crossmatched (takes 1 h)
Blood type specific (take 15 min)
O-ve (immediate)

If still bleeding

Hydrostatic balloon vaginally inflated with 200-400 ml water

If still bleeding

Intensive monitoring throughout and keep the patient warm
Urinary catheter (hourly)
Pulse, BP, temp and oxygen saturation
Consider a CVP line (hazardous if DIC)
Monitor for clotting disorders (and treat)

Take to theatre and perform a laparotomy
Can press on aorta and wait for surgical help
Uterine artery ligation
Compression of uterus using B-Lynch brace sutures
Hysterectomy (subtotal)
Embolization

If clotting disorder present give warmed fresh blood, fresh frozen plasma, cryoprecipitate
Platelets are rarely needed

Fig. 25.3 Large postpartum haemorrhage. BP, blood pressure; CVP, central venous pressure; DIC, disseminated intravascular coagulation; FBC, full blood count; FFP, fresh frozen plasma.

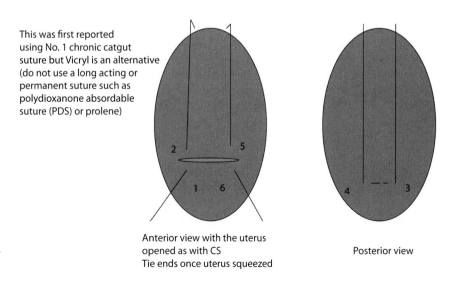

This was first reported using No. 1 chronic catgut suture but Vicryl is an alternative (do not use a long acting or permanent suture such as polydioxanone absordable suture (PDS) or prolene)

Fig. 25.4 B-Lynch 'brace' suture for treatment of bleeding due to uterine atony, but some uterine tone is needed.

Anterior view with the uterus opened as with CS
Tie ends once uterus squeezed

Posterior view

associated with problems [21–24]. Longer-term complications have also been reported [25,26] and it is worth reiterating that the suture should be of a rapidly absorbable material to avoid the prolonged presence of free loops of suture material after the uterus involutes [25].

Interventional radiology

Arterial embolization is increasingly reported in the management of postpartum haemorrhage [27,28]. It is especially effective in achieving haemostasis in cases of genital tract trauma where surgical control has failed or the injury is inaccessible. However, it can also help in more non-specific haemorrhage such as uterine atony, when the internal iliac and uterine arteries can be cannulated and their tributaries can be embolized. Developing links with, and knowing contact details of, an interventional radiology department in advance of the emergency scenario makes the urgent referral all the easier. There is a report suggesting that morbidity is better if embolization is carried out before rather than after hysterectomy [29], but this will clearly depend on local facilities and arrangements and the stability of the patient. Embolization is extremely difficult if the internal iliac arteries have been tied off and therefore this technique, which so threatens trauma to the internal iliac vein (a vascular surgeon's nightmare), should rarely be attempted by the obstetrician. Complications from embolization have been reported, including necrosis of uterus and bladder [30], but long-term follow-up has demonstrated fertility can be maintained but pregnancy outcomes are complicated by a 32% risk of recurrent severe postpartum haemorrhage [31].

Cell salvage

This technique of contemporary perioperative autologous blood salvage and retransfusion for use in obstetrics has been supported by NICE [32], the Obstetric Anaesthetists Association [33] and the Royal College of Obstetricians and Gynaecologists (RCOG) [34]. A recent review confirms is value and safety [35] and it is acceptable to Jehovah's witnesses [36,37].

Recombinant activated factor VII

There have now been a few case reports of the value of giving this in the presence of severe clotting disorders in obstetric haemorrhage [38] but these treatments are still largely research based. It is expensive and only works if the patient has been given other clotting factors on which this can work. Practically speaking, this tends to be on a named patient basis after discussion at consultant level between haematologist and obstetrician, whilst further evidence is collected, but initial reports are very encouraging and the subject has been well reviewed [39] and is mentioned in the RCOG guidelines on postpartum haemorrhage [34].

Obstetric causes of collapse

Eclampsia

Eclampsia can present with collapse due to the fitting and post-ictal phase of the disease, an intracerebral catastrophe, magnesium toxicity or pulmonary oedema. The principles of treatment are as for any collapse and, in addition, blood pressure control, magnesium sulphate and strict fluid balance to avoid fluid overload provide the basis of good care. If the patient is antenatal then the mother must be stabilized before delivery (see Chapter 11). A summary flow chart of acute management of this condition is shown in Fig. 25.5.

Uterine inversion and uterine rupture

Uterine inversion and uterine rupture can both contribute to maternal collapse as listed above and their management is illustrated in Figs 25.6 and 25.7. It is worth noting that 18 of the 42 cases of uterine rupture in the CESDI report had a laparotomy before a diagnosis was made [40]. Signs can be subtle and fetal heart abnormalities in the presence of a uterine scar should be taken extremely seriously and rarely, if ever, justify fetal blood sampling. Similarly, a multiparous patient with secondary arrest should arouse suspicion, and Syntocinon augmentation should only be decided after careful clinical assessment of the patient by the obstetrician to exclude obstructed labour.

Emergency obstetric deliveries

Most emergency operative deliveries (Caesarean section, instrumental delivery, breech and twin deliveries and interventions for fetal distress) together with neonatal resuscitation are mentioned in the relevant chapters, but the management of shoulder dystocia and cord prolapse are illustrated in Figs 25.8 and 25.9 and mentioned here.

Shoulder dystocia

Shoulder dystocia is every obstetrician's and midwife's nightmare, and rightly so. A lot of effort is now focused on practical training using sophisticated mannequins [41] and this has resulted in improved clinical outcomes [8]. The flow chart in Fig. 25.8 highlights the processes and sequences of its management, but additional points to note include the following.
- Always remember that the problem is at the pelvic brim and pulling on the baby or pushing down on the fundus are both unhelpful and dangerous.
- Time is deceptive and what feels like a lifetime is only a few minutes (try to glance at a clock or get someone to note timings).

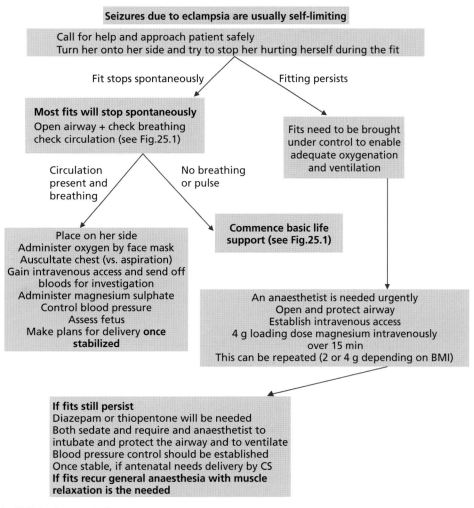

Fig. 25.5 Eclampsia. BMI, body mass index.

• There remains a place for cephalic replacement [42] and occasionally symphysiotomy can be life-saving [43]. Check if the posterior shoulder is still above the pelvic brim or has entered into the pelvis and can be felt in the sacral hollow to help decide which of these manoeuvres would best suit.
• Careful and precise documentation is essential after the event.

Cord prolapse

Figure 25.9 highlights the main features of this emergency. The principles of treatment are as follows.
• Handle the cord as little as possible.
• If an operative vaginal delivery is proposed, it should be simple and achieved quickly; if it is not, it should be abandoned early.
• If there is no fetal bradycardia this need not be a panic delivery under general anaesthesia, and regional block administered with the patient lying on her side may be appropriate.

• If the bladder has been filled up with saline, remember to empty it before surgery (just removing the spigot from the Foley catheter is not sufficient).

Summary

Good antenatal care, anticipating possible problems and preparing for them, and running a well-coordinated delivery suite are the mainstays of coping with obstetric emergencies. Training and drills helps to focus on teamwork and a supportive system to reduce adverse consequences. Keep things simple and focus on the problem to hand. The ABC principle is a good one for dealing with any ill patient, but is particularly useful in the apparently lifeless patient and those who require resuscitation, although it is crucial to remember to apply lateral tilt in anyone still pregnant. In any obstetric emergency keep the basic pathology in mind: why has this happened, where is the problem, and what can be done about it?

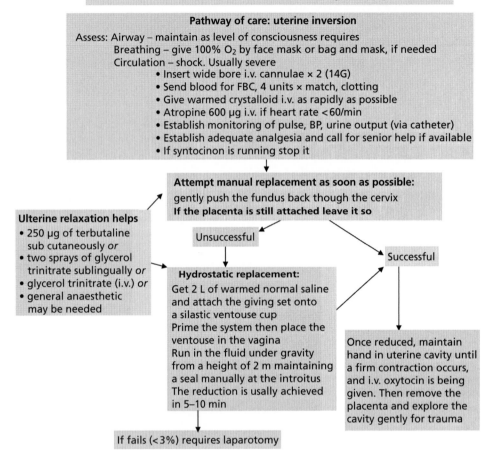

Uterine inversion presents with shock/haemorrhage

The main features of uterine inversion are shock out of proportion to blood loss and a bradycardia due to increased vagal tone. An urgent vaginal examination will reveal a mass in the vagina and the normally obvious post-partum uterus cannot be felt above the symphysis. Incomplete versions present more subtly with continuing PPH despite a contracted uterus: the fundus of the uterus may feel dimpled

Pathway of care: uterine inversion

Assess: Airway – maintain as level of consciousness requires
        Breathing – give 100% O₂ by face mask or bag and mask, if needed
        Circulation – shock. Usually severe
            • Insert wide bore i.v. cannulae × 2 (14G)
            • Send blood for FBC, 4 units × match, clotting
            • Give warmed crystalloid i.v. as rapidly as possible
            • Atropine 600 µg i.v. if heart rate <60/min
            • Establish monitoring of pulse, BP, urine output (via catheter)
            • Establish adequate analgesia and call for senior help if available
            • If syntocinon is running stop it

Attempt manual replacement as soon as possible:
gently push the fundus back though the cervix
If the placenta is still attached leave it so

Ulterine relaxation helps
• 250 µg of terbutaline sub cutaneously *or*
• two sprays of glycerol trinitrate sublingually *or*
• glycerol trinitrate (i.v.) *or*
• general anaesthetic may be needed

Unsuccessful

Successful

Hydrostatic replacement:
Get 2 L of warmed normal saline and attach the giving set onto a silastic ventouse cup
Prime the system then place the ventouse in the vagina
Run in the fluid under gravity from a height of 2 m maintaining a seal manually at the introitus
The reduction is usally achieved in 5–10 min

Once reduced, maintain hand in uterine cavity until a firm contraction occurs, and i.v. oxytocin is being given. Then remove the placenta and explore the cavity gently for trauma

If fails (<3%) requires laparotomy

Fig. 25.6 Uterine inversion. BP, blood pressure; FBC, full blood count; GTN, glyceryl trinitrate.

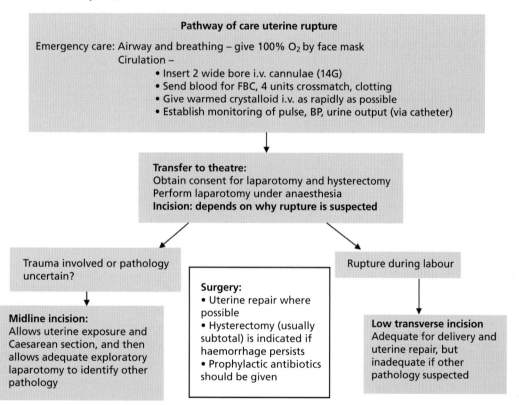

Uterine rupture
Presents with fetal bradycardia
maternal shock
haemorrhage (often concealed)

Anticipate: warning signs of pending rupture include:
- Cardiotocograph abnormalities (fetal blood sample rarely if ever indicated with scarred uterus)
- Failure of cervical effacement or dilatation despite regular uterine activity
- Scar pain or vaginal bleeding

Avoid:
- Actively look for warning signs and act on them
- Do not hyperstimulate a scarred uterus (or any other uterus)

Symptoms and signs which may be present:
- Abdominal pain changes from intermittent to continuous
- Vaginal bleeding and/or shoulder tip pain
- Fetal heart abnormal on cardiotocograph and uterine contraction trace changes
- Abdominal palpation may reveal high presenting part and obvious fetal parts
- Post-partum bleeding with apparently contracted uterus

Differential diagnosis: when presenting antenatally:
- **Spontaneous intra-abdominal bleed from ruptured vessel (usually splenic)**

Pathway of care uterine rupture

Emergency care: Airway and breathing – give 100% O$_2$ by face mask
Cirulation –
- Insert 2 wide bore i.v. cannulae (14G)
- Send blood for FBC, 4 units crossmatch, clotting
- Give warmed crystalloid i.v. as rapidly as possible
- Establish monitoring of pulse, BP, urine output (via catheter)

Transfer to theatre:
Obtain consent for laparotomy and hysterectomy
Perform laparotomy under anaesthesia
Incision: depends on why rupture is suspected

Trauma involved or pathology uncertain?

Rupture during labour

Midline incision:
Allows uterine exposure and Caesarean section, and then allows adequate exploratory laparotomy to identify other pathology

Surgery:
- Uterine repair where possible
- Hysterectomy (usually subtotal) is indicated if haemorrhage persists
- Prophylactic antibiotics should be given

Low transverse incision
Adequate for delivery and uterine repair, but inadequate if other pathology suspected

Fig. 25.7 Uterine rupture. BP, blood pressure; CTG, cardiotocography; FBC, full blood count; FBS, fetal blood sampling;

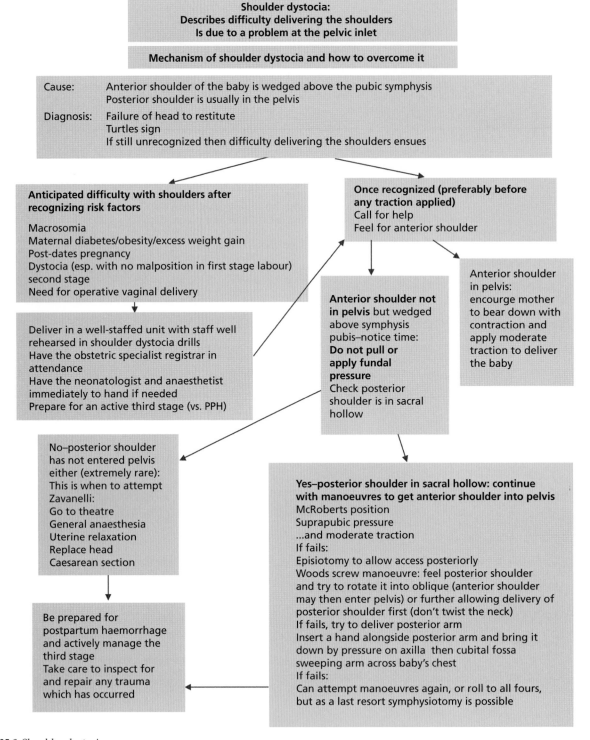

Shoulder dystocia:
Describes difficulty delivering the shoulders
Is due to a problem at the pelvic inlet

Mechanism of shoulder dystocia and how to overcome it

Cause: Anterior shoulder of the baby is wedged above the pubic symphysis
          Posterior shoulder is usually in the pelvis

Diagnosis: Failure of head to restitute
            Turtles sign
            If still unrecognized then difficulty delivering the shoulders ensues

Anticipated difficulty with shoulders after recognizing risk factors

Macrosomia
Maternal diabetes/obesity/excess weight gain
Post-dates pregnancy
Dystocia (esp. with no malposition in first stage labour)
second stage
Need for operative vaginal delivery

Deliver in a well-staffed unit with staff well rehearsed in shoulder dystocia drills
Have the obstetric specialist registrar in attendance
Have the neonatologist and anaesthetist immediately to hand if needed
Prepare for an active third stage (vs. PPH)

Once recognized (preferably before any traction applied)
Call for help
Feel for anterior shoulder

Anterior shoulder not in pelvis but wedged above symphysis pubis–notice time:
Do not pull or apply fundal pressure
Check posterior shoulder is in sacral hollow

Anterior shoulder in pelvis: encourge mother to bear down with contraction and apply moderate traction to deliver the baby

No–posterior shoulder has not entered pelvis either (extremely rare):
This is when to attempt Zavanelli:
Go to theatre
General anaesthesia
Uterine relaxation
Replace head
Caesarean section

Yes–posterior shoulder in sacral hollow: continue with manoeuvres to get anterior shoulder into pelvis
McRoberts position
Suprapubic pressure
...and moderate traction
If fails:
Episiotomy to allow access posteriorly
Woods screw manoeuvre: feel posterior shoulder and try to rotate it into oblique (anterior shoulder may then enter pelvis) or further allowing delivery of posterior shoulder first (don't twist the neck)
If fails, try to deliver posterior arm
Insert a hand alongside posterior arm and bring it down by pressure on axilla then cubital fossa sweeping arm across baby's chest
If fails:
Can attempt manoeuvres again, or roll to all fours, but as a last resort symphysiotomy is possible

Be prepared for postpartum haemorrhage and actively manage the third stage
Take care to inspect for and repair any trauma which has occurred

Fig. 25.8 Shoulder dystocia.

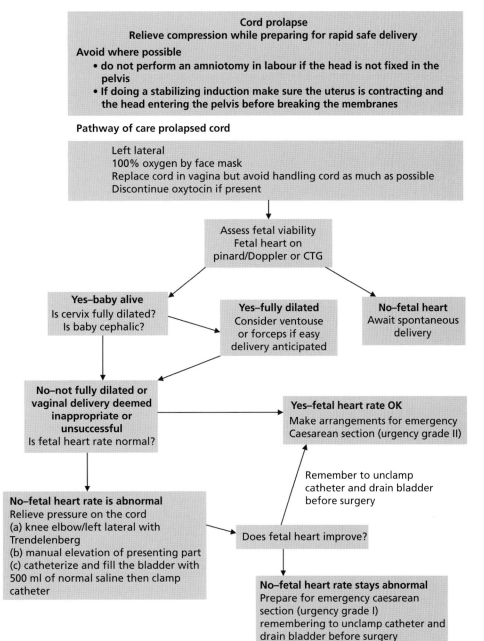

Fig. 25.9 Cord prolapse. CTG, cardiotocography.

References

1 Centre for Maternal and Child Enquiries. Saving Mothers' Lives: Reviewing Maternal Deaths to Make Motherhood Safer 2006–2008. The Eigth Report on Confidential Enquiries into Maternal Deaths in the United Kingdom. *Br J Obstet Gynecol* 2011;118:Suppl. 1. Available at: www.cmace.org./

2 National Institute for Health and Clinical Excellence. *Antenatal Care. Routine Care for the Healthy Pregnant Woman.* Clinical Guidelines CG62, 2008. Available at http://guidance.nice.org.uk/CG62

3 Grady K, Howell C, Cox C. *Managing Obstetric Emergencies and Trauma: The MOET Course Manual.* London: RCOG Press, 2007.

4 Sen R, Paterson-Brown S. Prioritisation on the labour ward. *Curr Obstet Gynaecol* 2005;15:228–236.

5 Crofts JF, Ellis D, Draycott TJ, Winter C, Hunt LP, Akande VA. Change in knowledge of midwives and obstetricians following obstetric emergency training: a randomised controlled trial of local hospital, simulation centre and teamwork training. *BJOG* 2007;114:1534–1541.

6 Ellis D, Croft JF, Hunt LP, Read M, Fox R, James M. Hospital, simulation centre, and teamwork training for eclampsia management. *Obstet Gynecol* 2008;111:723–731.

7 Draycott T, Sibanda T, Owen L *et al.* Does training in obstetric emergencies improve neonatal outcome? *BJOG* 2006;113:177–182.

8 Draycott TJ, Crofts JF, Ash PA et al. Improving neonatal outcome through practical shoulder dystocia training. *Obstet Gynecol* 2008;112:14–20.

9 Siassakos D, Crofts JF, Winter C, Weiner CP, Draycott TJ. The active components of effective training in obstetric emergencies. *BJOG* 2009;116:1028–1032.

10 Thompson S, Neal S, Clark V. Clinical risk management in obstetrics: eclampsia drills. *BMJ* 2004;328:269–271.

11 Morris S, Stacey M. Resuscitation in pregnancy. *BMJ* 2003;327:1277–1279.

12 Katz VL, Dotters DJ, Droegemueller W. Perimortem cesarean delivery. *Obstet Gynecol* 1986;68:571–576.

13 Perel P, Roberts I, Pearson M. Colloids versus crystalloids for fluid resuscitation in critically ill patients. *Cochrane Database Syst Rev* 2007;(4):CD000567.

14 Resuscitation Council (UK). Guidelines 2010. Available at www.resus.org.uk/pages/guide.htm

15 Brace V, Penney G, Hall M. Quantifying severe maternal morbidity: a Scottish population study. *BJOG* 2004;111:481–484.

16 Paterson-Brown S, Singh C. Developing a care bundle for the management of suspected placenta accreta. *Obstetrician and Gynaecologist* 2010;12:21–27.

17 Kayani SI, Walkinshaw SA, Preston C. Pregnancy outcome in severe placental abruption. *BJOG* 2003;110:679–683.

18 Baglin T. Disseminated intravascular coagulation: diagnosis and treatment. *BMJ* 1996;312:683–687.

19 Johanson R, Kumar M, Obhrai M, Young P. Management of massive postpartum haemorrhage: use of a hydrostatic balloon catheter to avoid laparotomy. *BJOG* 2001;108:420–422.

20 B-Lynch C, Coker A, Lawal AH, Abu J, Cowen MJ. The B-Lynch surgical technique for the control of massive postpartum haemorrhage: an alternative to hysterectomy? Five cases reported. *British Journal of Obstetrics and Gynaecology* 1997;104:372–375.

21 B-Lynch C. Partial ischemic necrosis of the uterus following a uterine brace compression suture. *BJOG* 2005;112:126–127.

22 El Hamamy E. Partial ischemic necrosis of the uterus following a uterine brace compression suture. *BJOG* 2005;112:126.

23 Joshi VM, Shrivastava M. Partial ischemic necrosis of the uterus following a uterine brace compression suture. *BJOG* 2004;111:279–280.

24 Treloar EJ, Anderson RS, Andrews HS, Bailey JL. Uterine necrosis following B-Lynch suture for primiary postpartum haemorrhage. *BJOG* 2006;113:486–488.

25 Cotzias C, Girling J. Uterine compression suture without hysterotomy: why a non-absorbable suture should be avoided. *J Obstet Gynaecol* 2005;25:150–152.

26 Kumara YS, Marasinghe JP, Condous G, Marasinghe U. Pregnancy complicated by a uterine fundal defect resulting from a previous B-Lynch suture. *BJOG* 2009;116:1815–1817.

27 Hansch E, Chitkara U, McAlpine J, El-Sayed Y, Dake MD, Razavi MK. Pelvic arterial embolisation for control of obstetric haemorrhage: a five-year experience. *Am J Obstet Gynecol* 1999;180:1454–1460.

28 Doumouchtsis SK, Papageorghiou AT, Arulkumaran S. Systematic review of conservative management of postpartum hemorrhage: what to do when medical treatment fails. *Obstet Gynecol Surv* 2007;62:540–547.

29 Bloom AI, Verstandig A, Gielchinsky Y, Nadiari M, Elchalal U. Arterial embolisation for persistent primary postpartum haemorrhage: before or after hysterectomy? *BJOG* 2004;111:880–884.

30 Porcu G, Roger V, Jacquier A et al. Uterus and bladder necrosis after uterine artery embolisation for postpartum haemorrhage. *BJOG* 2005;112:122–123.

31 Sentilhes L, Gromez A, Clavier E, Resch B, Verspyck E, Marpeau L. Fertility and pregnancy following pervic arterial embolisation for postpartum haemorrhage. *BJOG* 2009;117:84–93.

32 National Institute for Health and Clinical Excellence. *Intra-operative blood cell salvage in obstetrics*. Intervention Procedure Guidance No. 144, 2005. Available at http://guidance.nice.org.uk/IPG144

33 Obstetric Anaesthetists Association and the Association of Anaesthetists of Great Britain and Ireland. *Guidelines for Obstetric Anaesthetic Services*, revised edition, 2005. Available at www.aagbi.org/publications/guidelines/docs/obstetric05.pdf

34 Royal College of Obstetricians and Gynaecologists. *Prevention and Management of Postpartum Haemorrhage*. Green-top Guideline No. 52, 2009. Available at www.rcog.org.uk/files/rcog-corp/GT52PostpartumHaemorrhage0411.pdf

35 Allam J, Cox M, Yentis SM. Cell salvage in obstetrics. *Int J Obstet Anesth* 2008;17:37–45.

36 de Souza A, Permezel M, Anderson M, Ross A, McMillan J, Walker S. Antenatal erythropoietin and intra-operative cell salvage in a Jehovah's Witness with placenta praevia. *BJOG* 2003;110:524–526.

37 Currie J, Hogg M, Patel N, Modgwick K, Yoong W. Management of women who decline blood and blood products in pregnancy. *Obstetrician and Gynaecologist* 2010;12:13–20.

38 Boehlen F, Morales MA, Fontana P, Ricou B, Irion O, de Moerloose P. Prolonged treatment of massive postpartum haemorrhage with recombinant factor VIIa: case report and review of the literature. *BJOG* 2004;111:284–287.

39 Franchini M, Lippi G, Franchi M. The use of recombinant activated factor VII in obstetric and gynaecological haemorrhage. *BJOG* 2007;114:8–15.

40 Confidential Enquiry into Stillbirths and Deaths in Infancy. *5th Annual Report. Focus Group on Ruptured Uterus*. London: Maternal and Child Health Consortium, 1998.

41 Crofts JF, Attilakos G, Read M, Sibanda T, Draycott TJ. Shoulder dystocia training using a new birth training mannequin. *BJOG* 2005;112:997–999.

42 Vaithilingham N, Davies D. Cephalic replacement for shoulder dystocia: three cases. *BJOG* 2005;112:674–675.

43 Wykes CB, Johnston TA, Paterson-Brown S, Johanson RB. Symphysiotomy: a lifesaving procedure. *BJOG* 2003;110:219–221.

Chapter 26
Malpresentation, Malposition, Cephalopelvic Disproportion and Obstetric Procedures

Sabaratnam Arulkumaran
St George's Hospital Medical School, London, UK

Malpresentation and malposition

Definitions

At term 95% of fetuses present to the lower segment of the uterus with the vertex and hence *vertex* is the normal presentation. The vertex is the diamond-shaped area of the skull between the two biparietal eminences laterally and the anterior and the posterior fontanelle. When the presentation is other than vertex, i.e. breech, brow, face or shoulder, it is termed *malpresentation*. Malpresentations may be due to fetal or maternal reasons but in the vast majority the definitive aetiology is not known. Known associations include a large baby, polyhydramnios, multiple pregnancy, low-lying placenta, preterm labour, and anomalies of the fetus (neck tumours), uterus (congenital or acquired, e.g. lower segment fibroids) or pelvis (contracted or deformed).

Position is defined by the relationship of the denominator of the presenting part to fixed points of the maternal pelvis. The fixed points of the maternal pelvis are the sacrum posteriorly, sacro-iliac joint posterolaterally, ileopectineal eminences anterolaterally and symphysis pubis anteriorly. The denominator is the most definable peripheral point in the presenting part, i.e. occiput in vertex, mentum in face and sacrum in breech presentation. In about 90% of women in the late first stage of labour at term, the vertex presents in the occipito-anterior (OA) position, i.e. occiput in the anterior half of the pelvis (right, left or direct OA), and hence this is called the normal position. In these cases the head is well flexed and is synclitic (i.e. both parietal eminences are at the same level in the pelvis) allowing the smallest anteroposterior (suboccipito-bregmatic) and lateral (biparietal) diameters (both 9.5 cm) to pass through the pelvis. If the occiput presents in the lateral position or in the posterior half of the pelvis, this is considered a malposition. Malpositions

are characterized by minor degrees of deflexion of the head and thus present a larger anteroposterior diameter (occipito-frontal) of 11.5 cm (Fig. 26.1). They are also associated with anterior or posterior asynclitism: anterior asynclitism is when the parietal eminence is more palpable in the anterior half of the pelvis and lower than the posterior parietal eminence; posterior asynclitism presents with the opposite features. Asynclitism is diagnosed on vaginal examination when the sagittal suture is felt more posteriorly or anteriorly (Fig. 26.2). The larger diameter associated with malposition is the cause of longer and difficult labours and more operative deliveries.

With effective uterine activity malposition corrects to normal position with flexion of the head at the atlanto-occipital joint and rotation forwards of the occiput. This is due to the thrust of the spinal column of the fetus on one side of the oval-shaped head, which lies on the medially downwards sloping pelvic floor musculature of the levator ani. This natural mechanism promotes spontaneous vaginal deliveries.

Malpresentation (breech, face, brow, shoulder) in labour

Breech presentation

At term the fetus presents with the head because of its relative heaviness and because the smaller diameter of the head matches the lower segment – this is not the case with the breech presentation. The incidence of breech presentation varies according to gestation: 40% at 20 weeks but 6–8% at 34 weeks and about 3% by term [1]. Although most breech presentations have no aetiological factor, some may be associated with known factors and an ultrasound examination may reveal bicornuate uterus, uterine fibroids, low-lying placenta, multiple pregnancy, polyhydramnios, oligohydramnios, spina bifida or hydrocephaly.

Dewhurst's Textbook of Obstetrics & Gynaecology, Eighth Edition. Edited by D. Keith Edmonds.
© 2012 John Wiley and Sons, Ltd. Published 2012 by John Wiley and Sons, Ltd.

Types of breech presentation

Most cases of breech present with flexion at the hip and extension at the knees (extended breech). The next most common breech presentation is with flexion at the hips and knees (flexed or complete breech). Occasionally one leg is flexed and the other extended (incomplete breech) or one or two feet may present (footling breech). Knee presentation is rare (Fig. 26.3). Because of the smaller and irregular presenting part of a breech compared with a vertex labour, there is a greater incidence of cord prolapse and this is higher with footling presentation when it may be as high as 10%. Most breech presentations are recognized on antenatal clinical examination, identification being easier at later gestations and if the mother is multiparous or has a thin abdominal wall. The fetus will be in a longitudinal lie with the head palpable as a spherical hard mass in the upper pole. The head is usually to one or other side under the hypochondrium and is tender to deep palpation. In such cases the lower fetal pole is broader and is felt above or within the pelvis. In an extended breech there is difficulty in locating the head, but the diagnosis is aided by eliciting the ballotment sign: pushing on the round hard head causes it rebound back

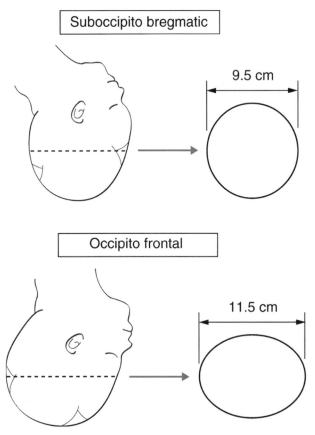

Suboccipito bregmatic

9.5 cm

Occipito frontal

11.5 cm

Fig. 26.1 Anteroposterior diameters of the vertex in the well-flexed head (suboccipito-bregmatic, usually OA position) and slightly deflexed head (occipito-frontal, usually occipito-posterior or occipito-transverse positions).

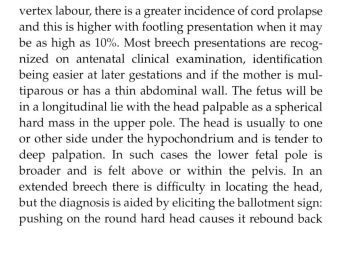

Asynclitism

The sagittal suture is lying behind the symphysis pubis

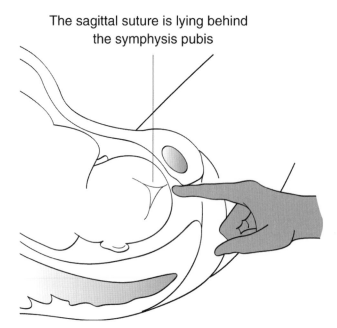

Fig. 26.2 Posterior asynclitism of the vertex: posterior parietal bone is prominent and the sagittal suture is shifted much anterior in the pelvis.

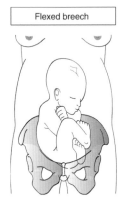

Flexed breech

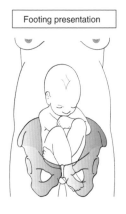

Footing presentation

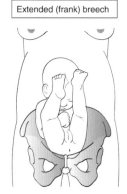

Extended (frank) breech

Fig. 26.3 Types of breech presentation.

to the hand similar to a ball being pushed under water. An extended breech engaged in the pelvis may mimic a deeply engaged head. Clinically, vaginal and ultrasound examination can help to identify the head that is engaged in the pelvis. Auscultation with a stethoscope locates the fetal heart in the maternal upper abdomen because of the higher position of the chest in a breech presentation. However, the fetal heart may also be heard from below the umbilicus when the transducer of a Doptone is directed upwards.

Antenatal management

Perinatal mortality and morbidity is marginally increased with breech presentation. In the developed countries prenatal screening for congenital malformation is routine between 19 and 22 weeks and cases with lethal malformations that may cause morbidity or mortality are offered termination. Prematurity, cord accidents and trauma are the main causes of morbidity and mortality with breech presentation. Although current literature recommends elective Caesarean section (CS) for term breeches [2], the study did not address those women in established labour with a breech presentation, preterm breeches or breech presentation in multiple pregnancies and hence training in assisted breech delivery is essential. In some women, breech presentation may be a manifestation of underlying pathology and in these cases the mode of delivery may not alter neonatal or long-term outcome [3]. However, the majority of cases do not have significant abnormality and delivery as a cephalic presentation or elective CS may reduce morbidity and mortality associated with vaginal breech delivery.

External cephalic version (ECV) is encouraged after 36+ weeks as the chances of spontaneous version from breech to cephalic presentation after 37 weeks is estimated as 1 in 20 [1]. Couples should receive counselling about the procedure and its success rates and complications, and the subsequent management of persistent breech presentation. ECV is contraindicated in those with placenta praevia, multiple pregnancies and history of antepartum haemorrhage, whilst intrauterine growth restriction, previous uterine scar, pre-eclampsia and hypertension are relative contraindications.

ECV should be performed in a setting where urgent CS is available should there be evidence of fetal compromise during or soon after ECV. The procedure should commence only after confirming by ultrasound examination that the fetus is in breech presentation and noting the type of presentation, fetal attitude, position of the placenta and the quantity of amniotic fluid. Cardiotocography (CTG) for 30–40 min prior to and after ECV should provide confirmation of fetal health. The chance of success is greater with multiparity, flexed breech presentation, adequate liquor volume and a breech that is mobile above the brim. The success rate may also be improved by placing the mother in the Trendelenberg position, by intravenous hydration just prior to ECV to increase amniotic fluid volume, use of vibroacoustic stimulation, and uterine relaxation with a short-acting tocolytic [4,5].

The first step in ECV involves disengaging the breech by moving the fetus up and away from the pelvis and shifting it to a sideways position, followed by a forward somersault to move the head to the lower pole; if this fails a backward somersault can be tried. The success rate in most centres is about 60% [5]. Complications are extremely rare but include cord accidents, pre-labour rupture of membranes, feto-maternal transfusion, placental separation and fetal compromise or death. Mothers who are rhesus-negative should receive anti-D after the procedure, and a Kleihauer–Betke test is useful for determining the need for additional doses of anti-D. The mother can be reassured by performing CTG for 30–40 min after the procedure. CTG should be reactive with normal baseline variability and no uterine irritability. There should be no bleeding or leaking of amniotic fluid per vagina and uterine tenderness or irritability prior to discharge. Women in whom ECV is unsuccessful need counselling about the option of an elective CS or assisted vaginal breech delivery.

Intrapartum management

Appropriate selection of women for assisted vaginal delivery ensures optimal outcome for mother and baby. Women with frank and complete breech presentations (fetal weight < 4000 g) encounter minimal problems, while those with footling presentations should be advised about the increased risk of cord prolapse and elective CS. Estimation of pelvis size by clinical methods is acceptable when planning vaginal delivery, and there is no evidence that CT or X-ray pelvimetry increases the chance of success. Spontaneous onset of labour is preferred. Induction of labour should be undertaken only if there are definitive indications and in such cases discussion must include the option of elective CS.

Mothers are advised to come to the labour ward when membranes rupture or with onset of painful contractions so that cord presentation or prolapse may be excluded. Management of labour is the same as for a vertex presentation. Successful outcome depends on a normal rate of cervical dilatation, descent of the breech and a normal fetal heart rate (FHR) pattern. Where progress of labour is poor and uterine contractions are inadequate, feto-pelvic disproportion should be excluded followed by a limited period of oxytocin augmentation. If progress is slow (<0.3 cm/hour) in the first few hours of augmentation, it may be best to advise CS.

The second stage of labour requires the full cooperation of the mother for a successful conclusion. Epidural anaesthesia provides pain relief in labour and prevents the mother bearing down before the cervix is fully dilated.

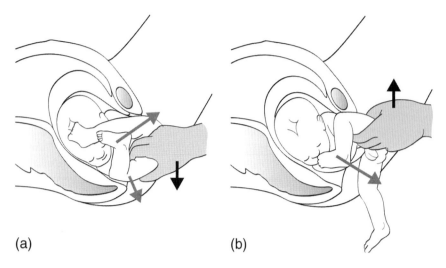

(a)   (b)

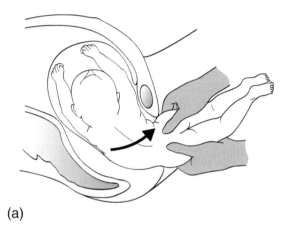

Fig. 26.4 Delivery of the extended legs by slight abduction of the thigh and flexion at the knees.

The mother should be encouraged to bear down only when the breech has reached the perineal phase of the second stage. Early intervention leads to poor outcome, so the mother should not be placed in lithotomy until the anterior buttock and anus of the baby are in view over the mother's perineum with no retraction between contractions. In the multiparous woman the perineum is distensible to allow easy delivery, but a primigravida may require episiotomy with regional or pudendal block and local infiltration of the perineum.

The buttocks of the fetus are delivered in the sacrolateral position. The mother should be encouraged to bear down with uterine contractions to ensure unassisted delivery of the fetus beyond the level of the umbilicus. Assistance, if required, should be in the form of lateral manipulation, with traction only for delivery of the head. In presentations where the legs are extended (frank breech), delivery is by abduction at the hip and flexion at the knees (Fig. 26.4). The dorsum of the fetus should always be facing upwards after each manoeuvre.

When the scapulae are seen at the introitus and the arms are flexed, the forearms can be delivered by sweeping them in front of the fetal chest. If the arms are extended, slight abduction and flexion of the shoulder followed by extension at the elbow delivers the forearm and hand. If the scapulae are not seen, the arms may be extended and the shoulders high in the pelvis. This presentation can be resolved using the Lovset manoeuvre: the posterior shoulder, which is below the level of the sacral promontory, is brought anterior and below the symphysis pubis by rotating the fetus clockwise by holding the baby with the thumbs on the sacrum and index fingers on the anterior superior iliac spines (Fig. 26.5). After delivery of the rotated extended arm which has come anterior, the fetus is turned in an anticlockwise direction to facilitate descent of the opposite shoulder. After delivery of the shoulders the dorsum of the fetus should face upwards, and vaginal examination should confirm that the chin is facing the sacrum and the occiput is behind the symphysis pubis.

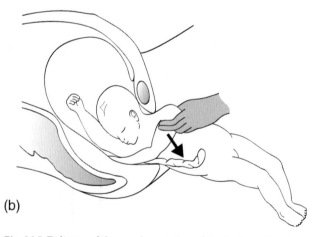

(a)

(b)

Fig. 26.5 Delivery of the arm by rotation of the body so that the posterior shoulder, which was below the sacral promontory, becomes anterior and below the pubic symphysis.

The slow descent of the head is assisted by the weight of the fetus, which is gently supported until the nape of the neck is seen under the symphysis pubis. At this point, delivery of the head is assisted by one of three methods.

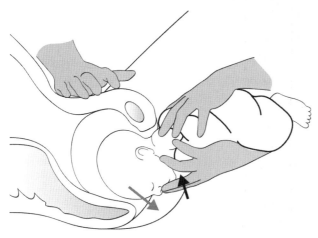

Fig. 26.6 Delivery of the head by jaw flexion and shoulder traction.

1 The body of the baby is swung over the maternal abdomen until the mouth and nose of the fetus become visible.

2 Two fingers are pressed over the maxilla to flex the head and delivery is accomplished by shoulder traction (Mauriceau–Smellie–Veit manoeuvre, Fig. 26.6).

3 Forceps are applied to the head from below while an assistant holds the baby just below the horizontal. Once it is checked that the blades lock easily, downwards traction is applied.

Delivery of the head is also assisted by 'ironing' the perineum beyond the forehead. Once delivery is completed, the oropharynx and nasopharynx are cleared by suction.

Conclusion

Elective CS is recommended for women with term breech presentation, but there is inadequate evidence to recommend the mode of delivery for preterm breeches. Morbidity and mortality are profoundly affected by gestation at birth and birthweight, and this is compounded by difficulties encountered at delivery. It is important that the parents receive counselling and consult with the paediatrician in order to make an informed decision about mode of delivery.

Some women prefer assisted vaginal breech delivery or present with breech in advanced labour, and their requests should be respected. The skills required to deliver a breech vaginally can be acquired by assisting others or by practising assisted breech delivery at the time of CS or on mannequins. Delivery may be carried out by a senior midwife or a doctor, provided they have experience with assisted breech delivery.

Brow presentation

In brow presentation the head is half extended and presents to the pelvis with the largest anteroposterior diameter (mento-vertical, 13 cm). The lower-most part of the head that is palpable on vaginal examination is the forehead, but because the orbital ridges and the bridge of the nose are the next most definable part of the presentation it is called 'brow' presentation. The incidence is about 1 in 1500–3000 deliveries.

The brow presentation may correct to vertex during labour by flexion of the neck or undergo further extension and present as a face, which can be delivered vaginally if in mento-anterior position. Persistence of brow presentation with slow progress of labour at term is not compatible with vaginal delivery and necessitates CS; augmentation of labour with oxytocin is not advisable. In extreme prematurity, the fetus descends in a brow presentation and delivers as a brow or, occasionally, converts to a face or vertex after it reaches the pelvic floor. Although vaginal delivery is possible in the preterm fetus, there is a small risk of spinal cord injury and CS is preferred. Because the presenting part of the fetus does not fit the pelvis, there is greater incidence of cord prolapse with membrane rupture and the possibility of uterine rupture in neglected cases. In cases of intrauterine fetal death in the extreme preterm period, where injury to the fetus is not a concern, labour may be allowed if there is good progress in anticipation of vaginal delivery. In the setting of lethal anomaly, destructive operations and vaginal delivery are still practised in some countries, but CS is preferred in the UK for fear of genital tract trauma in the hands of those not familiar with the type of instruments used.

Face presentation

Face presentation occurs in approximately 1 in 500–1000 deliveries. The general causes of malpresentation apply for face presentation, but the presence of anencephaly or thyroid goitre also needs to be excluded by ultrasound. The most frequent cause in a normal fetus is extension of the head: on abdominal examination the prominence of the head is palpable at a higher level on the opposite side of the fetal spine. In a multiparous woman with a thin abdominal wall, a deep groove may be palpable between the occiput and the back. On vaginal examination, palpation of the nose, eyes and the hard gum margins should confirm the presentation. Recognizing the presentation may be difficult when the membranes are intact and the presenting part is high or in the presence of oedema due to a few hours of labour.

At the onset of labour the transverse submento-bregmatic diameter enters the pelvis. With progressive contractions, when the face reaches the pelvic floor it rotates forwards to the mento-anterior position with the chin behind the symphysis pubis. The transverse biparietal diameter (9.5 cm) and the anteroposterior submento-bregmatic diameter (9.5 cm) are compatible with normal vaginal delivery (Fig. 26.7). Descent in the mento-anterior position is possible because of the large space in the posterolateral sacral area. The head emerges with the chin under the pubic arch followed by the forehead over the perineum. If the face rotates to a mento-posterior position, even though the diameters are the same as mento-anterior, the dimensions of the large frontal bones prevent descent behind the narrow retropubic arch, and in this situation CS is advisable.

The mento-lateral or mento-anterior position is more favourable, but poor progress in the first or early second stage indicates that the safer option is CS. Once the face is at the outlet in the mento-lateral or mento-anterior position, forceps delivery can be performed by skilled personnel.

Shoulder presentation

The incidence of shoulder presentation at term is 1 in 200. Shoulder presentation is diagnosed when the fetus is in the transverse lie and is associated with the lax abdominal wall and uterus in multiparous women. Other known associations include preterm, congenital fetal or uterine malformation, fibroids, placenta praevia and polyhydramnios. With the onset of labour most cases of transverse lie convert to a longitudinal lie due to increased muscular tone of the uterus, and this outcome should be anticipated. However, should rupture of the membranes occur with the fetus in the transverse lie or with cord or arm prolapse, CS should be performed to avoid injury to

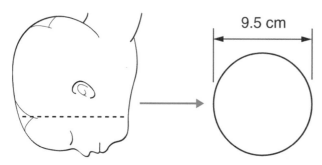

Fig. 26.7 The anteroposterior submento-bregmatic diameter of face presentation.

the fetus or uterus. In cases where the diagnosis is made late, the fetus may be impacted in the transverse lie and CS with a midline vertical incision is advisable to avoid trauma to the fetus, with extension of a transverse uterine incision. Delivery via a low transverse incision has been described with acute tocolysis using a short-acting uterine relaxant (0.25 mg terbutaline in 5 mL saline given intravenously over 5 min) [6]. After delivery if the uterus is still relaxed despite the use of oxytocics, a beta-blocker (e.g. propranolol 1 mg i.v.) may be needed to contract the uterus to avoid postpartum haemorrhage [7]. Spontaneous vaginal delivery is possible in early preterm fetuses by extreme flexion of the body.

Cephalopelvic disproportion

Cephalopelvic disproportion should be a retrospective diagnosis after a well-conducted trial of labour. The possibility of disproportion may be suggested by the poor progress of cervical dilatation despite optimal uterine activity for several hours, marked caput and moulding, prolonged variable decelerations on CTG suggestive of head compression, and appearance of fresh meconium. Failure to progress may be due to problems with the passage, the passenger or the power, or a combination of these. When the rate of cervical dilatation is less than 0.3 cm/hour over 6–8 hours despite oxytocin augmentation (leading to optimal uterine activity of four to five contractions every 10 min each lasting >40 s), one should exclude problems of power and instead look for problems related to the passage or passenger. Obvious problems with the passenger such as hydrocephalus, large baby or brow presentation should have been excluded prior to augmentation. Similarly, congenitally small pelvis or deformed pelvis due to accident are rare and should have been detected before onset of labour. The shape of the pelvis may also influence the outcome of labour and in some women may be android or platypelloid (Fig. 26.8). The next common cause of slow labour (after poor uterine contractions) relates to different degrees of deflexion or asynclitism of the head presenting a larger diameter.

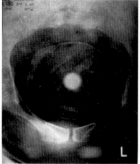
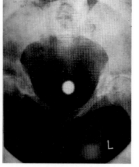
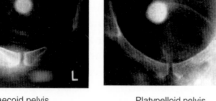

Gynaecoid pelvis   Platypelloid pelvis   Android pelvis

Fig. 26.8 The different shapes of pelvis.

Optimal uterine activity for 6–8 hours may help in flexion and correction of asynclitism resulting in presentation of a smaller diameter of the head. Moulding, caused by overlapping of the skull bones, and pelvic elasticity, caused by separation of the symphysis pubis, are dynamic changes that facilitate progress of labour and delivery.

In the second stage of labour, poor progress is diagnosed when there is failure of descent of the head with increasing caput and moulding despite optimal uterine activity. If spontaneous contractions are assessed to be inadequate and the head is in the 'pelvic phase', oxytocin augmentation may be tried for 1 hour. If the head is in the 'perineal phase' (i.e. reasonably low), then the woman should be encouraged to bear down for 1 hour.

Summary box 26.1

- Minor degrees of disproportion are due to deflexion of the head, malposition, and asynclitism compounded by inadequate uterine activity.
- Adequate uterine activity with oxytocin augmentation may help to promote flexion and rotation to OA position.

Failure of descent suggests disproportion. If this is due to malposition or asynclitism and if the station is below spines, it may be possible to deliver by forceps or ventouse. Failure to progress due to cephalopelvic disproportion in the first stage and in the second stage when the station is high is best managed by CS.

Instrumental vaginal deliveries

The incidence of instrumental vaginal delivery (IVD) varies from 6 to 12% and is greater in women with epidural analgesia for pain relief in labour. Common indications for IVD include delay in the second stage of labour due to inadequate uterine activity, mild disproportion due to malposition, poor maternal effort and fetal distress. Women with severe cardiac, respiratory or hypertensive disease or intracranial pathology where bearing down may not be conducive to health (e.g. arteriovenous malformations that are known to have bled) benefit from IVD.

Women undergoing epidural analgesia show decreased uterine activity in the second stage of labour secondary to inhibition of Ferguson's reflex, which normally causes release of oxytocin due to stretching of the upper vagina [8]. Inadequate uterine activity in these women can be improved by oxytocin infusion, leading to reduction in use of IVD [9].

The condition of the mother and fetus and the progress of labour should be assessed prior to performing IVD. Medical personnel should introduce themselves to the woman and her partner and explain the reason for IVD. Use of a chaperone in such situations is essential. The findings and plan of action and the procedure should be explained. Verbal or written consent should be obtained after explaining the indication, advantages and disadvantages, which should be recorded. It is important to remember that the mother and her partner may be physically and emotionally exhausted and hence the utmost care should be exercised in terms of behaviour, communication and medical action.

The woman should be given adequate pain relief and be well hydrated. Pudendal block and local perineal infiltration (20 mL of 1% plain lidocaine) may be adequate for low forceps or ventouse deliveries. Epidural anaesthesia is advisable for mid-cavity instrumental delivery or for a trial of IVD. In the absence of a pre-existing epidural, spinal anaesthesia may be more suitable. Abdominal and vaginal examination and CTG should provide adequate clinical information and reassurance to proceed with IVD. Cord prolapse, intrapartum bleeding and prolonged deceleration are acute emergencies and immediate delivery should be undertaken.

On abdominal examination the fetus should not be excessively large (>5 kg), none or less than one-fifth of the head should be palpable, and uterine contractions should be optimal. If uterine contractions are inadequate (less than four in 10 min, each lasting <40 s), oxytocin infusion should be considered in the absence of signs of fetal compromise. The bladder should be emptied by asking the woman to void. If this is difficult, the bladder should be catheterized. If the baby is large, extra care should be taken to avoid a prolonged period of traction and possible shoulder dystocia should be anticipated.

Vaginal examination should confirm that the cervix is fully dilated with membranes absent. The colour and quantity of amniotic fluid should be noted. Excessive caput (soft-tissue swelling) and moulding may suggest the possibility of disproportion. Overlapping of skull bones and inability to reduce it with gentle pressure is designated *moulding* +++; overlapping of the bones that can be reduced by gentle digital pressure is designated *moulding* ++ and meeting of the bones without any overlap is designated *moulding* +. Identification of position, station and degree of deflexion or asynclitism will help decide whether to perform IVD, where and by whom. Station below spines with descent of the head with every contraction and bearing down is likely to result in successful IVD.

The female pelvis accommodates the fetal head at term. Therefore when the head is 0/5th palpable above the pelvic brim, the leading part of the head is below the ischial spines. In an obese mother and in those with occipito-posterior positions, palpation of the fifths above the brim may be difficult and may be deceptive. If 1/5th or 0/5th of the head was palpable above the brim but on vaginal examination the head was above spines, then the small amount of head palpated may have been the fetal chin and the vertex may be in occipito-posterior position. When the head is more than 1/5th palpable and/or when the station is above spines, it is not advisable to undertake IVD.

The size of the fetus, fifths of head palpable, station and position will determine whether to proceed with IVD and the type of instrument to be used. Position is determined by identification of suture lines, posterior fontanelle and occiput. The posterior fontanelle can be identified by the inverted Y-shaped suture lines caused by overlapping of the parietal bones over the occipital bone. The posterior fontanelle is small and identification may be difficult when there is marked caput. Anterior fontanelle is easily identified as a soft diamond-shaped depression at the junction of the two parietal bones with the two frontal bones If the anterior fontanelle is felt easily around the centre of the pelvis, this indicates a deflexed head. If the head is well flexed, the anterior fontanelle faces the side wall of the pelvis. It is helpful to confirm the position by by palpating and flicking the fetal ear. The finger has to be moved from direction of the occiput for the ear to flick. Palpation of the ears also indicates that the largest diameter of the head (i.e. biparietal eminences) has descended below the mid pelvic strait. When the head is synclitic, the sagittal suture cuts the pelvis into halves. If the sagittal suture is far posterior or anterior, there is asynclitism and this suggests a reason for poor progress of labour and warns of possible difficulties with IVD. Significant descent and rotation of the head with contraction and bearing down effort is a good predictor of successful IVD.

IVD can be performed with the mother in the dorsal position with the legs flexed and abducted or in the left lateral position. Normally, however, the woman is placed in lithotomy. The procedure is performed with good anaesthesia under antiseptic and aseptic conditions. The vulva and perineum should be cleansed and the bladder catheterized if the woman is unable to void urine and the bladder is palpable.

Regional epidural or spinal anaesthesia is best for *mid-cavity IVD*, i.e. when the head is engaged and the station is 0 to +2cm below the ischial spines [10]. IVD at station +2cm or below is termed *low-cavity IVD* and regional or pudendal block with local infiltration of the perineum may be adequate. *Outlet IVD* is performed when the head is on the perineum with the scalp visible without any separation of the labia. Descent of the head to this level is associated with direct, right or left OA position that requires no rotation or rotation of less than 45°. Pudendal block anaesthesia and local infiltration of perineum may be adequate but some prefer regional anaesthesia.

If the head is above the ischial spines, CS should be considered. When the vertex is below the spines, IVD is carried out with different types of forceps and vacuum equipment, depending on the position and station of the vertex and the familiarity and experience of the doctor. In order to make comparisons of outcome, there have been proposals to use the terminology of the specific station and position at the time of instrumentation, e.g. right occipito-transverse (ROT) at +2 or left occipito-posterior (LOP) at +3, instead of the broad categories of mid, low and outlet IVD [11].

Choice of instruments: forceps or ventouse

The choice of instrument depends on the operator's experience, familiarity with the instrument, station and position of the vertex. Therefore, knowledge of the station and the position of the vertex is essential. The fetus in the OA position in the mid or low cavity or low direct occipito-posterior position (face to pubis) can be delivered by Neville Barnes forceps with or without axis traction handle or by Simpson's forceps. Wrigley's forceps is preferred by many for outlet deliveries. For the fetus in the occipito-lateral or occipito-posterior position, Keilland's forceps can be used to rotate the head without inflicting trauma to the fetus or the maternal passages. Vacuum devices made of Silc or Silastic or metal cups with the suction tubing arising from the dorsum of the cup (i.e. anterior cup) can be used for the fetus in OA position. A posterior metal cup or rigid plastic cup with the suction tubing coming from the circumference of the cup is needed for an occipito-posterior or occipito-lateral position so that the cup can be manipulated between the head and the vaginal wall to reach the flexion point that is 3cm in front of the occiput on the sagittal suture.

Forceps delivery

Most forceps have a pair of fenestrated blades with a cephalic and pelvic curve between the heel and toes (at the distal end) of the blades. The heel continues as a shank which ends in the handle. The handles of the two blades sit together so that they can be held by one hand and are kept in place by a lock on the shank. The cephalic curve is constructed to grasp the fetal head, with the toes of the blades over the maxilla or malar eminences while the length of the blade grasps the sides of the head from the malar area along the side of the head in front of the ear and the parietal bones in front of the occiput. This bimalar biparietal application exerts uniform pressure on the head. In this position the shank is over the flexion point and thus allows the correct direction of traction. If the posterior fontanelle is further backwards, the blades can be slightly disengaged, lifted upwards and locked so that the downwards pull will cause flexion. The pelvic curve fits the pelvis and is minimal in those forceps used for rotation as in cases with malposition (e.g. Kielland's forceps).

Prior to application of forceps the blades should be assembled to check whether they fit together as a pair.

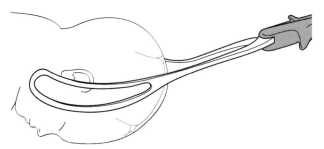

Fig. 26.9 Biparietal bimalar application offers uniform grip on the two sides. The occiput is 3 cm above the shank and the sagittal suture bisects the shank perpendicularly.

When the handle is held in the left hand, the left blade should sit comfortably in the palm of the right hand with the toes facing upwards because of the cephalic curve. In cases of direct or left OA positions, the left blade is inserted first, negotiating the pelvic and cephalic curve with a curved movement of the blade between the fetal head and the operator's right hand kept along the left vaginal wall. The right blade is held by the right hand and is applied between the left hand protecting the vagina and the head by negotiating the cephalic and pelvic curve. If the blades were applied correctly, the handles should lie horizontally, right on top of left and lock easily. The three *essential* features that should be satisfied before traction are (i) sagittal suture should be in the midline (i.e. no asynclitism), cutting the shank perpendicularly, (ii) occiput 3–4 cm above the shank (i.e. traction will be along the flexion point) and (iii) not more than one finger space between the head and the heel of the blade. Confirmation of these features guarantee that there is no asynclitism and that application is optimal with uniform pressure on the head from the malar to the parietal area (Fig. 26.9). Traction is in the direction of the pelvic curve and is synchronized with contractions and maternal bearing-down efforts. An episiotomy is usually needed when the head is crowning at the vulva. The direction of traction is upwards once the biparietal eminences emerge from underneath the pubic arch and the head is born by extension.

Keilland's forceps

Keilland's forceps has a cephalic curve but minimal pelvic curve that facilitates rotation of the head with little trauma to the maternal lower genital tract. The sliding lock helps to correct asynclitism. Abdominal and vaginal examination to identify position, station and asynclitism helps with correct application of Keilland's forceps. Palpation of the fetal ear will help to identify the position more accurately and will also indicate the possible level of descent.

The two sides of the forceps should be assembled to confirm that they fit each other. The forceps are then applied so that the knobs on the handles face the occiput of the baby. The blades can be applied directly to the side of head and face if space permits. Alternatively, the anterior blade can be positioned by the reverse or classical and wandering method. The blade is slid, or 'wandered', over the face to lie in a parietal and malar position. The posterior blade is usually applied directly because of the space in the pelvis posteriorly. Once locked, any asynclitism can be corrected by sliding the shanks over each other until the knobs come to the same level. The absence of asynclitism should be confirmed by checking that the sagittal suture lies equidistant from the two blades. If the blades cannot be locked or there is difficulty in application, forceps delivery should be abandoned. Rotation should only take place between contractions and only gentle force should be applied.

The position of the knobs should indicate whether the fetus is occipto-lateral or occipito-posterior. The handles of the forceps blades are rotated so that the occiput becomes anterior and just below the subpubic arch. Once the application has been checked to ensure that the sagittal suture is perpendicular to the shank, the occiput 3–4 cm above the shank and that only one finger can be inserted between the heel of the blade and the head, downwards traction is applied. If there is no descent with traction during the course of three contractions and maternal bearing-down effort, then forceps should be abandoned. Trial of IVD can lead to unexpected consequences for the mother and baby and is best performed by an experienced practitioner or under supervision in an operating theatre to allow conversion to CS should the procedure be abandoned.

Complications of forceps

Perineal lacerations, including third- and fourth-degree tears, are more common with forceps than with vacuum deliveries. Infra-levator haematomas may occur occasionally and these should be drained if symptomatic. Facial and scalp abrasions are usually minor and heal in a few days. Unilateral facial nerve palsy is rare and usually resolves within days or weeks; it is not due to poor technique. Cephalhaematomas and fracture of the skull are rare and most need no treatment, except depressed fracture which requires elevation by surgery.

Ventouse delivery

Ventouse or vacuum delivery is increasingly favoured over forceps delivery for similar indications in the second stage of labour. The conditions that must be satisfied before any instrumental delivery need to be checked prior to application of vacuum. The cups come in different sizes, usually 4, 5 or 6 cm in diameter. The cup is applied over the flexion point, which is 3–4 cm in front of the occiput on the midline indicated by the sagittal suture. Traction on this point promotes flexion that permits the minimal diameters for the vertex to descend through the pelvis. Application at the flexion point is termed a *flexing*

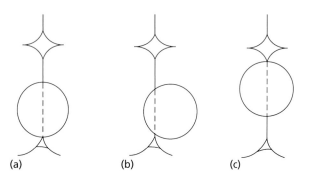

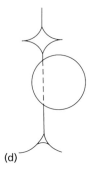

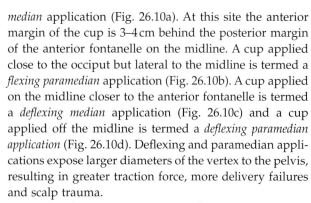

(a)   (b)   (c)   (d)

Fig. 26.10 Possible placement of the vacuum cup, from most favourable (a) to unfavourable (d). (a) Flexing median; (b) flexing paramedian; (c) deflexing median; (d) deflexing paramedian.

median application (Fig. 26.10a). At this site the anterior margin of the cup is 3–4 cm behind the posterior margin of the anterior fontanelle on the midline. A cup applied close to the occiput but lateral to the midline is termed a *flexing paramedian* application (Fig. 26.10b). A cup applied on the midline closer to the anterior fontanelle is termed a *deflexing median* application (Fig. 26.10c) and a cup applied off the midline is termed a *deflexing paramedian application* (Fig. 26.10d). Deflexing and paramedian applications expose larger diameters of the vertex to the pelvis, resulting in greater traction force, more delivery failures and scalp trauma.

It is therefore important to identify the position of the head and to determine whether it is synclitic so that the cup can be applied accurately over the flexion point. A specially designed cup should be used for occipito-lateral and occipito-posterior positions. The tubing should emerge from the lateral aspect of the cup (posterior metal cup) or through a groove in the cup (e.g. posterior rigid plastic cup, OmniCup), allowing the cup to be inserted and moved between the vaginal wall and the head to reach the flexion point [12]. The soft Silc, Silastic or anterior metal cup, where the tubing is attached in the centre of the cup, are not suitable for occipito-lateral or occipito-posterior positions as the lateral vaginal wall does not permit the central stem or suction tubing on the dorsum to be shifted to the flexion point. These cups are suitable for the OA position as the flexion point is in the midline.

Once the cup is placed firmly on the fetal scalp, a hand-held or mechanical pump creates a vacuum of up to 0.2 bar (150 mmHg or 0.2 kg/cm² negative pressure). It is essential to check that the cup has been correctly positioned over the flexion point and that maternal tissue has not been trapped in the cup. The vacuum is then increased to 0.7–0.8 bar (500–600 mmHg or 0.8 kg/cm²) before starting traction in concert with uterine contractions and bearing-down effort. There is no need to increase the vacuum stepwise (0.7–0.8 bar can be generated immediately) or for the release of vacuum between traction efforts. Traction in a downwards direction causes flexion of the head and descent along the axis of the pelvis. This promotes auto-rotation of the head to the OA position and hence the optimal diameter at the pelvic outlet.

Summary box 26.2

- It is important to identify the position and synclitism of the head in order to facilitate accurate cup application over the flexion point.

In most countries ventouse deliveries are on the increase over forceps deliveries because of less perineal trauma, including third-degree tears [13]. The tissue sucked into the cup leaves a circumscribed soft-tissue swelling called a 'chignon'. This settles over the following 2–3 days and the parents should be given this reassurance. In the neonate, scalp abrasions, retinal haemorrhages, haematoma confined to one of the skull bones, neonatal jaundice and, rarely, subgaleal haemorrhage may cause minor or severe morbidity and rarely mortality [14]. Follow-up of women who had low or outlet instrumental deliveries shows normal physical and neurological outcome of the newborn infant [13].

Vacuum is not used to deliver very preterm babies (<34 weeks) and those fetuses with possible haemorrhagic tendencies for fear of causing subgaleal haemorrhage. Ventouse is best done when the cervix is fully dilated, but application in multiparous women whose cervix is 7–8 cm dilated may be performed by experienced personnel, although CS is preferable in such situations. In those with cardiac, respiratory or neurological disease, where maternal expulsive efforts may cause compromise, forceps delivery is preferred over vacuum delivery [15].

Trial of instrumental delivery

Because the injudicious use of instrumental delivery may result in fetal and maternal injury, it is sometimes difficult to judge whether IVD should be undertaken in cases with malposition. In such cases a trial of IVD should be done in theatre under good epidural or spinal anaesthesia and with the theatre team, anaesthetist and paediatrician present. The intention is to abandon IVD should there be any difficulty and proceed immediately to CS in the interest of the baby and the mother. The couple should be advised of this strategy and appropriate consent obtained prior to the procedure, which should be undertaken by the most senior obstetrician available. Signs of fetal compromise on CTG are an indication for CS rather than persevering with a difficult IVD.

Caesarean section

The rise in rates of CS are partly a result of better surgical techniques and availability of blood transfusion and antibiotics, and partly because of social factors such as fear of litigation should there be any fetal or maternal morbidity and womens' aspiration to have a healthy baby. A very small proportion of the increase is due to maternal request for non-medical reasons [21] or to monetary incentives [22]. The incidence of CS varies between 10% and 25% in most developed countries.

Indications
The indications for CS are grouped into four categories depending on the urgency of the procedure [23].
• *Category 1 or emergency CS.* There is an immediate threat to the mother or the fetus. Ideally, CS should be done within the next 30 min. Examples include abruption, cord prolapse, scar rupture, scalp blood pH below 7.20, and prolonged FHR deceleration below 80 bpm.
• *Category 2 or urgent CS.* There is maternal or fetal compromise but it is not immediately life-threatening. The delivery should be completed within 60–75 min. Examples include those with FHR abnormalities of concern.
• *Category 3 or scheduled CS.* The mother needs early delivery but currently there is no maternal or fetal compromise. However, there is concern that continuation of pregnancy is likely to affect the mother or fetus in hours or days. This group has a wide range of indications. Examples include failure to progress, where CS is planned within the next hour or two; a growth-restricted fetus in the preterm period with absent end-diastolic flow but normal CTG; or pre-eclampsia where liver or renal function tests are gradually deteriorating, where CS is planned within hours to days. The timing of CS would vary but some plan should be in place to deliver before further deterioration occurs.
• *Category 4 or elective CS.* The delivery is timed to suit the mother and staff. These are cases where there is an indication for CS but there is no urgency. Examples include placenta praevia with no active bleeding, malpresentations (e.g. brow, breech), history of previous hysterotomy or vertical incision CS, past history of repair of vesico-vaginal or recto-vaginal fistulae or stress incontinence, or HIV infection.

Placenta accreta is more common with anterior placenta praevia in women with a scar. This may result in massive haemorrhage and rarely the need for a hysterectomy and hence consent and preparation should be appropriate. Placement of an intra-arterial catheter for embolization of uterine arteries at the time of CS should be considered where facilities exist.

Elective CS is generally done around 39 weeks as the incidence of tachypnoea of the newborn is much less after this gestation. However, the medical or obstetric condition determines the gestation at which the elective CS is planned, the main principle being to carry out CS as late as possible in gestation without compromising maternal or fetal health.

Types of Caesarean section
The type of CS is based on the type of incision of the uterus.

Lower uterine segment incision
Lower segment CS involves a horizontal incision on the lower segment after reflecting the visceral peritoneum. This is the commonest CS procedure. The abdomen is opened by a low midline, paramedian and, more commonly, by a Pfannenstiel (suprapubic horizontal) incision and the peritoneal cavity opened. The bladder is reflected from the lower segment and a transverse incision is made on the lower uterine segment, care being taken not to injure the fetus. The presenting part is delivered through the lower segment. A forceps can be used to assist delivery in a cephalic presentation.

Traditionally, the lower uterine segment muscle is closed in two layers followed by closure of the visceral peritoneum. The merits of single versus two-layer closure of the muscle and closure versus non-closure of the visceral peritoneum was investigated by the CAESAR randomized controlled study. Nonclosure of visceral peritoneum did not influence infectious morbidity [24]. Lower segment CS is the commonest procedure because it is easier to incise the lower segment, deliver the fetus from the point of incision and to approximate the layers because of the thin muscle layers compared with the upper segment. In addition, the peritoneal layer can be closed and was thought to provide an advantage against infection. Blood loss and infection rate is much less with lower segment CS compared with upper segment CS.

After delivery of the fetus, the uterine cavity should be cleaned so as not to leave any retained tissue and the cervical os must be open to allow drainage of blood. Closure of the uterine wound is followed by peritoneal toilet when any blood or liquor in the abdomen and pelvis is removed using suction or gauze swabs on a sponge holder. The opportunity is taken at this stage to inspect the ovaries and tubes. Prophylactic antibiotics and low-molecular-weight heparin to prevent thromboembolism are routinely administered intraoperatively by the anaesthetist. If the mother is rhesus-negative and the baby rhesus-positive, a dose of anti-D should be given and a Kleihauer–Betke test performed to determine the adequacy of the dose of anti-D. Care of the mother should be similar to that after any major abdominal surgery.

Midline vertical incision

The midline vertical incision could be in the lower or upper segment of the uterus. Commonly, it starts in the lower segment as a small buttonhole incision until the uterine cavity is reached and is extended upwards. The midline incision is reserved for specific indications because of the difficulty in making the incision, increased blood loss, inadequate approximation at closure, increased postoperative morbidity, and inability to offer a trial of vaginal delivery in the next pregnancy due to possible higher incidence of scar rupture.

A midline approach is used when the lower segment approach is difficult because of fibroids or anterior placenta praevia with large vessels in the lower segment. Other indications include preterm breech with poorly formed lower segment, impacted transverse lie with ruptured membranes or transverse lie with congenital anomaly of the uterus. An extreme example is peri-mortem CS.

In special circumstances a lower or upper segment (or spanning both segments) vertical or inverted T incision is made.

Complications associated with Caesarean section

Morbidity and mortality associated with the procedure cannot be totally avoided. The common complications are haemorrhage, anaesthesia-related complications and infection. Prophylactic antibiotics are administered to reduce the incidence of infection. Occasionally there is injury to bowel, bladder, ureters or the fetus. Thromboembolism is rare but could be fatal and hence preoperative, intraoperative and postoperative precautions should be taken to avoid it. Intraoperatively, pneumatic inflatable boots are used for the legs and prophylactic doses of heparin administered. Postoperatively, the use of heparin, graduated elastic stockings, mobilization and chest and leg physiotherapy are advocated to reduce the incidence of deep venous thrombosis. Late complications of infection and secondary haemorrhage are not that uncommon. Vesico-vaginal or uretero-vaginal fistulae due to visceral injury are extremely rare.

Anaesthetic complications are extremely rare because of the availability of experienced anaesthetists and because most Caesareans are performed under regional anaesthesia. Women sometimes complain of light general anaesthesia causing awareness that goes unnoticed by the anaesthetist because the patients are paralysed. Other problems include vomiting on induction of anaesthesia and postoperative lung atelectasis following general anaesthesia. Aspiration of gastric contents leads to Mendelson's syndrome, which can result in maternal mortality. To reduce such an event, gastric contents are neutralized with 20 mL of 0.3 mol/L sodium citrate and gastric emptying promoted with metoclopramide 10 mg i.v. For elective CS, a histamine H_2-receptor antagonist such as ranitidine 150 mg is administered 2 hours before surgery. In those who have had a recent meal or who have had opiates preoperatively, emptying of the stomach is advocated to minimize risk of postoperative aspiration.

Caesarean hysterectomy is indicated for uncontrollable postpartum haemorrhage, placenta accreta or uterine rupture and is performed for cervical malignant disease as part of planned treatment. Maternal mortality with CS is rare and is usually related to the reason for which CS is done or because of anaesthetic or haemorrhagic complications and is estimated to be less than 0.33 per 1000.

Episiotomy and perineal lacerations

Perineal lacerations may occur with normal or instrumental vaginal delivery. Vulval and anterior vaginal tears do occur with vaginal delivery, but posterior vaginal and perineal injury is more common and occurs with delivery of the head or shoulders. Perineal tears are classified based on the involvement of the perineum.

First-degree tear involves the skin only, while second-degree tear involves the perineal muscle. Injury to the anal sphincter is classified as third-degree tear and is subdivided based on the degree of involvement. If less than half the thickness of the external anal sphincter is involved, it is categorized as 3a; it becomes 3b if there is full-thickness involvement and 3c when the internal sphincter becomes involved. When the tear damages the sphincter and involves the anal epithelium, it is termed fourth-degree tear.

Episiotomy

Episiotomy is an intentional surgical incision of the perineum after informed consent with the aim of increasing the soft-tissue outlet dimensions to help with childbirth. It is not advocated for every delivery and the rate of episiotomy depends on the philosophy and judgement of the caregiver.

At the time of vaginal delivery the perineum may tear. Episiotomy should be considered when anterior tears that bleed or multiple perineal tears appear or when the presence of pathological CTG indicates the need for expeditious spontaneous or instrumental delivery. Episiotomy facilitates IVD, although the need for an episiotomy is less with ventouse deliveries and with a distensible perineum. Where delivery is delayed by the presence of a rigid perineum, an episiotomy may help. Whenever internal rotation manoeuvres are needed, such as in some assisted breech deliveries and in shoulder dystocia, an episiotomy may be useful. Those women who have had previous pelvic floor or perineal surgery may benefit from episiotomy.

In the USA, a midline episiotomy starting from the fourchette and extending for a few centimetres towards the anus is popular, whereas a mediolateral episiotomy starting from the fourchette and extending mediolaterally to 45° is preferred in other countries. It is a single incision and the length varies according to the size of the perineum. The superficial perineal muscles are incised similar to a second-degree tear. If episiotomy is performed with normal vaginal delivery, local infiltration to the perineum may be adequate. If episiotomy is perfomed for IVD, women are best treated with epidural or spinal anaesthesia or pudendal block and perineal infiltration. It is important to check whether the woman can feel pain prior to the incision, and if so, additional local infiltration is needed.

Midline episiotomies cause minimal bleeding, the two sides of the perineum are easier to approximate, and less pain relief is needed postoperatively compared with mediolateral episiotomy. However, there is a higher incidence of third- and fourth-degree tears and this is probably due to the close proximity to the anus. Blood loss is minimized by performing the episiotomy when the head crowns and does not recede between contractions. Early repair after removal of placenta and membranes and ligation of profusely bleeding vessels help to reduce blood loss.

Perineal repair

Although pain relief is given at the time of episiotomy, the perception of pain should be checked again prior to repair. If there are additional tears that need suturing, further local infiltration should be given. Good light and optimal exposure are essential to achieve a good repair. Bleeding from the uterus may cause difficulty in visualizing the edges of the wound but this can be overcome by inserting a tampon or vaginal swab with a tail before commencing repair. The vagina is very vascular and profuse bleeding can occur from arteries under the vaginal skin; these vessels may retract, so the apex of the tear or episiotomy should be secured by a suture above the apex. The vaginal walls should then be approximated with sutures placed at intervals of 0.5–1 cm with a continuous locking pattern using a synthetic material such as Vicryl Rapide. Close suturing helps to achieve haemostasis and prevents vaginal shortening. The distance between sutures on the medial wall is shorter than that on the lateral wall in order to bring about good approximation so that the fourchette, the hymenal membrane and the junction of pink and pigmented vaginal skin at the introitus are well reconstructed.

If there is minimal bleeding from the perineal wound, the perineal muscles can be approximated by continuous suture. Interrupted sutures may be preferable in the presence of bleeding. The perineal skin is approximated by subcuticular suture, which is reported to heal well and cause less pain. Continuous, loose, non-locking sutures to approximate perineal muscles and subcuticular structures has been found to be a suitable method, with less pain and no need for removal of sutures [25]. When the apex of the tear or episiotomy extends closer to the anal orifice, rectal examination may be helpful for identifying a third- or fourth-degree tear. Once this has been repaired, rectal examination should also be performed to exclude accidental suture involvement of the rectum or anal canal.

It is imperative to count instruments, needles and swabs at the end of the repair. Remember that retention of vaginal swabs after repair is a common cause for litigation, so vaginal examination is essential to exclude inadvertent retention. The notes should document estimated total blood loss and details of repair. Medication for pain relief should be prescribed and postoperative care carefully described.

Women should be observed for 1–2 hours after repair because the procedure may rarely be complicated by bleeding, pain and haematoma formation that may necessitate additional medical or surgical intervention. Late complications including infection, breakdown of repair, pain, scarring and dyspareunia are not uncommon. Vesico-vaginal or recto-vaginal fistula is rare following surgery. Endometriosis of the scar is exceptional but should be considered when the woman presents with cyclical pain at the site of the tear or episiotomy wound and may require excision.

Third- and fourth-degree tears

Unrecognized third- and fourth-degree tears can give rise to flatus and/or faecal incontinence. Proper vaginal examination should help to identify and classify the injury as 3a, 3b, 3c or fourth-degree tear. Third- or fourth-degree tears are best repaired in the operating theatre under adequate anaesthesia to relax the sphincter muscle. Good lighting, appropriate instruments, experienced assistance and an experienced surgeon are essential for successful repair. Dissection and mobilization of the muscle without adequate relaxation may tear the muscle. Anal epithelium is repaired with 3/0 Vicryl Rapide sutures with the knots inside the lumen. The muscle is repaired using 3/0 PDS suture on a round-bodied needle. An end-to-end or overlapping method can be used [26]. Many prefer end-to-end repair for 3a and overlap repair for 3b, 3c and fourth-degree tears.

Postoperative care should include antibiotics to prevent infection and laxatives for softening the stools in order to avoid stretching the repair site. At follow-up, the success of the repair should be evaluated by enquiring about symptoms of faecal incontinence or flatus and, where facilities exist, by endo-anal ultrasound and/or anal manometry. If symptoms persist and cannot be improved by physiotherapy and conservative measures, repair by an experienced colorectal surgeon may be of benefit.

Conclusion

The NICE intrapartum care guidelines provides useful information about the management of abnormal labour [27]. There are number of controversies that need to be addressed by properly conducted randomized trials. There is preliminary evidence that combined spinal/epidural anaesthesia compared with epidural anaesthesia alone does not increase the chances of instrumental or Caesarean delivery but this needs further evaluation [28]. Determination of position by trans-perineal ultrasound is claimed to be better and more accurate than manual palpation [29], but this technique requires equipment, expertise and training. Similarly, the degree of descent appears best assessed by ultrasound rather than by digital examination [30]. Trial of instrumental delivery is better performed in theatre rather than the delivery room for logistical reasons but significant benefits have not been demonstrated [31]. Although such studies may improve practice, we need to concentrate on simulation training to teach intrapartum procedures, with better supervision by a senior clinician and proper assessment by objective structured assessment of technical skills before a doctor is allowed to practise independently. Intrapartum procedures can be stressful to the couple, the fetus and the clinician. Adequate knowledge, training, communication skills before and after the procedure, and accurate record keeping are essential components to alleviate the stress.

> ### Summary box 26.3
>
> - Knowledge of the female pelvis, fetal anatomy and mechanisms of normal labour are prerequisites for performing skilled operative deliveries.
> - Instrumental vaginal delivery and Caesarean section account for 20–40% of deliveries in the UK.
> - Decisions about why and when to perform an operative delivery, communication of the procedure and expected outcome should be conveyed to the woman and her partner.
> - Birth injuries, complaints and litigation are not uncommon with operative deliveries.
> - Proper training and assessment of knowledge, technique and communication skills will lead to competence to execute the delivery with no or minimal complications.
> - The ability to perform a skilful operative delivery is the hallmark of a good obstetrician.

References

1 Westgren M, Edvall H, Nordstrom L, Svalenius E, Ranstam J. Spontaneous cephalic version of breech presentation in the last trimester. *Br J Obstet Gynaecol* 1985;92:19–22.

2 Hofmeyer GJ, Hannah ME. Planned Caesarean section for term breech delivery. *Cochrane Database Syst Rev* 2001;(1):CD000166. Update in *Cochrane Database Syst Rev* 2003;(3):CD000166.

3 Ingemarsson I, Arulkumaran S, Westgren M. Breech delivery: management and long term outcome. In: Tejani N (ed.) *Obstetrical Events and Developmental Sequelae*. Boca Raton, FL: CRC Press, 1989: 143–159.

4 Annapoorna V, Arulkumaran S, Anandakumar C, Chua S, Montan S, Ratnam SS. External cephalic version at term with tocolysis and vibroacoustic stimulation. *Int J Obstet Gynecol* 1997;59:13–18.

5 Hofmeyer G, Kulier R. External cephalic version for breech presentation at term. *Cochrane Database Syst Rev* 2000;(2):CD000083.

6 Chandraharan E, Arulkumaran S. Acute tocolysis. *Curr Opin Obstet Gynecol* 2005;17:151–156.

7 Anderson KE, Ingemarsson I, Persson CGA. Effects of terbutaline on human uterine motility at term. *Acta Obstet Gynecol Scand* 1975;54;165–172.

8 Ferguson JKW. A study of the motility of the intact uterus at term. *Surg Gynecol Obstet* 1941;73:359–366.

9 Goodfellow CF, Studd C. The reduction of forceps in primigravidae with epidural analgesia: a controlled trial. *Br J Clin Pract* 1979;33:287–288.

10 American College of Obstetricians and Gynecologists. Operative vaginal delivery. Clinical management guidelines for the obstetrician. ACOG Practice Bulletin No. 17, 2000. Washington, DC: ACOG.

11 Hale RW. Forceps classification according to station of head in pelvis. In: Hale RW (ed.) *Dennen's Forceps Deliveries*, 4th edn. Washington, DC: American College of Obstetricians and Gynecologists, 2001: 11–29.

12 Hayman R, Gilby J, Arulkumaran S. Clinical evaluation of a 'handpump' vacuum delivery device. *Obstet Gynecol* 2002;100:1190–1195.

13 Johanson RB, Menon BKV. Vacuum extraction versus forceps for assisted vaginal delivery. *Cochrane Database Syst Rev* 2000;(2):CD000224.

14 Uchil D, Arulkumaran S. Neonatal subgaleal hemorrhage and its relationship to delivery by vacuum extraction. *Obstet Gynecol Surv* 2003;58:687–693.

15 Patel RP, Murphy DJ. Forceps review in modern obstetric practice. *BMJ* 2004;328:1302–1305.

16 Gonik B, Stringer CA, Held B. An alternative maneuver for managing shoulder dystocia. *Am J Obstet Gynecol* 1983;145:882–884.

17 Woods CE. A principle of physics as applicable to shoulder delivery. *Am J Obstet Gynecol* 1943;45:796–805.

18 Goodwin TM, Banks E, Miller LK, Phelan JP. Catastrophic shoulder dystocia and emergency symphysiotomy. *Am J Obstet Gynecol* 1997;177:463–464.

19 Sandberg EC. Zavanelli maneuver: 12 years of recorded experience. *Obstet Gynecol* 1999;93:312–317.

20 Bruner JP, Drummond SB, Meenan AL, Gaskin IL. All fours maneuver for reducing shoulder dystocia during labor. *J Reprod Med* 1998;43:439–443.

21 Penna L, Arulkumaran S. Cesarean section for non-medical reasons. *Int J Gynaecol Obstet* 2003;82:399–409.

22 Finger C. Caesarean section rates skyrocket in Brazil. *Lancet* 2003;362:628.

23 Royal College of Obstetricians and Gynaecologists Clinical Effectiveness Support Unit. *The National Sentinel Caesarean Section Audit Report*. London: RCOG Press, 2001: 49–53.

24 CAESAR Study Collaborative Group. Caesarian section surgical techniques: a randomised factorial trial (Caesar). *Br J Obstet Gynaecol* 2010;117:1366–1376.

25 Kettle C, Hills RK, Jones P, Darby L, Grey R, Johanson R. Continuous versus interrupted perineal repair with standard or rapidly absorbed sutures after spontaneous vaginal birth: a randomised controlled trial. *Lancet* 2002;359:2217–2223.

26 Thakar R, Sultan AH. The management and prevention of obstetric perineal trauma. In: Arulkumaran S, Penna LK, Bhasker Rao K (eds) *The Management of Labour*. Chennai: Orient Longmans, 2005: 252–268.

27 National Institute for Health and Clinical Excellence. *Intrapartum Care: Management and Delivery of Care to Women in Labour*. Clinical Guideline CG55, 2007. Available at: http://guidance.nice.org.uk/CG55/Guidance/pdf/English.

28 Aneiros F, Vazquez M, Valiño C *et al.* Does epidural versus combined spinal–epidural analgesia prolong labor and increase the risk of instrumental and cesarean delivery in nulliparous women? *J Clin Anesth* 2009;21:94–97.

29 Molina FS, Nicolaides KH. Ultrasound in labor and delivery. *Fetal Diagn Ther* 2010;27:61–67.

30 Duckelmann AM, Bamberg C, Michaelis SA *et al.* Measurement of fetal head descent using the 'angle of progression' on transperineal ultrasound imaging is reliable regardless of fetal head station or ultrasound expertise. *Ultrasound Obstet Gynecol* 2010;35:216–222.

31 Majoko F, Gardener G. Trial of instrumental delivery in theatre versus immediate caesarean section for anticipated difficult assisted births. *Cochrane Database Syst Rev* 2008;(4):CD005545.

Further reading

Bahl R, Strachan B, Murphy DJ. Outcome of subsequent pregnancy three years after previous operative delivery in the second stage of labour: cohort study. *BMJ* 2004;328:311–315.

Baskett TF, Arulkumaran S (eds). Operative delivery and intrapartum surgery. *Best Pract Res Clin Obstet Gynaecol* 2002;16(1).

Baskett TF, Arulkumaran S. *Intrapartum Care for the MRCOG and Beyond*, 2nd edn. London: RCOG Press, 2011.

Hale RW (ed.) *Dennen's Forceps Deliveries*, 4th edn. Washington, DC: American College of Obstetricians and Gynecologists.

Johanson RB, Menon BKV. Soft versus rigid vacuum extractor cups for assisted vaginal delivery. *Cochrane Database Syst Rev* 2000;(2): CD000446.

Murphy D, Lebling R, Veruty L, Swingler R, Patel R. Early maternal and neonatal morbidity associated with operative delivery in second stage of labour: a cohort study. *Lancet* 2001;358: 1203–1207.

Society of Obstetricians and Gynaecologists of Canada. *Guidelines for Operative Vaginal Birth*. Clinical Practice Guideline No. 148, 2004. Available at: www.sogc.org/guidelines/public/148E-CPG-August2004.pdf.

Chapter 27
Fetal Monitoring During Labour

Sara Paterson-Brown
Queen Charlotte's and Chelsea Hospital, London, UK

What this chapter cannot do is provide a comprehensive manual of fetal physiology, fetal heart rate interpretation and fetal monitoring techniques. While the main principles of these are discussed here, the reader is referred to other learning tools for fetal monitoring, including standard textbooks, the forthcoming RCOG e-learning programme currently in development and the online K2 fetal monitoing training system [1]. This latter system is divided into three interactive chapters: the first explains physiology, the second describes the fetal heart rate and cardiotocography and the third comprises a wealth of cases that can be worked through, and decisions made by the learner can be compared with those of three experts.

Fetal physiology

Normal

The fetus is sustained by the uteroplacental unit and under normal circumstances provision is surplus to requirements, enabling the fetus to thrive, grow and build up energy reserves. Aerobic metabolism of glucose provides the fetus with its energy, and the oxygen which is vital for this process is usually plentiful. Thus in normal pregnancy there is more oxygen supplied by the uteroplacental unit than needed by the fetus and energy reserves in the form of glycogen are stored by the fetus.

Fetal compromise

The fetus can be compromised by a reduction in oxygen supply, an increase in oxygen requirements (e.g. in sepsis) or a reduced capacity to transport oxygen (severe fetal anaemia, e.g. rhesus disease or some intrauterine infections). The severity and duration of the insult will vary according to the cause, and similarly the effects on the fetus are equally wide-ranging, but the principal fetal responses are described below.

• *Acute.* If oxygen delivery falls, there is reduced oxygen in the fetal circulation (hypoxaemia); if levels fall further, hypoxia occurs (reduced oxygen in the fetal tissues). Two things occur in response to hypoxaemia and hypoxia: the circulation adapts to maintain supplies to vital organs (brain and heart) and anaerobic metabolism utilizing glucose released from the stored glycogen reserves to provide continued energy supplies. The main consequences of anaerobic metabolism, which is almost 20 times less efficient than aerobic metabolism, are that fetal reserves are used up relatively quickly and that lactic acid is the waste product of this metabolism, resultimg in a metabolic acidosis that can be harmful.

• *Chronic.* If there is uteroplacental disease and fetal supplies are compromised, then glycogen stores may not accumulate and fetal reserves will be lacking. In chronic cases of reduced supply, the fetal circulation adapts as mentioned above with cranial sparing, and the peripheral circulation is effectively reduced. Depending on the severity and duration of this compromise, the pathophysiology results in decreased renal perfusion which in turn produces oligohydramnios (and, when more severe, anhydramnios) and reduced fetal growth. If there is further deterioration, anaerobic metabolism occurs and a metabolic acidosis develops.

• *Acute on chronic.* If an acute insult occurs in a fetus already compromised, it can withstand less hypoxia than a well-nourished fetus because it has less reserve and may have already made adaptations to conserve vital cerebral perfusion.

Thus the response and vulnerability of any fetus to a hypoxic insult will be largely dictated by (i) the condition of the fetus at the onset of that insult, (ii) the severity of that insult, (iii) the duration of that insult and (iv) the fact that fetal condition can deteriorate extremely quickly. Defining the period of time beyond which damage will be sustained is impossible due to the individual circumstances of each fetus and each insult, but a normal well-grown and mature fetus that has good reserves can tolerate a short period of severe hypoxia, whereas the same insult can be catastrophic for a growth-restricted fetus.

Dewhurst's Textbook of Obstetrics & Gynaecology, Eighth Edition. Edited by D. Keith Edmonds.

Summary box 27.1

Progressive hypoxia with metabolic acidosis is accelerative. Hypoxia that has led to metabolic acidaemia indicates that:
- fetal reserves are spent;
- tissue hypoxia and acidaemia will be rapidly progressive;
- fetal damage becomes increasingly likely.

Metabolic acidaemia

Paired umbilical cord blood samples at delivery enable direct measurements of uteroplacental function (umbilical vein) and fetal acid–base status (umbilical artery). There are now a number of published series of routine paired cord samples [1–4] and results largely conform and are approximated in Table 27.1. The base deficit in the umbilical artery indicates the degree of fetal metabolic acidosis and values above 12 mmol/L suggest that there has been significant hypoxia and subsequent fetal damage may occur [5]. If venous pH and base deficit are normal, this rules out chronic hypoxia. The mean pH difference between artery and vein is 0.08 and if this difference is less than 0.03, it is likely that both samples have been taken from the umbilical vein.

Fetal and neonatal consequences of hypoxia

The damage that results from hypoxic insults varies according to the vulnerability of the fetus and the nature and duration of the insult, as described above, ranging from minimal clinical signs through brain damage to death. While neonatal complications tend to increase as cord arterial pH falls [6], especially at values below 7.0 [7,8], many born with such values do well [7,9] while approximately one-quarter suffer neurological morbidity or mortality [10].

Death

Intrapartum deaths do occur as a result of hypoxia. The incidence in the UK is approximately 0.6 per 1000 and this has remained unchanged over the last decade [11,12]. While scrutiny of these cases has identified elements of substandard care, many cases are managed well and

Table 27.1 Routine paired umbilical cord values.

	pH (median)	pH (2.5–97.5 centile)	Median base deficit (mmol/L)	Base deficit (mmol/L) (2.5–97.5 centile)
Umbilical vein	7.35	7.17–7.48	3.7	9.0–0.5
Umbilical artery	7.25	7.05–7.38	4.3	11.1–0.5

yet death still results. Confidential enquiries have shown that approximately half of intrapartum stillbirths are considered to be avoidable [12,13], with errors in care extending from a failure to recognize problems in the antenatal period and/or in labour to recognizing but failing to act on signs of fetal compromise [13].

Neonatal pathology

The paired umbilical cord gas results provide an objective measure of *in utero* fetal metabolism, reflecting the presence or absence of intrauterine hypoxia, but although they are associated with neonatal outcomes they are not predictive and do not indicate neonatal resuscitative needs. Indeed many babies born with low cord gases are vigorous at birth. On the other hand, the Apgar score is a subjective assessment of the need for neonatal resuscitation but does not indicate the cause of the problem. Resuscitation therefore occurs according to clinical need and the possible cause may then be clarified by the cord gases. A variety of neonatal problems can follow on from intrauterine hypoxia, including hypoglycaemia, disturbed thermoregulation and necrotizing enterocolitis, but the main worry is that of brain damage due to the long-term morbidity associated with it.

Hypoxic–ischaemic encephalopathy

Neonatal encephalopathy is associated with a multitude of causes but hypoxic–ischaemic encephalopathy (HIE) is neonatal encephalopathy specifically caused by peripartum hypoxia. The centiles listed in Table 27.1 demonstrate that 2.5% of neonates are born with a cord arterial pH below 7.05. The incidence of more severe acidaemia (cord arterial pH <7.0) is approximately 3.7 per 1000 live births, while that of HIE at term is approximately 2.5 per 1000 live births [10]. The diagnosis of HIE requires evidence of intrapartum hypoxia and although there are various definitions [14–16], in essence there needs to be evidence of:
- an intrapartum insult (e.g. a sentinel event in labour or a pathological fetal heart recording);
- a metabolic acidosis at birth (pH <7.0 and base excess >12 mmol/L);
- moderate or severe neonatal encephalopathy;
- specific features on imaging in the neonatal period.

If cerebral palsy occurs as a result of HIE, it is of the spastic quadriplegic or dyskinetic type [14,16]. The incidence of cerebral palsy is 1–2 per 1000 deliveries and although the majority of these are due to antenatal complications, at least 10–15% result from events in labour [10].

Treatment and outcome of HIE

Severe acidaemia at birth (pH <7.0) does not always result in HIE, which in turn does not automatically result in cerebral palsy, but the more severe the metabolic acidosis at delivery and the more severe the HIE, the worse the prognosis for the baby. Individual clinical features and responses of the baby help inform the likely outcome as does cerebral imaging.

The greatest advance in this field is that of controlled total body cooling of neonates with HIE. The cooling needs to start within 6 hours of birth and has been shown to improve intact neonatal survival (relative risk of cerebral palsy 0.67, 95% CI 0.47–0.96) with number needed to treat of 8 (95% CI 5–17) [17,18]. The obstetrician's role in this process is one of early communication and frank discussion with neonatal colleagues to help clarify the obstetric history and the likely diagnosis, which should help to promote early cooling or referral to a centre that provides this treatment if it is not available locally (see Chapter 31).

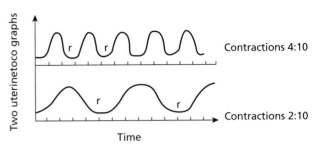

Fig. 27.1 Number of uterine contractions versus their duration in each 10-min period and how this influences the period of fetal recovery during uterine relaxation (r), both similar at approximately 4 min.

 Summary box 27.2

Factors that reduce oxygen delivery to the fetus:

Uteroplacental pathology
- Maternal demographics (age, smoking).
- Maternal diseases (hypertension, diabetes, sickle cell).
- Intrauterine growth retardation.
- Placental separation (marginal bleeds and abruptions).
- Post maturity.

Fetal pathology
- Fetal anaemia: rhesus isoimmunization, parvovirus infection.

Labour
- Uterine contractions (especially if hypertonic or with prolonged labour).
- Cord compression.
- Maternal hypotension (aortocaval compression).
- Obstetric emergencies (uterine rupture, abruptions, cord prolapse).

Midwives and obstetricians
- Injudicious use of prostaglandins or Syntocinon.

Labour

The rest of this chapter focuses on the normal physiology of labour and the fetal responses to labour, before highlighting abnormal labour patterns that increase fetal challenges and the problems which can arise from them. Without knowledge of the physiology and pathophysiology of labour, the anticipation and recognition of early signs of hypoxia may be missed. Failure to recognize the fetus at risk on entry to labour or failure to look for and then recognize early signs of hypoxia in labour can compromise the opportunity for prompt and timely action that may be crucial in avoiding irreversible damage.

The challenges of normal labour

Uterine contractions

In normal labour, the fetus is stressed due to uterine contractions. The uteroplacental circulation is a low-pressure system and its perfusion ceases at the height of a uterine contraction in the first stage of labour (where intra-uterine pressures reach about 90 mmHg) and throughout practically all of a contraction in the second stage of labour (intrauterine pressures up to 250 mmHg). Oxygen delivery to the fetus therefore effectively ceases during contractions.

A fetus in a normal pregnancy has adequate reserves of oxygen and can cope with this temporary insult as long as the uterus relaxes enough between contractions for gas transfer to occur. The interval between the contractions is *crucial* to allow this recovery (Fig. 27.1).

A less well-nourished fetus does not have adequate reserves even when the uterus is relaxed, and may have reduced or minimal energy reserves, so may not manage the episodic oxygen deprivation associated with each uterine contraction.

Head compression

The fetal head is subjected to pressure as it is compressed onto the cervix and through the pelvis by uterine contractions, and latterly this is exacerbated by maternal effort. Head compression can produce a reflex bradycardia due to changes in intracranial pressure. This is a normal autonomic response, but clearly during any bradycardic episode the fetal circulation is reduced, so once again a baby already compromised will be more affected by this temporary insult to oxygen delivery to the tissues.

Cord compression

The umbilical cord lies in random fashion around the fetus *in utero* and can wrap around or lie in close proximity to any part of the fetus so that during a contraction it can become squashed. This is increasingly likely once the membranes have broken. The normal autonomic

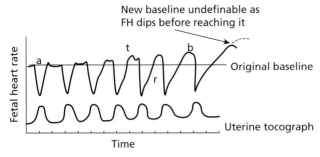

Fig. 27.2 Variable decelerations associated with cord compression demonstrating a typical dip (a). A rising baseline (b), a rebound tachycardia (t) and delayed recovery (r) are all suspicious signs.

responses of a healthy fetus to an episode of cord compression is the result of baroreceptor and chemoreceptor stimulation and proceed as follows.

• Umbilical vein obstructs, resulting in decreased cardiac return which stimulates baroreceptors that cause a tachycardia.
• Hypoxia from umbilical vein obstruction stimulates the chemoreceptors to trigger a parasympathetic response which produces a bradycardia.
• Umbilical artery obstruction raises peripheral resistance, exacerbating the bradycardia.
• As the contractions wear off, the process is reversed.

Thus cord compression, which is common, produces a fairly classic pattern of fetal heart rate (FHR) decelerations as a normal autonomic response in a healthy fetus (Fig. 27.2, pattern 'a'). However, as mentioned above, every time a deceleration occurs the fetal circulation is reduced and therefore adequate uterine relaxation between contractions is vital to allow recovery of the fetal circulation with subsequent tissue perfusion. Prolonged or repetitive decelerations can have a cumulative effect (Fig. 27.2). Moreover, cord compression is more common when there is reduced Wharton's jelly to protect the umbilical vessels, as with a premature or growth-restricted fetus, and these are therefore more likely to suffer cord compression as well as being already compromised.

The challenges of abnormal labour

Infection

Pyrexia in labour is associated with an increased risk of fetal hypoxic damage and cerebral palsy [19]. The two processes of hypoxia and sepsis seem to potentiate each other rather than being simply additive, and this process can escalate quickly needing early recognition and appropriate action. One problem is that epidural anaesthesia is associated with a rise in core temperature and therefore mild pyrexias in labour are now relatively common. This seems to be causing a rather relaxed attitude to fevers

in labour rather than raising alarm bells. Clinical vigilance is needed, with proper assessment and appropriate treatment.

• If there are clinical signs of infection, even a mild pyrexia is significant.
• If there is no regional blockade, pyrexia of 37.5°C is significant.
• Pyrexia of 38°C with regional blockade is significant.
• Paracetamol alone is not a treatment for infection: it may lower the temperature by nature of its antipyretic effect, and this is useful, but it does not mean that the infection is treated. 'Hiding' one of the signs of infection in this way can be dangerous.

In all the above situations appropriate microbiology cultures should be taken and antibiotic treatment started. Clinical awareness of the infection and what it might mean to fetal condition, fetal reserve and the likely tolerance of the fetus to the remaining labour will all play a part in timing the delivery.

Prolonged labour

A fetus has to tolerate more uterine contractions during prolonged labour. This is common with fetal malpositions and, as such, is also associated with induced labour for post-term pregnancies or prolonged rupture of membranes, both of which increase the risks to the fetus (added risk of uteroplacental insufficiency or infection, respectively).

Hypertonic uterine activity

This can occur spontaneously or be iatrogenic. When hypertonic uterine activity occurs spontaneously, it can be extremely concerning because it is likely to be associated with bleeding (which may be concealed retroplacental separation) and in such cases there is the added insult of placental separation as well as failure of adequate uterine relaxation for the fetus to contend with. This situation is very dangerous and fetal deterioration is likely to be rapid.

Conversely, iatrogenic hypertonic uterine contractions are reversible if recognized and acted upon. These can result from prostaglandin sensitivity or overdose as well as oxytocin overdose. A common obstetric and midwifery aim when stimulating labour with oxytocin is for a certain number of contractions every 10 min but as this focuses attention on the contraction and not the relaxation, it is easy to see why hyperstimulation is a relatively common problem [20–22]. If contractions last 1 min, then aiming for four contractions in 10 min is reasonable, but if they last 2 min squeezing four into 10 min will cause fetal hypoxia (see Fig. 27.1). The added problem here is that oxytocin tends to be used in abnormal labour (e.g. prolonged rupture of membranes, post-term inductions, prolonged labour) so there are many other risk factors for fetal compromise. Hyperstimulation often goes unrecognized, with the Syntocinon infusion continuing or even being increased further until FHR abnormalities develop.

Uterine rupture

This results in catastrophic interruption to fetal oxygenation and delivery needs to be effected within minutes. However, even with this dramatic pathology, signs other than fetal distress on heart rate monitoring may be minimal and the diagnosis is often not made until laparotomy [23]. Keeping the possibility in mind during problems with progress in labour or in those at increased risk may help to anticipate the diagnosis and lead to rapid action if needed.

Placental abruption

This may also be missed clinically as bleeding may be concealed and pain can be difficult to distinguish from labour, especially with a posterior placenta. Hypertonic uterine activity is a sign that is often missed because the focus of attention tends to be on the fetal heart and not the clinical signs and the tocograph. Therefore again the relatively later sign of an abnormal FHR pattern is often the only indication that there is something wrong.

Cord prolapse

Cord prolapse can also cause severe catastrophic cessation of fetal oxygenation requiring urgent delivery and is usually confirmed on vaginal examination after fetal heart abnormalities have been heard.

Detecting the fetus with hypoxia

Recognizing fetal risk

As the ability of any fetus to cope with labour depends on its condition on entry to labour, antenatal recognition of risk is vital in planning safe delivery. Any woman identified as high risk for fetal compromise in labour can then be cared for accordingly, while those of low risk can be monitored less intensively. Whichever technique is used, the aim of intrapartum monitoring of the fetus is to 'screen' for early signs of hypoxia in order to allow timely intervention and safe delivery before irreversible damage has been sustained. The priority with a low-risk pregnancy would be to have a detection system with a low false-positive rate so that unnecessary intervention is kept to a minimum; conversely, the priority for an at-risk fetus would be to have a detection system with a low false-negative rate and good sensitivity to identify the problem early.

The different techniques available for monitoring the fetus in labour are discussed below but it is worth pointing out that inevitably not all high-risk cases are detected antenatally and the unknown 'high-risk' fetus is especially vulnerable in labour because the index of suspicion

is absent. It is therefore important that with every woman and fetus admitted in labour, there is a deliberate effort to re-screen using history and examination to confirm normality before proceeding with the planned birth.

Summary box 27.3

Clinical scrutiny on admission in labour – be alert to clues for risk
- Antenatal risk factors may have been missed (revisit antenatal history).
- Risk factors may have developed since last seen (prolonged latent phase/rupture of membranes or bleeding).
- Examine carefully: fetal growth, liquor volume and colour, pyrexia.
- Labour characteristics: pattern of uterine contractions, fetal presentation.

Liquor and the passage of meconium

A good liquor volume is a reassuring sign that the fetus has not been subjected to chronic hypoxia in the antenatal period (discussed above). If no liquor is seen in labour after amniotomy (spontaneous or artificial), the safe assumption must be that there is oligohydramnios/anhydramnios. All practising midwives and obstetricians will have seen the thick 'green-pea soup' meconium following the delivery of a baby who had not previously been recognized as being compromised. The clinical secret is to think about this possibility and be clear that absence of liquor indicates oligohydramnios/anhydramnios until proved otherwise (e.g. in the labour ward setting this can be assessed by an ultrasound scan).

The other sign in labour is that of the colour of the liquor. The National Institute for Health and Clinical Excellence (NICE) guidelines on intrapartum care discusses whether the presence of particulate meconium is significant or not [24], but working from pathophysiological principles seems a more logical way to interpret the signs.
- A term fetus may have passed meconium by nature of its maturity, but if this is 'innocent' the meconium should be diluted by adequate liquor.
- If the fetus is preterm, the passage of meconium is not normal and may suggest infection or hypoxia.
- If the meconium is thick, then by definition the liquor volume is reduced and reflects uteroplacental insufficiency and possible fetal compromise.
- If the liquor has been clear and then becomes meconium stained during labour, it suggests that the fetus may be compromised and this could be due to either hypoxia or infection.

Fetal monitoring in labour

Searching for signs and understanding the condition of the fetus and the normal stresses or pathophysiological insults it is exposed to is the single most important part of fetal monitoring in labour. Omitting this fundamental process on admission in labour and proceeding directly to FHR monitoring assumes that all babies have the same reserves and vulnerabilities. The above discussions demonstrate how wrong such assumptions are: having an informed index of suspicion for a particular fetus and an understanding of any likely pathophysiology from the antenatal period and during labour increases the chance that signs of compromise will be detected early. Waiting until events are obvious is unthinking and dangerous as it may be too late to correct. To expect any monitoring system to dictate clinical decisions is unrealistic, illogical and hazardous.

The other point worth making before exploring the different techniques for monitoring the fetus in labour is that of the margin of error between the extremes of failing to recognize a fetus in difficulty (which will therefore sustain damage/death) and mistakenly identifying a healthy fetus as being in difficulty and subjecting it and the mother to an unnecessary operative delivery. When reviewing the different techniques of monitoring it is interesting to note that the trade-off is usually between increased operative delivery and increased neonatal morbidity, and the relative risks of these will depend on the background prevalences of pathology; hence the recommendation from NICE that low-risk women be monitored differently to high-risk women [24]. This does not remove an obligation to discuss the advantages and disadvantages with the pregnant woman in the antenatal period, so that she is informed and involved in the decisions surrounding her care in labour, particularly the fetal monitoring plan. The long-term outcomes of cerebral palsy and death are rare, and statistically significant differences have yet to be shown from the different monitoring modalities in low-risk pregnancies, although neonatal seizures are a significant concern and should not be ignored.

Historically, listening to the fetal heart has been the main method of monitoring the fetus in labour, but this is a step removed from the important information, which is whether oxygen supply is adequate for fetal tissue metabolism. If not and anaerobic metabolism has commenced, then by definition fetal hypoxia exists and is likely to get worse. The problem is that there is no direct continuous measure of fetal tissue pH, and even if there were it would be invasive and as such likely to be impractical for routine monitoring. Periodic fetal blood sampling (FBS) can be done in those showing signs of possible compromise, and to date this has been used when FHR pattern abnormalities have been found (discussed in more detail below). Fetal pulse oximetry has been explored as a means of measuring fetal oxygen saturation and is used in combination with FHR monitoring but randomized trials have failed to provide convincing evidence that it is helpful [25–27]. Near-infrared spectroscopy has also been explored [28,29] but has not been subjected to randomized clinical trials [30].

Fetal heart rate

FHR monitoring is the main technique used to supplement clinical scrutiny in intrapartum fetal monitoring. FHR is influenced by numerous factors that act largely through the two opposing divisions of the autonomic nervous system: the sympathetic nervous system, stimulation of which speeds up the rate, and the parasympathetic nervous system, stimulation of which slows it down. As such the heart rate is in a constant state of variation as these two influences oppose each other to maintain homeostasis. Both are responsive to the many stresses of labour, including changes in oxygen levels (via chemoreceptors), changes in fetal circulation (via baroreceptors) and infection, and these stresses are indirectly reflected in the FHR pattern. In addition, myocardial ischaemia also produces a fetal bradycardia. It is for these reasons that the FHR provides a reasonable indicator of fetal condition. This subject is well covered in the online K2 teaching programme.

> ### 💡 Summary box 27.4
>
> Fetal heart rate characteristics:
> - Baseline variability is the single most helpful parameter in screening for fetal hypoxia.
> - Baseline heart rate rises with chronic stresses including infection and hypoxia.
> - Baseline heart rate should not fall during labour; if it does, this reflects hypoxia.
> - Accelerations are a healthy sign.
> - Decelerations occur owing to:
>   - head compression (uniform and should be early);
>   - cord compression (variable and should be early; see Fig. 27.2); and
>   - hypoxia (late and either uniform or exist as extensions of the above dips)
> - What happens to the right-hand side of the deceleration shows how the fetus is coping with the stress (Fig. 27.3).

The NICE intrapartum care guidelines [24] classify features of the heart rate to assist with interpretation of fetal well-being. Table 27.2 summarizes the features defined by

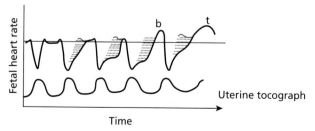

Fig. 27.3 Suspicious signs that the fetus is becoming compromised. The recovery phase from each deceleration (right-hand side of each dip) takes longer with successive contractions (shaded areas) and the baseline rises (b) with a rebound tachycardia (t).

Table 27.2 Summary of the NICE classification of fetal heart features.

Feature	Baseline (bpm)	Variability (bpm)	Decelerations	Accelerations
Reassuring	110–160	≥5	None	Present
Non-reassuring	100–109/161–180	<5 for 40–90 min	Variable for >90 min in >50% contractions Single prolonged dip for <3 min	Absence of unclear significance if all other features are normal
Abnormal	<100/>180 Sinusoidal for >10 min	<5 for >90 min	Atypical or late dips in >50% contractions for >30 min Prolonged dip for >3 min	

Table 27.3 Action required with abnormalities of the fetal heart.

Definition	Features	Action required
Normal	All four feautures are reassuring	Continue
Suspicious	One feature is non-reassuring but all other features are reassuring	Obstetric review and treat cause/change position
Abnormal	Two or more features are non-reassuring or one feature is abnormal	Fetal blood sampling or expedite delivery

NICE, but it should be remembered that the normal baseline values are taken from *populations* of healthy babies; it does not mean than the baseline of one fetus remains normal if it changes from, for example, 110 to 160bpm or from 160 to 110bpm over the course of labour. A small rise in the baseline (~20bpm) during the course of labour is common due to sympathetic stimulation (via adrenaline) but more than this suggests it is secondary to stresses such as hypoxia or infection; baselines rarely fall in labour (unless sepsis is treated for example) and hypoxia should be suspected.

These baseline changes are important and worthy of a word of caution: paper cardiotocograph traces are usually folded up as they print and then are neatly tucked away, while computerized traces only display a short section of the heart rate pattern at any one time. In both situations proper review of a trace requires deliberate unfolding or scrolling back to the preceding trace in order to evaluate it fully. The consequence of failure to do this is that important signs of deterioration may be overlooked.

The NICE classification [24] relates these parameters to definitions of normal, suspicious and pathological as shown in Table 27.3, where suggested actions for each are included.

Heart rate monitoring techniques

How is it best to monitor the fetal heart? The options are between intermittent auscultation (directly using a Pinard stethoscope or via an ultrasound transducer using Doppler) or continuous recording via Doppler transducer or fetal scalp electrode.

Intermittent auscultation

Listening directly to the fetal heart with a Pinard has been useful in the past, but although the device is small and cheap it has the disadvantage of only being heard by the person using it and the rate needs to be calculated by the listener. The hand-held Doppler machine is also small and portable but has the added advantages of magnifying the sound so that the woman and any other attendants can also hear the heart beat and it can also digitally display the heart rate. The only recording of these heart rates is done manually in the case notes. Listening should be after a contraction for a full minute on each occasion: every 15min in the first stage of labour and at least every 5min in the second stage. There is insufficient evidence to support one technique over the other, but one trial in Zimbabwe found more obstetric interventions and fewer neonatal complications when using the Doppler device compared with the Pinard stethoscope [31].

There are problems with intermittent auscultation: firstly, in clinical practice listening is often performed for less than 1min [32] and, secondly, because the heart rate varies during the course of the minute, the recommendation is that the rate is averaged [24]. This latter point is worthy of comment: baseline variability and changes in the baseline are of paramount importance in assessing fetal well-being and thus averaging the heart rate removes both. Recording a range is common practice (e.g 120–150 with accelerations and no decelerations) but a range without defining a baseline is not ideal; even on a trace it is difficult to distinguish accelerations and decelerations and it is much more difficult when just listening. This may explain why randomized controlled trials have consistently shown an increase in neonatal seizures in low-risk pregnancies monitored using intermittent auscultation compared with continuous electronic fetal monitoring (EFM) [24,33] (Table 27.4). However, as there is no statistically significant difference in rates of cerebral palsy or infant mortality, this disadvantage has to be weighed against the decreased risk of operative delivery associated with intermittent auscultation.

Admission cardiotocography

Because of the importance of assessment and risk stratification on admission in labour, and the potential disadvantages of intermittent auscultation, the concept of 'snapshot' cardiotocography (CTG) on admission to help differentiate the high-risk from the low-risk fetus is logical. Unfortunately, admission CTG in clinically low-risk pregnancies is not beneficial because they are associated with increased interventions without improved outcomes [34].

Cardiotocography

Electronic recording of the FHR with printout allows contemporaneous continuous recordings of the heart rate and a permanent record. The baseline and its variability are fairly easy to define and accelerations or decelerations from the baseline can be studied. As such it is a sensitive tool to document heart rate changes. Compared with intermittent auscultation its use improves fetal outcomes, with fewer neonatal seizures [33], but it impedes maternal mobility (unless telemetry transducers are used) and it tends to distract care from the woman to the monitor [32] and is associated with increased obstetric interventions (all forms of operative delivery).

The advantage of EFM is that it is very sensitive and detects the fetus at possible risk, but its poor specificity means that an abnormal trace does not mean the fetus is necessarily hypoxic. The need to improve the predictive value of EFM and reduce the disadvantage of increased operative delivery rates has focused research on additional techniques to supplement EFM when the trace is non-reassuring. Pulse oximetry and near-infrared spectroscopy have already been mentioned briefly as not yet being clinically useful [26–30]. Vibroacoustic stimulation for fetal assessment in labour in the presence of a non-reassuring FHR would be a logical tool to explore, but there are no randomized controlled trials of this [35]. The more invasive technique of intermittent FBS from the fetal scalp during labour is well integrated into intrapartum care as an adjunct to EFM and has been subject to clinical trials.

Fetal blood sampling

The reduction in operative delivery previously found when EFM was used with FBS is not supported by the most recent Cochrane review [33], but is still an integral part of intrapartum fetal monitoring and recommended

Table 27.4 Randomized controlled trials that have compared electronic fetal monitoring and intermittent auscultation (values are relative risk with 95% confidence interval in parentheses).

	All women*	Low-risk pregnancies[†]
Neonatal fits	0.5 (0.31–0.80)	0.36 (0.16–0.81)
Perinatal mortality	0.85 (0.59–1.23)	1.02 (0.31–3.31)
Instrumental vaginal delivery	1.16 (1.01–1.32)	
Caesarean section	1.66 (1.30–2.13)	
Total operative deliveries		1.35 (1.09–1.67)

*In over 37 000 pregnancies (12 trials) [33].
[†]NICE subset of three trials of low-risk pregnancies [24].

by NICE [24] except in acute fetal compromise where emergency delivery is needed, maternal infection (e.g. HIV and hepatitis), fetal bleeding disorders and prematurity (<34 weeks).

Most FBS measurements examine pH and gas values, but more recently fetal lactate has been measured. This needs a smaller blood volume and so has potential advantages to pH estimation. This comparison between pH and lactate measurements using fetal blood has now been the subject of two randomized controlled trials involving over 3348 women. While there were no differences in fetal outcomes or operative delivery rates, the success of FBS was greater in the lactate group due to the smaller volume of blood needed for analysis [36]. All FBS samples should be taken with the woman in the left lateral position to avoid aortocaval compression during the technique [24].

Interpretation of FBS results

The interpretation of the FBS result must include the clinical condition and the risk factors affecting the mother and fetus, and must allow for the fact that one result only reflects the pH/lactate at that moment. An isolated reading, even if normal, must not be taken as meaning there is no problem as the process of metabolic acidosis might only be starting (after hypoxaemia has proceeded to hypoxia, as described in detail earlier) and could yet accelerate quickly, depending on the cause. A pathological CTG requires repeat FBS even if the previous result was normal, to help assess the trend of fetal deterioration, and the timing of the repeat sample will depend on the nature of the CTG, the original result and, most importantly, the clinical features of the case. The NICE intrapartum guidelines describe the following classification and actions [24] (Table 27.5).

The aim is to achieve delivery before irreversible fetal damage, and to wait until severe acidaemia occurs in order to justify intervention is illogical if the chance of vaginal delivery is remote and the fetal condition is

Table 27.5 Fetal blood sample classification.

pH	Interpretation	Action suggested by NICE [24]	Appropriate clinical action
≥7.25	Normal	Repeat within 1 hour if trace stays pathological or sooner depending on trace	Clinical features should also influence this timing and falling results indicate compromise (see text)
7.21–7.24	Borderline	Repeat within 30 min or sooner depending on trace	Clinical features will determine whether this repeat sample is sensible or whether delivery should be expedited (see text)
≤7.20	Abnormal	Ask for consultant obstetric advice	Delivery is needed and consultant should be informed but this should not delay delivery

already deteriorating. Hence two successive fetal blood samples, an hour apart, with pH of 7.35 and 7.25 should not be reassuring: this fetus is deteriorating rapidly and in another hour it is likely that the next pH value will be below 7.20. The clinical decision here will be largely determined by whether the woman is 9 cm dilated and progressing quickly (in which case repeat FBS within the next 30 min might allow progress to full dilatation and vaginal delivery) or whether she is still 4 cm dilated despite Syntocinon for the last 4 hours (in which case expediting delivery by Caesarean section is likely to be more appropriate). This is why clinical judgement has to complement the basic rules suggested for guidance: such rules should not be followed unthinkingly.

Fetal blood sampling dilemmas
FHR abnormalities and oxytocin infusions cause enormous problems, and practice varies between stopping the oxytocin infusion to halt the FHR anomalies, stopping oxytocin until FBS is performed and found normal, or continuing the infusion and performing FBS. It should be remembered that contractions are needed for labour to progress, so the key decision is assessing the uterine contractions. The oxytocin infusion should continue if uterine contractions and relaxations are appropriate (see above) but if the fetal heart requires FBS, then proceed with it. NICE recommends stopping oxytocin if the trace is pathological until the FBS result is known; if it is normal, the oxytocin infusion can be restarted [24]. It needs to be remembered that FBS will need repeating to check that the fetus is not deteriorating with the augmented contractions.

FBS is rarely indicated at full dilatation as delivery is usually indicated for a pathological CTG, but a normal result can allow time for descent and rotation to convert what would have been a more complex operative delivery into a more straightforward one. If this is the plan, however, it should be remembered that the fetal condition deteriorates more quickly in second stage than in first stage (because of maternal effort) and such a policy is fairly high risk so the obstetrician should be on hand to effect delivery if the CTG deteriorates.

FBS is rarely supported in the presence of a uterine scar because fetal heart anomalies are often the first sign of problems with scar integrity and FBS can be falsely reassuring prior to what might be very rapid fetal demise. This decision should be taken at consultant level.

Fetal ECG

ST analysis
A relatively recent advance in intrapartum fetal heart monitoring has been the introduction of computerized analysis of the fetal ECG, particularly the ST segment. The fetal ECG is detected by means of an internal electrode (screwed into the fetal scalp) and the printout highlights when there is an ST event, namely elevation of the ST segment suggesting myocardial hypoxia. The original randomized trials [37–39] supporting this supplement to CTG monitoring suggested better neonatal outcomes with fewer operative deliveries, but the reality has been disappointing with a number of reports of problems when using this technique in routine clinical practice [40–42]. Furthermore, the most up-to-date Cochrane review suggests great caution in the interpretation of the results as one of the five trials included may not be completely reliable and is currently undergoing investigation by its relevant university [43]. The statistics from this meta-analysis are therefore not repeated here but suggest no difference in severe metabolic acidosis, rate of Caesarean section, Apgar scores below 7 at 5 min, or admission to the neonatal unit, while there appears to be fewer fetal blood samples and fewer operative vaginal deliveries.

The difficulties with this method of monitoring arise because of the following.
• ST events are frequent among controls (50%) with normal CTG and normal cord gas values [42].
• ST events, together with abnormal CTG patterns, appear late in the hypoxic process and are inconsistent (50% in moderate metabolic acidaemia, 67% in severe acidaemia) [42].
• If the ST event precedes the start of monitoring, it may not register [41].

A review of the first 1502 cases monitored in a teaching hospital in the UK showed no improvement in emergency operative delivery or neonatal encephalopathy rates [40]. The crux of the argument is that clinical decision-making when using this tool should include accurate CTG interpretation as well as registering the ST event, but the problem is that ST analysis has been marketed as reducing intervention because it is 'better' than CTG and it is therefore unsurprising that users have a tendency to disregard a pathological CTG if the ST event does not trigger [44].

Non-invasive fetal ECG

The other disadvantage of ST analysis is the internal spiral scalp electrode, which risks scalp trauma and transmission of infection. Work is currently underway exploring the signal pick-up and feasibility of external electrodes placed on the maternal abdomen [45]. This would avoid the spiral electrode problem, but difficulties remain with ST analysis and how to relate it to CTG interpretations in clinical practice.

The future

The conflict between the need to detect the fetus in danger and to expedite delivery while avoiding unnecessary intervention remains. The following suggestions or research examples demonstrate where further developments may improve this inexact science.

• Antenatal detection of growth restriction can be improved by the use of customized charts, and thorough antenatal care and admission assessments in labour will further help stratify women and their babies into lower- or higher-risk groups.

• Intermittent auscultation techniques for low-risk pregnancies could be further explored to establish whether neonatal outcomes can be improved by critically specifying the baseline (and variability from that baseline) rather than just recording an average rate or a range for FHR.

• Computerized CTG analysis is well established in, and has improved the accuracy of, antenatal EFM (where failing to fulfil the Dawes and Redman criteria is associated with acidaemia and intrauterine deaths) [46,47]. Development of this tool for intrapartum CTG application has had promising results [48] and further trials of intelligence systems are underway.

• Clinical flags that alert the clinician in real time during EFM and which take into account clinical factors as well as CTG parameters may all improve the detection of fetal compromise, but will never replace clinical acumen. Maintaining an alert, enquiring, critical review of the whole clinical picture will always be needed and highly valued. There is no place for complacency and the hope that machines will tell clinicians what to do is unrealistic.

Summary

Intrapartum fetal monitoring must start from a clinically inquisitive stance where all antenatal factors are assimilated and added to observations on presentation in labour. Distinguishing between low- and high-risk pregnancies will then tend towards one particular approach to fetal monitoring but it should be remembered that whichever technique is chosen, none is foolproof, and continued vigilance and awareness of clinical developments in labour are needed. This anticipation of hypoxia should help early recognition of problems so that appropriate action can avoid both unnecessary intervention and inappropriate inactivity which could lead to irreversible damage to the fetus.

References

1 K2 fetal monitoring training system. Available at: https://training.k2ms.com.

2 Eskes TK, Jongsma HW, Houx PC. Percentiles for gas values in human umbilical cord blood. *Eur J Obstet Gynecol Reprod Biol* 1983;14:341–346.

3 Westgate J, Garibaldi JM, Greene KR. Umbilical cord blood gas analysis at delivery: a time for quality data. *Br J Obstet Gynaecol* 1994;101:1054–1063.

4 Arikan GM, Scholz HS, Petru E, Haeusler MCH, Haas J, Weiss PAM. Cord blood oxygen saturation in vigorous infants at birth: what is normal? *BJOG* 2000;107:987–994.

5 Low JA, Lindsay BG, Derrick EJ. Threshold of metabolic acidosis associated with newborn complications. *Am J Obstet Gynecol* 1997;177:1391–1394.

6 Malin GL, Morris RK, Khan KS. Strength of association between umbilical cord pH and perinatal and long term outcomes: systematic review and meta-analysis. *BMJ* 2010;340:1471.

7 Goldaber KG, Gilstrap LC III, Leveno KJ, Dax JS, McIntire DD. Pathologic fetal acidemia. *Obstet Gynecol* 1991;78:1103–1107.

8 Sehdev HM, Stamilio DM, Macones GA, Graham E, Morgan MA. Predictive factors for neonatal morbidity in neonates with an umbilical arterial cord pH less than 7.00. *Am J Obstet Gynecol* 1997;177:1030–1034.

9 Goodwin TM, Belai I, Hernandez P, Durand M, Paul RH. Asphyxial complications in the term newborn with severe umbilical acidemia. *Am J Obstet Gynecol* 1992;167:1506–1512.

10 Graham EM, Ruis KA, Hartman AL, Northington FJ, Fox HE. A systematic review of the role of intrapartum hypoxia–ischemia in the causation of neonatal encephalopathy. *Am J Obstet Gynecol* 2008;199:587–595.

11 Chief Medical Officer. *On the State of Public Health: Annual Report of the Chief Medical Officer 2007*. Available at: www.dh.gov.uk/en/Publicationsandstatistics/Publications/AnnualReports/DH_086176.

12 Confidential Enquiry into Maternal and Child Health. *Perinatal Mortality 2007*. London: CEMACH, 2009. Available at: www.cemach.org.uk/getattachment/bc6ad9f0-5274-486d-b61a-8770a0ab43e7/Perinatal-Mortality-2007.aspx.

13 Maternal and Child Health Research Consortium. *Confidential Enquiry into Stillbirths and Deaths in Infancy, 4th Annual Report,*

1 January–31 December 1995. London: Maternal and Child Health Research Consortium, 1997.

14 MacLennan A. A template for defining a causal relation between acute intrapartum events and cerebral palsy: international consensus statement. *BMJ* 1999;319:1054–1059.

15 ACOG Committee Opinion. Use and abuse of the Apgar score. Number 174, July 1996 (replaces No. 49, November 1986). Committee on Obstetric Practice and American Academy of Pediatrics: Committee on Fetus and Newborn. American College of Obstetricians and Gynaecologists. *Int J Gynaecol Obstet* 1996;54:303–305.

16 American Congress of Obstetricians and Gynecologists Task Force on Neonatal Encephalopathy and Cerebral Palsy. *Neonatal Encephalopathy and Cerebral Palsy: Defining the Pathogenesis and Pathophysiology.* Washington, DC: ACOG, 2011.

17 Azzopardi DV, Strohm B, Edwards AD *et al.* Moderate hypothermia to treat perinatal asphyxial encephalopathy. *N Engl J Med* 2009;361:1349–1358.

18 Edwards AD, Brocklehurst P, Gunn AJ *et al.* Neurological outcomes at 18 months of age after moderate hypothermia for perinatal hypoxic ischaemic encephalopathy: synthesis and meta-analysis of trial data. *BMJ* 2010;340:c397.

19 Grether JK, Nelson KB. Maternal infection and cerebral palsy in infants of normal birth weight. *JAMA* 1997;278:207–211.

20 Jonsson M, Norden SL, Hanson U. Analysis of malpractice claims with a focus on oxytocin use in labour. *Acta Obstet Gynecol Scand* 2007;86:315–319.

21 Berglund S, Grunewald C, Pettersson H, Cnattingius S. Severe asphyxia due to delivery-related malpractice in Sweden 1990–2005. *BJOG* 2008;115:316–323.

22 Jonsson M, Norden-Lindeberg S, Ostlund I, Hanson U. Metabolic acidosis at birth and suboptimal care: illustration of the gap between knowledge and practice. *BJOG* 2009;116:1453–1460.

23 Maternal and Child Health Research Consortium. *Confidential Enquiry into Stillbirths and Deaths in Infancy: 5th Annual Report: Focus on Ruptured Uterus.* London: Maternal and Child Health Research Consortium, 1998.

24 National Institute for Health and Clinical Excellence. *Intrapartum Care: Management and Delivery of Care to Women in Labour.* Clinical Guideline CG55, 2007. Available at: http://guidance.nice.org.uk/CG55/Guidance/pdf/English.

25 Garite TJ, Dildy GA, McNamara H *et al.* A multicentre controlled trial of fetal pulse oximetry in the intrapartum management of non-reassuring fetal heart rate patterns. *Am J Obstet Gynecol* 2000;183:1049–1058.

26 Kuhnert M, Schmidt S Intrapartum management of non-reassuring fetal heart rate patterns: a randomised controlled trial of fetal pulse oximetry. *Am J Obstet Gynecol* 2004;191:1989–1995.

27 East CE, Chan FY, Colditz PB, Begg L. Fetal pulse oximetry for fetal assessment in labour. *Cochrane Database Syst Rev* 2007;(2): CD004075.

28 Peebles DM, Edwards AD, Wyatt JS. Changes in human fetal cerebral haemoglobin concentration and oxygenation during labour measured by near-infrared spectroscopy. *Am J Obstet Gynecol* 1992;166:1369–1373.

29 Aldrich CJ, D'Antona D, Wyatt JS, Spencer JA, Peedles DM, Reynolds EO. Fetal cerebral oxygenation measured by near-infrared spectroscopy shortly before birth and acid–base status at birth. *Obstet Gynecol* 1994;84:861–866.

30 Mozurkewich EL, Wolf FM. Near-infrared spectroscopy for fetal assessment during labour. *Cochrane Database Syst Rev* 2000; (3):CD002254.

31 Mahomed K, Nyoni R, Mulambo T *et al.* Randomised controlled trial of intrapartum fetal heart rate monitoring. *BMJ* 1994; 308:497–500.

32 Altaf S, Oppenheimer C, Shaw R, Waugh J, Dixon-Woods M. Practices and views on fetal heart monitoring: a structured observation and interview study. *BJOG* 2006;113:409–418.

33 Alfirevic Z, Devane D, Gyte GML. Continuous cardiotocography (CTG) as a form of electronic fetal monitoring (EFM) for fetal assessment during labour. *Cochrane Database Syst Rev* 2006; (3):CD006066.

34 Blix E, Reiner LM, Klovning A *et al.* Prognostic value of labour admission test and its effectiveness compared with auscultation only: a systematic review. *BJOG* 2005;112:1595–1604.

35 East CE, Smyth RMD, Leader LR, Henshall NE, Colditz PB, Tan KH. Vibroacoustic stimulation for fetal assessment in labour in the presence of a non-reassuring fetal heart rate trace. *Cochrane Database Syst Rev* 2005;(2):CD004664.

36 East CE, Leader LR, Sheehan P, Henshall NE, Colditz PB. Intrapartum fetal scalp lactate sampling for fetal assessment in the presence of a non-reassuring fetal heart rate trace. *Cochrane Database Syst Rev* 2010;(3):CD006174.

37 Westgate J, Harris M, Curnow JS, Greene KR. Plymouth randomised trial of cardiotocogram only versus ST waveform plus cardiotocogram for intrapartum monitoring in 2400 cases. *Am J Obstet Gynecol* 1993;169:1151–1160.

38 Amer-Wahlin I, Hellsten C, Noren H *et al.* Cardiotocography only versus cardiotocography plus ST analysis of fetal electrocardiogram for intrapartum fetal monitoring: a Swedish randomised controlled trial. *Lancet* 2001;358:534–538.

39 Ojala K, Vaarasmaki M, Makikallio K, Valkama M, Tekay A. A comparison of intrapartum automated fetal electrocardiography and conventional cardiotocography: a randomised controlled study. *BJOG* 2006;113:419–423.

40 Doria V, Papageorghiou AT, Gustafsson A, Ugwumadu A, Farrer K, Arulkumaran S. Review of the first 1502 cases of ECG-ST waveform analysis during labour in a teaching hospital. *BJOG* 2007;114:1202–1207.

41 Westerhuis ME, Kwee A, van Ginkel AA, Drogtrop AP, Gyselaers WJ, Visser GH. Limitations of ST analysis in clinical practice: three cases of intrapartum metabolic acidosis. *BJOG* 2007;114:1194–1201.

42 Melin M, Bonnevier A, Cardell M, Hogan L, Herbst A. Changes in the ST-interval segment of the fetal electrocardiogram in relation to acid–base status at birth. *BJOG* 2008;115: 1669–1675.

43 Neilson JP. Fetal electrocardiogram (ECG) for fetal monitoring during labour. *Cochrane Database Syst Rev* 2006;(3):CD000116.

44 Apantaku OO. Review of the first 1502 cases of ECG-ST waveform analysis during labour in a teaching hospital [Letter]. *BJOG* 2008;115:922–923.

45 Cleal JK, Thomas M, Hanson MA, Paterson-Brown S, Gardiner HM, Greene LR. Noninvasive fetal electrocardiography following intermittent umbilical cord occlusion in the preterm ovine fetus. *BJOG* 2010;117:438–444.

46 Dawes GS, Moulden M, Redman CWG. Short-term fetal heart-rate variation, deceleration and umbilical flow velocity waveforms before labour. *Obstet Gynecol* 1992;80:673–678.

47 Street P, Dawes GS, Moulden M, Redman CWG. Short-term variation in abnormal antenatal fetal heart rate records. *Am J Obstet Gynecol* 1991;165:515–523.

48 Schiermeier S, Pildner von Steinburg S, Thieme A *et al*. Sensitivity and specificity of intrapartum computerised FIGO criteria for cardiotocography and fetal scalp pH during labour: multicentre, observational study. *BJOG* 2008;115:1557–1563.

Further reading

Confidential Enquiry into Maternal and Child Health. *Perinatal Mortality 2007*. London: CEMACH, 2009. Available at: www.cemach.org.uk/getattachment/bc6ad9f0-5274-486d-b61a-8770a0ab43e7/Perinatal-Mortality-2007.aspx.

K2 fetal monitoring training system. Available at: https://training.k2ms.com.

National Institute for Health and Clinical Excellence. *Intrapartum Care: Management and Delivery of Care to Women in Labour*. Clinical Guideline CG55, 2007. Available at: http://guidance.nice.org.uk/CG55/Guidance/pdf/English.

Royal College of Obstetricians and Gynaecologists. *Intrauterine Infection and Perinatal Brain Injury*. Scientific Advisory Committee Opinion Paper 3, 2007. Available at: www.rcog.org.uk/files/rcog-corp/uploaded-files/SAC3IntrauterineInfection2007.pdf.

Chapter 28
Preterm Labour

Phillip Bennett
Imperial College London, London, UK

Epidemiology

Definitions

Preterm birth is defined as delivery of a baby before 37 completed weeks of pregnancy. Legally, in the UK, the 1992 Amendment to the Infant Life Preservation Act defined the limit of viability as 24 weeks. However, a small number of infants born at 23 weeks will survive. Mortality and morbidity in preterm babies born after 32 weeks' gestation is similar to that of babies born at term. The risk of neonatal mortality or survival with handicap becomes significant in very preterm infants, defined as those born between 28 and 32 weeks, but is most significant in extremely preterm infants, defined as those born before 28 weeks. In modern obstetric practice assessment of gestational age is based on both the date of the last menstrual period and ultrasound fetal biometry. In the past, however, assessment of gestational age was not always accurate and paediatric statistics may be based on birthweight rather than gestational age data. Low birthweight is defined as less than 2.25 kg, very low birthweight as less than 1.5 kg and extremely low birthweight as less than 1 kg. Using these definitions to describe outcome data leads to blurring of the distinction between preterm babies and small-for-gestational age babies, particularly in the low birthweight category, and also fails to differentiate the normally grown preterm neonate from the neonate who is both preterm and small for gestational age [1,2].

Incidence

The incidence of preterm birth in the developed world is 7–12%. There has been a small gradual rise in the incidence of preterm birth associated with assisted reproduction causing multiple pregnancies and an increased tendency to obstetric intervention. The rate of preterm birth prior to 32 weeks has remained relatively stable at 1–2%. About one-quarter of preterm births are elective deliveries, usually for pre-eclampsia, intrauterine growth restriction or maternal disease. The remainder are due to preterm labour and delivery. Of these, up to 30% are associated with preterm pre-labour rupture of the fetal membranes. The incidence of spontaneous preterm labour is at its lowest in women in their twenties. The risk is increased in teenagers and in women over 30. There is a higher incidence of preterm labour in first pregnancies. Higher parity alone is not a risk factor for preterm labour. Indeed there is a progressively lower risk with each successive term birth. Marital status, cigarette smoking, environmental stress, poor nutrition and use of alcohol, coffee and street drugs (especially cocaine) have all been linked to an increased risk of preterm birth. Many of these factors are interlinked and are all factors associated with social disadvantage.

There does appear to be an association between race and risk of preterm delivery. In the UK, the risk of preterm birth is 6% in white Europeans but 10% in Africans or Afro-Caribbeans but it is also difficult to differentiate genetic variation from social deprivation. In studies of populations where black and white women have similar lifestyles, levels of income and access to medical care (e.g. in US Army personnel) preterm delivery rates show a less marked ethnic variation. The recent identification of specific genetic polymorphisms that increase the risk of preterm labour does suggest that there may be genetic as well as environmental factors which explain the increased risk of preterm labour in certain ethnic populations. Intervention studies have shown that antenatal smoking cessation programmes reduce the risk of preterm birth. However, there is no evidence currently that other interventions such as increased frequency of antenatal care, dietary advice or an increase in social support reduce the risk.

Neonatal outcomes after preterm birth

Survival rates for preterm babies have improved steadily over the past two decades due to the introduction of surfactant therapy, improvements in neonatal respiratory management and more widespread use of antenatal steroids. Although the number of babies above 24 weeks who

Dewhurst's Textbook of Obstetrics & Gynaecology, Eighth Edition. Edited by D. Keith Edmonds.
© 2012 John Wiley and Sons, Ltd. Published 2012 by John Wiley and Sons, Ltd.

Table 28.1 Survival rates and birth centiles at gestational ages between 23 and 34 weeks.

Gestational age (weeks)	Weight 50th centile (g)	Weight 10th centile (g)	Weight 90th centile (g)	Survival (%)	Survival percent without major morbidity
23	600	450	970	6	2
24	700	550	1180	15	5
25	790	620	1250	45	15
26	880	700	1350	60	20
27	960	780	1450	75	50
28	1080	820	1600	85	60
29	1220	940	1720	90	80
30	1400	1050	1900	93	85
31	1600	1180	2100	96	90
32	1760	1300	2300	97	92
33	1980	1480	2500	97	95
34	2200	1650	2700	98	97

survive has increased, there has been no improvement in survival at the lower limits of viability below 23 weeks. The Epicure study [3] reported mortality rates of 100, 90 and 80% for preterm infants admitted to the neonatal unit at 21, 22 and 23 weeks' gestation respectively. Improved survival for very preterm infants has been associated with an increase in the proportion of children with cerebral palsy who were born preterm. Neonatal mortality rises gradually between 32 and 28 weeks from 2 to 8% and then more dramatically and exponentially to 80% at 23 weeks (Table 28.1).

In the past, surfactant deficiency leading to neonatal respiratory distress syndrome (RDS) was the major cause of morbidity and mortality in preterm infants. Alveolar surfactant production begins at 30–32 weeks' gestation. Therefore preterm infants born prior to 30 weeks are at highest risk. The impact of RDS on neonatal morbidity and mortality has been dramatically reduced in the past two decades through use of antenatal corticosteroids and exogenous surfactant replacement. However, the risk of chronic lung disease, defined as a need for ventilation or oxygen supplementation at 36 weeks after conception, has continued to rise because of the increased survival of extremely preterm infants. The fetal and neonatal brain is especially susceptible to injury between 20 and 32 weeks after conception. The greatest risk of long-term neural developmental problems is in infants born before 28 weeks or at birthweights of less than 1 kg. The Epicure study showed that in infants born before 26 weeks' gestation, approximately half had some disability at 30 months and approximately one-quarter had severe disability (Fig. 28.1).

Cerebral palsy may be related to periventricular haemorrhage, post-haemorrhagic hydrocephalus and periventricular leucomalacia. Hypoxia–ischaemia is a major risk factor for neonatal cerebral damage. However, there is growing evidence for a strong link between chorioamnio-

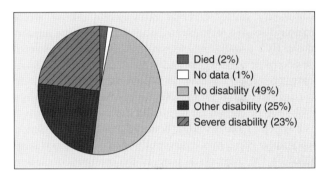

Died (2%)
No data (1%)
No disability (49%)
Other disability (25%)
Severe disability (23%)

Fig. 28.1 Outcomes for surviving infants born before 26 weeks' gestation when assessed at 30 months. (Adapted from Wood *et al.* [6] and Colvin *et al.* [7].)

nitis, fetal inflammation and the risk of periventricular leucomalacia [4,5].

Germinal matrix and intraventricular haemorrhage

Intraventricular haemorrhage is principally a feature of preterm babies born before 34 weeks' gestation since it arises in the subependymal germinal matrix (an area containing cells that will eventually migrate to other parts of the brain), which is found lining the cerebral ventricles and is only present between 24 and 34 weeks. Germinal matrix haemorrhage may be limited to germinal matrix itself or, in more severe cases, bleeding will occur into the cerebral ventricles. It is thought that germinal matrix haemorrhage occurs as a result of the combination of vulnerable immature cerebral development, the increased tendency to bleeding in the preterm neonate, and some form of interruption to cerebral vascular flow. Risk factors for germinal matrix haemorrhage are therefore those factors which increase the risk of prematurity, haemodynamic events and bleeding. Prenatal risk factors include maternal aspirin therapy. Factors at the time of delivery include severe prematurity, vaginal breech delivery, birth trauma and birth asphyxia. Postnatal factors include RDS, particularly if complicated by pneumothorax, acidosis or hypoxia, disturbance of blood clotting, bruising and episodes of hypotension [8,9].

Periventricular leucomalacia

Periventricular leucomalacia (Greek *malakia*, softening and *leukos*, white) is softening of the white matter of the brain and is seen adjacent to the cerebral ventricles at post-mortem examination of some preterm neonates. In the human brain, periventricular cerebral white matter is at especially increased risk of injury between 23 and 34 weeks' gestation. More than 80% of preterm infants develop white matter abnormalities. The two common patterns, cystic periventricular leucomalacia (PVL) and diffuse white matter disease, are characterized by reduced white matter volume, reduced brain growth and abnormal myelination on magnetic resonance imaging. PVL commonly causes cerebral palsy while diffuse white matter disease is thought to cause neurocognitive impairment. PVL usually therefore has its cause in the preterm period prior to 34 weeks and is most often seen in infants born preterm. However, it is possible for the insult to occur preterm but for the child to be born at term. Rarely PVL may be caused by insults occuring nearer to term.

It was previously widely believed that PVL represented a hypoxic–ischaemic injury to an area of the brain supplied by the most distal parts of the cerebral circulation in what is termed a 'watershed' area. The earliest descriptions of PVL associated the condition with hypoxic events, severe hypertensive pre-eclampsia, and in women who had seizures during their pregnancy. More recently significant doubt has been cast upon the concept that all cases of PVL are due to a hypoxic–ischaemic episode. Firstly, more modern and sophisticated anatomical studies have suggested that the areas affected by PVL are not in fact boundary zones between the most distal regions of the cerebral circulation. More importantly, a significant body of recent literature has found a strong association between bacterial infection and/or chorioamnionitis and white matter injury. It is now thought that cytokines released by inflammation and bacterial endotoxins released by infection may lead indirectly to cerebral injury by producing hypotension and intravascular coagulation and directly to cerebral injury through destruction of oligodendrocytes and proliferation of astrocytes. It seems likely that the periventricular areas represent white matter regions that are sensitive to injury from both hypoxia–ischaemia and inflammation and in some cases it may be that both mechanisms function together [9].

Visual and auditory impairment

The risk of visual impairment due to retinopathy of prematurity is inversely related to gestational age and directly related to the concentration and duration of oxygen treatment. Despite improvements in the management of oxygen therapy, most infants born before 28 weeks' gestation will develop some form of retinopathy. The risk of retinopathy of prematurity rises dramatically from less than 10% at 26 weeks to above 50% in infants born at 24 weeks. About 3% infants born before 28 weeks' gestation will require a hearing aid and 50% will be found to have learning difficulties at school requiring additional educational support [10].

Endocrinology and biochemistry of labour

To effectively predict and prevent labour requires a good understanding of the endocrinology and biochemistry underlying the onset of labour in humans, both at term and preterm. Unfortunately our understanding of the mechanisms leading to the onset of human labour is incomplete, partly because the mechanisms in different species appear to have evolved differently, making direct extrapolation of data from animal models to the human not necessarily valid.

Labour as an inflammatory process

Throughout pregnancy the uterine cervix needs to remain firm and closed whilst the body of the uterus grows by hypertrophy and hyperplasia but without significant fundally dominant contractions. For labour to be successful the cervix is converted into a soft and pliable structure that can efface and dilate and the uterus becomes a powerful contractile organ. There is no single endocrinological or biochemical switch in the human which changes the uterus from its no-labour state to its labour state. The onset of labour is a gradual process that begins several weeks before delivery with changes in the lower pole of the uterus that cause cervical ripening and effacement. The onset of clinically identifiable contractions is a relatively late event in this process. Cervical ripening occurs through breakdown of collagen, changes in proteoglycan concentrations and an increase in water content. The lower segment of the uterus also stretches and relaxes and behaves physiologically more like the cervix than the contractile upper segment of the uterus. These changes in the lower segment of the uterus are associated with an increase in the production of inflammatory cytokines, particularly interleukin (IL)-1, IL-6 and IL-8, and prostaglandins in the overlying fetal membranes and decidua and in the cervix itself. Cervical ripening is associated with an influx of inflammatory cells into the cervix that release matrix metalloproteins which contribute to the anatomical changes associated with ripening. The later increase in fundally dominant contractility in the upper segment of the uterus is associated with an increase in the expression of receptors for oxytocin and prostaglandins, in gap junction proteins that mediate electrical connectivity between myocytes, and in more complex changes in intracellular signalling pathways that increase the contractility of the myocytes [11].

Roles of progesterone, corticotrophin-releasing hormone and oxytocin

Progesterone is considered to play a major role in the maintenance of pregnancy. In 1956 Csapo proposed that the essential role of progesterone in pregnancy is to 'block' myometrial contractility and that the onset of labour therefore requires withdrawal of progesterone. In the majority of mammals labour is preceded by a decline in circulating progesterone concentrations. The mechanism for progesterone withdrawal varies among species [12].

So, in the rodent for example, prostaglandin-mediated regression of the corpus luteum leads to a fall in progesterone concentrations immediately prior to the onset of labour. In the sheep increased production of cortisol from the fetal adrenal signals fetal maturation and induces placental 17α-hydroxylase, which increases synthesis of oestrogen at the expense of progesterone, again leading to progesterone withdrawal prior to the onset of labour. There is no systemic withdrawal of progesterone in the human prior to labour, although there is an increase in the expression of genes formerly repressed by progesterone, which has led to the hypothesis of 'functional progesterone withdrawal' mediated by changes in the expression of progesterone receptors or of cofactors needed for the function of the progesterone receptor [13]. Another hypothesis is that inflammatory events seen within the uterus at the time of labour are associated with increased activity of nuclear factor (NF)-κB, a transcription factor strongly associated with inflammation in other contexts such as asthma, inflammatory bowel disease and arthritis [14]. NF-κB is known to repress the function of the progesterone receptor and so could mediate functional progesterone withdrawal. Although in the mouse progesterone concentrations fall due to luteolysis just prior to labour, there is still sufficient circulating progesterone to activate progesterone receptors. In the mouse it appears that the final event leading to parturition is the increased production of surfactant protein A from the fetal lung, which stimulates the activity of NF-κB within the uterus leading to an influx of inflammatory cells, an increase in inflammatory cytokine synthesis and depression of the residual function of the progesterone receptor. It is an attractive hypothesis that pulmonary maturation in the human may also signal the final phase of the onset of labour but there is at present no direct evidence that this mechanism applies in the human [15].

Progesterone is widely thought to inhibit contractions principally by repressing contraction-associated proteins such as gap-junction proteins, oxytocin and prostaglandin receptors and prostaglandin-metabolizing enzymes. However, it is now emerging that progesterone plays a more complex role in myometrial physiology during pregnancy via phenotypic modulation of myocytes during the synthetic phase of myometrial differentiation in the last third of pregnancy, during which there is myometrial hypertrophy and synthesis and deposition of interstitial matrix [16].

Circulating levels of corticotrophin-releasing hormone (CRH), synthesized in the placenta, increase progressively throughout pregnancy and especially during the weeks prior to the onset of labour. CRH-binding protein concentrations fall with advancing gestational age such that, approximately 3 weeks prior to the onset of labour, the concentration of CRH exceeds that of its binding protein. Unlike in the hypothalamus, placental CRH is upregulated by cortisol. Several studies have linked placental production of CRH with the timing of birth and have demonstrated that a premature rise in CRH is associated with preterm delivery [17].

In the monkey, uterine contractions occur only at night. In the days preceding labour and delivery there are nocturnal non-fundally dominant contractions that have been termed 'contractures'. The conversion from contractures to contractions is mediated by an increase in the production of oxytocin from the maternal posterior pituitary gland. In the monkey therefore whilst the fetus might signal its general readiness to be born through increased cortisol production from the adrenal, the precise timing of birth is signalled by the mother. This may be a mechanism of defence against predators which ensures that delivery is always at night. Contrary to the experience of many obstetricians, this phenomenon does not apply to the human. There is no increase in the production of oxytocin associated with the onset or progression of either preterm or term labour. However, there is an increase in the expression of oxytocin receptors within the uterus and there is local production of oxytocin in the uterus, decidua and fetal membranes. Although oxytocin probably does not play an important role in the precise timing of parturition in the human, an increase in the density of oxytocin receptors suggests that oxytocin does play a role in mediating contractility. Nevertheless, it remains possible that the principal physiological function of oxytocin receptor expression in myometrium is to mediate contraction and involution during breast-feeding [18].

However, there is now evidence that oxytocin receptor is expressed in the fetal membranes, particularly the amnion, and that expression increases in parallel with the expression of prostaglandin synthetic enzymes. In the amnion oxytocin clearly has no contractile function but does increase the synthesis of prostaglandin E₂. The source of the oxytocin which binds to amnion oxytocin receptors is not known but neurohypophysial oxytocin may diffuse from the maternal circulation across the amnion to the epithelium. Although the amnion is avascular, large amounts of oxytocin have been found to be present in decidua, chorion and amnion where the placenta was delivered shortly after administration of a bolus of exogenous Syntocinon to the mother, suggesting that oxytocin can diffuse from the maternal circulation to the amnion. It has been proposed that the fetus may secrete oxytocin into the amniotic fluid and that the chorion/decidua is capable of synthesizing the full neurophysin/oxytocin peptide directly. This suggests a clear role for oxytocin in the initiation of parturition, although the source of the relevant oxytocin may be largely local rather than systemic [19].

Causes of preterm labour

Preterm labour is not a single disease entity but is a symptom or syndrome that may have one or more causes (Fig. 28.2). Preterm labour has been linked to cervical incompetence, abnormalities of haemostasis, infection within the uterus, placental abruption or decidual haemorrhage, fetal or maternal stress and multiple pregnancy. In some cases several of these factors may act together to increase the likelihood of preterm delivery or to affect the gestational age at which preterm delivery occurs. So, for example, twin pregnancies deliver at 35 weeks. Multiple pregnancy probably leads to preterm delivery through at least two mechanisms and may increase the risk where other risk factors are present. Over-distension of the uterus leads to premature upregulation of contraction-associated proteins and of factors that mediate cervical ripening, all of which have been shown to be sensitive to mechanical stretch. Multiple pregnancy is associated with multiple placentae and therefore with an earlier rise in placental CRH concentrations in the circulation. A preterm delivery in twins at 28 weeks will not be due simply to the multiple pregnancy and must have another aetiology associated with it, for example infection or cervical weakness. Had the same pregnancy been a singleton preg-

nancy it is probable that the preterm delivery would have occurred at a later gestational age.

Cervical function

With improved survival at early gestational ages, there is now overlap between second-trimester pregnancy loss and early preterm delivery. Historically, cervical incompetence was diagnosed in women who experienced persistent, often rapid and painless, late second-trimester pregnancy loss. More recently the concept of cervical competence as a continuum has evolved. It is probable that cervical length and strength together with the quality of the cervical mucus contribute to function of the cervix, both to retain the pregnancy within the uterus and to exclude potential bacterial pathogens from ascending from the vagina. Numerous studies have demonstrated a strong relationship between cervical length and the risk of preterm delivery. The cervix may be damaged (or completely removed) by surgery in the treatment of cervical cancer or, rarely, during a difficult instrumental vaginal delivery or Caesarean section at full dilatation. There are also associations between exposure to diethylstilbestrol *in utero* and developmental anomalies in the genital tract and cervical weakness. However, this is less of a problem now that the women who were exposed to diethylstilbestrol are now generally beyond childbearing age. A short or partially dilated cervix may allow bacteria to ascend into the lower pole of the uterus where, acting through Toll-like receptors of the innate immune system, they stimulate activation of NF-κB, production of inflammatory cytokines and prostaglandins and the inflammatory response. This then leads to cervical ripening and shortening, which in turn decreases the ability of the cervix to act as a mechanical or a microbiological barrier and, ultimately, leads to the development of either localized or generalized chorioamnionitis and to preterm delivery. A short or weak cervix may therefore contribute to preterm delivery not only by leading to simple second-trimester miscarriage but also by contributing to a risk of ascending infection that leads to a more classical spontaneous preterm labour.

Common clinical experience shows that cervical 'incompetence' is not simply a matter of mechanical strength. A common manifestation of cervical incompetence is a woman who presents with vague pelvic pain, minimal bleeding and vaginal dampness. On taking a more detailed history many women will report previous cervical surgery, usually for cervical intraepithelial neoplasia (CIN), and speculum examination will show the cervix to be open and the membranes bulging through it. In these cases it is clear the cervix has not simply opened but has changed physically and is usually very thin and ripe. In some cases it is possible to completely reverse this cervical change following rescue cervical cerclage, whereas it is almost impossible to halt the progression of

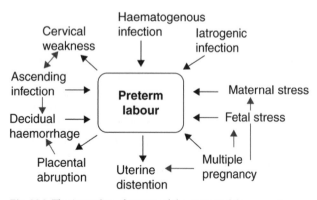

Fig. 28.2 The interplay of causes of the preterm labour syndrome.

labour and delivery once contractions have started (see below).

Cervical surgery

There is a strong correlation between extensive cervical surgery or damage and preterm delivery [20]. Radical trachelectomy confers a very high risk. Although it is now usual practice to place a high cervical cerclage at the time of trachelectomy, only 50% of such patients will take a pregnancy to term, about 15% will experience second-trimester pregnancy loss and 35% will deliver preterm. Other treatments for cervical malignancy and intraepithelial neoplasia are associated with a risk of preterm delivery. Cold knife conization increases the risk threefold, whilst loop excision of the transformation zone doubles the risk. Cervical damage associated with failed instrumental delivery or Caesarean section at full dilatation where disimpaction of the fetal head may cause a cervical tear may also lead to preterm labour in subsequent pregnancies.

Genital tract infection

There is a strong correlation between infection within the uterus and the onset of spontaneous preterm labour. As discussed above, infection within the uterus has the potential to activate all the biochemical pathways ultimately leading to cervical ripening and uterine contractions. A scenario has been described above where it is cervical weakness or shortness which is the primary factor leading to a risk of ascending bacterial infection. However, it is also possible that with a high number of virulent pathogens in the vagina, bacteria may gain access to the lower pole of the uterus through a normally functioning cervix, where they activate inflammatory mediators leading to cervical ripening and shortening. Bacteria may also gain access to the amniotic cavity through haematogenous spread or by introduction at the time of invasive procedures. Following preterm delivery, histological chorioamnionitis is usually more common and severe at the site of membrane rupture than elsewhere. In virtually all cases of congenital pneumonia, inflammation of the fetal membranes is also present. The bacterial species identified in the majority of cases of congenital infections are usually also found in the maternal lower genital tract. Following twin preterm delivery, chorioamnionitis is more common and severe in the presenting twin than in the second twin. These factors all suggest that ascending infection from the lower genital tract is the commonest mechanism for chorioamnionitis. However, there is also evidence that haematogenous spread of oral bacteria may play a key role in some cases of preterm labour, although studies of intensive dental hygiene in pregnancy have not shown it to reduce the risk [21,22].

Romero and Mazor [22] have proposed a four-stage sequence in chorioamnionitis: (i) overgrowth of potential pathogens in the vagina or cervix possibly associated with bacterial vaginosis; (ii) presence of the organisms in the uterine cavity, particularly in the decidua of the lower segment; (iii) a localized inflammatory reaction leading to deciduitis, chorionitis and extension through the amnion into the amniotic cavity; and (iv) infection of the fetus itself by aspiration and swallowing of infected amniotic fluid. The most common microbial isolates from the amniotic cavity of women in preterm labour are *Ureaplasma urealyticum*, *Fusobacterium* and *Mycoplasma hominis*. More than 50% of patients in preterm labour will have more than one microorganism isolated from the amniotic cavity. Microorganisms can be identified in the fetal membranes of the majority of women delivering both preterm and at term. It is probable that some cases of spontaneous preterm delivery are due to the generation of an excessive inflammatory response and, to a lesser degree, to bacterial invasion of the amniotic cavity. So, for example, it has recently been demonstrated that bacterial vaginosis (see below) may be a greater risk factor for preterm labour in women who carry a high secretory form of the gene for tumour necrosis factor (TNF)-α.

Haemorrhage

Placental abruption may lead to the onset of preterm labour. This is thought to be through release of thrombin, which stimulates myometrial contractions by protease-activated receptors but independently of prostaglandin synthesis. This may explain the clinical impression that preterm labour associated with chorioamnionitis is often rapid, whereas that associated with placental abruption is less so because there is no pre-ripening of the uterine cervix. Generation of thrombin may also play a role in preterm labour associated with chorioamnionitis when it is released as a consequence of decidual haemorrhage [23].

Fetal and maternal stress

There is evidence that both fetal and maternal stress may be risk factors for preterm labour. Fetal stress may arise in association with abnormal placentation and growth restriction. Maternal stress could be due to environmental factors. In both cases it is postulated that over-secretion of cortisol leads to upregulation of CRH production in the placenta [24].

 Summary box 28.1

- Preterm labour is a syndrome with multiple causes, not a single disease.
- Infection/inflammation is strongly associated with perinatal brain injury.
- Preterm labour before 30 weeks is more likely to be associated with infection/inflammation.

Prediction of preterm labour

In many cases of preterm labour obstetric management consists principally of attempting to suppress contractions in women who are already in established labour. As discussed in more detail below, this strategy is essentially ineffective. Strategies to reduce perinatal morbidity and mortality associated with preterm labour should involve the early identification of women at risk and the use of prophylactic therapies. Attempts have been made to devise risk scoring systems based on socio-demographic characteristics, anthropomorphic characteristics, past history, patient behaviour and habits and factors in the current pregnancy. None of these systems has been found to have positive predictive values or sensitivities that make them clinically useful. Most systems rely heavily on past obstetric history and are therefore irrelevant to women having their first baby. At present there are no screening tests which are routinely applied to primigravid women, or to multigravid women who are not at high risk for preterm labour.

Past obstetric history

Women at high risk of preterm labour will initially be detected based on past obstetric history [25] (Table 28.2). A single previous preterm delivery increases the risk of preterm delivery in a subsequent pregnancy fourfold compared with a previous delivery at term. Interestingly, a past obstetric history of a term delivery followed by a preterm delivery confers a higher risk of preterm delivery in the third pregnancy than a past obstetric history of a preterm delivery followed by a term delivery. This may be because the latter group contains a disproportionate number of women whose preterm delivery was for 'non-recurring' causes such as placental abruption, whereas in the former group some cases of preterm delivery following the term delivery may be due to damage to the cervix during the original term delivery.

Table 28.2 Effect of past obstetric history on relative risk of preterm delivery.

First delivery	Second delivery	Relative risk of preterm labour
Term		1
Preterm		4
Term	Term	0.5
Preterm	Term	1.3
Term	Preterm	2.5
Preterm	Preterm	6.5

Source: adapted from Hoffman & Bakketeig [25].

Bacterial vaginosis

The principal organism in the normal vaginal flora is *Lactobacillus*, a bacterium that produces lactic acid from glycogen and leads to an acid pH in vaginal secretions. The combination of large numbers of lactobacilli and the low pH is a protective mechanism against colonization with potential pathogens. Many important potential pathogens can be found in the vagina of healthy women, although in normal healthy pregnancies the numbers of lactobacilli increase as pregnancy progresses. Bacterial vaginosis is an abnormality of the normal vaginal flora characterized by a reduced number of lactobacilli, a higher pH and increased numbers of potential pathogens including *Gardenerella vaginalis*, *Escherichia coli*, group B *Streptococcus* and the anaerobes *Peptostreptococcus*, *Bacteroides* and *Mycoplasma hominis*. Since the presence of large numbers of lactobacilli and a low vaginal pH are important mechanisms that protect against the growth of potential pathogenic organisms, bacterial vaginosis represents a risk factor for preterm delivery. Diagnosis of bacterial vaginosis can be made by Gram staining or gas–liquid chromatography of vaginal fluid, or on clinical grounds based on high vaginal pH, a fishy odour in a thin homogeneous vaginal discharge and the presence of clue cells in the discharge on a wet mount (Table 28.3). There is no significant difference in the ability of each of these diagnostic tests to predict preterm birth. Studies of the risk of preterm labour associated with bacterial vaginosis have reported widely varying results. However, it appears that, overall, bacterial vaginosis approximately doubles the risk of preterm delivery.

Although there is evidence that bacterial vaginosis is a risk factor for preterm delivery, it is less clear that treating bacterial vaginosis with antibiotics is beneficial. This may be partly because various studies of bacterial vaginosis have used different antibiotics in different regimens and at different times, although it may also reflect the fact that antibiotics may not necessarily result in the re-establishment of normal bacterial flora. The two antibiotics commonly used in the treatment of bacterial vaginosis are metronidazole administered orally or clindamycin given either orally or vaginally. Clindamycin may have advantages over metronidazole since it has better activity against the anaerobic bacteria *M. hominis* and *U. urealyticum*, which are often associated with bacterial vaginosis. The current evidence is that screening can be justified in pregnant women who are at high risk for preterm delivery based on their past obstetric history or other factors and treatment of bacterial vaginosis but there is not currently strong evidence to recommend the routine screening and treatment of the general obstetric population [26].

Ultrasound measurement of cervical length

There is now good evidence that transvaginal sonographic measurement of cervical length can be used to

Table 28.3 Identification of bacterial vaginosis (BV).

Nugent's criteria

Scoring system: BV diagnosed if score >7

0	No morphotypes per oil-immersion field
1+	<1 morphotype per oil-immersion field
2+	1–4 morphotypes per oil-immersion field
3+	5–30 morphotypes per oil-immersion field
4+	>30 morphotypes per oil-immersion field

Score	Large Gram-positive rods*	Small Gram-variable or Gram-negative rods[†]	Curved Gram-variable rods[‡]
0	4+	0+	0
1	3+	1+	1–2+
2	2+	2+	3–4+
3	1+	3+	
4	0+	4+	

* *Lactobacillus acidophilus.*
[†] *Gardnerella vaginalis* and *Bacteroides* species.
[‡] *Mobiluncus* species.

Spiegel's criteria

Normal: Gram stain shows predominance of *Lactobacillus acidophilus* (3+ or 4+), with or without *Gardnerella vaginalis*

Bacterial vaginosis: Gram stain shows mixed flora (Gram-positive, Gram-negative or Gram-variable bacteria) and absent or decreased *L. acidophilus* (zero to 2+)

L. acidophilus: large Gram-positive bacilli

G. vaginalis: small Gram-variable rods

Scoring for each of the above bacterial morphotypes

0	No morphotypes per oil-immersion field
1+	<1 morphotype per oil-immersion field
2+	1–5 morphotypes per oil-immersion field
3+	6–30 morphotypes per oil-immersion field
4+	>30 morphotypes per oil-immersion field

Amsel's diagnostic criteria

Thin homogeneous discharge

Positive 'whiff' test

Clue cells present on microscopy (highly significant criterion)

Vaginal pH >4.5

Three of four criteria must be met

Gas–liquid chromatography

Succinate to lactate ratio >4

predict the risk of preterm labour in both low- and high-risk pregnancies and in women who are symptomatic. Transabdominal measurement of cervical length is unreliable because of the need for a full bladder, which may compress the cervix leading to an overestimate of its length, and because it is more difficult to obtain adequate views of the cervix with this technique. Transvaginal measurement of cervical length is performed with the bladder empty. A sagittal long-axis view of the entire endocervical canal is obtained with the probe in the anterior fornix of the vagina. The probe should be withdrawn until the image is blurred, and enough pressure reapplied to restore the image and so avoid excessive pressure on the cervix, which can elongate it. The cervical length is measured from the internal to the external os along the endocervical canal which may require several calliper sets to account for a non-linear canal. It is usual to obtain at least three measurements and record the shortest best measurement in millimetres. Fundal pressure is then applied to determine whether there is any further funnelling and shortening [27] (Fig. 28.3).

Two strategies are currently in common use: serial measurement of cervical length throughout the second and early third trimester of pregnancy or a single measurement of cervical length usually at the time of the routine ultrasound at 18–22 weeks. At any given gestational age there is a direct relationship between cervical length and the risk of preterm delivery. So, for example,

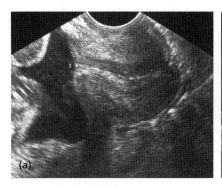
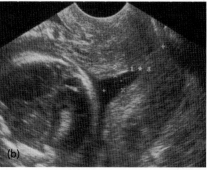

Fig. 28.3 Transvaginal measurement of cervical length. Top panel: normal cervix. Bottom panel: cervix showing funnelling and associated shortening.

Table 28.4 Risk of preterm delivery in asymptomatic women at high risk of preterm labour following measurement of cervical length.

Cervical length before 20 weeks (mm)	Risk of preterm labour	Cervical length between 20 and 24 weeks (mm)	Risk of preterm labour
15	62	15	56
20	28	20	30
22	20	22	15
25	12	25	9
27	10	27	6
30	6	30	4.6

> **Summary box 28.2**
>
> - Preterm labour may be predicted from past history, ultrasound measurement of cervical length and detection of fibronectin in cervicovaginal secretions.
> - At present there are no screening tests that are routinely applied to primigravid women, or to multigravid women who are not at high risk for preterm labour.
> - Bacterial vaginosis is a risk factor for preterm delivery, but it is not clear that treating bacterial vaginosis with antibiotics is beneficial.

a cervical length of 15 mm or less at 20–24 weeks predicts a 50% risk of preterm delivery prior to 34 weeks in a low-risk population. In multiple pregnancies the risk of preterm labour is higher at any given cervical length than in a singleton pregnancy with the same cervical length. A large number of studies have examined the relationship between gestational age, cervical length and the risk of preterm delivery (see review by Honest *et al.* [28]) (Table 28.4). It appears that it is the absolute cervical length rather than the presence or absence of funnelling that is the principal predictor of spontaneous preterm birth. If a screening strategy using a single ultrasound measurement of cervical length is used, then assessment between 21 and 24 weeks' gestation appears to be a better predictor of preterm labour than cervical length prior to 20 weeks. However, it is arguable that identification of a risk of preterm labour as late as 23 weeks may be too late for any potential prophylactic therapies to be effective. Serial measurement of cervical length is more costly but appears to be superior to a single measurement in assessing the risk of preterm delivery [29].

In continental Europe it is common practice to perform a vaginal assessment of cervical length at each antenatal consultation. However, multicentre trials have shown that this policy is of no benefit in predicting the risk of preterm delivery.

Prevention of preterm delivery

In primigravid women with no other significant risk factors for preterm delivery there is currently no effective method for the prediction of preterm labour and therefore management can only be instituted at the time of acute presentation with contractions. However, it is possible to identify a subgroup of women who can be identified as being at risk of preterm delivery based on their past obstetric history, the presence of abnormalities of the genital tract, and the use of screening tests such as measurement of cervical length and detection of fetal fibronectin in vaginal secretions. At present no prophylactic therapy has been demonstrated to be unequivocally beneficial in preventing the onset of preterm labour in a high-risk population. There is no evidence that oral beta-sympathomimetic drugs reduce the risk of preterm delivery and their use has generally been abandoned in UK obstetric practice. Commonly used therapies include cervical cerclage, non-steroidal anti-inflammatory drugs (NSAIDs) and progesterone.

Cervical cerclage

As discussed above, cervical competence is not a discrete entity but should be considered to be on a continuum. Abnormalities of cervical function may be a major factor or a minor contributor to the biochemical and mechanical events that lead to preterm delivery. There is probably considerable overlap between the mechanisms of second-trimester pregnancy loss and early preterm delivery. It is clear that in women whose history strongly suggests cervical weakness, for example those with a past history of cervical surgery or those with recurrent episodes of rapid relatively painful second-trimester fetal loss, cervical cerclage will significantly improve the prospects for success in subsequent pregnancies. Where the aetiology of previous second-trimester pregnancy loss or preterm delivery points less clearly to an obvious role for cervical weakness, then whether to insert a cervical cerclage is largely a matter for individual clinical judgement. A short cervix prior to pregnancy or in early pregnancy, relatively rapid or painless early preterm delivery and absence of symptoms of dysmenorrhoea all point to the possibility that cervical dysfunction may contribute to preterm delivery. An association between preterm delivery and chorioamnionitis does not necessarily discount a cervical problem since, as discussed above, there is interplay between cervical function and genital tract microbiology which means that, even in cases where cervical function is undoubtedly abnormal, there is likely to be a degree of chorioamnionitis associated with preterm delivery. Preterm deliveries which are later (beyond 32 weeks) or which are associated with major placental abruption, fetal growth restriction or pre-eclampsia are less likely to have a cervical element in their aetiology.

There have been few studies of the benefit of cervical cerclage in reducing the risk of preterm delivery partly because the views of obstetricians in this area are polarized and because it has been difficult to persuade clinicians to randomize their patients into trials. The RCOG/MRC trial [30] showed that cervical cerclage does reduce the risk of preterm delivery but that 25 patients would need to receive a cerclage for it to benefit one patient. Although it was previously widely believed that cervical cerclage increased the risk of genital tract infection, there is no good evidence for this. Nevertheless, there are clearly risks associated with the actual insertion of cervical cerclage and there has therefore been interest in trying to more precisely target cervical cerclage. There have been several studies where women previously defined as at high risk of preterm delivery have had serial ultrasound measurements of cervical length performed, with cerclage being performed when cervical length reached a predetermined cut-off. The CIPRACT study [31] randomized women found to have a cervical length of 25 mm or less before 27 weeks to either cervical cerclage and bed rest or bed rest alone. This study showed a significant benefit of cerclage in reducing the preterm delivery rate and improving neonatal morbidity. Rust and Roberts [32] randomly assigned 138 women whose cervical length was less than 25 mm between 16 and 24 weeks to cerclage or no cerclage and showed no benefit of cerclage. However, in this study there was a delay in the introduc-tion of cerclage to allow the results of amniocentesis to be obtained and a higher incidence of placental abruption.

To *et al.* [33] randomized 255 women from a low-risk population whose cervical length was found to be 15 mm or less at a single ultrasound examination at 22–24 weeks to either cerclage or no cerclage and found that although the strategy identified a group of women who were at high risk of early preterm birth, cervical cerclage did not reduce that risk. However, the screening event in this study was relatively late in pregnancy. The study therefore inevitably excluded any women having late second-trimester pregnancy loss or very early preterm delivery and the failure of cervical cerclage to be beneficial may have been due to the fact that those women who had the potential to benefit from cerclage had already developed biochemical and mechanical changes in the lower pole of the uterus which made their preterm delivery inevitable.

If ultrasound-indicated cervical cerclage is to be used, the appropriate threshold has not yet been established. Groom *et al.* [34] have shown that the presence of visible fetal membranes at the time of cervical cerclage is a strong prognostic indicator of preterm delivery. Visible fetal membranes are never seen at a cervical length greater than 15 mm. The threshold for cervical cerclage should therefore probably be greater than 15 mm, which may also explain the lack of positive findings in the large study of To *et al.* [33]. Given that the data on ultrasound-indicated cervical cerclage is currently limited and variable in its conclusions, further evaluation of this strategy is required before it is used widely in routine clinical practice.

It is not yet proven but is probable that cervical cerclage will improve the outcome in women with cervical dysfunction following surgery for cancer or CIN, although the great majority (85–90%) of women who have a cone biopsy LLETZ (large loop excision of the transformation zone) procedure will deliver at term. It may be in this group that measurements of cervical length may be used to more appropriately target these women for cervical cerclage. If cerclage was not perfomed at the time of the original surgery, trachelectomy would be an indication for cerclage. Because this may be technically difficult, it would be better to perform the procedure prior to pregnancy if possible since this allows for safer dissection and the suture may be nore accurately placed at the level of the internal os.

Emergency 'rescue' cerclage

Rescue cervical cerclage may be performed when a woman is admitted with silent cervical dilatation and bulging of the membranes into the vagina but without the onset of uterine contractions. Characteristically such women present with slight vaginal bleeding, a watery vaginal discharge, or vague pelvic or vaginal pain. One small, prospective, non-randomized study has suggested

Summary box 28.3

- Progesterone therapy has been shown to reduce the risk of preterm labour in women at high risk with a singleton pregnancy but long-term benefit for the neonate has not yet been proven.
- Progesterone therapy has not been shown to reduce the risk of preterm birth in multiple pregnancy.
- A short cervix prior to pregnancy, rapid or painless preterm deliveries and absence of symptoms of dysmenorrhoea point to the possibility that cervical dysfunction may contribute to preterm delivery.
- Cervical surgery for cancer or CIN is a risk factor for preterm delivery.

that rescue cervical cerclage improves birthweight and is not associated with a significant increase in the frequency of chorioamnionitis, maternal morbidity or perinatal mortality. The median pregnancy prolongation following emergency cervical cerclage is approximately 7 weeks. Poor outcome in these cases is usually due to chorioamnionitis and so rescue cerclage should not be performed where there is clinical evidence of sepsis, including elevated white cell count or C-reactive protein (CRP). This applies particularly at gestational ages close to the limit of viiality because of the risk of prolonging pregnancy in the presence of chorioamnionitis and so increasing the risk of the birth of a viable baby but with cytokine-mediated CNS damage. Whether antibiotics are beneficial in such cases has not been established. NSAIDs have been given during the procedure to reduce prostaglandin release stimulated by manipulation of the cervix and fetal membranes, but again there is currently no evidence that NSAID treatment improves outcome.

Non-steroidal anti-inflammatory drugs

The central role for prostaglandins and inflammatory cytokines in the aetiology of preterm labour suggests that NSAIDs may be beneficial in preventing preterm delivery. NSAIDs work largely by inhibition of the cyclooxygenase enzymes that catalyse the synthesis of prostaglandins. However, various NSAIDs also have other mechanisms of action, including effects on intracellular signalling pathways and on transcription factors including NF-κB. There are two major isoforms of the cyclooxygenase enzyme termed COX-1 and COX-2. COX-1 is constitutively expressed in the majority of cells whereas COX-2 is inducible and catalyses the synthesis of prostaglandins at the sites of inflammation. COX-2 is the principal cyclooxygenase associated with the increased prostaglandin synthesis that occurs at the time of labour. NSAIDs may be divided into three classes: those that are non-selective, those selective for COX-2 but which still have some action against COX-1, and those specific for COX-2.

Although there are several studies of the use of NSAIDs in the acute management of preterm labour, there are few good randomized trials of their use as prophylaxis. NSAIDs are associated with significant fetal side effects, in particular oligohydramnios and constriction of the ductus arteriosus. Oligohydramnios occurs in up to 30% of fetuses exposed to indometacin. The effect is dose dependent and may occur with both short-term and long-term exposure. Discontinuation of therapy usually results in rapid return of normal fetal urine output and resolution of the oligohydramnios.

Constriction of the ductus arteriosus occurs in up to 50% of fetuses exposed to indometacin at gestational ages greater than 32 weeks. There is a relationship between dose and duration of therapy and gestational age. Ductal constriction is seen less commonly below 32 weeks and rarely below 28 weeks. Long-term indometacin therapy, particularly after 32 weeks, is therefore associated with a significant risk of neonatal pulmonary hypertension.

It has been suggested that the use of NSAIDs which are selective or specific for COX-2 might be associated with a lower risk of fetal side effects. However, nimesulide, which is approximately 100-fold more effective at inhibiting COX-2 than COX-1, is nevertheless associated with an incidence of fetal oligohydramnios similar to that seen in fetuses exposed to indometacin and there have been isolated case reports of fetal renal failure. Groom *et al.* [35] studied the use of the COX-2 specific NSAID rofecoxib used prophylactically in a cohort of women at high risk of preterm delivery. Rofecoxib was associated with less effect on fetal renal function and the ductus arteriosus than that seen with indometacin or nimesulide. Unfortunately, the risk of preterm delivery prior to 32 weeks was not reduced by rofecoxib therapy and once rofecoxib was discontinued at 32 weeks, the rate of preterm delivery then increased in the rofecoxib-exposed patients. At present therefore there is no good evidence that NSAIDs confer benefit when used as prophylaxis for preterm labour. They are associated with a significant risk of potentially life-threatening side effects. If NSAIDs such as indometacin are to be used, for example as short-term therapies in association with cervical cerclage, then it is essential that there should be ultrasound surveillance of fetal urine production or amniotic fluid index and of the ductus arteriosus and that therapy should be stopped when fetal side effects become evident.

Progesterone

Progesterone is thought to inhibit the production of proinflammatory cytokines and prostaglandins within the uterus and to inhibit myometrial contractility. Although a meta-analysis in 1990 by Kierse [36] suggested that progesterone may be beneficial in reducing the risk of preterm delivery, it was not until the publication of two trials in 2003 that there was more widespread interest in the possibility that progesterone might be used as a prophylactic treatment in women at high risk of preterm delivery. In 2003, Da Fonseca *et al.* [37] reported that women who were at high risk of preterm delivery and were randomized to receive a 100-mg vaginal suppository daily between 24 and 33 weeks had a lower rate of preterm delivery (13.8% at 37 weeks, 2.8% before 34 weeks) compared with the placebo group (28% before 37 weeks, 18.6% before 34 weeks). In a similar study Meis *et al.* [38] used weekly injections of 250 mg of 17α-hydroxyprogesterone caproate between 16 and 36 weeks and this reduced the preterm delivery rate from 55 to 36% before 37 weeks and from 19 to 11% before 32 weeks. In this study the neonates of mothers treated with progesterone also had lower rates of necrotizing enterocolitis, intraventricular haemorrhage and the need for supplemental oxygen.

Although progesterone appears to be beneficial in singleton pregnancies at risk of preterm birth, two large studies have shown that it does not decrease the rate of preterm birth where the principal risk factor is multiple pregnancy [39,40]. Furthermore, it is not clear that short-term neonatal benefits translate into improved longer-term outcome. There are now a number of randomized controlled trials being conducted in various countries some of which have long-term paediatric primary outcomes and, ideally, patients at high risk of preterm labour should be enrolled in one of these studies.

However, the weight of both basic science and clinical evidence currently points to progesterone being potentially beneficial in women at high risk of preterm delivery, except where the only risk factor is multiple pregnancy, and there appear to be few if any side effects.

Management of acute preterm labour

Diagnosis
As discussed in more detail below, there is little evidence to suggest that use of tocolytic drugs, intended to suppress uterine contractions, confers any real benefit in cases of preterm labour. However, there is good evidence that the antenatal administration of corticosteroids to the mother and *in utero* transfer from a peripheral unit to a hospital with neonatal intensive care facilities significantly improves the outcome for the preterm neonate. It is therefore essential that a diagnosis of preterm labour should not be overlooked. It is usual to define the onset of labour at term as being when regular uterine contractions lead to cervical change or dilatation. To leave a woman with preterm contractions until there is cervical dilatation without either administering steroids or arranging an *in utero* transfer may be disadvantageous to the neonate. Preterm labour is therefore generally diagnosed solely on the basis of the presence of uncomfortable or painful regular uterine contractions. All the placebo-controlled trials of tocolytic drugs show a very high placebo response rate. From these it can be concluded that of women who attract a diagnosis of preterm labour sufficient to result in treatment with tocolytic drugs, some 60% will remain undelivered after 48 hours and close to 50% will deliver at term. Trials comparing tocolytic therapies often have apparent response rates of 80–90%, which are not consistent with the results of placebo-controlled trials. This is usually because comparison trials have recruited mostly women with contractions who were not genuinely in preterm labour and who would have delivered much later or at term. The results of such trials are therefore unreliable except for comparison of side-effect profiles. Tocolytic drugs may be potentially harmful or expensive. Unnecessary *in utero* transfer consumes healthcare resources and there is growing concern about the possible long-term side effects of exposure of the fetus to high-dose corticosteroid therapy. It is therefore highly desirable that obstetricians have some form of test which can differentiate the woman genuinely in preterm labour from the woman with preterm contractions who will not go on to deliver preterm. Tests based on the spectrum of electrical activity in the uterus are currently in development and are yielding encouraging results. At present, however, the two tests best able to differentiate true from false preterm labour are transvaginal measurement of cervical length and detection of fetal fibronectin in the vagina. In the UK, the lack of availability of a transvaginal ultrasound machine on the labour ward, and of an appropriately qualified or experienced clinician to perform the procedure, but the ready availability of bedside testing for fetal fibronectin means that fetal fibronectin testing is probably the optimal diagnostic test.

Fetal fibronectin testing
Fetal fibronectin is a glycoprotein present in amniotic fluid, placenta and the extracellular substance of the decidua. Its synthesis and release is increased by the mechanical and inflammatory events that occur prior to the onset of labour. Fetal fibronectin may normally be detected in vaginal secretions up to 20 weeks' gestation (at which time the amnion and chorion become fused) and is then normally undetectable until about 36 weeks' gestation.

The presence of fibronectin in vaginal secretions between 20 and 36 weeks may be used to predict a risk of preterm labour [41]. Fibronectin testing may be used to assess risk in asypomatic women at high risk of preterm labour. However, it is distinguishing true from false preterm labour in symptomatic women where fibronectin testing is probably of most value. Whilst a positive fibronectin test in a symptomatic woman only predicts a risk of preterm delivery within the next 7 days for approximately 40%, a negative fetal fibronectin test

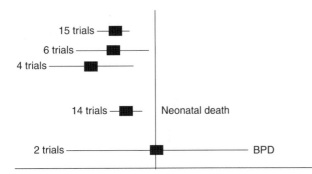

Fig. 28.4 Meta-analysis of the effect of antenatal corticosteroid administration on neonatal outcomes. (Adapted from Roberts & Dalziel [42].)

reduces the risk to less than 1%. This is a level of risk at which it would be reasonable to withhold *in utero* transfer and treatment.

Acute tocolysis

The maximum benefit to the preterm neonate from antenatal corticosteroid administration is from 24 hours to 7 days after the first dose (Fig. 28.4). *In utero* transfer has also been shown to improve neonatal morbidity and mortality and clearly time would be required to move a mother in preterm labour from one hospital to another. Suppression of uterine contractions may therefore be an obvious solution to the problem of preterm labour. However, meta-analysis of the effect of tocolytic administration on preterm delivery and neonatal outcomes shows that although tocolysis may delay preterm birth, this does not appear to be associated with any improvement in neonatal outcome (Fig. 28.4). Nevertheless, although it is unproven, the rationale for using tocolysis is that delaying preterm birth allows time for steroid adminstration and *in utero* transfer and that this will improve outcome.

Sympathomimetics

With the introduction beta-sympathomimetics into obstetric practice in the 1970s, accompanied by small clinical trials that suggested great efficacy in inhibiting preterm contractions, most obstetricians developed the impression that tocolysis with ritodrine or salbutamol was an effective therapy for acute preterm labour. This impression was strengthened because of the very high placebo response rate. More modern studies have shown that ritodrine will delay preterm delivery in a minority of patients for 24–48 hours but that its use is not associated with any improvement in any marker of neonatal morbidity or in neonatal mortality rates [43]. Ritodrine and salbutamol are associated with significant, potentially life-threatening maternal side effects (particularly if given in combination with corticosteroids) that include fluid overload, pulmonary oedema, myocardial ischaemia, hyperglycaemia and

hypocalcaemia. Numerous maternal deaths have been reported in which tocolysis using sympathomimetic drugs has played a role. Sympathomimetics as tocolytics are now rarely used in the UK and because safer though not necessarily more effective tocolytic drugs are now available, their use should now be completely abandoned.

Non-steroidal anti-inflammatory drugs

The NSAID most widely studied as an acute tocolytic is indometacin. Randomized placebo-controlled studies suggest that indometacin may significantly delay preterm delivery for 24 and 48 hours and for 7 days. However, the total number of women enrolled in all three randomized placebo-controlled trials is only 90 [44]. As discussed above, indometacin has a major effect on fetal renal function and on the fetal cardiovascular system, in particular the fetal ductus arteriosus. Use of indometacin for tocolysis has also been associated with higher incidences of necrotizing enterocolitis, intraventricular haemorrhage and abnormalities in neonatal haemostasis. In experimental animals the combination of a COX-2-specific NSAID and a tocolytic (either a calcium channel blocker or an oxytocin antagonist) appears to be superior to the use of a tocolytic alone, although this type of combination therapy has not yet been properly evaluated in the human. At present there is no evidence that indometacin or any other NSAID has any advantage as a first-line tocolytic over calcium channel blockers or oxytocin antagonists, each of which has a much better maternal and fetal side-effect profile.

Magnesium sulphate

Prior to the 1980s magnesium sulphate was widely used in the USA in the intrapartum management of pre-eclampsia and eclampsia and the clinical impression that magnesium sulphate made induction of labour more difficult led to its evaluation as a tocolytic agent [45]. With the withdrawal of sympathomimetic drugs from the American market and the failure of atosiban, an oxytocin antagonist, to obtain the approval of the Food and Drug Administration, there are no licensed tocolytic drugs available for American obstetricians to use and magnesium sulphate is therefore in common use. However, randomized placebo-controlled trials of magnesium sulphate show no significant short-term delay of delivery, increase in birthweight or difference in perinatal mortality compared with placebo. Studies where magnesium has been compared with sympathomimetics have suggested equal efficacy. As discussed above, these two apparently contradictory findings can probably be explained by the lack of power of the studies to detect a significance difference between drugs with little or no efficacy but a high placebo response rate. Although magnesium sulphate does not appear to be effective in preventing preterm delivery, evidence has been growing over the past decade that its administration to the mother is neuroprotective for the preterm neonate [46,47]. The evidence is now sufficiently strong that it is being widely introduced for this indication in the USA, Europe and the rest of the world.

Oxytocin antagonists

Although there is no good evidence for an increase in circulating concentrations of oxytocin in either term or preterm labour, both term and preterm labour are associated with an increase in the expression of oxytocin receptors in the myometrium and oxytocin is synthesized within the uterus itself, in both the myometrium and the decidua. This has led to the exploration of drugs that antagonize the oxytocin receptor as tocolytics. At present no specific oxytocin antagonist is available for clinical use. However, atosiban, which is principally an arginine vasopressin receptor antagonist but which also binds the oxytocin receptor at appropriate therapeutic concentrations, has a European licence for the treatment of preterm labour. Atosiban has been the subject of both placebo comparison trials and comparisons with sympathomimetic drugs. The placebo-controlled trial undertaken in the USA [48] was relatively flawed in that randomization at early gestational ages was skewed, resulting in an increase in neonatal deaths among very preterm babies whose mothers were treated with atosiban. The primary outcome of the placebo-controlled trial (i.e. the time between the initiation of treatment and therapeutic failure defined as either preterm delivery or the need for an alternative tocolytic) showed that atosiban was no better than placebo. However, there were statistically significant differences in the number of women who remained undelivered and did not require an alternative tocolytic at the specific 24 and 48 hour and 7 day time points. As with all previous trials of tocolytic drugs, this trial was complicated by a very high placebo response rate. Analysis of the data shows that at, for example, 48 hours, although 70% of women randomized to receive atosiban appeared to respond to it, in reality the majority of these represent placebo responses and that in fact only 11% had a genuine clinical response. This represents one-quarter of those women who were genuinely in preterm labour and had the potential to have a genuine clinical response (Fig. 28.5).

Trials comparing atosiban with sympathomimetic drugs showed equal clinical efficacy to beta-sympathomimetics but with atosiban having a dramatically improved maternal side-effect profile [49,50]. However, the clinical response rate to either atosiban or sympathomimetic drugs in those trials was so high (over 90%) that it is probable that the majority of patients enrolled in the study were not genuinely in preterm labour. Neither the placebo-controlled trial nor the sympathomimetic comparison trials demonstrated any improvement in any aspect of neonatal morbidity or neonatal mortality associated with the use of atosiban.

Calcium channel blockers

The central role of calcium in the biochemistry of myometrial contractions led to the exploration of the use of calcium channel blockers, specifically nifedipine, as a tocolytic drug. Because there has been no interest from the pharmaceutical industry in promoting nifedipine for this indication, there have only been small locally funded comparison trials of nifedipine versus sympathomimetics. There are no placebo-controlled trials of nifedipine as a tocolytic. Meta-analysis of the sympathomimetic comparison trials [51] suggests that nifedipine may be superior in its ability to delay delivery and is associated with a reduction in the rate of RDS and intraventricular haemorrhage in preterm neonates, although not with any improvement in perinatal mortality. This conclusion may be somewhat unsafe since in the largest trial comparing nifedipine with sympathomimetics [52] 13% of the patients randomized to ritodrine were excluded from the analysis because maternal side effects led to them being switched to nifedipine. It is unlikely that there will ever be any large-scale placebo-controlled trials of nifedipine nor any large trials comparing nifedipine with atosiban. There has been one study that indirectly compared atosiban with nifedipine by taking advantage of the fact that each had been compared with sympathomimetic drugs [53]. This study suggested that nifedipine is superior to atosiban in delaying delivery and, unlike atosiban, is associated with a reduction in the risk of RDS (Fig. 28.6).

At present the British obstetrician has a choice between atosiban and nifedipine and it is probably reasonable, in our current state of knowledge, not to use tocolytic

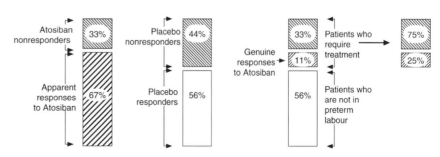

Fig. 28.5 Analysis of the 48-hour outcome data from the placebo-controlled trial of atosiban [48]. Of all patients allocated to atosiban treatment, only 11% showed a genuine clinical response, which represents one-quarter of those with the potential to benefit.

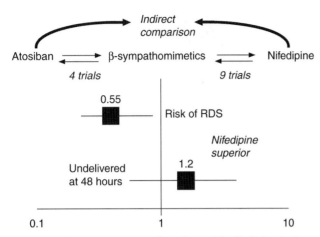

Fig. 28.6 Indirect comparison of atosiban with nifedipine in the acute management of preterm labour. (Adapted from Coomarasamy *et al.* [53].)

therapy at all. More specific oxytocin antagonists are in development, although barusiban, a more specific oxytocin antoginst than nifedipine, was found to be no better than placebo in preventing later preterm birth. Drugs which target other receptors, such as prostaglandin receptors, are in preclinical studies. It is probable that the disappointing results of tocolytics in trials to date may be because of poor trial design and, in particular, the high placebo response rates. In future, trials that are able to target tocolytic drugs more specifically at women genuinely in preterm labour, for example by taking advantage of fetal fibronectin testing, may more properly define the potential value of tocolytic therapy.

💡 Summary box 28.4

- Tocolytic drugs, intended to inhibit established contractions, will only delay preterm birth in a minority of women who are genuinely in preterm labour.
- Tocolytic drugs may be used to give steroids and achieve *in utero* transfer but there is no evidence that their use improves neonatal outcome.
- High placebo response rates give the impression in general clinical practice that tocolytic drugs are more effective than they really are.
- Magnesium sulphate is not an effective tocoytic but is neuroprotective for the fetus/neonate.
- Beta-sympathomimetics have serious maternal side effects and because safer though not necessarily more effective tocolytic drugs are now available, their use should be completely abandoned.
- Atosiban will delay preterm birth in a minority of women who are genuinely in preterm labour but there is no evidence that this benefits the neonate.
- Nifedipine has been shown to improve neonatal outcome although this conclusion should be treated with caution.

Corticosteroid therapy

The potential for antenatally administered corticosteroids to accelerate lung maturity was discovered by Liggens using experiments in which preterm labour was induced in sheep by injection of corticosteroids. A large number of randomized trials took place during the 1970s and 1980s which, taken together, have shown that a single course of either betamethasone or dexamethasone administered up to 7 days before preterm delivery in pregnant women at 24–34 weeks' gestation has a significant effect on neonatal morbidity and mortality. Although the paediatric use of surfactant has had a major impact on the incidence and consequences of RDS, nevertheless antenatal corticosteroid therapy is still associated with a reduction in neonatal mortality principally due to a significant reduction in rates of RDS and intraventricular haemorrhage. Antenatal corticosteroids have a receptor-mediated effect on all the components of the surfactant system in type 2 pneumocytes. However, they also have effects on structural development of the lungs and lead to accelerated maturation of the fetal intestine and have effects on the myocardium and on catecholamine responsiveness, which may explain the reduced incidence of necrotizing entocolitis and intraventricular haemorrhage seen in extremely preterm infants that appears to be independent of the effect on RDS.

The dramatic effects of a single course of corticosteroids unfortunately led in the past to the routine prescription of multiple courses of steroids, often at weekly intervals, in women deemed to be at risk of preterm delivery, especially those with multiple pregnancies. Recent concern about the long-term consequences of recurrent exposure to high-dose steroids suggesting adverse effects on development and behaviour has generally led to an abandonment of this policy. However, the Canadian Multiple Courses of Antenatal Corticosteroids for Preterm Birth Study [54] has shown that corticosteroid therapy, given every 14 days, did not increase or decrease the risk of death or neurological impairment at 18–24 months of age, compared with a single course of prenatal corticosteroid therapy. Both dexamethasone and betamethasone have been explored in randomized trials, with each having similar effects on rates of RDS. Studies in France suggested that betamethasone reduced the incidence of periventricular leucomalacia whereas dexamethasone had no such protective effect, although this may be explained by the presence of sulphating agents used as preservatives in French preparations of dexamethasone. It is probably the case that either steroid is suitable, provided that the preparation is non-sulphated.

Antibiotics

Meta-analysis of the use of antibiotics in symptomatic preterm labour is dominated by the ORACLE trial [55,56]. These show that administration of antibiotics to the mother do not delay delivery or improve any aspect of neonatal morbidity or mortality. The only positive health benefit is a reduction in maternal infection rates. However, the 7-year follow-up of the ORACLE I trial [57] showed that prescription of either erythromycin or co-amoxiclav for women in spontaneous preterm labour with intact membranes was associated with an increase in functional impairment among their children at 7 years of age, with the risk being higher for erythromycin. Interestingly, these children were actually born at term, suggesting that it is either exposure to antibiotics *in utero* or the combination of biochemical changes causing risk of preterm labour and antibiotics that increases the risk of cerebral palsy. While antibiotics should not therefore be given to a woman whose only presentation is preterm contractions, it remains essential that women who are actually in labour and have known group B *Streptococcus* colonization or women who have any established infection should receive appropriate effective antibiotics.

Conduct of preterm delivery

Rates of neonatal morbidity and mortality are higher in babies transferred *ex utero* to neonatal intensive care units compared with those born in a tertiary referral centre. Every effort should therefore be made to transfer a woman to an obstetric unit linked to a neonatal intensive care unit prior to a preterm delivery. The introduction of fetal fibronectin testing may reduce the numbers of unnecessary *in utero* transfers that currently take place. Except at the extremes of prematurity, there should be continuous electronic fetal heart rate monitoring once preterm labour is clearly established. There is no evidence for benefit of routine delivery by Caesarean section where the presentation is cephalic. However, hypoxia is a major risk factor for the development of periventricular leucomalacia and there should therefore be a relatively low threshold for delivery by Caesarean section in the presence of abnormal fetal heart rate patterns. The preterm delivery of a breech continues to be an obstetric dilemma. Although it is now established that elective Caesarean section is preferable for the term breech, it has proved impossible to undertake randomized trials of Caesarean section for the preterm breech. One potential disadvantage of planning to deliver the preterm breech (or indeed the cephalic presentation preterm) by elective Caesarean section is the high incidence of 'threatened' preterm labour that does not lead to preterm delivery. An aggressive policy of delivering preterm babies by Caesarean section has the potential to lead to iatrogenic preterm deliveries. At the other end of the spectrum, Caesarean section preterm where the breech is already in the vagina may be more traumatic than a vaginal delivery. At present, until further evidence becomes available, the mode of delivery of the preterm breech will need to be made on a case-by-case basis by the obstetrician. There is no evidence for the old practice of elective forceps delivery to protect the fetal head during preterm delivery and episiotomy is rarely required.

Preterm pre-labour rupture of membranes

Preterm pre-labour rupture of membranes (PPROM) occurs in approximately 2% of all pregnancies and accounts for up to one-third of preterm deliveries. The most frequent consequence of PPROM is preterm delivery, with some 50% delivering within a week, 75% within 2 weeks and 85% within 1 month. There appears to be an inverse relationship between gestational age and latency, with a shorter interval between membrane rupture and preterm labour at later gestational ages. As with preterm labour, postnatal survival following PPROM is directly related to gestational age at delivery and birthweight. However, there is the additional complication that where PPROM occurs prior to 23 weeks' gestation, there may be neonatal pulmonary hypoplasia leading to an increased risk of neonatal death, even if delivery occurs at gestational ages at which the outcome would usually be good. The risk of pulmonary hypoplasia following PPROM is approximately 50% at 19 weeks falling to about 10% at 25 weeks. The retention of amniotic fluid within the uterus is associated with better outcome. A pool of amniotic fluid greater than 2 cm is associated with a low incidence of pulmonary hypoplasia.

Once PPROM has been confirmed, by history, identification of the pool of liquor in the vagina and of oligohydramnios on ultrasonography, the management is a balance between the risks of prematurity if delivery is encouraged and the risks of maternal and fetal infection if there is conservative management. The ORACLE study showed that the use of erythromycin improves neonatal morbidity and is associated with a longer latency period, whilst co-amoxiclav increases the risk of necrotizing enterocolitis and should therefore be avoided. Management of PPROM continues to be controversial. However, many obstetricians will institute conservative management in PPROM before 34 weeks and would induce labour relatively early in women whose membrane rupture occurs subsequent to 37 weeks. There is currently no good evidence as to what ideal management should be between 34 and 37 weeks.

Conservative management should include clinical surveillance for signs of chorioamnionitis, including regular recording of maternal temperature and heart rate and cardiotocography. A rising white cell count or a rising CRP level may indicate the development of chorioamnionitis. However, neither of these are highly specific and many cases of histologically proven chorioamnionitis are associated with normal white cell counts and CRP concentrations. Lower genital tract swabs are routinely taken in women with PPROM. Positive cultures for potential pathogens do not correlate well with the risk of chorioamnionitis, although they are useful in determining the causative organisms once chorioamnionitis develops and in directing antibiotic therapy for both the mother and the preterm neonate.

Experiments have been performed in which amnioinfusion has been used in PPROM in an attempt to reduce the risk of pulmonary hypoplasia and/or orthopaedic abnormalities. Unfortunately, the literature contains only a few case reports. In the majority of cases it is likely that fluid infused into the amniotic cavity will simply leak out. If it is retained then it is probable that the amniotic fluid would reaccumulate in any case because of fetal urine production. Similarly there have been isolated case reports of the use of fibrin glue, or special catheters to attempt to seal ruptured membranes but there is no good evidence for any benefit and probably a high risk of introducing infection.

The onset of regular contractions and the establishment of preterm labour in cases of PPROM may be the first evidence of chorioamnionitis. The potential benefits of tocolytic drugs do not apply in the majority of cases of PPROM since there is usually time for administration of corticosteroids and *in utero* transfer before the onset of preterm labour itself. The few studies of the use of tocolysis in pregnancies complicated by PPROM show no improvement in perinatal outcome and suggest that long-term tocolysis may be associated with an increase in the risk of maternal and fetal infection [58,59].

References

1 Tucker J, McGuire W. Epidemiology of preterm birth. *BMJ* 2004;329:675–678.

2 Murphy DJ. Epidemiology and environmental factors in preterm labour. *Best Pract Res Clin Obstet Gynaecol* 2007;21: 773–789.

3 Wood NS, Costeloe K, Gibson AT, Hennessy EM, Marlow N, Wilkinson AR. The EPICure study: associations and antecedents of neurological and developmental disability at 30 months of age following extremely preterm birth. *Arch Dis Child* 2005; 90:F134–F140.

4 Wu YW, Colford JM Jr. Chorioamnionitis as a risk factor for cerebral palsy: a meta-analysis. *JAMA* 2000;284:1417–1424.

5 Leviton A, Paneth N, Reuss ML *et al.* Maternal infection, fetal inflammatory response, and brain damage in very low birth weight infants. *Pediatr Res* 1999;46:566–575.

6 Wood NS, Marlow N, Costeloe K, Gibson AT, Wilkinson AR. Neurologic and developmental disability after extremely preterm birth. EPICure Study Group. *N Engl J Med* 2000;343: 378–384.

7 Colvin M, McGuire W, Fowlie PW. Neurodevelopmental outcomes after preterm birth. *BMJ* 2004;329:1390–1393.

8 Takashima S, Itoh M, Oka A. A history of our understanding of cerebral vascular development and pathogenesis of perinatal brain damage over the past 30 years. *Semin Pediatr Neurol* 2009; 16:226–236.

9 Volpe JJ. Brain injury in premature infants: a complex amalgam of destructive and developmental disturbances. *Lancet Neurol* 2009;8:110–124.

10 Boot FH, Pel JJ, van der Steen J, Evenhuis HM. Cerebral visual impairment: which perceptive visual dysfunctions can be expected in children with brain damage? A systematic review. *Res Dev Disabil* 2010;31:1149–1159.

11 Smith R. Parturition. *N Engl J Med* 2007;356:271–283.

12 Zakar T, Mesiano S. How does progesterone relax the uterus in pregnancy? *N Engl J Med* 2011;364:972–973.

13 Mesiano S, Welsh TN. Steroid hormone control of myometrial contractility and parturition. *Semin Cell Dev Biol* 2007;18: 321–331.

14 Lindström TM, Bennett PR. The role of nuclear factor kappa B in human labour. *Reproduction* 2005;130:569–581.

15 Mendelson CR, Condon JC. New insights into the molecular endocrinology of parturition. *J Steroid Biochem Mol Biol* 2005;93: 113–119.

16 Shynlova O, Mitchell JA, Tsampalieros A, Langille BL, Lye SJ. Progesterone and gravidity differentially regulate expression of extracellular matrix components in the pregnant rat myometrium. *Biol Reprod* 2004;70:986–992.

17 Smith R, Nicholson RC. Corticotrophin releasing hormone and the timing of birth. *Front Biosci* 2007;12:912–918.

18 Nathanielsz PW. Comparative studies on the initiation of labor. *Eur J Obstet Gynecol Reprod Biol* 1998;78:127–132.

19 Terzidou V, Blanks AM, Kim SH, Thornton S, Bennett PR. Labor and inflammation increase the expression of oxytocin receptor in human amnion. *Biol Reprod* 2011;84:546–552.

20 Kyrgiou M, Koliopoulos G, Martin-Hirsch P, Arbyn M, Prendiville W, Paraskevaidis E. Obstetric outcomes after conservative treatment for intraepithelial or early invasive cervical lesions: systematic review and meta-analysis. *Lancet* 2006;367: 489–498.

21 Vrachnis N, Vitoratos N, Iliodromiti Z, Sifakis S, Deligeoroglou E, Creatsas G. Intrauterine inflammation and preterm delivery. *Ann NY Acad Sci* 2010;1205:118–122.

22 Romero R, Mazor M. Infection and preterm labor. *Clin Obstet Gynecol* 1988;31:553–584.

23 Buhimschi CS, Schatz F, Krikun G, Buhimschi IA, Lockwood CJ. Novel insights into molecular mechanisms of abruption-induced preterm birth. *Expert Rev Mol Med* 2010;12:e35.

24 Lockwood CJ. Stress-associated preterm delivery: the role of corticotropin-releasing hormone. *Am J Obstet Gynecol* 1999;180: S264–S266.

25 Hoffman HJ, Bakketeig LS. Risk factors associated with the occurrence of preterm birth. *Clin Obstet Gynecol* 1984;27:539–552.

26 McDonald HM, Brocklehurst P, Gordon A. Antibiotics for treating bacterial vaginosis in pregnancy. *Cochrane Database Syst Rev* 2007;(1):CD000262.

27 Mella MT, Berghella V. Prediction of preterm birth: cervical sonography. *Semin Perinatol* 2009;33:317–324.

28 Honest H, Bachmann LM, Coomarasamy A, Gupta JK, Kleijnen J, Khan KS. Accuracy of cervical transvaginal sonography in predicting preterm birth: a systematic review. *Ultrasound Obstet Gynecol* 2003;22:305–322.

29 Sinno A, Usta IM, Nassar AH. A short cervical length in pregnancy: management options. *Am J Perinatol* 2009;26:761–770.

30 MRC/RCOG Working Party on Cervical Cerclage. Final report of the Medical Research Council/Royal College of Obstetricians and Gynaecologists multicentre randomised trial of cervical cerclage. *Br J Obstet Gynaecol* 1993;100:516–523.

31 Althuisius SM, Dekker GA, Hummel P, Bekedam DJ, van Geijn HP. Final results of the Cervical Incompetence Prevention Randomised Cerclage Trial (CIPRACT): therapeutic cerclage with bed rest versus bed rest alone. *Am J Obstet Gynecol* 2001; 185:1106–1112.

32 Rust OA, Roberts WE. Does cerclage prevent preterm birth? *Obstet Gynecol Clin North Am* 2005;32:441–456.

33 To MS, Alfirevic Z, Heath VC *et al.* Cervical cerclage for prevention of preterm delivery in women with short cervix: randomised controlled trial. Fetal Medicine Foundation Second Trimester Screening Group. *Lancet* 2004;363:1849–1853.

34 Groom KM, Shennan AH, Bennett PR. Ultrasound-indicated cervical cerclage: outcome depends on preoperative cervical length and presence of visible membranes at time of cerclage. *Am J Obstet Gynecol* 2002;187:445–449.

35 Groom KM, Shennan AH, Jones BA, Seed P, Bennett PR. TOCOX: a randomised, double-blind, placebo-controlled trial of rofecoxib (a COX-2-specific prostaglandin inhibitor) for the prevention of preterm delivery in women at high risk. *BJOG* 2005;112:725–730.

36 Keirse MJ. Progestogen administration in pregnancy may prevent preterm delivery. *Br J Obstet Gynaecol* 1990;97:149–154.

37 Da Fonseca EB, Bittar RE, Carvalho MH, Zugaib M. Prophylactic administration of progesterone by vaginal suppository to reduce the incidence of spontaneous preterm birth in women at increased risk: a randomised placebo-controlled double-blind study. *Am J Obstet Gynecol* 2003;188:419–424.

38 Meis PJ, Klebanoff M, Thom E *et al.* Prevention of recurrent preterm delivery by 17 alpha-hydroxyprogesterone caproate. National Institute of Child Health and Human Development Maternal-Fetal Medicine Units Network. *N Engl J Med* 2003; 348:2379–2385.

39 Rouse DJ, Caritis SN, Peaceman AM *et al.* A trial of 17 alpha-hydroxyprogesterone caproate to prevent prematurity in twins. National Institute of Child Health and Human Development Maternal-Fetal Medicine Units Network. *N Engl J Med* 2007; 357:454–461.

40 Norman JE, Mackenzie F, Owen P *et al.* Progesterone for the prevention of preterm birth in twin pregnancy (STOPPIT): a randomised, double-blind, placebo-controlled study and meta-analysis. *Lancet* 2009;373:2034–2040.

41 Honest H, Bachmann LM, Gupta JK, Kleijnen J, Khan KS. Accuracy of cervicovaginal fetal fibronectin test in predicting risk of spontaneous preterm birth: systematic review. *BMJ* 2002; 325:301.

42 Roberts D, Dalziel S. Antenatal corticosteroids for accelerating fetal lung maturation for women at risk of preterm birth. *Cochrane Database Syst Rev* 2006;(3):CD004454.

43 Anotayanonth S, Subhedar NV, Garner P, Neilson JP, Harigopal S. Betamimetics for inhibiting preterm labour. *Cochrane Database Syst Rev* 2004;(4):CD004352.

44 King J, Flenady V, Cole S, Thornton S. Cyclo-oxygenase (COX) inhibitors for treating preterm labour. *Cochrane Database Syst Rev* 2005;(2):CD001992.

45 Crowther CA, Hiller JE, Doyle LW. Magnesium sulphate for preventing preterm birth in threatened preterm labour. *Cochrane Database Syst Rev* 2002;(4):CD001060.

46 Doyle LW, Crowther CA, Middleton P, Marret S. Antenatal magnesium sulfate and neurological outcome in preterm infants: a systematic review. *Obstet Gynecol* 2009;113:1327–1333.

47 Costantine MM, Weiner SJ. Effects of antenatal exposure to magnesium sulfate on neuroprotection and mortality in preterm infants: a meta-analysis. Eunice Kennedy Shriver National Institute of Child Health and Human Development Maternal-Fetal Medicine Units Network. *Obstet Gynecol* 2009; 114:354–364.

48 Romero R, Sibai BM, Sanchez-Ramos L *et al.* An oxytocin receptor antagonist (atosiban) in the treatment of preterm labor: a randomised, double-blind, placebo-controlled trial with tocolytic rescue. *Am J Obstet Gynecol* 2000;182:1173–1183.

49 The Worldwide Atosiban versus Beta-agonists Study Group. Effectiveness and safety of the oxytocin antagonist atosiban versus beta-adrenergic agonists in the treatment of preterm labour. *BJOG* 2001;108:133–142.

50 French/Australian Atosiban Investigators Group. Treatment of preterm labor with the oxytocin antagonist atosiban: a double-blind, randomised, controlled comparison with salbutamol. *Eur J Obstet Gynecol Reprod Biol* 2001;98:177–185.

51 Tsatsaris V, Papatsonis D, Goffinet F, Dekker G, Carbonne B. Tocolysis with nifedipine or beta-adrenergic agonists: a meta-analysis. *Obstet Gynecol* 2001;97:840–847.

52 Papatsonis DN, Van Geijn HP, Adèr HJ, Lange FM, Bleker OP, Dekker GA. Nifedipine and ritodrine in the management of preterm labor: a randomised multicenter trial. *Obstet Gynecol* 1997;90:230–234.

53 Coomarasamy A, Knox EM, Gee H, Song F, Khan KS. Effectiveness of nifedipine versus atosiban for tocolysis in preterm labour: a meta-analysis with an indirect comparison of randomised trials. *BJOG* 2003;110:1045–1049.

54 Asztalos EV, Murphy KE, Hannah ME *et al.* Multiple courses of antenatal corticosteroids for preterm birth study: 2-year outcomes. Multiple Courses of Antenatal Corticosteroids for Preterm Birth Study Collaborative Group. *Pediatrics* 2010;126: e1045–e1055.

55 Kenyon SL, Taylor DJ, Tarnow-Mordi W. Broad-spectrum antibiotics for spontaneous preterm labour: the ORACLE II randomised trial. *Lancet* 2001;357:989–994.

56 Kenyon SL, Taylor DJ, Tarnow-Mordi W. Broad-spectrum antibiotics for preterm, prelabour rupture of fetal membranes: the ORACLE I randomised trial. *Lancet* 2001;357:979–988. Erratum in *Lancet* 2001;358:156.

57 Kenyon S, Pike K, Jones DR *et al.* Childhood outcomes after prescription of antibiotics to pregnant women with preterm rupture of the membranes: 7-year follow-up of the ORACLE I trial. *Lancet* 2008;372:1310–1318.

58 Aagaard-Tillery KM, Nuthalapaty FS, Ramsey PS, Ramin KD. Preterm premature rupture of membranes: perspectives surrounding controversies in management. *Am J Perinatol* 2005;22: 287–297.

59 Simhan HN, Canavan TP. Preterm premature rupture of membranes: diagnosis, evaluation and management strategies. *BJOG* 2005;112(Suppl 1):32–37.

Chapter 29
Analgesia, Anaesthesia and Resuscitation

Felicity Plaat
Queen Charlotte's & Chelsea Hospital, Imperial College School of Medicine, London, UK

In consultant-led units more than 70% of obstetric patients require anaesthetic input. This includes labour analgesia, anaesthesia for Caesarean delivery and other surgical interventions, input into management of patients requiring critical care, and resuscitation. Because the role of the anaesthetist has expanded, current guidelines suggest that as a minimum there should be dedicated consultant anaesthetic input during the working week, although this likely to be revised upwards [1].

Pain

The International Association for the Study of Pain defines pain as 'an unpleasant, subjective, sensory and emotional experience associated with real or potential tissue damage, or described in terms of such damage'. In simple terms, pain is what hurts. More than 95% of women report pain in labour. Melzac [2] measured pain in parturients using the McGill Pain Questionnaire and showed that although scores ranged from mild to excruciating, on average only pain associated with digit amputation and causalgia was equal to or greater than labour pain, which outscored cancer, post-herpetic neuralgia and pain of fracture.

Although pain may be considered the physiological consequence of normal labour, it may also be the harbinger of pathological processes, such as obstructed labour, fetal malposition, uterine hyperstimulation, uterine rupture or extant pathology such as fibromas or other tumours, haemorrhoids, and adhesions or scarring from previous surgery.

Severe pain stimulates a sympathetic autonomic response the magnitude of which reflects the severity of pain, and is exacerbated by dehydration and exhaustion. It is characterized by hyperventilation, tachycardia, hypertension, increased oxygen and glucose consumption, and vasoconstriction with decreased blood flow across the placenta. Maternal plasma adrenaline and noradrenaline concentrations increase 200% and 600%,

respectively, during labour without analgesia. Increased maternal catecholamine levels have been associated with dysfunctional labour [3]. In the presence of maternal disease and/or fetal compromise, such effects are undesirable and in some may even be life-threatening.

> ## Summary box 29.1
>
> Severe and prolonged pain is associated with sympathetic automomic hyperactivity, increased maternal heart rate and blood pressure, vasoconstriction, increased oxygen consumption and reduced fetal oxygenation.

Non-regional analgesia for labour

Non-pharmacological methods of pain relief include antenatal education, aromatherapy, hypnotherapy ('hypnobirthing'), acupuncture, water immersion, massage and other relaxation techniques (this list is not exhaustive). A recent review suggests that the presence of a trained support person or 'doula' reduces analgesic requirements, shortens labour and increases satisfaction [4]. The evidence for other techniques is generally of poor quality, although some, such as birthing pools, are very popular and may reduce analgesia requirements.

Entonox® (50% N_2O in oxygen) is very widely used in the UK. Although 80% of women who use it would do so again, the evidence for its efficacy is conflicting [5]. Although the use of sevoflurane and other inhalation anaesthetics has been studied, currently they are not part of mainstream clinical practice. Systemic opioids are almost universally available in birthing units in the UK, although there is evidence that their effect is sedative rather than analgesic [6]. Diamorphine may be slightly more effective and may have less effect on the neonate than pethidine and is slowly replacing pethidine in some units in the UK.

Dewhurst's Textbook of Obstetrics & Gynaecology, Eighth Edition. Edited by D. Keith Edmonds.
© 2012 John Wiley and Sons, Ltd. Published 2012 by John Wiley and Sons, Ltd.

Table 29.1 Contraindications to regional analgesia.

Absolute
Maternal refusal
Lack of personnel/facilities
Pre-existing coagulopathy
Local infection at insertion site
Raised intracranial pressure (risk of coning)
Drug allergy

Relative
Haemodynamic instability
Anatomical abnormalities
Neurological disorders (medicolegal implications)
Systemic infection

Table 29.2 Single-shot spinal, combined spinal–epidural and epidural techniques.

	Single-shot spinal*	Epidural	Combined spinal–epidural
Onset of action (min)	Fast (1–5)	Slow (10–20)	Fast (1–5)
Median pain score 60–90 min	0	0–3	0
Total drugs dose	Low	High	Low
Observable leg weakness (%)[†]	100	5–50	0–40
Postdural puncture headache (%)	1–2	0.3–1.0	0.2–0.7
Hypotension (%)[†]	20–80	5–10	5–10
Failure (i.e. GA is required) (%)[†]	1.7–6.0	2–6	0.3–0.7
Pruritus (%)[†]	50–80	20–80	20–80
Duration (min)	60–240		

* Single-shot spinal anaesthesia dose is two to three times subarachnoid dose of combined spinal–epidural.
[†] These side effects are dose-dependent with epidural and combined spinal–epidural techniques. High ranges associated with full anaesthesia doses.
Source: modified from Paech M. Newer techniques of labor analgesia. *Anesthesiol Clin North Am* 2003;21:1–17, with permission.

Patient-controlled intravenous analgesia (PCA) may be used if regional analgesia is contraindicated. The ultra-short-acting opioid remifentanil has theoretical advantages over other opioids owing to its short latency and rapid metabolism. However, when remifentanil PCA is used for labour, pulse oximetry and the continuous presence of trained personnel is mandatory as respiratory depression and sedation occur [7].

Regional analgesia

There is no question that neuraxial blockade (epidural or intrathecal) provides the most effective form of pain relief in labour, and very few women cannot benefit from this form of analgesia (Table 29.1). Based on data from 81% of obstetric units in the UK, the Obstetric Anaesthetists' Association (www.oaa-anaes.ac.uk) estimated that the average regional analgesia rate in 2007 was 22%, although this varied between 0% and 47%. Modern regional techniques aim to provide pain relief whilst preserving sensation, minimizing motor blockade (muscle weakness) and reducing the effects on labour. The basis for providing this is to reduce the dose of local anaesthetic used. Such techniques are frequently referred to as 'low-dose' or 'mobile' epidurals. In 2008, 80% of UK units were using low-dose techniques [8]. Methods for reducing local anaesthetic consumption include combining the local anaesthetic with an opioid (commonly fentanyl), avoiding conventional test doses (usually high concentrations of local anaesthetics) and using a combined spinal–epidural technique. The latter involves injection of an initial dose into the intrathecal space (a spinal injection) prior to placing an epidural catheter. The intrathecal dose requires one-tenth of the amount of local anaesthetic to be effective and provides almost instantaneous pain relief. The combined spinal–epidural technique is therefore particularly useful in the later stages of labour and in multiparous women in whom rapid labour is antici-

pated. It may also provide more reliable analgesia (Table 29.2) throughout labour and the use of combined spinal–epidural analgesia for labour is growing [9].

There continues to be concern about the effect of regional analgesia on the progress and outcome of labour. Systematic review of randomized controlled trials comparing regional and non-regional (opioid) analgesia shows that regional analgesia does not increase the risk of Caesarean delivery [10], whether started early or later in labour [11]. Regional analgesia appears to prolong the first and second stages of labour (by 30 and 15 min, respectively) and increases the need for augmentation and the use of instrumental vaginal delivery [12]. However, such reviews include few studies using low-dose techniques, which randomized studies show are associated with decreased instrumental deliveries compared with conventional epidural analgesia [13]. Concerns about impaired maternal effort in the second stage of labour have resulted in the widespread habit of discontinuing regional analgesia in late labour [14]. However, a recent review concludes that in the absence of large trials the evidence suggests that all this achieves is poor analgesia in the second stage of labour [15]. Other side effects of regional analgesia include increased use of urinary catheterization, maternal fever (non-infective and believed to be a result of the local anaesthetic) and pruritus due to neuraxial opioids.

Table 29.3 Requirements for safe 'mobile epidurals' in labour.

Cooperative understanding parturient
Presenting part of fetus engaged and well applied to cervix
Minimal or no motor and proprioceptive block
No postural hypotension
Continuous fetal monitoring (cardiotocography) when indicated
Suitable conditions
   Good epidural catheter fixation
   Attending midwife
   Disconnection of intravenous line (bung inserted)
   No shoes
   Safe, even floor without cables, steps or mats

Ambulation in labour has not been shown to signifi- cantly affect the mode of delivery, However, mobility may decrease analgesic requirements and avoids the risks associated with prolonged recumbency. However, mobi- lizing with regional anaesthesia has been shown to be safe and is viewed positively by women who undertake it [16]. To permit safe ambulation, all delivery unit staff must be appropriately trained and certain conditions must be met (Table 29.3). Motor and proprioceptive block must be excluded. Studies have demonstarated that women them- selves can reliably tell if they can ambulate safely [17].

 Summary box 29.2

In the UK, 80% of units now use 'low-dose' epidurals. Reduced doses of local anaesthetics decrease the incidence of motor block, allow ambulation and may diminish the effects on progress of labour and need for assisted vaginal delivery.

Apart from pain, there are several obstetric and medical indications for neuraxial block in labour. (Table 29.4). Cases considered at high risk of requiring intervention for delivery benefit from an indwelling epidural catheter (which has been tested and shown to be effective) that can be rapidly replenished (e.g. in the case of an after-coming twin). Maternal disease in which the effects of pain or the Valsalva manoeuvre associated with pushing may be det- rimental will also benefit from regional analgesia in labour. Obesity per se may become a major indication for this type of analgesia, since the whole spectrum of obstet- ric complications are increased in this group. Difficulties in siting neuraxial blocks make its early use advisable.

Table 29.5 lists the serious complications of regional blockade. A recent national survey carried out by the Royal College of Anaesthetists found that serious compli- cations associated with death or pernenent sequelae were rarer than previously estimated [18]. Although approxi-

Table 29.4 Indications for regional analgesia for labour.

Pain relief
   Avoid the deleterious effects of pain (maternal exhaustion, raised
   catecholamines, maternal and fetal acidosis)
Reduce premature urge to push
Manual removal of placenta
Reduce need for emergency general anaesthesia
   Multiple pregnancy
   Breech
   Suspected cephalopelvic disproportion/macrosomia
   ? Previous Caesarean section
   ? Obesity
Improve uteroplacental flow/fetal condition
   Pre-eclampsia
   Preterm labour
   Impaired uteroplacental function (poor Doppler/non-reassuring
   CTG)
Improve maternal condition
   Reduced oxygen demand (especially women with cardiac/
   respiratory disease)
   Reduced circulating catecholamines (especially maternal fixed
   cardiac output states)
   Avoid Valsalva manoeuvre in second stage

Table 29.5 Serious complications of regional blockade.

Complication	Incidence
Cardiovascular collapse	
High total spinal (relative/absolute overdose of local anaesthetic)	
Local anaesthetic toxicity (inadvertent intravenous administration)	
Infection (epidural abscess)	1 in 145 000
Meningitis	
Epidural haematoma	1 in 168 000
Trauma (direct damage to spinal cord/nerve root damage)	
Permanent	1 in 240 000
Transient	1 in 6700

Source: incidence data from Ruppen W, Derry S, McQuay H, Moore RA. Incidence of epidural hematoma, infection, and neurologic injury in obstetric patients with epidural analgesia/anesthesia. *Anesthesiology* 2006;105:394–399, with permission.

mately 50% of all blocks performed are in the obstetric population, the incidence in this population was even lower possibly due to the general good health of this population. There were no deaths. Overall the incidence of permenent harm in the obstetric population resulting from neuraxial blockade was between 0.3 and 1.24 per 100 000; combined spinal–epidural analgesia was associ- ated with the highest incidence (3.9 per 100 000) and epi- durals with the lowest (0.62 per 100 000).

Anaesthesia for Caesarean section

The increased use of regional anaesthesia for Caesarean section has contributed to the fall in anaesthetic-related maternal mortality. The great majority of anaesthetic-related maternal deaths are due to general anaesthesia, particularly in the emergency situation. General anaesthesia is particularly hazardous in obstetrics because of changes associated with pregnancy increasing the risk of difficult or failed intubation, hypoxia and aspiration. General anaesthesia is frequently reserved for the extremely urgent section when the anaesthetist, who may not have previously met the patient, has very little time for assessment. There are concerns that as general anaesthesia is used less and less in obstetrics, skills will dwindle increasing the risks of this type of obstetric anaesthesia. The Royal College of Anaesthetists suggests that more than 95% of elective and more than 85% of emergency cases should be performed under regional anaesthesia [19]. In 2007, only 10% of Caesarean sections in the UK were performed under general anaesthesia.

The four-grade classification of urgency of Caesarean section, endorsed by the Royal College of Obstetricians and Gynaecologists and the Royal College of Anaesthetists and used in the National Sentinel Audit of Caesarean sections, should be universally adopted to improve communication especially in the emergency situation [20]. Prior to scheduled surgery, regardless of the type of anaesthetic planned, patients should be fasted (6 hours for solids, 2 hours for clear fluids) and given premedication (oral ranitidine and metoclopramide). Labouring women at risk of Caesarean section should be limited to sips of water and given ranitidine 150 mg 6-hourly throughout labour. Intravenous ranitidine 50 mg may be given within 30 min of induction whereas sodium citrate, which is only effective for 15–30 min, should be given immediately before induction of general anaesthesia. In the emergency situation, intrauterine resuscitation of the fetus (Table 29.6) should be undertaken during preparation for anaesthesia [21]. Oxygen therapy in the presence of profound fetal distress is still recommended, although the evidence is not compelling [22].

Table 29.6 Intrauterine resuscitation.

Relieve aortocaval compression: left lateral position ≥15° tilt, uterine displacement
Ensure effective analgesia: top up epidural (decreases maternal catecholamine levels and improves uteroplacental blood flow)
Rapid intravenous infusion (transiently decreases uterine activity)
Stop Syntocinon infusion (often overlooked)
Tocolysis (terbutaline/glyceryl trinitrate)
High-flow maternal oxygen (optimize oxygen delivery

Regional anaesthesia is recommended in severe pre-eclampsia as haemodynamic stability is better maintained than in the normotensive patient and because the risks of general anaesthesia are further increased. Abnormal placentation is also no longer seen as an absolute indication for general anaesthesia. A combination of general and neuraxial anaesthesia allows the mother to be awake for delivery, after which general anaesthesia can be induced for Caesarean hysterectomy or other complicated surgery. Similarly for fetal surgery, or other surgery during pregnancy, combined general anaesthesia and regional blockade is frequently used. The combined spinal–epidural technique allows effective anaesthesia to be prolonged as long as required and the epidural component can be used to provide postoperative analgesia.

Summary box 29.3

The great majority of direct anaesthetic-related maternal deaths are associated with emergency general anaesthesia. The Royal College of Anaesthetists recommends that more than 85% of emergency and more than 95% of elective Caesarean sections should be performed under regional anaesthesia.

Cardiopulmonary resuscitation and critical care

Cardiac arrest occurs in approximately 1 in 30 000 pregnancies [23]. As the obstetric population becomes older with more complex medical problems and the incidence of obesity continues to increase, it may become more common [24]. Reliable data on cardiopulmonary collapse per se in the obstetric population are missing. In the obstetric patient, pulseless electrical activity/asystole is more common than ventricular fibrillation arrest. Hypovolaemia due to haemorrhage is probably the commonest cause. Pulmonary embolism is another cause of pulseless electrical activity. Amniotic fluid embolism appears to be causing an increasing number of maternal deaths in the UK, and typically presents with sudden cardiovascular collapse often associated with profound hypoxia. Local anaesthetic toxicity and magnesium overdose are other causes in this population. Lack of knowledge of resuscitation (both basic and advanced) among healthcare professionals caring for maternity patients has recently been highlighted [25]. In consecutive reports on maternal mortality in the UK, resuscitation skills were judged to be poor in a significant number of cases. One of the 'top ten' recommendations of the 2003–5 report was that 'All staff must undertake regular, written, and audited training for the improvement of basic, immediate and advanced life support skills'. A growing number of courses are available. Training should be supplemented by regular practice of cardiac arrest drills to ensure appropriate care is delivered [26].

Resuscitation in pregnancy is different from resuscitation in the non-pregnant adult. There are several reasons why cardiopulmonary resuscitation is both more difficult to perform and less effective in the obstetric patient. Occlusion of the inferior vena cava is the norm in the supine position at term and results in a more than 60% reduction in venous return. In order to reduce this, pelvic tilt is required. However, cardiac compressions become progressively more difficult to perform effectively the more the patient is tilted, so a tilt of 15–30° is suggested. Hypoxia develops more quickly due to increased oxygen requirements and decreased oxygen reserves. Artificial ventilation becomes more difficult due to enlarged breasts and decreased lung compliance resulting from the enlarging uterus. Reduced lower oesophageal sphincter tone increases the risk of regurgitation, requiring endotracheal intubation as early as possible.

Speed of response is crucial to the outcome for both the woman and her child [27]. Minimizing aortocaval compression, airway protection, modified hand position for cardiac compressions and early uterine evacuation form the basis for resuscitation of the pregnant patient at term (Table 29.7). It is now recommended that early (within 5 min) evacuation of the uterus should be considered, regardless of fetal viability, to improve chances of successful resuscitation, from about 24 weeks. Uterine evacuation in this situation will not require haemostasis until circulation is restored. The delay caused by aseptic precautions may itself be fatal. A scalpel and a pair of forceps plus gloves for the operator's protection may be all that is required [28]. A midline incision has been recommended as it is helped by the separation of the recti abdomini muscles that occurs in later pregnancy; however, if staff involved are more familiar with a Pfannenstiel incision, then this should be used.

A recent report on obstetric admissions to intensive care indicates that the majority of obstetric admissions are postpartum (>80%). Of these, much the most common cause was haemorrhage (>30%). In contrast, among antenatal admissions, non-obstetric conditions predominated, with pneumonia being the single most common cause [29]. The early provision of critical care to the sick parturient can reduce morbidity and mortality. The anaesthetist on the delivery suite must identify as early as possible when transfer to intensive care is required (Table 29.8).

The limits to what care can be safely provided on the delivery suite will be determined to some extent by local resources. The effects of intensive care management on the fetus must be considered. Maternal oxygen-carrying capacity should be optimized, the effects of pharmacological agents on uteroplacental blood flow considered, adequate maternal nutrition ensured and radiological investigations minimized. The role of the obstetric anaesthetist in neonatal resuscitation is poorly defined. There is general agreement that the first responsibility is to the mother [30]. However, since up to one-third of cases where neonatal resuscitation is required occur apparently without warning, there is also consensus that all those likely to be present at delivery, including the obstetric anaesthetist, should have undergone training in neonatal resuscitation.

 Summary box 29.4

During cardiopulmonary resuscitation in the pregnant patient, aortocaval compression must be minimized, the airway protected from aspiration by intubation, and the uterus emptied within 5 min of cessation of circulation to maximize chances of maternal and fetal survival.

Table 29.7 Cardiopulmonary resuscitation in the pregnant patient.

Basic life support
Left uterine displacement (tilt/wedge/manual displacement)
Hands higher on sternum
Cricoid pressure to prevent regurgitation

Advanced life support
Secure airway early
Early evacuation of uterus (within 5 min of cardiac arrest)
Remove fetal monitors prior to defibrillation
Avoid lower limb intravenous access
(Drug doses should not be altered)

Table 29.8 Indications for transfer to an intensive care facility.

General
 Lack of trained staff/facilities on delivery suite
Cardiovascular
 Use of inotropes
 Management of pulmonary oedema
Respiratory
 Mechanical ventilation
 Airway protection
 Tracheal toilet
Renal
 Renal replacement therapy
Neurological
 Significantly depressed conscious level
Miscellaneous
 Multiorgan failure
 Uncorrected acidosis
 Hypothermia

Summary

The majority of parturients require anaesthetic input. Regional analgesia has been modified to reduce adverse effects on the progress and outcome of labour. By increasing consultant anaesthetic presence on the delivery suite and by minimizing the use of general anaesthesia for emergencies, anaesthetic-related maternal mortality and morbidity has been reduced. This requires identification of at-risk parturients with antenatal anaesthetic input. The anaesthetist plays a key role in the provision of critical care for the obstetric patient.

References

1 Association of Anaesthetists of Great Britain and Ireland (AAGBI)/Obstetric Anaesthetists' Association (OAA). *Guidelines for the provision of obstetric anaesthetic services*. London: AAGBI, 2005.

2 Melzack R. The myth of painless childbirth. *Pain* 1984;19: 321–337.

3 Lederman RP, Lederman E, Work B Jr, McCann DS. Anxiety and epinephrine in multiparous women in labor: relationship to duration of labor and fetal heart rate pattern. *Am J Obstet Gynecol* 1985;153:870–877.

4 Hodnett ED, Gates S, Hofmeyr GJ, Sakala C. Continuous support for women during childbirth. *Cochrane Database Syst Rev* 2011;(2):CD003766.

5 Carstoniu J, Levytam S, Norman P, Daley D, Katz J, Sandler AN. Nitrous oxide in early labor. Safety and analgesic efficacy assessed by a double-blind, placebo-controlled study. *Anesthesiology* 1994;80:30–35.

6 Olofsson C, Ekblom A, Ekman-Ordeberg G, Hjelm A, Irestedt L. Lack of analgesic effect of systemically administered morphine or pethidine on labour pain. *Br J Obstet Gynaecol* 1996; 103:968–972.

7 Balki M, Kasodekar S, Dhumne S, Bernstein P, Carvalho JC. Remifentanil patient-controlled analgesia for labour: optimizing drug delivery regimens. *Can J Anaesth* 2007;54:626–633.

8 Prabhu A, Plaatm F. Regional analgesia for labour: a survey of UK practice. *Int J Obstet Anesth* 2009;18:S28.

9 Plaat F. The dura is too vulnerable to be reached routinely in labour. *Int J Obstet Anesth* 1999;8:58–61.

10 Anim-Somuah M, Smyth R, Howell C. Epidural versus non-epidural or no analgesia in labour. *Cochrane Database Syst Rev* 2005;(4):CD000331.

11 Wong CA, Scavone BM, Peaceman AM *et al*. The risk of cesarean delivery with neuraxial analgesia given early versus late in labor. *N Engl J Med* 2005;352:655–665.

12 Leighton BL, Halpern SH. The effects of epidural analgesia on labor, maternal, and neonatal outcomes: a systematic review. *Am J Obstet Gynecol* 2002;186(5 Suppl Nature):S69–S77.

13 Comparative Obstetric Mobile Epidural Trial (COMET) Study Group UK. Effect of low-dose mobile versus traditional epidural techniques on mode of delivery: a randomised controlled trial. *Lancet* 2001;358:19–23.

14 Rathinam S, Plaat F. Pain relief in the second stage of labour: room for improvement? *Int J Obstet Anesth* 2008;17:S25.

15 Torvaldsen S, Roberts CL, Bell JC, Raynes-Greenow CH. Discontinuation of epidural analgesia late in labour for reducing the adverse delivery outcomes associated with epidural analgesia. *Cochrane Database Syst Rev* 2004;(4):CD004457.

16 Plaat F. Ambulatory analgesia in labour. In: Collis R, Plaat F, Urquhart J (eds) *Textbook of Obstetric Anaesthesia*. London: Greenwich Medical Media, 2002: 99–112.

17 Plaat F, Singh R, Al Saud SM, Crowhurst JA. Selective sensory blockade with low dose combined spinal/epidural allows safe ambulation in labour: a pilot study. *Int J Obstet Anesth* 1996;5:220.

18 Cook TM, Counsell D, Wildsmith JA. Major complications of central neuraxial block: report on the Third National Audit Project of the Royal College of Anaesthetists. *Br J Anaesth* 2009; 102:179–190.

19 Russell IF. Technique of anaesthesia for caesarean section. In: Kinsella M (ed.) *Raising the Standards: A Compendium of Audit Recipes*. London: Royal College of Anaesthetists, 2006.

20 Lucas DN, Yentis SM, Kinsella SM *et al*. Urgency of caesarean section: a new classification. *J R Soc Med* 2000;93:346–350.

21 Thurlow JA, Kinsella SM. Intrauterine resuscitation: active management of fetal distress. *Int J Obstet Anesth* 2002;11:105–116.

22 Fawole B, Hofmeyr GJ. Maternal oxygen administration for fetal distress. *Cochrane Database Syst Rev* 2003;(4):CD000136.

23 Mallampalli A, Powner DJ, Gardner MO. Cardiopulmonary resuscitation and somatic support of the pregnant patient. *Crit Care Clin* 2004;20:261–274.

24 Lewis G (ed.) *Saving Mothers' Lives: Reviewing Maternal Deaths to Make Motherhood Safer 2003–2005. The Seventh Report on Confidential Enquiries into Maternal Deaths in the United Kingdom*. London: Confidential Enquiry into Maternal and Child Health, 2007. Available at: www.cmace.org.uk/getattachment/26dae364-1fc9-4a29-a6cb-afb3f251f8f7/Saving-Mothers'-Lives-2003-2005-(Full-report).aspx.

25 Einav S, Matot I, Berkenstadt H *et al*. A survey of labour ward clinicians' knowledge of maternal cardiac arrest and resuscitation. *Int J Obstet Anesth* 2008;17:238–242.

26 Clarke J, Butt M. Maternal collapse. *Curr Opin Obstet Gynecol* 2005;17:157–160.

27 Katz V, Balderston K, DeFreest M. Perimortem caesarean delivery: were our assumptions correct? *Am J Obstet Gynecol* 2005; 192:1916–1920.

28 Grady K, Prasad BGR, Howell C. Cardiopulmonary resuscitation. In: Cox C, Grady K, Howell C (eds) *Managing Obstetric Emergencies and Trauma. The MOET Course Manual*. London: RCOG Press, 2007.

29 Harrison DA, Penny JA, Yentis SM, Fayek S, Brady AR. Case mix, outcome and activity for obstetric admissions to adult, general critical care units: a secondary analysis of the ICNARC Case Mix Programme Database. *Crit Care* 2005;9(Suppl 3): S25–S37.

30 Gaiser RR. Newborn resuscitation and anesthesia responsibility post-cesarean section. *J Clin Anesth* 1999;11:69–72.

Part 7
Postnatal Care

Chapter 30
Puerperium and Lactation

D. Keith Edmonds
Queen Charlotte's & Chelsea Hospital, London, UK

The puerperium is the period from delivery of the placenta to 6 weeks after delivery. It is a time of enormous importance to the mother and her baby and yet it is an aspect of maternity care that has received relatively less attention than pregnancy and delivery. During the puerperium the pelvic organs return to the non-gravid state, the metabolic changes of pregnancy are reversed and lactation is established. In the absence of breast-feeding, the reproductive cycle may start again within a few weeks. The puerperium is a time steeped in cultural customs and rituals in many different countries, and indeed many of the medical recommendations about the puerperium have developed as adaptations of socially acceptable traditions rather than science.

The puerperium is also a time of psychological adjustment and while most mothers' enjoyment of the arrival of a newborn baby is obvious, the transition to becoming a responsible parent and anxiety about the child's welfare will influence the mother's ability to cope. These anxieties may be compounded if she has had a difficult labour or if she has any medical complications. However, the majority of women are subject to another problem that new mothers find very difficult to cope with and this is the plethora of well-meaning but conflicting advice from doctors, midwives, relatives and friends. Here again, the cultural influences may be at conflict with the mother's own beliefs. It is extremely important that an atmosphere be created whereby a mother can learn to handle her baby with confidence, and here the influence of midwifery and obstetric staff plays an important role in trying to establish what will be an important part of their lives. In caring for a woman during the early puerperium, the role of the obstetrician and midwife is to monitor the physiological changes of the puerperium, to diagnose and treat any postnatal complications, to establish infant feeding, to give the mother emotional support and to advise about contraception and other measures that will contribute to continuing health. It is important to bear in mind that maternal death may still occur in the puerperium and hence its importance cannot be understated.

Physiology of the puerperium

Two major physiological events occur during the puerperium: the establishment of lactation and the return of the physiological changes of pregnancy to the non-pregnant state. During the first 2 weeks after childbirth, some changes are quite rapid but others take 6–12 weeks to complete.

The uterus
The crude weight of the pregnant uterus at term is approximately 1000 g while the weight of the non-pregnant uterus is 50–100 g. By 6 weeks after birth the uterus has returned to its normal size, and from a clinical perspective the uterine fundus is no longer palpable abdominally by 10 days after delivery. The cervix itself is very flaccid after delivery but within a few days returns to its original state. The placental site in the first 3 days after delivery is infiltrated with granulocytes and mononuclear cells and this reaction extends into the endometrium and the superficial myometrium. By the seventh day, there is evidence of regeneration of endometrial glands and by day 16 the endometrium is fully restored. Decidual necrosis begins on the first day and by the seventh day a well-demarcated zone exists between necrotic and viable tissue. The presence of mononuclear cells and lymphocytes persists for about 10 days and it is presumed that this acts as some form of antibacterial barrier. Haemostasis immediately after birth is accomplished by arterial smooth muscle contraction and compression of vessels by the uterine muscle. The vessels in the placental site are characterized during the first 8 days by thrombosis, hyalinization and obliterative fibrinoid endarteritis. Immediately after delivery, bleeding lasts for several hours and then rapidly diminishes to a red-brown discharge by the third or fourth day after birth. This vaginal discharge is known as lochia and after the third or fourth day the discharge becomes mucopurulent and sometimes malodorous. This is known as the lochia serosa and it has a mean duration of 22–27 days. However,

10–15% of women will have lochia serosa for at least 6 weeks [1]. Not infrequently, there is a sudden but transient increase in uterine bleeding between 7 and 14 days after delivery. This corresponds to the shedding of the slough over the placental site and as myometrial vessels are still at this stage larger than normal, it accounts for the dramatic bleeding that can occur with this phenomenon. However, it is self-limiting and subsides within 1–2 hours. A new endometrium will grow from the basal layers of the decidua but this is influenced by the method of infant feeding. If lactation is suppressed, the uterine cavity may be covered by new endometrium within 3–4 weeks, but if lactation is established, endometrial growth may be suppressed for many months.

Ovarian function

Women who breast-feed their infants will be amenorrhoeic for long periods, often until the child is weaned. However, in non-lactating women, ovulation may occur as early as 27 days after delivery, although the mean time is approximately 70–75 days. Among those women who are breast-feeding, the mean time to ovulation is 6 months. Menstruation resumes by 12 weeks after birth in 70% of women who are not lactating and the mean time to first menstruation is 7–9 weeks. The risk of ovulation within the first 6 months after delivery in women exclusively breast-feeding is between 1 and 5% [2]. The hormonal basis of puerperial ovulation suppression in lactating women appears to be the persistence of elevated serum prolactin levels. Prolactin levels fall to the normal range by the third week after birth in non-lactating women but remain elevated to 6 weeks after birth in lactating women.

Cardiovascular and coagulation systems

Changes take place in the cardiovascular and coagulation systems that have practical and clinical implications and these are summarized in Table 30.1. Although both heart rate and cardiac output fall in the early puerperium, there may be an early rise in stroke volume and, together with the rise in blood pressure due to increased peripheral resistance, it is a time of high risk for mothers with cardiac disease. Such mothers require extra supervision at this time (see Chapter 12). Although it is assumed that by 6 weeks the woman's body has changed physiologically back to the non-pregnant state, it can be seen from Table 30.1 that cardiac output may remain elevated for up to 24 weeks after birth. During the immediate postnatal period, fibrinolytic activity is increased for 1–4 days before it returns to normal by 1 week. Platelet counts are normal during pregnancy but there is a sharp rise in platelets after delivery, making it a time of high risk for thromboembolic disease [3].

Urinary tract

During the first few days, the bladder and urethra may show evidence of mild trauma sustained at delivery and

Table 30.1 Changes in the cardiovascular and coagulation systems during the puerperium.

	Early puerperium	Late puerperium
Cardiovascular		
Heart rate	Falls: 14% by 48 hours	Normal by 2 weeks
Stroke volume	Rises over 48 hours	Normal by 2 weeks
Cardiac output	Remains elevated and then falls over 48 hours	Normal by 24 weeks
Blood pressure	Rises over 4 days	Normal by 6 weeks
Plasma volume	Initial increase and then falls	Progressive decline in first week
Coagulation		
Fibrinogen	Rises in first week	Normal by 6 weeks
Clotting factors	Most remain elevated	Normal by 3 weeks
Platelet count	Falls and then rises	Normal by 6 weeks
Fibrinolysis	Rapid reversal of pregnancy inhibition of tissue plasminogen activator	Normal by 3 weeks

Source: adapted from Dunlop W. The pueperium. *Fetal Med Rev* 1989;1:43–60, with permission.

these changes are usually associated with localized oedema. These are transient and do not remain in evidence for long. The changes that occur in the urinary tract during pregnancy disappear in a similar manner to other involutional changes and within 2–3 weeks the hydroureter and pelvic dilatation in the kidney are almost eliminated and completely return to normal by 6–8 weeks after birth.

Weight loss

There is an immediate loss of 4.5–6 kg following birth due to the baby, the placenta, amniotic fluid and blood loss that occurs at delivery. By 6 weeks after delivery, 28% of women will have returned to their pre-pregnancy weight; those women who did not have excessive weight gain in pregnancy should have returned to their normal pre-pregnancy weight by 6 months after delivery. Women with excessive weight gain in pregnancy (>15 kg) are likely to find that at 6 months they still have net gain of 5 kg, which may persist indefinitely [4]. Breast-feeding has no effect on postpartum weight loss unless lactation continues for 6 months [5]. Diet and exercise have no effect on the growth of infants who are being breast-fed and women can therefore be encouraged to return to normal activity and to regain their weight even though they are lactating [6].

Thyroid function

Thyroid volume increases by approximately 30% during pregnancy and this returns to normal over a 12-week period. Thyroxine and triiodothyronine return to normal within 4 weeks after birth.

Table 30.2 Percentage of mothers having major, intermediate and minor morbidity after childbirth.

	Women in hospital (0–5 days) (N = 1249)	Women at home (up to 8 weeks) (N = 1116)
Minor	67 (95% CI 64–69)	74 (95% CI 71–77)
Intermediate	60 (95% CI 58–63)	48 (95% CI 46–57)
Major	25 (95% CI 22–27)	31 (95% CI 29–34)

Minor problems: tiredness, backache, constipation, piles, headache. Intermediate problems: perineal pain, breast problems, tearfulness/depression. Major problems: hypertension, vaginal discharge, abnormal bleeding, stitch breakdown, voiding difficulties/incontinence, urinary infection, side effects of epidural.
Source: Glazener *et al.* [16] with permission.

Hair loss

Hair growth slows in the puerperium and women will often experience hair loss as temporarily more hair is lost than regrown. This is a transient phenomenon but it is important for women to realize that this may take between 6 months and a year to return to normal.

Management of puerperium

The morbidity associated with the puerperium is underestimated and an important review shows that mothers have high levels of postpartum problems (Table 30.2). Nearly one-third (31%) of women felt that they had major problems for up to 8 weeks after birth. In trying to reduce the impact of this morbidity, there are a number of principles which need to be applied in planning postnatal care.

1 *Continuity of care.* An ideal pattern of care is one that offers continuity from the antenatal period through childbirth and into the puerperium involving the smallest team of health professionals with which the mother can empathize.

2 *Mother–infant bonding.* It is now well established that mothers and their partners should be able to hold and touch their babies as soon as possible after delivery. Good postnatal facilities that allow rooming-in, privacy and the opportunity for close contact play an important part in helping parents to have a good experience of early parenting.

3 *Flexible discharge policies.* The optimum duration of postnatal stay varies with the needs of the individual mother and her baby. Some mothers will elect to have a home confinement, some will elect to have early discharge at 6 hours postnatally and others may have greater needs, particularly those who have had complicated deliveries and those who wish to establish breast-feeding before going home. The current pressure on maternity services in the Western world means that any length of stay in hospital to respond to maternal needs as opposed to medical necessity has meant that this flexibility has been curtailed. While this has not had an impact on successful breast-feeding, the psychological morbidity may have increased.

4 *Emotional and physical support.* Mothers require help and support after childbirth and this may come from partners, relatives and friends. Good professional support is also important and good communication between hospital staff, community midwives, general practitioner (GP) and health visitor is essential.

Routine observations

During the patient's stay in hospital, regular checks are made of her pulse, temperature, blood pressure, fundal height and lochia and any complaints noted. The perineum should be inspected daily if there has been any trauma and the episiotomy or other wounds checked for signs of infection. It is also important that urinary output is satisfactory and that the bladder is being emptied completely. These observations are necessary to give the earliest warning of any possible complications.

Ambulation in the puerperium

It is now well established that early mobilization after childbirth is extremely important. Once the mother has recovered from the physical rigours of her labour, she should be encouraged to mobilize as soon as possible. The physiotherapist has an important role to play in returning the patient to normal health during the puerperium, and limb exercises will be particularly important to encourage venous flow in the leg veins of any mother who has been immobilized in bed for any reason. Exercises to the abdominal and pelvic floor muscles are most valuable in restoring normal tone, which may have been lost during pregnancy.

Complications of the puerperium

Serious and sometimes fatal complications may arise during the puerperium. The most serious complications are thromboembolism, infection and haemorrhage, as well as mental disorders and breast problems.

Thrombosis and embolism

The Confidential Enquiry into Maternal and Child Health 2003–2005 [7] shows that pulmonary embolism is still a major cause of death in the puerperium. Of a total of 33 deaths during the triennium, 15 occurred in the postnatal period. Table 30.3 illustrates how the rate of pulmonary embolism as a cause of death has remained static since 1985. The report identifies three major areas that give rise

Table 30.3 Deaths from pulmonary embolism reported by the Confidential Enquiry into Maternal and Child Health.

Triennium	Total deaths	Rate per 100 000	Postnatal	Rate per 100 000
1985–1987	30	1.3	13	0.6
1988–1990	24	1.0	11	0.5
1991–1993	30	1.3	17	0.7
1994–1996	46	2.1	25	1.1
1997–1999	31	1.5	13	0.6
2000–2002	25	1.3	16	0.8
2003–2005	33	1.56	15	0.8

Table 30.4 Deaths from puerperal sepsis as reported in the Confidential Enquiry into Maternal and Child Health.

Triennium	Total deaths	Rate per million	Postnatal	Rate per million
1985–1987	09	4	2	0.9
1988–1990	17	7.2	4	1.7
1991–1993	15	6.5	4	1.7
1994–1996	16	7.3	11	5.0
1997–1999	18	8.5	4	1.9
2000–2002	13	6.5	5	2.5
2003–2005	18	8.5	3	1.4

to this increased risk of pulmonary embolism: increased maternal age, a family history of thromboembolism, and obesity with its associated lack of mobility. Of the 15 deaths, seven occurred within 7 days of delivery and five in the subsequent 2 weeks. The other three deaths occurred after this time. Women who have had a Caesarean section are given prophylactic subcutaneous low-molecular-weight heparin in the puerperium, but attention must be given to any high-risk mother and prophylactic heparin given in the puerperium following vaginal delivery.

Puerperal infection

Puerperal pyrexia may have several causes but it is an important clinical sign that merits careful investigation. Infection may occur in several sites and each needs to be investigated in the presence of elevated temperature.

Genital tract infection

Genital tract infection continues to be a life-threatening problem for women and Table 30.4 shows the risk of puerperal sepsis and maternal death over the last years of maternal death reports. The most virulent organism is β-haemolytic *Streptococcus* but more commonly *Chlamydia*, *Escherichia coli* and other Gram-negative bacteria will be the infective agents. Table 30.5 summarizes the main

Table 30.5 Causes of postnatal pyrexia.

Urinary tract infection
Genital tract infection
  Endometritis
  Infected episiotomy
Mastitis
Wound infection following Caesarean section
Deep venous thrombosis
Other infection, e.g. chest infection, viral infections

causes of postnatal pyrexia. Early diagnosis and treatment are imperative if the long-term sequelae are to be avoided. Of importance in the three deaths that occurred between 2000 and 2002, two became ill in the community and it is important that healthcare professionals who are caring for women after discharge from hospital should be aware of the dangers of puerperal sepsis and the need for early treatment.

Urinary tract infection

This is a common infection in the puerperium following the not infrequent use of catheterization during labour. Some women will also develop urinary retention and require indwelling catheters. *Escherichia coli* is the commonest pathogen and again early treatment is advised.

Respiratory infection

These are now seen less commonly during the puerperium as fewer women have general anaesthesia for delivery. However, chest symptoms may be a sign of pulmonary embolism and in all women who present with a chest problem, a possible diagnosis of pulmonary embolism should be considered.

Other causes

Any surgical wound should be examined for evidence of infection and this is obviously important following Caesarean section. Wound infection may manifest itself as a reddened tender area deep to the incision, which may be surrounded by induration. Treatment will depend on the extent and severity of the infection. If the infection is well localized, it may discharge spontaneously but an abscess may require incision and drainage. Broad-spectrum antibiotics will be required and bacteriological specimens should be sent for examination. It is occasionally necessary to re-suture wounds after infection but often wounds will granulate from the base and heal spontaneously. The legs should always be inspected if a puerperal pyrexia is present because of the risk of thrombophlebitis and it may also be a sign of deep venous thrombosis. The breasts should be examined for signs of breast infection, although breast abscess formation is very unusual before 14 days after birth.

Urinary complications

Other than infection, urinary retention is the commonest complication following delivery, especially if there has been any trauma to the urethra and resulting oedema round the bladder neck. A painful episiotomy may make it very difficult for women to spontaneously micturate and retention of urine may occur. Following epidural anaesthesia, there may be temporary interruption of the normal sensory stimuli for bladder function and over-distension of the bladder may occur. It is extremely important that in the immediate postnatal period urinary retention is avoided as over-distension may lead to an atonic bladder, which is then unable to empty spontaneously. If the bladder is distended, it is usually palpable abdominally but if this is not the case or the clinician is uncertain of the abdominal findings, an ultrasound scan should be performed to determine the volume of urine retained in the bladder. The treatment of urinary retention is to leave an indwelling catheter on continuous drainage for 48 hours. The patient can be ambulant during this time. After the bladder has been continuously emptied, the catheter can be removed and then the volumes of urine passed can be monitored. If there is any suspicion that further retention is occurring, then a suprapubic catheter should be inserted so that the bladder can undergo a further period of continuous drainage and then intermittent clamping of the catheter can be instituted until normal bladder function returns.

Incontinence of urine

Urinary incontinence will occur in many women immediately following delivery and approximately 15% of women will have urinary incontinence that persists for 3 months after birth [8]. However, a recent study by Glazener *et al.* [9] showed that three-quarters of women with urinary incontinence 3 months after childbirth still have this 6 years later. Urinary incontinence is more frequently seen following instrumental delivery and least frequently after elective Caesarean section. Urinary fistulae are uncommon in obstetric practice today, although direct injury from obstetric forceps may occasionally occur. Complications to the ureter are most commonly seen after a complicated Caesarean section, when ureteric injury may either result in a ureteric fistula or ureteric occlusion. Women with this type of urinary problem should not be managed by obstetricians but should be referred to a urological colleague for surgical management.

Incontinence of faeces

It is now recognized that 35% of women undergoing their first vaginal delivery develop anal sphincter injury [10,11]. Approximately 10% will still have anal symptoms of urgency or incontinence at 3 months after birth. Again, in the 6-year follow-up study by Glazener *et al.* [9], there was no improvement in this anal incontinence rate over time

and at 6 years the faecal incontinence rate actually increased to 13%. The aetiology of this type of anal sphincter trauma is complex in the same way as the mechanisms that maintain continence are complex. Instrumental delivery is a recognized cause of trauma and randomized trials suggest that the use of vacuum extraction is associated with less perineal trauma than forceps delivery [12,13]. The incidence figures confirm this: forceps delivery is associated with a 32% incidence of anal incontinence compared with a 16% incidence for vacuum extraction. The incidence of third- and fourth-degree tears varies enormously from centre to centre, suggesting that the clinical ability to recognize this type of trauma may vary. In those women who have a recognized anal sphincter rupture, 37% continue to have anal incontinence despite primary sphincter repair [14]. A recent Cochrane review of the role of Caesarean section to avoid anal incontinence concluded that there is insufficient evidence to recommend this [15].

Secondary postpartum haemorrhage

Delayed postpartum bleeding occurs in 1–2% of patients. It occurs most frequently between 8 and 14 days after birth and in the majority of these cases it is due to sloughing of the placental site. However, if this bleeding is not self-limiting, further investigation will be required. Ultrasound examination of the uterine cavity will usually determine whether there is a significant amount of retained products, although it can be difficult to distinguish between blood clot and retained placental tissue. Suction evacuation of the uterus is the treatment of choice and, if this is required, it is imperative that antibiotic cover is given. If curettage is not required immediately to arrest bleeding, it is best to start antibiotics at least 12 hours beforehand. This will reduce the risk of endometritis leading to uterine synechae. A combination of metronidazole and co-amoxiclav can be used in those patients who have endometritis without retained products of conception. In those who do have retained products who require curettage, intravenous antibiotics in the form of metronidazole and a cephalosporin or clindamycin are the antibiotics of choice. Great care must be taken at the time of curettage as the infected uterus is soft and easy to perforate. Rarely, these measures do not result in cessation of bleeding, and in life-threatening circumstances embolization of the uterine arteries may be effective in controlling the bleeding, as may the use of uterine tamponade using a Foley catheter balloon.

Puerperal psychological disorders

Mild psychological disturbance and transient depression are extremely common in the few days after birth. This transient state of tearfulness, anxiety, irritation and restlessness has been variously described as the 'blues' and it may occur in up to 70% of women. It is usually resolved

Table 30.6 Risk factors for postnatal depression.

Unmarried
Age <20 years
Brought up by single parent
Poor parental support in childhood
Poor relationship with partner
Socially disadvantaged
Poor achievement educationally
Low self-esteem
Previous emotional problems
Previous depressive illness

---

by day 10 after delivery and is probably associated with disruptive sleep patterns and the adaptation and anxiety of having a newborn baby. The changes in steroid hormone levels that occur immediately following delivery are not correlated with this transient depressive state, and because it is transient no therapy is needed. Postpartum depression occurs in approximately 8–15% of women and may vary in severity from mild to suicidal depression [16]. The signs and symptoms of postnatal depression are no different from those of depression in non-pregnant women and there are a number of antenatal factors that increase the risk of major postpartum depression (outlined in Table 30.6). There is a high incidence of recurrence of postpartum depression in subsequent pregnancies (around 50%). Mode of delivery has not been associated with an increased risk of postpartum depression but early recognition of this condition is extremely important. When diagnosed early and treated, the prognosis is extremely good, although symptoms may persist for up to a year. Unfortunately, there may be delays in the diagnosis as this type of depression occurs most commonly when the mother has returned home and is in the community. A worrying trend over the last few years has been that suicide is now the leading cause of maternal mortality. In the Confidential Enquiry into Maternal and Child Health 2003–2005 [7], there were 37 deaths in the postnatal period related to psychiatric disorders. Of these, 19 deaths were the result of suicide by hanging, jumping from a height, cutting of the throat or overdose. It is therefore obvious that patients at risk must be identified in the antenatal period and communication between the hospital, obstetrician, midwife, GP, healthcare worker and the psychiatric liaison services must be improved if we are to reduce the level of suicide.

Postnatal psychosis

Approximately 0.1% of women may exhibit some signs of psychosis after birth. Postpartum psychosis is usually characterized by an increased degree of anxiety, a combination of mania and depression, suicidal thoughts, an expression of delusion and a wish to self-harm or to harm the baby. Women manifesting signs of postpartum psychosis should be referred immediately to a psychiatrist and transferred to a mother and baby unit where they can be appropriately cared for, as 5% of these women may commit suicide and the infanticide rate is also 5% if they are not treated.

Counselling of patients after perinatal death

When a woman and her family experience a loss associated with pregnancy, special attention must be given to the grieving process. Mourning is an extremely important part of coping and it is essential that the clinical signs and symptoms of grief are recognized so that healthcare workers can be sympathetic to this grieving process. These symptoms include sleeplessness, fatigue, poor eating habits, preoccupation with pictures of the baby, feelings of guilt, hostility and anger, and general disruption in the normal pattern of daily life. Unless clinicians are aware of these changes, misunderstandings may occur and the ability to help the process of grieving will be lost. These families require a sympathetic person so that they have the opportunity to express and discuss their feelings openly. The establishment of identified individuals who are trained to deal with perinatal death is extremely important and centres should have doctors, midwives and counsellors available to help the grieving families. It is also extremely important that trained individuals are able to help the family with the legal and administrative processes associated with the death so that they are not overburdened, which will interfere with their ability to grieve. Counselling and support for these families may need to go on for many weeks or months after the event and appropriate staff must be available to help them.

Drugs during lactation

Drugs taken by a breast-feeding mother may pass to the child, and it is important to consider whether particular drugs will have any effect on the fetus. This is often a difficult problem and the reader is referred to Schaefer *et al.* [17] for more information.

Infant feeding

The major physiological event of the puerperium is the establishment of lactation. Some mothers in developed countries still reject breast-feeding in favour of artificial feeding but there is increasing evidence of the important short- and long-term benefits of breast-feeding.

Advantages of breast-feeding

Nutritional aspects of breast milk

Human milk does not have a uniform composition: colostrum differs from mature milk and the milk of the early

Table 30.7 Comparison of the constituents of human and cows' milk.

Constituent	Human milk	Cows' milk
Energy (kcal/100 mL)	75	66
Protein (g/100 mL)	1.1	3.5
Fat (g/100 mL)	4.5	3.7
Lactose (g/100 mL)	6.8	4.9
Sodium (mmol/L)	7	2.2

puerperium differs from the milk of late lactation. Indeed, the content of milk varies at different stages of the same feed. Nevertheless, there are substantial differences in the constituent concentrations of human milk and cows' milk (Table 30.7), with human milk having less protein but more fat and lactose. Human milk and milk formulae also differ with respect to a number of specific components, for example the long-chain polyunsaturated fatty acids, and this has important neurodevelopmental consequences for the baby [18]. There is no doubt that breast milk is the ideal nutrition for the human baby.

Protection against infection

One of the most important secondary functions of breast-feeding is to protect the infant against infection. This is particularly important in developing countries, where it has been estimated that in each year there are 500 million cases of diarrhoea in infants and children and about 20 million of these are fatal. However, the extent to which breast-feeding protects against infection in infants in developed countries has been a matter of dispute. In a study from Dundee, Scotland, it was found that babies who had been breast-fed for at least 3 months had greatly reduced incidences of vomiting and diarrhoea compared with babies who were either bottle-fed from birth or completely weaned within a short time of delivery [19]. This study also found that the protection against gastrointestinal illness in breast-fed babies persisted beyond the period of breast-feeding itself and, in the developed country setting at least, was not undermined by the early introduction of at least some supplements. There was a smaller protection against respiratory tract infections but not against other illnesses.

A number of mechanisms contribute to the anti-infective properties of breast milk. Breast milk contains lactoferrin which binds iron, and because *E. coli* requires iron for growth, the multiplication of this organism is inhibited. Breast-feeding also encourages colonization of the gut by non-pathogenic flora that competitively inhibit pathogenic strains. In addition, there are bactericidal enzymes, such as lysozyme, present in breast milk that contribute to its protective effect.

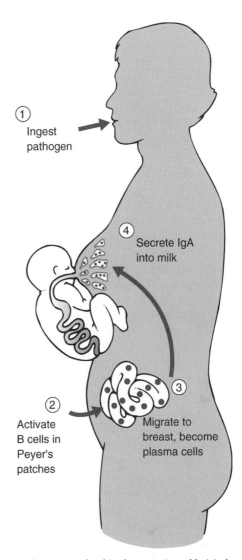

Fig. 30.1 Pathways involved in the secretion of IgA in breast milk by the enteromammary circulation. (Courtesy of Professor R.V. Short, Melbourne, Australia.)

However, the most specific anti-infective mechanism is an immunological one. If a mother ingests a pathogen that she has previously encountered, the gut-associated lymphoid tissue situated in the Peyer's patches of the small intestine will respond by producing specific IgA, which is transferred to the breast milk via the thoracic duct (Fig. 30.1). This immunoglobulin, which is present in large amounts in breast milk, is not absorbed from the infant's gastrointestinal tract but remains in the gut to attach to the specific offending pathogen against which it is directed. In this way the breast-fed infant is given protection from the endemic infections in the environment against which the mother will already have immunity [20]. Breast milk also contains living cells, such as polymorphs, lymphocytes and plasma cells and although their functions are not yet fully understood they may also be active against invading pathogens.

Breast-feeding and neurological development

A number of studies have shown positive associations between breast-feeding and improved childhood cognitive functions, such as increased IQ, which persist even after allowing for potential confounding variables. For example, one study found that, at 2 years of age, babies who had been breast-fed for more than 4 months had a 9.1 point advantage in the Bayley score [21]. Other studies have shown similar but smaller benefits and preterm babies also have improved neurological development if exposed to breast milk [22,23].

The mechanism for the improved neurological development is not fully understood but the presence of long-chain ω-3 fatty acids in breast milk, particularly docosahexanoic acid, may be important. The composition of the infant brain is sensitive to dietary intake but the relationship between the biochemical composition of brain lipid and cognitive function is not yet known. Nevertheless, the possible beneficial effect of breast-feeding on cognitive function is a topic of great potential importance.

Breast-feeding and atopic illness

There are a number of reports that show a lower incidence of atopic illness such as eczema and asthma in breast-fed babies. This effect is particularly important when there is a family history of atopic illness [24]. When the atopic illness is present, it is commonly associated with raised levels of IgE, especially cows' milk protein. Oddy *et al.* [24] suggest that apart from a positive family history, the most important predisposing factor for atopic illness is the early introduction of weaning foods. The protective effect of breast-feeding against atopic illness may therefore be secondary rather than primary, because breast-feeding mothers tend to introduce supplements at a later stage. Nevertheless, mothers with a family history of atopic illness should be informed of the advantages of breast-feeding and of the dangers of introducing supplements too quickly.

Breast-feeding and disease in later life

Breast-feeding may be associated with reduced juvenile-onset diabetes mellitus [25] and neoplastic disease in childhood [26]. It is possible that some of these benefits are related to the avoidance of cows' milk during early life rather than to breast-feeding per se, for example it is possible that early exposure to bovine serum albumin could trigger an autoimmune process leading to juvenile-onset diabetes. Breast milk is a particularly important ingredient in the diet of preterm infants as it appears to help prevent necrotizing enterocolitis among these particularly vulnerable babies.

Breast-feeding and breast cancer

There is an epidemic of breast cancer among women in developed countries of the Western world. A number of recent studies have shown a reduced risk of breast cancer among women who have breast-fed their babies [27]. Because breast-feeding appears to have no effect on the incidence of postmenopausal breast cancer, its overall protective effect will be relatively small but the protection offered by lactation still represents an important advantage against a much feared and common disease.

Breast-feeding and fertility

The natural contraceptive effect of breast-feeding has received scant attention in the Western world because it is not a reliable method of family planning in all cases. Nevertheless, on a population basis, the antifertility effect of breast-feeding is large and of major importance in the developing world. It has to be remembered that the majority of women in the developing world do not use artificial contraception and rely on natural checks to their fertility. By far the most important of these natural checks is the inhibition of fertility by breast-feeding. In many developing countries, mothers breast-feed for 2 years or more, with the effect that their babies are spaced at intervals of about 3 years. In the developing world, more pregnancies are still prevented by breast-feeding than by all other methods of family planning combined. The current decline in breast-feeding in the developing world is a cause for great concern because, without a sharp rise in contraceptive usage, the loss of its antifertility effect will aggravate the population increase in these countries.

Mechanisms of lactational amenorrhoea

The mechanisms of lactational amenorrhoea are complex and incompletely understood. The key event is a suckling-induced change in the hypothalamic sensitivity to the feedback effects of ovarian steroids. During lactation, the hypothalamus becomes more sensitive to the negative feedback effects and less sensitive to the positive feedback effects of oestrogen. This means that if the pituitary secretes enough follicle-stimulating hormone and luteinizing hormone to initiate the development of an ovarian follicle, the consequent oestrogen secretion will inhibit gonadotrophin production and the follicle will fail to mature. During lactation there is inhibition of the normal pulsatile release of luteinizing hormone from the anterior pituitary gland which is consistent with this.

From a clinical standpoint, the major factor is the frequency and duration of the suckling stimulus, although other factors such as maternal weight and diet may be important confounding factors. If supplementary food is introduced at an early stage, the suckling stimulus will fall and early ovulation and a return to fertility will be the consequence.

Breast-feeding and obesity

Artificially fed children have twice the risk of childhood obesity compared with breast-fed children [28]. Breast-

Table 30.8 Prevalence of breast-feeding from birth until 9 months, 1985–2005.

	1985	1990	1995	2000	2005
Birth	63	62	66	69	76
6 weeks	41	42	42	42	41
4 months	26	28	27	28	27
6 months	23	22	21	21	22
9 months	14	14	14	13	12

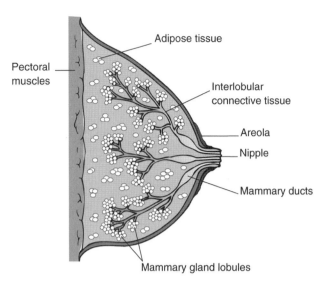

Fig. 30.2 Structure of the lactating breast.

fed children also have a significantly reduced blood pressure [29]. These children have a significantly reduced chance of being obese as adults and dying prematurely from cardiovascular disease.

Trends in infant feeding in the UK

Because of the many advantages of breast-feeding, it is important that mothers are given accurate information and encouraged to breast-feed successfully whenever possible. Conversely, mothers who choose to bottle-feed should be given proper instructions on best practice and be supported in their decision. In the UK, about 69% of mothers overall start to breast-feed but many discontinue after a short time. The prevalence of breast-feeding in the UK in 2005 is shown in Table 30.8 and the figures have shown no significant change over the previous 10 years, although a small increase in breast-feeding at birth is noted. Factors associated with higher breast-feeding prevalence include higher social class, primiparity, older age of mother and place of residence (mothers in the south of the UK have a higher prevalence). In attempting to improve these disappointingly low rates of successful breast-feeding, it is important that health professionals should understand the physiology of lactation.

Physiology of lactation

At puberty, the milk ducts that lead from the nipple to the secretory alveoli are stimulated by oestrogen to sprout, branch and form glandular tissue buds from which milk-secreting glands will develop (Fig. 30.2). During pregnancy, this breast tissue is further stimulated so that pre-existing alveolar–lobular structures hypertrophy and new ones are formed. At the same time milk-collecting ducts also undergo branching and proliferation. Both oestrogen and progesterone are necessary for mammary development in pregnancy but prolactin, growth hormone and adrenal steroids may also be involved. During pregnancy only minimal amounts of milk are formed in the breast despite high levels of the lactogenic hormones prolactin and placental lactogen. This is because the actions

of these lactogenic hormones are inhibited by the secretion of high levels of oestrogen and progesterone from the placenta and it is not until after delivery that copious milk production is induced.

Milk production

Two similar but independent mechanisms are involved in the establishment of successful lactation (lactogenesis): the first mechanism causes release of prolactin, which acts on the glandular cells of the breast to stimulate milk secretion (Fig. 30.3), and the second induces release of oxytocin, which acts on the myoepithelial cells of the breast to induce the milk ejection reflex (Fig. 30.4). Although these two mechanisms are similar, in that they can both be activated by suckling, they are mediated through two entirely different neuroendocrinological pathways. As can be seen in Figs 30.3 and 30.4, the key event in lactogenesis is suckling and the sensitivity of the breast accommodates itself to this important activity. During pregnancy the skin of the areola is relatively insensitive to tactile stimuli but becomes much more sensitive immediately after delivery. This is an ingenious physiological adaptation which ensures that there is an adequate stream of afferent neurological stimuli from the nipple to the hypothalamus to initiate and maintain the release of prolactin and oxytocin, both of which are required for successful lactation.

Milk ejection reflex

Successful breast-feeding depends as much on effective milk transfer from the breast to the baby as on adequate milk secretion. The milk ejection reflex is mediated by the release of oxytocin from the posterior pituitary gland (see Fig. 30.4). Oxytocin causes contraction of the sensitive myoepithelial cells that are situated around the

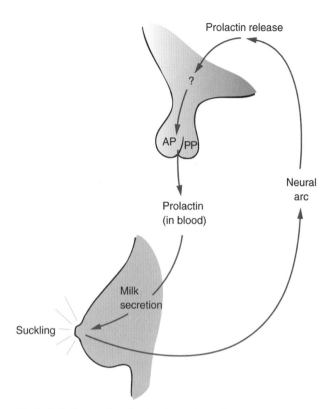

Fig. 30.3 Pathway of prolactin release from the anterior pituitary (AP).

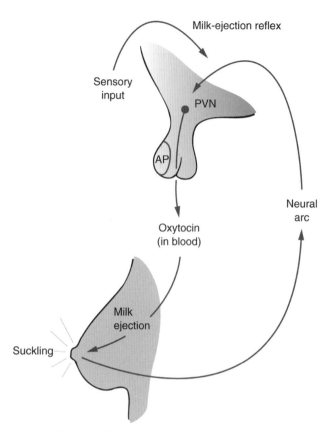

Fig. 30.4 Pathway of oxytocin release from the posterior pituitary. PVN, paraventricular nucleus.

milk-secreting glands and also dilates the ducts by acting on the muscle cells that lie longitudinally in the duct walls. Contraction of these cells therefore has the dual effect of expelling milk from the glands and of encouraging free flow of milk along dilated ducts. This is recognized by the mother as milk 'let-down' and she may be aware of milk being ejected from the opposite breast from which the baby is suckling. In contrast to prolactin, which is secreted only in response to suckling, oxytocin can be released in response to sensory inputs such as the mother seeing the baby or hearing its cry. Oxytocin has a very short half-life in the circulation and is released from the posterior pituitary in a pulsatile manner. As shown in Fig. 30.5 the highest levels of oxytocin may be released prior to suckling in response to the baby's cry, while prolactin is released only after suckling commences. The milk ejection reflex is readily inhibited by emotional stress and this may explain why maternal anxiety frequently leads to failure of lactation. Successful breast-feeding depends on engendering confidence in the mother and ensuring correct fixing and suckling at the breast.

Another factor is of potential physiological importance as an inhibitor of breast milk: if the milk is not effectively stripped from the breast at each feed, this will inhibit lactopoiesis and lead to a fall in milk production.

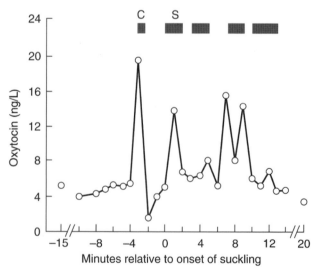

Fig. 30.5 Pattern of oxytocin release in response to the infant's cry (C) and to suckling (S). Redrawn from McNeilly AS, Robinson IC, Houston MJ, Howie PW. Release of oxytocin and prolactin in response to suckling. *BMJ* 1983;286:257–259, with permission.

Volumes of breast milk

During the first 24 hours of the puerperium the human breast usually secretes small volumes of milk, but with regular suckling milk volumes steadily increase and, by the sixth day of the puerperium, an average volume of 500 mL will be taken by the baby. Once lactation is fully established, an average daily milk volume is about 800 mL. In well-established lactation, it is possible to sustain a baby on breast milk alone for 4–6 months.

Management of breast-feeding

Despite the fact that it is a physiological event, many women experience difficulties in establishing breast-feeding. The greatest asset that a nursing mother can have is the support of an experienced and sympathetic counsellor. This counsellor may be a midwife, a health visitor or a lay person but the creation of a relaxed and confident environment is vital for successful breast-feeding. Babies are individuals, so there is no simple strategy that works in every case; mothers should be encouraged to learn to respond to their own babies but all too often well-meaning but dogmatic and conflicting advice is given. The best approach is to give mothers all the options and let them make their own decisions; they will soon learn by trial and error what is best for their own babies. As an important stimulus to the promotion of effective breast-feeding, the concept of 'baby-friendly' hospitals has been developed, with breast-feeding an important part of that assessment. The Baby-Friendly Initiative has adopted 10 successful steps to breast-feeding as its central strategy and these are outlined in Table 30.9. Support for the breast-feeding mother is both an art and a science and the reader is referred to some of the detailed texts on the subject [30].

Table 30.9 Ten steps to successful breast-feeding.

1	Have a written breast-feeding policy
2	Train all staff
3	Inform all pregnant women about the benefits and management of breast-feeding
4	Help mothers to initiate breast-feeding within 30 min of birth
5	Show mothers how to breast-feed
6	Foster the establishment of breast-feeding support groups
7	Practice 24-hour rooming-in
8	Encourage breast-feeding on demand
9	Give newborn infants no other food or drink, unless medically indicated
10	Use no artificial teats

Source: UNICEF UK Baby Friendly Initiative [31].

Summary box 30.1

- The physiological changes that occur during pregnancy are reversed after birth and return to their normal pre-pregnancy state over a period that varies from 6 weeks to 6 months.
- Thromboembolism remains a major cause of maternal death, which in the majority of cases is avoidable with prompt and appropriate treatment.
- Puerperal infection remains a major cause of maternal death worldwide and in the majority of cases is avoidable with prompt recognition of the clinical symptoms and signs and subsequent treatment.
- Postpartum monitoring of urinary function is essential to avoid urinary retention and subsequent long-term bladder dysfunction.
- Postnatal suicide is an increasing cause of maternal death and there is therefore a need for antenatal and postnatal vigilance in detecting at-risk mothers and ensuring they receive appropriate psychiatric support.

References

1 Oppenheimer LW, Sheriff EA, Goodman JD *et al.* The duration of lochia. *Br J Obstet Gynaecol* 1986;93:754–757.

2 Kovacs GT. Post-partum fertility: a review. *Clin Reprod Fertil* 1985;3:107–114.

3 Greer IA. Prevention of venous thromboembolism in pregnancy. *Best Pract Res Clin Haematol* 2003;16:261–278.

4 Rooney BL, Schauberger CW. Excess pregnancy weight gain and long-term obesity: one decade later. *Obstet Gynecol* 2002;100: 245–252.

5 Dewey KG. Impact of breastfeeding on maternal nutritional status. *Adv Exp Med Biol* 2004;554:91–100.

6 Larson-Meyer DE. Effect of postpartum exercise on mothers and their offspring: a review of the literature. *Obes Res* 2002;10: 841–853.

7 Lewis G (ed.) *Saving Mothers' Lives: Reviewing Maternal Deaths to Make Motherhood Safer 2003–2005. The Seventh Report on Confidential Enquiries into Maternal Deaths in the United Kingdom.* London: Confidential Enquiry into Maternal and Child Health, 2007. Available at: www.cmace.org.uk/getattachment/ 26dae364-1fc9-4a29-a6cb-afb3f251f8f7/Saving-Mothers'-Lives-2003-2005-(Full-report).aspx.

8 Chaliha C, Stanton SL. Urological problems in pregnancy. *BJU Int* 2002;89:469–476.

9 Glazener CM, Herbison GP, Macarthur C, Grant A, Wilson PD. Randomised controlled trial of conservative management of postnatal urinary incontinence and faecal incontinence: six year follow up. *BMJ* 2005;330:337.

10 Donnelly VS, Fynes M, Campbell D. Obstetric events leading to anal sphincter damage. *Obstet Gynecol* 1998;92:955–961.

11 Sultan AH, Kamm MA, Hudson CN, Thomas JM, Bartram CI. Anal-sphincter disruption during vaginal delivery. *N Engl J Med* 1993;329:1905–1911.

12 Bofill JA, Rust OA, Schorr SJ *et al.* A randomized prospective trial of the obstetric forceps versus the M-cup vacuum extractor. *Am J Obstet Gynecol* 1996;175:1325–1330.

13 Johansson RB, Rice C, Doyle MA. A randomised prospective study comparing the new vacuum extractor policy with forceps delivery. *Br J Obstet Gynaecol* 1993;100:524–530.

14 Sultan AH. Third degree tear repair. In: McJean AB (ed.) *Incontinence in Women*. London: RCOG Press, 2002: 379–390.

15 Nelson RL, Furner SE, Westercamp M, Farquhar C. Cesarean delivery for the prevention of anal incontinence. *Cochrane Database Syst Rev* 2010;(2):CD006756.

16 Glazener CM, MacArthur C, Garcia J. Postnatal care: time for a change. *Contemp Rev Obstet Gynaecol* 1993;5:130–136.

17 Schaefer C, Peters PW, Miller RK. *Drugs During Pregnancy and Lactation*, 2nd edn. San Diego: Academic Press, 2007.

18 Anderson JW, Johnstone BM, Remley DT. Breastfeeding and cognitive development: a meta-analysis. *Am J Clin Nutr* 1999; 70:525–535.

19 Howie PW, Forsyth JS, Ogston SA, Clark A, Florey CD. Protective effect of breast feeding against infection. *BMJ* 1990; 300:11–16.

20 Morrow-Tlucak M, Haude RH, Ernhart CB. Breastfeeding and cognitive development in the first 2 years of life. *Soc Sci Med* 1988;26:635–639.

21 Brandtzaeg P. The mucosal immune system and its integration with the mammary glands. *J Pediatr* 2010;156(2 Suppl):S8–S15.

22 Lucas A, Morley R, Cole TJ, Lister G, Leeson-Payne C. Breast milk and subsequent intelligence quotient in children born preterm. *Lancet* 1992;339:261–264.

23 Vestergaard M, Obel C, Henriksen TB, Sørensen HT, Skajaa E, Ostergaard J. Duration of breastfeeding and developmental milestones during the latter half of infancy. *Acta Paediatr* 1999; 88:1327–1332.

24 Oddy WH, Peat JK, de Klerk NH. Maternal asthma, infant feeding, and the risk of asthma in childhood. *J Allergy Clin Immunol* 2002;110:65–67.

25 Gerstein HC. Cow's milk exposure and type I diabetes mellitus. A critical overview of the clinical literature. *Diabetes Care* 1994; 17:13–19.

26 Davis MK. Review of the evidence for an association between infant feeding and childhood cancer. *Int J Cancer Suppl* 1998;11: 29–33.

27 Collaborative Group on Hormonal Factors in Breast Cancer. Colloborative group on breast cancer and breastfeeding: collaborative reanalysis of individual data from 47 epidemiological studies in 30 countries, including 50302 women with breast cancer and 96973 women without the disease. *Lancet* 2002;360: 187–195.

28 von Kries R, Koletzko B, Sauerwald T *et al.* Breast feeding and obesity: cross sectional study. *BMJ* 1999;319:147–150.

29 Martin RM, Ness AR, Gunnell D, Emmett P, Davey Smith G. Does breastfeeding in infancy lower blood pressure in childhood? The Avon Longitudinal Study of Parents and Children (ALSPAC). *Circulation* 2004;109:1259–1266.

30 NHS Choices. Breastfeeding. Available at: www.nhs.uk/planners/breastfeeding/pages/breastfeeding.aspx.

31 UNICEF. Baby Friendly Initiative. Available at: www.babyfriendly.org.uk.

Chapter 31
Neonatal Care for Obstetricians

Glynn Russell

Division of Neonatology, Imperial College Healthcare NHS Trust, London, UK

Management decisions during pregnancy and labour require knowledge of neonatal care and outcome. The informed obstetrician will thus more confidently deal with prospective parent's questions and be more engaged in the collaborative planning of perinatal care, particularly in high-risk pregnancies or where the fetus is at high risk of neonatal complications. This chapter therefore focuses on the basic neonatal knowledge required by the practising obstetrician but also provides a personal perspective gained from experience of some of the determinants of success and occasional failure of perinatal care. A neonatal reference text should be consulted for more detail on transitional physiology, neonatal resuscitation, neonatal conditions and management to augment the brief notes included later in this chapter.

Anticipation and levels of neonatal care

After birth, 90% of babies are cared for by their mothers and healthcare professionals should aim to facilitate this natural process. Approximately 8–10% of babies require more than normal care and about 2–3% need intensive care (level III) following delivery; the majority of these may be anticipated because of impending prematurity, fetal abnormalities or concerns about fetal well-being. Care in complex cases requires multidisciplinary involvement, good planning and handover of respective responsibilities and duties of care from obstetrician and midwife to the neonatal team. Anticipating potential problems during the antenatal period facilitates the achievement of excellent care and helps avoid the unexpected becoming an uncontrolled emergency.

Other care categories are special care (level I) or high dependency care (level II). Levels I–III are delivered in the neonatal unit. If the baby's condition allows, a level of care sometimes referred to as 'transitional care' is delivered usually on a postnatal ward and aims to avoid separation of mother and baby and to promote breast-feeding.

Healthcare professionals support the mother to deliver medical care that may not be safely provided at home. Promotion of and support for breast-feeding is essential at all levels of neonatal care.

Summary box 31.1

Promoting good neonatal outcome in high-risk deliveries:
- Anticipation and management of potential problems requiring specialist neonatal care is facilitated by multidisciplinary communication.
- Explicit, detailed and well-documented explanation of anticipated neonatal scenarios after delivery allows clear pathways of care to be agreed with parents before birth.
- Consider a late karyotype to inform early neonatal management. This may prevent active resuscitation when a more appropriate plan may be to provide compassionate care and support for the family.

Antenatal communication and care plans

Anticipation and management of potential problems requiring specialist neonatal care is facilitated by multidisciplinary communication. The essential role of the neonatologist in antenatal discussions is to ensure that a comprehensive plan for delivery (timing, mode and place) and clear plans for resuscitation and stabilization are in place. The possible scenarios following birth need to be clearly discussed with parents to ensure their views and aspirations are fully taken into account when plans are agreed. The neonatal management plan will include the personnel and expertise of staff required at the delivery and the level of resuscitation deemed appropriate.

Documentation
The neonatal plan for complex babies should be clearly documented and copies made available in the maternal

Dewhurst's Textbook of Obstetrics & Gynaecology, Eighth Edition. Edited by D. Keith Edmonds.
© 2012 John Wiley and Sons, Ltd. Published 2012 by John Wiley and Sons, Ltd.

case record, the hand-held maternal notes and the neonatal service pending file. These plans will involve resuscitation, specialist management (e.g. cardiac or surgical) and likely scenarios that may require different pathways of care. The plans should also detail the mother's feeding intention, particularly if feeding after birth is anticipated to be problematic (e.g. extreme prematurity and some surgical cases). In some cases where only compassionate care is required, detailed plans should include pain relief and comfort feeds and may also include hospice care plans.

Antenatal counselling and late karyotype

Knowledge of the karyotype can reduce uncertainty when considering the longer-term prognosis of the high-risk fetus. Not always considered is the value to the neonatologist of knowing the karyotype for planning the extent of resuscitation even if parents are unwilling to terminate the pregnancy on the basis of an abnormal karyotype. In such cases, a late karyotype specifically to inform early neonatal management is invaluable and may prevent active resuscitation when a more appropriate plan may be to provide compassionate care and support for the family.

Timing of delivery

Consideration of the multidisciplinary management of the baby after elective delivery facilitates team coordination. It is essential to ensure appropriate members, equipment, investigations and theatres are available if these should be required. In addition anxious parents should not have their expectations and confidence dashed by unrealistic or non-existent perinatal plans.

Resuscitation plan for high-risk deliveries

Formal resuscitation plans are required for certain high-risk deliveries, such as extreme prematurity at the margins of viability, some serious fetal malformations that may require specialist intervention and stabilization, or if there is uncertainty about survival and long-term outcome. Explicit, detailed and well-documented explanation of anticipated neonatal scenarios after delivery allows clear pathways of care to be agreed with parents before birth. A well-meaning reassurance that the paediatrician or neonatologist will be present at delivery is inadequate and unhelpful. Therefore it is essential that engagement and timely communication between professionals involved antenatally (obstetrician, midwife, fetal medicine specialists, clinical geneticists, fetal cardiologists or surgeons) and a senior neonatologist is required in all cases where neonatal resuscitation and early stabilization may be needed before definitive management can be started. Such engagement will provide full and detailed information to the family and permit a written plan to be agreed with the parents and other professionals. The plans help to avoid confusion, especially if spontaneous labour and delivery occurs after-hours or pre-empts planned delivery.

Resuscitation guidelines

Plans for resuscitation need to take into consideration the various resuscitation guidelines that have been produced by international and national bodies such as the International Liaison Committee on Resuscitation (ILCOR) and the Royal Colleges. The ethical and practical issues of starting, withholding or withdrawing (or redirecting) resuscitation and neonatal intensive care should be explicitly considered and discussed with the family [1,2]. Palliative care may be a positive option but needs to be discussed and planned in detail. These discussions help prepare families and staff for the different outcomes following birth.

In the UK the guidelines are heavily reliant on data obtained by the population-based EPICure study of 1996 [3]. There have been significant advances in health service organization and perinatal management including use of antenatal steroids, surfactant and ventilation techniques. The 2-year outcome data of the EPICure 2 study performed in 2006 are awaited but preliminary data suggest that survival has increased in babies born at 23–26 weeks' gestation.

Guidelines need to be continually reviewed in the light of advances in care. Of interest is the recent national population-based study in Sweden which suggests that 1-year survival in extremely preterm infants (23–26 weeks) is improved with active perinatal care (see section Active perinatal care, p. 381) [4,5]. Although long-term morbidity data are not yet available, these preliminary data could inform future guidelines if long-term outcome is also improved.

Compassionate and palliative care

Palliative care after birth may be the preferred option for some babies. There is increasing awareness of the need for palliation, improving management and increasing availability of resources for neonatal palliative care. Planning before birth for such a care pathway helps parents establish links with caring staff and plan visits to palliative care centres if needed and avoids delays in hospital.

Communication following neonatal death

In circumstances where neonatal death is the outcome, family support by neonatal staff should include the antenatal team wherever possible. Continuing engagement by the obstetric staff in the postnatal care of the baby and family is especially helpful when the outcome is death or significant early morbidity. This ongoing communication between the antenatal and postnatal teams improves quality of care for the individual family and for all babies in general as open dialogue fosters respect and support.

Organization of neonatal services

Providing the appropriate level of care for the mother and/or her baby requires careful planning and well-organized and integrated health services.

Perinatal networks

Managed health service networks aim to deliver appropriate healthcare to a defined local population in the most effective and efficient manner. Specialized neonatal care is a high-cost, low-volume service that is increasingly delivered in managed networks. Neonatal or perinatal networks were developed in England as a result of recommendations from the Department of Health's National Strategy for Improvement in 2003.

Within each network, different hospitals provide a range of care as agreed by that network. The level of care provided by each hospital is based on resources, capacity, geography and the availability of appropriately skilled and trained staff. A network consists of at least one level III unit providing intensive care facilities, with specialist staff and facilities. The various network hospitals collaborate to ensure that every infant has access to the most appropriate level of care. The development of coterminous maternity networks would enhance the organization of perinatal services.

In the UK, level III neonatal intensive care units provide care for extremely preterm babies and the sickest term babies requiring all levels of advanced respiratory support and parenteral nutrition. These units have 24-hour cover from specialized nursing staff and neonatal specialist doctors. Level II units provide respiratory support for babies of 28 weeks' gestation or more and level I units provide care for babies that do not require respiratory support for prolonged periods (usually 24–48 hours only).

Neonatal transport

Ensuring that babies receive the appropriate level of care ideally requires delivery in the correct place if delivery is predictable and safe antenatal transfer of mother is possible. Postnatal transfer of babies to the correct level of unit after delivery also needs to be available. Specialist neonatal transfer services are evolving that have the expertise and equipment and thus help to avoid depleting specialist staff from the either the referral unit or the specialist centre.

Birth and postnatal adaptation

Neonatal resuscitation

Only 1% of normal birthweight babies require active resuscitation after birth and only 0.2% require advanced resuscitation including endotracheal intubation. Although the need for resuscitation may be predictable based on risk factors, 30% of babies requiring resuscitation are not predicted. Babies who may be at risk of not making a successful adaptation without assistance include those in the following groups: preterm births (usually <36 weeks), those with known fetal complications, fetal distress, fresh meconium-stained liquor, malpresentation and breech, multiple pregnancies, Caesarean section under general anaesthesia or for fetal distress, risk of fetal infection and instrumental delivery.

In the UK, the Royal College of Paediatrics and Child Health (RCPCH), the Royal College of Obstetrics and Gynaecology (RCOG) and the Royal College of Midwives (RCM) have published their recommendation that all professionals present at the time of birth are proficient in resuscitation of the newborn [6]. Basic neonatal resuscitation is now a requirement of training for obstetricians and midwives and advanced resuscitation for neonatal paediatricians and practitioners.

Antenatal and newborn screening

Antenatal screening continues after birth with newborn screening programmes. In the UK, antenatal screening includes the National Health Service (NHS) fetal anomaly, infectious diseases in pregnancy and sickle cell and thalassaemia screening programmes. These results influence antenatal management of mother and fetus and, in some cases, postnatal management of the newborn. The NHS National Screening Committee recommendations for systematic neonatal population screening include the following.

• NHS Newborn and Infant Physical Examination (NIPE) Screening Programme carried out within 72 hours and then repeated at 6–8 weeks. The specific areas included are the detection of congenital cataracts (red reflex), congenital heart disease, developmental dislocation of the hip and cryptorchidism in boys.

• Newborn Hearing Screening Programme (NHSP) carried out within 2 weeks by automated otoacoustic emission (AOAE) in well babies and automated auditory brainstem response (AABR) in babies following neonatal intensive or special care.

• NHS Newborn Blood Spot Screening Programme involves taking a blood sample at 5–8 days after birth in term babies. There are currently differences in the tests included in the different countries within the UK (Table 31.1).

In other countries, such as Australia and New Zealand, multiple metabolic disorders are included in their newborn screening programmes. Table 31.2 shows the conditions not currently recommended for systematic neonatal screening in the UK, although these are kept under review.

	England	Wales	Scotland	Northern Ireland
Congenital hypothyroidism	√	√	√	√
Cystic fibrosis (newborn)	√	√	√	√
Medium-chain acyl dehydrogenase deficiency	√	√	From 2011	√
Phenylketonuria	√	√	√	√
Sickle cell disease (newborn)	√	–	From 2011	√
Duchenne muscular dystrophy (males)	–	√	–	–
Homocystinuria	–	–	–	√
Tyrosinaemia	–	–	–	√

Table 31.1 NHS Newborn Blood Spot Screening Programme.*

* Blood sample taken at 5–8 days after birth.

Table 31.2 NHS National Screening Committee: systematic neonatal population screening not currently recommended in the UK with date for review of recommendation.

Amino acid metabolism disorders: 2011–2012
Biliary atresia: 2011–2012
Biotinidase deficiency: 2011–2012
Canavan's disease: 2009–2010
Congenital adrenal hyperplasia: 2010–2011
Fatty-acid oxidation disorders: 2008–2009
Galactosaemia: 2009–2010
Gaucher's disease: 2010–2011
Kernicterus: 2010–2011
Muscular dystrophy: 2010–2011
Neuroblastoma: 2010–2011
Organic acid metabolism disorders: 2010–2011
Thrombocytopenia (newborn): 2010–2011
Thrombophilia (newborn): 2012–2013

Neonatal outcome

 Sumary box 31.2

Neonatal outcome in developed countries:
- The majority of deaths before 1 year of age (infant mortality) follow preterm birth (66%).
- Advances in perinatal care have resulted in a significant increase in survival of preterm babies.
- Neurodevelopmental sequelae of prematurity present during the first 5 years after birth and include cerebral palsy, poor cognitive performance and sensory impairments (visual and auditory deficits).

Prematurity

Prematurity is the major determinant of outcome in developed countries. The preterm birth rate (live births occurring before 37 weeks' gestational age) is 5–9% in Europe and 12–13% in the USA and is increasing. In the USA there has been a 31% increase in prematurity since 1981 [7]. In England and Wales, there were 640000 live-born babies in 2005, 7.5% preterm and 1.3% less than 32 weeks' gestation [8].

The majority of deaths before 1 year of age (infant mortality) follow preterm birth (66%) and nearly half (44%) of babies that die before 1 year of age are born at less than 32 weeks' gestation. However, published survival rates of preterm births vary widely. Variation may be due to methodological differences such as case ascertainment, selection bias, and varying outcome definitions and follow-up duration. Reports from geographically defined population-based studies show lower survival rates than single-centre selective studies that are subject to bias.

Variation in preterm birth rates (all births) also appears to have a major influence on reported neonatal mortality rates between populations. Compared with other European regions, the delivery rate per 1000 births between 22 and 31+6 weeks in two regions in England (Trent: 16.8, 95% CI 15.7–17.9; Northern: 17.1, 95% CI 15.6–18.6) was significantly higher compared with a group mean of 13.2 (95% CI 12.9–13.5) [9]. Live birth rates showed similar trends. When comparisons were made between regions after adjustment for prematurity rates, the variation in survival outcomes was reduced.

Perinatal management policies and differences in perinatal healthcare provision as determinants of survival are inadequately quantified. The extent to which obstetricians use antenatal steroids and active management of delivery and neonatologists perform resuscitation and redirection of care during intensive care all potentially have effects on reported survival and outcome.

At the extremes of viability, biological variation and ethical considerations are important in determining management policies. Policies based simply on gestation at birth are inadequate and prediction of outcome may be more accurate if gender, exposure to antenatal steroids, single or multiple births and birthweight are considered with gestation.

Survival

Advances in perinatal care have resulted in a significant increase in survival of preterm babies. Tables 31.3–31.9 provide essential details on important population-based epidemiological studies from which meaningful and informative data can be obtained for use by both obstetricians and neonatologists.

Survival in late preterm babies (32–36 weeks) is 98–99% (Tables 31.5 and 31.6). There are limited data on longer-term morbidity in this group but recent reports suggest this neglected area should be studied in greater detail. There are five times more late preterm babies born than babies born before 32 weeks' gestation and therefore as a group require considerable healthcare resources.

Babies born before 28 weeks' gestation have shown the greatest increase in survival since the advent of modern perinatal care. Few babies less than 28 weeks' gestation survived until techniques were developed to provide respiratory support during the 1960s and 1970s. Over the following two decades, the use of antenatal corticosteroids, use of surfactant and improvements in respiratory support have resulted in striking improvements in reported survival.

The EPICure study of all births between 22 and 25 weeks' gestation in the UK and the Republic of Ireland during 1995 provided important population-based information on babies born at the borderline of viability [3,10]. During the study regionalized neonatal care was poorly developed. This study was repeated in the UK during 2006 and although full outcome results are awaited, survival has apparently increased. The development of more regionalized neonatal care delivery in the UK, with increasing use of managed neonatal networks during the period between the two studies, may have contributed to the improvement. This increase in survival in the UK is supported by studies in the Trent region during 1994–1999 and 2000–2005 that show that at least in the 24 and 25 week group there has been an improvement [11].

While there are differences in survival between studies, the most dramatic survival figures are reported from Sweden during 2004–2007 [4]. Compared with survival of all births of less than 10% at 23 weeks in all the other studies in Table 31.3, survival in Sweden was 29%. This survival advantage is seen in all gestation weeks from 22–26 weeks, with 50% survival at 24 weeks and 67% survival at 25 weeks. The survival end-point was 1 year compared with the other studies that reported survival to discharge from neonatal care.

Survival of live births also shows differences between countries and decades and apparent improvement in later studies within the same region. Of note is the survival improvement in England and Wales reported by the Office of National Statistics (ONS) in 2005 that shows improvements in survival to 1 year between 22 and 25 weeks compared with the EPICure study of 1995. The Swedish study shows significantly higher live birth survival, with 10% surviving at 22 weeks, 52% at 23 weeks, 67% at 24 weeks and 82% at 25 weeks and has been attributed to active perinatal care policies.

Active perinatal care

Active perinatal care for extremely preterm babies compared with an expectant and individualized care approach was increasingly adopted in Sweden following a report on regional differences in outcome during 1985–1999. The population of Sweden has a high standard of general health, there is general health insurance cover, pregnancy care is standardized and free of charge with a high uptake and each healthcare region has a regional level III hospital. Active perinatal care includes regionalized delivery of extremely preterm babies, antenatal steroids, Caesarean section delivery if indicated by maternal or fetal condition, specialist neonatologists at the delivery, use of early surfactant and admission to a level III neonatal intensive care unit.

The active care of babies at the limits of viability is controversial. Such controversy arises from concerns about risks of later disability, possible long-term complications such as hypertension and diabetes in adult survivors and the high costs of neonatal intensive care at the limits of viability. However, it is argued that misconceptions regarding survival and neurodevelopmental outcome may result in suboptimal care being offered and thus a self-fulfilling poor survival and adverse neurodevelopmental outcome.

While the survival results from Sweden are important, the later neurodevelopmental outcome results are eagerly awaited. Major neonatal morbidity, such as periventricular leucomalacia, severe intraventricular haemorrhage, retinopathy of prematurity and bronchopulmonary dysplasia (BPD), all increase the risk of poor long-term outcome morbidity. In the Swedish study, the proportions of survivors free of such early predictors of long-term morbidity were 17% at 23 weeks, 31% at 24 weeks, 45% at 25 weeks and 63% at 26 weeks. Increased survival without improvements in the complications and sequelae of prematurity will result in an absolute increase in the number of cases of cerebral palsy and other neurocognitive deficits within a population.

Neonatal mortality and early morbidity

Neonatal death in preterm births is largely due to respiratory complications, periventricular haemorrhage and infection. Antenatal steroids, the use of early surfactant and continuous positive airway pressure are all associated with a reduction in death and morbidity.

Childhood morbidity

Neurodevelopmental sequelae of prematurity present during the first 5 years after birth and include cerebral

Table 31.3 Survival of all births (22–27 weeks).

Study	N	Outcome	22 weeks N	%	23 weeks N	%	24 weeks N	%	25 weeks N	%	26 weeks N	%	27 weeks N	%
All births														
EPICure 1 (1995) [3,10]	4004	Survival of all births to discharge	(2/2112) (20–22 weeks)	0.1	(26/622)	4.2	(100/636)	15.7	(186/634)	29.3				
EPIPAGE (1997) [23]	1086	Survival of all births to discharge	(0/102)	0	(0/137)	0	(13/115)	11.3	(59/204)	28.9	(89/239)	37.2	(164/289)	57.0
Sweden (2004–07) [4]	1011	Survival of all births to 1 year	(5/142)	3.5	(53/183)	29.0	(96/191)	50.3	(167/250)	66.8	(176/245)	71.8		
*All births (alive at labour onset)**														
EPIBEL (1999–2000) [24]	525	Survival of all births to discharge	(0/72)	0	(1/71)	1.4	(19/101)	18.8	(50/115)	43.5	(105/166)	63.3		
Trent (1994–99) [11]	855	Survival of all births to discharge	(0/142)	0	(15/206)	7.3	(40/237)	16.9	(119/270)	44.1				
Trent (2000–05) [11]	797	Survival of all births to discharge	(0/119)	0	(12/164)	7.3	(82/258)	31.8	(142/256)	55.5				

* In these three studies the population was defined as all births known to be alive at labour onset.
EPICure, Extremely Premature Infant: Curosurf Study (UK and Ireland); EPIPAGE, Epidémiologique sur les Petits Ages Gestationnels, in nine French regions; EPIBEL, Extremely Premature Infants in Belgium, in all 19 perinatal centres in Belgium.

Table 31.4 Survival of live births (22–27 weeks).

Study	N	Outcome	22 weeks N	22 weeks %	23 weeks N	23 weeks %	24 weeks N	24 weeks %	25 weeks N	25 weeks %	26 weeks N	26 weeks %	27 weeks N	27 weeks %
EPICure 1 (1995) [3]	1289	Survival of live births to discharge	(2/142) (20–22 weeks)	1.4	(26/241)	10.8	(100/382)	26.2	(186/424)	43.9				
EPIPAGE (1997) [23]	595	Survival of live births to discharge	(0/16)	0	(0/30)	0	(13/42)	31.0	(59/119)	49.6	(89/158)	56.3	(164/230)	71.3
VICS (1991–92) [25]	438	Survival of live births to discharge	(0/37)	0	(5/52)	9.6	(21/63)	33.3	(51/88)	58.0	(72/98)	73.5	(78/100)	78.0
VICS (1997) [26]	223	Survival of live births to 2 years	(1/15)	6.7	(9/22)	40.9	(12/29)	41.4	(41/56)	73.2	(46/52)	88.5	(42/49)	85.7
Trent (1994–99) [3]	682	Survival of live births to discharge	(0/81)	0	(15/148)	10	(40/198)	20.2	(119/255)	46.6				
EPIBEL (1999–2000) [24]	322	Survival of live births to discharge	(0/2)	0	(1/18)	5.5	(19/65)	29.2	(50/90)	55.6	(105/147)	71.5		
Trent (2000–05) [11]	669	Survival of live births to discharge	(0/69)	0	(12/131)	9.2	(82/227)	36.1	(142/242)	58.7				
Sweden (2004–07) [4]	707	Survival of live births to 1 year	(5/51)	9.8	(53/101)	52.5	(96/144)	66.7	(167/205)	81.5	(176/206)	85.4		
VICS (2005) [27]	288	Survival of live births to 2 years	(1/33)	3.0	(7/35)	20.0	(22/43)	51.2	(31/46)	67.4	(47/59)	79.7	(64/72)	88.9
ONS (2005) [8]	2866	Survival of live births to 1 year	(8/152)	5.3	(44/283)	15.6	(198/474)	41.8	(322/499)	64.7	(537/704)	76.3	(648/754)	85.9

Survival end-points vary between discharge and 2 years although deaths after discharge are uncommon.
ONS, Office for National Statistics; VICS, Victorian Infant Collaborative Study (Australia). For other abreviations, see Table 31.3.

Table 31.5 Survival of live births (28–32 weeks).

Study	N	Outcome	28 weeks		29 weeks		30 weeks		31 weeks		32 weeks	
			N	%	N	%	N	%	N	%	N	%
EPIPAGE (1997) [23]	2306	Survival of live births to discharge	(222/285)	77.9	(244/273)	89.4	(385/419)	91.9	(526/551)	95.5	(757/778)	97.3
ONS (2005) [8]	8579	Survival of live births to 1 year	(967/1072)	90.2	(1136/1213)	93.7	(1542/1605)	96.1	(1876/1935)	97.0	(2692/2754)	97.8

Table 31.6 Survival of live births (33–40 weeks).

Study	N	Outcome	33–36 weeks		37–40 weeks	
			N	%	N	%
ONS (2005) [8]	475 444	Survival of live births to 1 year	(36 426/36 784)	99.0	(437 803/438 660)	99.8
British Columbia (1999–2002) [28]	95 248	Survival of live births to 1 year	(6345/6381)	99.4	(88 725/88 867)	99.8

Table 31.7 Follow-up of live births (22–27 weeks) at 2–2.5 years: disability.*

Study	Gestation range (weeks)	Live birth survival (%)	Age (years)	Survivors	Follow-up survivors		No disability		Other disability						Severe disability	
					N	%	N	%	N		%				N	%
									Mild			Moderate				
									N	%		N	%			
EPICure 1 (1995) [3,10]	22–25	24.4	2.5	308	283	91.9	155	54.8	78		27.6				73	25.8
VICS (1991–92) [25]	22–27	56.1	2	225	221	98.2	119	54.3	54	24.7		29	13.2		17	7.8
VICS (1997) [26]	22–27	69.6	2	151	149	98.7	72	48.3	35	23.5		19	12.8		23	15.4
VICS (2005) [27]	22–27	63.7	2	172	163	94.8	83	50.9	47	28.8		27	16.6		6	3.7

*Disability reported in studies usually refers to one or more severe functional impairments, including non-ambulatory cerebral palsy, developmental quotient or IQ of less than −2 or −3 standard deviations from the norm, blindness and hearing impairment not improved with aids. VICS, Victorian Infant Collaborative Study (Australia).

palsy, poor cognitive performance and sensory impairments (visual and auditory deficits). During later years, academic underachievement and behavioural sequelae may occur. The definitions used for neurodevelopmental impairments and disability between studies are not uniform but more rigorous definitions are evolving. Disability reported in studies usually refers to one or more severe functional impairments, including non-ambulatory cerebral palsy, developmental quotient or IQ of less than −2 or −3 standard deviations from the norm, blindness and hearing impairment not improved with aids. Tables 31.5 and 31.6 show that disability rates at 2–2.5 years and at 5 years are considerably higher in the EPICure study compared with the other comparable

Table 31.8 Follow-up of live births (22–32 weeks) at 5–6 years: disability.*

Study	Gestation range (weeks)	Live birth survival (%)	Age (years)	Survivors	Follow-up survivors N	%	No disability N	%	Mild disability N	%	Moderate disability N	%	Severe disability N	%
EPICure 1 (1995) [10,29]	22–25	24.4	6	308	241	78.0	48	19.9	83	34.4	57	23.7	53	22
VICS (1991–92) [25]	22–27	56.1	5	225	221	98.2	119	54.3	54	24.7	29	13.2	17	7.8
EPIPAGE (1997) [23]	22–28	62.2	5	547	402	73.5	207	51.5	105	26.1	58	14.4	32	8.0
	(No survivors 22–23 weeks)													
	29–32	94.6	5	1912	1198	62.7	757	63.2	293	24.5	97	8.1	51	4.3

*Disability reported in studies usually refers to one or more severe functional impairments, including non-ambulatory cerebral palsy, developmental quotient or IQ of less than –2 or –3 standard deviations from the norm, blindness and hearing impairment not improved with aids.

Table 31.9 Follow-up of live births (22–32 weeks) at 5–6 years: neurocognitive.

Study	Gestation range (weeks)	Live birth survival (%)	Age (years)	Survivors	Follow-up survivors N	%	Cerebral palsy Severe N	%	Other motor N	%	Sensorineural Blind N	%	Deaf N	%	Cognitive N	%	
EPICure 1 (1995) [10,29]	22–25	24.4	6	308	241	78.0	15	6.2	43	17.8	7	2.9	5	2.1	50*	20.7	(<–2 SD)*
VICS (1991–92) [25]	22–27	56.1	5	225	221	98.2	15	6.8	10	4.5	4	1.8	2	0.9	34	15.4	(<–2.5 SD)
EPIPAGE (1997) [23]	22–28	62.2	5	547	402	73.5							4	1.0	71	17.7	(<–2 SD)
	(No survivors 22–23 weeks)						30†	1.9	129	8.1	12†	0.8					
	29–32	94.6	5	1912	1198	62.7							4	0.3	111	9.3	(<–2 SD)

*27 (11.2%) were less than –3 SD.
†The EPIPAGE study reported combined rates of cerebral palsy and blindness for the two groups comparable to the EPICure and VICS studies.

studies in Australia, France and Belgium. The lack of perinatal organization that existed in the UK in 1995 has been suggested as one possible explanation for the differences.

Neuromotor domain

Although cerebral palsy is the most commonly quoted outcome after very preterm birth, developmental and cognitive impairments are more common. The term refers to static injury to the developing brain that affects motor function. Different patterns are described and most commonly after preterm birth spastic diplegia is found. Of very low birthweight babies, 8–10% are affected with increasing proportions at lower gestation and it is more commonly seen in boys. Overall rates do not appear to be changing significantly as survival increases, but there is concern that the absolute prevalence will increase with increased survival of the most immature babies.

Developmental domain

The most common disability at 2 years is developmental or cognitive impairment, affecting up to 50% of extremely preterm babies. During the school years this domain of impairment is even more significant.

Sensory and communication domain

The prevalence of severe impairment of hearing and vision in very preterm babies is relatively low (hearing impairment not improved with aids <2%, blindness <3%). Less severe impairments are more common and include squints and refractive errors.

Academic attainment

Cognitive impairment appears to be the major determinant of school performance. At 8–9 years, approximately 20% of very low birthweight babies require special education and for those in regular schools, 25% repeat a year and 11–15% receive special help. At 11 years, the EPICure cohort showed significantly lower academic attainment compared with controls [12]. The proportions requiring special educational support was 62% of the extremely preterm group compared with 11% for the term controls (OR 13.1, 95% CI 7.4–23.3). Statements of Special Educational Needs were issued for 34% of the preterm cohort compared with 0.7% for controls (OR 76, 95% CI 10–552).

Behavioural/psychiatric sequelae

There is an excess of attention deficit hyperactivity disorder (ADHD) among preterm survivors. A meta-analysis of six follow-up studies revealed a relative risk of 2.64 (95% CI 1.85–3.78) among preterm babies. The EPICure study found ADHD in 11.5% of preterm babies and in 2.9% of term controls (OR 4.3, 95% CI 1.5–13) and autism spectrum in 8% compared with 0% in term controls [13].

Outcome in teenage and adult survivors

Various functional limitations occur in 86% of early teenage survivors with birthweight below 750 g. Growth disorders (49%), mental or emotional problems (58%), restrictions on physical activity (32%) and visual impairment (31%) are found and 75% use aids such as spectacles and medication. However, in a study of health-related quality of life in adolescent survivors with birthweight below 1000 g, the proportion that scored within the normal range was similar to normal-birthweight adolescents. Although fewer adult very low birthweight survivors go on to higher education than their peers, they are less likely to engage in risk-taking behaviour and social integration is not impaired.

Health and social care and educational resource utilization

There is a significant increase in utilization of public health, social and educational services by extremely preterm survivors. During the 11th year of life, the EPICure study estimates of public sector costs were £4007 (SD £2537) for controls and £6484 (SD £2537) for the preterm cohort, a significant mean cost difference of £2477 (95% CI 1605–3360; P < 0.001) [14].

Other morbidity

Many preterm survivors experience less severe problems such as clumsiness, visual impairment (squints, refractive errors, etc.), growth disorders and respiratory problems.

Respiratory

More than 50% of extremely low birthweight babies require hospital readmission during the first 12 months after discharge from the neonatal unit. These admissions are usually due to respiratory illness precipitated by lower respiratory infections. Chronic lung disease of prematurity or BPD has been reported in up to 40% of very low birthweight survivors. The rate is higher as birthweight and gestation falls. Significant airflow limitation on lung function tests are found in adolescent survivors.

Growth

Growth failure is common during infancy and early childhood but adult stature within the normal range is achieved. Despite this catch-up, extremely low birthweight babies remain at a height disadvantage to normal birthweight controls. In the longer term, there are concerns that accelerated weight gain may lead to increased risk of hypertension and other cardiovascular diseases as well as type 2 diabetes.

Effect on family

The psychological distress that parents of high-risk preterm babies experience is greatest during the first month after birth and persists for the first 2 years. The greatest effect of stress is found in families of low income and lower parental education and the more severe the child's functional disability. By adolescence, despite the preceding years of emotional distress, families report positive interactions with friends and within the family, they experience enhanced personal feelings of accomplishment and both positive and negative effects on the marital relationship.

Important clinical conditions in neonatology

The most common reasons for babies to require neonatal management or admission are management of prematurity, respiratory distress and possible infection.

Common problems in neonatal care

Prematurity

Infants born significantly before term usually require neonatal care until around the expected date of delivery. Mortality in extremely preterm babies has been significantly reduced by the use of modern perinatal practices including use of antenatal steroids, early use of surfactant and avoiding hypothermia after delivery (Fig. 31.1).

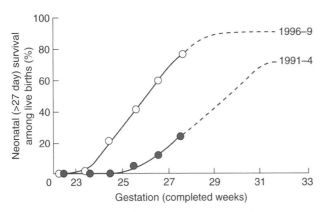

Fig. 31.1 Neonatal survival among registered live births. Redrawn from Tin *et al. Br Med J* 1997;314:107–110.

The stress on parents and family of having a baby who undergoes intensive care can be immense. They have to suffer prolonged uncertainty about the infant's survival as well as loss of control over their baby's and their own lives. Careful preparation of parents with visits to the intensive care unit and meetings with unit staff may help, but the difficulties for families in this situation should not be underestimated.

Hypoglycaemia

Conditions commonly associated with transient low blood glucose are hypothermia, infection, prematurity, intrauterine growth retardation and maternal diabetes. Some infants develop transient hyperinsulinaemia, particularly infants of diabetic mothers with poor antenatal control or those with severe rhesus disease. Rare causes include Beckwith–Wiedemann syndrome and metabolic defects such as cortisol deficiency, galactosaemia and other enzyme defects of glycogenolysis, gluconeogenesis or fatty acid oxidation. Preterm infants are much less able to mount a ketotic response and hypoglycaemia should be treated promptly. Treatment is initially to give calories in the form of milk or as intravenous glucose infusion. If hypoglycaemia persists, investigations including insulin and counter-regulatory hormone measurements are required.

Jaundice

Jaundice is the most common clinical condition needing medical attention in newborn babies. It occurs in 60% of term and 80% of preterm babies during the first week. Jaundice beginning in the first 24 hours after birth is always pathological. It is usually unconjugated and the commonest causes are haemolytic anaemia or infection. Jaundice beginning on days 2–5 is commonly physiological, but unconjugated hyperbilirubinaemia may have many causes including haemolytic disease, ABO incompatibility and glucose 6-phosphate dehydrogenase deficiency.

Phototherapy is the mainstay of treatment where treatment is indicated. Failure to control bilirubin levels with phototherapy may necessitate an exchange blood transfusion to avoid neurotoxicity such as kernicterus and hearing impairment. In the UK, the National Institute for Health and Clinical Excellence (NICE) guidelines for the screening and management of neonatal jaundice have recently been published [15]. Conjugated hyperbilirubinaemia signifies liver disease and requires urgent specialist investigation. These infants may be at risk of complications such as significant bleeding and neurological damage.

Respiratory conditions

Respiratory distress

Respiratory distress is one of the commonest problems encountered in the neonatal period. It is manifest by the clinical signs of tachypnoea (persistently over 60 breaths/min), intercostal recession, grunting, nasal flaring and tachycardia. If the baby becomes hypoxic, then cyanosis, apnoea and bradycardia may result. The presence of any signs of respiratory distress needs further evaluation and investigation. Tachypnoea with recession and nasal flaring is frequently the presentation of respiratory or cardiac disorders, while apnoea may be the presentation of a great many systemic disorders such as septicaemia, meningitis, gastrointestinal obstruction or heart disease.

Respiratory distress syndrome (surfactant deficiency)

The respiratory distress syndrome caused by inadequate surfactant production is mainly a disease of the preterm infant. However, it can occur in term infants, particularly those of diabetic mothers or after Caesarean section without labour. Affected infants may require mechanical ventilation and intensive care. The classical clinical presentation is an infant with tachypnoea, subcostal and intercostal recession and nasal flaring that becomes progressively worse over the first 60 hours after birth, and chest radiography shows a ground-glass appearance with air bronchograms. It can be associated with pneumothorax and intraventricular haemorrhage, although in more mature infants it normally resolves without sequelae. The combined use of antenatal corticosteroids and surfactant modify the illness, improving survival and reducing the rates complications but have little effect on reducing the incidence of BPD or chronic lung disease, which occurs mainly in preterm babies.

Congenital pneumonia

Congenital pneumonia is a relatively common problem associated with a variety of microorganisms. The infant presents with respiratory distress and chest radiography shows patchy inconsistent shadowing. Treatment is with antibiotics and intensive care as required.

Meconium aspiration

Inhalation of meconium before or during delivery can be an extremely severe problem if pulmonary hypertension with reduced lung perfusion and severe hypoxaemia develop. Meconium may block large or small airways or both and lead to a ventilatory deficit. Although meconium aspiration may be apparent at birth, severe disease may present an hour or more later and it is important that babies suspected of having aspirated are carefully observed.

Treatment of meconium aspiration and associated pulmonary hypertension requires expert intensive care. Early surfactant administration may be beneficial, while high-frequency oscillatory ventilation and the administration of nitric oxide reduce mortality. When other measures fail, extracorporeal membrane oxygenation should be considered.

Transient tachypnoea of the newborn

Transient tachypnoea of the newborn is due to delayed reabsorption of lung liquid and leads to a moderate degree of intercostal recession and tachypnoea. In the preterm infant this can lead to marked respiratory distress, but in a term baby needing high inspired oxygen concentrations, other causes of respiratory distress should be excluded.

Bronchopulmonary dysplasia/chronic lung disease of prematurity

This is a chronic condition affecting up to 50% of infants born at 26 weeks or less. Premature delivery, prenatal and postnatal inflammation and infection, ventilation, oxygen and poor nutrition are among the many factors contributing to the development and persistence of BPD. The underlying problem is an arrest in alveolar and peripheral vascular development. The severity is variable, ranging from the need for supplemental oxygen for several weeks to prolonged respiratory support with a ventilator or continuous positive airways pressure and even death. A small proportion of babies are discharged home on supplemental oxygen; most outgrow the need by 12 months of age. All babies born prematurely have an increased risk of respiratory illness within the first few years of life. This is increased in the group with BPD and respiratory problems may persist into adult life.

Infections

Newborn infants are particularly prone to perinatal infection. Risk factors include low birthweight, prolonged ruptured of membranes, maternal fever or chorioamnionitis. Indwelling cannulae, central venous lines and invasive mechanical ventilation increase the risk of nosocomial infection in those who require neonatal intensive care. Organisms responsible for later neonatal infection frequently come from the skin or gut. Breast-feeding helps promote normal gut flora and reduces the risk of acquired neonatal infections. Adherence to good hand-washing practices by all staff, parents and visitors can significantly reduce the risk of acquired infection.

Septicaemia

The signs of systemic sepsis are non-specific. Infants may present with apnoea, bradycardia or cyanotic episodes and poor feeding is a common association. They may be lethargic and hypotonic and are hyperthermic or hypothermic. Sepsis frequently presents as a metabolic acidosis or shock and occasionally causes petechial skin rash or severe jaundice.

Organisms that commonly cause infection in the newborn period include group B *Streptococcus* (GBS) and Gram-negative organisms such as *Escherichia coli* or *Klebsiella*. The prolonged use, or multiple changes, of antibiotics in the antenatal period may increase the risk of infection with resistant organisms. Rapid treatment with antibiotics, immediate resuscitation and, frequently, mechanical ventilation is required. Investigations include chest radiography, blood cultures, urine culture, and examination and culture of the placenta. A lumbar puncture is performed once the baby is stable and will tolerate the procedure. The mortality of infants who develop septicaemia in the neonatal period is high, with a significant number of survivors developing subsequent impairment.

Group B *Streptococcus* infection

Mortality due to maternal colonization by GBS is reduced by antibiotic therapy to the mother during labour and early treatment of infants with evidence of infection. About 2% of infants of colonized mothers develop infections, and 70% of these manifest risk factors at birth such as preterm labour, prolonged rupture of membranes or meconium-stained liquor. Urgent antibiotic therapy is indicated for these infants. Well infants shown by surface cultures to be colonized do not require treatment. Recurrent GBS infection can occur, but more commonly GBS infection occurs later in infancy when meningitis is the presenting problem.

Meningitis

Signs of meningitis in newborn infants are non-specific. Meningitis usually presents as septicaemia and can be complicated by cerebral oedema, cerebral infarction, brain abscess or deafness. Common causal organisms are GBS and *E. coli*. *Listeria monocytogenes* is a rare cause of perinatal infection in the UK.

Eye infection

The majority of sticky eyes are not infected but are due to a blocked nasolacrimal duct. In the absence of conjunctival redness or swelling, investigation for infection and treatment with topical antibiotics is not required. Simple measures such as cleaning with boiled water and lacrimal duct massage suffice, with symptoms usually resolving in 3–6 months. Neonatal conjunctivitis can be caused by such organisms as *Staphylococcus aureus*, *Chlamydia trachomatis*, *Haemophilus influenzae*, *Streptococcus pneumoniae* and *Neisseria gonorrhoeae*. Gonococcal ophthalmia usually presents within 24 hours of delivery with profuse purulent conjunctival discharge, and immediate diagnosis and treatment (systemic and topical) is required to prevent damage to the cornea.

Chlamydial ophthalmia, which is now among the commonest causes of neonatal conjunctivitis, presents between 5 and 12 days postnatal age; some babies infected as neonates will develop chlamydial pneumonia later in infancy. Corneal scarring is rare. Two weeks systemic and topical treatment is required. The identification of either *N. gonorrhoeae* or *Chlamydia* in the baby requires referral of mother and her sexual partner for investigation and treatment.

Skin infection

Simple hygienic methods such as bathing and handwashing can prevent many skin infections. The infant's skin is vulnerable to infection by staphylococci, which usually leads to small pustules or lesions but which can also cause scalded skin syndrome with severe exfoliation. Staphylococcal infections should therefore be treated with antibiotics after appropriate cultures have been taken. Streptococci can also cause skin infection and both may cause systemic illness.

Infection of the umbilical cord is commonly limited to periumbilical redness with a small amount of discharge. The presence of oedema indicating cellulitis can occasionally lead to complications such as spreading cellulitis of the abdominal wall, fasciitis and septicaemia and requires treatment with systemic antibiotics.

Candidiasis usually presents after the first week with napkin dermatitis with or without oral thrush. Topical and oral treatment is required to prevent the candidiasis returning as the gut is colonized with *Candida*. Maternal nipple candidial infection can occur in breast-feeding mothers.

Tuberculosis

Tuberculosis is a re-emergent disease and many hospitals now offer bacille Calmette–Guérin (BCG) immunization to newborn infants. Infants born to mothers infected with active tuberculosis should be vaccinated with isoniazid-resistant BCG vaccine and kept with the mother while both receive treatment with appropriate drugs. Breast-feeding should be encouraged.

Tetanus

Neonatal tetanus due to infection of the umbilical stump by *Clostridium tetani* is the result of poor hygiene and is a distressing and severe condition with extremely high mortality. Opisthotonus and muscle spasms of the jaw and limbs are presenting features and can appear very rapidly after birth. Prevention centres on maternal vaccination during pregnancy and education to improve hygiene and change of local cultural practices.

Neurological conditions

Neonatal encephalopathy

Neonatal encephalopathy can be caused by hypoxic ischaemia due to birth asphyxia but also by other conditions including metabolic disorders and infections. These conditions should be excluded before a confident diagnosis of hypoxic–ischaemic encephalopathy (HIE) due to birth asphyxia can be accepted.

Hypoxia–ischaemia followed by resuscitation may lead to apparent recovery followed by inexorable deterioration beginning 6–8 hours later and ending in severe cerebral injury. Consequently, it is frequently difficult to determine the prognosis soon after birth on clinical grounds alone. However, if asphyxia is severe or happened some time before delivery, the infant will not develop spontaneous breathing; therefore, if despite advanced life support there is no sign of spontaneous breathing 20 min after birth, the outcome is extremely poor.

HIE is graded clinically and a frequently used grading system was described by Sarnat and Sarnat [16]. Infants with grade 1 encephalopathy have a very good prognosis whereas infants with grade 3 almost all die or are severely impaired. About half the infants with grade 2 have severe neurodevelopmental impairment. Unfortunately a large number of infants at risk fall into grade 2, limiting the utility of the system.

Moderate hypothermia for perinatal HIE

The recent publication of studies using therapeutic hypothermia for 72 hours for HIE confirms a significant reduction in death and disability. The Treatment of Perinatal Asphyxial Encephalopathy (TOBY) study has also shown that the treated group had a significantly increased survival without neurological abnormality at 18 months (relative risk 1.57, 95% CI 1.16–2.12; $P = 0.003$) [17]. The risk of cerebral palsy in survivors was reduced (relative risk 0.67, 95% CI 0.47–0.96; $P = 0.03$) and there were significant improvements in both the Mental Development Index (MDI) and the Psychomotor Development Index (PDI) of the Bailey Scales of Infant Development 11 and also in the Gross Motor Function Classification System. A meta-analysis of three trials (767 patients) confirmed the significant reduction in death and severe disability at 18 months (risk ratio 0.81, 95% CI 0.71–0.93; $P = 0.002$), with a number needed to treat of 8 (95% CI 5–17) [18].

Therapeutic hypothermia is now accepted by most neonatologists in the UK as the standard of care for perinatal HIE. Research is progressing to find additional interventions to augment the benefit of hypothermia. It is important that eligible babies (36 weeks or more) are considered soon after birth for treatment as cooling should be commenced before 6 hours of age. The British Association of Perinatal Medicine has recently published recommendations for the use of therapeutic hypothermia in the UK [19].

> **Summary box 31.3**
>
> Hypoxic–ischaemic encephalopathy:
> - Neonatal encephalopathy can be caused by hypoxia–ischaemia due to birth asphyxia but other causes have to be excluded.
> - The severity of HIE is graded clinically.
> - Therapeutic hypothermia is effective in significantly reducing death and disability following perinatal HIE.

Cerebral palsy

Cerebral palsy is an umbrella term that describes the consequences of a non-progressive injury to the developing brain. The clinical manifestations include motor, sensory and cognitive deficits that may not be apparent until after 1 year of age and cannot be confidently diagnosed at birth. Although there is an association between neonatal encephalopathy and cerebral palsy, population-based studies have shown that only about 10% of all cases of moderate to severe neonatal encephalopathy in term babies are associated with intrapartum risk factors. Other risk factors for cerebral palsy are preterm birth or very low birthweight, perinatal infection, congenital malformations or multiple pregnancies [20–22].

Convulsions

Convulsions occurring just after delivery in term infants may be due to HIE, metabolic disorders, infections, hypoglycaemia, hypocalcaemia, and hypomagnesaemia or pyridoxine deficiency. Many otherwise idiopathic fits are caused by focal cerebral infarction, which have a much better prognosis than generalized hypoxic–ischaemic injury but are difficult to diagnose without magnetic resonance imaging.

Brain injury in preterm babies

Preterm infants are at high risk of cerebral injury and consequent neurodevelopmental impairment. The proportion of preterm babies that have injury and impairment is inversely related to gestational age. There are two major patterns of brain injury.

1 Intraventricular haemorrhage may affect only the germinal layers or ventricles in which case the prognosis is good; however, haemorrhage into the brain parenchyma is caused by haemorrhagic infarction and is associated with neurodevelopmental impairment.

2 Parenchymal injury is referred to as periventricular leucomalacia and defines general loss of white matter, sometimes with cavitation. Whereas haemorrhagic parenchymal infarctions can usually be seen by cerebral ultrasonography, periventricular leucomalacia is difficult to see and is probably under-diagnosed.

Both these conditions seem to be becoming less common than a more subtle loss of cerebral matter. The usefulness of cerebral ultrasonography alone to predict neurological prognosis in extremely preterm infants is therefore limited. The more mature preterm infants with normal ultrasound scans at discharge from intensive care have a very low risk of neurodevelopmental impairment, whereas those with definable loss of brain tissue from whatever cause have a greater than 50% chance of long-term impairment.

Brachial plexus injury

Brachial plexus injury occurs in 0.4–2.5 per 1000 live births. The commonest type, Erb's palsy, involves C5 and C6 nerve roots. The incidence has not declined over the past few decades but the prognosis for recovery has improved, with full recovery expected in the majority of babies with Erb's palsy. A fracture to the clavicle may also be present. Careful neurological examination is needed to determine the level of the lesion as this affects the prognosis for recovery of function. Associated Horner's syndrome is a bad prognostic sign.

Effects of maternal drug use

Infants of mothers who take drugs such as opiates, cocaine, amphetamines, barbiturates, benzodiazepines and some other medical drugs may develop a withdrawal syndrome, with irritability, poor feeding, apnoea and fits. The babies of mothers who have high alcohol or nicotine intake may also exhibit withdrawal. Wherever possible the mother and baby should be kept together; in many cases breast-feeding is not contraindicated. If a history of maternal drug abuse was known antenatally, a plan of management can be agreed before birth and referral to the social work team may be appropriate. Management of a baby at risk of drug withdrawal involves careful observation and skilled nursing. If withdrawal is severe, treatment with opiates may be required. Naloxone should never be given to infants at risk of opiate withdrawal as it can provoke convulsions. Many labour wards no longer stock naloxone for fear it will be given inadvertently to an infant of a substance-abusing mother.

Gastrointestinal conditions

Necrotizing enterocolitis

This poorly understood inflammatory disease is primarily a condition of preterm infants and those with congenital heart disease. It presents as an acute abdomen in the days or weeks after birth and varies in severity from mild to fatal. Diagnosis is clinical, aided by characteristic radiographic changes such as air in the bowel wall or biliary tree. Treatment is conservative, with antibiotics or surgery and cessation of enteral feeding.

Congenital abnormalities

Cardiac

Some form of congenital heart disease affects between 7 and 9 per 1000 live births, of whom approximately one-quarter will present in the newborn period. Fetal anomaly ultrasound can detect many lesions but some are more difficult to diagnose. Neonatal presentation is normally due to cyanosis, heart failure and respiratory distress, and shock. Some conditions present with asymptomatic findings on neonatal examination such as a murmur, absent femoral pulses or tachyarrhythmia.

Cyanosis

Causes of cyanotic heart disease include transposition of the great arteries and conditions that reduce pulmonary blood flow such as tetralogy of Fallot and pulmonary or tricuspid atresia. Pulmonary blood flow in these conditions depends on arterial ductal patency and the degree of blood mixture between heart chambers. For those presenting in the neonatal period, immediate treatment is required to prevent the arterial duct (ductus arterious) from closing (by infusion of prostaglandin E_1) and transfer to a specialist paediatric cardiac centre.

Cardiorespiratory distress and heart failure

Causes of cardiorespiratory distress due to increased pulmonary blood flow or heart failure include left-to-right shunting though septal defects. The commonest causes are large ventricular septal defect and persistent patent arterial duct.

Shock

Neonatal shock is usually due to major sepsis, significant hypovolaemia or blood loss or congenital heart disease. Congenital heart diseases causing shock include major interruption to the systemic circulation such as hypoplastic left heart syndrome, critical aortic stenosis and severe coarctation of the aorta or complex cardiac defects.

The asymptomatic murmur

Murmurs are common in newborn infants and are frequently innocent. A thorough search for other signs of cardiac disease should be made and an expert opinion arranged where appropriate. It is important to remember that the mention of a heart murmur can strike panic into even the calmest of parents and the situation needs to be handled with great tact. Rapid definitive diagno-

sis by echocardiography is the mainstay of successful management.

Respiratory

Congenital diaphragmatic hernia

Herniation of the abdominal contents into the hemithorax leads to severe respiratory difficulties with persistent pulmonary hypertension. Most cases present with respiratory distress and cyanosis at birth. Essential early management is the passage of a large-bore nasogastric tube into the stomach to prevent gaseous distension, ventilation and rapid transfer to intensive care. All these infants require tertiary-level intensive care, with access to sophisticated mechanical ventilation and modern vasodilator therapy such as nitric oxide. Surgery is delayed until the infant's respiratory status has been stabilized. Survival depends on the degree of underlying pulmonary hypoplasia and the presence of associated congenital anomalies such as cardiac defects. Long-term complications include persistent gastro-oesophageal reflux and respiratory problem; neurodevelopmental problems can develop if neonatal hypoxia was severe.

Gastrointestinal and abdominal wall defects

Oesophageal atresia and tracheo-oesophageal fistula

These conditions should be suspected when there is polyhydramnios or excessive mucus from the mouth at birth. The baby may show rapid onset of respiratory distress and cyanosis particularly after the first feed. Radiography after a nasogastric tube has been inserted confirms the diagnosis, showing the nasogastric or orogastric tube curling up in the oesophageal pouch (if atresia is present). Associated congenital anomalies occur in 50% or more of infants. Survival is usually determined by the severity of associated congenital anomalies and not the defect itself.

Abdominal wall defects

Exomphalos, in which part or all of the intestine and abdominal organs are in a peritoneal sac outside the abdomen, should be differentiated from gastroschisis, where a congenital defect of the abdominal wall allows herniation of the abdominal contents without a peritoneal sac. The former is frequently associated with other congenital defects while the latter is not. Urgent surgery is required if the amniotic sac has broken and for gastroschisis; immediate management is to wrap the abdominal contents in a plastic wrapper taking care not to twist the bowel and disrupt its vascular supply. This should help prevent hypovolaemia due to fluid loss from the exposed bowel. The long-term outcome for most with exomphalos is determined by the presence of associated congenital anomalies. In gastroschisis 90% or more now survive. However, their postnatal course is often protracted and parenteral nutrition may be required for several weeks with its risks and complications. In addition, bowel atresia and necrotizing enterocolitis may develop.

Intestinal obstruction

High intestinal obstructions usually present with vomiting that may be bile stained, and this ominous sign demands urgent investigation. Plain radiography of the abdomen can confirm the presence of obstruction by showing a lack of air in the lower gut or a sign such as the 'double bubble' of duodenal atresia, but an upper gastrointestinal contrast study may be required to exclude malrotation and volvulus. Hypertrophic pyloric stenosis does not usually present until 2–6 weeks of age.

Lower intestinal obstruction usually presents as failure to pass meconium within 24 hours followed by abdominal distension with or without vomiting. Causes include Hirschsprung's disease, meconium ileus due to cystic fibrosis, low bowel atresia or hypoplasia and imperforate anus. A meconium plug can sometimes mimic obstruction especially in preterm infants.

Breast-feeding

The importance of breast milk and nutrition cannot be over-emphasized. Human breast milk is the preferred nutrition source for both term and preterm babies and is associated with a significant reduction in both morbidity and mortality. Every effort should be made to encourage a mother to breast-feed. Breast-feeding within 30 min of a normal birth and early breast massage and expression within 6 hours of a preterm delivery is essential to establish breast-feeding. All professionals who care for women and their babies need to offer support and expert council to promote successful breast-feeding in challenging conditions of stress and ill health.

There are few genuine contraindications to breast-feeding but include some rare inborn errors of metabolism in the baby such as galactosaemia. It is not the practice in the UK to encourage HIV-positive mothers to breast-feed, but this is not the case in developing countries. Breast-feeding is generally safe for the baby if the mother requires medication; rarely breast-feeding is absolutely contraindicated. Examples of drugs which require caution are given in Table 31.10. When prescribing for a breast-feeding mother it is wise to check that the drug prescribed is safe. Information can be found in the *British National Formulary*; if a contraindication, caution or a potential problem is identified, the advice of the local paediatric pharmacist or local drug information centre should be sought. Often alternative drugs can be prescribed and breast-feeding continued. Information is also available via websites such as www.ukmi.nhs.uk.

Table 31.10 Drugs and breast-feeding.

Breast-feeding contraindicated
Cytotoxics, immunosuppressants, ergotamine, lithium, phenindione, chloramphenicol, tetracyclines

Example of drugs to be used with caution during breast-feeding
Antiarrhythmic: amiodarone
Antibiotic: metronidazole
Anticonvulsant: gabapentin, levetiracetam, oxcarbazepine, phenobarbital, phenytoin, pregabalin, primidone, topiramate, vigabatrin
Antidepressant: doxepin, selective serotonin reuptake inhibitors (SSRIs)
Antihypertensive: beta-blockers
Anxiolytic: benzodiazepines, buspirone
Radioisotopes

Table 31.11 Frequently asked questions.

Is milk from the newborn infant's breast normal?
Answer: Normal in boys and girls

Is vaginal bleeding in girls normal?
Answer: Normal

What causes persistent sticky eye after culture and treatment of infection?
Answer: Blocked nasolacrimal duct. Will recannulate spontaneously. Does not need probing

How often should a baby feed 'on demand'?
Answer: Usually about 2–4 hours, but every 6 hours is not uncommon in healthy infants

My baby is squinting. Is this normal?
Answer: Yes, in the first week after birth

Is my breastfed baby getting enough milk?
Answer: If the baby is gaining weight properly, yes

Many minor alterations in physiology cause alarm to parents. Some common questions and responses to them are outlined in Table 31.11. In the absence of disease, reassurance is all that is required.

References

1 Nuffield Council on Bioethics. *Critical Care Decisions in Fetal and Neonatal Medicine: Ethical Issues.* Available at: www.nuffieldbioethics.org/publications.
2 Royal College of Paediatrics and Child Health. Withholding or withdrawing life sustaining treatment in children: a framework for practice. Available at: www.rcpch.ac.uk.
3 Wood NS, Marlow N, Costeloe K, Gibson AT, Wilkinson AR. Neurological and developmental disability after extremely preterm birth. The EPICure Study Group. *N Engl J Med* 2000;343: 378–384.

4 The EXPRESS Group. One-year survival of extremely preterm infants after active perinatal care in Sweden. *JAMA* 2009;301: 2225–2233.

5 Hakansson S, Farooqi A, Holmgren PA, Serenius F, Hogberg U. Proactive management promotes outcome in extremely preterm infants: a population-based comparison of two perinatal management strategies. *Pediatrics* 2004;114:58–64.

6 Royal College of Paediatrics and Child Health/Royal College of Obstetricians and Gynaecologists/Royal College of Midwives. *Training and Maintenance of Skills for Professionals Responsible for Resuscitation of Babies at Birth*. Available at: www.rcog.org.uk/womens-health/clinical-guidance/training-and-maintenance-skills-professionals-responsible-resuscitat.

7 Goldenberg RL, Culhane JF, Iams JD, Romero R. Epidemiology and causes of preterm birth. *Lancet* 2008;371:75–84.

8 Moser K, MacFarlane A, Chow YH, Hilder L, Dattani N. Introducing new data on gestation-specific infant mortality among babies born in 2005 in England and Wales. *Health Stat Q* 2007;(35):13–27.

9 Field D, Draper ES, Fenton A *et al.* Rates of very preterm birth in Europe and neonatal mortality rates. *Arch Dis Child* 2009;94: F253–F256.

10 Costeloe K, Hennessy E, Gibson AT, Marlow N, Wilkinson AR. The EPICure study: outcomes to discharge from hospital for infants born at the threshold of viability. *Pediatrics* 2000;106: 659–671.

11 Field DJ, Dorling JS, Manktelow BN, Draper ES. Survival of extremely premature babies in a geographically defined population: prospective cohort study of 1994–9 compared with 2000–5. *BMJ* 2008;336:1221–1223.

12 Johnson S, Hennessy E, Smith R, Trikic R, Wolke D, Marlow N. Academic attainment and special educational needs in extremely preterm children at 11 years of age: the EPICure study. *Arch Dis Child* 2009;94:F283–F289.

13 Johnson S, Hollis C, Kochhar P, Hennessy E, Wolke D, Marlow N. Psychiatric disorders in extremely preterm children: longitudinal finding at age 11 years in the EPICure study. *J Am Acad Child Adolesc Psychiatry* 2010;49:453–463.e1.

14 Petrou S, Abangma G, Johnson S, Wolke D, Marlow N. Costs and health utilities associated with extremely preterm birth: evidence from the EPICure Study. *Value Health* 2009; 12:1124–1134.

15 National Institute for Health and Clinical Excellence. *Neonatal Jaundice*. Clinical Guideline CG98, 2010. Available at: http://guidance.nice.org.uk/CG98.

16 Sarnat HB, Sarnat MS. Neonatal encephalopathy following fetal distress. A clinical and electroencephalographic study. *Arch Neurol* 1976;33:696–705.

17 Azzopardi DV, Strohm B, Edwards AD *et al.* Moderate hypothermia to treat perinatal asphyxial encephalopathy. *N Engl J Med* 2009;361:1349–1358.

18 Edwards AD, Brocklehurst P, Gunn AJ *et al.* Neurological outcomes at 18 months of age after moderate hypothermia for perinatal hypoxic ischaemic encephalopathy: synthesis and meta-analysis of trial data. *BMJ* 2010;340:c363.

19 British Association of Perinatal Medicine. Position statement on therapeutic cooling for neonatal encephalopathy. Available at: www.bapm.org/media/documents/publications/.

20 Nelson KB, Ellenberg JH. Antecedents of cerebral palsy. Multivariate analysis of risk. *N Engl J Med* 1986;315:81–86.

21 Badawi N, Kurinczuk JJ, Keogh JM *et al.* Intrapartum risk factors for newborn encephalopathy: the Western Australian case-control study. *BMJ* 1998;317:1554–1558.

22 Gaffney G, Sellers S, Flavell V, Squier M, Johnson A. Case-control study of intrapartum care, cerebral palsy, and perinatal death. *BMJ* 1994;308:743–750.

23 Larroque B, Ancel P, Marret S *et al.* Neurodevelopmental disabilities and special care of 5-year-old children born before 33 weeks of gestation (the EPIPAGE study): a longitudinal cohort study. *Lancet* 2008;371:813–820.

24 Vanhaesebrouck P, Allegaert K, Bottu J *et al.* The EPIBEL Study: outcomes to discharge from hospital for extremely preterm infants in Belgium. *Pediatrics* 2004;114:663–675.

25 The Victorian Infant Collaborative Study Group. Outcome at 2 years of children 23–27 weeks' gestation born in Victoria in 1991–92. *J Paediatr Child Health* 1997;33:161–165.

26 Doyle LW. Outcome at 5 years of age of children 23 to 27 weeks' gestation: refining the prognosis. Victorian Infant Collaborative Study Group. *Pediatrics* 2001;108:134–141.

27 Doyle LW, Roberts G, Anderson PJ. Outcomes at age 2 years of infants <28 weeks' gestational age born in Victoria in 2005. *J Pediatr* 2010;156:49–53.e1.

28 Khashu M, Narayanan M, Bhargava S, Osiovich H. Perinatal outcomes associated with preterm birth at 33 to 36 weeks' gestation: a population-based cohort study. *Pediatrics* 2009;123: 109–113.

29 Marlow N, Wolke D, Bracewell MA, Samara M. Neurologic and developmental disability at six years of age after extremely preterm birth. *N Engl J Med* 2005;352:9–19.

Further reading

Abman SH, Fox WW, Polin RA (eds) *Fetal and Neonatal Physiology*, 3rd edn. London: Saunders, 2003.

Brindley S, Richmond S. *Resuscitation at Birth. The Newborn Life Support Provider Manual*. London: Resuscitation Council, 2001.

Levene M, Evans DJ. Hypoxic–ischaemic brain injury. In: Rennie J (ed.) *Roberton's Textbook of Neonatology*, 4th edn. Philadelphia: Elsevier, 2005: 1128–1148.

Lissauer T, Fanaroff AA, Weindling AM. *Neonatology at a Glance*. Oxford: Blackwell Publishing, 2006.

Rennie JM (ed.) *Roberton's Textbook of Neonatology*, 4th edn. Philadelphia: Elsevier, 2005.

Chapter 32
Obstetric Statistics

James J. Walker
Department of Obstetrics and Gynaecology, St James's University Hospital, Leeds, UK

According to Mark Twain, the nineteenth-century British Prime Minister Benjamin Disraeli (1804–1881) stated that 'There are three kinds of lies: lies, damned lies, and statistics.' This suggests that statistics are used to mislead and support weak arguments. If things really are different, it should be obvious. However, as doctors we use numbers and statistics daily and in our everyday lives and accept them without question as they are often transparent to us. The problem is not with statistics themselves but when statistics are used in the wrong way or interpreted incorrectly.

Taking a patient's pulse, blood pressure and temperature provides numbers that we decide are normal or not. To help make these decisions, we learn the normal ranges and develop MEOWS (Modified Early Obstetric Warning System) charts, where white shading indicates normal, yellow is a warning and red demands escalation to prompt the recorder to respond. Similarly, when carrying out treatments or procedures, we assess the risks and benefits of interventions using our knowledge and experience or we follow guidelines where someone else has done the assessment for us. So we use statistics as part of everyday living; we embrace and welcome them as they give clarity to our thoughts and evidence for our decisions. To achieve this evidence we need to count and compare and use tools to support our theories. This produces evidence-based medicine.

It's all in the numbers

Ignaz Philipp Semmelweis was appointed the assistant professor in the Vienna General Hospital in 1846. While assessing the maternity cases prior to rounds, he noted that the mortality rate from puerperal sepsis was at least twice as high in patients seen in the morning clinic compared with those in the later clinic, with women who gave birth in the streets having the lowest rate of all (Table 32.1) [1]. He made this assessment by counting the number of women that died from puerperal fever against a standard denominator, in this case per 100 births or per cent in any given year. This allowed him to compare the death rates in the two groups by standardizing the results as an incidence (number of new cases per fixed population in a given time period). The earlier cases were cared for by medical students, who had come straight from the postmortem rooms, and the later cases were cared for by midwives who had not. From this he developed his theory of cadaveric contamination without knowing the infective organism. This led to his introduction of a strict hand-washing technique, which reduced the incidence of maternal death almost instantly. In this work he exemplified the importance of accurate counting and the appropriate denominator providing rates for comparison, followed by intervention and reassessment: the modern concept of 360-degree audit.

Counting

When counting anything, it is important to have an accurate classification of what it is that you are counting. Maternal death is a 'hard' end-point but puerperal sepsis is not. Semmelweis would have made a good clinical judgement but he may not have been 100% accurate. The fact that after hand-washing the incidence did not fall to zero means that some of the deaths may have been from other causes. However, his inaccuracies would have been present in both groups and would not have affected his study. This emphasizes the importance of proper definitions to classify cases as well as comparable groups for assessment.

Ascertainment

Not only is it important to know what you are meant to be counting but also to know whether you have counted them all. That is ascertainment. Differences in maternal and perinatal mortality between different countries may partly be due to the differences in the ascertainment of deaths in the countries concerned (Table 32.2). However, in order to compare figures in different countries, not only do we need accurate and complete counting but we also

Dewhurst's Textbook of Obstetrics & Gynaecology, Eighth Edition. Edited by D. Keith Edmonds.
© 2012 John Wiley and Sons, Ltd. Published 2012 by John Wiley and Sons, Ltd.

need to standardize the presentation of results, in a similar way to what Semmelweis did, as rates using a standard denominator.

Rate

Semmelweis counted deaths in his institution per 100 births or per cent. Current assessments of maternal death use specific definitions and a larger denominator due to the relatively low rates of maternal mortality in the developed world. The denominator should be independent of the factor or disease that is being measured and is therefore an independent standard. In pregnancy, this is easy and self-selecting: all pregnant women.

A maternal death is a death while pregnant or within 42 days of delivery, miscarriage, termination of pregnancy or ectopic pregnancy from any cause related to or aggravated by the pregnancy or its management, but not from accidental or incidental causes. There is also a late maternal death category, which is death from 42 days to 1 year. This is relevant in specific cases such as suicide, which tends to occur after 42 days. These deaths

must be assessed against an accepted denominator. However, the two different ones which are used can lead to confusion.

- *Maternal mortality ratio* (MMR) is easier to count, but excludes stillbirths from the denominator. This ratio is used for international comparisons (Table 32.2).
- *Maternal mortality rate* is used in the Confidential Enquiries into Maternal Death reports.

Maternal deaths are further categorized as direct, indirect and fortuitous as well as late deaths [2]. Similar assessments are made for perinatal deaths [3]. Because these assessments are repeated regularly, they are available for trend analysis and comparisons between institutions and geographical areas. Individual institutions can assess how they perform against the national figures, which is a driver for health improvement (Fig. 32.1).

However, simple counting of numbers may not be enough, as it does not give a complete picture of the causes behind the deaths. In the UK triennial reports,

Table 32.1 Puerperal fever mortality rates for the First and Second Clinic at the Vienna General Hospital [1].

Year	First clinic			Second clinic		
	Births	Deaths	Rate (%)	Births	Deaths	Rate (%)
1841	3036	237	7.8	2442	86	3.5
1842	3287	518	15.8	2659	202	7.6
1843	3060	274	9.0	2739	164	6.0
1844	3157	260	8.2	2956	68	2.3
1845	3492	241	6.9	3241	66	2.0
1846	4010	459	11.4	3754	105	2.8

Table 32.2 Maternal mortality ratio (MMR) for different countries and sources compared with that of the UK.

	MMR	Lower and upper estimates
Sweden	6	(3–8)
Germany	7	(6–9)
UK	7	
France	8	(5–14)
Canada	12	(7–20)
USA	24	(20–27)
Afghanistan	1400	(750–2600)

Not only do the ratios change dramatically but the range of estimates do as well. This emphasizes the difficulty of comparing figures from different sources [2].

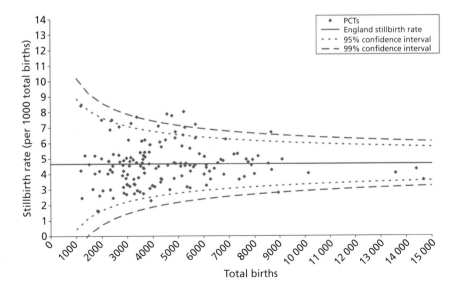

Fig. 32.1 Adjusted stillbirth rates per primary care trust compared with the English stillbirth rate and the 95% and 99% confidence intervals. These figures have to be assessed with care as each point has relatively wide confidence limits [3].

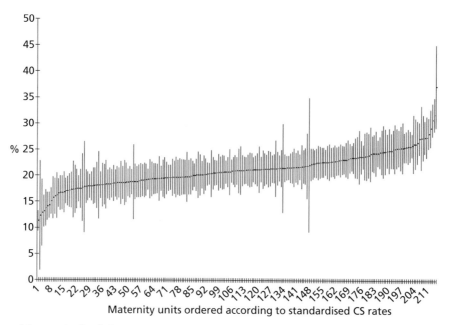

Fig. 32.2 The variation of the standardized Caesarean section rate between different units in the UK from the National Sentinel Caesarean Section Audit. The UK average Caesarean section rate was 21.3% showing that the rate is influenced by a small number of units with higher rates, with the majority of units having a rate less than this. This is a skewed distribution to the left with a median of just below 20% [4].

deaths related to different causes and associated factors are assessed individually to allow trend analysis of deaths due to these causes and the effects of interventions – a true 360-degree audit cycle [2]. This greatly enriches the process and the benefits gained and can assess the value of implementation of new guidelines.

Another common figure regularly assessed and used to measure outcome is the Caesarean section rate. This is usually calculated as a percentage of all deliveries in a given institution or geographical area. and comparisons can then be made. The National Sentinel Caesarean Section Audit did this across the UK and showed wide variation of the rates after standardization for case mix [4] (Fig. 32.2). In order to improve the ability to compare results, standardized groups can be used, as described by Robson and published in the audit (Table 32.3). This allows the Caesarean section rate to be assessed between units using standardized patient groups, specifically, the standard primigravida, standard multigravida or women undergoing labour after Caesarean section. These figures show the contribution of each of these groups to the overall rate and demonstrate that nulliparous women make up around 40% of Caesarean sections and a further 24% are multiparous women with a scar as a direct result of a nulliparous Caesarean section. This implies that for every Caesarean section carried out in a primigravida, there is an amplification factor of 60% on future figures due to repeat section. The reverse is also true in that any reduction will similarly be amplified.

These figures also demonstrate the danger of association and cause. The table would imply that the risk of a Caesarean section in induced women is twice as high as when labour is spontaneous. Although this is a true association, the interpretation of this is open to bias. Despite the fact that no randomized trial has demonstrated that induction of labour increases the risk of Caesarean section, it is a widely held belief, which leads people to change policy in an attempt to reduce Caesarean section rates. The association shown in these results do not demonstrate cause. It may be that the reason for induction is more relevant than the induction itself. Beware of preconceived bias and false assumptions of causation.

The rates or ratios described above are a variation of incidence and prevalence, which are widely used in audit of disease in the population.

Summary box 32.1

Definitions used in maternal death audits

- *Maternal mortality ratio* (MMR): number of maternal deaths per 100 000 live births.
- *Maternal mortality rate*: number of maternal deaths per 100 000 maternities.
- *Total number of maternities*: the number of pregnancies that result in a live birth at any gestation or stillbirths occurring at or after 24 completed weeks of gestation and are required to be notified by law. Multiple pregnancies are counted only once.
- *Direct maternal death*: the result of a complication of pregnancy, delivery or puerperium from interventions, omissions, incorrect treatment or from a chain of events resulting from any of the above.

- *Indirect maternal death*: a pregnancy-related death in a patient with a pre-existing or newly developed health problem that was not the result of direct obstetric causes but which was aggravated by the physiological effects of pregnancy.
- *Coincidental (fortuitous) maternal death*: other fatalities during, but unrelated to, pregnancy or the puerperium.
- *Late maternal death*: a death occurring after 42 days up to 1 year after abortion, miscarriage or delivery that is the result of direct or indirect maternal causes.

 Summary box 32.2

Classification of perinatal deaths
- *Stillbirth*: a baby born without signs of life after 23+6 weeks of pregnancy. This can be further divided into:
  - Intrapartum stillbirth: a baby known to be alive at the beginning of labour but stillborn.
  - Neonatal death: death of a liveborn baby occurring before 28 completed days after birth. This can be further divided into (i) early (0–6 completed days) and (ii) late (7–27 completed days).
- *Perinatal death*: death of a fetus or a newborn in the perinatal period, which commences at 24 completed weeks' gestation and ends before seven completed days after birth (total of stillbirths and early neonatal death).

Incidence and prevalence

Incidence is a measure of the risk of developing some new condition within a specified period of time. Although sometimes loosely expressed simply as the number of new cases during some time period, it is better expressed as a proportion or a rate within a specific denominator to allow meaningful comparison. Therefore, the incidence (rate) is usually given as the number of new cases per given population in a given time period. In the examples above in pregnancy, the population and time period is self-selecting, the population is pregnant women and the time period is pregnancy and the puerperium.

In the non-pregnant population it is more difficult. The time period is usually fixed at a year but the population denominator is more of a problem. Obviously in gynaecology only women should be used but, depending on the disease being studied, the at-risk female population may be different. Endometriosis is typically, but not absolutely, seen during the reproductive years; it has been estimated that it affects approximately 10% of all women at some point, but this is lifetime risk not incidence, which is risk of new cases within a risk group over a fixed period of time. Nor is it prevalence.

Table 32.3 Caesarean section rate according to the Robson groups [4].

	Robson group	Per cent total births	Caesarean section rate (% of group)	Per cent contribution to Caesarean section rate	Per cent total births
1	Nulliparous, single cephalic, >37 weeks' gestation, spontaneous labour	24.8	12.2	14.1	3
2	Nulliparous, single cephalic, >37 weeks' gestation:				
	Induced labour	9.7	27	12.3	2.7
	Caesarean section before labour	1.1	100	5.3	1.1
3	Multiparous, single cephalic, >37 weeks' gestation, no uterine scar, spontaneous labour	33	3.1	4.7	1
4	Multiparous, single cephalic, >37 weeks' gestation, no uterine scar:				
	Induced labour	9.5	7.8	3.5	0.8
	Caesarean section before labour	1.2	100	5.5	1.2
5	Multiparous, single cephalic, >37 weeks' gestation, with uterine scar	8	64.4	23.9	5.3
6	Nulliparous singleton breeches	1.9	91.7	8.1	1.7
7	Multiparous singleton breeches, including previous scar	1.7	83.9	6.6	1.4
8	Multiple pregnancies, including previous uterine scar	1.5	59.9	4.1	1
9	Singleton transverse, oblique or unstable lies, including previous uterine scar	0.4	99.7	1.8	0.4
10	Singleton cephalic, <37 weeks' gestation, including previous uterine scar	5.8	33	9	1.9
	Total	98.5		98.9	21.5

Prevalence is a measure of the total number of cases of disease in a specific population, rather than the rate of occurrence of new cases. This indicates the burden of the disease on society and is dependent on both the number of new cases and the length of time the disease is present (prevalence = incidence × duration). This equation demonstrates the relationship between prevalence and incidence: when the incidence goes up, prevalence must also rise. Incidence is more useful in understanding disease aetiology as it reflects disease occurrence. As in the case of puerperal fever, the higher incidence in one group suggested an aetiological factor related to that group alone and the fall in incidence that followed the hand-washing initiative demonstrated a successful intervention. Therefore, incidence will vary with changes in aetiological factors and prevention. Prevalence is dependent on the duration of disease and the availability of cure. The longer the duration of disease, the higher the prevalence.

So how does this relate to endometriosis? Estimates about its overall prevalence vary, but 5–10% is a reasonable. A study in asymptomatic women undergoing sterilization gave a figure of 6% but this rises to 21% in women with infertility and as high as 60% in those with pelvic pain [5]. Therefore, the prevalence is dependent on the denominator group. The incidence of endometriosis was investigated in the Nurses' Health Study II prospective cohort of 116 678 female registered nurses, ranging in age from 25 to 42 years [6]. During 10 years of follow-up (1989–1999), 1721 cases of laparoscopically confirmed endometriosis were reported among these women. This is an incidence of 1.5% over 10 years or 1.5 per 1000 new cases on average per year. At the end of the study, the prevalence *in this cohort* is the same as the cumulative incidence over 10 years, 1.5%, assuming no cures. However, the incidence of endometriosis is not constant, with the rates higher in the older age groups. Therefore, the incidence may have been higher in the later years of the study and will continue to rise in the years following it, leading to a higher prevalence in later years.

One way round this changing incidence is to use a Kaplan–Meier plot, which presents incidence data as a plot of cumulative incidence over time, taking into account variations in rate of events. This was used in a study of recurrent miscarriage where a comparison was made between low-dose aspirin and heparin and aspirin alone [7] (Fig. 32.3). The main results showed that the rate of live births was 71% (32/45 pregnancies) with low-dose aspirin and heparin and 42% (19/45 pregnancies) with low-dose aspirin alone (odds ratio 3.37, 95% CI 1.40–8.10). However, as can be seen from the graph, this difference related to the first trimester alone, with little difference in the slopes of the line after 12 weeks' gestation. These sorts of plots are also used in survival studies in cancer trials.

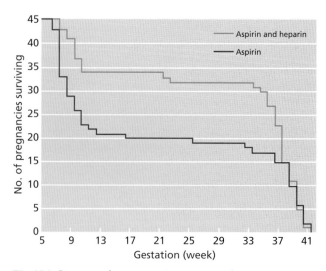

Fig. 32.3 Outcome of pregnancy in women with recurrent miscarriages and phospholipid antibodies who were given aspirin or aspirin and heparin. All pregnancies longer than 32 weeks' gestation resulted in live birth (From Rai *et al.* [7] with permission).

Pearl Index

The incidence of a disease or event is often quoted in rate per cent per year, for example the failure rate of contraceptives is quoted using the Pearl Index [8]. The following information is required to calculate the Pearl Index: the number of pregnancies and the total number of months or cycles of exposure of women. The index can then be calculated as follows:

• number of pregnancies in the study divided by the number of months of exposure and then multiplied by 1200;
• number of pregnancies in the study divided by the number of menstrual cycles experienced by the women and then multiplied by 1300; 1300 is used instead of 1200 because the average menstrual cycle is 28 days giving 13 cycles per year.

These are normally calculated over a trial period of 1–2 years and claims to give the risk of pregnancy in 100 women over 1 year of use or 10 women over 10 years. This assumes that the pregnancy risk is static over the years of use and based on the rate in the first 1–2 years. Also, some people think it gives a lifetime risk but it does not; it gives a percentage risk over 1 year of use, which needs to be multiplied by years of use to give a lifetime risk assuming the risk remains the same over time. Again a Kaplan–Meier plot could be used to test for accumulative pregnancy rates over time when comparing different methods of contraception rather than the Pearl Index alone.

Comparison

In the example given above relating to the treatment of recurrent miscarriage, the two treatment arms had success rates of 71% (32/45 pregnancies) in one and 42% (19/45 pregnancies) in the other. This is an example of binary classification where the groups can be classified into two. The results look different and most readers would assume that one treatment was better than the other but are they statistically different? Is the number of patients sampled enough to be sure this was not chance?

Statistical significance

A result is called statistically significant if it is unlikely to have occurred by chance alone. It is important to remember that being statistically significant does not mean the result is important or clinically relevant. In large studies small differences can be found to be statistically significant but have little clinical or practical relevance. Tests of correlation may show significant correlations but have no or minor causative relation. Tests of significance should always be accompanied by assessments of relevance and effect-size statistics, which assess the size and thus the practical importance of the difference.

Tested often enough, in theory any result is possible but the likelihood that any given result would have occurred by chance is known as the significance level or *P*-value. In traditional statistical testing, the *P*-value is the probability of observing data similar to that observed by chance alone. If the obtained *P*-value is small, then it can be said this is unlikely and the results are significantly different. To test whether the results are true or not, they are compared with those expected if the null hypothesis is true or there is no difference. So the basis of comparison of data is testing whether the null hypothesis is true and the level of significance desired.

The null hypothesis and statistical tests

Statistical convention assumes that the experimental hypothesis (e.g. that one treatment is better than another) is wrong and assumes the *null hypothesis*, or no difference, as correct and that testing will assess whether this is wrong (i.e. that the treatment is better). When the null hypothesis is nullified (not supported within accepted confidence limits), the *alternative hypothesis* (that one treatment is better than the other) is accepted. Therefore, the null hypothesis is generally a statement that a particular treatment has no effect or benefit or that there is no difference between two particular measured variables in a study. So in the study of recurrent miscarriage [7], the null hypothesis is that there is no difference between the treatment arms and the statistics are used to test the likelihood of this being correct. In this case, the null hypothesis was not supported and therefore it is accepted that one treatment was better than the other.

The result of the statistical test is given as a *P*-value. The size of the *P*-value relates to the likelihood of the result occurring by chance. The lower the *P*-value, the more likely the null hypothesis is nullified and the results

are significantly different. A result of *P* < 0.05 means that the probability of this result being due to chance is less than 5% so the results are different to a 95% probability. The nearer to unity the *P*-value, the more likely that the null hypothesis is accepted and that there is no difference, but it should be remembered that 'the null hypothesis is never proved or established, but is possibly disproved'. In other words, if no significant difference is found, the test has not proven that there is no difference but has failed to show difference.

The *P*-value of any test is dependent on the degree of difference in the test results and the number of people or values in the trial. If the trial is not of appropriate size, then two basic statistical errors can be made, type I and type II errors. Type I error, also known as the false positive, occurs when a statistical test falsely rejects a null hypothesis, for example where there is no difference between treatment arms in a trial as stated by the null hypothesis but the test rejects the hypothesis, falsely suggesting that there is benefit of treatment. The rate of type I error is denoted by the Greek letter alpha (α) and equals the significance level of the test, which by convention is usually taken as 0.05 or below. This means that any positive result is correct to a level of 95% probability.

Type II error, also known as the false negative, occurs when the test fails to reject a false null hypothesis, for example where there is a difference between treatment arms in a trial but the null hypothesis states that there is no difference and the test fails to reject the null hypothesis, falsely suggesting that there is no difference. The rate of type II error is denoted by the Greek letter beta (β) and is usually taken as 0.80, i.e. an 80% chance of rejecting a false null hypothesis.

Therefore when designing a trial, two considerations must be assessed:
• to reduce the chance of rejecting a true hypothesis to as low a value as possible;
• to devise the test so that it will reject the hypothesis tested when it is likely to be false.

The ability of a study to achieve this is assessed by the power. The power of a statistical test is calculated on the probability that the test will reject the null hypothesis when the null hypothesis is false and not produce a type II error or a false-negative result. As the power increases, the chance of a type II error occurring decreases as calculated by power = $1 - \beta$.

Statistical power may depend on a number of factors but, at a minimum, power nearly always depends on the following three factors:
• the statistical difference desired;
• the size of the effect of the treatment or difference between test groups;
• the sample size used to detect the effect.
The statistical difference desired is the chosen maximum *P*-value where the results are accepted as statistically

significant, which is usually 0.05 but may be less than this if multiple testing is to be carried out. Once this *P*-value is agreed, power analysis can be used to calculate the minimum sample size required that is likely to detect a specified effect size (or difference). Similarly, the reverse is true and power analysis can be used to calculate the minimum effect size that is likely to be detected in a study using a given sample size. In general, a larger sample size will allow testing for a larger effect size and boost statistical power.

The specificity of the test is equal to $1 - \alpha$ ($1 - 0.05 = 0.95$). Increasing the specificity of the test lowers the probability of false-positive errors, but raises the probability of false-negative errors, which is a reflection on the sensitivity of the test. There are no formal standards for power but it is mostly calculated against the agreed *P*-value of 0.05 (95% specificity) and a 0.80 chance of avoiding a type II error (80% sensitivity). This convention implies a four-to-one trade-off between type II (β) risk and type I (α) risk and can be changed depending on whether a false-positive or false-negative rate is thought to be more important.

Working example

Let us look at the study of therapy in recurrent miscarriage quoted above [7]. The study compared two treatments, aspirin alone and aspirin and heparin, in women who had a history of recurrent miscarriage. Prior risk from previous trial data suggested that in women with this history given aspirin alone, the success rate would be 30%. The trialists felt that an increase in success to 60% would be clinically significant considering the intervention of daily heparin injections. The power calculation gave a result of 42 patients per arm using standard power calculation programs based on a study power of 80% and a significance level of 0.05 (two-tailed test, i.e. one that makes no assumption about which arm of the study will show benefit).

In the trial, 45 patients were randomized to each arm allowing for drop-out. The relatively small numbers required for this trial is based on two factors: the low prior success rate and the magnitude of benefit desired. If the prior success rate was 50% and the desired success rate of the new therapy 60%, the study numbers would have been 388 in each arm or 776 in total for the same power and significance. In reality, the results showed that the difference was 42% in one arm and 71% in the other. Both arms did better than the a priori assumptions but the success difference of 29% was almost as predicted.

After the trial has been carried out, the results can be assessed for significance by using contingency or 2×2 tables similar to Fisher's exact test (Table 32.4). If more than two arms are studied, the chi-squared test can be used using the same principles. Contingency tables are used to investigate binary classification tests where there are two groups to study and each group has two possible

Table 32.4 Contingency (2 × 2) table to test for significance in the rates of two populations.

	Positive	Negative	Total
Group 1	*a*	*b*	*a + b*
Group 2	*c*	*d*	*c + d*
Total	*a + c*	*b + d*	*a + b + c + d = N*

results. Depending on the investigation being carried out various variables can be calculated. The one used in this case is the odds ratio (OR), which tells us the significance of the difference in the two treatment arms. As published in the paper the OR was 3.37.

Summary box 32.3

Statistical terms (see Table 32.4)

Specificity
Relates to the ability of the test to identify negative results:

True negatives / total condition negatives $= d / b + d$

where *d* is true negatives correctly identified and *b* is false positives. A high specificity implies a high probability that a positive result is positive and there is a low type I (α) error rate.

Sensitivity
Relates to the ability of the test to identify positive results:

True positives / total condition positives $= a / a + c$

where *a* is true positives correctly identified and *c* is false negatives. A high sensitivity implies a high probability that a negative result is negative and there is a low type II (β) error rate.

Power
Relates to the probability that the test will not produce a type II error:

$=$ Sensitivity $= 1 - \beta$

Positive predictive value (PPV)
The ratio of positives that are truly positive:

True positives / total test outcome positives $= a / a + b$

A high positive predictive value gives an estimate of the chances that a positive result is truly positive.

Negative predictive value (NPV)
The ratio of negatives that are truly negative:

True negatives / total test outcome negatives $= d / c + d$

A high negative predictive value gives an estimate of the chances that a negative result is truly negative.

Positive likelihood ratio
A measure of the change in the likelihood of a positive result from the prior test likelihood of positivity:

$$= \text{Sensitivity}/(1-\text{specificity}) = [a/(a+c)]/1-[d/(b+d)]$$

It is commonly used in assessments of treatments or predictors of disease. The odds of positivity equals the pre-test odds multiplied by the positive likelihood ratio.

Negative likelihood ratio
A measure of the change in the likelihood of a negative result from the prior test likelihood of negativity:

$$= (1-\text{sensitivity})/\text{specificity} = 1-[a/(a+c)]/[d/(b+d)]$$

It is commonly used in assessments of treatments or predictors of disease. The odds of negativity equals the pre-test odds multiplied by the negative likelihood ratio.

Odds ratio
A test of effect size as measured by the ratio of the positive odds in one arm against the positive odds in the other arm of the study.

$$OR = (a/b)/(c/d) = ad/bc$$

Relative risk
A test of the probability of an event occurring relative to the risk in the comparative group

$$RR = [a/(a+b)]/[c/(c+d)]$$

Terms of significance

The OR is a test of effect size. In the example we are analysing, the chances or odds of a successful pregnancy if given aspirin and heparin was 32/13 or 2.46 and the chances or odds of success with aspirin alone was 19/26 or 0.73; therefore the OR is 2.46/0.73 = 3.37. How certain are we that this result is correct? It has been stated that 'statistics means that we never have to say we are certain'. Statistics is about probability not certainty. This is measured by confidence intervals. Confidence intervals are the range of probability (usually 95%) that if the test is repeated many times the result will always fall within that given range. For ORs, the plot of the potential results is not normally distributed as the there is skewness (see below) and it is calculated using logarithmic conversion. All good statistical packages can provide this. In this study, the results are presented as an OR of 3.37, with a 95% confidence interval (CI) of 1.40–8.10. This means that if repeated many times, in 95% of the tests the result would fall between 1.4 and 8.1. However, the majority

will fall nearer the OR of 3.37, which is the best estimate of the result using this data. The skewness can be observed by noting that the difference between the OR and the limits of the confidence interval is more in one direction than the other. What is important is that the confidence intervals do not cross 1 (or unity), meaning that in all cases the direction of difference is the same – that aspirin and heparin is better than aspirin alone. The results indicate that with aspirin and heparin the odds of success are 3.37 times that of the odds with aspirin alone. Another way, and probably more appropriate in this study, of assessing statistical difference would be the relative risk.

The relative risk (RR) is simply the probability of an event occurring relative to the risk in the comparative group. This measure of effect size differs from the OR in that it compares probabilities instead of odds. For small probabilities, the RR and OR are similar. Using the example above, the probabilities of success in the aspirin group and aspirin/heparin group are 19/45 (or 0.42) and 32/45 (or 0.71), respectively. The effect size can be computed the same as above, but using the probabilities instead. Therefore, the RR is 0.71/0.42 or 1.68 (CI 1.14–2.4) implying that, with the addition of heparin, the changes of a successful pregnancy is 68% higher. In medical research, the OR is favoured for case–control studies and retrospective studies, with the RR being used for randomized trials and cohort studies.

So was Semmelweis correct when he thought there was a difference in death rates between his groups? His was a retrospective study, looking back over the previous 6 years.

	Died	Survived	Total
First clinic	1989	18053	20042
Second clinic	691	17100	17791
Totals	2680	35153	37833

This produces a highly significant result of RR = 2.6 (CI 2.35–2.78), showing the greatly increased risk of dying from sepsis in the morning clinic, justifying his successful interventions.

Study definitions

As mentioned above, different types of studies are used in medical research, and the most common are defined below.

Retrospective studies

A retrospective study is one where the records are studied after all the events and outcomes have already occurred. The data are collected from a given population. Risk factors or disease outcomes are compared between subgroups that have different known outcomes. The study can be designed using a case–control or cohort model (see below). This differs from a *prospective study*, which is conducted by starting with two groups which are selected by risk factor or randomized and subsequent future outcomes are noted.

Retrospective studies have the following benefits: they are cheap, it is easier to collect large numbers and to select cohorts of disease and non-disease, and they are less time-consuming since the main effort required is the collection of data. In contrast, prospective studies follow populations over time to study outcome. In population risk studies, a large number of negative controls will be collected depending on the disease incidence.

Case–control studies

Case–control studies can be used for both retrospective and prospective studies. In a case–control study, people with a disease are matched as closely as possible with people who do not have the disease but who act as controls. Data are then collected in both groups and compared to find out any factor(s) which are different between the groups that may demonstrate an association. It does not prove cause. One of the most famous studies using this method was carried out by Sir Richard Doll showing the correlation of smoking with lung cancer [9]. Although a relative risk can be demonstrated between the groups, the control group is a sample of the total population and selected because they do not have the disease. To determine true population risk, a larger cross-sectional study is required.

A variation of this method is the nested case–control study, where cases with a disease in a defined cohort (the nest) are identified and, for each, a specified number of matched controls are selected from the same cohort who have not yet developed the disease. The nested case–control design is easier and less expensive than a full cohort approach.

Cross-sectional studies

Cross-sectional studies involve observation of a total population, or a random subset of it, at a defined time. They provide information on an entire population under study and can describe absolute risks and not just relative risks. They can also describe the prevalence of disease.

Cohort studies

Cohort studies are a form of longitudinal observational study used to analyse risk factors by studying groups of people who do not have the disease in retrospect or prospectively (the preferred method). The cohort is often selected by a specific event such their week of birth (a birth cohort). A comparison group, if required, is generally from the same general population as the cohort is drawn or is otherwise similar apart from a specific factor, such as place of birth.

Randomized controlled trials

Randomized controlled trials (RCTs) are the superior methodology in medical statistical research because they reduce the potential for bias by random selection of patients to one intervention arm or to another intervention, non-intervention or placebo arm. This minimizes the possibility that confounding variables will differ between the two groups. However, not all studies are suitable for RCTs and the methodologies mentioned above may be more suitable. In order to further reduce bias, the randomized trial may be designed as a double-blind RCT, where neither the clinician nor the participant knows which treatment arm the participant is in, or a single-blind RCT, where the clinician knows but the participant does not. In some circumstances an open label trial is carried out, where it is not possible to blind either the clinician or the patient but randomization is performed without bias at time of therapy.

Meta-analysis

The trial we analysed above on women who suffered recurrent miscarriage was a powerful but small RCT. It showed statistical significance. However, if it had not, or if greater power is desired, several trials testing the same research hypothesis can be combined into a meta-analysis. By doing this, a weighted average of the combined effect size can be produced. The weighting is generally related to sample sizes within the individual studies but other differences need to be allowed for. The purpose of the meta-analysis is to produce a more powerful estimate of the true effect size, rather than the smaller effect size derived in a single small study. The confidence limits of the single study showed a range from 1.40 to 8.10, so although the OR was quoted as 3.37, the result could have been between 1.4 and 8.1, a wide range. This process of meta-analysis can be part of a systematic review, for example those reported to the Cochrane Collaboration. Figure 32.4 demonstrates the results of a meta-analysis that includes the study quoted above [10]. This is a forest (Peto) plot, a graphical display of the relative strength of treatment effects in the different trials. Down the left-hand side are the trials included. The trial quoted above is the last of the four trials listed (first author Rai). On the right-hand side is a plot of the risk ratio (not OR) for each of these studies incorporating confidence intervals represented by horizontal lines. The graph is plotted on a logarithmic scale so that the confidence intervals are symmetrical about the means to prevent apparent exaggeration in ratios greater than 1 when compared to those less than 1. The area of each square is proportional to the study's weight. The overall meta-analysed measure of effect is represented as the diamond on the bottom and the lateral points indicate the confidence intervals.

A vertical line is plotted at unity and if the confidence intervals for individual studies or the total effect overlap

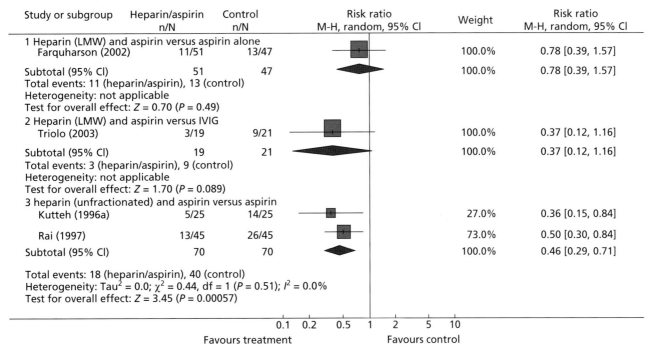

Review: Prevention of recurrent miscarriage for women with antiphospholipid antibody or lupus anticoagulant
Comparison: 1 All interventions-pregnancy loss
Outcome: 2 Heparin (LMW and unfractionated) and aspirin versus aspirin or IVIG

Fig. 32.4 Meta-analysis of heparin and aspirin compared with aspirin alone in the treatment of recurrent miscarriage in women with antiphospholipid syndrome. The results did not change the effect of the Rai paper but gives tighter confidence limits [10]. (With permission from Wiley.)

with this line, then the results are not significant. In this case the top two studies did not reach significance but the last two did, giving an overall significant result. The meta-analysis used miscarriage as the event so the results are reversed (reduction in miscarriage not increased live birth) and our original study gave an RR of 0.5 (CI 0.3–0.84), halving the risk of miscarriage, and the meta-analysis gave an RR of 0.46 (CI 0.29–0.71), which is a slightly increased benefit (reduction of repeat miscarriage) but with far tighter confidence intervals. This result shows an increased confidence that the quoted RR approximates to the expected benefit.

Prediction testing

Another use for contingency tables is in studies evaluating potentially new tests that screen for disease. Each individual taking the test either does or does not develop the disease. The test can be assessed for its value in predicting the disease.
- True positive: correctly predicts those who will develop the disease.
- False positive: does predict disease but the patient does not get it.
- True negative: does not predict the disease and the patient does not get it.
- False negative: does not predict the disease and the patient does get it.

An example this would be the detection of Down's syndrome babies by combination screening in the first trimester. Modern techniques are said to detect at least 85% of affected babies (sensitivity) with a 5% false-positive rate (specificity) [11]. This sounds very impressive. However, since the incidence of Down's syndrome in the population is approximately 1 in 1000, in a screened population of 100000 there will be 100 Down's syndrome babies of which 85 will be detected by the test.

	Down's syndrome baby	Normal	Total
Positive test	85	4995	5080
Negative test	15	94905	94920
	100	99900	100000

The 5% false-positive value means that there are over 5000 screen positives, of which which only 1/59 will be positive, and nearly 5000 amniocentesis or chorionic villous sampling procedures will be done with the accompanying complications, with the majority being negative. However, the specificity is high and negative predictive value is approaching 100%, which is very reassuring. Although the Down's screening test 'detects' 85% of babies with Down's syndrome, it only in fact selects a high-risk group that requires further invasive testing.

The current cut-off risk used in counselling of women is 1 in 250 and the reasons for choosing this number are historical. However, it can be seen that in this population if the screen is positive, the average risk is 1 in 60 that the invasive testing will find a positive result and that the mother is therefore carrying a Down's syndrome baby.

The Down's syndrome screening test uses an accepted level of sensitivity and specificity that are partly dependent on the desired level of positive screening requiring invasive testing (specificity) and a an accepted false-negative rate (sensitivity). This balance between sensitivity and specificity can be assessed using the receiver operating characteristic (ROC) curve. The ROC curve is a graph of the sensitivity or true positive rate plotted against the false-positive rate (1 – specificity). It is called the ROC curve because it compares the two operating characteristics, the true positive rate and the true negative rate with changing cut-off levels. This allows the optimum cut-off level of a predictive or diagnostic test for any given disease to be determined by finding the optimum sensitivity and specificity for that test (Fig. 32.5).

In a study of a diagnostic test that seeks to diagnose a disease, a cut-off point for the test will determine the number of true disease cases diagnosed but also the number of false positives. Generally, if the number of true positives is increased, then the number of false positives will also increase. Plotting the true positive rate against the false-positive rate for the different cut-off points will give the ROC curve. In Fig. 32.5, the straight line running from zero to 1 is no better than chance alone. Any curve

to the left of the line is better than chance. The more to the left, and the nearer the 'perfect' upper left-hand corner, the better the test. In this example the left-hand curve gives the best result for sensitivity 80–90% and specificity 80–90% (false-positive rate = 1 – sensitivity). Our previous example of Down's syndrome screening was better than this, with a sensitivity of 85% and specificity of 95% and, if plotted, would give a line to the left of those demonstrated. What cut-off point is used depends to some extent of whether it is better to capture the maximum or miss the fewest in the disease being investigated.

Descriptive statistics

Up to now we have discussed the assessment of rates and incidence of a given problem in a population but statistics are also used to describe a population and what values fall outwith the normal range that could be used for diagnostic purposes.

What is normal?
The term 'normal' is one of the most misunderstood terms in medical statistics and epidemiology. In its pure sense, it is the whole population, good and bad, and this should contribute to the normal range. However, in medical testing, normal is often taken as all individuals who are not abnormal, i.e. do not have the disease under study. This produces problems when comparisons are being made or predictors are being assessed as 'not abnormal' is a post-test value and when using a predictor it is important to test it against the whole population including those who will develop the disease or other diseases as this is how it will function in the real world. Without doing this, the value of most predictive tests is overstated.

Normal distribution
The graph of most 'normal' populations is a bell-shaped curve demonstrating a Gaussian distribution with the mean in the middle and a mirror-image distribution on either side (Fig. 32.6). It is one of the statistical standards and implies that, in most populations, there is an even spread (symmetrical) around the mean or average. The mean is calculated by taking the sum of all the measurements and dividing it by the total number of measurements taken. It is the same as the average. If the dataset were based on a series of observations obtained from a sample of the population, it is known as the sample mean, which will relate to, but may not be exactly the same as, the true population mean. Knowing the mean of a population is only the start. Different populations will have different ranges of measurements, some with a far wider range of values making up the population.

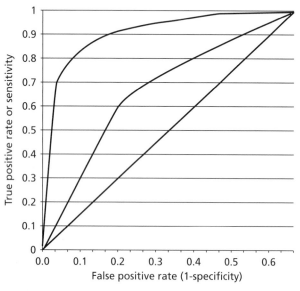

Fig. 32.5 Receiver operating characteristic (ROC) curve. As the lines move further left, the more discriminate the test with a higher sensitivity and low false-positive rate.

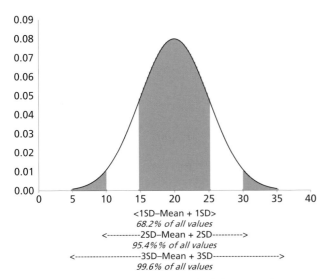

Fig. 32.6 Normal distribution and standard deviation: the mean is 20 and the SD 5. The bands correspond to 1, 2 and 3 SDs from the mean. Mean ±1SD takes in 68.2% of all values; mean ±2SD takes in 95.4% of all values and is equivalent to 95% CI; mean ±3SD takes in 99.6% of all values and is equivalent to the range.

The range is calculated by subtracting the smallest measurement (minimum) from the greatest (maximum) and provides an indication of sample spread. It is measured in the same units as the data. For example, if in a given dataset the mean body mass index (BMI) was 29.6, the lowest value 15.2 and the highest 47.3, the range would be 47.3 – 15.2 = 32.1. Because it is calculated from two measurements, the lowest and the highest, it is a weak statistical measure of distribution as it gives no indication of how the measurements are distributed throughout the range. Also, since it is often a measurement of a sample of a larger population, it does not necessarily give the full potential range of the population as a whole.

The measure of variation or spread around the mean can be assessed in many ways but the most common is the standard deviation. The mean and standard deviation describe a sample population and can be used to assess differences with other sample populations. The standard deviation (SD) is the assessment of variability of each individual measurement from the mean and is calculated by taking the average difference of each measurement from the calculated mean. A low SD indicates that the measurements tend to be very close to the mean as the variation is small and the distribution tight, producing a narrow peaked curve, whereas a high SD indicates that the data are spread out over a large range of values, giving a wider flatter curve.

Figure 32.6 shows the graph for a normal distribution and the SD. In a normal distribution, about 68% of the measurements will be within one standard deviation from the mean, while two standard deviations from the

mean account for about 95% and three standard deviations for about 99.7%. Therefore, the range of the mean ±1SD will contain the majority of the measurements; the 95% confidence interval of the population will lie within the mean ±2SDs and the mean ±3SDs approximates to the range. This 68/95/99.7 rule holds for all normal distributions irrespective of the size of the range. Therefore, if a sample lies more than 2SDs from the mean of a sample set, it is statistically not part of the set to a level of 95% confidence. Similarly, if two populations are being compared and the means of the populations are further apart than the addition of each population's SD, then the probability is that they are statistically different although more formal testing should be done.

In scientific experimentation, the standard error of the mean (SEM) is sometimes used instead of the SD. The SEM is the SD of the estimated mean of the study sample compared with the true population mean. Therefore, whereas the SD demonstrates the spread or range of the individual sample measurements around the sample mean, the SEM gives the spread or range of the calculated sample mean. The mean ±2SEMs is the 95% confidence range of the sample mean. Therefore if another sample population was studied, the calculated mean will fall within that range 95% of the time. The SEM can be calculated by dividing the SD by the square root of the sample size. Therefore, it is dependent on both the sample range and the sample size.

Comparing sample groups

The most common method of testing two sample populations is Student's *t*-test. The name comes from the pen-name of its introducer, William Gosset, who worked for Guinness Brewery in Dublin [12]. It was originally used to monitor the quality of Guinness. The test requires that the populations being compared are normally distributed. It can be used in one of two forms, the unpaired or the paired *t*-test.

The unpaired *t*-test is used when two separate unlinked normal populations are compared. For example, if you are studying two methods of induction of labour and you enrol 100 subjects into your study and randomize half into each treatment group, there are two independent samples to compare the outcomes, in this case the induction to delivery interval. The test used would be the unpaired form of the *t*-test. It does not need to be two randomized groups, just two groups that differ by a single parameter, e.g. primigravida and multiparous women, where the same induction agent is used and the results of the primigravida are compared with those of the multiparous women.

A paired *t*-test consists of matched pairs where a group of patients are tested twice, e.g. once before an intervention and repeated afterwards. An example would be to test for changes in the Bishop's score after application of vaginal prostaglandin. An unpaired *t*-test can be converted to a dependent *t*-test when the individuals in the two groups are assessed for similarities using measured variables that demonstrate similarities. This could be done in a cohort study looking at the effect of smoking on birthweight and matching each smoker with a matched control, matched for parity, BMI and gestation at delivery.

The *t*-test should be used when the population groups are assumed to be normal in distribution. Normality tests can assess any given dataset for the likelihood that it comes from a normal distribution, allowing the *t*-test to be used. If the data are not normally distributed or are skewed, a non-parametric test should be used. The most common simple tests are the Wilcoxon signed rank test for paired samples and the Mann–Whitney *U* test for independent populations.

Skewness is a measure of the asymmetry of the population distribution around the mean due to a larger and longer tail on one side or the other (Fig. 32.7) This can be positive or negative, indicating on which side of the mean the skewness lies. A negative skew indicates that the tail on the left side is longer than that on the right side and vice versa. The tail affects the mean, moving it towards the side of the tail and indicating that it is no longer representative of the sample as a whole and thus will overestimate or underestimate the 'average' of the population. The better measure of this is the median.

The median is the value separating the higher half of the population sampled from the lower half. It is calculated by ranging all the sample values from the lowest to the highest and finding the value in the middle (see Fig. 32.2). If there is an even number of values, then the median is defined to be the mean of the two middle values. In this case half the population have values less than the median and half have values greater than the median.

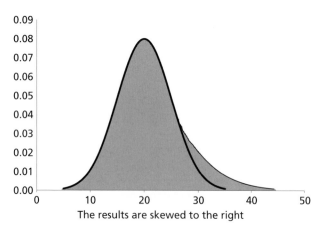

Fig. 32.7 This graph is similar to the normal distribution apart from a skewness to the right. This will make the mean higher than 20 and thus no longer halfway through the distribution. The median is a better measure of this in this case.

In a skewed population, the SD is not an accurate value of the distribution of the population around the median and in this case a better descriptor is the centile range. Just as the median is the value which describes the middle value within the range, the centile describes the percentage of the values contained within a given value range. In this case the median is the 50th centile as it describes the point where 50% of the population lie below and 50% above that value. Similarly, the 90th centile describes the value where 90% of the population are below and 10% above and the 10th centile the value where 10% are below and 90% are above.

It has to be remembered that the normal range statistically is the population range including all values, not a range of those who are designated 'normal' or disease-free. For example, if intrauterine growth restriction is classified as babies less than the 10th centile, then 10% of the normal baby population will fall into that category as well as those who may be truly growth restricted. Further evaluations are required to assess whether the baby is truly growth restricted or just a small normal baby. However, if the 5th centile is used, the baby lies outside the 95% confidence limit of what would be expected; similarly, the 3rd centile would make the baby even more likely to fall into the growth-restricted range as 97% of babies would be expected to be heavier. The 3rd centile is the equivalent of 2SDs from the population mean of a normal distribution. If two skewed or asymmetric populations are to be compared, then non-parametric tests are required.

Comparing asymmetric populations

The Mann–Whitney *U* test (also called Wilcoxon rank-sum test) is a non-parametric test for assessing two independent populations. It is variation of the original Wilcoxon test that is used to study populations of equal size. The Mann–Whitney *U* test is performed by putting all the values from each group into one ranked column from highest to lowest. The sum of the ranks for each group is compared and used to calculate the value *U*. If the samples are different, then one group will have a smaller value of *U*, implying a higher average ranking. This is then used to consult significance tables to assess whether the groups are statistically significant. Most statistical packages will do this automatically.

The Wilcoxon signed-rank test is a paired non-parametric test for assessing two populations which are related, e.g. a single population tested twice, once before and once after an intervention. It is used as an alternative to the paired Student's *t*-test where the population is not normally distributed. Since this is a paired test, the value from test 2 is subtracted from the value from test 1, giving a value Z. These values are ranked similarly to the Mann–Whitney *U* test, rank 1 being given to the smallest absolute value of Z. The ranks of the positive values for Z and the negative values of Z are summed. The smaller of the two rank sums is then used to compare against a table of critical values for a given sample size to assess whether there is a significant difference, with either an increase or decrease after the intervention. This test is powerful as it is less dependent on the size of individual pair changes and is a measure of a population shift, although the problem with this is that the changes could be very small but still statistically significant. As with all statistics, the results must be interpreted with clinical relevance.

Correlation and dependence

All the tests above have looked at ways of studying populations if they are different. Other tests look for the correlation between values within the population studied. These tests study the changes between two or more values to see if the changes in these values are linked, for example studies on the effect of maternal BMI on the incidence of Caesarean section. In the National Sentinel Caesarean Section Audit, the higher the BMI, the higher the Caesarean section rate in those women. Logic tells us that rising BMI affects Caesarean section rate and not Caesarean section rate affecting BMI. However, the statistics cannot make this assumption and this has to be interpreted by the investigator. Correlations can demonstrate a predictive relationship, for example a rise in BMI of x should be associated with a rise of $y\%$ in the Caesarean section rate, and this can be used to predict how the BMI of women presenting in pregnancy would affect the Caesarean section rate in an institution. Similarly, it may also suggest that a reduction in BMI might reduce the risk of Caesarean section in any given woman. However, just because the values are linked does not mean that they are causative; statistical dependence is not sufficient to demonstrate the presence of such a relationship. The two variables may both be influenced independently by a common third factor.

The result of a test for correlation is given as the correlation coefficient, usually denoted by r, which is a measure of the degree of correlation. The most common test is the Pearson correlation test, which tests for linear correlation. The nearer r is to 1 or -1, the closer the correlation, implying that for each unit rise in one variable there is an equal unit rise ($r = 1$) or fall ($r = -1$) in the other variable. A value P can be given, similar to other statistical tests, stating the confidence that the test is accurate (e.g. 95% confidence if $P < 0.05$) but does not assess how closely correlated the two variables are. The square of the r value gives an approximation of the percentage effect the change of one variable has on the other. Therefore, a test that gives an result of $r = 0.5$ and $P < 0.01$ indicates that there is a statistically valid correlation but only 25% (r^2) of any given change in variable 2 is associated with a change in variable 1. It is only when r is greater than 0.7

that the variable in 1 has over a 50% effect on the variable in 2.

What has been described above is standard statistics and what is seen as statistical significance. It has also been suggested that it is important to assess the results obtained from a clinical viewpoint to assess reality and how the results influence accepted pre-test thinking. This is part of the thinking behind Bayesian inference.

Bayesian inference

Bayesian inference is the use of a priori belief or probability about a test result to determine the probability that a new test result is true. In other words knowing what we know from experience or belief, can this new result be true? In day-to-day terms, this is the basis on how we change our beliefs and practices. If a study confirms our preconceived beliefs, we will accept it without question but if it disagrees, then we may struggle to accept it and only change our practice to a degree. However, as more evidence accumulates, the degree of confidence in a test result changes. With enough evidence, the degree of confidence should become either very high or very low. This means that results will naturally be biased due to pre-test prejudices but it allows the changing of that bias with more confirmatory evidence. This is really how we practise in the real world. Many observational studies suggested an increased risk of vaginal breech delivery but many practitioners did not accept these results due to their pre-existing prejudices. The Term Breech Trial, with its large randomized format, convinced those who already believed and some of those who were sceptical but others still found flaws in the study so they did not have to change their beliefs. In a statistical form, Bayesian inference estimates the degree of pre-test belief before any evidence is collected, and then re-estimates the degree of confidence after a set of evidence has been observed by combining the pre-test values with the test results. This process is then repeated whenever additional evidence is obtained, leading to a changing probability that the results are true or false.

 Summary box 32.4

Descriptive statistics
- Mean: the sum of all the measurements divided by the total number of measurements taken.
- Range: calculated by subtracting the smallest measurement (minimum) from the greatest (maximum).
- Standard deviation (SD): the assessment of variability of each individual measurement from the mean, calculated by taking the average difference of each measurement from the calculated mean.

(Continued)

- Standard error of the mean (SEM): standard deviation of the estimated mean of the study sample compared with the true population mean.
- Student's *t*-test: used to compare normally distributed populations. The populations can be paired or unpaired.
- Skewness: a measure of the asymmetry of the population distribution around the mean.
- Median: the value separating the higher half of the population sampled from the lower half.
- Centiles: describe the percentage of values contained within a given value range.
- Mann–Whitney *U* test: a non-parametric test for assessing two independent populations.
- Wilcoxon signed-rank test: a paired non-parametric test for assessing two populations which are related.
- Correlation: studies the changes between two or more values within a population to see if the changes in these values are linked.
- Bayesian inference: a method that uses a priori belief or probability about a test result to determine the probability that a new test result is true.

How we use statistics

The above are all examples of how we use statistics. Whatever the results, all are interpreted in the light of our own experience. If we have no preconceived beliefs, we are open to the results of any trial. If we have a preconceived idea and the trial shows a null result, it confirms to us that what we do is correct, but that is also true of people with a preconceived idea opposite to our own. The Term PROM trial showed no difference between immediate induction of labour or delay in cases of pre-labour rupture of the membranes. This indicates that there is no evidence to support either action. This allowed people to continue to act as they previously did, believing themselves to be correct, but it should have told people that there is no correct answer and that women should be offered a choice of action.

Statistics is a powerful tool in medical research and epidemiology, but it is important to use it at the right time in the right way. If the wrong question is asked, the result is worthless irrespective of the outcome and statistical significance. It is important to think through the problem being addressed carefully and set the correct hypothesis and test it with a study of the appropriate power. Statistics will not cover up for a poorly designed trial with insufficient numbers testing the wrong hypothesis. It is also important to assess the results for clinical relevance and the consequences of changing actions potentially resulting in unforeseen consequences that were not tested for.

References

1 Semmelweis IP. Die Aetiologie, der Begriff und die Prophylaxis des Kindbettfiebers. [The aetiology, concept, and prophylaxis of childbed fever.] Budapest and Vienna, 1961.
2 Cantwell R, Clutton-Brock T, Cooper G *et al.* Saving Mothers' Lives: Reviewing maternal deaths to make motherhood safer: 2006–2008. The Eighth Report of the Confidential Enquiries into Maternal Deaths in the United Kingdom. *BJOG* 2011; 118(Suppl 1):1–203.
3 Centre for Maternal and Child Enquiries. *Perinatal Mortality 2009: United Kingdom.* London: CMACE, 2011.
4 Thomas J, Paranjothy S. *The National Sentinel Caesarean Section Audit Report.* London: RCOG Press, 2001.
5 Mahmood TA, Templeton A. The impact of treatment on the natural history of endometriosis. *Hum Reprod* 1990;5:965–970.
6 Missmer SA, Hankinson SE, Spiegelman D, Barbieri RL, Marshall LM, Hunter DJ. Incidence of laparoscopically confirmed endometriosis by demographic, anthropometric, and lifestyle factors. *Am J Epidemiol* 2004;160:784–796.
7 Rai R, Cohen H, Dave M, Regan L. Randomised controlled trial of aspirin and aspirin plus heparin in pregnant women with recurrent miscarriage associated with phospholipid antibodies (or antiphospholipid antibodies). *BMJ* 1997;314:253–257.
8 Shelton JD, Taylor RN Jr. The Pearl Pregnancy Index reexamined: still useful for clinical trials of contraceptives. *Am J Obstet Gynecol* 1981;139:592–596.
9 Doll R, Hill AB. Mortality in relation to smoking: ten years' observations of british doctors. *BMJ* 1964;1:1460–1467.
10 Empson M, Lassere M, Craig J, Scott J. Prevention of recurrent miscarriage for women with antiphospholipid antibody or lupus anticoagulant. *Cochrane Database Syst Rev* 2005;(2): CD002859.
11 Cuckle HS, Malone FD, Wright D *et al.* Contingent screening for Down syndrome: results from the FaSTER trial. *Prenat Diagn* 2008;28:89–94.
12 Hanley JA. The statistical legacy of William Sealy Gosset ('Student'). *Community Dent Health* 2008;25:194–195.

Section 2

Gynaecology

Part 8
Gynaecology

Chapter 33
Clinical Anatomy of the Pelvis and Reproductive Tract

Alan Farthing
Imperial College NHS Trust, London, UK

This chapter aims to summarize important aspects of the anatomy of the abdomen and the pelvis that should be known to the obstetric or gynaecological specialist. Many of the investigations and treatments we order on a daily basis require good anatomical knowledge in order to be properly understood.

Surface anatomy

The anterior abdominal wall can be divided into four quadrants by lines passing horizontally and vertically through the umbilicus (Fig. 33.1). In the upper abdomen is the epigastrium, which is the area just inferior to the xiphisternum, and in the lower abdomen lie the right and left iliac fossae and the hypogastrium.

The cutaneous nerve supply of the anterior abdominal wall arises from the anterior rami of the lower thoracic and lumbar vertebrae. The dermatomes of significant structures on the anterior abdominal wall are T7 (xiphisternum), T10 (umbilicus) and L1 (symphysis pubis).

The blood supply is via the superior epigastric (branch of the internal thoracic artery) and the inferior epigastric (branch of the external iliac artery) vessels. During laparoscopy, the inferior epigastric vessels can be seen between the peritoneum and rectus muscle on the anterior abdominal wall and commence their journey superiorly from approximately two-thirds of the way along the inguinal ligament closer to the symphysis pubis. Care needs to be taken to avoid them while using accessory trochars during laparoscopy and to ensure that they are identified when making a Maylard incision of the abdominal wall.

The anterior abdominal wall

Beneath the skin and the fat of the superficial anterior abdominal wall lies a sheath and combination of muscles including the rectus abdominis, external and internal oblique and tranversalis muscles (Fig. 33.2). Where these muscles coalesce in the midline, the linea alba is formed. Pyramidalis muscle is present in almost all women, originating on the anterior surface of the pubis and inserting into the linea alba. The exact configuration of the muscles encountered by the surgeon depends on exactly where any incision is made.

The umbilicus

The umbilicus is essentially a scar made from the remnants of the umbilical cord. It is situated in the linea alba and in a variable position depending on the obesity of the patient. However, the base of the umbilicus is always the thinnest part of the anterior abdominal wall and is the commonest site of insertion of the primary port in laparoscopy. The urachus is the remains of the allantois from the fetus and runs from the apex of the bladder to the umbilicus. Occasionally this can remain patent in newborns. In early embryological life, the vitelline duct also runs through the umbilicus from the developing midgut. Although the duct is severed long before delivery, a remnant of this structure is found in 2% of the population as a Meckel's diverticulum.

The aorta divides into the common iliac arteries approximately 1–2 cm below the umbilicus in most slim women (Fig. 33.3). The common iliac veins combine to form the inferior vena cava just below this and all these structures are a potential hazard for the laparoscopist inserting ports at the umbilicus.

Epithelium of the genital tract

The anterior abdominal wall including the vulva, vagina and perineal areas are lined with squamous epithelium. The epithelium lining the endocervix and uterine cavity is columnar and the squamocolumnar junction usually

---

Dewhurst's Textbook of Obstetrics & Gynaecology, Eighth Edition. Edited by D. Keith Edmonds.
© 2012 John Wiley and Sons, Ltd. Published 2012 by John Wiley and Sons, Ltd.

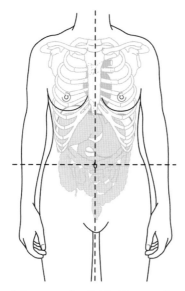

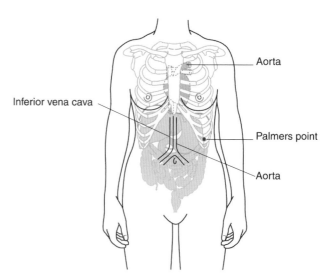

Fig. 33.1 The abdomen can be divided into quadrants.

Fig. 33.3 The umbilicus in relation to the underlying vasculature in a thin patient.

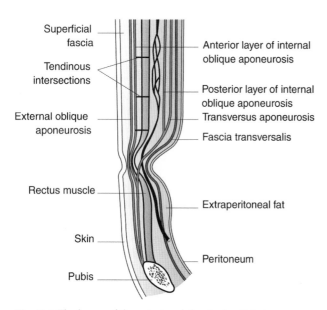

Fig. 33.2 The layers of the anterior abdominal wall in tranverse section.

arises at the ectocervix in women of reproductive age. This is an important site as it is the area from which cervical intraepithelial neoplasia (CIN) and eventually cervical malignancy arises. The bladder is lined by transitional epithelium that becomes columnar as it lines the urethra. The anal margin is still squamous epithelium but this changes to columnar immediately inside the anus and into the rectum.

The genital tract, from the vagina, through the uterus and out through the fallopian tubes into the peritoneal cavity, is an open passage. This is an essential route for sperm to traverse in the process of fertilization but unfor-

tunately it also allows the transport of pathological organisms that may result in ascending infection.

The peritoneum

The peritoneum is a thin serous membrane that lines the inside of the pelvic and abdominal cavities. In simplistic terms, it is probably best to imagine the pelvis containing the bladder, uterus and rectum (Fig. 33.4) and note that the peritoneum is a layer placed over these organs in a single sheet. This complete layer is then pierced by both the fallopian tubes and the ovaries on each side. Posteriorly the rectum also pierces the peritoneum where it connects to the sigmoid colon, and the area between the posterior surface of the uterus and its supporting ligaments and the rectum is called the pouch of Douglas. This particular area is important in gynaecology as the place where gravity-dependent fluid collects. As a result this is where blood is found in ectopic pregnancies, pus in infections and endometriosis caused by retrograde menstruation.

Vulva

The vulva is the area of the perineum comprising the mons pubis, labia majora and minora and the opening into both the vagina and urethra (Fig. 33.5). The labia majora are areas of skin with underlying fat pads which bound the vagina. Medial to these are the labia minora, which consist of vascular tissue that engorges with blood during sexual arousal. Anteriorly they come together to form the prepuce of the clitoris and posteriorly they form

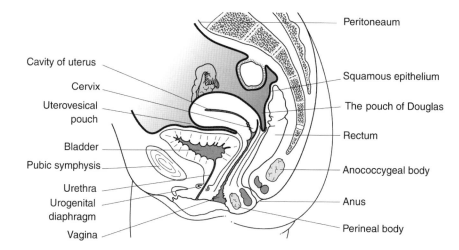

Fig. 33.4 Transverse view of the pelvic organs.

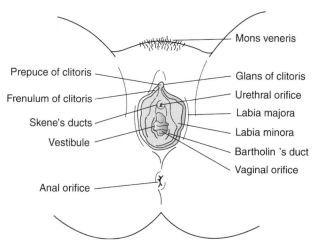

Fig. 33.5 Surface anatomy of the vulva.

the fourchette. The hymen is a fold of mucosa at the entrance to the vagina. It usually has a small opening in virgins and is only seen as an irregular remnant in sexually active women. To each side of the introitus are the ducts of the vestibular glands commonly known as Bartholin's glands, which produce much of the lubrication during sexual intercourse.

The vulval blood supply comes from the pudendal artery and lymphatic drainage is through the inguinal lymph nodes. The nerve supply comes mostly from the pudendal nerve and pelvic plexus, with branches of the perineal nerves and posterior cutaneous nerve of the thigh important in the posterior region.

The clitoris

The clitoris corresponds to the male penis and consists of the same three masses of erectile tissue (Fig. 33.6). The bulb of the vestibule is attached to the underlying urogenital diaphragm and splits into two because of the pres-

ence of the vagina. The right and left crura become the corpora cavernosa and are covered by the ischiocavernosus muscles.

Bony pelvis

The bony pelvis consists of two hip bones (comprising ilium and ischium) that are joined together by the sacrum posteriorly and the symphysis pubis anteriorly (Figs 33.7 and 33.8). In addition, the coccyx lies on the inferior aspect of the sacrum. A plane drawn between the sacral promontory and the superior aspect of the symphysis pubis marks the pelvic inlet and a similar plane drawn from the tip of S5 to the inferior aspect of the symphysis pubis marks the pelvic outlet.

Clinically the ischial spine is important as it can be felt vaginally and progress in labour can be measured using it as a landmark. Additionally, it is an insertion point of the sacrospinous ligament, which also attaches to the lower lateral part of the sacrum. Together with the sacrotuberous ligament and the bony pelvis, it forms the borders of the greater sciatic foramen (through which the sciatic nerve passes) and the lesser sciatic foramen (through which the pudenal nerve enters the pelvis).

The sacrum and ilium are joined by the very strong sacro-iliac joint. This is a synovial joint and is supported by the posterior and interosseous sacro-iliac ligaments. The symphysis pubis is a cartilaginous joint with a fibro-cartilaginous disc separating the two bones, which are firmly bound together by the supporting ligaments. There should be virtually no movement of this joint.

Pelvic floor

The obturator internus muscle sits on the medial side of the ischial bone and, together with the body of the pubis, forms a wall that supports the origins of the pelvic floor.

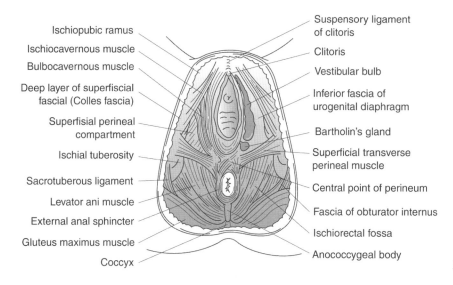

Ischiopubic ramus

Ischiocavernous muscle

Bulbocavernous muscle

Deep layer of superfiscial fascial (Colles fascia)

Superfisial perineal compartment

Ischial tuberosity

Sacrotuberous ligament

Levator ani muscle

External anal sphincter

Gluteus maximus muscle

Coccyx

Suspensory ligament of clitoris

Clitoris

Vestibular bulb

Inferior fascia of urogenital diaphragm

Bartholin's gland

Superficial transverse perineal muscle

Central point of perineum

Fascia of obturator internus

Ischiorectal fossa

Anococcygeal body

Fig. 33.6 The deeper vulval tissues.

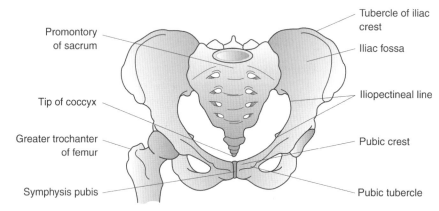

Promontory of sacrum

Tip of coccyx

Greater trochanter of femur

Symphysis pubis

Tubercle of iliac crest

Iliac fossa

Iliopectineal line

Pubic crest

Pubic tubercle

Fig. 33.7 Bony pelvis.

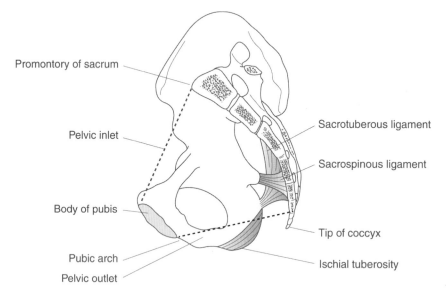

Promontory of sacrum

Pelvic inlet

Body of pubis

Pubic arch

Pelvic outlet

Sacrotuberous ligament

Sacrospinous ligament

Tip of coccyx

Ischial tuberosity

Fig. 33.8 Bony pelvis.

The pelvic floor itself is a sling of various muscles that are pierced by the urethra, the vagina and the anal canal. Posterior to the vagina these muscles form the perineal body. The puborectalis muscle forms a sling around the junction of the anus and rectum and posterior to the anus, and these fibres consist of the pubococcygeus that forms the anococcygeal body in the midline (Fig. 33.9). The collection of muscles is variously referred to as the pelvic diaphragm or levator ani muscles (Fig. 33.10). These muscles support the pelvic organs, holding them in position and resisting the forces created when the intraperitoneal pressure is raised as in coughing or straining. The

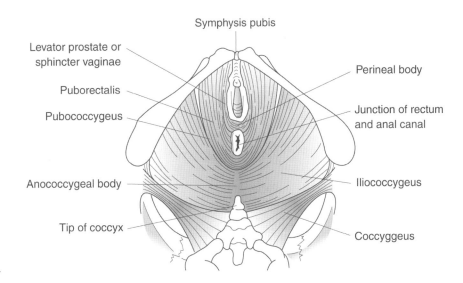

Fig. 33.9 Pelvic floor muscles.

Symphysis pubis

Levator prostate or
sphincter vaginae

Puborectalis

Pubococcygeus

Anococcygeal body

Tip of coccyx

Perineal body

Junction of rectum
and anal canal

Iliococcygeus

Coccyggeus

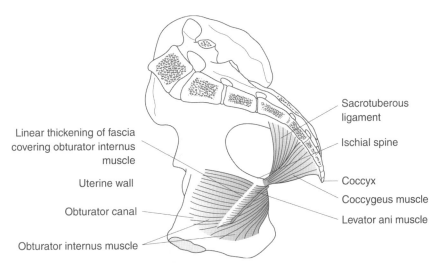

Fig. 33.10 Transverse view of the pelvic
floor muscles.

Linear thickening of fascia
covering obturator internus
muscle

Uterine wall

Obturator canal

Obturator internus muscle

Sacrotuberous
ligament

Ischial spine

Coccyx

Coccygeus muscle

Levator ani muscle

nerve supply is from the fourth sacral nerve and pudendal nerve.

Pelvic organs (Fig. 33.11)

Vagina

The vagina is a distensible muscular tube that passes from
the introitus to the cervix. It pierces the pelvic floor and
then lies flat on its posterior surface using it as support.
It is approximately 8 cm long and the anterior and posterior walls oppose each other. Anatomical textbooks can
give a confusing impression when showing this structure
as an open tube with a lumen. However, on imaging, the
normal vagina should not be distended and does not
contain air. Projecting into the top of the vagina is the
uterine cervix. The areas of the vagina that border the
cervix are referred to as the fornices and are labelled as
anterior, posterior, right or left.

The vaginal wall consists of outer and inner circular
layers of muscles that cannot be distinguished from each

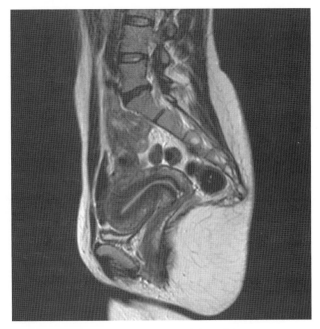

Fig. 33.11 Magnetic resonance image of the pelvis.

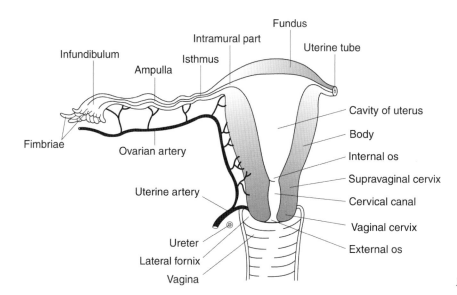

Fig. 33.12 Uterus and fallopian tubes.

other. The epithelium contains no glands but is rich in glycogen in the premenopausal woman. The normal commensal, *Lactobacillus acidophilus*, breaks down this glycogen to create an acid environment.

Uterus

The uterus is approximately the size and shape of a pear with a central cavity and thick muscular walls (Fig. 33.12). The serosal surface is the closely applied peritoneum, beneath which is the myometrium. The myometrium is smooth muscle supported by connective tissue and comprises three layers of muscle: external, intermediate and internal layers. Clinically this is important as fibroids leave the layers intact and removal through a superficial incision leaves the three layers intact. The three layers run in complimentary directions, encouraging vascular occlusion during contraction, an important aspect of menstrual blood loss and postpartum haemostasis. The mucous membrane overlying the myometrium and which lines the cavity is the endometrium. Glands of the endometrium pierce the myometrium and a single layer of columnar epithelium on the surface changes cyclically in response to the menstrual cycle.

The uterus consists of a fundus superiorly, a body, an isthmus (internal os) and inferiorly the cervix (external os). The cervix is a cylindrical structure that is muscular in its upper portions but comprises fibrous connective tissue in its lower part where it connects with the vagina. The cervix is lined by columnar epithelium which secretes alkaline mucus that neutralizes the effects of vaginal acidity.

The cervix and uterus do not always lie in the same plane and when the uterine body rotates anteriorly it is referred to as 'anteflexed'; when rotated posteriorly, it is referred to as 'retroflexed'. The axis of the entire uterus can be anteverted or retroverted in relation to the axis of the vagina (Fig. 33.13).

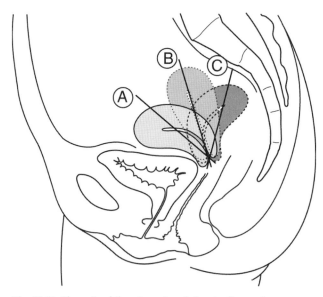

Fig. 33.13 The axis of the uterus in relation to the vagina.

The uterus is supported by the muscles of the pelvic floor together with three supporting condensations of connective tissue. The pubocervical ligaments run from the cervix anteriorly to the pubis, the cardinal ligaments pass laterally from the cervix and upper vagina to the lateral pelvic side walls, and the uterosacral ligaments run from the cervix and upper vagina to the sacrum. These uterosacral ligaments can be clearly seen posterior to the uterus in the pouch of Douglas and are a common site for superficial and deep infiltrating endometriosis.

The uterine blood supply is derived mainly from the uterine artery, a branch of the anterior division of the internal iliac artery. An anastomosis occurs with the blood supply delivered through the ovarian ligament and derived direct from the ovarian artery.

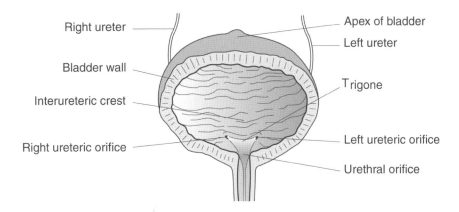

Fig. 33.14 The bladder.

The round ligament is the remains of the gubernaculum and extends from the uterus laterally to the pelvic side wall and then into the inguinal canal before passing down into the labia majora. It holds the uterus in anteversion, although it is a highly elastic structure in pregnancy. It is usually the first structure divided at hysterectomy, allowing the surgeon to open the overlying folds of peritoneum known as the broad ligament.

Fallopian tubes

The fallopian tubes are delicate tubular structures that allow transport of the ovum or sperm between the ovary and uterine cavity. The tubes are divided into named regions, most medially the cornu and interstitial portion within the uterine wall, then the isthmus followed by the infundibulum, ampulla and finally fimbrial ends. They are lined by columnar epithelium and cilia which, together with the peristaltic action of the surrounding smooth muscle, propel the fertilized ovum towards the uterine cavity. The blood supply of the fallopian tubes arises from both the uterine and ovarian arteries through the mesosalpinx which is covered by peritoneum.

Ovaries

The ovaries vary in size depending on age and their function. They measure approximately 2 × 4 cm, with the long axis running vertically, and are attached to the posterior leaf of the broad ligament by the mesovarium. In addition they are fixed in position by the ovarian ligament (to the uterus medially) and the infundibulopelvic ligament, which contains the ovarian blood supply direct from the aorta. Venous drainage is to the ovarian veins which drain directly into the inferior vena cava on the right and into the renal vein on the left. The aortic nerve plexus also accompanies the ovary in its descent from around the level of the first lumbar vertebra.

The lateral pelvic side wall is covered by peritoneum that is folded to form the ovarian fossa. Pathological adhesions around the ovary will often cause it to become fixed into the ovarian fossa, causing cyclical pain or dyspareunia. The ovary is not covered by peritoneum but is surrounded by a thin membranous capsule, the tunica albuginea, which in turn is covered by the germinal epithelium.

Bladder

The urinary bladder is situated immediately behind the pubic bone and anterior to the uterine cervix and upper vagina. It has a strong muscular wall consisting of three layers of interlacing fibres, which together are known as the detrusor muscles (Fig. 33.14). The trigone is the only smooth part of the bladder as it is fixed to the underlying muscle. At the superior margins of the trigone lie the ureteric openings and at the inferior aspect the urethra. An inter-ureteric ridge can often be visualized horizontally between the ureters at cystoscopy and is useful for orientation. The rest of the bladder is highly distensible, ensuring that as it is expanded by urine, the pressure of its contents remains the same.

The bladder receives its blood supply from the superior and inferior vesical arteries, which originate from the internal iliac artery. The nerve supply is from the inferior hypogastric plexus. Sympathetic nerves arise in the first and second lumbar ganglia and the parasympathetic supply from the splanchnic nerves of the second, third and fourth sacral nerves.

Urethra

The urethra is approximately 4 cm long in the female adult, starting at the internal meatus of the bladder and passing through the pelvic floor to the vestibule. The epithelium is squamous near the external meatus but changes to transitional epithelium approximately 2.5 cm from the meatus. The deeper tissue is muscular and this maintains urethral tone. There are no anatomical sphincters but the muscle fibres of the bladder at the internal meatus act as an 'internal sphincter' and the pelvic floor as a voluntary external sphincter.

Ureters

The ureters run from the renal hilum to the trigone of the bladder and are approximately 30 cm in length. They enter the pelvis by passing over the common iliac bifurcation at the pelvic brim. They then pass along the lateral pelvic side wall before passing anteriorly and medially under the uterine artery as it originates from the internal iliac artery and into the base of the bladder. The ureter comes close to the ovarian artery and vein and can be adherent to these vessels or the overlying ovary in pathological cases. By passing close to the uterine artery it can be mistakenly clamped and divided as a rare complication of hysterectomy.

The ureters are muscular tubes lined by transitional epithelium. The blood supply varies during its course but small vessels along the surface of the ureter require careful preservation when dissecting it free from other structures.

Rectum

The rectum is approximately 12 cm in length and starts at S3 as a continuation of the sigmoid colon. The puborectalis part of the pelvic floor forms a sling around the lower end at the junction with the anal canal. The rectum is commonly depicted in anatomical drawings as being dilated, causing the other pelvic organs to be pushed forward. This is because the original drawings were taken from cadavers but in the live patient the rectum is often empty, allowing the other structures to lie supported on the pelvic floor. The mucosa of the rectum is columnar and this is surrounded by inner circular and outer longitudinal fibres of smooth muscle. The serosal surface is covered by peritoneum.

The blood supply is from the superior rectal artery from the inferior mesenteric artery, and the middle and inferior rectal arteries arise from the posterior division of the internal iliac artery. The nerve supply is from the inferior hypogastric plexus and ensures the rectum is sensitive to stretch only.

Conclusion

A clear knowledge of anatomy is required for many gynaecological diagnoses and certainly for surgery. Many clinicians do not gain a full understanding of pelvic anatomy until they start operating and then rarely refer back to anatomical textbooks. The advent of more sophisticated pelvic floor surgery and especially minimal access surgery has modified the skills required of a gynaecological surgeon, necessitating the need for greater practical anatomical knowledge.

Further reading

The Interactive Pelvis and Perineum: Female. Available at www. primalpictures.com/Male_Female_Pelvis.aspx

Snell RS. *Clinical Anatomy for Medical Students*, 6th edn. Philadelphia: Lippincott, Williams and Wilkins, 2000.

Chapter 34
Normal and Abnormal Development of the Genital Tract

D. Keith Edmonds
Queen Charlotte's & Chelsea Hospital, London, UK

Sexual differentiation and its control are vital to the continuation of our species, and for the gynaecologist an understanding of the development of the genital organs is clearly important. Our knowledge of this process has greatly increased in recent years and with it an appreciation of normal and abnormal sexual development. Following fertilization the normal embryo contains 46 chromosomes, including 22 autosomes derived from each parent. The basis of mammalian development is that a 46XY embryo will develop as a male and a 46XX embryo as a female. However, it is the presence or absence of the Y chromosome which determines whether the undifferentiated gonad becomes a testis or an ovary.

Although the sequence of genes required for differentiation of the gonads and development of the genital tract remains to be clearly defined, sex determination equates to gonadal development. This is then followed by a second process known as sex differentiation. Studies of the genetic control of gonadal development are based on animal data. The Y chromosome contains a region known as *SRY* (sex-determining region of the Y chromosome) and it has been shown that the testis-determining factor is on chromosome Yp11.31. In males this gene triggers testis formation from the undifferentiated gonad [1] but *SRY* is only one member of a family of genes that exist within the homeobox known as HMG. These genes, known as *SOX* genes, act in combination to differentiate the gonad to a testis. Mutations of *SRY* cause pure gonadal dysgenesis or hermaphroditism. Ovarian development is also dependent on genes on the short arm of the X chromosome, although the exact mechanism by which these genes invoke ovarian development remains to be defined.

Ovarian differentiation seems to be determined by the presence of two X chromosomes and the ovarian determinant is located on the short arm of the X chromosome; this was discovered by observing that the absence of the short arm results in ovarian agenesis [2]. At present, it is believed that *DAX1* is the gene which determines that the bipotential gonad will become an ovary. Other autosomal loci are certainly involved in ovarian development and development of the Wolffian and Müllerian structures is also under genetic control; this is thought to be a polygenic multifactorial inheritance, although autosomal recessive genes may also be involved [3]. The influence of the differentiated gonad on the development of other genital organs is thus fundamental and the presence of a testis will lead to male genital organ development and its absence means the individual will develop female genital organs whether ovaries are present or not.

Summary box 34.1

Mammalian development depends on the chromosome complement: a 46XY embryo develops as a male but the default state is female if the chromosome complement is anything other than male.

Development of the genital organs

Most embryological accounts agree on the principles of genital tract development, although some different views are held on the development of the vagina. The genital organs and those of the urinary tract arise in the intermediate mesoderm on either side of the root of the mesentery beneath the epithelium of the coelom (Fig. 34.1). The pronephros, a few transient excretory tubules in the cervical region, appears first but quickly degenerates. The duct, which begins in association with the pronephros, persists and extends caudally to open at the cloaca, connecting as it does so with some of the tubules of the mesonephros shortly to appear. The duct is called the mesonephric (Wolffian) duct. The mesonephros itself, the second primitive kidney, develops as a swelling bulging into the dorsal wall of the coelom of the thoracic and upper lumbar regions. The mesonephros in the male persists in part as the excretory portion of the male genital

Dewhurst's Textbook of Obstetrics & Gynaecology, Eighth Edition. Edited by D. Keith Edmonds.
© 2012 John Wiley and Sons, Ltd. Published 2012 by John Wiley and Sons, Ltd.

system; in the female only a few vestiges survive (Fig. 34.2). The genital ridge in which the gonad of each sex is to develop is visible as a swelling on the medial aspect of the mesonephros; the paramesonephric (Müllerian) duct from which much of the female genital tract will develop forms as an ingrowth of the coelomic epithelium on its lateral aspect; the ingrowth forms a groove and then a tube and sinks below the surface.

Uterus and fallopian tubes

The two paramesonephric ducts extend caudally until they reach the urogenital sinus at about 9 weeks' gestation. The blind ends project into the posterior wall of the sinus to become the Müllerian tubercle (Fig. 34.3). At the beginning of the third month the Müllerian and Wolffian ducts and mesonephric tubules are all present and capable of development. From this point onwards in the female there is degeneration of the Wolffian system and marked growth of the Müllerian system. In the male the opposite occurs as a result of production of Müllerian inhibitory substance by the fetal testis. The lower ends of the Müllerian ducts come together in the midline, fuse and develop into the uterus and the cervix. The cephalic ends of the duct remain separate to form the fallopian tubes. The thick muscular walls of the uterus and cervix develop from proliferation of mesenchyme around the fused portion of the ducts.

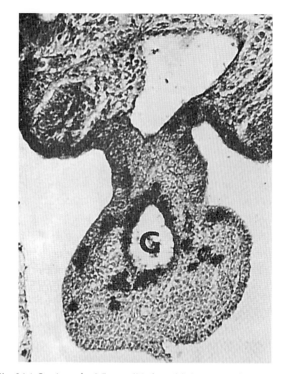

Fig. 34.1 Section of a 3.5-mm (28-day-old) human embryo stained with alkaline phosphatase showing the primitive gut (G), above which is the root of the mesentery. Above this again on either side is the intermediate mesoderm in which the genital organs develop. Germ cells are stained black and seen on either side of the primitive gut. (From Leigh Simpson [4] with permission.)

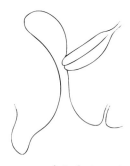

Fig. 34.3 Paired paramesonephric ducts protruding into the urogenital sinus as the Müllerian tubercle at 9 weeks of intrauterine life.

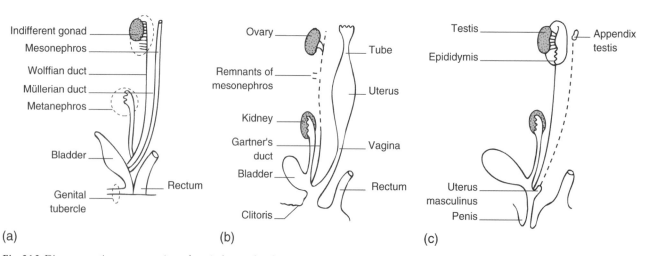

Fig. 34.2 Diagrammatic representation of genital tract development: (a) indifferent stage; (b) female development; (c) male development.

Vagina

At the point where the paramesonephric ducts protrude their solid tips into the dorsal wall of the urogenital sinus as the Müllerian tubercle there is marked growth of tissue from which the vagina will form, known as the vaginal plate. This plate grows in all dimensions, greatly increasing the distance between the cervix and the urogenital sinus, and later the central cells of this plate break down to form the vaginal lumen. The complete canalization of the vagina does not usually occur until around weeks 20–24 of pregnancy and failure of complete canalization may lead to a variety of septae, which cause outflow tract obstruction in later years. The debate which continues concerns that portion of the vagina formed from the Müllerian ducts and that from the urogenital sinus by the growth of the sinovaginal bulb. Some believe that the upper four-fifths of the vagina is formed by the Müllerian duct and the lower fifth by the urogenital sinus, while others believe that sinus upgrowth extends to the cervix displacing the Müllerian component completely and the vagina is thus derived wholly from the endoderm of the urogenital sinus. It seems certain that some of the vagina is derived from the urogenital sinus, but it has not been determined whether or not the Müllerian component is involved.

External genitalia

The primitive cloaca becomes divided by a transverse septum into an anterior urogenital portion and a posterior rectal portion. The urogenital portion of the cloacal membrane breaks down shortly after division is complete and this urogenital sinus develops into three portions (Fig. 34.4). There is an external expanded phallic part, a deeper narrow pelvic part between it and the region of the Müllerian tubercle and a vesico-urethral part connected superiorly to the allantois. Externally in this region the genital tubercle forms a conical projection around the anterior part of the cloacal membrane. Two pairs of swellings, a medial part (genital folds) and a lateral pair (genital swellings), are then formed by proliferation of mesoderm around the end of the urogenital sinus. Development up to this time (10 weeks' gestation) is the same in the male and the female. Differentiation then occurs. The bladder and urethra form from the vesico-urethral portion of the urogenital sinus, and the vestibule from the pelvic and phallic portions. The genital tubercle enlarges only slightly and becomes the clitoris. The genital folds become the labia minora and the genital swellings enlarge to become the labia majora. In the male greater enlargement of the genital tubercle forms the penis and the genital folds fuse over a deep groove formed between them to become the penile part of the male urethra. The genital swellings enlarge, fuse and form the scrotum.

The final stage of development of the clitoris or penis and the formation of the anterior surface of the bladder and anterior abdominal wall up to the umbilicus is the result of the growth of mesoderm, extending ventrally around the body wall on each side to unite in the midline anteriorly.

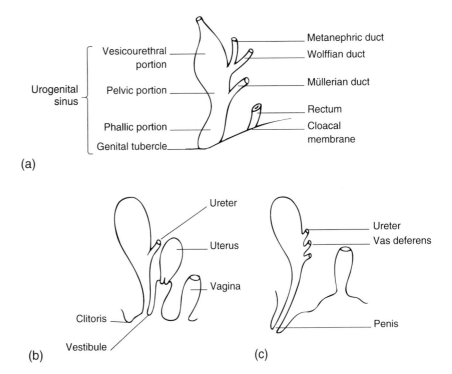

Fig. 34.4 Diagrammatic representation of lower genital tract development: (a) indifferent stage; (b) female development; (c) male development.

Gonads

The primitive gonad appears in embryos at around 5 weeks' gestation. At this time coelomic epithelium develops on the medial aspect of the urogenital ridge and following proliferation leads to the establishment of the gonadal ridge. Epithelial cords then grow into the mesenchyme (primary sex cords) and the gonad now possesses an outer cortex and an inner medulla. In embryos with an XX complement, the cortex differentiates to become the ovary and the medulla regresses. The primordial germ cells develop by the fourth week in the endodermal cells of the yolk sac and during the fifth week they migrate along the dorsal mesentery of the hindgut to the gonadal ridges, eventually becoming incorporated into the mesenchyme and the primary sex cords by the end of the sixh gestational week.

The differentiation of the testis is evident at about 7 weeks by the disappearance of germ cells from the peripheral zone and gradual differentiation of remaining cells into fibroblasts, which form the tunica albuginea. The deeper parts of the sex cords give rise to the rete testis and the seminiferous and straight tubules. The first indication that the gonad will become an ovary is failure of these testicular changes to appear. The sex cords below the epithelium develop extensively with many primitive germ cells evident in this active cellular zone (Fig. 34.5). The epithelial cells in this layer are known as pregranulosa cells. The active growth phase then follows, involving the pregranulosa cells and germ cells, which are now very much reduced in size. This proliferation greatly enlarges the bulk of the gonad and the next stage (by 20 weeks onwards) shows the primitive germ cells, now known as oocytes, becoming surrounded by a ring of pregranulosa cells; stromal cells develop from the ovarian mesenchyme later, surround the pregranulosa cells and become known as granulosa cells and follicle formation is complete (Fig. 34.6). An interesting feature of the formation of follicles and the development of stroma is the disintegration of those oocytes which do not succeed in encircling themselves with a capsule of pregranulosa cells.

The number of oocytes is greatest during pregnancy and thereafter declines. Baker [5] found that the total population of germ cells rose from 600000 at 2 months to a peak of 7 million at 5 months. At birth the number falls to 2 million, of which half are atretic. After 28 weeks or so of intrauterine life, follicular development can be seen at various stages and various sizes of follicles are also seen (Figs 34.7 and 34.8).

Disorders of sexual development

Disorders of sexual development (DSD) have been reclassified by Hughes [6] and this has now been adopted as the best way of classifying these disorders (Table 34.1).

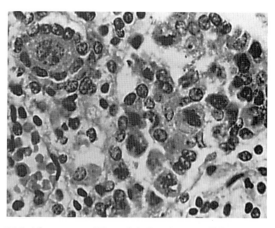

Fig. 34.6 A later ovary (31 weeks) showing a well-formed primary follicle (top left) and a germ cell (centre right) which is not yet completely surrounded by granulosa cells.

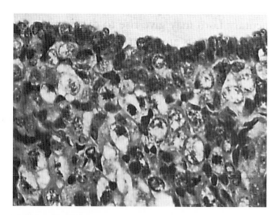

Fig. 34.5 Detail of immature ovary showing small epithelial cells (pregranulosa cells) and larger germ cells.

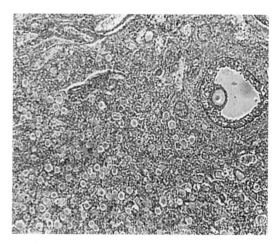

Fig. 34.7 Numerous primary follicles and one showing early development in the ovary of a child stillborn at 38 weeks.

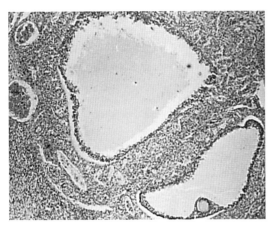

Fig. 34.8 Ovary from a child stillborn at 41 weeks showing a mature Graafian follicle, and a cystic follicle. (Courtesy of the *Journal of Pathology and Bacteriology*.)

Sex chromosome disorders

This group of disorders includes Turner's syndrome (46XO), which is the most important in this group of disorders and the most common. Patients with Turner's syndrome have gonads that contain no oocytes and merely fibrous tissue and as a result of this they have no secondary sexual development (see Chapter 37).

46XY

This group of disorders is divided up into three groups.

Disorders of gonadal (testicular) development

The gynaecologist may occasionally come across a case of ovotesticular DSD where ovarian and testicular tissue exist within the same individual. These patients are rare in Europe and the USA but are notably more common in South Africa. They present with varying degrees of sexual ambiguity and maleness predominates in some patients while female changes are more apparent in others. In the majority the uterus and vagina are present and the karyotype is usually normal female (46XX); in the largest series reported Van Niekirk [7] found 58% of cases had a normal karyotype, 13% had 46XX/XY, followed by 46XY (11%) and 46XY/47XXY in 6% with other mosaics accounting for 10%. Gonadal differentiation is interesting in that the commonest combination of ovotestis is for an ovotestis to be on one side and an ovary on the other, with a testis on one side and an ovary on the other being almost as frequent. Ovotestes can be bilateral or combined with a testis but this is much rarer. Diagnosis of true ovotesticular DSD can only be made after gonadal biopsy, and sex of rearing should be determined on the functional capability of the external genitalia after which inappropriate organs should be removed. In some cases it may be possible to identify the ovarian and testicular portions of an ovotestis for certain and to remove only that part that is unwanted.

Table 34.1 Proposed classification of disorders of sexual development (DSDs).

Sex chromosome DSD

A 47XXY (Klinefelter's syndrome and variants)
B 45X (Turner's syndrome and variants)
C 45X/46XY (mixed gonadal dysgenesis)
D 46XX/46XY (chimerism)

46XY DSD

A *Disorders of gonadal (testicular) development*
   1 Complete or partial gonadal dysgenesis
   2 Ovotesticular DSD
   3 Testis regression
B *Disorders of androgen synthesis or action*
   1 Disorders of androgen synthesis
      LH receptor mutations
      Smith–Lemli–Opitz syndrome
      Steroidogenic acute regulatory protein mutations
      Cholesterol side-chain cleavage
      3β-hydroxysteroid dehydrogenase
      17β-hydroxysteroid dehydrogenase
      5α-reductase
   2 Disorders of androgen action
      Androgen insensitivity syndrome
      Drugs and environmental modulators
C *Other*
   1 Syndromic associations of male genital development (e.g. cloacal anomalies, Robinow, Aarskog, hand–foot–genital, popliteal pterygium)
   2 Persistent Müllerian duct syndrome
   3 Vanishing testis syndrome
   4 Isolated hypospadias
   5 Congenital hypogonadotrophic hypogonadism
   6 Cryptorchidism
   7 Environmental influences

46XX DSD

A *Disorders of gonadal (ovarian) development*
   1 Gonadal dysgenesis
   2 Ovotesticular DSD
   3 Testicular DSD
B *Androgen excess*
   1 Fetal
      3β-hydroxysteroid dehydrogenase
      21-hydroxylase
      P450 oxidoreductase
      11β-hydroxylase
      Glucocorticoid receptor mutations
   2 Fetoplacental
      Aromatase deficiency
      Oxidoreductase deficiency
   3 Maternal
      Maternal virilizing tumours (e.g. luteomas)
      Androgenic drugs
C *Other*
   1 Syndromic associations (e.g. cloacal anomalies
   2 Müllerian agenesis/hypoplasia (e.g. MRKH)
   3 Uterine abnormalities (e.g. MODY5)
   4 Vaginal atresia (e.g. McKusick–Kaufman)
   5 Labial adhesions

If this is not possible, both must be removed and then the patient needs to be brought up in the gender role for whichever is appropriate and hormone replacement therapy instituted at puberty.

Disorders of androgen synthesis

There are two conditions which need to be considered. In group B1 (see Table 34.1), the most commonly seen, though rare, is 5α-reductase deficiency. These patients are genetic males who show ambiguous genitalia at birth and at puberty begin to virilize like normal males. This results in penile enlargement, increased facial hair and muscular hypertrophy but breast development does not occur. The phallus is rather small and a perineal urethral orifice is present. The disorder of androgen synthesis relates to deficiency of 5α-reductase, the enzyme responsible for the conversion of testosterone to dihydrotestosterone, which results in virilization of the external genitalia during embryogenesis. Testosterone is unable to induce virilization during fetal life but at puberty androgen receptors become sensitive to circulating levels of testosterone and therefore a degree of virilization can occur. Management of these patients after puberty can be difficult as they themselves may find sexual orientation difficult and may wish to change their gender role but they must be fully assessed before any permanent decisions are made.

Androgen insensitivity syndromes

In these conditions the individual has a chromosome complement of 46XY but an absence of functional androgen receptors. This is known as complete androgen insensitivity syndrome and during fetal life female external genitalia develop but as the testis produces Müllerian inhibitor the internal structures of the Müllerian duct regress. However, the Wolffian duct cannot develop as it also lacks androgen receptors. These individuals usually present at puberty with failure of menstruation. They are shown to have bilateral testes and a blind-ending vagina and they may well feminize as testicular production of oestrogen induces breast growth. Absence of the androgen receptor means that pubic hair and axillary hair growth is sparse and the diagnosis is often easy to make clinically. The testes are usually normal in size and located either in the abdomen or the inguinal canal and can present as inguinal hernias. These sometimes present in childhood when the diagnosis is made on surgical excision of the mass. Height is slightly increased compared with normal women. Testicular neoplasia is increased though very rare under the age of 30. It is therefore perfectly acceptable to leave the gonads *in situ* until pubertal development has been completed and then to remove them.

Partial androgen insensitivity occurs when the androgen receptor has a mutation and has partial function. At puberty therefore individuals feminize as do patients with complete androgen insensitivity but their external genitalia change, with phallic enlargement and partial labioscrotal fusion. Again, bilateral testes are present within the abdominal cavity or the inguinal canal and there are normal circulating levels of testosterone equivalent to male. At birth phallic enlargement may already be present due to incomplete virilization and the intersex state at birth needs to be assessed and the sex of rearing determined.

Summary box 34.2

- Androgen insensitivity may be complete or partial depending on the defect in the androgen receptor.
- Phenotypic changes depend on the degree of function of the androgen receptor.

46XX

Patients with this group of disorders will most commonly present with congenital adrenal hyperplasia (CAH). Deficiency of 21-hydroxylase is the most common and this leads to elevated levels of androstenedione, 17-hydroxyprogesterone and testosterone. As this is a disorder which is present during fetal life, the elevated levels of androgen lead to virilization of the fetus and therefore clinically female fetuses show clitoral hypertrophy and labioscrotal fusion. The urethral orifice is displaced usually along the dorsal surface of the clitoris and the extent of virilization can vary considerably. Müllerian duct development is normal as are the ovaries. The most severe form at birth is a salt-losing syndrome that can be life-threatening and the administration of mineralocorticoids and sodium are usually needed to correct the hyperkalaemia. Cortisol administration remains necessary throughout life although requirements may diminish with age.

These patients must be diagnosed at birth and this is done by noting elevated levels of 17-hydroxyprogesterone. Little attention needs to be paid to the anatomy unless there is marked virilization, in which case discussion with the parents about surgical intervention should be considered. However, debate continues about whether or not surgical intervention should occur in infancy or at puberty when the individual can be involved in the decision-making process. Further discussion of this is outside the remit of this chapter.

46XX Müllerian agenesis

The most common of this group of disorders is Mayer–Rokitansky–Küster–Hauser (MRKH) syndrome and here congenital absence of the vagina in a 46XX individual is generally associated with absence of the uterus. These patients usually present with primary amenorrhoea at the age of 12–16 years with normal secondary sexual characteristics as the ovaries are normally developed and functional. The combination of normal secondary sexual characteristics and primary amenorrhoea suggests an anatomical cause but inspection of the vulva will reveal that this is normal but there is a short vagina which is blind-ending. The diagnosis of an absent vagina can generally be made without difficulty but subsequent ultrasound of the abdomen will define the absence of Müllerian structures. It must be remembered that a very short vagina may also occur in patients with androgen insensitivity but the assessment of karyotype will differentiate these two groups of patients. In all patients found to have MRKH syndrome, the renal tract should be investigated using ultrasound as some 40% of patients will have renal anomalies, with 15% having an absent kidney. If further investigation is required, intravenous urography can be used to delineate any other renal anomalies [8]. It is extremely rare for laparoscopy to be required to determine the diagnosis but if undertaken must be used with great care as a pelvic kidney may be present. Once the diagnosis is certain, management can be divided into two phases. The first is devoted to the psychological counselling of patients and the second involves the correction of the vaginal anatomy. Some patients may present having already attempted intercourse and this may in fact be entirely satisfactory and therefore no attention needs to be paid to the anatomical side of their management. However, it is important that all patients with MRKH syndrome are assessed with great care so that appropriate therapy can be instigated at the correct time. A full psychological assessment must be carried out before any treatment is commenced or success will be extremely limited.

Psychological counselling in these patients is imperative as they will manifest problems that are devastating and profound. They have feelings of fear and confusion, particularly around their sexual orientation, and may express feelings of rejection and isolation. They have understandable concerns about the ability to embark on heterosexual relationships and of their feeling of inadequacy as they are infertile. The help of a skilled psychologist in managing these patients and a multidisciplinary approach means that the outcome will be successful in a holistic way, not merely an anatomical success. Until patients are deemed psychologically capable of undergoing the rigours of treatment, all attempts to coerce the clinical team to begin treatment prior to this should be resisted [9,10].

> **Summary box 34.3**
>
> - MRKH syndrome is the second most common cause of primary amenorrhoea.
> - Turner's syndrome is the most common.

Non-surgical management

The creation of a vagina should always be attempted by a non-surgical method as the treatment of first choice and only in the rare cases of failure should a surgical solution be considered. This technique was pioneered by Frank [11] and a recent review by Edmonds [8] suggests that success rates in excess of 95% can now be achieved. The principle of the method is that the vaginal dimple should be stretched into a potential space filled with comparatively loose connective tissue and this is capable of considerable indentation. The patient is instructed to use graduated glass dilators that are placed against the introitus and the blind vagina and gentle pressure is exerted in a posterior direction for approximately 10–20 min twice a day. Gradually the dilator distends the space and then increasing sizes of dilators are used until a neovagina is created. In general it takes between 8 and 10 weeks of repeated use to achieve a satisfactory result. The sexual satisfaction associated with this non-surgical technique far exceeds that of operative vaginoplasty.

> **Summary box 34.4**
>
> Vaginal dilator therapy is the therapy of choice for patients with MRKH syndrome.

Surgical techniques

In those patients who fail a non-surgical technique, vaginoplasty will need to be considered. A large number of techniques have been devised to create a vagina surgically, the most widely used being that of McIndoe and Banister [12]. In this procedure a cavity is created between the bladder and the bowel at the site where the natural vagina would have been and the cavity is then lined by a split-thickness skin graft from the thigh and applied to the space on a plastic mould. The anatomical result can be very successful and remarkably good sexually. A review of 1311 reported cases gave a success rate of 92% [8].

However, there are a number of difficulties and disadvantages of this technique, not least the postoperative period which is painful and somewhat protracted. The graft does not always take well and granulation may form over part of the cavity giving rise to discharge. Pressure necrosis between the mould and urethra, bladder or rectum may lead to fistula formation but the most important disadvantage is the tendency for the vagina to retract unless a dilator is worn or the vagina used for intercourse regularly. It is therefore best to perform this procedure when sexual intercourse is desired soon afterwards because failure of the patient to maintain the vagina means there will be surgical failure. A further disadvantage of this technique is the graft donor site, which remains visible as evidence of the vaginal problem and most women prefer not to have any external scarring. In order to avoid the use of skin grafts a number of other materials have been used including amnion, although this material is no longer desirable due to the risk of transmission of infection. Other reported techniques include the use of bowel [13] and skin flaps [14] and these have their own individual complications. A procedure known as Vecchietti's operation has been popular in Europe for many years and this involves the use of a small olive placed in the dimple of the absent vagina [15,16]. Laparoscopically, wires are then brought through from the dimple to the anterior abdominal wall and then pressure exerted on a spring device, thereby creating a neo-vagina in a way that mimics the non-surgical technique of Frank. However, it does not require the woman herself to use the dilators but after 7–9 days the olive is removed and the stretched vaginal skin needs to be further dilated with glass dilators. A recent review of this technique revealed success rates approximating to 90% [8].

Other anatomical anomalies

Fusion anomalies
Fusion anomalies of various kinds are not uncommon (Fig. 34.9) and may present clinically either in association with pregnancy or not. The lesser degrees of fusion defects are quite common, the cornual parts of the uterus remaining separate, giving the organ a heart-shaped appearance known as a bicornuate uterus. There is no

evidence that such minor degrees of fusion defect give rise to clinical signs or symptoms. However, the presence of a septum extending over some or all of the uterine cavity is likely to give rise to clinical features. Such a septate or subseptate uterus may be of normal external appearance or of bicornuate outline. Clinically, it may present with recurrent spontaneous abortion or malpresentation. A persistent transverse lie of the fetus in late pregnancy may suggest a uterine anomaly since the fetus tends to lie with its head in one cornu and the breech in the other.

In more extreme forms of failure of fusion the clinical features may be less, rather than more, marked. Two almost separate uterine cavities with one cervix are probably less likely to be associated with abnormalities than are the lesser degrees of fusion defect. Complete duplication of the uterus and cervix (uterus didelphys), if associated with a clinical problem, may prevent descent of the head in late pregnancy, or obstruct labour by the non-pregnant horn.

Rudimentary development of one horn may give rise to a very serious situation if a pregnancy is implanted there. Rupture of the horn with profound bleeding may occur as the pregnancy increases in size. The clinical picture will resemble that of a ruptured ectopic pregnancy, with the difference that the amenorrhoea will probably be measured in months rather than weeks, and shock may be profound. A poorly developed or rudimentary horn may give rise to dysmenorrhoea and pelvic pain if there is any obstruction to communication between the horn and the main uterine cavity or the vagina. Surgical

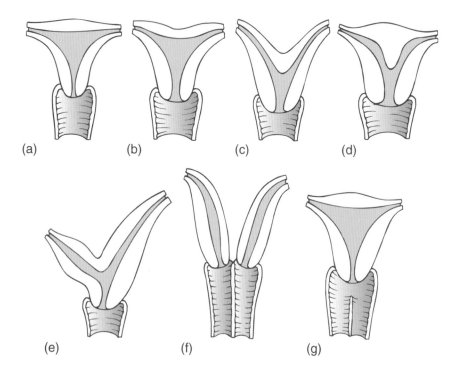

Fig. 34.9 Various fusion abnormalities of the uterus and vagina. (a) Normal appearance; (b) arcuate fundus with little effect on the shape of the cavity; (c) bicornuate uterus; (d) subseptate uterus with normal outline; (e) rudimentary horn; (f) uterus didelphys; (g) normal uterus with partial vaginal septum.

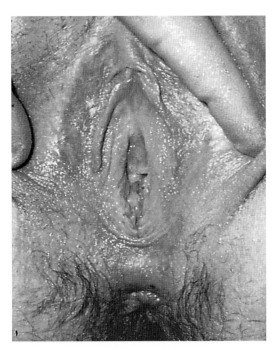

Fig. 34.10 Vulval appearances in a case of absence of the vagina.

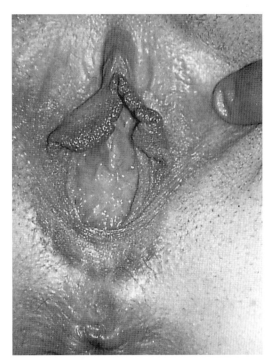

Fig. 34.12 An imperforate membrane occluding the vaginal introitus in a case of haematocolpos. Note the hymen clearly visible immediately distal to the membrane.

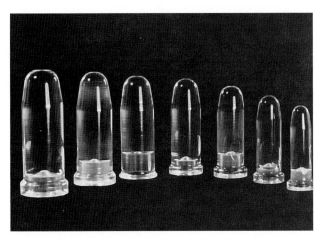

Fig. 34.11 Graduated glass dilators.

removal of this rudimentary horn is then indicated (Figs 34.10 and 34.11).

Transverse vaginal septum/imperforate hymen

An imperforate membrane may exist at the lower end of the vagina, which is loosely referred to as imperforate hymen, although the hymen can usually be distinguished separately (Fig. 34.12). These abnormalities of vertical fusion are seldom recognized clinically until puberty when retention of menstrual flow gives rise to the clinical features of haematocolpos, although rarely they may present in the newborn as hydrocolpos. The features

of haematocolpos are predominantly abdominal pain, primary amenorrhoea and occasionally interference with micturition. The patient is usually 14–15 years old but may be older, and a clear history may be given of regular cyclical lower abdominal pain for several months previously. The patient may also present as an acute emergency if urinary obstruction develops. Examination reveals a lower abdominal swelling, and per rectum a large bulging mass in the vagina may be appreciated (Fig. 34.13). Vulval inspection may reveal the imperforate membrane, which may or may not be bluish in colour depending on its thickness. Diagnosis may be more difficult if the vagina is imperforate over some distance in its lower part or if there is obstruction in one-half of a septate vagina.

Treatment may be relatively simple or rather complex. If the membrane is thin, then simple excision of the membrane and release of the retained blood resolves the problem. Redundant portions of the membrane may be removed but nothing more should be done at this time. Fluid will then drain naturally over some days. Examination a few weeks later is desirable to ensure that no pelvic mass remains that might also suggest haematosalpinx. In fact, haematosalpinx is most uncommon except in cases of very long standing and is associated with retention of blood in the upper vagina. On these rare occasions when a haematosalpinx is discovered, laparoscopy is desirable, the distended tube being removed or preserved as seems

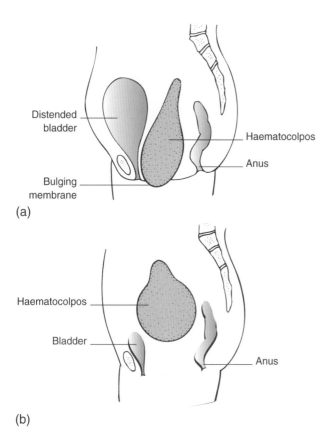

Distended
bladder

Bulging
membrane

Haematocolpos

Anus

(a)

Haematocolpos

Bladder

Anus

(b)

Fig. 34.13 (a) Haematocolpos: note how the blood collecting in the vagina presses against the urethra and bladder base, ultimately causing retention of urine. (b) Haematocolpos associated with absence of the lower portion of the vagina. Note that the retained blood is now above the bladder base and retention of urine is unlikely.

best. Haematometra scarcely seems to be a realistic clinical entity, the thick uterine walls permitting comparatively little blood to collect therein. The subsequent menstrual history and fertility of patients who are successfully treated are probably not significantly different from those of unaffected women, although patients who develop endometriosis may have some fertility problems.

When the obstruction is more extensive than a thin membrane and a length of vagina is absent, diagnosis and management are less straightforward and the ultimate interference with fertility is greater. Resection of the absent segment and reconstruction of the vagina may be done by an end-to-end anastomosis of the vagina or by a partial vaginoplasty.

The combination of absence of most of the lower vagina together with a functioning uterus presents a difficult problem. The upper part of the vagina will collect menstrual blood and a clinical picture similar in many ways to haematocolpos will be seen. However, urinary obstruction is rare because the retained blood lies above the level of the bladder base (Fig. 34.13). Diagnosis is more difficult

and it may not be at all certain how much of the vagina is absent or how extensive the surgery would need to be to release the retained fluid and recreate the normal anatomy. Imaging may be by ultrasound or magnetic resonance imaging (MRI), and both these techniques may be successful in determining the exact anatomical relationships prior to surgery being performed. However, in the clinical situation the surgical approach is rarely entirely through the perineum and usually involves a laparotomy to establish finally how best the anatomy can be recreated.

Treatment is difficult and a dissection upwards is made as in the McIndoe–Read procedure. The blood is released, but its discharge for some time later may interfere with the application for a mould and skin graft. If possible, the upper and lower portions of the vagina should be brought together and stitched so that the new vagina with its own skin is created, obviating the risk of contraction. However, the upper fragment tends to retract upwards resulting in a narrow area of constriction some way up the vagina, and this results in subsequent dyspareunia.

> ### 💡 Summary box 34.5
>
> - Transverse vaginal septae cause primary amenorrhoea and cyclical abdominal pain.
> - The most common septae are low and surgical treatment usually restores total reproductive function.
> - High septae have a higher rate of fertility failure.

Longitudinal vaginal septum

A vaginal septum extending throughout all or part of a vagina is not uncommon; such a septum lies in the sagittal plain in the midline, although if one side of the vagina has been used for coitus the septum may be displaced laterally to such an extent that it may not be obvious at the time of examination. The condition is found in association with a completely double uterus and cervix or with a single uterus and double cervix. In obstetrics this septum may have some importance if vaginal delivery is to be attempted. In these circumstances the narrow hemivagina may be inadequate to allow passage of the fetus and serious tears may occur if the septum is still intact at this time. It is therefore prudent to arrange to remove the vaginal septum as a formal surgical procedure whenever one is discovered, either before or during pregnancy. The septum may occasionally be associated with dyspareunia, when similar management is indicated.

Occasionally, a double vagina may exist in which one side is not patent, and a haematometra and haematocolpos may occur in a single side. Under these circumstances the vaginal septum must be removed to allow drainage

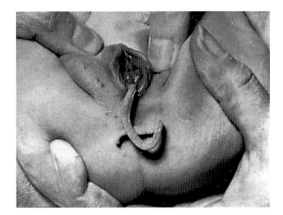

Fig. 34.14 Ectopic opening of the anus at the fourchette.

of the obstructed genital tract and the results are generally excellent.

Vulval anomalies

Rarely, anomalies in the development of bowel or bladder may give rise to considerable abnormality in the appearance of the vulva. The anus may open immediately adjacent to the vulva or just within it (Fig. 34.14). Bladder exstrophy will give rise to a bifid clitoris and anterior displacement of the vagina, in addition to bladder deformities themselves. Further discussion of these complex problems may be found in Edmonds [17].

Wolffian duct anomalies

Remnants of the lower part of the Wolffian duct may be evident as vaginal cysts, whereas remnants of the upper part are evident as thin-walled cysts lying within the layers of the broad ligament (paraovarian cysts). It is doubtful if the vaginal cyst per se calls for surgical removal, although removal is usually undertaken. The cysts may cause dyspareunia and this is the most likely reason for their discovery and surgical removal. Cysts situated at the upper end of the vagina may be found to burrow deeply into the region of the broad ligament and the base of the bladder and should be approached surgically with considerable caution. A painful and probably paraovarian cyst will require surgical exploration and its precise nature will be unknown until the abdomen is opened. Such cysts normally come out easily from the broad ligament.

Renal tract abnormalities

The association between congenital malformations of the genital tract and those of the renal tract is mentioned above. When a malformation of the genital organs of any significant degree presents, some investigation to confirm or exclude a renal tract anomaly would be wise. An ultrasound scan can be arranged without any upset to the patient and will probably be sufficient in the first instance;

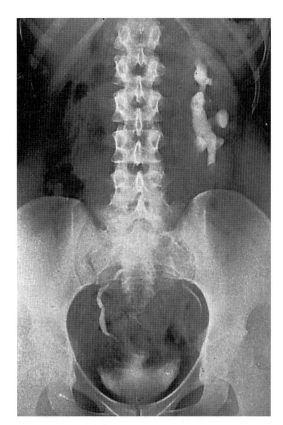

Fig. 34.15 An intravenous pyelogram in a patient with absence of the vagina, showing a single kidney and a gross abnormality of the course of the ureter.

however, if any doubt arises, an intravenous pyelogram may be performed. Lesions such as absence of a kidney, a double renal element on both or one side, a double ureter or a pelvic kidney (Fig. 34.15) may not call for immediate treatment but may do so later; moreover, it is as well to be aware of such abnormalities if the abdomen is to be opened for exploration or treatment of the genital tract lesion itself.

Ectopic ureter

One abnormality which apparently presents with gynaecological symptoms is the ectopic ureter (Fig. 34.16). A ureter opening abnormally is usually an additional one, although sometimes a single one may be ectopic. The commonest site of the opening is the vestibule, followed closely by the urethra and then the vagina. Other sites are less common. The main symptom is uncontrollable wetness. However, the amount of moisture appearing at the vulva may be small and is sometimes mistaken for a vaginal discharge. This confusion, together with difficulties in confirming the diagnosis of an ectopic ureter, even when one is suspected, may lead to many patients being investigated for years before the condition is recognized. Diagnosis can sometimes be easy but is usually not so.

The orifice at the vestibule may be clearly visible but more often careful search is necessary to locate it, if it can be seen at all. Cystoscopy and urethroscopy may be necessary to establish if normal ureteric openings exist in the bladder. Radiological study may be helpful by indicating a double element on one or both sides. Treatment will involve the help of a urological surgeon, and partial nephrectomy and ureterectomy or reimplantation of the ectopic ureter into the bladder may be undertaken.

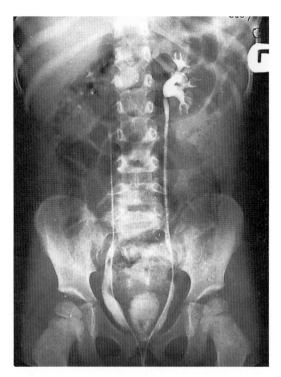

Fig. 34.16 An intravenous pyelogram in a child with an imperforate vagina. Both ureters open ectopically into the posterior urethra.

XY females

Faults in androgen production
In this group of patients androgen production may fail from either anatomical or enzymatic testicular failure.

Anatomical testicular failure
Failure of normal testicular differentiation and development may be the result of a chromosome mosaicism affecting the sex chromosomes or possibly associated with an abnormal isochromosome [18], but usually the sex chromosomes appear normal and the condition is referred to as pure gonadal dysgenesis. Clinically such cases show variable features depending on how much testicular differentiation is present. Since differentiation is often poor, most patients have mild masculinization or none at all, and the uterus, tubes and vagina are generally present. The presence of the uterus in this condition contrasts with the other forms of XY female described below.

Management of this group of patients is concerned with the reconstruction of the external genitalia in the manner described previously and removal of the streak or rudimentary gonads in view of their raised potential for cancer. The degree of masculinization of such patients is often minimal and if it is limited to a minor degree of clitoral enlargement with little or no fusion of the genital folds, surgery need not be undertaken. The risk of malignancy in the rudimentary testes is probably in the order of 30% and gonadal removal during childhood would be wise. Around the age of puberty replacement oestrogen–progestogen therapy must be started in order to initiate secondary sexual development and menstruation.

Enzymatic testicular failure
Several metabolic steps are necessary for the complete formation of testosterone from cholesterol (Fig. 34.17). A number of biosynthetic defects have been reported at each stage of the process. As a result, clinical features are

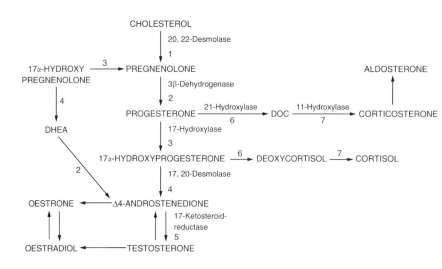

Fig. 34.17 The enzyme steps necessary to convert cholesterol through its various intermediate stages to aldosterone, cortisol and testosterone. Note that 3β-dehydrogenase (labelled 2) is active at two points, as are 17-hydroxylase (labelled 3), 17,20-desmolase (labelled 4), 21-hydroxylase (labelled 6) and 11-hydroxylase (labelled 7).

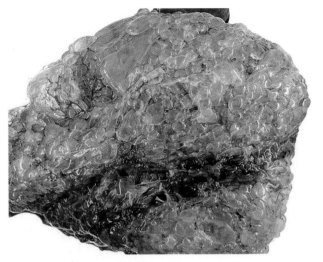

Plate 8.1 The macroscopic appearance of a complete molar pregnancy from early in the second trimester.

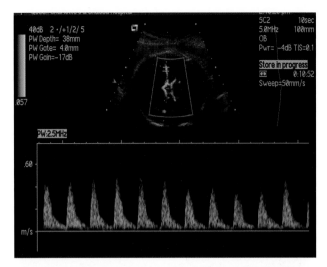

Plate 17.1 Colour Doppler flow pattern of the circle of Willis in the fetal brain. The callipers are placed with a 0° angle on the middle cerebral artery and the pulse wave Doppler flow pattern demonstrated.

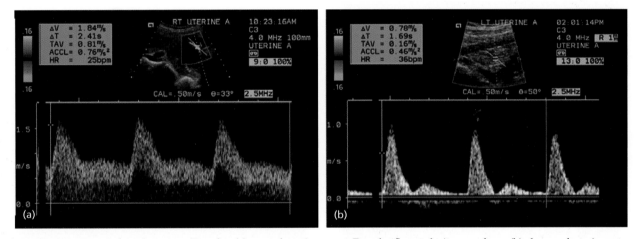

Plate 18.1 Assessment of uterine artery Doppler: (a) normal uterine artery Doppler flow–velocity waveform; (b) abnormal uterine artery Doppler flow–velocity waveform.

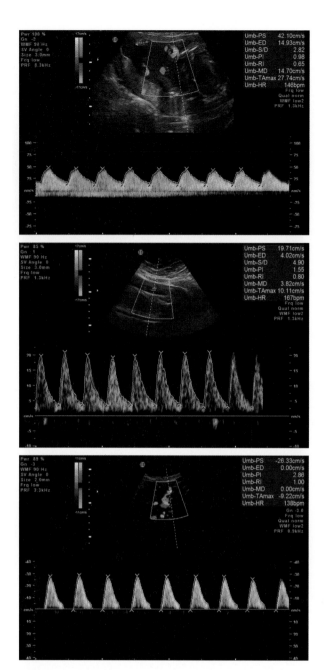

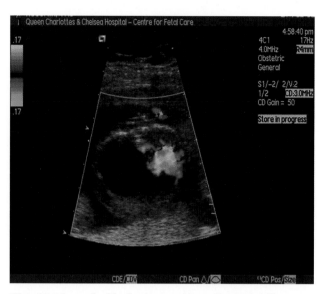

Plate 20.1 Large fetal hydrothorax with mediastinal shift.

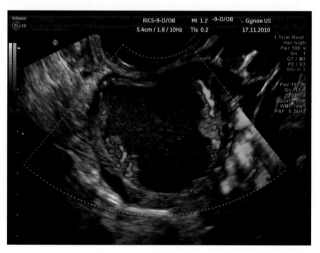

Plate 35.1 An endometrioma that has undergone decidualization at 12 weeks' gestation. Note the solid projections into the cyst cavity with ground-glass contents.

Plate 18.2 Assessment of umbilical artery Doppler: (a) normal umbilical artery Doppler flow–velocity waveform; (b) reduced end-diastolic flow; (c) absent end-diastolic flow.

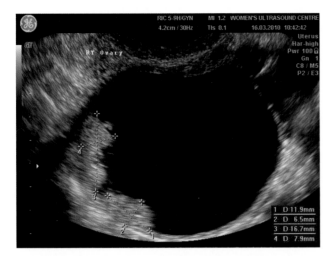

Plate 35.2 Borderline ovarian cyst illustrating solid projections into the cyst cavity.

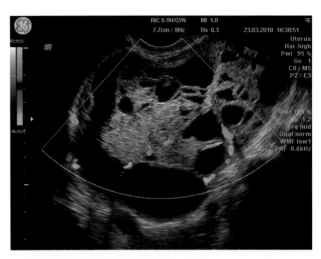

Plate 35.3 Multilocular cystic-solid ovarian tumour with a high colour score. These are all features of ovarian malignancy.

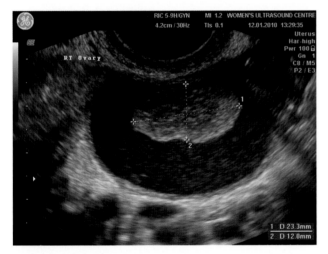

Plate 35.4 Physiological ovarian cyst: the apparent solid area is retracting blood clot in the cyst.

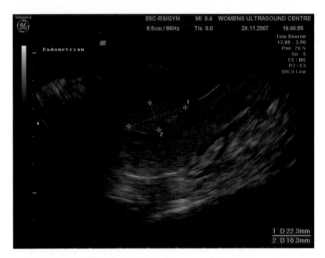

Plate 35.5 Characteristic appearance of an endometrial polyp: note the hyperechogenic nature of the polyp with bright outline.

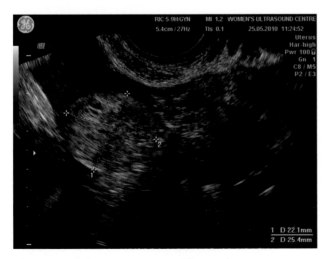

Plate 35.6 Tubal ectopic pregnancy. Most are homogeneous 'blobs'; in this case there is some blood surrounding the mass.

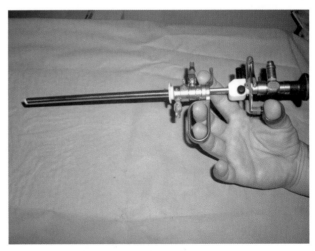

Plate 36.1 A continous flow resectoscope with a passive handle mechanism.

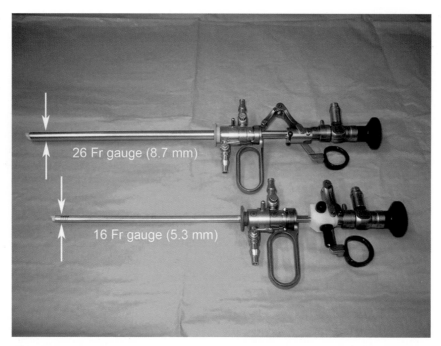

Plate 36.2 Mini-resectoscope.

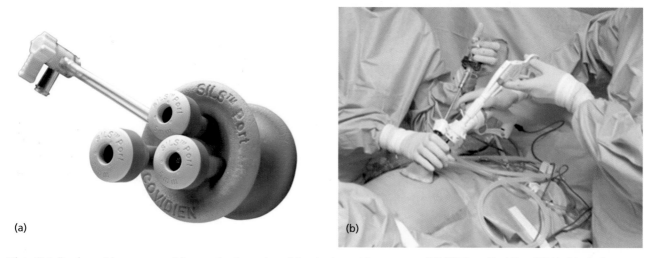

(a)

(b)

Plate 36.3 Single-port laparoscopy: (a) example of a port used for single-port laparoscopy (SILS™ Port, Covidien, USA); (b) single-port laparoscopy being carried out. (With permission from Elsevier.)

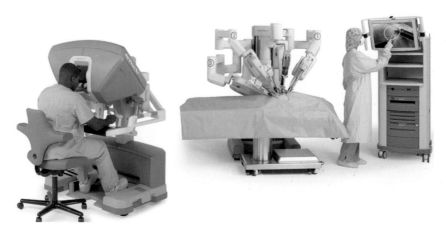

Plate 36.4 da Vinci Surgical System.

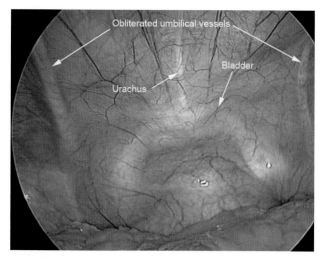

Plate 36.5 Laparoscopic view of the 'safe triangle'.

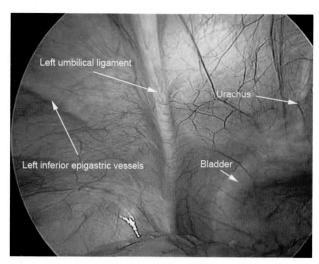

Plate 36.6 Laparoscopic view of the left inferior epigastric vessels lateral to the umbilical ligament (obliterated umbilical vessels).

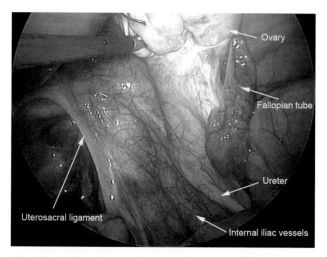

Plate 36.7 View of the right lateral pelvic side wall after elevation and rotation of the ovary.

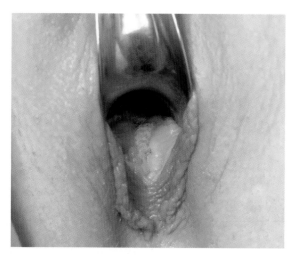

Plate 50.1 Illustration of mesh erosion.

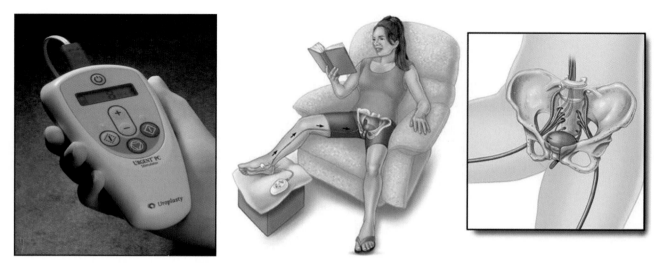

Plate 51.1 Posterior tibial nerve stiimulation. (a) PTNS stimulator (Urgent PC, Uroplasty, Minneapolis, MN, USA). (b) PTNS treatment showing needle placement.

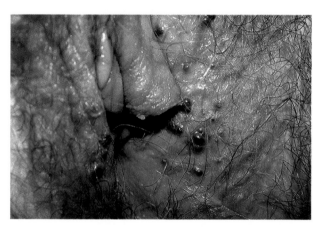

Plate 52.1 Angiokeratomas – dark red papules seen on the labia majora.

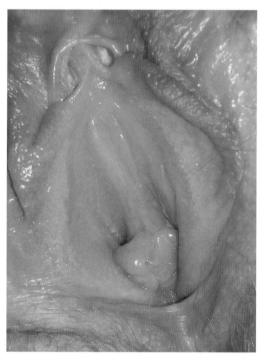

Plate 52.2 Hart's line demarcating the junction between the keratinized skin of the labia minora and the non-keratinized mucosa of the vestibule.

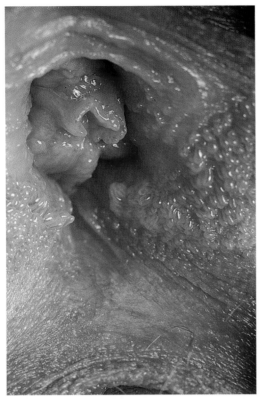

Plate 52.3 Vestibular papillae – filamentous projections of the vestibular epithelium.

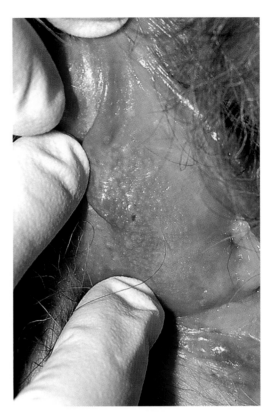

Plate 52.4 Fordyce spots – tiny yellow papules on the inner labium minus.

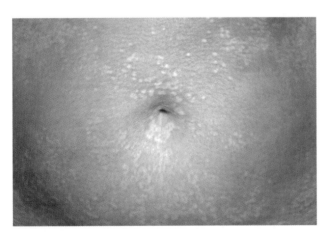

Plate 52.5 Extragenital lichen sclerosus – 'white spot disease'. Flat white lesions which can coalesce into plaques. Follicular plugging may be seen.

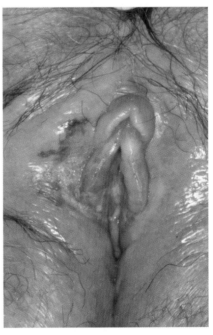

Plate 52.6 Vulval lichen sclerosus – early established disease showing rubbery oedema of labia minora and clitoral hood and stark whitening extending to perianal skin. Note currently healed fissure at 6 o'clock position.

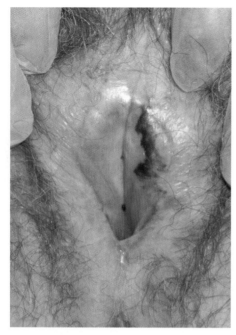

Plate 52.7 Advanced vulval lichen sclerosis. Stark whitening, complete burying of the clitoris and total replacement of architecture with 'plastering' down and resorption of labia. Gross ecchymoses and narrowing of vaginal introitus.

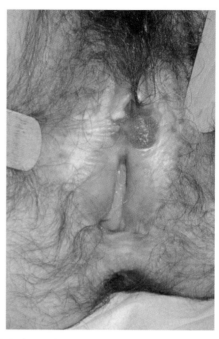

Plate 52.9 Lichen sclerosus complicated by squamous carcinoma. Note the classical cigarette-paper scarring and stark background whitening. Here the squamous cell carcinoma presents as a fleshy nodule, but persistent erosion should also prompt biopsy.

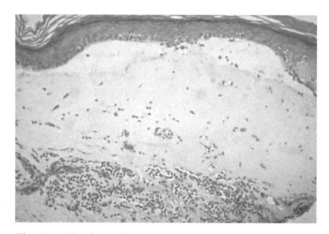

Plate 52.8 Histology of lichen sclerosus (haematoxylin and eosin ×40). An atrophic epidermis is seen over the homogenized band of collagen and, below this, a lymphocytic infiltrate.

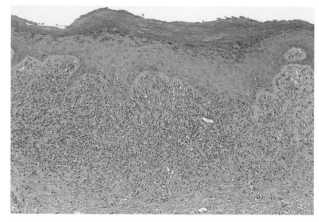

Plate 52.10 Histology of lichen planus showing saw-toothing of the epidermis, with a dense lymphocytic infiltrate and liquefactive degeneration of the basement membrane (courtesy of Dr E. Calonje).

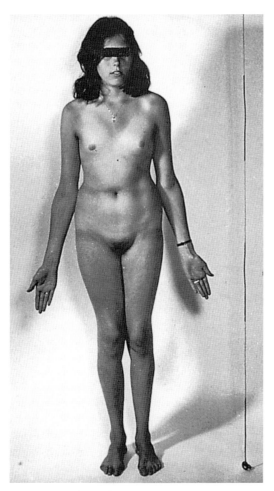

Fig. 34.18 A patient with enzymatic testicular failure believed to be due to 17-ketosteroid reductase deficiency. (From Dewhurst [19] with permission.)

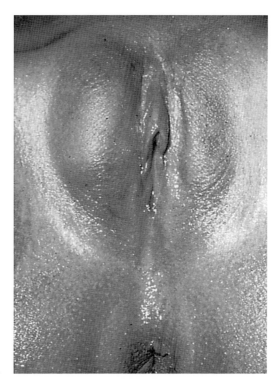

Fig. 34.19 The external genitalia of a 10-year-old 46XY child with a 5α-reductase deficiency. Reproduced from Edmonds [17] with permission.

somewhat varied but since such enzyme defects are generally incomplete there is external genital ambiguity of varying degrees, the uterus, tubes and upper vagina being absent since the production of Müllerian-inhibiting substance by the testes is normal.

The decision on the sex of rearing will depend on the degree of masculinization of the external genitalia but the female role is often the chosen one (Fig. 34.18). Surgical management is as already described. The identification of the precise enzyme defect can be difficult, but may be approached through human chorionic gonadotrophin stimulation of the gonads and measurement of various androgens to determine where the enzyme block occurs (Fig. 34.19).

References

1 Sinclair AH, Berta P, Palmer MS *et al*. A gene from the human sex determining region encodes a protein with homology to DNA-binding motif. *Nature* 1990;346:240–244.

2 Simpson JL. Genetic control of sex differentiation. *Semin Reprod Med* 1987;5:209–220.

3 Elias S, Simpson JL, Carson SA *et al*. Genetic studies in incomplete Müllerian fusion. *Obstet Gynecol* 1984;63:276–281.

4 Leigh Simpson J. *Disorders of Sexual Differentiation: Etiology and Clinical Delineation*. New York: Academic Press, 1976.

5 Baker TG. A quantitative and cytological study of germ cells in human ovaries. *Proc R Soc Lond B* 1963;158:417–433.

6 Hughes IA. Disorders of sexual development: new definition and classification. *Best Pract Res Clin Endocrinol Metab* 2008;22:119–134.

7 Van Niekerk W. True hermaphroditism. *Am J Obstet Gynecol* 1976;126:890–907.

8 Edmonds DK. Congenital malformations of the genital tract and their management. *Best Pract Res Clin Obstet Gynaecol* 2003;17:19–40.

9 Heller-Boersma JG, Schmidt UH, Edmonds DK. Psychological distress in women with uterovaginal agenesis (Mayer–Rokitansky–Küster–Hauser syndrome, MRKH). *Psychosomatics* 2009;50:277–281.

10 Heller-Boersma JG, Schmidt UK, Edmonds DK. A randomised controlled trial of a cognitive-behavioural group intervention versus waiting-list control for women with uterovaginal agenesis (Mayer–Rokitansky–Küster–Hauser syndrome: MRKH). *Hum Reprod* 2007;22:2296–2301.

11 Frank RT. The formation of the artificial vagina without operation. *Am J Obstet Gynecol* 1938;35:1053–1056.

12 McIndoe AH, Banister JB. An operation for the cure of congenital absence of the vagina. *J Obstet Gynaecol Br Commonwealth* 1938;45:490–495.

13 Parsons JK, Gearhart SL, Gearhart JP. Vaginal reconstruction using sigmoid colon. *J Pediatr Surg* 2002;37:629–633.

14 Wee JT, Joseph VT. A new technique of vaginal reconstruction using neurovascular pudendal thigh flaps. *Plast Reconstr Surg* 1989;83:701–709.

15 Borruto F. Mayer–Rokitansky–Küster syndrome: Vecchietti's personal series. *Clin Exp Obstet Gynecol* 1992;19:273–274.

16 Fedele L, Bioanchi S, Zanconato G *et al*. Laparoscopic creation of a neovagina in patients with Rokitansky syndrome. *Fertil Steril* 2000;74:384–389.

17 Edmonds DK. Sexual developmental anomalies and their reconstruction: upper and lower tracts. In: Sanfilippo JS (ed) *Pediatric and Adolescent Gynecology*, 2nd edn. Philadelphia: Saunders, 2001: 553–583.

18 Simpson JL. *Disorders of Sexual Differentiation: Etiology and Clinical Delineation*. New York: Academic Press, 1976:199.

19 Dewhurst CJ. *Practical Paediatric and Adolescent Gynaecology*. New York: Marcel Dekker.

Further reading

Gidwani G, Falconi T. *Congenital Malformations of the Female Genital Tract. Diagnosis and Management*. Philadelphia: Lippincott, Williams and Wilkins, 1999.

Sanfilippo J, Lara-Torre E, Edmonds K, Templeman C. *Clinical Paediatric and Adolescent Gynaecology*. New York: Informa Healthcare, 2008.

Chapter 35
The Role of Ultrasound in Gynaecology

Tom Bourne
Queen Charlotte's & Chelsea Hospital, London, UK

The introduction of ultrasound has changed the approach to the diagnosis and management of many disorders in gynaecology. It has redefined the diagnostic criteria and management of problems in early pregnancy, decreased the need for more invasive procedures for many women with postmenopausal and dysfunctional uterine bleeding, enabled the accurate characterization of ovarian pathology and allowed significant advances in the management of infertility with ultrasound-guided techniques in *in vitro* fertilization (IVF). Ultrasound is becoming increasingly important in urogynaecology and oncology. An ultrasound examination of the pelvis is one of the most common procedures used in gynaecology, with most women presenting to a gynaecology department undergoing a scan at some point in their management pathway.

It is important to remember that a scan is performed as part of the overall assessment of the patient. It is an adjunct to history and examination and a clinician must always make sure that management decisions about a patient take into account all relevant information and that they do not fall into the trap of 'treating the scan result'.

Ultrasound techniques

The term 'ultrasound' describes sound waves of such a high frequency that they cannot be heard by humans. The higher the probe frequency, the narrower the beam width. This results in improved resolution, but with the trade-off of poorer penetration. As a result such probes need to be used close to the area of interest. In gynaecology, transabdominal (TA) probes tend to range from 3 to 5 MHz and transvaginal (TV) probes from 5 to 8 MHz. However, improvements in probe design have led to them being significantly more adaptable than in the past. Along with the probe, facilities for capturing digital images are required, although thermal print images can be used if no other archiving facility is available. Although not essential in most situations, the use of Doppler is useful, in particular for evaluating the vascularity of ovarian masses. In almost all cases in gynaecology, impedance indices are of little value and power or colour Doppler is used to make a subjective evaluation of both the amount of blood flow and the pattern of any blood vessels present. The option of three-dimensional ultrasound is a further advance. This is helpful for the characterization of uterine congenital abnormalities and use of the 'four-dimensional' view of the pelvic floor is gaining significance in urogynaecology [1]. The facility to store a 'volume' for later review is also becoming of increased clinical significance. It is important to note that most gynaecological scanning can be carried out on relatively low specification equipment and a portable laptop-type scanner will be more than adequate for the majority of examinations both in early pregnancy and general gynaecology.

The relative merits of TA versus TV ultrasound scanning have been well rehearsed. TV ultrasound is usually the method of choice; however the quality of abdominal probes is now such that often very good views of the pelvic organs can be achieved both with and without a full bladder. TA scanning is the technique of choice when examining women who are unable to tolerate a vaginal (or rectal) examination. It is also important for assessing large pelvic masses arising from the pelvis. A complete abdominal scan should also be performed when assessing any oncology patient in order to assess possible lymph node, omental or liver metastasis. In the event of suspected blood loss, looking for fluid in Morrison's pouch (hepatorenal space) is a quick way to estimate the volume of blood in the abdomen (if there is fluid it is likely that more than 750 mL of blood are in the abdomen and pelvis). Thus, it is important that any practitioner performing ultrasound examinations is familiar with both approaches (Fig. 35.1). A full bladder is not required for the majority of abdominal scans in gynaecology. The technique involves following the blood vessels in the pelvis starting at the femoral vessels and moving cranially.

The uterus should generally be assessed in the sagittal plane and examination should include the cervix, the body of the uterus, the fundus and the endometrial cavity. Views obtained in the oblique transverse plane (coronal view) may help establish the location of focal pathology.

Dewhurst's Textbook of Obstetrics & Gynaecology, Eighth Edition. Edited by D. Keith Edmonds.
© 2012 John Wiley and Sons, Ltd. Published 2012 by John Wiley and Sons, Ltd.

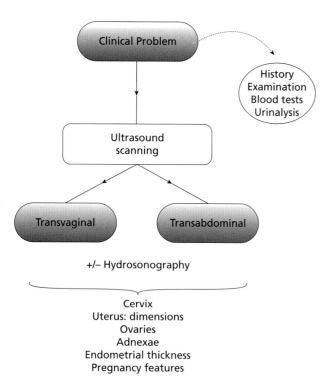

Fig. 35.1 Use of ultrasound to solve a clinical problem.

The detection of congenital uterine abnormalities is best achieved using three-dimensional ultrasound whereby the unique coronal view allows most anomalies to be characterized relatively easily [2].

The endometrial thickness, defined as the maximal measurement across the lumen of the endometrial cavity from one endometrial–myometrial interface to another, is an important assessment. Prior to the menopause, endometrial thickness generally varies from 4 to 8 mm in the follicular phase and from 7 to 14 mm in the secretory phase. In general, however, the endometrium must be thought of as a dynamic structure that undergoes cyclical changes that are synchronous with the variations of the menstrual cycle. There are no clear cut-off values to define abnormalities in premenopausal women. The ideal time to perform an ultrasound scan is either just after a period or in the middle of the cycle as focal pathology is easily identified against a background of peri-ovulatory endometrium. The main application of endometrial thickness measurements relates to postmenopausal women, where an endometrial thickness of 4 mm or less is associated with endometrial atrophy [3]. A recent consensus document has outlined proposed terminology to describe both the endometrium itself and any intra-cavity pathology that may be present [4].

Transvaginal ultrasound: practical points
Excess gel must be wiped off the probe and the transducer cleaned to prevent cross-infection. Using alcohol-based wipes is no longer considered sufficient for this purpose and a chlorine dioxide generator is a good option. An appropriate cover must be placed over the transducer; this should preferably be latex free. Normal hygiene measures, such as hand-washing after each case, apply as always. A small amount of gel is applied to the transducer tip before it is covered and a small amount of lubricant gel is then used to allow insertion of the probe. During TV ultrasound always remember you have two hands: the hand not holding the probe can be used to press on the abdomen and help optimize the image. The vaginal probe can also be used to assess the mobility of pelvic organs as well as the presence of site-specific tenderness. These may be soft markers for the presence of endometriosis [5].

Transabdominal ultrasound: practical points
Although a full bladder can be useful for TA scanning, in many cases it is not required, and can be positively unhelpful. In particular when examining the pelvic side wall the femoral vessels may be indentified and these are followed upwards to the iliac vessels and finally to the bifurcation of the aorta. An ovarian mass and any lymphadenopathy present can be assessed in this way. A gynaecologist learning to scan should be aware that an examination of the abdomen does not stop in the pelvis and the examiner should be familiar with the normal appearances of the organs of the upper abdomen and the likely sites of metastatic disease in the event of gynaecological malignancy. These might include the vicinity of the coeliac trunk, hilus of the spleen, and the liver or omentum.

When performing a scan it is useful to be aware of important landmarks in the pelvis: the cervix, iliac vessels, bladder and body of the uterus. These can be used for immediate orientation, the iliac vessels being particularly helpful when trying to locate the ovaries. Once the area of interest has been located the image can be magnified in order to obtain maximum detail.

Saline infusion sonography
Saline infusion sonography (SIS) is a relatively simple technique involving the instillation of sterile saline into the uterine cavity [6]; the saline acts as a negative contrast agent to outline any focal intra-cavity pathology. The saline is injected into the uterine cavity using a catheter passed through the cervix. A paediatric nasogastric feeding tube is an inexpensive option as a catheter, although it can be useful to have a balloon on the catheter in some instances to prevent backflow from the cervical canal. Possible indications for SIS include a thickened or irregular endometrium, poor views of the endometrium (e.g. due to axial position of uterus) and further characterization of focal intra-cavity pathology such as polyps, submucous fibroids and adhesions [7]. Some examiners advise that prophylactic antibiotics should be administered prior to the procedure in all potentially fertile women to avoid pelvic inflammatory disease. There is a large amount of data to suggest that SIS is comparable to hysteroscopy for the assessment of most focal endome-

trial pathology. Ultrasound without saline instillation is significantly less accurate for this purpose [8]. In the event of uncertainty regarding the endometrial findings SIS is always a good option to consider. It is also important to remember that the endometrium in premenopausal women is a dynamic structure and so simply repeating a scan after menstruation will often clarify whether there is focal intrauterine pathology or not.

> ## 💡 Summary box 35.1
>
> - A full bladder is not required for many transabdominal scans.
> - The use of Doppler can be useful, but indices of impedance have no value in the assessment of ovarian pathology.
> - Power or colour Doppler is used to make a subjective evaluation of both the amount of blood flow and the pattern of any blood vessels present.
> - Clinicians performing gynaecological ultrasound should be able to assess the entire abdomen and pelvis abdominally in the event of suspected malignancy.
> - Endometrial thickness data are unreliable in premenopausal women but important after the menopause for women with bleeding.

The role of ultrasound in a non-pregnant patient

Ultrasound should be considered an extension of the bimanual clinical examination; indeed it is unlikely that a woman with a normal pelvic examination and a negative ultrasound scan has any significant gynaecological pathology. This is true in both the acute and chronic setting. In a study by Haider *et al.* [9] of women attending an acute gynaecology unit, a normal scan was found to be associated with resolution of symptoms in 94.5% of cases. Okaro *et al.* [5] found that for women with chronic pelvic pain and a normal scan, a subsequent laparoscopy was abnormal in 20% of cases compared with the 58% of cases that would be expected. In medicine we are generally taught that a test should only be ordered if it will help change the management of the patient (Fig. 35.2). In modern gynaecology the majority of women who present will need a scan at some point in their investigative pathway.

Investigation of a pelvic mass

Ultrasonography is the principal first-line investigation when evaluating a woman presenting with a possible pelvic mass.

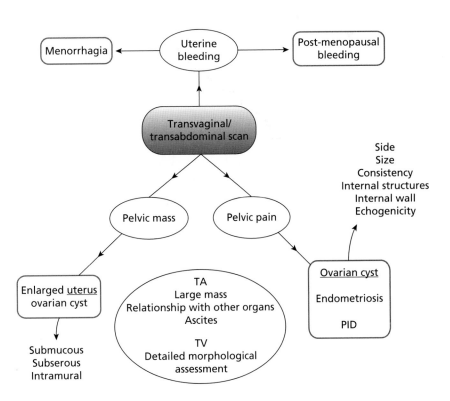

Fig. 35.2 Investigating a gynaecological symptom.

Uterine pathology

Fibroids are a common finding in the non-pregnant uterus. They can be usefully divided into the following groups:

- Intramural: within the myometrium without distorting the endometrial cavity or serosal surface of the uterus.
- Subserous: distorting the serosal surface of the uterus.
- Pedunculated or broad ligament.
- Submucous: protruding into and distorting the endometrial cavity.

An ultrasound scan that describes fibroids should define their number, size and perhaps most importantly their location. This is important as these factors will significntly impact on the choice of intervention should one be needed, and in particular for laparoscopic surgery. When there are multiple fibroids, determining their number and relationships may be very difficult in practice. In the event of a submucous fibroid, it is necessary to estimate the percentage of the fibroid protruding into the cavity in order to establish whether hysteroscopic resection is possible. Leone *et al.* [4] have described in detail terms and definitions that might be used when describing fibroids projecting into the uterine cavity. Fibroids are generally well-circumscribed lesions and typically contain foci of calcification with characteristic acoustic shadowing (Fig. 35.3). Power Doppler usually reveals a blood supply around the periphery of the lesion. The diagnostic difficulty with fibroids relates to their discrimination from adenomyosis. The features of adenomysis are myometrial asymmetry, cystic areas within the myometrium, a heterogeneous-looking myometrium, and blood vessels passing through the abnormal-looking area as opposed to around the lesion as is seen with fibroids. More recently an evaluation of the endometrial–myometrial junctional zone imaged using three-dimensional ultrasound in the coronal plane has been reported to have a high diagnositic accuracy for adenomyosis [10].

The calcification associated with fibroids can make it more difficult to visualize other structures in the pelvis and in particular the ovaries. Moving from the vaginal approach to the abdominal is often helpful in this circumstance. Pedunculated and broad ligament fibroids present their own problems. These principally relate to how confident the examiner is that he or she is not looking at a solid ovarian lesion. The demonstration of two normal ovaries is the obvious solution to this problem. The use of Doppler to demonstrate that the blood supply originates from the uterus may identify the lesion as uterine in origin and acoustic shadowing is a reassuring sign.

Fibroids can undergo degeneration and this may lead to frankly bizarre-looking appearances, including large cystic areas, hyperechogenicity and large amounts of calcification. Fortunately leiomyosarcomas are relatively rare. Unfortunately, however, there are no specific ultrasound markers to enable the examiner to define them. In general, sarcomas are more likely to be solitary, large (>8.0 cm) and cystic and have increased vascularity [11].

Ovarian masses

Having established that an ovarian or other adnexal mass is present, ultrasound may then be used to discriminate between cysts that are physiological, pathological and benign, or pathological and malignant. Whilst the focus of attention usually relates to predicting whether a mass is likely to be benign or malignant, in most cases a reasonably accurate evaluation of the likely histological outcome should also be possible. The overwhelming consensus is that ultrasound is the best imaging technique for the assessment of ovarian pathology. In 2001, a consensus document was published by the International Ovarian Tumor Analysis (IOTA) group, which aimed to standardize the terms and definitions used to characterize ovarian pathology. These terms are now becoming standard in many countries and represent the most appropriate approach to describing ovarian masses [12]. The IOTA study has recruited over 3000 ovarian or other adnexal masses and this has allowed a comprehensive evaluation of the features associated with different types of adnexal tumour. Recently the IOTA group published a set of simple rules that may be used to define whether a lesion is benign or malignant. Table 35.1 shows the rules that may be presented as a simple tick box system to usefully assess a mass. If no rule applies to a mass or there are both malignant and benign rules present, then a further second-stage test is needed to evaluate the mass. In this study about 75% of masses could be correctly evaluated using simple rules with any residual masses needing a further test to clarify the nature of the pathology.

Certain ultrasound features can be used to predict the histological diagnosis of a specific mass [13]. Generally,

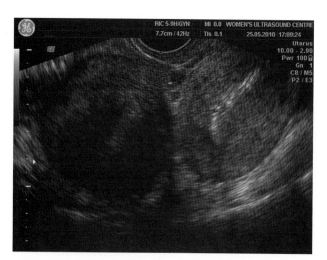

Fig. 35.3 Sagittal section of a uterus with a fundal pedunculated fibroid, with characteristic acoustic shadowing.

Table 35.1 Ten simple rules to identify a benign or malignant tumour.

Rules for predicting a malignant tumour (M-rules)
M1 Irregular solid tumour
M2 Presence of ascites
M3 At least four papillary structures
M4 Irregular multilocular solid tumour with largest diameter ≥100 mm
M5 Very strong blood flow (colour score 4)

Rules for predicting a benign tumour (B-rules)
B1 Unilocular
B2 Presence of solid components where the largest solid component has a largest diameter <7 mm
B3 Presence of acoustic shadows
B4 Smooth multilocular tumour with largest diameter <100 mm
B5 No blood flow (colour score 1)
If one or more M-rules apply in the absence of a B-rule, the mass is classified as malignant
If one or more B-rules apply in the absence of an M-rule, the mass is classified as benign
If both M-rules and B-rules apply, the mass cannot be classified
If no rule applies, the mass cannot be classified

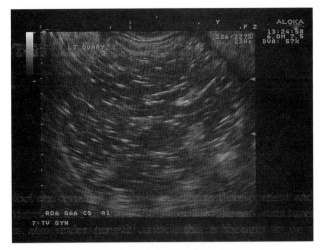

Fig. 35.4 Dermoid cyst showing characteristic bright echoes secondary to hair in the cyst.

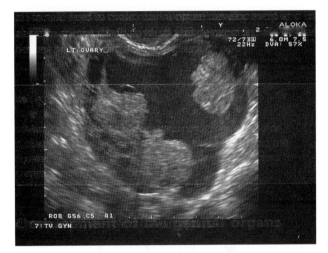

Fig. 35.5 Borderline ovarian carcinoma: note the large solid papillary projections into the cyst.

dermoid cysts are relatively easily recognized on ultrasound owing to their fat and hair content, although if they mainly contain fat they can appear isoechogenic with bowel and be easily missed. Dermoid cysts usually show mixed echogencity and are characterized by acoustic shadowing (Fig. 35.4). The typical 'white ball' or Rokitansky nodule is a very specific finding and corresponds to hair and sebum. Hair that is free within the cyst shows up as long echoic lines or bright dots [14]. Endometriomas tend to be unilocular and have a characteristic ground-glass appearance, although this may not always be the case (Plate 35.1). This classic ground-glass appearance has a very high predictive value for endometriomas. However, a significant number of endometriomas have atypical appearances and sometimes appear quite complex. The age of the patient is also important because the morphological features of an endometrioma are not common in postmenopausal women and the risk of malignancy in such lesions is significant [15].

There is no doubt that the most accurate approach to characterizing ovarian pathology is subjective impression of the morphology and vascularity of a mass by an experienced operator (Plate 35.2). This was first shown by Timmerman [16] and subsequently confirmed by Valentin *et al.* [17,18]. Experienced gynaecological ultrasonographers can reliably differentiate benign from malignant cysts and are probably better at predicting malignancy than mathematical models [16]. Markers of malignancy are described in Table 35.1 relating to simple rules. These confirm the findings of Granberg *et al.* [19] who found the frequency of malignancy in unilocular cysts to be 0.3%.

Although Doppler studies of vascularity have been suggested as a useful adjunct for assessing the possibility of malignancy in ovarian tumours, previous studies focused on the use of impedance indices to predict cancer but these have now been shown to be of no value. The optimal approach is a simple colour score based on the amount of colour that can be seen when the Doppler settings are at an agreed level (Plate 35.3). The 'colour score' has been shown to be a significant variable in most mathamatical models used to predict malignancy [12].

Other markers have been investigated as indicators of the benign or malignant nature of a mass. In 2004 it was suggested that the absence of visible normal ovarian tissue in conjunction with a cyst was a marker of malignancy (Fig. 35.5) [20]. However, a subsequent large study by the IOTA group confirmed that the presence of normal ovarian tissue or an ovarian crescent sign (OCS) had a very high predictive value for a benign lesion and that an absent OCS was not a reliable predictor of malignancy, thus explaining the poor overall test performance of the OCS overall [21].

In general, individual features of ovarian masses have not proved to be useful as predictors of the likely histology. Accordingly, attention turned to different mathamatical models using multiple variables. The ultrasound findings can be used in conjunction with menopausal status/age and serum CA-125 levels to give a risk of cancer, a score termed the risk of malignancy index (RMI); this can be used as a triage for suspected ovarian cancers. A meta-analysis in 2009, comprising 109 studies reporting on 21750 adnexal masses, assessed the accuracy of prediction models in the preoperative assessment of an adnexal mass [22]. RMI I, originally described by Jacobs *et al.*, and RMI II, modified by Tingulstad *et al.*, appeared to be the best predictors [23,24]. However, this review did not include data from the IOTA trial in the analysis. RMI is based heavily on the serum CA-125 level so it suffers from the inherent problems associated with that marker: a relatively low sensitivity for early stage and borderline disease and relatively poor specificity. The logistic regression models (LR1 and LR2) developed in the IOTA study perform significantly better than the RMI and have been validated both temporarily, using centres that were also involved in model development, and externally, using unrelated clinical centres. Both models provide excellent discrimination between benign and malignant masses [12]. It is important to note that in a series of three reports the IOTA group has also shown that measurement of serum CA-125 does not add any value to the diagnostic performance of an ultrasound scan carried out by an expert examiner [17,25,26].

Investigation of pelvic pain

It is important to take a history of the nature and location of pelvic pain prior to performing an ultrasound examination. There are many causes of pelvic pain, many of which may be non-gynaecological, and ultrasound findings taken in isolation may be misleading. For example, the majority of simple ovarian cysts, tubal cysts and sometimes hydrosalpinges are an incidental finding; however, ultrasound can help select those patients in whom surgical intervention is required. For acute pain, a normal scan is highly reassuring. The commonest pathologies where ultrasound may be of use are cyst accidents, the sequelae of pelvic infection and endometriosis.

Ovarian cysts

Ovarian cysts are relatively common. An ovarian cyst in isolation may not cause pain and there are few data to tell us what size of cyst is significant in this respect. However, cyst accidents such as haemorrhage, rupture or torsion may lead to varying degrees of pelvic pain.

Haemorrhage within a cyst can have a variety of ultrasound appearances and there is a natural history in the

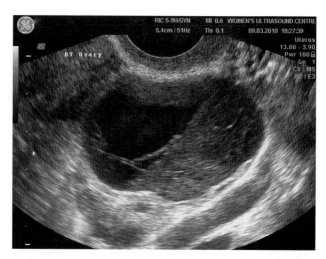

Fig. 35.6 Haemorrhagic luteal cyst with typical 'cobweb' strands secondary to resolving haemorrhage.

morphology. Initially the cyst contents will appear 'ground glass' in nature. Then, as clotting (Plate 35.4) and retraction occur, the clot will give a typical 'spiders web' appearance or wobble like jelly when the ovary is moved by the ultrasound probe (Fig. 35.6). Haemorrhagic luteal cysts are a common cause of pain in women of reproductive age. Even when large (up to 10cm in maximum diameter) they usually resolve spontaneously, although laparoscopy may still sometimes be required.

Torsion of the adnexae may occur when there is a mass in the ovary, most commonly a dermoid cyst. However, it may occur with both normal and polycystic ovaries. A torted ovary appears congested, enlarged and oedematous; multiple small cysts may be seen at the periphery of a markedly enlarged ovary. It also appears 'ghost like' and loses its normal architecture. Doppler is often misleading as venous flow is lost first with torsion but arterial flow will still be seen. Free fluid will be present in about one-third of cases. Prompt action is self-evident and management should be laparoscopic detorsion, even where the ovary appears to be infarcted and non-viable. When dealing with torsion it is important not to be misled as symptoms resolve. Most torsions are characterized by acute severe pain with nausea and often vomiting; however the pain often resolves due to nerve damage. Even at this stage detorsion is likely to lead to a good outcome [27]. Table 35.2 summarizes the above information.

Endometriosis

Chronic pelvic pain may be caused by endometriosis. Making a diagnosis of endometriosis may be challenging with ultrasound (Fig. 35.7); however, Okaro *et al.* [5] have shown that site-specific pelvic tenderness and reduced ovarian mobility (known as soft markers) are associated with the presence of endometriosis at laparoscopy. Significant attention has recently been given to the detec-

Table 35.2 Ultrasound markers in ovarian cyst events.

Diagnosis	Probable ultrasound findings
Adnexal torsion	Adnexal mass with thickened wall, possible free fluid and reduced or absent Doppler flow
Haemorrhagic cyst	Ovarian cyst with typical mixed, often bizarre, internal echoes suggestive of blood clot
Ovarian cyst rupture	Normal ovaries but site-specific tenderness and free fluid in the pouch of Douglas

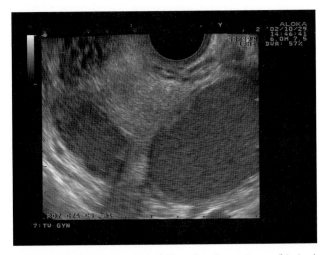

Fig. 35.7 Severe endometriosis: bilateral endometriomas 'kissing' in the midline.

tion of deep pelvic endometriotic nodules using ultrasound [28]. Nodules in the rectovaginal septum can be detected with resonable accuracy with both transvaginal, transrectal and perineal ultrasound. The addition of fluid contrast in the vagina in the form of saline may improve diagnostic performance further [29]. The characteristics of endometriotic cysts (endometriomas) within the ovary have been discussed above.

Pelvic inflammatory disease

Acute pelvic infection is a clinical diagnosis and should be considered in any sexually active woman with a history of pelvic pain, vaginal discharge or intermenstrual bleeding. Ultrasound features may include the presence of fluid both in the endometrial cavity and within the pelvis. As a result pelvic organs can often be seen to slide easily over each other. Tenderness throughout the pelvis is not unusual when carrying out a vaginal scan. A normal fallopian tube may be tracked using ultrasound but often cannot be visualized. As the tube becomes inflamed and oedematous it becomes more prominent and the accumulation of either pus or exudate within it makes visualization easier still. A pyosalpinx has a sausage-shaped

structure, thicker walls, echogenic fluid within the tube and incomplete septa. Depending on the section, an infected tube has been described as both retort-shaped or having a 'cogwheel' appearance. The term 'beads on a string' has also been used to describe the mural nodules in the tube when imaged in cross-section. Timor-Tritsch *et al.* [30] usefully suggested a list of criteria corresponding to these classic features and concluded that the best marker of tubal inflammatory disease, either acute or chronic, was the presence of an incomplete septum of the tubal wall, which was present in 92% of the total cases studied.

Timor-Tritsch and colleagues suggested that the degree of ovarian involvement should be documented. No involvement means the ovaries can be indentified and move seperately to the tube. A tubo-ovarian complex implies the ovaries can be seen, but cannot be moved when pressure is applied with the probe. For an abscess there is total breakdown of the normal architecture with loculations of particulate material (pus and exudate). For both an abscess and ovarian complex, the patient should have acute clinical features of pelvic inflammatory disease including tenderness during the examination. Ultrasound-guided treatment is an important option for tubo-ovarian abscesses. In a study of 302 women, a total of 282 (93.4%) were successfully treated by TV aspiration of purulent fluid, together with antibiotic therapy. In the other 20 women (6.6%), surgery was performed [31].

Ultrasound and abnormal uterine bleeding
Menorrhagia

Menorrhagia is relatively common, and in secondary care a scan is indicated in all women to exclude focal endometrial pathology.

Endometrial polyps

Terms and definitions used to describe polyps have been published by the IETA group [4]. Polyps are often hyperechoic and sometimes have an echogenic bright rim (Plate 35.5). The finding of a pedical artery is diagnostic [32]. There is some debate regarding the relevance of endometrial polyps. It seems unlikely that small polyps in asymptomatic menstruating women are significant and in practice a repeat scan after a period sometimes shows that they disappear in any event.

Postmenopausal bleeding

TV ultrasound is now the first-line investigation for women attending wth bleeding after the menopause. The scan is used to assess the presence or absence of endometrial, cervical, tubal, ovarian or bladder pathology. A number of studies have shown that a thin atrophic-looking endometrium is associated with a very low risk of underlying endometrial pathology. A reasonable definition of a thin endometrium is one where thickness is less than 5.0 mm. After this point the risk of pathology increases roughly in proportion to the thickness and an endometrial biopsy is advised. A measurement of endometrial thickness includes both layers and is thus the total thickness across the cavity, excluding any free fluid that may be present [33,34].

Other possible causes of postmenopausal bleeding should be considered. An advantage of TV ultrasound is that it enables the examiner to investigate the entire pelvis. Bladder pathology may be obvious. Therefore, if no endometrial pathology is detected, an examination of the bladder should be considered [35].

Investigation of infertility

Ultrasonography is now integral to both the investigation and subseqent management of women presenting with subfertility.

Baseline infertility scan

Transvaginal ultrasound can be used as a screening test for women presenting with subfertility. Strandell *et al.* [36] showed that a simplified ultrasound-based investigation protocol could helpfully be used and may be associated with reduced costs and avoid extended investigations. The use of ultrasound contrast to facilitate tubal patency testing has removed the need for hysterosalpingography or laparoscopy in many cases and there are several studies to suggest it is at least comparable to hysterosalpingography [37]. Ultrasound contrast in this context traps air bubbles and it is the air that acts as reflective contrast media. The contrast is injected through a balloon catheter into the endometrial cavity and then tracked through the tubes.

Ultrasound assessment of the ovaries has long been a significant part of the assessment of women with irregular or absent periods. The principal aim is to identify polycystic ovaries. This has been defined according to the Rotterdam criteria as the presence of 12 or more follicles measuring 2–9 mm in one or both ovaries and an ovarian volume greater than 10 mL [38]. The definition makes no mention of the distribution of the follicles or the amount of stroma seen in the ovary. There is some debate over the clinical relevance of this ultrasound-based definition of polycystic ovaries. Other authors have found that ovaries of this appearance are a common finding in the normal population [39]. For the moment, however, the Rotterdam criteria remain the basis on which the ultrasound-based diagnosis of polycystic ovaries is made.

Ultrasound has also become important for the assessment of ovarian reserve, as this is reflected in the number of small (2–6 mm) or antral follicles within the ovary [40]. The facility that now exists to automatically count follicles has further stimulated interest in this area and seems likely to give us more information about the number and distribution of follicles in varous clinical situations [41]. There are many studies that have detailed the changes in both the morphology and vascularity of the ovary and uterus in the menstrual cycle [42,43]. Ultrasound

can be used to detect normal follicular development and ovulation as well as measure endometrial thickness as a means of assessing the likelihood of successful implantation. More recently attention has focused on the endometrial–myometrial junction (or junctional zone) and how this may relate to implantation and early pregnancy (Fig. 35.8) [44].

Summary box 35.2

- Ultrasonography is the first-line investigation for evaluating a woman presenting with a possible pelvic mass.
- Subjective impression of a mass by an experienced examiner is the most accurate way of characterizing ovarian pathology.
- The IOTA terms and definitions used to characterize ovarian pathology are becoming increasingly used in clinical practice.
- Dermoid cysts are characterized by acoustic shadowing, their fat and hair content and Rokitansky nodule.
- Endometriomas tend to be unilocular and have a characteristic ground-glass appearance of the cyst contents.
- Measurements of serum CA-125 do not add diagnostic value to the assessment of a mass with ultrasound by an experienced clinician.
- A torted ovary appears congested, enlarged and oedematous; follicles may be seen peripherally. Blood flow may still be detected despite the torsion.
- A pyosalpinx has a sausage-shaped structure, thicker walls, echogenic fluid within the tube and incomplete septa.
- In postmenopausal women, a reasonable definition of a thin endometrium is one of thickness below 5.0 mm.
- Currently, the Rotterdam criteria are used to define the ultrasound features of polycystic ovaries.

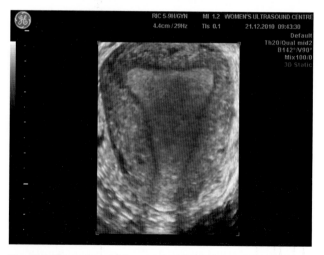

Fig. 35.8 The endometrial–myometrial junction or junctional zone imaged in the coronal plane with three-dimensional ultrasound.

Role of ultrasound in early pregnancy

Normal pregnancy

Transvaginal ultrasonography is the principal dignostic tool for assessing women in early pregnancy. Many women attend for a scan to reassure themselves that all is well with the pregnancy and it is probably best to carry out these scans after 49 days' gestation in order to avoid inconclusive outcomes [45]. An early pregnancy can be dated by comparing the crown–rump length of the embryo with established reference curves derived from large numbers of apparently normal pregnancies [46]. It has commonly been thought that the size of an embryo in the first trimester can be translated into a gestational age value with impunity. Recent publications have shown that the size and growth of the first-trimester embryo are affected by maternal age, ethnicity, chromosomal abnormalities in the embryo and imminent miscarriage [47,48]. Finding a smaller than expected embryo is not necessarily a reflection of inaccurate dating and it is often wise to schedule a follow-up scan in these circumstances in view of the risk of miscarriage.

Miscarriage

Nearly every woman with a possible miscarriage has this diagnosis confirmed or otherwise with ultrasound. In view of this it might be expected that the ultrasound-based definitions of miscarriage are clear-cut and not open to interpretation. However, the American College of Radiologists (ACR) guideline, updated in 2009 [49], states that 'the embryo will initially appear as a thickened, linear echogenic structure between the yolk sac and the gestational sac, possibly seen at 8mm sac size, but definitely by 16mm' and that 'embryonic demise may be diagnosed with an embryo >5mm without cardiac activity'. In contrast one of the few prospective studies on the subject shows us a different picture. Elson *et al.* [50] examined 200 pregnancies with an empty gestation sac with a mean sac diameter (MSD) of less than 20mm. They found a considerable overlap between the MSD in viable and non-viable pregnancies. Also two pregnancies with an empty sac of more than 18 but less than 20mm were subsequently shown to be viable. A further concern was raised by Pexsters *et al.* [51] who suggested that if one operator measures the MSD as 20mm, another operator may measure the same gestation sac as being between 16 and 24mm. Anecdotally it is not unusual to see women who have had a miscarriage diagnosed incorrectly on the basis of just one measurement of gestation sac diameter or where MSD has been measured incorrectly. Currently the UK guidelines [52] state:

Pregnancy of 'uncertain viability': Intrauterine sac (<20mm mean diameter) with no obvious yolk sac or fetus or >6mm crown–rump length with no obvious fetal heart activity. In order to confirm or refute viability, a repeat scan at a minimal interval of 1 week is necessary.

It is important for anyone carrying out a scan in early pregnancy to always remember that doctors should do no harm, and so repeating an ultrasound scan after an interval is mandatory if there is any doubt about the outcome. The Cardiff report put it best by stating 'the death of an early pregnancy should be regarded as of equal significance to that occurring at a later stage' [53]. If examiners approach things with this attitude, they are unlikely to go far wrong.

> ### 💡 Summary box 35.3
>
> - Missed miscarriage (early fetal demise): crown–rump length of at least 6mm with no cardiac activity or no change in size on weekly serial scanning.
> - Blighted ovum (empty sac): mean diameter of gestational sac of at least 20mm with no embryonic/extraembryonic structures present.
> - There is significant interobserver error when measuring MSD. When the gestation sac size is near the decision boundary, repeat the scan at an interval.

Ectopic pregnancy

Each year ectopic pregnancy remains an avoidable cause of death in a number of women. It is important to emphasize the long-held maxim that every fertile woman has a potential ectopic pregnancy until proved otherwise. Over the years we have seen women referred for ultrasound with indications ranging from intermenstual bleeding, amenorrhoea, pelvic discomfort and diarrhoea in whom an ectopic pregnancy has been found at the time of a scan. The list is not exhaustive, so if in doubt carry out a pregnancy test. Risk factors in the patient's history, for example previous ectopic pregnancy, pelvic infection, tubal surgery or use of an intrauterine contraceptive device, may raise the clinician's index of suspicion.

At one time the assessment of women with possible ectopic pregnancy was built on the principle of 'failing to identify an intrauterine pregnancy', that is a diagnosis of exclusion. In most cases the diagnosis is now based on the positive visualization of the ectopic pregnancy. Condous *et al.* [54] have reported that the sensitivity and specificity of TV ultrasound to detect an ectopic pregnancy prior to surgery were 90.9 and 99.9%, respectively. The morphological findings suggesting an ectopic pregnancy were (i) an inhomogeneous mass or blob sign adjacent to the ovary and moving separately from the ovary; (ii) a mass with a hyperechoic ring around the gestational sac or 'bagel' sign; or (iii) a gestational sac with a fetal pole with or without cardiac activity [55]. These data are slightly misleading as they relate to the diagnosis of ectopic pregnancy immediately prior to surgery. In a further paper Kirk *et al.* [56] found that the sensitivity and specificity of ultrasound to diagnose ectopic pregnancy at the time of initial presentation to an early pregnancy unit were 73.9 and 99.9% respectively. In a number of cases an early pregnancy is categorized as 'pregnancy of unknown location', before the ectopic pregnancy mass is subsequently seen using ultrasonography. This appears to be simply a reflection of the gestational age of the pregnancy; at early gestations the ectopic mass may simply be too small to visualize with ultrasound or even in some cases by laparoscopy [57]. Ectopic pregnancy is covered in further detail elsewhere in this book. However, it is clear that most ectopic pregnancies should be visualized before surgery (Plate 35.6). Conversely, it should be relatively uncommon for a laparoscopy performed when an ectopic pregnancy has been identified using ultrasound to find no pathology.

Ultrasound can usefully be applied to assess the amount of blood in the pelvis; if blood in the pelvis is above the uterus or in the utero-vesical fold, then there is significant bleeding. As detailed above, use of FAST (focused assessment with sonography in trauma) for patients with blunt abdominal trauma has been transferred to emergency gynaecology [57]. An abdominal transducer is used to image Morrison's pouch, and the presence of fluid there suggests at least 750 mL of blood in the abdomen (Fig. 35.9).

The morphology of an ectopic pregnancy when imaged with ultrasound is important. The majority are inhomogeneous masses. However, visualizing a yolk sac or fetal embryonic heart beat has management implications as these cases tend to do badly when treated medically with methotrexate.

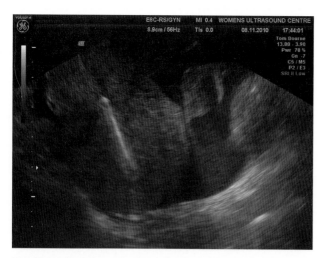

Fig. 35.9 A large amount of blood in the pouch of Douglas. Note the uterus containing an IUCD anteriorly. This patient had a ruptured ectopic pregnancy.

Pregnancy of unknown location

For a proportion of women attending for an ultrasound scan in early pregnancy, no evidence of a pregnancy can be seen either inside or outside the uterus. The number of cases of pregnancy of unknown location (PUL) in any given unit is likely to reflect the quality of the ultrasonography in that unit, and a rate of about 15% is probably reasonable. In many cases the inability to locate a pregnancy is simply a reflection of gestational age. It may be possible to reduce this. Bottomley *et al.* [45] showed that in asymptomatic women, restricting scans until 49 days' gestation would optimally reduce the PUL rate without missing ectopic pregnancies. In symptomatic women there was no gestational age cut-off value that could be used to restrict access to scanning.

Pregnancies classified as PUL include a very early intrauterine pregnancy, an ectopic gestation or a failing pregnancy, whether intrauterine or extrauterine. The management of these cases is based on knowledge of the behaviour of serum β human chorionic gonadotrophin (HCG) and progesterone. In general terms the HCG ratio, or change in HCG over time, is the most informative tool available. Care must be taken when comparing data from different institutions, as shown by a recent attempt to reach consensus on the terminology and definitions used [58].

The introduction of sensitive home pregnancy testing kits has led to women knowing they are pregnant at an early stage and often before the first missed period. This has led women to seek earlier scans and a consequent rise in the number of PUL being seen. To some extent the emphasis for the management of PUL has shifted from detection of ectopic pregnancies in the population to selection of pregnancies that are highly likely not to be an ectopic pregnancy in order to reduce follow-up [59]. In order to standardize and rationalize PUL management, a number of mathamatical models have been developed that have a high predictive value for failing and intrauterine pregnancies and reasonable performance for the prediction of ectopic pregnancy [60,61].

PUL will continue to be a major part of the workload in many gynaecology units, but this can be made significantly easier by adhering to straightforward protocols and avoiding ad hoc follow-up, whether using ultrasound or serum biochemistry.

> ### Summary box 35.4
>
> - Over 90% of ectopic pregnancies should be visualized prior to surgery. Most appear as homogeneous 'blobs'.
> - In 10–20% of pregnancies, no evidence of a pregnancy inside or outside the uterus will be seen. This is termed a pregnancy of unknown location or PUL.
> - The rate of PUL in a unit reflects the quality of the ultrasound.
> - PUL should be managed on the basis of changing serum HCG levels over time.

Conclusion

Ultrasound is now at the centre of many decisions in modern gynaecology. We have seen that the management of menstrual disturbances, ovarian cysts, infertility, pelvic pain, early pregnancy, urogynaecology and many other conditions now use ultrasound as an integral part of the patient care pathway. Increasingly, ultrasound is seen as a diagnostic tool that is carried out at the point of first contact with the patient, whether in the outpatient clinic, acute gynaecology unit or primary care. There is no doubt about the potential value of ultrasound in gynaecology, but there is a downside. An ultrasound scan frequently reveals structures that, though present, are clinically unimportant. Small simple cysts in postmenopausal women, physiological ovarian cysts, hydrosalpinges, small fibroids, Nabothian cysts and loculated fluid secondary to adhesions are all possible examples of this. It is as important to know how to recognize normality or insignificant pathology as it is to make a positive diagnosis.

Like all practical skills, becoming proficient at ultrasonography takes time and requires the operator to build up experience based on repetition, feedback and reinforcement for improvement to take place. This requires that clinicians carrying out ultrasound scans know the final outcomes of their patients. The best way to learn to scan is to make the diagnosis and then reinforce the findings by being present at any surgery that then occurs. Any unit carrying out gynaecological scanning should have a clinical review meeting and outcomes must be followed up. In the future as ultrasound machines become more and more portable, the number will proliferate. Matching operator competency to the availability of ultrasound machines will continue to be a major challenge in the future.

References

1 Santoro GA, Wieczorek AP, Dietz HP *et al*. State of the art: an integrated approach to pelvic floor ultrasonography. *Ultrasound Obstet Gynecol* 2011;37:381–396.
2 Jurkovic D, Geipel A, Gruboeck K, Jauniaux E, Natucci M, Campbell S. 3D-ultrasound for the assessment of uterine anatomy and detection of congenital anomalies: a comparison with hysterosalpingography and two-dimensional sonography. *Ultrasound Obstet Gynecol* 1995;5:233–237.
3 Karlsson B, Granberg S, Wikland M *et al*. Transvaginal ultrasonography of the endometrium in women with postmenopausal bleeding: a Nordic multicenter study. *Am J Obstet Gynecol* 1995;172:1488–1494.
4 Leone FP, Timmerman D, Bourne T *et al*. Terms, definitions and measurements to describe the sonographic features of the endometrium and intrauterine lesions: a consensus opinion from the International Endometrial Tumor Analysis (IETA) group. *Ultrasound Obstet Gynecol* 2010;35:103–112.
5 Okaro E, Condous G, Khalid A *et al*. The use of ultrasound-based 'soft markers' for the prediction of pelvic pathology in women with chronic pelvic pain: can we reduce the need for laparoscopy? *BJOG* 2006;113:251–256.
6 Parsons AK, Lense JJ. Sonohysterography for endometrial abnormalities: preliminary results. *J Clin Ultrasound* 1993;21:87–95.
7 Leone FP, Bignardi T, Marciante C, Ferrazzi E. Sonohysterography in the preoperative grading of submucous myomas: considerations on three-dimensional methodology. *Ultrasound Obstet Gynecol* 2007;29:717–718.
8 Schwärzler P, Concin H, Bösch H *et al*. An evaluation of sonohysterography and diagnostic hysteroscopy for the assessment of intrauterine pathology. *Ultrasound Obstet Gynecol* 1998;11:337–342.
9 Haider Z, Condous G, Khalid A *et al*. Impact of the availability of sonography in the acute gynaecology unit. *Ultrasound Obstet Gynecol* 2006;28:207–213.
10 Exacoustos C, Brienza AL, Di Giovanni A *et al*. Adenomyosis: three dimensional (3D) sonographic findings of the junctional zone and correlation to histology. *Ultrasound Obstet Gynecol* 2010 [Epub ahead of print].
11 Exacoustos C, Romanini ME, Amadio A *et al*. Can gray-scale and color Doppler sonography differentiate between uterine leiomyosarcoma and leiomyoma? *J Clin Ultrasound* 2007;35:449–457.
12 Timmerman D, Van Calster B, Testa AC *et al*. Ovarian cancer prediction in adnexal masses using ultrasound-based logistic regression models: a temporal and external validation study by the IOTA group. *Ultrasound Obstet Gynecol* 2010;36:226–234.
13 Timmerman D, Schwarzler P, Collins WP *et al*. Subjective assessment of adnexal masses using ultrasonography: an analysis of intraobserver variability and experience. *Ultrasound Obstet Gynecol* 1999;13:11–16.
14 Jermy K, Luise C, Bourne T. The characterisation of common ovarian cysts in premenopausal women. *Ultrasound Obstet Gynecol* 2001;17:140–144.
15 Van Holsbeke C, Van Calster B, Guerriero S *et al*. Endometriomas: their ultrasound characteristics. *Ultrasound Obstet Gynecol* 2010;35:730–740.
16 Timmerman D (2004) The use of mathematical models to evaluate pelvic masses, can they beat an expert operator? *Best Pract Res Clin Obstet Gynecol* 18, 91–104.
17 Valentin L, Jurkovic D, Van Calster B *et al*. Adding a single CA 125 measurement to ultrasound imaging performed by an experienced examiner does not improve preoperative discrimaination between benign and malignant adenxal masses. *Ultrasound Obstet Gynecol* 2009;34:345–354.
18 Valentin L, Hagen B, Tingulstad S, Eik-Nes S. Comparison of 'pattern recognition' and logistic regression models for discrimination between benign and malignant pelvic masses: a prospective crossvalidation. *Ultrasound Obstet Gynecol* 2001;18:357–365.
19 Granberg S, Wikland M, Jansson I. Macroscopic characterisation of ovarian tumours and the relation to the histological diagnosis: criteria to be used in ultrasound evaluation. *Gynecol Oncol* 1989;35:139–144.
20 Hillaby K, Aslam N, Salim R, Lawrence A, Raju KS, Jurkovic D. The value of detection of normal ovarian tissue (the 'ovarian crescent sign') in the differential diagnosis of adnexal masses. *Ultrasound Obstet Gynecol* 2004;23:63–67.

21 Van Holsbeke C, Van Belle V, Leone FP *et al.* Prospective external validation of the 'ovarian crescent sign' as a single ultrasound parameter to distinguish between benign and malignant adnexal pathology. *Ultrasound Obstet Gynecol* 2010;36:81–87.

22 Geomini P, Kruitwagen R, Bremer G, Cnossen J, Mol BWJ. The accuracy of risk scores in predicting ovarian malignancy: a systematic review. *Obstet Gynecol* 2009;113:384–394.

23 Jacobs I, Oram D, Fairbanks J, Turner J, Frost C, Grudzinskas JG. A risk of malignancy index incorporating CA 125, ultrasound and menopausal status for the accurate preoperative diagnosis of ovarian cancer. *Br J Obstet Gynaecol* 1990;97: 922–929.

24 Tingulstad S, Hagen B, Skjeldestad FE *et al.* Evaluation of a risk of malignancy index based on serum CA 125, ultrasound findings and menopausal status in the pre-operative diagnosis of pelvic masses. *Br J Obstet Gynaecol* 1996;103:826–831.

25 Van Calster B, Timmerman D, Bourne T *et al.* Discrimination between benign and malignant adnexal masses by specialist ultrasound examination versus serum CA-125. *J Natl Cancer Inst* 2007;99:1706–1714.

26 Timmerman D, Van Calster B, Jurkovic D *et al.* Inclusion of CA-125 does not improve mathematical models developed to distinguish between benign and malignant adnexal tumours. *J Clin Oncol* 2007;25:4194–4200.

27 Bottomley C, Bourne T. Diagnosis and management of ovarian cyst accidents. *Best Pract Res Clin Obstet Gynaecol* 2009;23: 711–724.

28 Guerriero S, Ajossa S, Gerada M, Virgilio B, Angioni S, Melis GB. Diagnostic value of transvaginal 'tenderness-guided' ultrasonography for the prediction of location of deep endometriosis. *Hum Reprod* 2008;23:2452–2457.

29 Bignardi T, Condous G. Sonorectovaginography: a new sonographic technique for imaging of the posterior compartment of the pelvis. *J Ultrasound Med* 2008;27:1479–1483.

30 Timor-Tritsch IE, Lerner JP, Monteagudo A, Murphy KE, Heller DS. Transvaginal sonographic markers of tubal inflammatory disease. *Ultrasound Obstet Gynecol* 1998;12:56–66.

31 Gjelland K, Ekerhovd E, Granberg S. Transvaginal ultrasound-guided aspiration for treatment of tubo-ovarian abscess: a study of 302 cases. *Am J Obstet Gynecol* 2005;193:1323–1330.

32 Timmerman D, Verguts J, Konstantinovic ML *et al.* The pedicle artery sign based on sonography with color Doppler imaging can replace second-stage tests in women with abnormal vaginal bleeding. *Ultrasound Obstet Gynecol* 2003;22:166–171.

33 Smith-Bindman R, Kerlikowske K, Feldstein VA *et al.* Endovaginal ultrasound to exclude endometrial cancer and other endometrial abnormalities. *JAMA* 1998;280:1510–1517.

34 Karlsson B, Milsom I, Granberg S. Can ultrasound replace dilatation and curettage? A longitudinal evaluation of postmenopausal bleeding and transvaginal sonographic measurement of the endometrium as predictors of endometrial cancer. *Am J Obstet Gynecol* 2003;188:401–408.

35 Betsas G, Van Den Bosch T, Deprest J, Bourne T, Timmerman D. Picture of the Month: The use of transvaginal ultrasonography to diagnose bladder carcinoma in women presenting with postmenopausal bleeding. *Ultrasound Obstet Gynecol* 2008;32: 959–960.

36 Strandell A, Bourne T, Bergh C, Granberg S, Thorburn J, Hamberger L. A simplified ultrasound based infertility inves-

tigation protocol and its implications for patient management. *J Assist Reprod Genet* 2000;17:87–92.

37 Strandell A, Bourne T, Bergh C, Granberg S, Asztely M, Thorburn J. The assessment of endometrial pathology and tubal patency: a comparison between the use of ultrasonography and X-ray hysterosalpingography for the investigation of infertility patients. *Ultrasound Obstet Gynecol* 1999;14: 200–204.

38 Balen AH, Laven JS, Tan SL, Dewailly D. Ultrasound assessment of the polycystic ovary: international consensus definitions. *Hum Reprod Update* 2003;9:505–514.

39 Kristensen SL, Ramlau-Hansen CH, Ernst E *et al.* A very large proportion of young Danish women have polycystic ovaries: is a revision of the Rotterdam criteria needed? *Hum Reprod* 2010;25:3117–3122.

40 Jayaprakasan K, Deb S, Batcha M *et al.* The cohort of antral follicles measuring 2–6 mm reflects the quantitative status of ovarian reserve as assessed by serum levels of anti-Müllerian hormone and response to controlled ovarian stimulation. *Fertil Steril* 2010;94:1775–1781.

41 Raine-Fenning N, Jayaprakasan K, Deb S *et al.* Automated follicle tracking improves measurement reliability in patients undergoing ovarian stimulation. *Reprod Biomed Online* 2009;18: 658–663.

42 Bourne TH, Hagström H, Hahlin M *et al.* Ultrasound studies of vascular and morphological changes in the human corpus luteum during the menstrual cycle. *Fertil Steril* 1996;65: 753–758.

43 Bourne TH, Hagström HG, Granberg S *et al.* Ultrasound studies of vascular and morphological changes in the human uterus after a positive self-test for the urinary luteinising hormone surge. *Hum Reprod* 1996;11:369–375.

44 Naftalin J, Jurkovic D. The endometrial–myometrial junction: a fresh look at a busy crossing. *Ultrasound Obstet Gynecol* 2009;34:1–11.

45 Bottomley C, Van Belle V, Mukri F *et al.* The optimal timing of an ultrasound scan to assess the location and viability of an early pregnancy. *Hum Reprod* 2009;24:1811–1817.

46 Pexsters A, Daemen A, Bottomley C *et al.* New crown–rump length curve based on over 3500 pregnancies. *Ultrasound Obstet Gynecol* 2010;35:650–655.

47 Bottomley C, Daemen A, Mukri F *et al.* Assessing first trimester growth: the influence of ethnic background and maternal age. *Hum Reprod* 2009;24:284–289.

48 Mukri F, Bourne T, Bottomley C, Schoeb C, Kirk E, Papageorghiou AT. Evidence of early first-trimester growth restriction in pregnancies that subsequently end in miscarriage. *BJOG* 2008;115:1273–1278.

49 American College of Radiologists. First trimester bleeding. American College of Radiologists (ACR) appropriateness criteria. Originated 1996, updated in 2009.

50 Elson J, Salim R, Tailor A, Banerjee S, Zosmer N, Jurkovic D. Prediction of early pregnancy viability in the absence of an ultrasonically detectable embryo. *Ultrasound Obstet Gynecol* 2003;21:57–61.

51 Pexsters A, Luts J, Van Schoubroeck D *et al.* Clinical implications of intra- and inter-observer reproducibility of first trimester measurements performed with transvaginal ultrasound between 6 and 9 weeks gestation. *Ultrasound Obstet Gynecol* 2010 [Epub ahead of print].

52 Royal College of Obstetricians and Gynaecologists. *The Management of Early Pregnancy Loss*. Green-top Guideline No. 25, 2006. Available at: www.rcog.org.uk/files/rcog-corp/uploaded-files/GT25ManagementofEarlyPregnancyLoss2006.pdf.

53 Hately W, Case J, Campbell S. Establishing the death of an embryo by ultrasound: report of a public enquiry with recommendations. *Ultrasound Obstet Gynecol* 1995;5:353–357.

54 Condous G, Okaro E, Khalid A *et al*. The accuracy of transvaginal ultrasonography for the diagnosis of ectopic pregnnacy prior to surgery. *Hum Reprod* 2005;20:1404–1409.

55 Kirk E, Papageorghiou AT, Condous G, Tan L, Bora S, Bourne T. The diagnostic effectiveness of an initial transvaginal scan in detecting ectopic pregnancy. *Hum Reprod* 2007;22:2824–2828.

56 Kirk E, Daemen A, Papageorghiou AT *et al*. Why are some ectopic pregnancies characterised as pregnancies of unknown location at the initial transvaginal ultrasound examination? *Acta Obstet Gynecol Scand* 2008;87:1150–1154.

57 Tsui CL, Fung HT, Chung KL, Kam CW. Focused abdominal sonography for trauma in the emergency department for blunt abdominal trauma. *Int J Emerg Med* 2008;1:183–187.

58 Barnhart K, van Mello NM, Bourne T *et al*. Pregnancy of unknown location: a consensus statement of nomenclature, definitions, and outcome. *Fertil Steril* 2011;95:857–866.

59 Kirk E, Condous G, Van Calster B, Van Huffel S, Timmerman D, Bourne T. Rationalising the follow-up of pregnancies of unknown location. *Hum Reprod* 2007;22:1744–1750.

60 Condous G, Kirk E, Van Calster B, Van Huffel S, Timmerman D, Bourne T. Failing pregnancies of unknown location: a prospective evaluation of the human chorionic gonadotrophin ratio. *BJOG* 2006;113:521–527.

61 Bignardi T, Condous G, Alhamdan D *et al*. The HCG ratio can predict the ultimate viability of the intrauterine pregnancies of uncertain viability in the pregnancy of unknown location population. *Hum Reprod* 2008;23:1964–1967.

Chapter 36
Hysteroscopy and Laparoscopy

Adam Magos
Royal Free Hospital, London, UK

It is perhaps even truer today than in 2007 when the previous edition of this textbook was published that hysteroscopy and laparoscopy are playing an increasingly important role in the care of our patients. This is for a number of reasons. New instruments, techniques and procedures continue to be introduced. For instance, hysteroscopic sterilization, for so long an aspiration, has become a reality. The use of robots at laparoscopic surgery, although relatively cumbersome at this time, is likely to be the future as the technology improves and costs come down to a reasonable level. In the mean time, novel approaches such as single port laparoscopy and natural orifice transluminal endoscopic surgery are being developed to lessen the trauma of modern surgery even further. The scientific basis of minimal access surgery (MAS) is vouched for by the ever-growing library of evidence from organizations such as the Cochrane Database and, in the UK, the National Institute of Health and Clinical Excellence (NICE) to name but two, a trend which is seen worldwide. For instance, since the publication of the last edition of this book, the Cochrane Database has issued guidance on endometrial ablation, laparoscopic surgery for endometriosis, including pain, subfertility and endometriomas, benign ovarian tumours, ectopic pregnancy, tubal infertility, ovarian drilling, hysterectomy, and even laparoscopic entry techniques. Arguably most importantly, many of the new cadre of gynaecologists are becoming trained in operative laparoscopy and hysteroscopy, so not surprisingly more patients are undergoing endoscopic surgery.

Nonetheless, it is important to acknowledge the past and important role played by the early pioneers of this new surgery, such as Semm and Lindemann from Germany, Bruhat and Hamou from France, Sutton from England, and Reich, Neuwirth and Goldrath from the USA to name but a few. It is thanks to them and others that gynaecological surgery has undergone a revolution since the 1970s and 1980s, a revolution characterized by the realization that many patients formerly treated by laparotomy can be managed by laparoscopic or hysteroscopic surgery. It is not an exaggeration to claim that in many respects gynaecologists were the leaders in this change of practice; whereas laparoscopic procedures such as ovarian cystectomy, salpingo-oophorectomy and myomectomy were described by Semm as early as 1979, the first comparable general surgical procedure, laparoscopic cholecystectomy, was only described several years later. Indeed, it was Semm, a gynaecologist, who carried out the first laparoscopic appendicectomy in 1983 [1].

Since those early days, MAS has continued to affect every area of gynaecology, from diagnosis to therapy, from reproductive medicine to urogynaecology and oncology. The advantages seemed obvious: less postoperative pain, shorter hospitalization and faster return to normal activities. While it has to be admitted that the widespread adoption of endoscopic surgery has not always been based on proof of its efficacy and safety compared with traditional surgery, it is equally true to say that MAS has introduced a scientific rigour into surgical practice which was rarely seen with the 'old' surgery. As a result, the medical literature on MAS across all surgical specialities is extensive and growing by the day, and randomized controlled trials, cost–benefit analysis and quality-adjusted life-years have become common currency among surgeons just as they have been for many years for physicians.

Instruments and equipment for endoscopy

Much more than is the case with conventional surgery, endoscopic surgery relies heavily on not only the skill of the surgeon but also technology. The vision of the early pioneers would have been but nothing without technical developments in optics, illumination, video technology and instrumentation. There has always been a close link between the endoscopic surgeon and industry, and it is

---

Dewhurst's Textbook of Obstetrics & Gynaecology, Eighth Edition. Edited by D. Keith Edmonds.
© 2012 John Wiley and Sons, Ltd. Published 2012 by John Wiley and Sons, Ltd.

not an exaggeration to claim that the instruments and equipment for MAS is an inherent part of the surgery. It is therefore essential that the surgeon fully understands all aspects of their use if he or she is to be a safe and effective operator, from basic physical principles to how equipment is assembled and connected, from when and how to use a particular instrument to what to do when it appears to be malfunctioning.

Equipment common to hysteroscopy and laparoscopy

Light source and light lead

Without adequate illumination, endoscopic surgery becomes an impossibility. Illumination is primarily a function of the power of the light source and the light transmission properties of the light lead, but is also influenced by the size and tissue properties of the structure being illuminated. For instance, laparoscopy requires a brighter light to sufficiently illuminate a larger cavity at a greater distance compared with hysteroscopy, and the same is true in the presence of bleeding as blood absorbs light.

Older tungsten and metal halide light sources have been superseded by more powerful xenon generators. When used with modern auto-aperture cameras it is generally recommended that they should be set to maximum illumination during surgery. Conversely, the light source should not be switched off between cases but merely put on standby to prolong the life of the bulb. Although modern light bulbs are guaranteed for several hundred hours use, a spare one should be available in the operating theatre in case the bulb fails in the middle of a procedure.

Light leads are of two types, fibreoptic or liquid. The former are more common because they are cheaper, but the fibres are prone to breaking with gradual deterioration in light transmission. Rough handling (e.g. kinking, knotting or tight rolling) should be avoided as this will tend to damage the delicate light fibres. The state of the fibres is easily checked by aiming one end at a light and looking at the other end for dark areas. Liquid light cables do not suffer from this problem but can be irreversibly damaged if the outer casing is punctured.

Whatever the power of the light source or the type of light lead, and despite the common use of the term 'cold light fountain' to describe medical light systems, the light produced at the end of the light lead is actually relatively 'hot' even in standby mode to the extent that it can burn drapes as well as the patient if inadvertently left in contact.

Camera and monitor system

There is little doubt that the introduction of video cameras and high-resolution colour monitors in the 1980s played a major role in popularizing endoscopic surgery. Until then, only the surgeon could see the surgery, and it was difficult for assistants to play a useful role as they were blind to the procedure. An optical teaching aid could be attached to the telescope, but this merely limited movement of the endoscope and reduced illumination, and was not really a solution. Then, suddenly, after years of working in the dark as far as the rest of the operating theatre staff were concerned, everyone could see the operation. Assistants could assist, the surgeon could teach, and even the anaesthetist felt more involved.

Early tube cameras were superseded by single CCD (charged coupled device) chip cameras, which in turn have been superseded by current three-chip cameras. Videolaparoscopes are now also available where the chips are built into the end of the optic, as are three-dimensional camera systems, but these have still not achieved widespread popularity. Apart from focus, various other functions can usually be controlled through the camera itself (e.g. white balance, taking a still image), and it is useful to be able to have a zoom facility. Some cameras can be autoclaved, the alternative being to place the camera and lead in a sterile sleeve.

The camera is connected to a control unit and thence to a high-resolution colour monitor; an ordinary television, which has a relatively low resolution, would provide a far inferior image.

Electrosurgical generator

Electrosurgery, often referred to as 'diathermy', has been used in surgery for over 100 years for haemostasis or cutting, and has become a very important component of both hysteroscopic and laparoscopic surgery. The modern solid-state generator safely and reliably delivers a high-frequency current at low voltage and is a very different machine from the spark generators of years gone by. It can be used in one of three modalities: bipolar, monopolar cutting (including pure cut and blended cut) and monopolar coagulation (including desiccation, fulguration and spray). Bipolar coagulation, for instance, is often used in laparoscopy for haemostasis, whereas the resectoscope is traditionally a monopolar instrument.

There is insufficient space here to discuss the principles of electrosurgery fully, but the following are useful practical points for the endoscopic surgeon that are not always appreciated.

1 The bipolar, monopolar cut and monopolar coagulation are three independent circuits within the generator. For instance, blending a monopolar cut waveform is not influenced at all by the setting on the monopolar coagulation circuit.

2 Bipolar electrosurgery is inherently safer than monopolar as the current only has to travel between the prongs of the electrodes and not between the electrode and the

patient plate. It should therefore be used in preference to monopolar electrosurgery whenever possible.

3 The minimum power and voltage should be used that will achieve the desired end result. Remember that the current produced when activating the bipolar circuit has the lowest voltage while monopolar coagulation the highest, monopolar cut being intermediate. Voltage drives the current and also causes sparking. From this point of view as well, bipolar electrosurgery is the safest and monopolar coagulation the most dangerous when working in a confined space such as the pelvis.

4 As the bipolar electrodes are in effect composed of the active and return electrodes, a patient plate is not required for bipolar electrosurgery.

5 The terms 'cut' and 'coagulation' are in some respects a misnomer. Electrosurgical cutting depends on electrical arcing between the electrode and tissue resulting in vaporization and cell explosion, whereas coagulation is achieved with the electrode in contact with tissue causing heating and coagulation. As these effects are independent of the current waveform, it is possible to achieve both cutting and coagulation with a cutting current by simply altering the position of the electrode; keeping the electrode off the tissue will result in cutting while deliberately touching the tissue will produce coagulation. As the cutting current is at a lower voltage, coagulating with monopolar cut is inherently safer than using monopolar coagulation, although it may not be as effective.

6 Some other practical aspects of electrosurgery are addressed later in the chapter. However, electrosurgery is such a useful and powerful tool that I urge the reader to study the subject in greater depth (see Further reading).

Lasers

The laser, an acronym for *l*ight *a*mplification by *s*timulated *e*mission of *r*adiation, has always had a mystique, perhaps because it is expensive and therefore available only to a few. The wider utilization of newer and, above all, cheaper technologies such as the harmonic scalpel and improved electrosurgical instruments has meant that lasers are now even less important than previously.

Nonetheless, a little background knowledge is useful. While there is no evidence that lasers produce a better end result, certain lasers represent a safer surgical modality because (i) thermal spread tends to be less (e.g. using a CO_2 laser for cutting or tissue vaporization) and (ii) the classic problems associated with electrosurgery such as distant burns, insulation failure and capacitive coupling just cannot happen. Conversely, lasers tend to be less efficient at haemostasis than diathermy.

Several different lasers have been used for endoscopy over the years, but of these CO_2, Nd:YAG (neodymium: yttrium–aluminium–garnet), argon and KTP (potassium titanyl phosphate) lasers tended to be used for laparoscopy, and the Nd:YAG laser for hysteroscopy. The CO_2 laser is an optical laser delivered through a tubular arm containing mirrors. The beam is almost completely absorbed by water, and is therefore suited to laparoscopy because it cuts accurately with minimal thermal spread. On the negative side, CO_2 lasers are relatively poor haemostats, and the need for an optical arm makes it cumbersome to operate and prone to misalignment. The Nd:YAG laser is a fibreoptic laser which makes it easier to use, and as the energy is poorly absorbed by water, this type of laser is suitable for hysteroscopic procedures as well as laparoscopy. For the same reason, the thermal spread with Nd:YAG is greater, making it more suited to tissue coagulation rather than vaporization. However, tissue penetration can be reduced and precision increased by using a sapphire tip at the end of the fibreoptic cable. The argon and KTP lasers are also fibre lasers with tissue effects intermediate between those of CO_2 and Nd:YAG lasers.

Photo and video documentation

The universal use of video cameras at endoscopic surgery lends itself to recording still images, short excerpts of procedures or even whole procedures. Photographs are useful clinical records that can be discussed with the patient as well as colleagues if a second opinion is sought. Video recordings are excellent for teaching, and can also be used for research, to measure performance and to assess new instruments and techniques. Review of recordings can also help with the understanding of operative complications.

There are numerous recording systems available. Digital systems have replaced analogue recording, and typically consist of a modified computer with a touch screen, DVD writer and colour printer. Although convenient, commercial systems are expensive and still have limited continuous recording capabilities at least if the intention is to record whole procedures, which in the case of complex laparoscopic surgery can last several hours. However, it is possible to construct a digital recording system based around a standard personal computer whose recording capacity is hundreds of times greater, limited only by the size of the hard disk inside [2]. For those less technologically minded or wishing for ultimate convenience, personal portable digital recorders are an ideal tool for recording one's surgery [3].

It must be remembered that local guidelines have to be followed when any visual recordings are made of patients. In the UK, for instance, the General Medical Council has issued guidelines which state that, in the case of laparoscopic images or images of internal organs, permission or consent is not required from patients provided the recording are effectively anonymized by removal of any identifying marks.

Equipment for hysteroscopy

Hysteroscopes

Both rigid and flexible hysteroscopes are available, the majority of gynaecologists preferring the former because the image tends to be superior, the equipment is more robust, it can be used with a resectoscope and, not least, the purchase cost is significantly less. Rigid hysteroscopes generally have a Hopkins rod-lens optical system whereas flexible and very narrow rigid hysteroscopes contain optical fibres.

Rigid hysteroscopes come in different sizes in terms of their outer diameter, 2.7, 2.9 and 4 mm being popular sizes. They are available at 0°, 12°, 15° and 30° angles of view, the oblique view ones being most suited to working within the uterine cavity. For any procedure other than contact hysteroscopy, at least a single sheath has to be fitted to the optic to allow uterine distension, while continuous flow sheaths permit simultaneous irrigation/suction and tend to be used for surgery (inner sheath for inflow, outer sheath for outflow).

Uterine distension

The uterine cavity is a potential space and has to be distended at relatively high pressure to afford a panoramic view. To achieve this, gas (CO_2), low-viscosity fluids (e.g. normal saline, 5% dextrose, 1.5% glycine, 3% sorbitol, 5% mannitol) or high-viscosity fluid (e.g. Hyskon, which is 32% dextran 70 in dextrose) can be used. Diagnostic hysteroscopy typically uses CO_2, or more commonly normal saline, operative hysteroscopy with mechanical instruments or laser uses normal saline, and resectoscopic surgery uses electrolyte-free solutions such as glycine, sorbitol or mannitol.

The pressure required to provide an adequate view of the uterine cavity depends on a number of factors, but tends to be around 100 mmHg (13.3 kPa). An enlarged non-compliant uterus, leakage of distension medium through the cervix or excessive suction when using a continuous flow system will mean that a higher inflow pressure is required. To achieve the desired distension, gravity, pressure bags or special hysteroscopic pumps are available. Modern pumps designed for low-viscosity fluids can not only control the intrauterine pressure with the press of a button but also monitor fluid balance, thereby reducing the risk of fluid overload. Pumps which control flow rather than pressure should not be used for hysteroscopy as they tend to over-distend and promote fluid overload.

Similarly, if using CO_2 for diagnostic hysteroscopy, a special hysteroscopic insufflator must be used as laparoscopic insufflators produce too high a pressure and too fast a flow rate of gas and risk cardiac arrhythmias or gas embolism.

Mechanical instruments

Miniature flexible or semi-rigid mechanical instruments such as scissors, grasping and biopsy forceps and monopolar electrodes can be used with operating sheaths for minor procedures such as target biopsy or polypectomy. These instruments tend to be fragile because of their size, typically 7 or 5 French gauge (3 Fr = 1 mm), so replacements should be available should they break. On the plus side, they are very unlikely to injure the patient.

Resectoscope

The resectoscope was introduced into gynaecology by Robert Neuwirth in 1978 when he described its use to resect small submucous fibroids [4]. It has since proved itself to be a highly efficient and versatile operative tool for gynaecologists just as it has been for urologists, not just for myomectomy, but for polypectomy, metroplasty, adhesiolysis and endometrial resection/ablation.

The modern resectoscope consists of five components: the optic, handle mechanism, inflow and outflow sheaths and an electrode (Plate. 36.1). The handle mechanism can be active or passive in design; for hysteroscopy, a passive handle is preferable as it maintains the electrode inside the sheathing system out of view and out of harms way. A typical resectoscope has an outer diameter of 26 or 27 Fr (8.7–9 mm), uses a 4-mm oblique view optic, and is designed for use with electrolyte-free low-viscosity distension media (remember to connect the inflow tubing to the inner sheath and the outflow to the outer sheath). Narrower 'mini' resectoscopes are now also available, essentially a paediatric instrument with a lengthened sheathing system, and this makes office/outpatient resectoscopy possible (Plate. 36.2) [5].

Traditionally, resectoscopes are monopolar instruments, but bipolar resectoscopes are gradually replacing them for reasons of safety. The electrodes themselves come in different designs, but the cutting loop (for polypectomy, myomectomy and endometrial resection), rollerball or rollerbar (for endometrial ablation or tissue vaporization) and the knife electrode (for metroplasty) are the most popular. The power settings for monopolar electrosurgery depend on the characteristics of the electrosurgical generator, the resectoscope and the patient's tissues, so it is difficult to be prescriptive, but 100–120 W pure cut or blend 1 cut if using a monopolar resectoscope is usually sufficient to avoid too much drag or charring. As always, the lowest power setting should be used to minimize the risks of electrosurgical injury.

Versapoint

Although bipolar resectoscopes are beginning to be introduced, the Gynecare Versascope™ Hysteroscopy System and Versapoint™ Bipolar Electrosurgery System (Ethicon, USA) are now widely used for office diagnostic and minor operative procedures [6]. The basic sheath of the Versascope™ is only 3.5 mm in diameter, which means that cervical dilatation is rarely necessary. The 5 Fr Versapoint™ electrodes are available in different designs (e.g. spring, twizzle, ball) and can be used for polypectomy, myomectomy of small intra-cavity fibroids, and metroplasty. As the electrodes are bipolar, physiological solutions such as normal saline and Hartmann's solution can be used for uterine distension, but a dedicated electrosurgical generator is required.

Laser hysteroscope

The clinical application of laser for intrauterine surgery was first reported by Goldrath *et al.* in 1981 [7]. The use of laser energy for hysteroscopic surgery also has the advantage over the monopolar resectoscope that distension media such as normal saline can be used. Nd:YAG is the preferred laser energy, the fibre being passed down the operating channel of a standard hysteroscope and used in contact or non-contact mode to vaporize or coagulate, respectively. As with laparoscopy, and partly because of capital and running costs and longer operating times, laser intrauterine surgery is now rarely done.

Intrauterine morcellator

In 2005, Emanual and Wamsteker described a morcellator for hysteroscopic polypectomy and myomectomy [8]. The instrument has the dual advantages that thermal energy is not required and, arguably more importantly, the tissue chips which can easily obscure the operative view with traditional instruments is not an issue. A subsequent comparative study by the same group reported that unlike with resectoscopy, there was no learning curve with the intrauterine morcellator [9]. Although a seemingly promising technique, there have been no other reports of its use.

Equipment for laparoscopy

Laparoscopes

As with rigid hysteroscopes, most laparoscopes are built around a rod-lens system and come in a range of diameters (3–12 mm) and angles of view (00–300), with 10-mm 0° scopes being the most widely used; fibreoptic microlaparoscopes are also available but are much more fragile and provide an inferior image. Operating laparoscopes have an additional operating channel for instruments or lasers but are less popular, most gynaecologists preferring to use a multipuncture approach with instruments inserted through ancillary ports. Videolaparoscopes, with CCD chips built into the tip of the instrument and three-dimensional laparoscopes are still too expensive for widespread use.

Veress needle

Traditionally, gynaecologists use a Veress needle to insufflate the abdomen with gas at the start of laparoscopy. Veress was a Hungarian chest physician who, in the 1930s [10], invented the special needle which takes his name for draining chest empyemas; when used at laparoscopy, the Veress needle's design is meant to reduce the risk of intra-abdominal injury to bowel or major blood vessels. The Veress needle is usually inserted transabdominally, but in obese patients can be introduced through the uterine fundus [11]. It is available in reusable and disposable forms.

Trocars and cannulae

Trocars and cannulae act as a conduit for the laparoscope and other instruments. They come in a variety of sizes depending on the diameter of the instrumentation to be accommodated, with 5 mm and 10–12 mm ports being the most commonly used. Traditionally, trocars and cannulae were made of surgical steel and were non-disposable, but as with most laparoscopic instruments there is growing trend for plastic disposables, coupled to an ever-growing array of designs incorporating safety shields, optical cannulae, expanding sleeves, various shaped tips and different methods of anchoring to name but a few. Of the disposable instruments, pyramidal trocar–cannula systems require the least force for insertion, while blunt conical cannulae and those with expanding sleeves produce the smallest fascial defect [12–14]. Disposable instruments are of course more expensive, but if non-disposable trocars and cannulae are being used it is important that the trocar tips are regularly sharpened to avoid having to use too much force during insertion. Non-disposable cannulae typically contain a flap or trumpet valve to prevent the leakage of gas. However, such valves can damage instruments and make laparoscopic suturing difficult, so modern disposable cannulae generally have a simple diaphragm valve.

A recent development has been single-port laparoscopic surgery variously known as SILS (single incision laparoscopic surgery), LESS (laparo-endoscopic single-site surgery), SPA (single port access) laparoscopy or eNOTES (embryonic natural orifice transumbilical endoscopic surgery). A special port is utilized that can accept up to three instruments (e.g. 5 mm × 3 or 5 mm × 2 and 12 mm × 1), and which is inserted into the peritoneal cavity via a 2–3 cm incision in the base of the umbilicus (Plate 36.3). Initially described for cholecystectomy and prostatectomy in 2008, the approach has been adopted by gynaecologists for procedures such as salpingectomy for ectopic pregnancy [15], the treatment of ovarian cysts [16], benign adnexal disease and endometriosis [17,18] and even oncologic cases [19]. Although any comparative data with conventional laparoscopic surgery is understandable limited, the early studies have put SILS and

LESS in a favourable light, although it has to be noted that all our current knowledge comes from a single unit [20–22].

Robotic laparoscopic surgery

Preceding single-port laparoscopy, but now sometimes combined, is robotic laparoscopic surgery. Robots were first used by neurosurgeons to improve the accuracy of CT-guided stereotactic brain surgery as long ago as 1988. Within a few years, robots were designed to help with transurethral prostatectomy and hip replacement. These early robots functioned in a passive manner, but their role has since evolved to a more active one commonly referred to as robotic telepresence. Originally developed to facilitate the treatment of wounded soldiers on the battlefield, the robotic telepresence technology was first utilized for cardiac surgery at the end of the 1990s, and was introduced to gynaecological laparoscopy soon afterwards.

Examples of early robots used in gynaecology included Aesop (Computer Motion Inc., USA), used to manoeuvre the laparoscope during surgery, and the more complex ZEUS (Computer Motion Inc., USA), which added two additional arms to control instruments as well as the optic. These robots have been superseded by the da Vinci surgical system (Intuitive Surgical, USA), which is currently the only robot approved by the Food and Drug Administration in the USA (Plate 36.4). The da Vinci consists of three components: the console, which allows the surgeon to control the robot remotely; the inSite vision system, which provides a three-dimensional image of the operative field via a 12-mm laparoscope; and the patient-side cart fitted with three to four robotic arms to control Endowrist instruments. The unique property of the Endowrist instruments is their ability for 7° of movement, which replicates the full range of motion of the human hand but without the fulcrum effect seen with conventional laparoscopic surgery. The claimed advantages of this system include a stable camera platform that eliminates random hand movement; hand-like motion of the instruments within the peritoneal cavity, which is not possible with traditional straight laparoscopic instruments; a three-dimensional virtual operative field, which provides improved spatial awareness compared with standard two-dimensional imaging systems; and, not least, an ergonomically comfortable position at the remote console, thus reducing the shoulder and back fatigue associated with prolonged laparoscopic operations [23]. All this comes at a price, and not surprisingly the capital and running costs of the da Vinci robotic surgery system is considerable, although treatment costs can be less than with laparotomy but not standard laparoscopy [24]. Other drawbacks of the da Vinci system include its bulk and, just as with conventional laparoscopy, the absence of tactile feedback.

The use of robotic surgery is increasing across all specialities. In gynaecology, the da Vinci system has been used for laparoscopic procedures such as hysterectomy, myomectomy, radical hysterectomy, pelvic and aortic lymphadenectomy, trachelectomy, parametrectomy, tubal anastomosis, sacrocolpopexy, treatment of endometriosis, ovarian transposition, pelvic reconstructive surgery and cervical cerclage, but the list is no doubt incomplete [25]. There are limited comparative data with conventional laparoscopy and the results are variable in terms of operating time and outcome, but broadly similar [26]. However, it does seem that learning new skills such as laparoscopic suturing is easier with the help of a robot [24].

Laparoscopic insufflator

Although 'gasless' laparoscopy has its advocates [12], the overwhelming majority of gynaecologists operate within a CO_2 pneumoperitoneum. Most of the principles of safe abdominal insufflation were established by Kurt Semm in the 1970s, and modern fast-flow insufflators are merely faster, computerized versions of his original design. As in the case of hysteroscopy, these pumps control intra-abdominal pressure rather than flow, and this should be set at 12–15 mmHg (1.6–2.0 kPa) during surgery; a higher pressure of up to 25 mmHg (3.3 kPa) is recommended during the set-up phase as this has the effect of increasing the distance between any trocar being inserted and bowel or large blood vessels, thereby, in theory at least, reducing the risk of injury [27]. Some insufflators allow the CO_2 to be warmed prior to insufflation and others have smoke traps built into them, useful when using any instrument which produces heat (e.g. electrosurgery, laser surgery).

Suction/irrigation pump

An absolute requirement for operative procedures is a suction/irrigation pump. Not only can this be used to aspirate blood and clean the pelvis, but ovarian cysts can be quickly deflated, ectopic pregnancies sucked out, and hydrodissection used in difficult cases. While a basic system using pressure bags and ordinary theatre suction unit is usable, any serious laparoscopic surgeon benefits from the convenience of a dedicated high-pressure unit.

Ancillary instruments

There is an enormous range of disposable and non-disposable instruments available for laparoscopy of various designs and sizes. The usual starting points are 5-mm instruments, although some specialist instruments are only available in larger form (e.g. retrieval bags, morcellators, certain staplers).

If the laparoscope is the eye of the surgeon, grasping forceps are the surgeon's hands. A pair of atraumatic 5-mm grasping forceps is therefore indispensable, ideally ones which are easy to lock and unlock (Fig. 36.1). Sharp

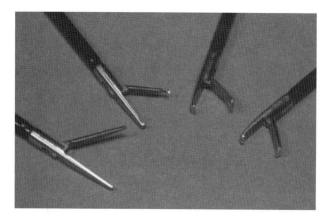

Fig. 36.1 5-mm laparoscopic grasping forceps.

Table 36.1 Methods for haemostasis at laparoscopy.

Electrosurgery
Suturing
Clips
Staples
Laser (e.g. Nd:YAG)
Harmonic scalpel
LigaSure™ (Covidien, USA)
BiClamp (ERBE Elektromedizin GmbH, Germany)
PK (Gyrus ACMI, Japan)
Argon beam coagulator
Dilute vasopressin

scissors are the other essential and the curved Mayo type are arguably the most versatile. Similarly, a suction/irrigation cannula is usually a basic requirement for surgery.

Laparoscopic surgery only became a reality once techniques were developed to control intraoperative bleeding, so it goes without saying that some method of haemostasis must be available for all but purely diagnostic procedures. There is a considerable choice of methods as listed in Table 36.1. Bipolar forceps remain the workhorse for haemostasis, and many gynaecologists use nothing else at laparoscopy. While scissors can be used electrosurgically to cut or coagulate, and may therefore be considered more convenient, they are generally monopolar instruments and require greater care to avoid unintended burns; monopolar electrosurgery is also insufficient for larger vessels (e.g. ovarian or uterine arteries).

Newer electrosurgical devices such as Ligasure, BiClamp and PK monitor the electrosurgical output to improve efficacy and efficiency but at the expense of increased costs due to the use of disposable instruments. The harmonic scalpel's attraction is that it is not an electrosurgical instrument, making distant burns an impos-

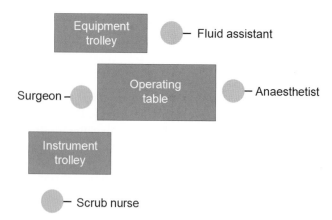

Fig. 36.2 Theatre set-up for hysteroscopic surgery.

sibility, but on the downside the instrument cuts as it coagulates and local unintended thermal injury is still a risk. Less used in gynaecology is the argon beam coagulator. Clips and staples are also available for haemostasis.

Pre-tied loop sutures, suture carriers and needle holders should be available for major procedures both for haemostasis and repair. Dilute vasopressin is used by some for myomectomy.

Retrieval bags are extremely useful and a better option than extending incisions for the removal of larger masses from the pelvis (e.g. intact ovarian cyst). Once the specimen is in the bag, it is sometimes easier to bring it out through a posterior colpotomy. The gynaecologist is fortunate that, unless the pouch of Douglas is obliterated, all patients have this exit route. Powered morcellators are an alternative, but small diameter ones tend to be time-consuming whereas large ones, although time efficient, leave a relatively large external scar.

Operating theatre organization

Hysteroscopy

While diagnostic hysteroscopy has become an outpatient procedure in most cases, and even minor operative procedures can be done under local anaesthesia, more major surgery (e.g. hysteroscopic myomectomy for a sizeable submucous fibroid) usually requires general anaesthesia. Wherever it is being done, there are a few basic principles to remember. It is best to have all the necessary equipment together on a surgical cart, with the monitor at a comfortable height and position for the operator (and patient if she is awake) (Fig. 36.2).

In the case of an operative procedure where fluid balance becomes an issue, a collecting drape should be placed under the buttocks to save any cervical leakage of irrigant. A member of staff should be appointed whose only duty is (i) to control and monitor fluid balance and

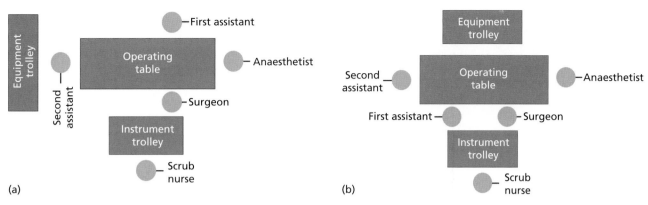

Fig. 36.3 Two schemes for theatre set-up for laparoscopic surgery: (a) first assistant holds camera (better with 0° optic); (b) operating surgeon holds camera (better with 30° optic unless first assistant is experienced).

(ii) ensure that air bubbles do not get into the inflow tubing as this risks air embolism.

Laparoscopy

The set-up for laparoscopy is more varied than for hysteroscopy partly because there tends to be more equipment and partly because laparoscopy is not 'solo' surgery but, as is the case with laparotomy, requires the help of assistants. Where they stand, where the surgical carts are placed, where the scrub nurse is situated with the ancillary instruments, and so on becomes largely a matter of personal preference.

As most gynaecologists prefer to use 0° optics, it is common for one of the assistants to stand on the contralateral side of the patient and control the laparoscope leaving the lead surgeon free to operate with two hands. Some, including myself, prefer to use a 30° laparoscope as the ability to 'look around the corner' often affords a better view when there are adhesions, fibroids or ovarian cysts. On the negative side, the use of an oblique view optic is more difficult, and I therefore prefer to control the laparoscope myself and operate single-handedly (except for suturing and tissue stripping); the first assistant's role is to hold and retract tissue (Fig. 36.3).

Diagnostic hysteroscopy

Diagnostic hysteroscopy has become a basic investigation in modern gynaecology and has replaced the time-honoured D&C (dilatation and curettage). It can be done as an outpatient procedure, and is an integral component of a one-stop approach to the management of menstrual symptoms [28]. Hysteroscopy provides a virtually instant diagnosis and is the logical precursor to operative hysteroscopy. The Royal College of Obstetricians and Gynaecologists (RCOG) recognized the importance of diagnostic hysteroscopy several years ago and it is now part of core training in our speciality. The indications and contraindi-

Table 36.2 Indications and contraindications for diagnostic hysteroscopy.

Indications
Abnormal menstruation (age >40 years)
Abnormal menstruation not responsive to medical treatment (age <40 years)
Intermenstrual bleeding despite normal cervical smear
Post-coital bleeding despite normal cervical smear
Postmenopausal bleeding (persistent or endometrial thickness ≥4 mm)
Abnormal pelvic ultrasound findings (e.g. endometrial polyps, submucous fibroids)
Subfertility
Recurrent miscarriage
Asherman's syndrome
Congenital uterine anomaly
Lost intrauterine contraceptive device

Contraindications
Pelvic infection
Pregnancy
Cervical cancer
(Heavy uterine bleeding)

cations, of which there are few, are summarized in Table 36.2. The hysteroscopic view is best in the immediate postmenstrual phase, but a diagnosis is usually possible at any time, even during menstruation. Liquid distension has several advantages over the use of CO_2 [29].

Technique

The patient should be in the correct position, i.e. lithotomy with the hips well flexed and the buttocks slightly over the edge of the table to allow unimpeded access irrespective of uterine position (Fig. 36.4). The perineum and vagina are usually washed with a warmed antiseptic solution, although there are those who do not clean the vagina. Full draping of the perineum, legs and lower abdomen is rarely required. A gentle bimanual

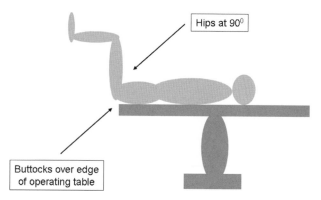

Fig. 36.4 Patient position for hysteroscopy.

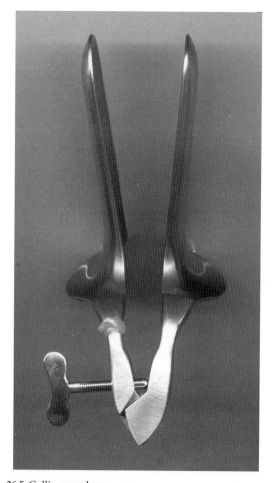

Fig. 36.5 Collin speculum.

examination should be done to determine the size and position of the uterus.

Conventional technique

The conventional approach to diagnostic hysteroscopy, and certainly the one that is quickest and easiest if the patient is asleep, is to insert a speculum into the vagina to visualize the cervix (a single-hinged Collin speculum is preferable to a Cuscoe as it can be removed once the

Table 36.3 Anaesthesia for hysteroscopy.

Intracervical local anaesthetic
Local anaesthetic spray
Local anaesthetic gel
Paracervical local anaesthetic
Regional anaesthesia
General anaesthesia
Nothing

hysteroscope has been inserted; Fig. 36.5), hold the anterior lip with a tenaculum, sound the cervix and uterine cavity, and then insert the hysteroscope with or without prior cervical dilatation depending on the calibre of the cervical canal. A similar technique can also be used in the outpatient setting, with the option of giving a local anaesthetic if required (Table 36.3); the injection of 2–4 mL of 2.2% lidocaine with 1 in 80 000 adrenaline via a dental syringe and needle is arguably the easiest and safest, but several methods of analgesia are available should the need arise [30]. Pre-emptive analgesia with non-steroidal anti-inflammatory drugs seems to make little difference to any discomfort during the procedure [31].

Unlike cystoscopy, it is better to guide the hysteroscope into the uterine cavity under direct vision rather than blindly by means of on obturator. When using an oblique-view optic, it is important to take account of this angulation by adjusting the approach accordingly (Fig. 36.6). Once in the uterine cavity, it is simply a matter of systematically inspecting the fundus, tubal areas and the four walls of the uterus by a combination of rotating (if using an oblique-view hysteroscope) and moving the hysteroscope up/down and left/right. If the view is poor, it is usually because the intrauterine pressure is too low, either because the distending medium is at a relatively low pressure or because of cervical leakage. Once the uterine cavity has been inspected, the hysteroscope is withdrawn and this is the best time to inspect the endocervical canal. A biopsy can then be taken, if indicated, using a small curette or a device such as a Pipelle, or a change made to an operative sheath for a target biopsy.

'No touch' (vaginoscopic) hysteroscopy and 'no touch' biopsy

An alternative approach to the above is 'no touch' or vaginoscopic hysteroscopy. This technique is ideally suited to the outpatient clinic as it minimizes patient discomfort by the simple fact that as no additional instruments (e.g. speculum and tenaculum) need to be inserted into the vagina, the procedure is quicker and less uncomfortable [32]. Instead, the tip of the hysteroscope is introduced into the vaginal introitus, the low-viscosity distension medium is turned on, and the hysteroscope is guided under direct vision to the external cervical os, along the cervical canal and thence the uterine cavity. This

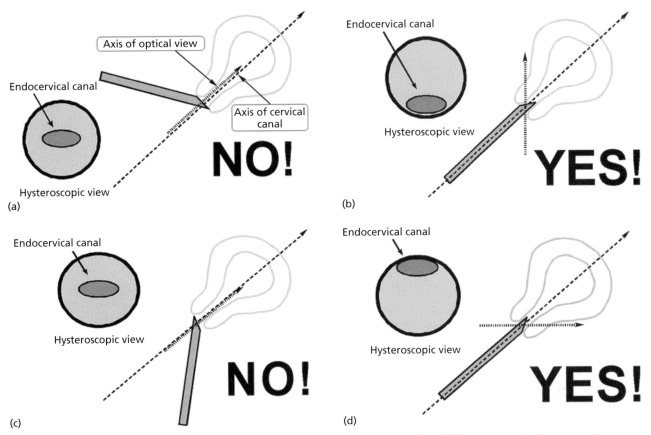

Fig. 36.6 How to insert an oblique-view hysteroscope into the uterus: (a) incorrect insertion with hysteroscope looking upwards; (b) correct insertion with hysteroscope looking upwards; (c) incorrect insertion with hysteroscope looking downwards; (d) correct insertion with hysteroscope looking downwards.

method works in the majority of cases unless there is cervical stenosis, and it is uncommon to have to stop to give local anaesthetic. As a result, this is now our default approach to outpatient hysteroscopy.

It is now also possible to take an endometrial biopsy using a 'no touch' technique without the need to instrument the uterus. Based on the Pipelle, the H Pipelle (Laboratoire C.C.D., France) is approximately twice as long but narrow enough to be passed through even a narrow diagnostic sheath. At the end of the hysteroscopy, the hysteroscope is not withdrawn from the uterus; instead the diagnostic sheath is unlocked and the optic removed to be replaced by the H Pipelle, which is pushed through the sheath into the uterine cavity (Fig. 36.7). Once the uterine fundus is reached, the sheath is pulled out of the cervix and an endometrial biopsy taken in the usual fashion [33,34].

Results

The medical literature is replete with studies of diagnostic hysteroscopy, and although arguments rage with those who favour ultrasound, it remains the gold standard technique for the assessment of the uterine cavity. Even outpatient hysteroscopy has been shown to have a success rate of well over 90%, particularly if a narrow hystero-

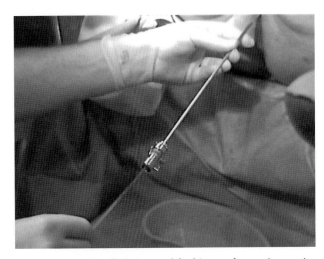

Fig. 36.7 The H Pipelle being used for biopsy after vaginoscopic or 'no touch' hysteroscopy.

scope and a 'no touch' technique is used [35]. The detection rate of pathology depends on the indication, but about 40–50% of women with menstrual symptoms will have positive findings, chiefly fibroids and polyps [36], and figures as high as 60% have been reported in infertility [37,38].

Complications

Diagnostic hysteroscopy is a safe procedure, and complications are uncommon [36]. Perhaps the most frequently seen problem is pain when negotiating the cervix or distending the uterine cavity, and a vasovagal reaction to cervical dilatation. The simple act of stopping and providing local anaesthesia is usually enough to solve the problem, and it is rare to have to resort to giving atropine for a bradycardia. Uterine perforation should not happen if the hysteroscope is introduced under direct vision unless there is extreme cervical stenosis; in this situation, insertion of the hysteroscope under ultrasound guidance is a useful ploy, as may be prior priming with misoprostol [39]. Infection and excessive bleeding are rarely seen.

Table 36.4 Operative hysteroscopic procedures.

Adhesiolysis
Endometrial ablation/resection
Metroplasty
Myomectomy
Polypectomy
Proximal fallopian tube cannulation
Removal of intrauterine contraceptive device
Target biopsy
Treatment of cervical and interstitial pregnancy
Treatment of missed abortion
Tubal sterilization

Summary box 36.1

Diagnostic hysteroscopy:

1. A vaginoscopic ('No touch') technique is ideal for outpatient/office diagnostic hysteroscopy as in most women it can be done without the need to insert a vaginal speculum, apply a tenaculum, sound the uterus or use local anaesthesia.
2. When using an oblique-view hysteroscope (e.g. 12° or 30°), you must make an allowance for the fact that the optic is angled, particularly during insertion of the hysteroscope through the cervical canal to avoid traumatizing the cervix or even perforating the uterus.
3. Liquid uterine distension with low viscosity fluids such as N/Saline has the advantage over gaseous distension with CO_2 that a special pump is not required, there are no bubbles, any menstrual blood is washed away and it is more suited to operative procedures.

Operative hysteroscopy

Hysteroscopic surgery has a number of well-defined indications (Table 36.4), and is the treatment of choice for polypectomy, myomectomy for intra-cavity or submucous fibroids, adhesiolysis and metroplasty. The various techniques of endometrial destruction have been superseded to some extent by the newer second-generation ablative techniques which are technically easier to perform [40]. Newer indications for hysteroscopic surgery include the treatment of missed abortion, cervical and interstitial pregnancies and, above all, tubal sterilization [41]. Devices such as the Essure Permanent Birth Control System (Conceptus, Inc., USA) and Adiana Permanent Contraception System (Hologic, Inc., USA) are already available and, as newer reversible procedures become available, are likely to replace laparoscopic sterilization [42].

Any of the modalities already discussed can be used for surgery, but the resectoscope remains the most versatile of instruments for more major intrauterine surgery, and is a skill well worth learning. The Versapoint system, and in my view the mini resectoscope, are useful alternatives for minor office procedures. Pretreatment to thin the endometrium and make it less fluffy is often worthwhile if surgery is likely to be relatively prolonged as it improves the operating conditions for the surgeon, although there is little advantage in terms of outcome and of course it adds to the cost of treatment [43]. If used, the choice is between GnRH analogues, danazol, a progestogen or the combined pill, usually for at least 6 weeks prior to surgery. The alternative is either to time the operation to just after menstruation, which can be difficult in a busy clinical service, or to curette the endometrium prior to hysteroscopy, but neither is as good as formal endometrial preparation.

Technique

Although minor procedures using mechanical instruments or Versapoint can be done under local anaesthesia, more major cases are generally managed under general anaesthesia. Even such cases, however, can be carried out under local anaesthesia combined with light sedation. For instance, our regimen still consists of premedication with diclofenac and temazepam, followed by small doses of midazolam and fentanyl or alfentanyl in the operating theatre, finished with intracervical, paracervical and intrauterine local anaesthetic injections, the latter given via an injection needle option on our resectoscope [44].

There is insufficient space here to describe how to use all the various instruments available to the hysteroscopic surgeon or how to carry out specific procedures, but because of its versatility and usefulness, it is worth discussing the principles of using the resectoscope safely and effectively.

Using a resectoscope

The resectoscope is a very powerful instrument that has to be used correctly to ensure the safety of the patient. The first step is to dilate the cervix sufficiently to allow easy insertion but not to over-dilate and risk excessive leakage of the uterine irrigant and poor distension; dilating to 1 mm above the diameter of the resectoscope is adequate for this, for example we dilate to Hegar 10 when using a 26 Fr (8.7 mm) diameter resectoscope. Once the resectoscope has been inserted and the decision made that hysteroscopic surgery can proceed, there are three cardinal rules to remember.

1 The electrode should only be activated as it is being moved into the resectoscope sheath, i.e. towards the cervix; activating the electrode as it is being pushed out risks uterine perforation, a potentially life-threatening complication. The only exception to this rule is metroplasty when the cut has to be made towards the uterine fundus.

2 The myometrium should not be cut too deeply, particularly at the cornu and in the cervix; if cut ends of arterioles become visible, the resection is too deep. Cutting deeply does not only risk uterine perforation, but also major haemorrhage.

3 Fluid balance should be monitored continuously. Several methods of fluid monitoring have been suggested (e.g. assessment of central venous pressure, serial measurement of serum sodium, osmolality or tracer substances such as 1% ethanol, weighing the patient), but the simplest is to keep an inflow/outflow chart. In any event, surgery should be stopped if fluid absorption exceeds 1.5–2 L to avoid serious fluid overload and a transurethral resection of prostate (TURP)-like syndrome [45].

Results

Provided the indication is appropriate, hysteroscopic surgery can be highly effective. The literature concerning polypectomy, whether intrauterine or cervical, is not extensive but, logically, removal of polyps under direct vision is likely to be superior to blind curettage [46–48]. In contrast, there are numerous series showing the efficacy of hysteroscopic myomectomy, particularly when the uterus is not grossly enlarged and the fibroid(s) are mainly intra-cavitary [49,50]. Metroplasty should no longer be done by laparotomy [51], and the same applies to the treatment of Asherman's syndrome [52,53]. Hysteroscopic endometrial resection and ablation have been subjected to numerous randomized trials and cost–benefit analyses showing that they are effective and useful alternatives to hysterectomy but are no more effective than the newer second-generation techniques [54]. The Mirena IUS (Schering) is of course another effective alternative for such patients [55].

Complications

Although complications are uncommon with operative hysteroscopy [56], anyone carrying out hysteroscopic surgery should be aware of the risks, their prevention and management (Table 36.5). Uterine perforation is the most

Table 36.5 Complications of operative hysteroscopy.

Early
Uterine perforation
Fluid overload
Haemorrhage
Gas embolism
Infection
Cervical trauma
Electrosurgical burn

Late
Intrauterine adhesions
Uterine rupture in pregnancy (after metroplasty or myomectomy)
Haematometra (after endometrial ablation)
Post-ablation sterilization syndrome (after endometrial ablation)
Pregnancy (after endometrial ablation)
Cancer (after endometrial ablation)

feared complication because if it occurs while the hysteroscope is being activated, major intra-abdominal trauma can result with haemorrhage and viscus injury. The first sign of perforation might be sudden loss of uterine distension or rapid absorption of fluid. A laparoscopy and arguably a laparotomy is mandatory to check the abdominal contents; if there is no injury, hysteroscopic surgery can continue once the perforation has been sutured. Perforation is most likely when using the resectoscope with a cutting loop, although proper technique can greatly reduce this risk [57].

Fluid overload with low-viscosity fluids, particularly those which are electrolyte-free, is the second fear of the hysteroscopic surgeon. Fluid is absorbed throughout surgery by intravasation and transtubal loss. Apart from the cardiac and pulmonary effects, major electrolyte imbalance can result with build-up of free fluid in the brain, hyponatraemia and dilutional hypo-osmolality, resulting in cerebral oedema, increased intracranial pressure and cellular necrosis [56]. This complication is totally avoidable by proper monitoring during surgery and stopping the procedure before the patient is placed at risk. We also catheterize the bladder and give a low dose of frusemide once fluid absorption exceeds 1.5 L to induce a diuresis, monitoring recovery by regular assay of serum sodium.

Intraoperative haemorrhage can accompany uterine perforation but is more often a sign of surgery deep in the myometrium. Electrocoagulation (or laser coagulation) of the offending vessel can be one solution, but if the bleeding persists at the end of the procedure, tamponade for a few hours with a balloon catheter usually works.

Air embolism is a rare but devastating complication [58]. It usually happens if air is allowed to enter the distension tubing, typically when bags of irrigant are being changed. Air embolism is therefore entirely preventable.

Infection is rare after hysteroscopic surgery. There is no evidence for routine use of antibiotics [59], although some surgeons prefer to administer them.

As noted earlier, cervical priming with misoprostol has been proposed as a means of facilitating insertion of the hysteroscope into the uterine cavity and reducing the risk of cervical lacerations during dilatation [39], but this is a very rare complication.

The late adverse consequences of endometrial ablation are all relatively rare. Cervical stenosis in the presence of functional endometrial tissue can lead to the development of haematometra, and women who have been sterilized can develop painful swellings of the fallopian tubes secondary to retrograde menstruation [60]. Pregnancies have been reported, many with complications [61]. A handful of cases of endometrial cancer have been described after endometrial ablation, but the majority of women had risk factors [62].

Summary box 36.2

Resectoscope surgery:
1. Passive and active resectoscopes require opposite hand movement for cutting, so get used to one or the other – passive resectoscopes are more suited to intrauterine surgery.
2. Bipolar resectoscopes should be used in preference to monopolar instruments because more physiological, electrolyte-containing fluid can be used for uterine distension and irrigation. Fluid overload can still occur, but the associated electrolyte disturbances will be less serious.
3. Small calibre, mini-resectoscopes are ideal for minor outpatient/office intrauterine surgery.

Diagnostic laparoscopy

Having replaced culdoscopy in the 1960s and 1970s, diagnostic laparoscopy has been an accepted part of gynaecological care even longer than diagnostic hysteroscopy. It is usually done as an inpatient procedure under general anaesthesia, although microlaparoscopes have been used with some success [63]. The main indication for diagnostic laparoscopy is the investigation of pelvic pain and subfertility (Table 36.6). While the list of contraindications is relatively long, few patients fall into these categories.

Technique

As with hysteroscopy, it is important to position the patient correctly on the operating table. Again, this means ensuring that the buttocks are over the edge of the table to allow full uterine anteversion. The legs are ideally placed in hydraulic leg supports with the thighs at about

Table 36.6 Indications and contraindications for diagnostic laparoscopy.

Indications
Acute or chronic pelvic pain
Ectopic pregnancy
Pelvic inflammatory disease (including TB)
Endometriosis
Adnexal torsion
Subfertility
Congenital pelvic abnormality
Abnormal pelvic scan
Unexplained pelvic mass
Staging for ovarian malignancy

Absolute and relative contraindications
Mechanical or paralytic bowel obstruction
Generalized peritonitis
Diaphragmatic hernia
Major intraperitoneal haemorrhage (e.g. shock)
Severe cardiorespiratory disease
Massive obesity
Inflammatory bowel disease
Large abdominal mass
Advanced pregnancy
Multiple abdominal incisions
Irreducible external hernia

45° to the horizontal while ensuring that the hips can be extended sufficiently to bring the thighs in line with the trunk should the need arise for any abdominal (cf. pelvic) surgery (Fig. 36.8).

After washing and draping, the bladder is checked and, if full, emptied with a catheter. Bimanual examination will also confirm the size, position and mobility of the uterus as well as any adnexal or rectovaginal pathology. The uterus is sounded and a uterine cannula inserted, firstly to permit effective uterine manipulation and secondly to allow for hydrotubation if required; should the uterus be retroverted, it is worthwhile attempting to forcibly antevert it by rotating the uterine cannula 180° as this will greatly improve access to the pouch of Douglas at laparoscopy.

Subumbilical insufflation

Although open and gasless laparoscopy have their proponents, for most gynaecologists laparoscopy starts with insufflation of the peritoneal cavity with CO_2 using a Veress needle (closed laparoscopy) [64]. The spring mechanism of the Veress needle should be checked as this is an essential safety feature. It is also useful to carry out a pressure test, i.e. check the flow of gas through the needle, making a note of the pressure in the tubing as this information can be used later to confirm proper intraperitoneal placement. The usual insertion point for the Veress needle is the inferior border of the umbilicus, via a verti-

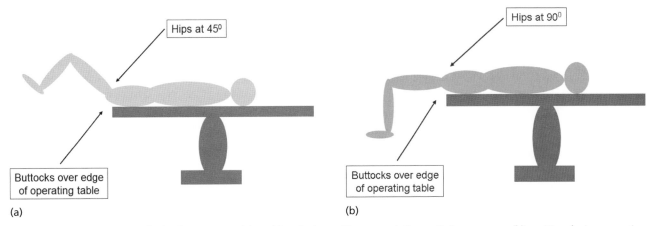

Fig. 36.8 Patient positioning during laparoscopy: (a) position during setting up and diagnostic laparoscopy; (b) position during operative laparoscopy which allows pelvic and abdominal surgery.

Table 36.7 Technique for subumbilical insufflation and insertion of the primary port.

1 Palpate for aorta
2 Elevate anterior abdominal wall (to increase distance between needle and bowel/major vessels)
3 Aim Veress needle and trocar and cannula towards the hollow of the sacrum (away from major vessels)
4 Create a high-pressure pneumoperitoneum prior to inserting umbilical trocar and cannula (to increase distance between needle and bowel/major vessels)
5 Insert trocar and cannula no more than a few centimetres into the peritoneal cavity (to reduce risk of bowel or vascular injury)
6 Avoid Trendelenburg tilt (head down) until laparoscope has been inserted (to avoid bringing major vessels closer to umbilicus)
7 Avoid excessive force during insertion (to limit the distance the instruments advance into the peritoneal cavity

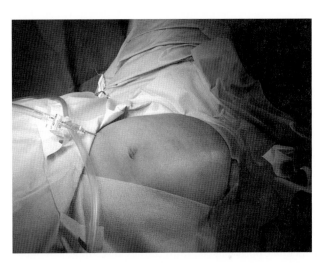

Fig. 36.9 CO_2 insufflation via Palmer's point.

cal midline incision long enough to accommodate the umbilical trocar and cannula.

The actual technique of inserting the Veress needle and subsequently the trocar and cannula for the laparoscope are summarized in Table 36.7. The aim is to instrument the peritoneal cavity without causing any unnecessary trauma; it should be remembered, for instance, that the aortic bifurcation is inferior to the umbilicus in a significant proportion of women, and umbilical instrumentation should take account of this [65].

Once the Veress needle is in place, correct positioning can be checked using Palmer's test; the basis of the test is that saline in a syringe should be sucked into the peritoneal cavity because of its negative pressure. Alternatively, the gas tubing can be connected and the initial Veress intraperitoneal pressure noted; a pressure greater than 10 mmHg (1.33 kPa) and slow flow of gas at high pressures once the insufflator is started both mean incorrect placement, and the Veress should be repositioned [64].

It is reasonable to insufflate to a relatively high intra-abdominal pressure, for example 20–25 mmHg (2.66–3.3 kPa) to reduce the risk of viscus injury during insertion of the primary trocar and cannula. Once the correct distension has been reached, the gas is switched off, the Veress needle removed and the trocar and cannula inserted, again taking care to aim towards the sacral hollow. Some gynaecologists manually elevate the lower abdominal wall at this time, others press the upper abdomen to increase the gas bubble in front of the oncoming trocar.

Insufflation via Palmer's point

A well-recognized alternative to subumbilical insufflation is the use of Palmer's point, which is situated in the left mid-clavicular line approximately 3 cm below the costal margin (Fig. 36.9). The left upper quadrant of the abdomen is the area least likely to be affected by adhesions, so Palmer's point is useful when there is concern about possible lower abdominal or periumbilical adhesions (e.g. previous laparotomy) or when faced with a large pelvic mass [66]. It is useful to remember that one study found periumbilical adhesions in 21.4% of women with a history of low transverse laparotomy and in 53.1% of those who had undergone midline laparotomy [67]. The technique of entry is similar to that already described.

Open laparoscopy

There is much debate about the relative safety of 'closed' and 'open' laparoscopy, which was in fact first described by Hasson, a gynaecologist, in 1970 (for an update and description of the technique see Hasson *et al.* [68]). While open laparoscopy is favoured by surgeons, and this approach is claimed to reduce the risk of vascular injury, the case is by no means proven [69,70]. However, there have been no large-scale randomized comparisons and, for now at least, the overwhelming majority of gynaecologists continue to use a Veress needle for insufflation [71].

Technique

Insertion of ancillary port(s)
Once the laparoscope has been inserted, the patient can be placed head down to encourage the bowel out of the pelvis and lower abdomen; the greater the tilt, the better the view of the pelvis but the more difficult it is for the anaesthetist to ventilate the patient. A quick check is made of the abdominal cavity, and one or two ancillary ports are inserted in the lower abdomen. Injury by the ancillary ports can be minimized by inserting them under direct vision, having identified the deep and superficial epigastric vessels and the bladder [72].

A useful concept here is that of the 'safe triangle', which is bounded by the umbilical ligaments (remnants of the umbilical vessels) laterally with the symphysis pubis as its base and the umbilicus as its apex (Plate 36.5); although the position of the inferior epigastric vessels can be variable [73], their course is always lateral to the safe triangle (Plate 36.6). Ports should therefore be placed either inside the safe triangle or lateral to the inferior epigastric vessels.

Inspecting the pelvis and abdomen
It is not possible to inspect the pelvis properly without using at least one probe or grasper to manipulate the pelvic organs. Once the upper abdomen has been checked, bowel in the cul-de-sac should be gently pushed cephalad. The best way to inspect the adnexa and pelvic side wall is to grasp, lift and rotate the ovary towards the ipsilateral round ligament, a manoeuvre which also reveals the course of the ureter (Plate 36.7). Do not forget to inspect the uterovesical fold, which can be the sole site of endometriosis. Tubal patency can then be checked by hydrotubation with dilute methylene blue solution.

Ending the procedure
The ancillary ports should be removed under direct vision followed by deflation of the abdomen via the port used for the optic. By keeping the laparoscope inside the cannula as it is being withdrawn, it is possible to check that this port site is not bleeding and has not caught a loop of bowel or omentum. The fascia in lateral ports greater than 10 mm should be formally closed to prevent herniation [74].

Results
The rate of detection of pathology very much depends on the indication for the laparoscopy. Some abnormalities will be obvious from preoperative investigation, usually ultrasound, where laparoscopy is merely used to confirm or clarify the diagnosis. Although diagnostic laparoscopy is no longer recommended as a standard investigation for all infertile couples [75], the detection rate for unexpected conditions such as endometriosis and pelvic adhesions is about 20% [76]. In the case of chronic pelvic pain, about two-thirds of cases will have a positive laparoscopy, endometriosis being found in one-third [77].

Complications
Diagnostic laparoscopy is a safe procedure with published complication rates of 2–4 per 1000 [78]. By definition, as no laparoscopic surgery is being done, most complications occur during the set-up phase of the procedure when the abdomen is being instrumented (e.g. injury to the inferior epigastric vessels or major retroperitoneal vessels, bowel injury). Bleeding from the inferior epigastrics should be avoidable with good technique, but if does occur a variety of instruments and techniques have been described to control the bleeding [79]. Injury to retroperitoneal vessels usually requires immediate laparotomy, whereas bowel injury can be managed laparoscopically provided the perforation is small and there is minimal faecal soiling [80].

Operative laparoscopy

Laparoscopy is becoming the preferred route of surgery for an increasing number of conditions traditionally carried out by laparotomy (Table 36.8). Provided there are no obvious contraindications, such as the presence of a large abdominal mass which would make access difficult or extensive malignancy requiring debulking, and provided the surgical skills and equipment are both available, there are few limits for the laparoscopic surgeon. This does not mean that laparoscopy is the best option or should be done in all these cases, and there is much debate about the more complex procedures in particular. In fact, only a few procedures have been subjected to prospective randomized comparisons (e.g. ectopic pregnancy, colposuspension, endometriosis, hysterectomy), so

Table 36.8 RCOG classification of laparoscopic procedures.

Level 1
Diagnostic laparoscopy
Sterilization
Aspiration of ovarian cyst
Ovarian biopsy

Level 2
Division of filmy adhesions
Linear salpingotomy or salpingectomy for ectopic pregnancy
Salpingostomy for infertility
Ovarian cystectomy
Treatment of endometrioma
Salpingo-oophorectomy
Ovarian drilling with laser or diathermy for polycystic ovaries
Treatment of AFS stage I and II endometriosis
Myomectomy for pedunculated subserous fibroid
Uterosacral nerve ablation (LUNA)
Laparoscopic-assisted vaginal hysterectomy without significant
    associated pathology

Level 3
Division of thick adhesions
Laparoscopic-assisted vaginal hysterectomy with significant
    associated pathology
Total laparoscopic hysterectomy
Myomectomy for intramural fibroids
Treatment of AFS stage III and IV endometriosis
Pelvic and aortic lymphadenectomy
Pelvic side wall and ureteric dissection
Presacral neurectomy
Incontinence procedures
Prolapse procedures

in many cases the decision about the route of surgery depends more on the particular skills of the gynaecologist, the presence of contraindications, and the relative risks of complications.

Technique

There is insufficient space to describe individual procedures, but the following considerations and techniques are generally applicable to operative laparoscopy.

Ancillary port placement

Operative laparoscopy inevitably requires multiple ports, and two to three ancillary ports are the norm. The ports are most usefully placed well lateral to the inferior epigastric vessels, and should be inserted high enough so that any instrument can be used on both sides of the pelvis. If there is to be anything more than the occasional suturing, a 10-mm port will allow the insertion of curved needles without having to remove the ports with each suture [81]; a larger cannula will also accept larger diameter instruments (e.g. SEMM's claw forceps).

Tissue dissection and hydrodissection

The principles of dissection and adhesiolysis are the same as at laparotomy, i.e. traction and counter-traction. Dissection can be done with scissors, and if any powered instruments are used (e.g. electrosurgery, harmonic scalpel, laser), care has to be taken to avoid thermal damage to nearby structures. High-pressure irrigation can sometimes facilitate dissection as well as protect underlying structures from thermal injury.

Safe use of electrosurgery

Electrosurgery is widely used at laparoscopy for haemostasis as well as cutting. As electrosurgical injury is one of the most feared complications, it is essential that gynaecologists understand how to use this modality safely [82]. Whatever instrument is used, it should only be activated when in view of the laparoscope, and the electrode(s) should be withdrawn fully into the cannula afterwards to avoid accidental injury. Electrosurgery should only be used close to bowel or other vital structures in short bursts, if at all. The surgeon should be aware of risks due to insulation failure, direct and capacitive coupling, and remember that the electrodes remain hot for a few seconds after activation.

Laparoscopic suturing

The ability to suture extracorporeally and intracorporeally is an extremely useful skill and can mean the difference between a successful laparoscopy and laparotomy. Pre-tied loop sutures are the easiest to use and are ideal for procedures such as salpingectomy. Untied ties can be used to tie off adhesions or vascular pedicles (e.g. infundibulo-pelvic ligament at hysterectomy or salpingo-oophorectomy) and are secured with slip knots (e.g. Roeder, Weston or surgeon's knot) and a knot pusher. Needle sutures are used to repair incisions (e.g. uterine repair at myomectomy), and can be tied extracorporeally or tied inside the body in the case of delicate tissue (e.g. ovarian repair after cystectomy).

Results

Laparoscopic surgery, for whatever indication, is typically associated with less postoperative discomfort, shorter hospitalization and faster return to normal activities than laparotomy [83]. On the downside, the more complex procedures tend to take longer, and the operating time is less predictable [84]. Cost comparisons produce variable results, a longer operating time and the use disposable instruments often outweighing any advantages of shorter hospitalization [85].

Complications

Laparoscopic surgery appears to be inherently safer than conventional surgery [86]. However, although the overall complication rate is generally less, this is not inevitable

Table 36.9 Complications of laparoscopic surgery.

Intraoperative
Bowel injury
Vascular injury
Bladder injury
Ureteric injury
Surgical emphysema
Anaesthetic complications

Postoperative
Unrecognized visceral or vascular injury
Venous thromboembolism
Infection
Port site hernia

[87] (Table 36.9). What is definitely true is that (i) major complications such as viscus injury and bleeding from retroperitoneal vessels are more common and (ii) many of the injuries are unfortunately not recognized during the procedure.

The reported rate of complications from major national surveys give an overall figure of 7–12.6 per 1000 procedures, with the more complex procedures having a greater risk of injury [88,89]. More specifically, the risk of intra-operative intestinal injury has been estimated as 1.6–2.4 per 1000, major vascular injuries as 0.3 per 1000, and damage to the urinary tract as 2–8.5 per 1000 cases. Laparoscopic hysterectomy, in particular, places the ureter at risk of injury [90]. About one-third to half of complications occur during the set-up phase, and one-quarter are not recognized during the surgery, including more than half of bowel and ureteric injuries [91]. Conversion to laparotomy is required, on average, in 2% of patients [92]. The mortality after gynaecological laparoscopy is 4.4 per 100 000, which compares with a mortality of 150 per 100 000 for hysterectomy for benign indications [93].

> **Summary box 36.3**
>
> Laparoscopy:
> 1. Palmer's point is the safest entry point if there is concern about adhesions from previous surgery.
> 2. Any instrument which produces heat (e.g. electrosurgery, laser, harmonic scalpel, etc.) should be used extremely carefully, if at all, close to vital structures such as bowel and ureter.
> 3. The course of the ureter must be identified when performing any surgery on the pelvic side wall to avoid accidental injury.
> 4. Most ureteric and bowel injuries are not recognised at the time of primary surgery. Excessive postoperative pain should be deemed as secondary to bowel injury unless proven otherwise.

Informed consent for endoscopy

There is still a common misconception among patients that keyhole surgery converts a 'major' surgical procedure into a 'minor' one, and not only is the cosmetic result better and recovery faster, but the risks are also lessened. The reality is that it is only the incision size which is different. It is not surprising therefore that if there is a problem, patients often assume there has been negligence. As a result, endoscopic surgery has become one of the major areas of medical litigation in gynaecology [94,95].

The Department of Health as well as the General Medical Council have issued guidelines regarding informed consent for surgery, and there is also much useful information available on the internet on this topic. While appropriate indications for surgery and good surgical technique are basic requirements for effective patient care, the patients also have to be provided with sufficient information on which to base their decision to undergo a particular procedure. All patients should be told not only what and why they are undergoing a particular procedure, but also warned about the relative risks of MAS compared with conventional surgery. In particular, patients need to be aware that any endoscopic operation may have to be converted to laparotomy and that bowel, bladder and ureteric injury are accepted risks with laparoscopy, and uterine perforation and fluid overload with hysteroscopy.

Training in endoscopic surgery

One area which MAS has changed for ever is surgical training. Endoscopic surgery is very different to conventional surgery and it probably takes longer to acquire the necessary skills to operate without the benefits of direct vision and tissue handling.

As an acknowledgement of the importance of hysteroscopic and laparoscopic surgery to modern gynaecological care, coupled to a wish to improve and structure training in this area, the RCOG, for instance, have made basic endoscopic surgery (Level 1 hysteroscopy and laparoscopy) a core curriculum subject for trainees. The RCOG has appointed preceptors and has developed Special Skills Modules for advanced hysteroscopic and laparoscopic surgery as a means of accreditation for those wishing to extend their skills. This is the first time that surgical proficiency in a particular area has been so tested and these modules may yet prove to be models for other surgical procedures.

Another aspect of surgical training which is undergoing a minor revolution is the use of video training and, more recently, virtual training (computer simulation) [96,97]. It is now accepted that apprentice-based learning is costly, time-consuming and of variable efficacy. Added to this, reduction in junior doctors' hours has been inevitably paralleled by a reduction in exposure to surgery. In such an environment, video and virtual reality training has been shown to have the capacity to improve the standard surgical training [98].

References

1 Semm K. Endoscopic appendectomy. *Endoscopy* 1983;15:59–64.

2 Magos A, Kosmas I, Sharma M, Buck L, Chapman L, Taylor A. Digital recording of surgical procedures using a personal computer. *Eur J Obstet Gynecol Reprod Biol* 2005;120:206–209.

3 Papadopoulos N, Polyzos D, Gambadauro P, Papalampros P, Chapman L, Magos A. Do patients want to see recordings of their surgery? *Eur J Obstet Gynecol Reprod Biol* 2008;138: 89–92.

4 Neuwirth RS. A new technique for and additional experience with hysteroscopic resection of submucous fibroids. *Am J Obstet Gynecol* 1978;131:91–94.

5 Papalampros P, Gambadauro P, Papadopoulos N, Polyzos D, Chapman L, Magos A. The mini-resectoscope: a new instrument for office hysteroscopic surgery. *Acta Obstet Gynecol Scand* 2008;88:227–230.

6 Garuti C, Luerty M. Hysteroscopic bipolar surgery: a valuable progress or a technique under investigation? *Curr Opin Obstet Gynecol* 2009;21:329–334.

7 Goldrath MH, Fuller TA, Segal S. Laser photovaporization of endometrium for the treatment of menorrhagia. *Am J Obstet Gynecol* 1981;140:14–19.

8 Emanuel MH, Wamsteker K. The Intra Uterine Morcellator: a new hysteroscopic operating technique to remove intrauterine polyps and myomas. *J Minim Invasive Gynecol* 2005;12:62–66.

9 van Dongen H, Emanuel MH, Wolterbeek R, Trimbos JB, Jansen FW. Hysteroscopic morcellator for removal of intrauterine polyps and myomas: a randomized controlled pilot study among residents in training. *J Minim Invasive Gynecol* 2008;15: 466–471.

10 Gordon AG, Magos AL. The development of laparoscopic surgery. *Baillieres Clin Obstet Gynaecol* 1989;3:429–449.

11 Pasic RP, Kantardzic M, Templeman C, Levine RL. Insufflation techniques in gynecologic laparoscopy. *Surg Laparosc Endosc Percutan Tech* 2006;16:18–23.

12 Tarnay CM, Glass KB, Munro MG. Entry force and intra-abdominal pressure associated with six laparoscopic trocar-cannula systems: a randomized comparison. *Obstet Gynecol* 1999;94:83–88.

13 Tarnay CM, Glass KB, Munro MG. Incision characteristics associated with six laparoscopic trocar-cannula systems: a randomized, observer-blinded comparison. *Obstet Gynecol* 1999;94: 89–93.

14 Yim SF, Yuen PM. Randomized double-masked comparison of radially expanding access device and conventional cutting tip trocar in laparoscopy. *Obstet Gynecol* 2001;97:435–438.

15 Savaris RF, Cavazzola LT. Ectopic pregnancy: laparoendoscopic single-site surgery. Laparoscopic surgery through a single cutaneous incision. *Fertil Steril* 2009;92:1170.e5–e7.

16 Fagotti A, Fanfani F, Marocco F, Rossitto C, Gallotta V, Scambia G. Laparoendoscopic single-site surgery (LESS) for ovarian cyst enucleation: report of first 3 cases. *Fertil Steril* 2009;92:168. e13–16.

17 Kim TJ, Lee YY, Kim MJ *et al.* Single port access laparoscopic adnexal surgery. *J Minim Invasive Gynecol* 2009;16:612–5.

18 Escobar PF, Bedaiwy MA, Fader AN, Falcone T. Laparoendoscopic single-site (LESS) surgery in patients with benign adnexal disease. *Fertil Steril* 2010;93:2074.e7–e10.

19 Fader AN, Escobar PF. Laparoendoscopic single-site surgery (LESS) in gynecologic oncology: technique and initial report. *Gynecol Oncol* 2009;114:157–161.

20 Yim GW, Jung YW, Paek J *et al.* Transumbilical single-port access versus conventional total laparoscopic hysterectomy: surgical outcomes. *Am J Obstet Gynecol* 2010;203:26.e1–e6.

21 Kim TJ, Lee YY, Cha HH *et al.* Single-port-access laparoscopic-assisted vaginal hysterectomy versus conventional laparoscopic-assisted vaginal hysterectomy: a comparison of perioperative outcomes. *Surg Endosc* 2010;24:2248–2252.

22 Lee YY, Kim TJ, Kim CJ *et al.* Single port access laparoscopic adnexal surgery versus conventional laparoscopic adnexal surgery: a comparison of peri-operative outcomes. *Eur J Obstet Gynecol Reprod Biol* 2010;151:181–184.

23 Ahmed K, Khan MS, Vats A *et al.* Current status of robotic assisted pelvic surgery and future developments. *Int J Surg* 2009;7:431–440.

24 Bell MC, Torgerson J, Seshadri-Kreaden U, Suttle AW, Hunt S. Comparison of outcomes and cost for endometrial cancer staging via traditional laparotomy, standard laparoscopy and robotic techniques. *Gynecol Oncol* 2008;111:407–411.

25 Schreuder HW, Verheijen RH. Robotic surgery. *BJOG* 2009;116:198–213.

26 Chen CC, Falcone T. Robotic gynecologic surgery: past, present, and future. *Clin Obstet Gynecol* 2009;52:335–343.

27 Reich H, Ribeiro SC, Rasmussen C, Rosenberg J, Vidali A. High-pressure trocar insertion technique. *JSLS* 1999;3:45–48.

28 Baskett TF, O'Connor H, Magos AL. A comprehensive one-stop menstrual problem clinic for the diagnosis and management of abnormal uterine bleeding. *Br J Obstet Gynaecol* 1996;103: 76–77.

29 Nagele F, Bournas N, O'Connor H, Broadbent M, Richardson R, Magos A. Comparison of carbon dioxide and normal saline for uterine distension in outpatient hysteroscopy. *Fertil Steril* 1996;62:305–309.

30 Cooper NA, Khan KS, Clark TJ. Local anaesthesia for pain control during outpatient hysteroscopy: systematic review and meta-analysis. *BMJ* 2010;340:c1130.

31 Nagele F, Lockwood G, Magos AL. Randomised placebo controlled trial of mefenamic acid for premedication at outpatient hysteroscopy: a pilot study. *Br J Obstet Gynaecol* 1997;104:842–844.

32 Cooper NAM, Smith P, Khan KS, Clark JT. Vaginoscopic approach to outpatient hysteroscopy: a systematic review of the effect on pain. *BJOG* 2010;117:532–539.

33 Di Spiezio SA, Sharma M, Taylor A, Buck L, Magos A. A new device for 'no touch' biopsy at 'no touch' hysteroscopy: the H Pipelle. *Am J Obstet Gynecol* 2004;191:157–158.

34 Madari S, Al-Shabibi N, Papalampros P, Papadimitriou A, Magos A. A randomized trial comparing the H Pipelle with the standard Pipelle for endometrial sampling at 'no touch' (vaginoscopic) hysteroscopy. *BJOG* 2009;116:32–37.

35 Di Spiezio Sardo A, Taylor A, Tsirkas P, Mastrogamvrakis G, Sharma M, Magos A. Hysteroscopy: a technique for all?

Analysis of 5,000 outpatient hysteroscopies. *Fertil Steril* 2008;89:438–443.

36 Nagele F, O'Connor H, Davies A, Badawy A, Mohamed H, Magos A. 2500 outpatient diagnostic hysteroscopies. *Obstet Gynecol* 1996;88:87–92.

37 Valle RF. Hysteroscopy in the evaluation of female infertility. *Am J Obstet Gynecol* 1980;137:425–431.

38 Preutthipan S, Linasmita V. A prospective comparative study between hysterosalpingography and hysteroscopy in the detection of intrauterine pathology in patients with infertility. *J Obstet Gynaecol Res* 2003;29:33–37.

39 Crane JM, Healey S. Use of misoprostol before hysteroscopy: a systematic review. *J Obstet Gynaecol Can* 2006;28:373–379.

40 Practice Committee of the American Society for Reproductive Medicine. Indications and options for endometrial ablation. *Fertil Steril* 2008;90(Suppl 1):S236–S240.

41 Vilos GA, Abu-Rafea B. New developments in ambulatory hysteroscopic surgery. *Best Pract Res Clin Obstet Gynaecol* 2005;19: 727–742.

42 Castaño PM, Adekunle L. Transcervical sterilization. *Semin Reprod Med* 2010;28:103–109.

43 Sowter MC, Lethaby A, Singla AA. Pre-operative endometrial thinning agents before endometrial destruction for heavy menstrual bleeding. *Cochrane Database Syst Rev* 2002;(3): CD001124.

44 Lockwood GM, Baumann R, Turnbull AC, Magos AL. Extensive hysteroscopic surgery under local anaesthesia. *Gynaecol Endosc* 1992;1:15–21.

45 Varol N, Maher P, Vancaillie T *et al.* A literature review and update on the prevention and management of fluid overload in endometrial resection and hysteroscopic surgery. *Gynecol Endosc* 2002;11:19–26.

46 Nathani F, Clark TJ. Uterine polypectomy in the management of abnormal uterine bleeding: a systematic review. *J Minim Invasive Gynecol* 2006;13:260–268.

47 van Dongen H, Janssen CA, Smeets MJ, Emanuel MH, Jansen FW. The clinical relevance of hysteroscopic polypectomy in premenopausal women with abnormal uterine bleeding. *BJOG* 2009;116:1387–1390.

48 Stamatellos I, Stamatopoulos P, Bontis J. The role of hysteroscopy in the current management of the cervical polyps. *Arch Gynecol Obstet* 2007;276:299–303.

49 Di Spiezio Sardo A, Mazzon I, Bramante S *et al.* Hysteroscopic myomectomy: a comprehensive review of surgical techniques. *Hum Reprod Update* 2008;14:101–119.

50 Agdi M, Tulandi T. Endoscopic management of uterine fibroids. *Best Pract Res Clin Obstet Gynaecol* 2008;22:707–716.

51 Homer HA, Li TC, Cooke ID. The septate uterus: a review of management and reproductive outcome. *Fertil Steril* 2000;73: 1–14.

52 Yu D, Wong YM, Cheong Y, Xia E, Li TC. Asherman syndrome: one century later. *Fertil Steril* 2008;89:759–779.

53 Thomson AJ, Abbott JA, Deans R, Kingston A, Vancaillie TG. The management of intrauterine synechiae. *Curr Opin Obstet Gynecol* 2009;21:335–341.

54 Lethaby A, Hickey M, Garry R, Penninx J. Endometrial resection/ablation techniques for heavy menstrual bleeding. *Cochrane Database Syst Rev* 2009;(4):CD001501.

55 Kaunitz AM, Meredith S, Inki P, Kubba A, Sanchez-Ramos L. Levonorgestrel-releasing intrauterine system and endometrial ablation in heavy menstrual bleeding: a systematic review and meta-analysis. *Obstet Gynecol* 2009;113:1104–1116.

56 Bradley LD. Complications of hystersocopy: prevention, treatment and legal risk. *Curr Opin Obstet Gynecol* 2002;14:409–415.

57 Overton C, Hargreaves J, Maresh M. A national survey of the complications of endometrial destruction for menstrual disorders: the MISTLETOE study. Minimally Invasive Surgical Techniques-Laser, EndoThermal or Endoresection. *Br J Obstet Gynaecol* 1997;104:1351–1359.

58 Brooks PG. Venous air embolism during operative hysteroscopy. *J Am Assoc Gynecol Laparosc* 1997;4:399–402.

59 Thinkhamrop J, Laopaiboon M, Lumbiganon P. Prophylactic antibiotics for transcervical intrauterine procedures. *Cochrane Database Syst Rev* 2007;(3):CD005637.

60 McCausland AM, McCausland VM. Frequency of symptomatic cornual hematometra and postablation tubal sterilization syndrome after total rollerball endometrial ablation: a 10-year follow-up. *Am J Obstet Gynecol* 2002;186:1274–1280; discussion 1280–1283.

61 Hare AA, Olah KS. Pregnancy following endometrial ablation: a review article. *J Obstet Gynaecol* 2005;25:108–114.

62 McCausland AM, McCausland VM. Long-term complications of endometrial ablation: cause, diagnosis, treatment, and prevention. *J Minim Invasive Gynecol* 2007;14:399–406.

63 Tu FF, Advincula AP. Miniaturizing the laparoscope: current applications of micro- and minilaparoscopy. *Int J Gynaecol Obstet* 2008;100:94–98.

64 Vilos GA, Ternamian A, Dempster J, Laberge PY. Laparoscopic entry: a review of techniques, technologies, and complications. *J Obstet Gynaecol Can* 2007;29:433–465.

65 Hurd WW, Bude RO, DeLancey JO, Pearl ML. The relationship of the umbilicus to the aortic bifurcation: implications for laparoscopic technique. *Obstet Gynecol* 1992;80:48–51.

66 Granata M, Tsimpanakos I, Moeity F, Magos A. Are we underutilizing Palmer's point entry in gynecologic laparoscopy? *Fertil Steril* 2010;94:2716–2719.

67 Audebert AJM. The role of microlaparoscopy for safer wall entry: incidence of umbilical adhesions according to past surgical history. *Gynecol Endosc* 1999;8:363–367.

68 Hasson HM, Rotman C, Rana N, Kumari NA. Open laparoscopy: 29-year experience. *Obstet Gynecol* 2000;96:763–766.

69 Jansen FW, Kolkman W, Bakkum EA, de Kroon CD, Trimbos-Kemper TC, Trimbos JB. Complications of laparoscopy: an inquiry about closed- versus open-entry technique. *Am J Obstet Gynecol* 2004;190:634–638.

70 Ahmad G, Duffy JMN, Phillips K, Watson A. Laparoscopic entry techniques. *Cochrane Database Syst Rev* 2008;(2):CD006583.

71 Varma R, Gupta JK. Laparoscopic entry techniques: clinical guideline, national survey, and medicolegal ramifications. *Surg Endosc* 2008;22:2686–2697.

72 Hurd WW, Amesse LS, Gruber JS, Horowitz GM, Cha GM, Hurteau JA. Visualization of the epigastric vessels and bladder before laparoscopic trocar placement. *Fertil Steril* 2003;80: 209–212.

73 Hurd WW, Bude RO, DeLancey JO, Newman JS. The location of abdominal wall blood vessels in relationship to abdominal landmarks apparent at laparoscopy. *Am J Obstet Gynecol* 1994;171:642–646.

74 Boike GM, Miller CE, Spirtos NM *et al.* Incisional bowel herniations after operative laparoscopy: a series of nineteen cases and

review of the literature. *Am J Obstet Gynecol* 1995;172:1726–1731; discussion 1731–1733.

75 National Institute for Health and Clinical Excellence. *Fertility: Assessment and Treatment for People with Fertility Problems.* Clinical Guideline CG11, 2004. Available at: http://guidance.nice.org.uk/CG11.

76 Henig I, Prough SG, Cheatwood M, DeLong E. Hysterosalpingography, laparoscopy and hysteroscopy in infertility. A comparative study. *J Reprod Med* 1991;36:573–575.

77 Howard FM. The role of laparoscopy as a diagnostic tool in chronic pelvic pain. *Baillieres Best Pract Res Clin Obstet Gynaecol* 2000;14:467–494.

78 Harkki-Siren P, Sjoberg J, Kurki T. Major complications of laparoscopy: a follow-up Finnish study. *Obstet Gynecol* 1999;94:94–98.

79 Chatzipapas IK, Magos AL. A simple technique of securing inferior epigastric vessels and repairing the rectus sheath at laparoscopic surgery. *Am J Obstet Gynecol* 1997;90:304–306.

80 Makai G, Isaacson K. Complications of gynecologic laparoscopy. *Clin Obstet Gynecol* 2009;52:401–411.

81 Reich H, Clarke HC, Sekel L. A simple method for ligating with straight and curved needles in operative laparoscopy. *Obstet Gynecol* 1992;79:143–147.

82 Advincula AP, Wang K. The evolutionary state of electrosurgery: where are we now? *Curr Opin Obstet Gynecol* 2008;20:353–358.

83 Owusu-Ansah R, Gatongi D, Chien PF. Health technology assessment of surgical therapies for benign gynaecological disease. *Best Pract Res Clin Obstet Gynaecol* 2006;20:841–879.

84 Shushan A, Mohamed H, Magos AL. A case-control study to compare the variability of operating time in laparoscopic and open surgery. *Hum Reprod* 1999;14:1467–1469.

85 Bijen CB, Vermeulen KM, Mourits MJ, de Bock GH. Costs and effects of abdominal versus laparoscopic hysterectomy: systematic review of controlled trials. *PLoS One* 2009;4:e7340.

86 Chapron C, Fauconnier A, Goffinet F, Breart G, Dubuisson JB. Laparoscopic surgery is not inherently dangerous for patients presenting with benign gynaecologic pathology. Results of a meta-analysis. *Hum Reprod* 2002;17:1334–1342.

87 Garry R, Fountain J, Mason S *et al.* The eVALuate study: two parallel randomised trials, one comparing laparoscopic with abdominal hysterectomy, the other comparing laparoscopic with vaginal hysterectomy. *BMJ* 2004;328:129.

88 Jansen FW, Kapiteyn K, Trimbos-Kemper T *et al.* Complications of laparoscopy: a prospective, multicentre, observational study. *Br J Obstet Gynaecol* 1997;104:595–600.

89 Chapron C, Querleu D, Bruhat MA *et al.* Surgical complications of diagnostic and operative gynecologic laparoscopy: a series of 29 966 cases. *Hum Reprod* 1998;13:867–872.

90 Saidi MH, Sadler RK, Vancaillie TG, Akright BD, Farhart SA, White AJ. Diagnosis and management of serious urinary complications after major operative laparoscopy. *Obstet Gynecol* 1996;87:272–276.

91 Wind J, Cremers JE, van Berge Henegouwen MI, Gouma DJ, Jansen FW, Bemelman WA. Medical liability insurance claims on entry-related complications in laparoscopy. *Surg Endosc* 2007;21:2094–2099.

92 Magrina JF. Complications of laparoscopic surgery. *Clin Obstet Gynecol* 2002;45:469–480.

93 Varol N, Healey M, Tang P, Sheehan P, Maher P, Hill D. Ten-year review of hysterectomy morbidity and mortality: can we change direction? *Aust NZ J Obstet Gynaecol* 2001;41:295–302.

94 Rein H. Complications and litigation in gynecologic endoscopy. *Curr Opin Obstet Gynecol* 2001;13:425–429.

95 Argent VP. Medico-legal problems in gynaecology. *Curr Obstet Gynaecol* 2003;13:294–299.

96 Gambadauro P, Magos A. Digital video technology and surgical training. *Eur Clin Obstet Gynaecol* 2007;3:31–34.

97 Botden SM, Jakimowicz JJ. What is going on in augmented reality simulation in laparoscopic surgery? *Surg Endosc* 2009;23:1693–1700.

98 Gurusamy KS, Aggarwal R, Palanivelu L, Davidson BR. Virtual reality training for surgical trainees in laparoscopic surgery. *Cochrane Database Syst Rev* 2009;(1):CD006575.

Part 9
Childhood and Adolescence

Chapter 37
Puberty and Its Disorders

D. Keith Edmonds
Queen Charlotte's & Chelsea Hospital, London, UK

The transition from childhood to adolescence and adulthood is one of the most dynamic changes that occurs during the life of a woman. The changes are not only physical but emotional, psychological, behavioural and sexual, and all these changes encompass the maturation of the female to become reproductively capable. There is enormous variation between individuals in the processes involved in puberty but the five major physical changes are growth, breast development, pubic hair development, axillary hair development and, ultimately, menstruation. Whilst these changes occur temporally at different rates, there may be changes that occur prematurely or in a delayed fashion which alter this process. Finally, some girls may undergo pubertal change without menstruation and others may fail to enter puberty entirely.

Control of the onset of puberty

The age of onset of puberty in girls ranges from 8.5 to 13.3 years and the appearance of secondary sexual characteristics before this age is known as precocious puberty; failure of appearance of any secondary sexual characteristics after 13.5 years in girls is considered delayed puberty. A number of factors are known to play a role in the timing of puberty. Genetics has a clear and dominant role and there is a clear correlation between age at puberty of a woman and that of her daughter. However, there are racial differences, with black females showing an earlier age of pubertal onset compared with white [1]. Furthermore, nutritional status in all ethnic groups seriously influences the age of onset of puberty. Children living in areas of malnutrition have significantly delayed onset of puberty and transfer of these girls to a socioeconomically superior environment reduces the age of onset of puberty significantly [2]. At the other extreme, evidence now exists to suggest that a high body mass index (BMI) is linked to earlier age of maturation, and the relationship between body fat and the onset of puberty is proposed to be linked to the release of leptin from adipose sites [3]. Leptin and kisspeptin would seem to act as a primary signal to the hypothalamus to allow puberty to commence [4].

The hypothalamus–pituitary–gonadal axis is active during fetal life and quiescent during childhood. It is the reactivation of this axis that leads to sexual maturation. The arcuate nucleus in the basal hypothalamus is responsible for secretion of gonadotrophin-releasing hormone (GnRH) into the hypothalamus–pituitary portal circulation. As puberty commences, the arcuate nucleus begins to secrete GnRH in a pulsatile manner, initially solely at night; however, as time progresses GnRH release adopts a low-frequency low-amplitude pulsatile pattern that starts to induce release of luteinizing hormone (LH) from the pituitary. The low-amplitude pulsatile pattern gradually extends to include daytime secretion and gonadotrophin levels themselves start to increase, reflecting higher pulse amplitude and increasing frequency of GnRH production. As the pattern of follicle-stimulating hormone (FSH) and LH release becomes established, so ovarian activity commences and initially this is totally chaotic as it is uncoordinated. This means that there is follicular growth without coordinated ovulation and although oestradiol levels start to rise, there is no evidence of ovulation. The ovary may have appearances that are multicystic due to this chaotic gonadotrophin stimulation and, over time (about 5–10 years), coordinated pulsatile release of GnRH leads to adult frequency of FSH release (approximately every 90 min). At this stage the ovulatory cycle is established.

From age 7, most girls will begin activation of adrenal androgen production, a phenomenon known as adrenarche. As with ovarian oestradiol production, androgen

---

production is initially at extremely low levels and increases over time.

Physical changes of puberty

Growth

An increase in vertical growth is the initial physical sign of the onset of puberty. Growth during infancy is relatively rapid until age 3–4 and then it rapidly decelerates when the childhood phase begins. Growth velocity during infancy is approximately 15 cm/year but in middle childhood, until the onset of puberty, slows to 5–6 cm/year. Interestingly, childhood growth rates are usually at their slowest in the 12–18 months immediately preceding puberty and thus if puberty is delayed this effect is exaggerated. At puberty, girls may reach a peak growth velocity of 10 cm/year and girls will gain approximately 25 cm of growth during puberty. Males in contrast have their growth spurt approximately 2 years later than females but eventually gain approximately 28 cm of added height. Once the final stage of growth velocity decreases, epiphyseal fusion occurs which prevents further growth. During the adolescent growth phase, bone density increases rapidly. Control of the growth spurt is primarily through growth hormone and its major secondary messenger insulin-like growth factor (IGF)-1. Oestradiol plays an important role in the increased secretion of growth hormone during puberty, particularly in the early stages. As bone growth and height are maximally achieved, oestradiol initiates epiphyseal fusion as it reaches its maximum towards the end of puberty. Thyroid hormone also plays a key role in growth and development as illustrated in severe childhood hypothyroidism, which results in a dramatic decrease in the velocity of growth.

Breast development

Although the growth spurt is usually the first sign of the onset of puberty, in females it is breast change that is usually used as an indicator of development. The initiation of breast development is known as thelarche and this has been classified by Tanner into five stages [5]. Breast growth is often unequal between the two breasts and Tanner stage 5 represents the mature end-stage of breast development. This takes approximately 5 years.

Pubic and axillary hair growth

The adolescent development of female pubic hair occurs in conjunction with androgen release and it is the presence of androgen that determines both pubic and axillary hair growth. In approximately 20% of females, pubic hair growth may precede breast development.

Summary box 37.1

Development of secondary sexual characteristics is characterized by:
- growth;
- breast development;
- pubic and axillary hair development;
- menstruation.

Precocious puberty

This phenomenon has received increased attention over the last few years with the belief that the age of onset of puberty has been falling. However, in accepting some guidance over age, the appearance of secondary sexual characteristics prior to 8 years should be considered precocious and prompt the clinician to carry out investigations.

Differential diagnosis of early onset of puberty

Premature adrenarche

This is due to the precocious increase in adrenal androgen secretion and is the most common cause of referral for precocious puberty. There seems to be an association between premature adrenarche and increased BMI [6], and in the overweight child referred with precocious puberty it is important not to assume that breast tissue is truly breast development and not adipose tissue. Signs of virilization such as clitoral enlargement, severe acne or increased muscle mass would lead to concerns of a virilizing ovarian or adrenal tumour or late-onset congenital adrenal hyperplasia (CAH). Late-onset CAH can present with pubic hair growth from the age of 1 and should be appropriately investigated.

Premature thelarche

Here, breast growth tends to appear earlier than age 8 and progresses very slowly and usually occurs in isolation of the growth spurt or any other secondary sexual characteristic. The cause of this condition remains unknown and although it is appropriate to exclude an ovarian cyst, these are rarely found.

Central precocious puberty

This refers to progressive breast development prematurely due to early activation of the hypophyseal–pituitary–ovarian axis and is accompanied by the growth spurt; pubic hair is frequently but not always found. This therefore mimics normal onset of puberty but at a very early age. A positive family history of early onset of puberty may be discovered but in the majority of cases the aetiology is idiopathic. Brain imaging is important, especially in girls with an onset of puberty before the age of 6, where 20% will be found to have a central nervous system (CNS) tumour.

Peripheral precocious puberty

This is far less common than central precocious puberty and is usually induced by excess production of sex steroids. Causes include the following.

- Androgen secretion from a virilizing adrenal tumour.
- Late-onset CAH.
- Oestrogen-secreting tumour causing rapid breast development. If a large ovarian cyst is present, this may be part of McCune–Albright syndrome, with associated classical features of irregular café-au-lait spots and cystic bone lesions called polyostotic fibroid dysplasia.
- Exposure to exogenous hormones, e.g. inadvertent ingestion of birth control pills by children causing excess levels of oestrogens; topical androgen exposure.

Investigations

A number of hormonal studies may be carried out in children with precocious puberty. However, they are of limited value and should be focused on specific clinical entities. LH may be used to distinguish between premature thelarche and central precocious puberty. FSH is of limited value. Oestradiol is usually elevated in girls with precocious puberty but very high levels may suggest a tumour. Dehydroepiandrosterone is always elevated in children with premature adrenarche; testosterone when markedly elevated would suggest an androgen-secreting tumour; and in those children who are considered to have late-onset CAH, the diagnosis can be confirmed by measuring 17-hydroxyprogesterone. Radiological studies have somewhat limited value, although pelvic ultrasound may be used if an abdominal tumour is suspected and brain magnetic resonance imaging (MRI) may be used in those children with extreme precocious puberty, where the chances of a positive finding are around 20%.

Treatment

The majority of girls with central precocious puberty do not require hormonal treatment, because most development is extremely slow and will result in maturity at an age which would be expected even though onset has been early. It is therefore prudent to review children with precocious development of secondary sexual characteristics 6 months later to see whether there has been rapid development of secondary sexual characteristics or not. In these cases, there is a high chance that sexual maturity will be reached by age 9 and therefore suppression of the progress of puberty would be sensible. While it is possible to suppress the pituitary, growth hormone cannot be suppressed and therefore treatment will result in adult height that is significantly greater than would be expected than if the child were left untreated. Children with extremely early puberty are often tall at the time of diagnosis and they tend to finish their growth early and achieve normal

adult height. It is therefore pertinent in these young children to suppress the development of secondary sexual characteristics. The standard treatment for central precocious puberty is GnRH analogues, which may be given nasally or by intramuscular injection. Three-monthly preparations are now available and therefore four injections a year is all that is required to suppress puberty. GnRH analogues can then be administered until such time as the child reaches approximately age 11, when withdrawal will result in the normal resumption of pubertal changes. Peripheral precocious puberty, when due to an ovarian or adrenal tumour, requires surgical intervention; however, for girls with androgen excess due to CAH, suppression of the adrenal with hydrocortisone will reverse the changes.

Delayed puberty

Delayed puberty is usually considered when girls have no secondary sexual characteristics by age 13.5 years. Delay in puberty occurs in only 2.5% of the population but the identification of those children who do have a significant aetiology for this may be extremely important. However, it is mandatory to take a detailed history as the presence of chronic medical conditions or excessive athletic participation may be an obvious explanation for delay in the onset of puberty. In females, approximately 50% will have constitutional delay that is presumably genetically based. In the presence of secondary sexual characteristics, menstruation ought to occur within 2 years of the establishment of Tanner stage 2 breast change. However, any child presenting at any stage because of concern over failure to establish either secondary sexual characteristics or menstruation should be investigated at that time. There are often extremely good reasons why a mother will bring her daughter for investigation and this often relates to the fact that a sibling completed her pubertal development at an earlier age or she herself went through puberty at an earlier age. While investigations may not lead to a diagnosis of abnormality, proof of normality is extremely important.

Summary box 37.2

Precocious puberty is usually idiopathic and requires treatment only if changes are accelerated such that completion of puberty will occur prematurely.

Aetiology of primary amenorrhoea

From a clinical point of view it is probably best to classify the aetiologies of primary amenorrhoea based on the presence or absence of secondary sexual characteristics. This is the basis of the classification system shown in

Table 37.1 Classification of primary amenorrhoea.

Secondary sexual characteristics normal

Imperforate hymen
Transverse vaginal septum
Absent vagina and functioning uterus
Absent vagina and non-functioning uterus
XY female: androgen insensitivity
Resistant ovary syndrome
Constitutional delay

Secondary sexual characteristics absent

Normal stature

Hypogonadotrophic hypogonadism
  Congenital
    Isolated gonodotrophin-releasing hormone deficiency
    Olfactogenital syndrome
  Acquired
    Weight loss/anorexia
    Excessive exercise
    Hyperprolactinaemia

Hypergonadotrophic hypogonadism
  Gonadal agenesis
    XX agenesis
    XX or XY agenesis
  Gonadal dysgenesis
    Turner mosaic
    Other X deletions or mosaics
    XY enzymatic failure
  Ovarian failure
  Galactosaemia

Short stature

Hypogonadotrophic hypogonadism
  Congenital
    Hydrocephalus
  Acquired
    Trauma
    Empty sella syndrome
    Tumours

Hypergonadotrophic hypogonadism
Turner syndrome
Other X deletions or mosaics

Heterosexual development

Congenital adrenal hyperplasia
Androgen-secreting tumour
5α-Reductase deficiency
Partial androgen receptor deficiency
True hermaphrodite
Absent Müllerian inhibitor

Table 37.1. Finally, there is the group of patients in whom there is heterosexual development.

Normal secondary sexual characteristics

Imperforate hymen

The imperforate hymen may present at two stages of development. It may present in early childhood when the infant presents with a bulging hymen behind which is a mucocele, the vagina expanded by vaginal secretions of mucus. This is easily released and does not subsequently cause any problems following hymenectomy. It may also present in later life when a pubertal girl complains of intermittent abdominal pain, which is usually cyclical. The pain is due to dysmenorrhoea associated with the accumulation of menstrual blood within the vagina. The vagina is a very distensible organ and can allow quite large quantities of blood to collect in some cases. This situation is known as haematocolpos. It is very unusual for blood to accumulate within the uterus as the uterus is a muscular organ that is difficult to distend. When some blood does accumulate within the cavity it is known as haematometra. As the vaginal mass enlarges there may be associated difficulty with micturition and defecation. Examination will occasionally reveal an abdominal swelling and observation of the introitus will display a tense bulging bluish membrane, which is the hymen.

Transverse vaginal septum

In circumstances where the vagina fails to cannulate, the upper and lower parts of the vagina are separate. These girls present with cyclical abdominal pain due to the development of haematocolpos, but the thickness of the transverse vaginal septum means that the clinical appearance is very different from that of an imperforate hymen. Again, an abdominal mass may be palpable but inspection of the vagina shows that it is blind-ending and, although it may be bulging, it is pink not blue. The hymenal remnants are often seen separately. Transverse vaginal septum may occur at three levels, known as a lower, middle or upper third septum. If the space between the upper and lower vagina is considerable, no introital swelling may be visible and rectal examination may disclose a mass. The management is very different from imperforate hymen and very careful assessment must be made before embarking on any management strategy.

Absent vagina and the functioning uterus

This is a rare phenomenon when embryologically the uterine body has developed normally but there is failure of development of the cervix. This leads to failure of the development of the upper vagina. The presenting symptom is again cyclical abdominal pain, but there is no pelvic mass to be found because there is no vagina to be distended. Although a small haematometra may be present, retrograde menstruation occurs leading to the development of endometriosis and in some patients pelvic adhesions.

Absent vagina and a non-functioning uterus

This is the second most common cause of primary amenorrhoea, second only to Turner's syndrome. Secondary sexual characteristics are normal as would be expected as ovarian function is unaffected. Examination of the genital area discloses normal female external genitalia but a blind-ending vaginal dimple which is usually not more than 1.5 cm in depth. This is known as Mayer–Rokitansky–Küster–Hauser (MRKH) syndrome and uterine development is usually absent. Often small uterine remnants (anlage) are found on the lateral pelvic side walls. It is important to remember that 40% of these patients have renal anomalies, 15% of which are major, for example an absent kidney, and there are also recognizable skeletal abnormalities associated with this syndrome [7].

XY female

There are a number of ways in which an individual may have an XY karyotype and a female phenotype, and these include failure of testicular development, enzymatic failure of the testis to produce androgen (particularly testosterone), and androgenic receptor absence or failure of function. In androgen insensitivity there is a structural abnormality of the androgen receptor, due to defects in the androgen receptor gene, which results in a non-functional receptor. This means that the masculinizing effect of testosterone during normal development is prevented and patients are therefore phenotypically female with normal breast development. This occurs because of peripheral conversion of androgen to oestrogen and subsequent stimulation of breast growth. Pubic hair is very scanty in these patients as there is no androgen response in target tissues. The vulva is normal and the vagina is usually short. The uterus and tubes are absent in this particular version of the XY female. The testes are usually found in the lower abdomen, but occasionally may be found in hernial sacs in childhood, which alerts the surgeon to the diagnosis [8]. Other versions of this syndrome are not associated with secondary sexual development (see below).

Resistant ovary syndrome

This is an extremely rare cause of primary amenorrhoea, but it has been described. There are elevated levels of gonadotrophin in the presence of apparently normal ovarian tissue; patients do have some development of secondary sexual characteristics, but never produce adequate amounts of oestrogen to result in menstruation. It is believed that these women have an absence or malfunction of FSH receptors in the ovarian follicles, and are unable to respond properly to FSH.

Constitutional delay

A number of girls have constitutional delay and normal secondary sexual characteristics, but there is no anatomical anomaly and endocrine investigations are all normal. If serial sampling is carried out over a 24-hour period, these young women are found to have immature pulsatile release of GnRH. This is the sole reason for their constitutional delay. These young women will eventually menstruate spontaneously as the maturation process proceeds.

Summary box 37.3

The management of primary amenorrhoea should be based on the presence or absence of secondary sexual characteristics and treatment appropriately instituted.

Absent secondary sexual characteristics (normal height)

Isolated GnRH deficiency (olfactogenital syndrome, Kallman's syndrome)

In this condition the hypothalamus lacks the ability to produce GnRH and there is therefore a hypogonadotrophic state. The pituitary gland is normal and stimulation with exogenous GnRH leads to normal release of gonadotrophins. This condition arises due to maldevelopment of neurones in the arcuate nucleus of the hypothalamus. These neurones are derived embryologically from the olfactory bulb and therefore some patients may also have failure of development of the ability to smell (anosmia). When this occurs it is known as Kallman's syndrome. The genetic basis of Kallman's syndrome is slowly being uncovered and so far two possibilities exist: there is either mutation of the *KAL1* gene (encoding anosmin) on the X chromosome or mutation of the fibroblast growth factor receptor 1 (*FGFR1*) gene, both of which lead to agenesis of the olfactory and GnRH-secreting neurones [9]. There may well be other mutations and other genes involved which still need to be discovered.

Weight loss/anorexia

Weight loss is more commonly associated with secondary amenorrhoea than primary amenorrhoea, but unfortunately it is increasingly apparent that young girls may suffer from anorexia nervosa in the prepubertal state. This leads to failure of activation of the gene which initiates GnRH release in the hypothalamus, and therefore a persistent hypogonadotrophic state exists. The growth spurt is not usually influenced by this, but secondary sexual characteristics are absent.

Excessive exercise

Over recent years it has become increasingly recognized that excessive exercise in pubertal children leads to decreased body fat content, without necessarily affecting body mass. Development of muscle contributes to overall weight, and therefore weight alone cannot be used as the parameter for deciding whether there is an aetiology for their amenorrhoea via this mechanism. A number of examples of this exist, including ballet dancers, athletes and gymnasts. These girls fail to menstruate and may actually develop frank anorexia nervosa.

Hyperprolactinaemia

This is an unusual cause of primary amenorrhoea and is much more commonly seen as a cause of secondary amenorrhoea. There may be a recognizable prolactinoma in the pituitary, but often no apparent reason is seen. Imaging may reveal an anomaly.

Gonadal agenesis

In this situation there is complete failure of development of the gonad. These girls may be either 46XX or 46XY. The 46XX pure gonadal dysgenesis is an autosomal recessive disorder and genes other than those located on the X chromosome are involved. The location of these genes remains unclear and in all these patients their genotype does not affect their phenotype, all of them being female. In 46XY or 45X/46XY, when the absence of testicular determining factor or its receptor is postulated as the cause of the failure of differentiation of the gonad, there is absence of testicular development. These individuals therefore fail to produce any androgen or Müllerian inhibitor. Therefore Wolffian structures regress and Müllerian structures persist and menstruation will occur when oestrogen is administered. The external genitalia reflect normal female phenotype. Height is normal as the growth spurt occurs at the normal time. However, in those girls who are 46XY, the failure of production of androgen or oestrogen means that their long bones do not undergo epiphyseal closure at the normal time and therefore final height may be excessive.

Ovarian failure

These unfortunate girls have ovarian failure as a result of either chemotherapy or radiotherapy for childhood malignancy.

Galactosaemia

This inborn error of galactose metabolism is due to deficiency of galactose-1-phosphate uridyltransferase. The aetiology of the association between this enzyme and hypogonadotrophic hypogonadism is still to be clarified but patients with galactose-1-phosphate uridyltransferase deficiency have an acute toxic syndrome that causes ovarian cellular destruction thought to be due to the accumulation of galactose metabolites, which may induce programmed cell death (apoptosis).

Gonadal dysgenesis

The gonad is described as dysgenetic if it is abnormal in its formation. This encompasses a spectrum of conditions which vary with the degree of differentiation. The commonest is Turner's syndrome, where there is a single X chromosome giving a 45X karyotype. The missing chromosome may be either X or Y. There are other circumstances in which the gonadal dysgenesis may be associated with a mosaic. Here two cell lines exist within one individual, the most common being 45X/46XX. Other structural chromosomal anomalies associated with gonadal dysgenesis involve deletions. If the deletion involves part of the long or short arm of the X chromosome, then loss of this genetic material may affect gonadal development. In Turner's syndrome ovarian development is normal until 20 weeks' gestation and at this stage oocytes are found in the ovaries. However, further maturation is impaired and massive atresia occurs during the latter part of pregnancy. The ovaries in most individuals consist solely of stroma and are unable to produce oestrogen. There is a normal female phenotype and internal genital development is also normal. The loss of an X chromosome results in short stature as the genes for height are on the short arm of the X chromosome. In mosaicism the proportion of each cell line determines the manifestation of the condition. The higher the percentage of 45X cells, the more likely the features of Turner's syndrome.

In XY individuals there may be a dysgenetic gonad associated with enzymatic failure. In this situation testosterone fails to be produced. This is usually associated with normal production of Müllerian inhibitor. Therefore internal development leads to Müllerian atrophy, but external development fails to masculinize due to the lack of testosterone. Wolffian structures also fail to develop. The external phenotype is therefore female with a short vagina.

Absent secondary sexual characteristics (short stature)

Congenital infection

The most common aetiology in this group is hydrocephalus, as a result of childhood or neonatal infection. It is believed that this damages the hypothalamus and renders the GnRH-secreting neurones functionless, thereby creating a hypogonadotrophic hypogonadic state.

Trauma

Trauma to the skull base may also damage the hypothalamus and prevent GnRH secretion.

Empty sella syndrome

In this unusual condition the sella turcica is found to be empty and there is congenital absence of the pituitary gland or at least part of it, leading to failure to produce gonadotrophins. Thus secondary sexual characteristics do not develop.

Tumours

A number of tumours have been described in the pituitary which may lead to destruction of the gland. The most common of these is craniopharyngioma. This is a tumour which usually arises in childhood and results in destruction of the pituitary gland. These children present already on maintenance therapy for other hormonal deficiencies and are hypogonadotrophic.

Turner's syndrome

In pure Turner's syndrome the chromosome complement is 45X and here a syndrome of short stature and ovarian failure lead to the typical features. These children usually present in the teenage years because of failure of development of secondary sexual characteristics or, more commonly, are referred from growth clinics for induction of secondary sexual characteristics. Attempts to improve height have proved difficult to achieve.

Heterosexual development

Congenital adrenal hyperplasia

This occurs as a result of an enzyme deficiency in the steroid pathway of the adrenal gland (see Chapter 34) and children with this condition require steroid replacement [10]. It is imperative that there is good control of CAH at puberty if the children are to develop secondary sexual characteristics at the appropriate time. However, many of these girls fail to comply with their steroid therapy and are therefore uncontrolled. As a result of this, they fail to establish the normal process of puberty. It is therefore quite common to find that puberty is delayed and steroid control needs to be addressed.

Androgen-secreting tumours

This is extremely rare and arises when the ovary contains an arrhenoblastoma. Here excessive production of androgen results in virilization and removal of the tumour resolves the problem.

5α-Reductase deficiency

This form of XY female results from an enzyme deficiency that prevents the conversion of testosterone to 5-hydroxytestosterone, which is a necessary biochemical step in the development of the external genitalia in the male. The cloaca can only respond to this testosterone derivative and not to testosterone itself. The external genitalia are therefore female, but the internal genitalia are normal male as secretion of Müllerian inhibitor leads to Müllerian agenesis. These patients are therefore amenorrhoeic.

True hermaphrodite

In this condition the child has both testicular and ovarian tissue. This may occur either in isolation, such that there is an ovary and a testis in the same individual, or the gonad may contain both ovarian and testicular tissue. This leads to intersex problems at birth (see Chapter 34) and subsequently, if not resolved at birth, amenorrhoea due to androgen production at puberty, thereby preventing the development of the normal menstrual cycle.

Absent Müllerian inhibitor

There is a rare condition in which an XY individual may not produce Müllerian inhibitory substance, which means that the internal genitalia are female with persistence of the Müllerian structures and also because testosterone is produced the Wolffian structures also persist. In this extremely rare syndrome there is dual internal organ persistence.

Evaluation and management

Having understood the classification of these syndromes, it becomes apparent that most of the conditions are rare and constitutional delay is undoubtedly the most common diagnosis. However, as the rest of the diagnoses have serious implications, this diagnosis of constitutional delay should only be made when all other syndromes have been excluded. It is important to record a full history and examination, including most importantly the development of secondary sexual characteristics and height. Secondary sexual characteristics should be classified according to the staging system of Tanner. Individuals can then be classified according to their secondary sexual characteristics.

Normal secondary sexual characteristics

The presence of normal secondary sexual characteristics should alert the clinician to the presence of outflow tract obstruction. This is the most common cause of primary amenorrhoea in the presence of normal secondary sexual characteristics. It is thus appropriate to carry out investigations to make this diagnosis. It is inappropriate to perform any physical pelvic examination on these young adolescents and imaging techniques should be used. It is simple to arrange a pelvic ultrasound scan to assess the pelvic anatomy, and only in rare circumstances where this cannot be delineated by ultrasound should it be necessary to use MRI or computed tomography (CT). If the uterus is absent, the karyotype should be performed; if this is 46XX, then MRKH syndrome is the most likely diagnosis. If the chromosome complement is 46XY, the patient is, by definition, an XY female. If the uterus is present on ultrasound, then there may be an associated haematocolpos and haematometra and appropriate reconstructive surgery should be carried out. If the pelvic anatomy is normal, then it is essential to assess gonadotrophin and prolactin levels as this would tend to indicate a hypothalamic cause for the amenorrhoea, so-called constitutional delay. In some conditions the LH to FSH ratio may be elevated (e.g. polycystic ovaries), and if resistant ovary syndrome is the diagnosis these gonadotrophin levels will be elevated. Elevation of prolactin levels suggests a prolactinoma.

Management

Patients with an absent uterus require special psychological counselling and their care should be managed in a centre able to offer the complete range of psychological, psychosexual and gynaecological expertise. These young girls will have major problems with future sexual activity and their infertility and require very careful counselling. At the appropriate time a vagina may be created either non-surgically or surgically. In 85% of cases the use of vaginal dilators is successful (see Chapter 34).

In girls found to have an XY karyotype, careful counselling is necessary over the malignant potential of their gonads, this being reported in around 30%. It is therefore necessary for them to have their gonads removed and this must be performed at a time when counselling is complete. Sharing the information of the karyotype with the patient should be entertained at that time when the relationship between the clinician and the patient warrants it. Not all women wish this information when they are young, but if directly requested it should be shared with them. All patients should be informed of their karyotype when appropriate.

In outflow tract obstruction, surgical management may occur at various levels. The simplest form is an imperforate hymen and in this condition a cruciate incision in the hymen allows drainage of the retained menstrual blood. Transverse vaginal septae are much more difficult to deal with and require specialist reconstruction to create a vagina which is subsequently functional (see Chapter 34) [7].

If investigations suggest constitutional delay and development of secondary sexual characteristics is complete, there is no need to suggest any treatment other than annual review. These young women very much appreciate the opportunity to return for monitoring until such time as their menstruation commences. In some circumstances it may be useful to promote a menstruation using the oral contraceptive pill for one cycle to prove that menstruation can occur and this can be extremely reassuring. If the diagnosis of resistant ovary syndrome is suspected, then diagnosis can really only be made by ovarian biopsy and subsequent histology confirming or illustrating the absence of oocytes. Finally, elevated prolactin levels should provoke the clinician to perform imaging of the pituitary fossa, probably best done by CT, to determine the presence or absence of a microadenoma and management subsequently with bromocriptine.

Absence of secondary sexual characteristics

In this particular situation, it is extremely important to make an assessment of the patient's height. If the patient is of normal height for age, measurement of gonadotrophin will reveal levels that are either low or high. Low levels of gonadotrophins confirm the diagnosis of hypogonadotrophic hypogonadism, while elevated levels should provoke the clinician to perform a karyotype. The 46XX patient will have premature ovarian failure, resistant ovary syndrome or gonadal agenesis while the XY female will have 46XY gonadal agenesis or testicular enzymatic failure. If stature is short, gonadotrophin levels will either be low (associated with an intracranial lesion) or high (which, following a karyotype, almost certainly indicates Turner's syndrome or a Turner mosaic).

Management

In patients with hypogonadotrophic hypogonadism, treatment should be to manage any avoidable problem or, in isolated GnRH deficiency, hormone replacement therapy will need to be instituted to induce development of secondary sexual characteristics. These patients can be informed that they are infertile and that ovulation induction in the future can be invoked using various fertility regimens. Hormone replacement therapy is essential and regimens exist for the induction of secondary sexual characteristics over 3–5 years. Oestrogen should be used alone for about 2 years, and then 2–3 years of gradual introduction of progestogens, thereby establishing normal breast growth over a time frame that is equivalent to normal. Any attempt to accelerate breast growth by using higher doses of oestrogen will result in abnormal breast growth and this should be avoided at all costs. Patients with an XY dysgenesis or enzymatic failure should have gonadectomies performed to avoid malignancy.

It must always be remembered that any chronic medical illness which prevents normal growth will result in delayed onset of puberty and these causes must be considered in any patient presenting in this way.

References

1 Sun SS, Schuber CM, Chumlea WC *et al.* National estimates of the timing of sexual maturation and racial differences among US children. *Pediatrics* 2002;110:911–919.
2 Martorell R. Physical growth and development of the malnourished child: contributions from 50 years of research at INCAP. *Food Nutr Bull* 2010;31:68–82.

3 Biro FM, Khoury P, Morrison JA. Influence of obesity on timing of puberty. *Int J Androl* 2006;29:272–277.

4 Roa J, Garcia-Galiano D, Castellano JM *et al.* Metabolic control of puberty onset: new players, new mechanisms. *Mol Cell Endocrinol* 2010;324:87–94.

5 Marshall WA, Tanner JM. Variations in pattern of pubertal changes in girls. *Arch Dis Child* 1969;44:291–303.

6 Maclaren NK, Gujral S, Ten S *et al.* Childhood obesity and insulin resistance. *Cell Biochem Biophys* 2007;48:73–78.

7 Edmonds DK. Congenital malformations of the genital tract and their management. *Best Pract Res Clin Obstet Gynaecol* 2003;17:19–40.

8 Dewhurst CJ, Spence JEH. The XY female. *Br J Hosp Med* 1977;17:498.

9 Karges B, de Roux N. Molecular genetics of isolated hypogonadotropic hypogonadism and Kallmann syndrome. *Endocr Dev* 2005;8:67–80.

10 Hindmarsh PC. Management of the child with congenital adrenal hyperplasia. *Best Pract Res Clin Endocrinol Metab* 2009;23:193–208.

Chapter 38
Gynaecological Disorders of Childhood and Adolescence

D. Keith Edmonds
Queen Charlotte's & Chelsea Hospital, London, UK

Gynaecological problems in the prepubertal child and at adolescence create great levels of anxiety in parents particularly, but fortunately very few of these disorders could be considered common. However, when they do present it is important that the clinician has an understanding so that appropriate advice may be given to the patient and management is frequently through simple means. The disorders fall into two groups: those related to pre-puberty and those of adolescence.

Summary box 38.1

- Vulvovaginitis is usually due to non-specific bacterial contamination.
- Child sexual abuse should always be borne in mind.
- Treatment is usually through hygiene techniques.

Prepubertal child

Examination of the prepubertal child requires cooperation from both the patient and the mother and requires extreme sensitivity if a successful examination is to be carried out. Positioning the child for examination may require considerable time to gain the confidence of the child to allow examination. External examination should be performed with minimal handling of the vulva and, in order to expose the vaginal orifice, gentle traction on the buttocks to expose the vaginal opening can be performed. Specimens can be obtained using syringes with flexible catheters or occasionally a swab may be inserted if the hymenal orifice allows. In adolescents, vaginal examination should be avoided unless there is good evidence that it is necessary in order to make a diagnosis. This is rarely so in the light of the ability to image using ultrasound which is by far the most preferred form of investigation.

Vulvovaginitis

This is the only gynaecological disorder of childhood which can be thought of as common. Its aetiology is based on opportunistic bacteria colonizing the lower vagina and inducing an inflammatory response. At birth the vulva and vagina are well oestrogenized due to the intrauterine exposure of the fetus to placental oestrogen. This oestrogenization causes thickening of the vaginal epithelium, which is entirely protective against any bacterial invasion. However, within 2–3 weeks of delivery the resultant hypo-oestrogenic state leads to changes in the vulval skin, which becomes thinner, and the vaginal epithelium also becomes much thinner. The vulval fat pad disappears and the vaginal entrance becomes unprotected. The vulval skin is thin, sensitive and easily traumatized by injury, irritation, infection or any allergic reaction that may ensue. The lack of labial protection and the close apposition of the anus mean that the vulva and lower vagina are constantly exposed to faecal bacterial contamination. The hypo-oestrogenic state in the vagina means that there are no lactobacilli and therefore the vagina has a resulting pH of 7, making it an ideal culture medium for low-virulence organisms. The childhood problems of poor local hygiene compound the risk of low-grade non-specific infection. Children also have the habit of exploring their genitalia and in some cases masturbating. This chronic habit may lead to vulvovaginitis, which can prove extremely difficult to treat. Vulvovaginitis may also occur in childhood in those who have an impaired local host defence deficiency due to the lack of an innate local protective response from neutrophils.

The causes of vulvovaginitis in children are shown in Table 38.1. The vast majority of cases are due to non-specific bacterial contamination, although the other causes should be remembered. Candidal infection in children is extremely rare, although because it is a common cause of vulvovaginitis in the adult, it is a common

Table 38.1 Causes of vulvovaginitis in children.

Bacterial
  Non-specific (common)
  Specific (rare)

Fungal (rare)
  Candida of vulva only

Viral (rare)

Dermatitis
  Atopic
  Lichen sclerosis
  Contact

Sexual abuse
Enuresis
Foreign body

misdiagnosis in children. *Candida* in children is usually associated with diabetes mellitus or immunodeficiency and almost entirely related to these two medical disorders. The presence of viral infections, for example herpes simplex or condyloma acuminata, should alert the clinician to the possibility of sexual abuse. Vulval skin disease is not uncommon in children, particularly atopic dermatitis in those children who also have eczema. Referral to a dermatologist is appropriate in these circumstances. Lichen sclerosis is also seen in children and may cause persistent vulval itching. The skin undergoes atrophy and fissuring and is very susceptible to secondary infection.

Sexual abuse in children may present with vaginal discharge. Any child who has recurrent attacks of vaginal discharge should alert the clinician to this possibility. However, as non-specific bacterial infection is a common problem in children, the clinician must proceed with considerable caution in raising the possibility of sexual abuse. Only those bacterial infections related to venereal disease, for example gonorrhoea, may be cited as diagnostic of sexual abuse.

It is important that the clinician remembers that many girls suffer from urinary incontinence, particularly at night, and this creates a moist vulva allowing secondary infection by bacteria leading to vulvovaginitis.

Diagnostic procedures

There are two aspects of the diagnosis in this condition in children. The first is inspection of the vulva and vagina. It is imperative that the clinician has good illumination, particularly if there is a history of a vaginal foreign body. It is usually possible to examine the vagina through the hymen using an otoscope. This may well allow the diagnosis of a foreign body to be made.

The second aspect of diagnosis involves the taking of bacteriological specimens. This can be extremely difficult

in a small child, as it is unlikely that the child will be cooperative. Any object which touches the vulva causes distress. The best way to take a bacteriological specimen is to use a pipette, which is much less irritating than a cottonwool swab. The pipette allows 1–2 mL of normal saline to be expelled into the lower part of the vagina, the tip of the pipette having been passed through the hymenal orifice. The fluid is then aspirated and sent for bacteriology. If a diagnosis of pinworms is to be excluded, then a piece of sticky tape over the anus early in the morning before the child gets out of bed will reveal the presence of eggs on microscopy.

Treatment

The vast majority of children do not have a pathological organism. The primary treatment in this group is advice about perineal hygiene. All parents of children with chronic vaginal disease are extremely worried that this may cause long-term detrimental effects to their daughters, particularly the fear of sexual dysfunction or subsequent infertility. There is no evidence that this is the case and therefore parents should be reassured that this is a local problem only. Management of these children is directed towards diligent hygiene of the perineum. The child must be taught to clean her vulva, particularly after defecation, from front to back, as this avoids the transfer of enterobacteria to the vulval area. After micturition the mother and child should be instructed to clean the vulva completely and not to leave the vulval skin wet, as this damp warm environment is an ideal culture surface for bacteria that cause vulvovaginitis. The mother must also be informed that vulval hygiene through daily washing should be performed, but that the soap should be gentle and not scented. Excessive washing of the vulva must be avoided as this leads to recurrent exfoliation and vulval dermatitis. During acute attacks of non-specific recurrent vulvovaginitis, children often complain of burning during micturition due to the passage of urine across the inflamed vulva. The use of barrier creams in these circumstances may be very useful. In the case of specific organisms being identified antibiotics can be prescribed and amoxicillin is probably the most effective.

Foreign body

Foreign bodies are occasionally found in the vagina and may lead to vaginal discharge. In patients who have persistent vaginal discharge despite treatment, an ultrasound scan may detect a foreign body or, if a history of a foreign body is forthcoming, it is probably best to carry out an examination under anaesthetic and remove any foreign body at that time.

Vaginal bleeding

Vaginal bleeding in childhood is extremely rare and should always be treated with extreme caution. The causes of genital bleeding in childhood include a vaginal foreign body, trauma, a neoplasm, premature menarche or urethral prolapse and the diagnosis can almost always be made on clinical inspection. Treatment should be appropriate but if trauma is suspected, sexual abuse must always be considered and referral to the appropriate team made.

Labial adhesions

Labial adhesions are usually an innocent finding and a trivial problem, but its importance is that it is frequently misdiagnosed as congenital absence of the vagina. The physical signs of labial adhesions are easily recognized. In the post-delivery hypo-oestrogenic state the labia minora stick together in the midline, usually from posterior to anterior until only a small opening is left through which urine is passed. Similar adhesions sometimes bind down the clitoris. It may be difficult to distinguish the opening at all. The vulva has the appearance of being flat, and there are no normal tissues beyond the clitoris evident. However, a translucent, dark, vertical line in the midline where the adhesions are thinnest can usually be seen, and these appearances are quite different from congenital absence of the vagina. There are usually no symptoms associated with this condition, although older children may complain that there is some spraying when they pass urine. The aetiology of the hypo-oestrogenic state means that they are never seen at birth, and instead occur during early childhood. As late childhood ensues and ovarian activity begins, there is spontaneous resolution of the problem. In the majority of cases no treatment is required and the parents should be reassured that their daughters are entirely normal. In those children in whom there are some clinical problems, local oestrogen cream can be applied for about 2 weeks. There is usually complete resolution of the labial adhesions. In some rare circumstances this will not resolve the problem, but at the end of the oestrogen therapy the midline is so thin that gentle separation of the labia may be undertaken using a probe, and this procedure causes no discomfort to the child. Application of a bland barrier cream at this stage will prevent further adhesion formation. Finally, in taking a history it is important to establish that there has not been any trauma to the vulva, as very rarely labial adhesions may be the result of sexual abuse.

Summary box 38.2

- Labial adhesions are frequently misdiagnosed as congenital abnormalities.
- Treatment is by topical oestrogen.

Adolescence

The adolescent gynaecological patient usually presents with one of three disorders: (i) problems associated with the menstrual cycle and menstrual dysfunction, dysmenorrhoea and premenstrual syndrome being the main group of disorders; (ii) primary amenorrhoea (see Chapter 37); and (iii) teenage hirsutism.

Menstrual problems

As can be seen in the description of puberty (Chapter 37), menstrual cycles are rarely established as normal ovulatory cycles from the beginning of puberty. It can take many years before the normal ovulatory menstrual cycle is established. It is extremely important that the gynaecologist understands this phenomenon, as the management of these cases is usually not active treatment but support and understanding of the condition and the child.

Heavy menstruation

Faced with a mother and her daughter giving a story of heavy menstrual loss, it is important that the clinician takes an accurate history from the child if possible. This is often difficult if the mother is present throughout and it must be remembered that the perception of heavy menstruation is often not reflected in studies that have looked at actual menstrual loss. Normal menstrual loss should not exceed 80 mL during a period, although in 5% of individuals it is heavier than this and causes no trouble. If a history of prolonged bleeding during surgical or dental procedures is obtained, screening for a coagulopathy is appropriate. Some reports suggest that 2–33% of these patients will have an underlying bleeding disorder [1]. The clinician is faced in these circumstances with attempting to assess whether the child truly has menstrual loss that is medically serious or menstrual loss that is irritating and distressing without being medically harmful. The best way to establish which of these is the case is by measuring the haemoglobin. If the haemoglobin level is normal (i.e. >12 g/dL), then an explanation should be given to the mother and child of the normal physiology of menstrual establishment, that the manifestation of the menstrual loss is normal and that it may take some time for the cycle to be established. This condition requires no active treatment. However, it is imperative that the child is followed up at 6-monthly intervals until the pattern of menstruation is established as reassurance is the most important part of the management process of these girls.

In those girls with haemoglobin levels between 10 and 12 g/dL, it is apparent that they are losing more blood at menstruation than is desirable. Again, an explanation is required so that the mother and daughter understand the cause of the problem and the child should be administered iron therapy to correct what will be mild iron deficiency anaemia. In terms of management, menstrual loss needs to be reduced and this may be achieved by using either progestogens cyclically for 21 days in every 28-day cycle or the combined oral contraceptive pill. It would be unusual for either of these therapies to be unsuccessful in controlling the menstrual loss. If these therapies are used, they should be stopped on an annual basis so that assessment may be made about whether or not the normal pattern of menstruation has been established by maturation of the hypothalamic–pituitary–ovarian axis. Thereafter, the child requires no further medication. Again follow-up is essential if reassurance is to be given appropriately.

Finally, in the child with a haemoglobin of less than 10 g/dL, it is obvious that serious anaemia has resulted from menstrual loss. This again requires an explanation but more urgent attention from a medical point of view. Blood transfusion should be given if clinically indicated. Progestogens are very much less likely to be effective in this group and the oral contraceptive pill is by far the treatment of choice. It may be given continuously for a short period of time so that the anaemia can be corrected using oral iron and then the pill may be used in the normal way so that menstrual loss occurs monthly, if desired.

Any girl who continues to have menstrual loss which is reported to be uncontrolled by these management strategies should have an ultrasound scan performed to exclude uterine pathology.

Summary box 38.3

- Menstrual disorders in adolescents are usually a reflection of normal physiology.
- Treatment should only be instigated if the adolescent is found to be anaemic.
- Treatments should be as simple as possible.

Primary dysmenorrhoea

Primary dysmenorrhoea is defined as pain which begins in association with menstrual bleeding. The management of dysmenorrhoea in the teenager is no different from that in the adult (see Chapter 34). The use of both non-steroidal anti-inflammatory drugs and the oral contraceptive pill is pertinent in teenagers, but again failure of these medications to control dysmenorrhoea should alert the clinician to the possibility of uterine anomaly and ultrasound imaging of the uterus should be performed to establish whether an anomaly exists.

Premenstrual syndrome

This is a difficult problem in adolescence as the psychological changes that are occurring during this time in a woman's life are often complex and stressful. It has been established that premenstrual syndrome is a stress-related disorder. Therefore in teenage girls undergoing puberty the stresses and emotional turbulence associated with this may, not surprisingly, lead to premenstrual problems. These are very difficult to manage and are usually not medically treated but addressed through the help of psychologists, if reassurance from the gynaecologist and an understanding of the process to the mother is not successful.

Hirsutism

Hair follicles cover the entire body and different types of hair are found in different sites. Androgens affect some areas of the human body and increase hair growth rate and also the thickness of terminal hairs. Androgens are also involved in sebum production and may cause this to be excessive. In some women excessive hair growth may occur on the arms, legs, abdomen, breasts and back such that it constitutes the problem of hirsutism. This may also be associated with acne, which may occur not only on the face but on the chest and back.

Differential diagnosis

There are four major groups of disorders that may cause hirsutism in adolescence (Table 38.2). Androgenic causes include congenital adrenal hyperplasia and its late-onset variant and also androgen-secreting tumours. The commonest group constitutes women with polycystic ovarian syndrome and while this is sometimes a difficult diagnosis to make in adolescents, it constitutes by far the greatest problem group. The diagnosis of XY gonadal dysgenesis is something that should be borne in mind when considering a child with hirsutism but a large percentage of patients have idiopathic hirsutism. It is important to remember that some girls will have a constitutional basis for their hirsutism and familial body hair patterns should be borne in mind when considering whether a young patient does in fact have hirsutism. Treatment for hirsutism is the same as in the adult and is covered in Chapter 41. In adolescence the mainstay in the treatment of androgen excess has been the oral contraceptive pill

Table 38.2 Causes of hirsutism in adolescents.

Androgenic causes
Congenital adrenal hyperplasia
Classic
Late onset
Androgen-secreting tumours
Polycystic ovarian syndrome
Idiopathic
XY gonadal dysgenesis

and without doubt this remains the main form of therapy. As the majority of these girls have some ovarian dysfunction, be that polycystic ovarian syndrome or an undefined problem, suppression of ovarian activity is very effective at lowering circulating androgens. If this is insufficient to gain control of hair growth, then the use of cyproterone acetate or spironolactone may be considered.

In those patients who are not considered to have hirsutism due to a medical disorder, drug therapies may be ineffective and supportive measures may be necessary for cosmetic benefit. These include hair removal by shaving, waxing or electrolysis of those areas which are particularly cosmetically sensitive and also the use of bleaches to change hair colour, thereby gaining cosmetic benefit.

 Summary box 38.4

Hirsutism in adolescents is often idiopathic or cultural. Treatment, as in the adult, is by cosmetic means or endocrine manipulation.

References

1 Wilkinson JP, Kadir RA. Management of abnormal uterine bleeding in adolescents. *J Pediatr Adolesc Gynecol* 2010;23(6 Suppl):S22–S30.

Further reading

Sanfilippo J, Lara-Torre E, Edmonds K, Templeman C. *Clinical Paediatric and Adolescent Gynaecology*. New York: Informa Healthcare, 2008.

Part 10
Menstruation

Chapter 39
The Menstrual Cycle

William L. Ledger
University of New South Wales, Royal Hospital for Women, Sydney, Australia

The human female is monotocous. The complex and highly regulated sequence of events that manifests as regular monthly menstruation exists in order to ensure that only one oocyte is ovulated in any one cycle, and that implantation of an early embryo can arrest the process of endometrial shedding and ensure its survival. Monthly menstruation is an obvious marker that the various levels of interaction between hypothalamus, pituitary, ovary and uterus are functional. Interruption of this axis at any point leads to disordered menses. Gynaecologists will frequently have to investigate and treat such disorders and a clear understanding of the regulation of the normal cycle is therefore necessary in order to guide rational management when things go wrong.

Although termed the 'menstrual cycle', since menstruation is the obvious monthly event during reproductive life, the normal menstrual cycle is mostly a reflection of ovarian events. The selection and growth of the dominant follicle leads to increasing concentrations of oestrogens in the blood, stimulating endometrial growth. Later, following the luteinizing hormone (LH) surge, ovarian oestrogens and progesterone from the corpus luteum induce endometrial secretory changes, and the decline in luteal steroid production in the absence of pregnancy leads to the onset of menstruation. Hence a description of clinical relevance of the menstrual cycle should focus on ovarian physiology, while not overlooking events in the hypothalamus and pituitary and at the level of the uterus.

The menstrual cycle is regulated at both endocrine and paracrine levels. Endocrinologically, there are classical feedback loops that modulate release of gonadotrophin hormones from the pituitary, with the ovarian steroids as the afferent arm. More recent studies have begun to elaborate a complex series of paracrine processes that operate within the tissues of the ovary and uterus to impose local regulation.

Step one: ensuring mono-ovulation

Folliculogenesis and the 'follicular phase'

At birth, the human ovaries contain approximately 1 million primordial follicles, arrested at prophase of the first meiotic division. This number already reflects considerable attrition from the maximum size of about 7 million in the follicle 'pool' at 5 months of fetal life [1]. Further depletion of the follicle pool will continue throughout reproductive life, with regular escape of follicles from the primordial 'resting phase' by re-entry into meiosis. The process of 'escape' from the resting state is not dependent on extra-ovarian influences: follicle depletion occurs before and after menarche, during use of the oral contraceptive pill and during pregnancy, and whether or not regular menstruation occurs. The majority of follicles will never develop beyond the pre-antral stage, travelling instead towards atresia. Of the original pool of 7 million primordial follicles, only about 400 will ever acquire gonadotrophin receptors and the possibility of ovulation. This dramatic attrition defines the female arm of natural selection, mirrored by the huge wastage of spermatogenesis in the male, in which millions of sperm are produced each day during fertile life, with only a tiny proportion ever fertilizing an oocyte (Fig. 39.1) [2].

The early stages of follicle development in the human are independent of gonadotrophins. Studies using transgenic animal species have begun to elucidate the contribution of locally acting intra-ovarian paracrine regulators of primordial follicle development, including bone morphogenetic proteins (BMPs), growth differentiation factor (GDF)-9, anti-Müllerian hormone (AMH) and the Bax family of regulators of apoptosis (Table 39.1).

Such studies are of more than theoretical interest: understanding the mechanisms regulating rate of entry into the pool of growing follicles should help to explain

Dewhurst's Textbook of Obstetrics & Gynaecology, Eighth Edition. Edited by D. Keith Edmonds.
© 2012 John Wiley and Sons, Ltd. Published 2012 by John Wiley and Sons, Ltd.

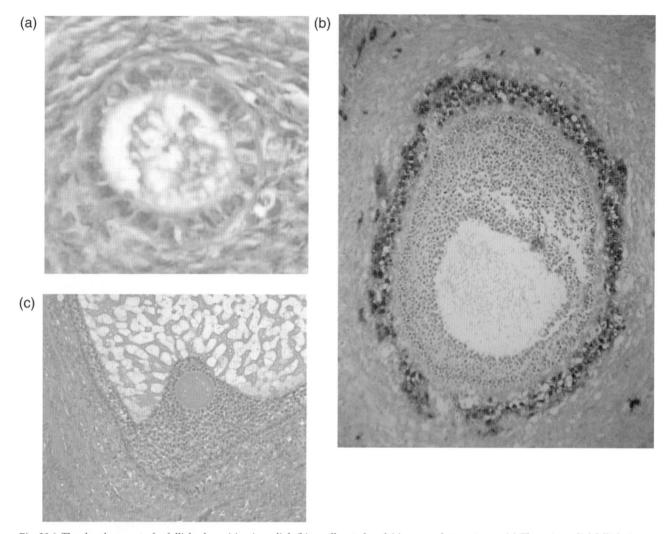

Fig. 39.1 The development of a follicle, from (a) primordial, (b) small antral and (c) pre-ovulatory stages. (a) The primordial follicle is surrounded by a single layer of undifferentiated epithelial cells, and is insensitive to gonadotropins. (b) The early antral follicle has well-differentiated theca (immunostained brown) and granulosa cell layers surrounding the developing antral cavity with the oocyte. (c) The pre-ovulatory follicle with the oocyte surrounded by the cumulus oophorus with well-differentiated granulosa and theca cell layers.

Table 39.1 Specific gene knockouts and their effects on ovarian function in the mouse.

Transgenic/mutant mouse	Ovarian phenotype
C-Kit deficiency, Kit ligand deficiency	Loss of germ cells (migration/proliferation failure)
WT1 knockout	Failure of gonadal development
BMP15/GDF9 knockout	Folliculogenesis arrest (primary stage)
IGF1 knockout	Folliculogenesis arrest (before antral follicle stage)
Kisspeptin/*GPPSU* knockout	Folliculogenesis alternation of LU stage
Oestrogen receptor gene knockout	Failure to ovulate
WNT4 knockout	Reduced germ cell number, masculinization

such common clinical problems as 'idiopathic' premature ovarian failure and early onset of menopause, as well as suggesting means of prolonging the reproductive lifespan. For example, some patients with premature ovarian failure have been found to carry mutations in the *BMP15* gene that lead to defective secretion of bioactive BMP15 dimer. BMPs are involved in the earlier stages of egress of follicles from the primordial pool, and such mutations may provide a diagnosis in cases of previously unexplained premature ovarian failure.

Once a developing follicle reaches the pre-antral stage of development, further progression to the antral and pre-ovulatory stages appears to be absolutely dependent on the presence of gonadotrophins. The temporary elevation in circulating concentration of follicle-stimulating hormone (FSH) seen in the early follicular phase of the ovarian cycle allows a limited number of pre-antral follicles to reach this stage of maturity, creating a cohort of practically synchronously developing follicles. However, only one 'lead' follicle will acquire significant aromatase enzyme activity within its granulosa cells, leading to increased synthesis and secretion of oestradiol from androgenic precursors. The 'two-cell, two gonadotrophin' hypothesis specifies the need for both LH, to stimulate production of precursor androgens, particularly androstenedione, by the theca cell layer, and FSH, to drive aromatization to oestradiol within the adjacent granulosa cell layer [3]. FSH, LH and human chorionic gonadotrophin (HCG) are structurally similar, sharing an identical α-subunit. Their specificity lies in structural differences in the β-subunit (Fig. 39.2). Hence assays for these molecules use antibodies directed against β-subunit epitopes.

The necessity for both LH and FSH at this stage of the cycle is demonstrated when exogenous gonadotrophin replacement is given to patients with Kallmann's syndrome. These patients are unable to secrete gonadotrophins into the circulation, but have normal ovarian physiology. The results of a study of such a patient are shown in Fig. 39.3. The patient had Kallmann's syndrome with anosmia, primary amenorrhoea and hypogonadal hypogonadism. Ovulation induction was undertaken using two different preparations of gonadotrophin. Treatment with both FSH and LH in the form of human menopausal gonadotrophins (HMG) induces both normal

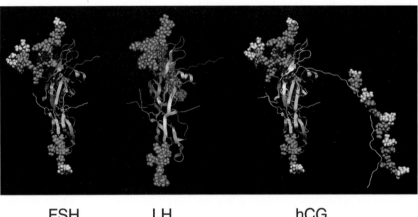

Fig. 39.2 Molecular structure of FSH, LH and HCG.

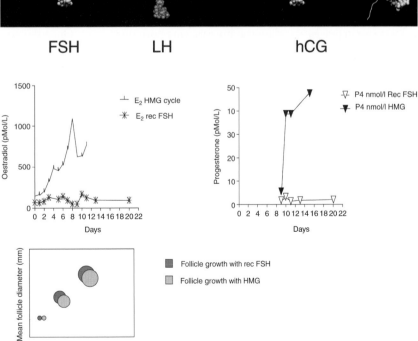

Fig. 39.3 Effects of FSH alone, and FSH and LH in combination, on follicle development in a hypogonadotrophic patient with Kallmann's syndrome.

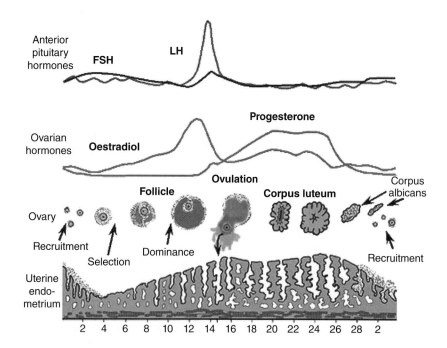

Fig. 39.4 Synchronization of the ovarian and endometrial cycles. Endocrine events seen in the peripheral circulation during the menstrual cycle.

follicle growth, monitored by transvaginal ultrasound (bottom panel), and oestradiol secretion (top left panel), leading to high luteal phase progesterone concentrations after an artificial LH surge with HCG injection. This indicates that successful ovulation and luteinization occurred. In contrast, treatment with FSH in the absence of LH, using a recombinant FSH preparation, led to identical follicle development on ultrasound but little elevation in circulating oestradiol concentration in the phase of follicular growth and no increase in progesterone after HCG injection.

The pituitary secretes the gonadotrophins LH and FSH in response to pulses of gonadotrophin releasing hormone (GnRH) from the hypothalamus, which travel to the anterior pituitary via the hypothalamo-hypophyseal portal tract. LH secretion appears to be closely regulated by GnRH pulsatility, while secretion of FSH is coregulated by hypothalamic GnRH and other factors which act directly on the pituitary, possibly including the inhibins and activins. In the normal follicular phase, GnRH pulse frequency is approximately once per 90 min. GnRH pulses are less frequent in the luteal phase, occurring approximately once in 4 hours. Disorders that slow GnRH pulsatility, such as anorexia nervosa, result in failure of secretion of pituitary gonadotrophins and a state of hypogonadal hypogonadism, with undetectable serum LH and FSH and amenorrhoea.

The genetic basis of hypogonadotrophic hypogonadism has recently been partially explained. Study of a patient with Kallman's syndrome and a deletion on the X chromosome led to the identification nearly 20 years ago of the *KAL1* gene as a cause of X-linked Kallman's syn-

drome. More than 10 other gene defects have been identified in cases of hypogonadal hypogonadism. The peptide kisspeptin acts as a potent stimulant to GnRH secretion in the human and mutations in *KISS1* have been identified as rare causes of hypogonadal hypogonadism. A second neuropeptide, neurokinin B, is also expressed on GnRH neurones and stimulates GnRH secretion and both kisspeptin and neurokinin B expression are downregulated by oestrogen. Hence it appears likely that kisspeptin and neurokinin B may participate in the relay of feedback from oestrogens, acting at the level of the hypothalamus, to GnRH production.

Once the concentration of serum oestradiol begins to rise in the mid-follicular phase, there is rapid suppression of pituitary FSH production by negative feedback (Fig. 39.4). Recent studies have suggested that suppression of pituitary FSH secretion in the follicular phase might be co-mediated by rising serum concentrations of inhibin B, a glycoprotein secreted by the granulosa cells of the developing dominant follicle. It is perhaps not surprising that a dual mechanism to control follicular phase FSH secretion has evolved [4]. The resulting decrease in circulating concentration of FSH withdraws gonadotrophin 'drive' from the remainder of the growing cohort of follicles. The result is progression to atresia for all but the dominant follicle, leading to mono-ovulation.

The mechanism by which this selection of a single dominant follicle occurs has been described by the 'threshold' concept, in which the rising concentration of FSH exceeds the threshold and thereby opens a 'window' that allows one follicle to continue growth and development. Suppression of FSH concentration then closes the

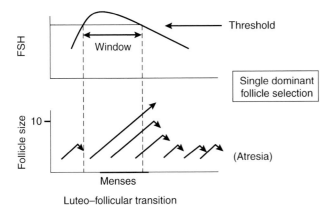

Figure 39.5 The threshold concept illustrating dependence of advanced follicle growth and maturation on a rise in circulating FSH concentration above an arbitrary 'threshold', with subsequent suppression of FSH preventing multiple follicle development. (With permission from Elsevier.)

window, preventing growth of multiple mature follicles (Fig. 39.5).

The threshold concept is useful in understanding the pitfalls of super-ovulation, in which daily injections of high doses of FSH are given as part of *in vitro* fertilization (IVF). The aim is to produce a cohort of eight or more mature follicles suitable for ultrasound-guided oocyte retrieval. However, if the follicle pool is small (e.g. if the patient is nearing menopause), then the yield of mature follicles will be disappointing, while if the follicle pool is large (e.g. if the patient has polycystic ovary syndrome), then there is a danger of over-response with hyperstimulation syndrome. Recent introduction of rapid ELISA assay for AMH has allowed measurement of this dimeric glycoprotein to be used in the estimation of ovarian response to super-ovulation induced by gonadotrophin injection. Serum AMH is high in patients with polycystic ovary syndrome who are in danger of over-response and hyperstimulation, and low in patients who are closer to menopause with low ovarian reserve. Measurement of AMH is proven to be clinically useful in IVF practice and also provides an indication of the size of the remaining pool of follicles in the ovaries. Recent studies have suggested that this can provide a reasonably accurate estimate of a woman's time to menopause, with clear clinical implications for management of infertility. The serum concentration of AMH varies little across the menstrual cycle and is not significantly affected by use of combined oral contraceptives, facilitating easy measurement in clinical practice.

Physiologically, AMH is secreted by small antral follicles and is not seen in large pre-ovulatory follicles. Hence measurement gives a direct assessment of the number of small antral follicles in the developing pool, which in turn depends on the size of the primordial follicle pool remaining in the ovaries.

Step two: ensuring maintenance of very early pregnancy

The LH surge and ovulation

Final maturation of the oocyte only occurs after initiation of the LH surge. This ensures that the oocyte is mature and ready for fertilization after release from the follicle. The LH surge represents a coordinated discharge of LH from the gonadotroph cells of the anterior pituitary. This occurs in response to the rapid rise in oestradiol during the latter days of the follicular phase of the ovarian cycle. Pulses of GnRH from the hypothalamus increase in both magnitude and frequency, triggering the LH surge with a rapid outpouring of LH and, to a lesser extent, FSH from the anterior pituitary.

The LH surge is also preceded by a rise in serum concentration of progesterone. The contribution of this rise to the peri-ovulatory phase of the cycle is unclear, but prevention of the pre-ovulatory rise in serum progesterone concentration using the progesterone receptor antagonist mifepristone prevents efficient ovulation. Compounds with effects similar to mifepristone are being tested as possible contraceptive agents, possibly acting by inhibiting both ovulation and implantation.

The LH surge initiates final maturation of the oocyte with completion of meiosis and extrusion of the first polar body, which contains one of the two haploid sets of chromosomes from the oocyte. The LH surge also induces an inflammatory-type reaction at the apex of the follicle adjacent to the outer surface of the ovarian cortex. A process of new blood vessel formation, with associated release of prostaglandins and cytokines, leads to rupture of the follicle wall and ovulation about 38 hours after the initiation of the LH surge. A chemotactic effect of ovarian cytokines draws the fimbria of the fallopian tube to within close proximity of the rupturing follicle. A thin mucus strand seems to join the mouth of the fallopian tube to the ovular follicle, forming a bridge for transit of the oocyte into the tube.

The 'empty' follicle rapidly fills with blood and the theca and granulosa cell layers of the follicle wall luteinize, with formation of the corpus luteum (Fig. 39.6). A rapid synthesis of progesterone, along with oestradiol, follows. Concentrations of progesterone in serum rise to above 25 nmol/L, one of the highest concentrations seen for any hormone in the circulation. These concentrations rise still further if pregnancy follows.

Endometrial development during the menstrual cycle and early pregnancy

Progression through the follicular phase of the cycle is characterized by the appearance of increasing amounts of oestradiol in the circulation. This acts on the basalis layer of endometrium, which persists from cycle to cycle in contrast to the monthly shedding of the more

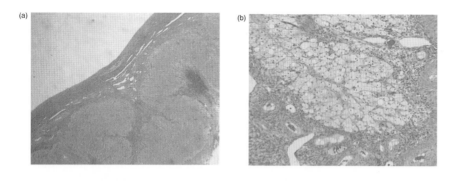

Fig. 39.6 The histological appearances of the corpus luteum, showing (a) an active corpus luteum and (b) regression of the corpus luteum with histiocyte infiltration.

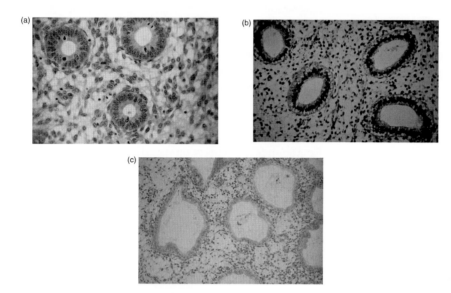

Fig. 39.7 The histological appearances of the endometrial cycle, showing the menstrual, proliferative and secretory phases.

superficial layers of endometrium. The new, proliferative endometrium grows rapidly under the influence of oestradiol, in synchrony with the growth and maturation of the oocyte and its follicle. An organized architecture appears, with endometrial glands and stromal compartments, in preparation for the development of secretory endometrium permissive of implantation following the LH surge, luteinization of the ruptured follicle and formation of the corpus luteum, with secretion of large amounts of progesterone (Fig. 39.7).

A key element in growth of healthy endometrium is formation of new blood vessels (endometrial angiogenesis), which seems to occur by elongation and expansion from pre-existing small vessels in the basalis. Endometrial angiogenesis can be divided into three stages: firstly, during menstruation, to reform the vascular bed; second, during the proliferative phase to develop endometrial vascular supply; and, finally, with spiral arteriole growth and coiling during the secretory phase, with the aim of providing an adequately vascularized site for implantation [6]. Therefore, in contrast to most vascular beds, which keep a persistent structure throughout life, the

endometrial vascular network grows and regresses during each menstrual cycle. Numerous angiogenic and angiostatic factors have been identified in the human endometrium. Most of these studies have focused on vascular endothelial growth factor (VEGF) and interleukins, which may be directly responsive to changing concentrations of ovarian steroids.

The development of a healthy secretory endometrium is essential for implantation and successful development of pregnancy. In the human, the oocyte is fertilized in the ampullary portion of the fallopian tube and then travels to enter the uterus on day 3, at the morula stage of development. The blastocyst, with distinct trophectoderm and inner cell mass, forms on day 4. The blastocyst sheds the zona pellucida and then adheres to the endometrial epithelium, beginning the process of implantation. Implantation is the first step in the interaction between the cells of the blastocyst and endometrium, i.e. between the mother and the fetus. Hence this interaction is critical to successful pregnancy, and a number of endometrial proteins have been identified as potential regulators of blastocyst development and implantation. These include endometrial integrins, glycosylated cell adhesion molecule (GlyCAM)-1 and osteopontin [7]. Continuous exposure of the endometrium to progesterone in early pregnancy downregulates progesterone receptors in the epithelia, a process associated with loss of the cell-surface mucin MUC1 and induction of secreted adhesion proteins. 'Rescue' of the corpus luteum by HCG secreted from the trophoblast of the developing pregnancy is essential for its continuance.

Interruption of progesterone synthesis and secretion by the corpus luteum, for example using the progesterone receptor antagonist mifepristone, is used in clinical practice to induce termination of early pregnancy. In contrast, luteal phase support in the form of HCG injection or injected or vaginal progestogens is used to maintain IVF pregnancies, since normal luteinization is interrupted by the GnRH agonist drugs used to prevent premature LH surges and unwanted ovulation.

Menstruation

Menstruation refers to the shedding of the superficial layers of the endometrium, with subsequent repair in preparation for regrowth from the basalis layer. Menstruation is initiated by a fall in the circulating concentration of progesterone that follows luteal regression, i.e. failure of 'rescue' of the corpus luteum by an implanted early pregnancy. Luteal progesterone synthesis is dependent on LH from the pituitary gland. During luteolysis, progesterone secretion falls despite maintained serum concentrations of LH, since the corpus luteum becomes less sensitive to gonadotrophic support and becomes increasingly unable to maintain production of progesterone. In contrast, in a conception cycle, the increasing block to progesterone synthesis is overcome by the rapidly increasing concentrations of HCG which act on the corpus luteum through its LH receptors.

In the immediate premenstrual phase, progesterone withdrawal activates a complex series of intrauterine signals, including expression of chemotactic factors that draw leucocytes into the uterus and expression of matrix metalloproteinase enzymes, prostaglandins and other compounds that act on the uterine vessels and smooth muscle. The 'invasion' of leucocytes and subsequent expression of inflammatory mediators has led to menstruation being likened to an inflammatory event [8,9]. The prostaglandins of the E and F series are present in high concentrations in the endometrium, and their synthesis is regulated by the ovarian steroids. Increased production of $PGF_{2\alpha}$ produces the myometrial contractions and vasoconstriction seen at menstruation, while E series prostaglandins increase pain and oedema, and are vasodilatory. PGE_2 also appears to induce synthesis of the cytokine interleukin (IL)-8, another key inflammatory and chemotactic mediator [10]. Pronounced vasoconstriction in turn leads to localized tissue hypoxia, further re-

inforcing release of inflammatory mediators. The end result of this cascade of events is constriction of the spiral arterioles with contraction of the uterine muscle, leading to expulsion of the shed tissue.

These studies have clear relevance to clinical management of menorrhagia and other menstrual disorders. Inhibitors of prostaglandin synthesis are widely used in these conditions, with good scientific basis. However, prostaglandin synthesis is also an important component of ovulation, and use of powerful inhibitors of prostaglandin synthesis, such as non-steroidal anti-inflammatory agents, can lead to anovular cycles and involuntary infertility.

Conclusion

Although complex, the endocrine and paracrine events that regulate the normal ovarian and uterine cycles are well understood. This chapter illustrates several examples by which understanding of the basic physiology of the cycle has led to scientifically based therapeutics. Further exploration of these regulatory mechanisms will produce new approaches to diagnosis and treatment for gynaecologists and their patients.

Summary box 39.1

The physiological events of the menstrual cycle represent the outcome of a complex system of inter-regulation by endocrine and paracrine factors.

Understanding of the physiology of the ovarian and menstrual cycle is critical before attempting to understand the various pathological states associated with anovulation and premature menopause.

New research into the genetic basis of regulation of re-entry of primordial follicles into the growing pool will provide new insights into the determination of ovarian reserve and timed menopause.

References

1 Baker TC. A quantitative and cytological study of germ cells in human ovaries. *Proc R Soc Lond B Biol Sci* 1963; 158:417–433.

2 Block E. Quantitative morphological investigations of the follicular system in women: variation in the different phases of the sexual cycle. *Acta Endocrinol* 1951;8:33–54.

3 Baird DT. A model for follicular selection and ovulation: lessons from superovulation. *J Steroid Biochem* 1987;27:15–23.

4 Groome NP, Illingworth PJ, O'Brien M *et al.* Measurement of dimeric inhibin B throughout the human menstrual cycle. *J Clin Endocrinol Metab* 1996;81:1401–1405.

5 Macklon NS, Fauser BCJM. Follicle-stimulating hormone and advanced follicle development in the human. *Arch Med Res* 2001;32:595–600.

6 Rogers PA, Gargett CE. Endometrial angiogenesis. *Angiogenesis* 1998;2:287–294.

7 Lessey BA. Adhesion molecules and implantation. *J Reprod Immunol* 2002;55:101–112.

8 Kelly RW. Pregnancy maintenance and parturition: the role of prostaglandin in manipulating the immune and inflammatory response. *Endocr Rev* 1994;15:684–706.

9 Kelly RW, King AE, Critchley HO. Cytokine control in human endometrium. *Reproduction* 2001;121:3–19.

10 Sales KJ, Jabbour HN. Cyclooxygenase enzymes and prostaglandins in pathology of the endometrium. *Reproduction* 2003;126:559–567.

Chapter 40
Contraception and Sterilization

Sharon T. Cameron[1] and Anna Glasier[2]

[1]Chalmers Sexual and Reproductive Health Service, Royal Infirmary of Edinburgh, Edinburgh, UK
[2]University of Edinburgh Clinical Sciences and Community Health, Edinburgh and School of Hygiene and Tropical Medicine, London, UK

The prevalence of contraception in the UK in the early twenty-first century is high. Only 4% of sexually active, potentially fertile women who were not wishing to conceive reported not using a method of contraception in 2008/2009 [1]. The average age of first intercourse in the UK for both men and women is 16 years, and the average age of first childbirth in 2008 was 30 years [2]. Since the mean age of menopause is 51 years, most women will need to use contraception for more than 30 years. Contraceptive choice varies with age, ethnicity, marital status, fertility intentions and education. In the UK in 2008/2009 the oral contraceptive pill (25% of women) and the male condom (25%) were the most popular methods of contraception (Table 40.1). Long-acting reversible (LARC) methods of contraception (injectables, ring, implants, intrauterine devices and systems) are used by 12% of women. The National Institute for Health and Clinical Excellence (NICE) recently produced guidance on LARC and recommended that increased uptake could lead to fewer unintended pregnancies [3].

Despite high contraceptive prevalence, unintended pregnancy is common. In England and Wales in 2008, 195 296 abortions were performed [4]. This corresponded to an abortion rate of 18 per 1000 women of reproductive age and 32 per 1000 for women aged 20–24 years [4]. Not all unintended pregnancies end in abortion; as many as 30% of pregnancies which end in childbirth are unplanned when they are conceived. Most data suggest that true method failure accounts for fewer than 10% of unintended pregnancies, the rest arising either because no method was used at the time of conception (30–50%) or because the method was used inconsistently or incorrectly.

Currently available reversible methods of contraception fall into two broad categories, hormonal and non-hormonal. Certain issues are common to all methods.

Efficacy and effectiveness

The effectiveness of a method of contraception is expressed by the failure rates associated with its use. The rates in Table 40.2 are based on studies in the USA and estimate the percentage of couples experiencing an unintended pregnancy during the first year of use of each method [5]. The effectiveness of a contraceptive depends on how it works and how easy it is to use. If a method prevents ovulation in every cycle in every woman, it should have an efficacy of 100%, since if there is no egg there can be no conception. Only if a mistake is made, or if the method is used inconsistently, will a pregnancy occur. The contraceptive implant and combined oral contraceptive pill both inhibit ovulation. Pregnancy rates for perfect use of the combined pill are around 1 in 1000, failures being due to incomplete inhibition of ovulation among women who metabolize the pill rapidly. However, if pills are missed ovulation can occur and typical-use failure rates are 8 per 100. In contrast the implant makes no demands on compliance, use can only ever be perfect, and perfect-use and typical-use failure rates are virtually the same. For implants and intrauterine devices (IUDs), typical-use failures occur because the provider has failed (e.g. the IUD perforated the uterus or the woman was already pregnant when the implant was inserted).

Pregnancy rates are still often described by the Pearl Index, the number of unintended pregnancies divided by the number of woman-years of exposure to the risk of pregnancy while using the method. Most rates are derived from clinical trials. There are some problems with this. The longer a cohort of couples using a method of contraception is followed, the lower the pregnancy rate is likely to be since the cohort increasingly comprises couples unlikely to fall pregnant (because they are highly motivated to avoid pregnancy, good at using the method or subfertile). Furthermore, failure rates in clinical trials are often underestimated because all the months of use of the

Table 40.1 Current use (%) of contraception by women aged 16–49 years in Great Britain 2008/2009 [1].

Pill*	25[†]
Progestogen-only	6
Combined pill	16
Male condom	25
Withdrawal	4
IUD	6
Injection	3
Implant	1
Patch	0
Natural family planning	2
Cap/diaphragm	0
Foams/gels	1
Hormonal IUS	2
Female condom	1
Emergency contraception	1
Total at least one method	58
Sterilized	6
Partner sterilized	11
Total of at least one method	75

* Includes women who did not know the type of pill used.
[†] Percentages sum to more than 100 as respondents could give more than one answer.

Table 40.2 Effectiveness of contraceptive methods: percentage of women experiencing an unintended pregnancy during the first year of use and percentage continuing use at the end of the first year (USA) [5].

Method	Per cent pregnant	
	Typical use	Perfect use
No method	85	85
Spermicides	29	18
Withdrawal	27	4
Periodic abstinence	25	
Calendar	9	
Ovulation method	3	
Sympto-thermal	2	
Cap		
Parous women	32	26
Nulliparous women	16	9
Diaphragm	16	6
Condom		
Female	21	5
Male	15	2
Combined pill and progestogen-only pill	8	0.3
Combined hormonal patch	8	0.3
Combined hormonal ring	8	0.3
Injectable (DMPA)	3	0.3
IUD, copper T	0.8	0.6
IUS (Mirena)	0.1	0.1
Implant	0.05	0.05
Female sterilization	0.5	0.5
Male sterilization	0.15	0.10

method are taken into account when calculating failure rates, regardless of whether or not intercourse has occurred during that cycle. Additionally people who participate in trials do not represent the general public and compliance is atypically good. For long-acting methods of contraception such as IUDs and implants, pregnancy rates with time (cumulative pregnancy rates) are reported.

Compliance/adherence/concordance

Many couples use contraception inconsistently and/or incorrectly. Some methods are easier to use than others. The IUD/IUS (intrauterine system) and implants are inserted and removed by a health professional and are entirely independent of compliance for efficacy. Depo-Provera lasts 12 weeks but correct use demands the motivation and organizational skills required to attend a clinic for repeat doses. Compliance with oral contraception is not easy. In one study, 47% of women reported missing one or more pills and 22% two or more pills per cycle [6]. In a study using electronic diaries to record compliance, 63% of women missed one or more pills in the first cycle, and 74% in the second cycle of use [7]. Typical-use failure rates are even higher with condoms, diaphragms, withdrawal and natural family planning, which rely on correct use with every act of intercourse.

Discontinuation

Discontinuation rates are higher for methods which do not require removal by a health professional as is clear from Table 40.3, which shows the percentage of couples in the USA still using each method at the end of 1 year [5]. In a US study, 50% of women discontinued the pill during the first 3 months of use [6]. Reasons for discontinuation are often associated with perceived risks and real or perceived side effects. The commonest reason for discontinuation is for bleeding problems. In a Swedish study of 656 women followed for 10 years, 28–35% of women (depending on age) stopped taking the pill because of fear of harmful side effects, 13–17% of women stopped because of menstrual dysfunction, 15–20% because of weight gain and 14–21% because of reported mood change [8].

Contraindications

Most contraceptive users are young and medically fit and can use any available method safely. However, a few medical conditions are associated with theoretical increased health risks with certain contraceptives, either

Table 40.3 Percentage of US women continuing to use each method at the end of the first year [5].

No method	
Spermicides	42
Withdrawal	43
Periodic abstinence	51
Cap	
Parous women	46
Nulliparous women	57
Diaphragm	57
Condom	
Female	49
Male	53
Combined pill and mini-pill	68
Combined hormonal patch	68
Combined hormonal ring	68
Injectable (DMPA)	56
IUD	
Copper T	78
Mirena (IUS)	81
Implant	84
Female sterilization	100
Male sterilization	100

Table 40.4 Common non-contraceptive benefits of selected methods of hormonal contraception.

Improved symptom	Combined oral contraceptive pill	IUS	DMPA
Heavy menstrual bleeding	✓	✓	✓
Acne and hirsutism	✓		
Premenstrual syndrome	✓		
Endometriosis	✓	✓	✓
Ovarian cancer risk	✓		Probably
Endometrial cancer risk	✓	Probably	Probably

IUS, levonorgestrel-releasing intrauterine system; DMPA, injectable (Depo-Provera).

because the method adversely affects the condition or because the condition, or its treatment, affects the contraceptive. The combined pill, for example, may increase the risk of a woman with diabetes developing cardiovascular complications; some anticonvulsants interfere with the efficacy of the combined pill. Since most trials of new contraceptive methods deliberately exclude subjects with serious medical conditions, there is little direct evidence on which to base sound prescribing advice. In an attempt to produce a set of international norms for providing contraception to women and men with a range of medical conditions that may contraindicate one or more contraceptive methods, the World Health Organization developed a system addressing medical eligibility criteria for contraceptive use. The Faculty of Sexual and Reproductive Healthcare (FSRH) have produced a UK version [9]. Using evidence-based systematic reviews, conditions are classified into one of four categories. Category 1 includes conditions for which there is no restriction for use of the method, while category 4 includes conditions that represent an unacceptable health risk if the contraceptive method is used (absolutely contraindicated). Classification of a condition as category 2 indicates that the method may generally be used but that more careful follow-up is required. Category 3 conditions are those for which the risks of the method generally outweigh the benefits (relatively contraindicated). Provision of a method to a woman with a category 3 condition requires careful clinical judgement since use of that method is not recommended unless there is no acceptable alternative.

Health benefits of contraception

Most couples use contraception for over 30 years. Additional health benefits beyond pregnancy prevention offer significant advantages and influence acceptability. In a nationwide sample of 943 US women, satisfaction with oral contraception was increased among women aware of the non-contraceptive benefits of the pill [10]. The commonest benefit of hormonal methods is an improvement in menstrual bleeding patterns (including amenorrhoea) which many women in the UK appreciate (Table 40.4). Barrier methods, particularly condoms, protect against sexually transmitted infections (STIs), including cervical cancer. When contraceptives are being used for their beneficial side effects or in the management of a medical problem such as menorrhagia, the risk–benefit ratio changes.

Combined hormonal contraception

The methods
Combined hormonal contraception can be administered orally (the combined oral contraceptive pill), transdermally (the contraceptive patch), systemically (combined injectables) and via the vaginal route (the combined contraceptive vaginal ring). All methods contain both oestrogen and a progestogen. Although there are far fewer data available on the other delivery systems, the mode of action, side effects and risks are similar.

Oral
Most of the combined oral contraceptive pills in the UK contain the oestrogen ethinylestradiol in a dose of 20–50 µg. Most women now use the so-called 'low-dose' pills containing 20–35 µg. Low-dose pills are potentially safer since the cardiovascular risks of the pill are mainly due to oestrogen. Although the lowest dose pill currently

available in Europe (15 μg ethinylestradiol) has the same efficacy as 30-μg pills, cycle control is less effective and breakthrough bleeding more common. The most recent preparation in the UK contains the oestrogen estradiol valerate. The progestogens used in currently available pills fall broadly into three groups: first- and second-generation progestogens (e.g. norethisterone and levonorgestrel), third-generation progestogens (gestodene, desogestrel and norgestimate) and newer progestogens with anti-androgenic activity such as drospirenone and dienogest. Co-cyprindiol is a preparation containing ethinylestradiol in combination with the anti-androgen cyproterone acetate, which is licensed for the treatment of severe acne and hirsutism. It is contraceptive and has over the years often been regarded as just another combined pill. It is useful for women with symptoms of hyperandrogenism who require contraception but should not be used routinely for other women, as some studies have suggested that it is associated with an increased risk of venous thrombosis compared with second-generation pills.

Most combined pill preparations are taken for 21 days followed by a 7-day break when withdrawal bleeding usually occurs. Everyday preparations in which a placebo tablet is taken during the pill-free interval may improve compliance but are more expensive and not widely used in the UK. Combined pills are available as monophasic preparations, in which every pill in the packet contains the same dose of steroids, and as biphasic, triphasic and, more recently, tetraphasic preparations in which the dose of both steroids changes during the cycle. Phasic pills were introduced in order to reduce the total dose of progestogens and in the belief that a regimen which mimicked the normal cycle would produce better cycle control. There is no evidence for better cycle control, and they are more expensive. Increasing number of women run packets of pills together for 3 months (tricycling because they like the associated amenorrhoea). This is particularly useful for women who experience symptoms associated with the withdrawal bleed such as dysmenorrhoea or menstrual migraine.

Transdermal

Only one contraceptive patch is currently available (20 cm^2 in size) and it delivers 20 μg ethinylestradiol and 150 μg norelgestromin daily. Each patch lasts 7 days, three patches being used consecutively with a placebo patch or patch-free interval in week 4 when withdrawal bleeding occurs. Contraceptive protection lasts for up to 10 days, allowing for errors in changing the patch. In a randomized trial comparing the patch with a combined pill, effectiveness was not significantly different: the overall Pearl Index for the patch was 1.24 per 100 woman-years and for the pill was 2.18 [11]. In a large non-randomized trial four of the six pregnancies that occurred were in women weighing over 90 kg, suggesting that efficacy may be reduced among heavier women. After the first few cycles of use, bleeding patterns and side effects are similar to those associated with the combined pill. Self-reported 'perfect use' was significantly better with the patch (88%) than with the pill (78%) in the randomized trial, although whether this is so with use outside a clinical trial remains to be seen.

Vaginal

A combined contraceptive vaginal ring releasing 15 μg ethinylestradiol and 120 μg etonorgestrel daily is licensed in the UK. The ring is made of soft ethylene-vinyl-acetate copolymer, has an outer diameter of 54 mm and a cross-sectional diameter of 4 mm. Designed to last for 3 weeks, a 7-day ring-free interval is associated with bleeding patterns that appear superior to those associated with the combined pill. In a comparison with a combined pill containing 30 μg ethinylestradiol and levonorgestrel 150 μg, the incidence of irregular bleeding with the ring was significantly less (<5% vs. 38.8% in each cycle). In all other respects, including efficacy, the ring is no different from the pill, although there may be advantages in terms of demands on compliance.

Mode of action

The principal mode of action of combined hormonal contraception is inhibition of ovulation. Oestrogen inhibits pituitary FSH, suppressing the development of ovarian follicles, while progestogen inhibits the development of the LH surge. Most pills, patches and rings are administered for 21 days followed by a 7-day hormone-free interval. In some women the 7-day interval is long enough to allow follicle growth and 25% of pill users have ultrasound evidence of follicles of 10 mm in diameter on the last day of the interval. If the interval is extended beyond 7 days, these follicles will continue to develop and, despite restarting contraception, ovulation may occur. If pills are missed, the chance that pregnancy will occur depends not only on how many pills were missed, but also on when those pills were missed. The risk of pregnancy is greatest when pills are missed at the beginning or at the end of the packet, i.e. when the hormone-free interval is extended. Current advice on when additional contraceptive precautions are required when pills are missed has been criticized as being too complicated and so this advice is likely to be readdressed and simplified by the FSRH in the near future [12]. Manufacturers of transdermal patch and ring advise use of barrier methods for 7 days if a patch is applied 48 hours late or a ring is removed for more than 3 hours during the 21 days of treatment.

Additional contraceptive properties of combined hormonal contraceptives include changes in characteristics of cervical mucus that interfere with sperm transport, a possible alteration in tubal motility, endometrial atrophy and impaired uterine receptivity.

Efficacy
See Table 40.2.

Contraindications
The absolute (UK MEC category 4 conditions) and relative (UK MEC category 3 conditions) contraindications to combined hormonal contraception (pill, patch and ring) are listed in Tables 40.5 and 40.6.

Risks and side effects

Minor side effects
Combined hormonal contraception affects almost every system in the body. Contraceptive steroids are metabolized by the liver and affect the metabolism of carbohydrates, lipids, plasma proteins, amino acids, vitamins and clotting factors.

Many of the reported side effects, particularly headache, weight gain and loss of libido, are common among women not using hormonal contraception. Those likely to be directly related to the contraceptive steroids include fluid retention, nausea and vomiting, chloasma, mastalgia and breast enlargement. All but chloasma (which gets worse with time) improve within 3–6 months. A different dose of oestrogen or type of progestogen or a different delivery system may help if time alone does not solve the problem. For women with persistent nausea on the pill,

Table 40.5 UK medical eligibility criteria (MEC) category 3 conditions (relative contraindications) for use of combined hormonal contraception [9].

Multiple risk factors for arterial disease (UK MEC 3/4)
Hypertension: systolic blood pressure 140–159 mmHg or diastolic pressure 90–99 mmHg, or adequately treated to below 140/90 mmHg
Some known hyperlipidaemias
Diabetes mellitus with vascular disease (UK MEC 3/4)
Smoking (even less than 15 cigarettes/day) and age 35 or over
Obesity (BMI ≥35 kg/m²)
Migraine, and age 35 and over
Past history of migraine, with aura more than 5 years ago or more
Breast cancer, with more than 5 years without recurrence
Breast-feeding until 6 months post partum
Post partum and not breast-feeding until 21 days after childbirth
Current or medically treated gallbladder disease
History of cholestasis related to combined oral contraceptives
Viral hepatitis (acute or flare) (UK MEC 3/4)
Continuing immobility unrelated to surgery (e.g. wheelchair)
Taking rifampicin (rifampin) or certain anticonvulsants
Taking certain antiretrovirals (ritonavir, protease-boosted inhibitors)
Family history of venous thromboembolism in first-degree relative under age of 45 years

Table 40.6 UK medical eligibility criteria (MEC) category 4 conditions (unacceptable health risk) for use of the combined oral contraceptive pill [9].

Breast-feeding <6 weeks postpartum
Smoking ≥15 cigarettes/day and age ≥35 years
Multiple risk factors for cardiovascular disease
Hypertension: systolic ≥160 mmHg or diastolic ≥100 mmHg
Hypertension with vascular disease
Current or history of deep vein thrombosis/pulmonary embolism
Major surgery with prolonged immobilization
Known thrombogenic mutations
Current or history of ischaemic heart disease
Current or history of stroke
Complicated valvular heart disease
Migraine with aura
Current breast cancer
Diabetes with vascular disease or nephropathy, retinopathy or neuropathy
Acute viral hepatitis (MEC 3/4)
Severe cirrhosis
Benign or malignant liver tumours
Raynaud's with lupus anticoagulant
Systemic lupus erythematosus with positive or unknown antiphospholipid antibodies

the patch may be indicated. Side effects (real or perceived) often lead to discontinuation; 73% of British women of all ages quote weight gain as being a disadvantage of the pill.

Serious side effects

Cardiovascular disease
The combined pill is extremely safe. Data from a large UK cohort study of over 46 000 women using the contraceptive pill for up to 39 years reported that oral contraception was not associated with an increased risk of death [13]. Indeed, 'ever users' of the contraceptive pill (predominantly combined pill) had a 12% reduction in the overall risk of death for all conditions compared with 'never users' (RR 0.88, 95% CI 0.82–0.93).

However, combined hormonal contraception does increase the tendency to thrombosis in both the venous and arterial circulation. The adverse effect on clotting is related to the dose of oestrogen and, for pills, lower doses are theoretically associated with reduced risk. There is a threefold to fivefold increase in the risk of venous thromboembolism (VTE) associated with combined pill use. Two recent studies have shown that reducing the dose of ethinylestradiol from 30 to 20 µg may reduce the risk of deep venous thrombosis (DVT).

The risk is unaffected by age, smoking or duration of pill use, but is higher in obese women [body mass index (BMI) >25 kg/m²] and in women with a history of pregnancy-induced hypertension. Four studies published in 1995 and 1996 demonstrated a differential risk of VTE depending on the type of progestogen in the pill. Combined pills containing a third-generation progestogen (gestodene or desogestrel) were shown to have a roughly twofold increased risk of VTE compared with first- or second-generation combined pills (containing levonorgestrel or norethisterone). Although often attributed to confounding or bias, there is some biological plausibility for this differential risk. Regarded as second choice in the UK, these pills should be prescribed only for women intolerant of other types of combined pill and prepared to accept the increased risk of VTE. Less data are available regarding the risk of DVT with pills containing the newer progestogens (drospirenone and dienogest). There is also ongoing debate about whether the risk of DVT with pills containing cyproterone acetate is greater than that of third-generation pills. However, whichever progestogen is used, the absolute risk of VTE is small (15 per 100000 woman-years for second-generation pill users compared with 5 per 100000 woman-years for non-users), and much less than that associated with pregnancy (60 per 100000 woman-years). The risk is greatest during the first year of use, possibly due to the unmasking of inherited thrombophilias such as factor V Leiden. Screening for known thrombophilias is not cost-effective and although asking about a family history of VTE is routine when prescribing the pill, this too fails to detect most women at risk of VTE. Although non-oral routes of administration avoid the first pass through the liver, thereby theoretically having less effect on clotting factors, in the absence of contrary evidence, the patch, ring and combined injectable methods carry the same warning as the combined pill.

Arterial disease is much less common but more serious. It is related to age, and the risk is strongly influenced by smoking. Pooled data from four large Phase II clinical trials suggest that the combined pill has a negligible effect on blood pressure [14]. The relationship between combined pill use and myocardial infarction (MI) is controversial. While there is widespread agreement that there is an increased risk of MI among women who smoke or have hypertension, some studies have demonstrated an increased risk among normotensive non-smokers while others have not. One study from the Netherlands reported a relative risk of MI of 2.8 (95% CI 1.3–6.3) among women with no known risk factors [15]. Another case–control study from the UK showed no significant association between combined oral contraceptive pill use and MI [16]. In a recent meta-analysis of 23 studies, the adjusted odds ratio of MI was 2.48 (95% CI 1.91–3.22) for current combined pill users compared with 'never users' [17]. The risk among past users was not significantly increased. The risk of MI was significant for users of second- but not third-generation pills. There

was also a dose–response relationship with ethinylestradiol, with pills containing 20 µg ethinylestradiol associated with no increase in risk. The risk of MI was significantly increased by smoking (OR 9.3, 95% CI 3.89–22.23) compared with non-smokers (many other studies have shown this) and in women with a history of hypertension (OR 9.9, 95% CI 1.83–53.53) and hypercholesterolaemia (OR 2.08, 95% CI 1.5–2.9). The absolute risk of MI in women of reproductive age, even those with known risk factors, is extremely small.

Use of the combined pill increases the risk of ischaemic stroke twofold, although the risk of haemorrhagic stroke is unchanged. Smoking and hypertension increase the risk of stroke by three to ten times. However, stroke is also rare in women of reproductive age.

The combined pill is also contraindicated in migraine with aura. In a recent meta-analysis of 17 good-quality observational studies, migraine was associated with a relative risk of stroke of 2.16 (95% CI 1.89–2.48) and users of oral contraceptives had an eightfold increase in the risk of stroke compared with non-users [18]. Many people describe their headaches as migraine, so it is important to make an accurate diagnosis of those severe headaches reported as migraines and, in addition, those complicated by aura. Aura occurs before the onset of headache and symptoms of aura include homonymous hemianopia, unilateral paraesthesia and/or numbness, unilateral weakness and aphasia or unclassifiable speech disorder. Visual symptoms progress from fortification spectra (a star-shaped figure near the point of fixation with scintillating edges) to scotoma (a bright shape which gradually increases in size). Flashing lights are not classified as aura.

Malignant disease

Breast cancer

Published data on combined hormonal contraception and breast cancer are difficult to interpret because pill formulations, patterns of reproduction (particularly age at first pregnancy and family size), diet and average weight have changed with time. A meta-analysis of 54 studies involving over 53000 women with breast cancer and 100000 control subjects concluded that use of the combined pill was associated with a small increase in the risk of breast cancer. The increased risk persists for 10 years after stopping the pill [19]. The relative risk for current users was 1.24; for those 1–4 years after stopping, 1.16; and for those 5–9 years after stopping, 1.07. After 10 years the relative risk was the same as that of non-users. Although the relative risk was higher for women who started the pill at a young age, there was little added effect from the duration of use, dose or type of hormone. Ever-users were significantly less likely (RR 0.88) to have metastatic disease even if they had stopped the pill more than 10 years earlier. A more recent case–control study involving 8000 women, including those over 35, suggested no increased risk of breast cancer (RR 1.0, 95% CI 0.8–1.3), although the upper limit of the confidence interval is in keeping with the much larger meta-analysis. It has been suggested that starting to use the pill may accelerate the appearance of breast cancer in susceptible women. Alternatively, women using the pill might have their tumours diagnosed earlier, although it is difficult to explain why a tendency to earlier diagnosis would persist for years after stopping. A biological effect of combined hormonal contraception remains a possibility.

Cervical cancer

Data on the risk of cervical cancer among pill users are also difficult to interpret since barrier methods confer some protection and any association identified in epidemiological studies may simply be the result of inadequate adjustment for sexual behaviour. In a recent meta-analysis of 10 case–control studies, women with persistent infection with human papillomavirus (HPV) using hormonal contraception (mainly combined) for more than 5 years had an increased relative risk of cervical cancer of 2.8. Hormonal contraceptive use for longer than 10 years increased the relative risk to 4.0. Thus, despite concerns that sexual behaviour among women using different methods of contraception may be confounding, evidence is mounting for a real association between the use of combined hormonal contraception and cervical cancer. However, women can be advised that the risk of cervical cancer can be reduced through condom use, HPV vaccination (young people) and regular cervical screening.

Ovarian, endometrial and colon cancer

There is substantial evidence that the oral contraceptive pill protects against ovarian, endometrial and colon cancer. For ovarian cancer, there is a 50% reduction in the risk of both epithelial and non-epithelial ovarian cancer after 5 years use of the combined pill. This effect may be related to the reduction in the total number of ovulations, and therefore rupture of the ovarian capsule, experienced in a lifetime. Epidemiological studies from 21 countries including 23257 women with ovarian cancer and 87303 controls have shown that this reduction in risk of ovarian cancer persists for 30 years after discontinuation of the contraceptive pill. Protection is also evident for women with a family history of breast cancer (who may thus be at higher risk of ovarian cancer). The effect of the combined pill on endometrial cancer is strongly related to the duration of use (20% reduction in risk after 1 year, 50% after 4 years) and is sustained for 15 years after stopping the pill. There is also evidence that current or recent use of the combined pill may confer protection against colon cancer.

Practical prescribing

The FSRH recommends a pill containing 30μg ethinylestradiol in combination with a second-generation progestogen as the pill of choice for new users on the grounds that such pills are the safest and cheapest (all pill types appear to be equally effective) [20].

Women should be carefully instructed how to use the pill, patch or ring and what to do when mistakes are made. Many women choose to have a break from hormonal contraception for a few months. While most cardiovascular risks decline when the method is stopped, they recur as soon as it is restarted and unplanned pregnancies commonly occur during such breaks. Most women who stop the pill regain normal fertility after stopping. Secondary amenorrhoea is almost always the result of abnormalities present before the method was started (such as polycystic ovarian syndrome) but regular withdrawal bleeds mask these conditions. There is no evidence for any adverse effect on the fetus as a result of past or current pill use.

A number of medicines (some anticonvulsants, antifungals, antiretrovirals and antibiotics) induce liver cytochrome P450 and will thus reduce the efficacy of low-dose hormonal contraception such as combined oral contraceptive pill, implant, patch, ring and progestogen-only pill (Table 40.7). These medicines are not thought to affect the efficacy of the injectable, IUD or IUS. If a woman using enzyme-inducing medication wishes to use a low-dose hormonal method, then the consistent use of condoms is also advised. In contrast to previously accepted advice about reduced efficacy of the combined pill with broad-spectrum antibiotics, there is intermediate-level evidence that the contraceptive effectiveness of the

Table 40.7 Drug interactions with low-dose hormonal contraception (pills, patch, ring and implant).

Type of drug	Liver enzyme induction
Anticonvulsant	Carbamazepine, eslicarbazepine, oxcarbazepine, phenobarbital, phenytoin, primidone, rufinamide, topiramate
Antibiotic	Rifampicin, rifabutin
Antifungal	Griseofulvin
Antiretroviral	*Protease inhibitors*
	Amprenavir, atazanavir, nelfinavir, lopinavir, saquinavir, ritonavir
	Non-nucleoside reverse transcriptase inhibitors
	Efavirenz, nevirapine
Gastrointestinal	Lansoprazole
Immunosuppressant	Tacrolimus
Respiratory	Bosentan
Central nervous system	Modafinil

combined oral contraceptive pill (and all other methods) is not affected by coadministration of most broad-spectrum antibiotics. While the antiepileptic lamotrigine is not an enzyme inducer, use of combined hormonal contraception increases the clearance of lamotrigine and reduces serum levels of this drug. Women using lamotrigine should be advised that seizure frequency may increase when initiating combined hormonal contraception and that lamotrigine side effects may increase in the pill-free interval or when discontinuing this method of contraception.

Summary box 40.1

- Combined hormonal contraception is available in a range of delivery systems.
- The main action is to suppress ovulation.
- The length of the pill-free interval is crucial to efficacy.
- The oral contraceptive pill reduces the risk of ovarian and endometrial cancer by 50%.
- Combined hormonal contraception is contraindicated in women with arterial and venous disease.
- Third-generation progestogens may increase the risk of VTE.
- Current users of the combined pill have an increased risk of breast cancer (RR 1.24).
- The perfect-use failure rate for the combined pill is 0.1 per 100 woman-years, but the typical-use failure rate is 8 per 100 woman-years.

Progestogen-only contraception

Progestogen-only contraception avoids the side effects of oestrogen. It is available in a wide variety of delivery systems including oral, injectables, implants and IUS. Implants and the IUS last for 3 and 5 years respectively. Progestogen-only contraception has in the past been less commonly used than combined hormonal contraception and so there are fewer data on the risks associated with long-term use.

The methods

Oral
A number of types of progestogen-only pills are available in the UK. The older formulations contain a very low dose of second-generation progestogen which does not consistently inhibit ovulation. A newer pill contains the third-generation progestogen desogestrel at a dose sufficient to inhibit ovulation in almost every cycle [21].

Injectable
Long-acting depot medroxyprogesterone acetate (DMPA) is given by deep intramuscular injection, 150 mg every 12 weeks. A new micronized preparation of DMPA that is administered subcutaneously is licensed but not yet marketed in the UK. This micronized preparation is a lower dose (104 mg DMPA), but has the same efficacy as the intramuscular preparation and is given at the same injection intervals. Since it is administered subcutaneously, this affords the possibility of self-administration.

Subdermal
The first contraceptive implant to become available was a six-rod system known as Norplant® but this is no longer available in the UK. The only currently available implant (Implanon®, Organon, UK) is a single rod, containing 68 mg 3-keto-desogestrel (a metabolite of desogestrel) providing contraception for 3 years. The initial release rate of 60–70 µg/day falls gradually to around 25–30 µg/day at the end of 3 years. The implant is preloaded into a sterile disposable inserter and is inserted subdermally on the inner aspect of the non-dominant arm above the elbow. It is inserted and removed using local anaesthetic. The insertion device has recently been redesigned to make insertion easier (Nexplanon®, Organon, UK)

Intrauterine
The intrauterine system (Mirena®, Bayer Schering, UK) has a T-shaped plastic frame with a reservoir on the vertical stem containing 52 mg levonorgestrel releasing 20 µg/day for at least 5 years. The IUS is inserted and removed using the same procedures as for copper IUD insertion (see below), although the stem of the IUS is bigger and difficulties with insertion may be experienced, particularly in women with a small uterus (such as following prolonged use of DMPA). The IUS is licensed for the management of heavy menstrual bleeding. In randomized controlled trials it has been associated with a reduction in menstrual blood loss of 71–96% [22], although the benefit is not usually seen until at least 6 months of treatment. The observed dramatic decrease (one-third) in the number of hysterectomies being performed in England over the last decade has been partly attributed to increased use of the IUS [23]. Increasingly, the IUS is being used to deliver the progestogen component of hormone replacement therapy, an indication for which it is licensed to be used for 4 years, but may be used 'off licence' in this way for up to 5 years [24].

Mechanism of action
All methods of progestogen-only contraception have a number of mechanisms of action. The injectable, implant and desogestrel-containing progestogen-only pill inhibit ovulation. Older progestogen-only pill formulations inhibit ovulation only inconsistently. All progestogen-only contraception, regardless of the route of administration, affect cervical mucus, reducing sperm penetrability and transport, and all (but particularly the IUS, which has

little effect on ovarian activity but causes marked endometrial atrophy) have an effect on the endometrium compromising implantation if ovulation and fertilization occur.

Efficacy

Failure rates for progestogen-only methods are shown in Table 40.2. The older progestogen-only pills (containing low doses of second-generation progestogens) have higher failure rates than the combined pill. The reduced efficacy is due partly to the fact that many women continue to ovulate, and partly because the pill has a shorter half-life in the circulation so that missing even just one pill may interfere with contraceptive efficacy. The desogestrel-containing pill is believed to have failure rates equivalent to those of the combined pill as ovulation is consistently inhibited. The IUS lasts for 5 years. Although not licensed beyond 5 years, the FSRH recommend that women who have an IUS inserted at 45 years or over can use the device for contraceptive purposes for 7 years, or if amenorrhoiec until the menopause. After this, the device should be removed [24]. The progestogen implant is effective (and licensed) for 3 years; there are no data on use beyond this time.

Indications and contraindications

Progestogen-only contraception is commonly prescribed for women in whom oestrogen is absolutely or relatively contraindicated, for example women with cardiovascular disease, migraine, diabetes or mild hypertension. In the UK, breast-feeding women are advised to use progestogen-only methods since oestrogen impairs milk production. There are few contraindications to use of progestogen-only methods. The UK MEC 4 conditions (unacceptable health risk if contraceptive is used) for use of progestogen-only methods include a history of breast cancer (within last 5 years) and postpartum sepsis or septic abortion (IUS method only). UK MEC conditions 3, which apply to all progestogen-only methods, are shown in Table 40.8.

Side effects

Minor side effects

Bleeding disturbances

The commonest side effect and cause for discontinuation of a progestogen-only method is an unacceptable bleeding pattern. This includes amenorrhoea if women have not been forewarned that it may happen or find that they do not like it. Low-dose progestogen-only methods (pills and implants) are associated with a high incidence of irregular vaginal bleeding. This is due partly to their effect on ovarian function. In the normal cycle, ovulation determines regular menstruation. Inconsistent ovulation and fluctuating endogenous oestrogen production from irregular follicle growth lead to irregular bleeding.

Table 40.8 UK medical eligibility criteria (MEC) category 3 conditions (relative contraindications) for use of progestogen-only methods [9].

Stroke (continuation of method only)
Breast cancer, past and with no evidence of disease for 5 years
Liver tumours
Cirrhosis
Current or history of ischaemic heart disease or stroke (continuation of method)
Unexplained vaginal bleeding (injections, implants and IUS)
Use of certain drugs: some antiretrovirals, some anticonvulsants (progestogen-only pills and implants)
Multiple risk factors for arterial cardiovascular disease (injectable only)
Vascular disease (injectable only)
Antiphospholipid antibody
Severe thrombocytopenia (injectable and implant only)
Diabetes with nephropathy, neuropathy, retinopathy, other vascular disease (injectable only)
Distorted uterine cavity (IUS only)

However, there is also evidence to suggest that progestogen-only methods directly affect the vasculature of the endometrium, increasing the chance of bleeding. Bleeding patterns differ according to the dose of progestogen and the route of administration. It is important to ensure that women with unscheduled bleeding are up to date with cervical smears and a speculum and pelvic examination should be performed to ensure that the cervix looks normal and uterus and adnexae feel normal. Testing for STIs such as *Chlamydia* should be considered, particularly for young women (<25 years) or women in high-risk groups. The FSRH have produced guidance on the investigation of women who present with bleeding problems on hormonal contraception [25].

There is limited evidence that the irregular bleeding associated with DMPA and the implant can be temporarily alleviated by the administration of oestrogens. The Clinical Effectiveness Unit of the FSRH therefore advise that, in women with unscheduled bleeding using an injectable, implant or IUS, the combined pill may be used (in medically eligible women) for up to 3 months as a short-term solution [25]. There is also limited evidence that mefenamic acid may reduce the duration of an episode of unscheduled bleeding in women using the injectable [25].

Oral

Around 50% of women using the classical progestogen-only pill continue to ovulate and therefore menstruate regularly, while 10% will experience complete suppression of follicular development and will have amenorrhoea. The rest will have inconsistent ovulation (often with a short luteal phase), or follicular development only and will bleed irregularly. Up to 20% of women using the desogestrel-containing pill will experience amenorrhoea while the rest are likely to have irregular bleeding since ovulation is inhibited.

Injectable

The high dose of progestogen in injectable DMPA inhibits ovulation and by the end of 1 year of use 70% of women will have either infrequent scanty vaginal bleeding or amenorrhoea. Heavy prolonged bleeding may be a problem in around 2% of women. The cause is unknown and often leads to discontinuation of the method.

Subdermal

Menstrual disturbance is the norm; up to 20% of users experience amenorrhoea and almost all the rest will have irregular unpredictable bleeding. Heavy bleeding is uncommon and measured blood loss is much less than that experienced during a normal menstrual cycle. Many women do not like the unpredictability of the bleeding; even very light bleeding is unacceptable if it lasts for days on end. Patterns do not become more regular with time as the dose of progestogen remains sufficient to inhibit ovulation for the full 3 years.

Intrauterine

While women using the IUS continue to develop ovarian follicles and ovulate, most have amenorrhoea or only very light occasional bleeding because the presence of high concentrations of levonorgestrel in the uterine cavity induces endometrial atrophy. However, it takes time for atrophy to occur and most women experience frequent and often persistent spotting for 3–6 months after IUS insertion. IUS users can be reassured that bleeding patterns usually improve with time.

Long-term use of implants and the IUS (for which upfront costs are high) is essential for cost-effectiveness, and careful counselling about menstrual irregularities is vital to avoid premature discontinuation.

Persistent follicles/follicular cysts

The effect of low-dose progestogen-only methods on ovarian activity also results in a relatively high incidence of functional ovarian cysts or, more accurately, persistent follicles. It has been estimated that one in five women using the progestogen-only pill will have a 'cyst' demonstrable by ultrasound, and they are common among IUS users. Usually asymptomatic, persistent follicles can cause abdominal pain or dyspareunia. Most will disappear with menstruation and so treatment should be conservative.

Other 'hormonal' side effects

These include headache, nausea, bloating, breast tenderness and weight and mood change, all common in women not using hormonal contraception. They often settle with time but if not may be alleviated by changing to a different progestogen. A Cochrane Review found that progestogen-only injectable users had a mean weight gain of 3 kg after 2 years of use. Weight gain may be predicted by BMI prior to use. In a prospective study of obese and non-obese adolescents, those who were obese had a greater weight gain (average 9.5 kg) than women of normal BMI (4 kg) [26]. Oily skin and acne can be a problem, particularly with the more androgenic progestogens levonorgestrel and norethisterone. Some studies have suggested an increased risk of ectopic pregnancy. This has not been confirmed, although methods of contraception that do not prevent ovulation are more likely to be associated with ectopic pregnancies than those which prevent ovulation.

Delay in the resumption of fertility

Fertility returns rapidly after stopping low-dose progestogen-only contraception. However, it may take up to 1 year for normal fertility to return following cessation of DMPA. Women can be assured that there is no permanent impairment of fertility but this delay makes DMPA an inappropriate method for women wishing short-term contraception.

Serious side effects

Because progestogen-only methods are much less widely used than the combined pill, data on long-term risks are sparse.

Cardiovascular disease

There is no evidence for an increase in the risk of stroke, MI or VTE in association with progestogen-only contraception. Any association between VTE and doses of progestogen used for the treatment of gynaecological conditions such as heavy menstrual bleeding may be due to prescriber bias since the combined pill, often the method of choice, may not be given to women with known risk factors for VTE.

Malignant disease

The injectable DMPA confers a high degree of protection against endometrial carcinoma but although it should theoretically also protect against ovarian cancer, there are as yet no data to support this. There are no data on risks of cervical cancer, although it is thought that all hormonal contraception may play a promoting role. Recent concern that the progestogen component of hormone replacement therapy may contribute to the increased risk of breast cancer has raised concerns about progestogen-only contraception. The large meta-analysis on breast cancer and hormonal contraception included a small percentage of progestogen-only pill (0.8%) and injectable (1.5%) users [17]. Use of the progestogen-only pill within the last 5 years was associated with a very small but statistically significant increase in relative risk of breast cancer (1.17%). However, the same increase among injectable users was not significant. For both methods the relative risk had returned to normal 5 years after stopping.

Bone mineral density

Complete inhibition of ovulation by the injectable DMPA causes hypo-oestrogenism and amenorrhoea. Hypo-oestrogenism is associated with a reduction in bone mineral density (BMD). It has been recognized for some time that current use of DMPA is associated with a loss of BMD compared with non-users. This may be more of an issue with very young women who have not yet achieved peak bone mass. Results of cross-sectional studies are limited and inconsistent, although two prospective studies have reported statistically significant decreases in BMD over 2 years among DMPA users aged between 12 and 21 compared with users of non-hormonal contraception [27,28]. While current DMPA users in older age groups do seem to have decreased BMD compared with non-users, limited evidence suggests that women who stop using DMPA before the menopause can regain lost bone mass. However, there is some concern about women over 40, who may not recover normal BMD after stopping DMPA before they inevitably lose more bone when they reach the menopause. While the data on BMD across all age groups is consistent, only one study has examined fracture risk and this was among women of a mean age of 21. There was no significant association between use of DMPA and the risk of stress fractures after adjusting for baseline BMD. In the UK the FSRH endorses the advice of the Medicines and Healthcare product Regulatory Agency (MHRA) [29,30] as listed below.

• DMPA may be used in women under the age of 18 years, as first-line contraception after consideration of other methods.

• In women of all ages who wish to continue using DMPA, re-evaluation of the risks and benefits of treatment should be carried out every 2 years.

• In women with significant lifestyle and/or medical risk factors for osteoporosis, other methods of contraception should be considered.

The MHRA does not advise how women who wish to continue DMPA should be evaluated after 2 years of use. However, the FSRH in the UK cautions against using BMD scans which are unlikely to help in the decision-making process.

There are no robust data which demonstrate an effect of low-dose progestogen-only methods on BMD. Whether women who experience amenorrhoea while using the implant or the progestogen-only pill are at any risk is unknown.

Summary box 40.2

- Progestogen-only contraception is available in a wide range of delivery systems.
- The dose of progestogen determines the mode of action and side effects.
- Irregular vaginal bleeding is a common reason for discontinuation of low-dose progestogen-only contraception, which does not inhibit ovarian activity completely.
- Despite normal ovarian activity, the IUS is associated with amenorrhoea because of endometrial atrophy.
- DMPA inhibits ovarian activity completely and most users have amenorrhoea.
- There are few data on long-term safety. Theoretically progestogen-only contraception is safer than combined hormonal contraception.
- Progestogen-only contraception does not increase the risk of cardiovascular disease.
- DMPA is associated with decreased BMD.

Intrauterine device

Most copper-containing IUDs currently available in the UK have a plastic frame with copper wire wound round the stem or copper sleeves on the end of the arms. In all devices a tail protrudes through the cervical canal into the upper part of the vagina allowing easy removal. A Cochrane Review showed that devices containing 380 mm^2 of copper have the lowest failure rates [31]. One IUD in the UK that contains 380 mm^2 of copper is licensed for 10 years of use, while those containing 300 mm^2 of copper are licensed for 5 years. The FSRH advises that any IUD inserted at or after the age of 40 can be retained until contraception is no longer required (i.e. beyond the licensed duration) [24]. Since the risks of uterine perforation, infection and device expulsion are all highest around the time of IUD insertion, it makes sense to discuss prolonged continuation with the user.

Efficacy

In a WHO sponsored study of an IUD containing 380 mm^2 copper, the failure rate was 1 per 100 women in the first year of use. Over 5 years of use, cumulative pregnancy rates for devices containing at least 300 mm^2 are around 2%.

Mechanism of action

IUDs stimulate a marked inflammatory reaction in the uterus. The concentrations of macrophages and leucocytes, prostaglandins and various enzymes in both uterine and tubal fluid increase significantly. It is thought that these effects are toxic to both sperm and egg and interfere with sperm transport. If a healthy fertilized egg reaches the uterine cavity implantation is inhibited.

Contraindications

There are very few women for whom an IUD is contraindicated. A history of malignant trophoblastic disease, endometrial cancer or pelvic tuberculosis and current STI or pelvic inflammatory disease are the only UK MEC category 4 conditions. Women at risk of STI and women with HIV can use an IUD but should be carefully counselled about safe sex and additional condom use should be promoted. Unexplained vaginal bleeding should be investigated before IUD insertion and a distorted uterine cavity (due for example to fibroids) may make insertion impossible.

Side effects

Menstrual disturbance

The effect of the IUD, particularly the effect on local prostaglandins, on the endometrium tends to cause increased menstrual bleeding and dysmenorrhoea. Bleeding can be both heavier and more prolonged, particularly during the first 3–6 months of use. In clinical trials up to 15% of women will discontinue for these reasons.

Dysmenorrhoea

The presence of an IUD in the uterus is associated with an increased incidence of dysmenorrhoea. There is no good evidence that dysmenorrhoea is less among women using the frameless device.

Ectopic pregnancy

A meta-analysis of case–control studies demonstrated no increase in the risk of ectopic pregnancy among current users, but the risk was increased among past users (OR 1.4, 95% CI 1.23–1.59) [32]. The absolute risk of *any* pregnancy is very low among IUD users and the annual ectopic pregnancy rate is 0.02 per 100 woman-years compared with 0.3–0.5 per 100 woman-years for women not using contraception.

Pelvic infection

The risk of pelvic infection associated with IUD use has been overestimated in the past. Infection is most likely to occur during the first 20 days following insertion and is estimated to occur in 1 in 100 women [33]. Thereafter the risk of developing infection is not significantly higher than that among women using no contraception (<1.5 per 1000 woman-years).

The risk can be reduced by using aseptic techniques during insertion and by restricting the method to women who do not have multiple partners and whose partners do not have multiple partners Screening for STI is recommended prior to insertion in areas where the prevalence of infection is high and among individual women with known risk behaviours (including women under 25).

Pelvic actinomycosis can rarely occur in association with IUD use. *Actinomyces* is a commensal organism in the vagina. Actinomycosis-like organisms are sometimes seen on cervical smears. Their role in infection in the presence of an IUD is unclear. If seen on a cervical smear in a symptom-free patient, the IUD can be left *in situ*. There is no indication for follow-up screening. If, however, there are symptoms, the IUD should be removed (avoiding contamination from the vagina and cutting off the tails) and sent for culture.

Insertion and removal

An IUD can be inserted at any time in the cycle if it is reasonably certain the woman is not pregnant. Otherwise insertion should be limited to the first 7 days of the cycle. Postpartum insertion should be delayed until 4 weeks after childbirth for all women including breast-feeding women. An IUD can be inserted immediately after miscarriage or induced abortion, although expulsion rates may be higher in the second-trimester uterus. Unless pregnancy is desired, removal should only be undertaken during menstruation or if one can be reasonably certain that there is no risk of pregnancy (no unprotected intercourse within 7 days). In menopausal women the IUD should be left in for 1 year after the last menstrual period, if menopause occurs at 50 or later. If menopause occurs in a woman's forties, then the IUD should be left for 2 years after the last menstrual period [24]. If the IUD threads are not visible or snap during removal, it may be possible to remove the device with a specially designed hook or a pair of artery forceps.

Perforation

Perforation of the uterus may occur at the time of insertion although it is often unnoticed. In large clinical trials it occurs in 1.3 per 1000 insertions. Absent threads should be investigated by ultrasound. If ultrasound confirms the absence of a device within the uterus, then abdominal radiography should be performed to confirm that the device is within the abdominal cavity, thus excluding the possibility of device expulsion. In most cases, the IUD can be retrieved laparoscopically. At insertion, the length of the uterine cavity should be measured using a sound and a tenaculum should be used at insertion in order to reduce the risk of perforation.

Expulsion

The risk of expulsion is around 1 in 20. It is most common in the first 3 months of use and usually occurs during menstruation. Many clinicians advise that IUD users should regularly check to feel the IUD strings in order to detect expulsion.

Summary box 40.3

- The IUD is a very effective method of contraception, lasting for at least 5 years, which can be used by unmarried nulliparous women.
- Devices containing less than 300 mm² copper have higher failure rates and should not be used routinely.
- If an IUD is inserted after age 40, it can be left in place until contraception is no longer required.
- The commonest side effect (and commonest reason for premature removal) is heavy bleeding.
- The risk of ectopic pregnancy is enormously reduced compared with women using no contraception.
- The risk of pelvic infection has been over-emphasized and by 3 weeks after insertion is not increased. Women with risk factors for STI should be screened before insertion but the IUD is not contraindicated.

Emergency contraception

Emergency contraception is defined as any drug or device used after intercourse to prevent pregnancy. There are three options for emergency contraception within the UK: a pill containing a progesterone receptor modulator (ulipristal acetate), a pill containing a progestogen (levonorgestrel) and the IUD. The most widely used hormonal method in the UK is levonorgestrel 1.5 mg (LNG-EC) and it can be obtained from community pharmacists in addition to contraceptive services. In 2008/2009, 42% of women using LNG-EC sought this from the pharmacy rather than their general practitioner or contraceptive clinic [1]. LNG-EC is taken as a single dose within 72 hours of intercourse. LNG-EC has replaced the formerly used 'Yuzpe' regimen (a combination of 100 μg ethinylestradiol and 0.5 mg levonorgestrel taken twice with the two doses separated by 12 hours), since studies demonstrated that the Yuzpe regimen had a lower efficacy and a higher incidence of adverse effects than LNG-EC.

Since 2009, ulipristal acetate, a progesterone receptor modulator, has been available in the UK for emergency contraception. Ulipristal acetate (UPA-EC) is licensed to be used up to 5 days after unprotected sex and is taken as a single oral dose (30 mg). A meta-analysis of the two randomized controlled trials that compared both LNG-EC and UPA-EC for emergency contraception (combined dataset of 3445 women) showed that UPA-EC almost halved the risk of pregnancy compared with LNG-EC for women presenting within 72 hours of unprotected sex (OR for the risk of pregnancy of 0.58, 95% CI 0.33–0.99) [34]. For women who presented within 24 hours of sex, treatment with UPA-EC reduced the risk of pregnancy by almost two-thirds (OR 0.35, 95% CI 0.11–0.93) compared with LNG-EC.

The IUD (but not IUS) is probably the most effective emergency contraceptive, with failure rates of less than 1%. In the UK it is used for up to 5 days after the estimated day of ovulation, which may be more than 5 days after intercourse. It is particularly appropriate for women who wish to continue the IUD as a long-term method of contraception. However, most women requesting emergency contraception are young and nulliparous and it can sometimes be difficult to insert a device. Simultaneous antibiotic prophylaxis against STI (with STI screening) is recommended for women at risk who have an IUD inserted for emergency contraception.

Mechanism of action

Both levonorgestrel 1.5 mg (LNG-EC) and ulipristal acetate (UPA-EC) have been shown to inhibit or delay ovulation if taken several days in advance of ovulation in the follicular phase of the cycle. However, if taken just immediately before ovulation, when the risk of pregnancy is greatest, LNG-EC appears to be ineffective in inhibiting ovulation. In contrast, UPA-EC is able to delay ovulation when given just before or on the day of ovulation. This is thought to account for the higher efficacy of UPA-EC compared with LNG-EC in the meta-analysis comparing both treatments [34]. It has been suggested that LNG-EC may interfere with sperm transport, although there is no evidence for this. There is no evidence that LNG-EC interferes with implantation. While UPA-EC has been shown to exert endometrial effects, it is unknown whether such effects are contraceptive.

Efficacy

Effectiveness of emergency contraception is estimated by calculating the number of pregnancies that might have occurred in the absence of treatment and such estimates of efficacy are difficult to make. Many women are unsure of the exact date of their last menstrual period and most do not ovulate on exactly the same day each cycle. The majority of women who use emergency contraception are of unproven fertility and many use it after an accident with a condom which may not in fact have resulted in the leakage of seminal fluid. The chance of conception following one act of intercourse at mid-cycle has been calculated to be around 27% per cycle, so that even without emergency contraception over 70% of women will not conceive. The effectiveness of oral emergency contraception has probably been overestimated in the past. In recent studies comparing UPA-EC and LNG-EC within 72 hours of sex, lower than previously accepted efficacy rates were reported [34]. In one of the randomized controlled trials comparing UPA-EC and LNG-EC, UPA-EC was calculated to prevent 85% of expected pregnancies and LNG-EC to prevent 69% of pregnancies [35].

Side effects

The side-effect profiles of UPA-EC and LNG-EC have been shown to be similar. Menses after LNG-EC normally occurs at the expected date or one day earlier, although the next menses after UPA-EC come on average 2 days later than expected.

Few data are available on the safety of LNG-EC but the FSRH advise that there are no contraindications to its use [36]. There is no evidence that LNG-EC is teratogenic should it fail to prevent pregnancy. Interactions between UPA-EC and hormonal contraception have not been studied but UPA-EC is a progesterone receptor modulator and so could in theory reduce the efficacy of progestogen-containing contraceptives. The manufacturer thus advises abstinence/condoms for the remainder of the menstrual cycle in which UPA-EC is used. While the outcome of the small number of babies born in women who have taken UPA-EC has been good, clearly UPA-EC is a new drug and so a European registry has been established to follow up the outcome of births occurring after its administration.

Use of emergency contraception

In 2008/2009, 7% of women of reproductive age had used emergency contraception at least once in the past year. Among women aged 16–19 that figure rose to 17% [1]. A number of studies suggest that around 11% of women presenting for abortion in the UK used emergency contraception to try to prevent the pregnancy. While increasing access to emergency contraception may be desirable, increased use of emergency contraception has not as yet been shown to reduce abortion rates.

 Summary box 40.4

- Ulipristal acetate is a progesterone receptor modulator that is available for emergency contraception.
- Ulipristal acetate has been shown in a meta-analysis to be more effective than levonorgestrel for emergency contraception.
- Ulipristal acetate can be given within 120 hours of unprotected intercourse.
- The most effective method of emergency contraception is an IUD (about 99% effective).
- An IUD can be inserted up to 5 days after ovulation for emergency contraception.

Sterilization

Female sterilization

Female sterilization involves blocking both fallopian tubes at laparoscopy, hysteroscopy or, less commonly, laparotomy or mini-laparotomy. A variety of techniques exists for occluding the tube. Filshie clips are the method of choice for laparoscopic sterilization and results in immediate tubal occlusion. The Pomeroy technique, where a loop of tube is tied and excised, is the preferred method of tubal occlusion during laparotomy and mini-laparotomy. Postpartum sterilization using mechanical occlusion with clips rather than partial salpingectomy has a much higher failure rate.

The hysteroscopic method of female sterilization offers the advantage of avoiding abdominal incisions and can be performed under local anaesthesia. This approach is particularly suitable for women who present a particular anaesthetic or operative risk (e.g. high BMI, coexisting medical conditions, previous abdominal or pelvic surgery). Using hysteroscopy under local anaesthesia or mild sedation in an outpatient setting, a micro-insert is placed in the proximal section of the fallopian tube. The micro-inserts induce a local inflammatory response and, eventually over the subsequent weeks, fibrosis of the intramural tubal lumen. A disadvantage of this method is that an additional method of contraception should be used until fibrosis of the lumen has been achieved and imaging (radiography, ultrasound or hysterosalpingography) at 3 months has confirmed satisfactory placement of the inserts. A number of different devices for hysteroscopic sterilization may be used for this procedure. One device, Essure® (Conceptus, UK), is an expanding spring measuring 2 mm in diameter and 4 cm in length made of titanium, stainless steel and nickel-containing Dacron fibres. Another device, Adiana® (Hologic, UK), uses radiofrequency ablation in conjunction with a silicone micro-insert.

Efficacy

Follow-up data available for the Filshie clip suggests a failure rate of 2–3 per 1000 procedures after 10 years. The Royal College of Obstetricians and Gynaecologists (RCOG) recommends telling women that the lifetime risk of failure is 1 in 200 [37]. In case series of hysterocopic sterilization procedures (Essure®), pregnancy prevention rates reported in a 1-year period were over 98%.

Timing of female sterilization

Should sterilization be undertaken in association with pregnancy, women should be made aware of the possibility of regret and of potential increased failure rates. The RCOG advise that consent for sterilization should be obtained at least 1 week prior to Caesarean section if the two procedures are to be combined [37]. It is seldom possible to arrange sterilization for a particular time of the cycle and women should continue using their current method of contraception until surgery. It is not necessary to stop the combined pill before sterilization as the risk of thromboembolic complications is negligible. If an IUD is *in situ*, it should be removed during the next menstrual period. The date of the last menstrual period should be checked preoperatively. The RCOG recommends a routine pregnancy test on the day of sterilization as this significantly reduces the rate of undetected pregnancies [37]. It has been suggested that the operative complication rate is higher when sterilization is done at the same time as an induced abortion. However, the complication rate is less than that of the two separate procedures added together. Nevertheless, there is an increase in the failure rate. A number of studies have demonstrated an increased incidence of gynaecological consultation and of hysterectomy following sterilization despite no demonstrable change in menstrual blood loss. Changes in menstrual bleeding patterns are inevitable with advancing age and after stopping hormonal contraception.

Although hysteroscopic sterilization can avoid the risks of a general anaesthetic, laparoscopy and abdominal scars, potential adverse events with the procedure include tubal perforation, infection, device migration, device expulsion and vasovagal and pelvic pain.

Vasectomy

Male sterilization is safer and cheaper than female sterilization and is more commonly performed under local anaesthesia than female sterilization. The ability to check for efficacy (with semen analysis) is a clear advantage when male is compared with female sterilization. Division or occlusion of the vas deferens prevents the passage of sperm. Division alone is associated with a high failure rate, so should be accompanied by fascial interposition or diathermy. The vas can be ligated or occluded with clips or by diathermy, but clips appear to be associated with a higher failure rate and are not recommended. No one method seems to be more effective than any other but the 'no-scalpel' vasectomy, which obviates the need for a skin incision, is associated with a reduced incidence of haemorrhage and infection. 'No-scalpel' vasectomy is recommended in the RCOG guidelines [37].

The success of the procedure is verified by the absence of sperm from two consecutive samples of ejaculate collected at least 4 weeks apart. Histological examination of the excised portion of the vas is not necessary unless there is doubt about their identity. The time for azoospermia to develop depends on the frequency of intercourse, but it is estimated that some 20 ejaculations are required and in the UK seminal fluid is usually examined at 12 and 16 weeks. Contraception must be continued until confirmation of two negative results has been received.

Efficacy

Even after azoospermia has been confirmed, there is a failure rate of around 1 in 2000 procedures. In a small number of men non-motile sperm persist after vasectomy. No pregnancies have been reported when less than 10 000 non-motile sperm per millilitre are found in a fresh specimen produced at least 7 months after the vasectomy.

Complications

Scrotal bruising occurs in almost everyone, and haematoma (1–2%) and wound infection (up to 5%) are common minor complications. The development of anti-sperm antibodies (thought to be in response to leakage of sperm) occurs in most men and appears to be harmless unless restoration of fertility is desired. Small inflammatory granulomas can form at the cut ends of the vas, presumably also in response to leaked sperm. Sperm granulomas may be painful and persistent but can be effectively excised. Chronic testicular pain of unknown cause can persist in a very small number of men for years after a vasectomy.

Concerns have been raised in the past linking vasectomy with an increased risk of atherosclerosis, testicular cancer and other, mainly autoimmune, diseases. Several large studies have failed to substantiate these concerns. However, an increased risk of prostate cancer has also been suggested. Only epidemiological evidence is available and there seems to be no biological plausibility for such a link, but further research is required.

Counselling for sterilization

Most couples seeking sterilization have been thinking about the operation for some considerable time. As many as 10% of couples may regret being sterilized and 1% request reversal. Couples sterilized at a young age, immediately after delivery or at the time of an induced abortion, are more likely to experience regret. A change of partner is the commonest reason for requesting reversal. Factors that should be explored during counseling are listed in Table 40.9.

Reversal of sterilization

Reversal of female sterilization involves laparotomy, does not always work (microsurgical techniques are associated with around 70% success), and carries a significant risk of

Table 40.9 Points to cover when counselling for male or female sterilization.

Age: those less than 30 years are more likely to regret the decision
Family size and the possibility of wanting children/more children
Previous and current contraception and any problems experienced: some women request sterilization because they are unable to find any other acceptable method of contraception. It is particularly important to discuss long-acting methods which are equally effective but reversible
Which partner should be sterilized
Stability of the relationship and the possibility of its breakdown
The procedure
Failure rate
Risks and side effects
Reversibility
Practical arrangements, e.g. continued use of interim contraception

ectopic pregnancy (up to 5%). Reversal of vasectomy is technically feasible in many cases, with patency rates of almost 90% being reported in some series. Pregnancy rates are much less (up to 60%), perhaps as a result of the presence of anti-sperm antibodies. Ovulation should be confirmed and a normal semen analysis obtained before reversal is undertaken.

Summary box 40.5

- Female sterilization has a failure rate of 1 in 200 and vasectomy 1 in 2000 after 10 years.
- Menstrual disorders are common after female sterilization but are related to cessation of other methods of contraception (which affect menstrual bleeding) and ageing and not to sterilization itself.
- There is no evidence to support the suggestion that vasectomy may be associated with an increased risk of prostate and testicular cancer.
- Reversal of sterilization is not always successful.

Barrier methods

Barrier methods work by preventing the passage of sperm into the female genital tract.

Male and female condoms

The male condom remains one of the most popular methods of contraception in the UK, with 25% of couples using it as their main method (Table 40.1). The latex condom is cheap, widely available over the counter and, with the exception of the occasional allergic reaction, is free from side effects. Polyurethane condoms offer an alternative for people with latex sensitivity. Condoms are effective in preventing STIs, including HIV. Spermicide alone is not recommended for prevention of pregnancy as it is only moderately effective. Nonoxynol 9 (N-9) is a spermicidal product sold as a gel, cream, foam, film or pessary for use with diaphragms or caps. In response to data suggesting that frequent use of N-9 might increase the risk of HIV transmission, it is recommended that women who have multiple daily acts of intercourse or who are at high risk of HIV infection should not use N-9 [38]. For women at low risk of HIV infection N-9 is probably safe. Since there is no evidence that lubricating male condoms with N-9 improves efficacy, such condoms should no longer be promoted.

The female condom is a polyurethane sheath, the open end of which is attached to a flexible polyurethane ring. A removable ring inside the condom acts as an introducer and helps keep the device inside the vagina. It comes in one size with a non-spermicidal lubricant. It is designed for single use and is expensive. Failure rates are similar to those of the male condom (Table 40.2). Designed primarily with the prevention of STIs in mind, the female condom has not become popular in the UK.

Diaphragm and cervical cap

The diaphragm (and cap) is much less popular than male condoms. Both must be fitted by a doctor or nurse and do not confer the same degree of protection against STIs since the vaginal mucosa is not covered. In order to select the correct size of diaphragm, a vaginal examination is conducted. The distance between the point at which the ulnar border of the index finger of the examining hand abuts the symphysis pubis and the tip of the middle finger corresponds to the appropriate size of diaphragm. Latex allergy, recurrent vaginal infections such as bacterial vaginosis or candida and recurrent urinary tract infection are possible side effects.

Caps fit snugly over the cervix but are very seldom used. Femcap® (FemCap Inc., USA) is a silicone rubber device designed to be easier to fit, and less likely to slip, than the traditional diaphragm. Since it is said to confer less pressure on the surrounding vaginal walls, it was also supposed to reduce the risk of urinary tract infection. In a randomized multicentre study comparing it with a traditional diaphragm, the failure rate of Femcap® was almost double (1.96 times that for diaphragm users). Although Femcap® users did have a lower risk of urinary tract infection (OR 0.6, 95% CI 0.4–1.0), they were much more likely to find the device difficult to insert and remove and much more likely to experience dislodgement.

Summary box 40.6

- All barrier methods have high failure rates when used typically.
- Diaphragms and caps must be fitted by a health professional.
- Male condoms reduce the risk of sexually transmitted disease including HIV.
- Spermicides should not be used alone and if used frequently and in large quantities may increase the risk of HIV transmission.

Fertility awareness methods/natural family planning

Few couples in the UK use so-called natural methods of family planning (NFP), although in some parts of the world these methods are common. All involve the avoidance of intercourse during the fertile period of the cycle (periodic abstinence). Methods differ in the way in which they recognize the fertile period. The simplest is the calendar or rhythm method in which the woman calculates the fertile period according to the length of her normal menstrual cycle. The first day of the fertile period is calculated as the length of the woman's shortest cycle minus 20 days, and the last day of the fertile period as the longest cycle minus 11 days. Therefore if cycle length varies from 25 to 31 days, the potential fertile period and days when intercourse should be avoided are days 5–20.

Others approaches use symptoms which reflect fluctuating concentrations of circulating oestrogen and progesterone. The mucus or Billings method relies on identifying changes in the quantity and quality of cervical and vaginal mucus. As circulating oestrogens increase with follicle growth, the mucus becomes clear and stretchy allowing the passage of sperm. With ovulation, and in the presence of progesterone, mucus becomes opaque, sticky and much less stretchy or disappears altogether. Intercourse must stop when fertile-type mucus is identified and can start again when infertile-type mucus is recognized. Progesterone secretion is also associated with a rise in basal body temperature of about 0.5°C. The basal body temperature method is thus able to identify the end of the fertile period. Other signs/symptoms, such as ovulation pain, position of cervix and degree of dilatation of the cervical os, can be used additionally to help define the fertile period.

Whatever method is used many couples find it difficult always to abstain from intercourse during the fertile period. Failure rates are high (Table 40.2) and most of the failures are due to conscious rule breaking.

Lactational amenorrhoea method

Breast-feeding delays the resumption of fertility after childbirth and the length of the delay is related to the frequency and duration of breast-feeding episodes and the timing of the introduction of food other than breast milk (e.g. solids). Prolonged breast-feeding can postpone ovulation and therefore the risk of pregnancy for more than a year. A woman who is fully or nearly fully breast-feeding and who remains amenorrhoeic has less than a 2% chance of pregnancy during the first 6 months after childbirth (lactational amenorrhoea method or LAM). In developed countries, where average durations of breast-feeding are short and where few women practice full or nearly full breast-feeding beyond 4 months after delivery, LAM is unlikely to be a practical method of contraception. In developing countries, however, where women breast-feed for much longer and where modern methods of contraception may be expensive and difficult to obtain, the potential to use LAM is much greater.

> ### Summary box 40.7
>
> - Periodic abstinence, using a variety of fertility awareness methods, can prevent pregnancy but depends heavily on compliance.
> - LAM is associated with a 2% pregnancy rate.

References

1 Lader D. Contraception and sexual health 2008/2009. A report on research using the ONS Omnibus Survey produced by the Office for National Statistics on behalf of the Department of Health, London. Office for National Statistics, 2009. Available at: www.statistics.gov.uk (accessed 31 August 2010).

2 Average age of mother at childbirth. In Social Trends 33. Available at: www.statistics.gov.uk (accessed 31 August 2010).

3 Long acting reversible contraception. Available at: www.evidence.nhs.uk (accessed 31 August 2010).

4 Abortion statistics England and Wales 2009. Available at: www.dh.gov.uk (accessed 31 August 2010).

5 Trussell J. The essentials of contraception: efficacy, safety, and personal considerations. In: Hatcher RA, Trussell J, Stewart F *et al.* (eds) *Contraceptive Technology*, 18th revised edn. New York: Ardent Media, 2004.

6 Rosenberg MJ, Waugh MS. Causes and consequences of oral contraceptive noncompliance. *Am J Obstet Gynecol* 1999;180: S276–S279.

7 Potter L, Oakley D, de Leon-Wong E, Canamanr R. Measuring compliance among oral contraceptive users. *Fam Plan Perspect* 1996;28:154–158.

8 Larsson G, Blohm F, Sundell G *et al.* A longitudinal study of birth control and pregnancy outcome among women in a Swedish population. *Contraception* 1997;56:6–16.

9 UK medical eligibility criteria for contraceptive use 2009. Available at: www.fsrh.org.uk (accessed 31 August 2010).

10 Rosenburg MJ, Waugh MS, Meehan TE. Use and misuse of oral contraceptives: risk indicators for poor pill taking and discontinuation. *Contraception* 1995;51:283–288.

11 Audet MC, Morean M, Koltun WD *et al.* Evaluation of contraceptive efficacy and cycle control of a transdermal contraceptive patch vs an oral contraceptive. A randomised controlled trial. *JAMA* 2001;285:2347–2354.

12 Missed pill advice. Available at: www.fsrh.org.uk (accessed 31 August 2010).

13 Hannaford PC, Iversen L, Macfarlane TV, Elliott AM, Angus V, Lee AJ. Mortality among contraceptive pill users: cohort evidence from Royal College of General Practitioners' Oral Contraception Study. *BMJ* 2010;340:c927.

14 Endrikat J, Gerlinger C, Cronin M, Ruebig A, Schmidt W, Düsterberg B. Blood pressure stability in a normotensive population during intake of monophasic oral contraceptive pills containing 20 µg ethinyl oestradiol and 75 µg desogestrel. *Eur J Contracept Reprod Health Care* 2001;6:159–166.

15 Tanis BC, Van der Bosch MAAJ, Kemmeren JM *et al.* Oral contraceptives and the risk of myocardial infarction. *N Engl J Med* 2001;345:1787–1793.

16 Dunn N, Thorogood M, Faragher B *et al*. Oral contraceptives and myocardial infarction: results of the MICA case control study. *BMJ* 1999;318:1579–1583.

17 Khader YS, Rice J, John L, Abueita O. Oral contraceptive use and risk of myocardial infarction: a meta-analysis. *Contraception* 2003;68:11–17.

18 Etminan M, Takkouche B, Isorna FC, Samii A. Risk of ischaemic stroke in people with migraine: systematic review and meta-analysis of observational studies. *BMJ* 2005:330:63–65.

19 Collaborative Group on Hormonal Factors in Breast Cancer. Breast cancer and hormonal contraceptives: a collaborative re-analysis of individual data on 53,297 women with breast cancer and 100,239 women without breast cancer from 54 epidemiological studies. *Lancet* 1996;347:1717–1727.

20 Faculty of Sexual and Reproductive Healthcare Clinical Effectiveness Unit. First prescription of combined oral contraception. Available at: www.fsrh.org.

21 Rice CF, Killick SR, Dieben T, Coelingh Bennink HC. A comparison of the inhibition of ovulation achieved by desogestrel 75 μg and levonorgestrel 30 μg daily. *Hum Reprod* 1999;14: 982–985.

22 Stewart A, Cummins C, Gold L *et al*. The effectiveness of the levonorgestrelreleasing intrauterine system in menorrhagia: a systematic review. *BJOG* 2001;108:74–86.

23 Reid PC, Mukri F. Trends in number of hysterectomies performed in England for menorrhagia: examination of health episode statistics, 1989 to 2002–3. *BMJ* 2005;330: 938–939.

24 Faculty of Sexual and Reproductive Healthcare Clinical Effectiveness Unit. Contraception for women aged over 40 years. Available at: www.fsrh.org.

25 Faculty of Sexual and Reproductive Healthcare Clinical Effectiveness Unit. Management of unscheduled bleeding in women using hormonal contraception. Available at: www.fsrh.org.

26 Lopez LM, Grimes DA, Schulz KF, Curtis KM. Steroidal contraceptives: effect on bone fractures in women. *Cochrane Database Syst Rev* 2009;(2):CD006033.

27 Cromer BA, Blair JM, Mahan JD, Zibners L, Naumovski Z. A prospective comparison of bone density in adolescent girls receiving depot medroxyprogesterone acetate (Depo-Provera). *J Pediatr* 1996;129:671–676.

28 Lara-Torre E, Edwards CP, Perlman S, Hertwick SP. Bone mineral density in adolescent females using depomedroxyprogesterone acetate. *J Pediatr Adolesc Gynecol* 2004;17:17–21.

29 Faculty of Sexual and Reproductive Healthcare Clinical Effectiveness Unit. Contraceptive choices for young people. Available at: www.fsrh.org.

30 Parenteral progestogen-only contraceptives. Available at: www.bnf.org (accessed 31 August 2010).

31 Kulier R, O'Brien PA, Helmerhorst FM, Usher-Patel M, D'Arcangues C. Copper containing, framed intra-uterine devices for contraception. *Cochrane Database Syst Rev* 2007;(4):CD005347.

32 Sivin I. Dose and age-dependent ectopic pregnancy risks with intrauterine contraception. *Obstet Gynecol* 1991;78:291–298.

33 Faculty of Sexual and Reproductive Healthcare Clinical Effectiveness Unit. Intrauterine contraception. Available at: www.fsrh.org (accessed 31 August 2010).

34 Glasier A, Cameron ST, Fine P *et al*. Ulipristal acetate versus levonorgestrel for emergency contraception: a randomised non-inferiority trial and meta-analysis of ulipristal acetate versus levonorgestrel. *Lancet* 2010;375:555–562.

35 Creinin MD, Schlaff W, Archer DF *et al*. Progesterone receptor modulator for emergency contraception: a randomised controlled trial. *Obstet Gynecol* 2006;108:1089–1097.

36 Faculty of Sexual and Reproductive Healthcare Clinical Effectiveness Unit. Emergency contraception. Available at: www.fsrh.org (accessed 31 August 2010).

37 Royal College of Obstetricians and Gynaecologists. *Male and Female Sterilisation*. Evidence-based Clinical Guideline No. 4, 2004. Available at: www.rcog.org.uk/files/rcog-corp/uploaded-files/NEBSterilisationFull060607.pdf.

38 Faculty of Sexual and Reproductive Healthcare Clinical Effectiveness Unit. Female barrier methods of contraception. Available at: www.fsrh.org (accessed 31 August 2010).

Chapter 41
Polycystic Ovary Syndrome and Secondary Amenorrhoea

Adam Balen
Leeds Teaching Hospitals and The Leeds Centre for Reproductive Medicine, Seacroft Hospital, Leeds, UK

Introduction: defining polycystic ovary syndrome and secondary amenorrhoea

The current understanding of polycystic ovary syndrome (PCOS) is that it is a condition that presents with ovarian dysfunction and endocrine problems and is also associated with hyperinsulinaemia and metabolic disease. PCOS is a heterogeneous condition which is defined by the presence of two out of the following three criteria: (i) oligo- and/or anovulation, (ii) hyperandrogenism (clinical and/or biochemical), or (iii) polycystic ovaries as seen by ultrasound scan, with the exclusion of other causes of androgen excess and menstrual cycle irregularity or amenorrhoea. PCOS therefore encompasses symptoms of menstrual cycle disturbance and as such is the commonest cause of secondary amenorrhoea. The second part of the chapter will discuss the pathophysiology and management of other causes of secondary amenorrhoea.

Amenorrhoea is the absence of menstruation, which may be temporary or permanent. Amenorrhoea may occur as a normal physiological condition such as before puberty, during pregnancy, lactation or the menopause, or as a feature of a systemic or gynaecological disorder. Primary amenorrhoea may be a result of congenital abnormalities in the development of the ovaries, genital tract or external genitalia, or a perturbation of the normal endocrinological events of puberty. Furthermore, most of the causes of secondary amenorrhoea can also cause primary amenorrhoea, if they occur before the menarche.

Examination and investigation of patients with polycystic ovary syndrome and secondary amenorrhoea

A thorough history and a careful examination should always be carried out before investigations are instigated, looking particularly at stature and body form, signs of endocrine disease, secondary sexual development and the external genitalia. A history of secondary amenorrhoea may be misleading, as the 'periods' may have been the result of exogenous hormone administration in a patient who was being treated with hormone replacement therapy (HRT) for primary amenorrhoea. In most cases, however, a history of secondary amenorrhoea excludes congenital abnormalities. A family history of fertility problems, autoimmune disorders or premature menopause may also give clues as to the aetiology.

Exclude pregnancy

It is always important to exclude pregnancy in women of any age, and whereas some may think this statement superfluous, there are regularly women who present with amenorrhoea who are pregnant despite denying the possibility.

Examination

Measurement of height and weight should be performed in order to calculate the patient's body mass index (BMI). The normal range is 20–25 kg/m^2, and a value above or below this may suggest a diagnosis of weight-related amenorrhoea (which is a term usually applied to underweight women).

Signs of hyperandrogenism [acne, hirsutism, balding (alopecia)] are suggestive of PCOS, although biochemical screening helps to differentiate other causes of androgen excess. It is important to distinguish between hyperandrogenism and virilization, which is also with high circulating androgen levels and causes deepening of the voice, breast atrophy, increase in muscle bulk and cliteromegaly (see Summary box 41.1). A rapid onset of hirsutism suggests the possibility of an androgen-secreting tumour of the ovary or adrenal gland. Hirsutism can be graded and given a 'Ferriman Gallwey Score' by assessing the amount of hair in different parts of the body (e.g. upper lip, chin, breasts, abdomen, arms, legs). It is useful to monitor the

Dewhurst's Textbook of Obstetrics & Gynaecology, Eighth Edition. Edited by D. Keith Edmonds.
© 2012 John Wiley and Sons, Ltd. Published 2012 by John Wiley and Sons, Ltd.

Table 41.1 Endocrine normal ranges.

FSH*	1–10 IU/L (early follicular)
LH*	1–10 IU/L (early follicular)
Prolactin*	<400 mIU/L
TSH*	0.5–5.0 IU/L
Thyroxine (T4)	50–150 nmol/L
Free T4	9–22 pmol/L
Tri-iodothyronine (T3)	1.5–3.5 nmol/L
Free T3	4.3–8.6 pmol/L
TBG	7–17 mg/L
Testosterone (T)*	0.5–3.5 nmol/L
SHBG	16–120 nmol/L
Free androgen index [(T x 100) ÷ SHBG]	<5
Dihydrotestosterone	0.3–1 nmol/L
Androstenedione	2–10 nmol/L
Dehydroepiandrosterone sulphate	3–10 µmol/L
Cortisol	140–700 nmol/L
8 a.m.	0–140 nmol/L
Midnight	<400 nmol/24 h
24-hour urinary	
Oestradiol	250–500 pmol/L
Oestrone	400–600 pmol/L
Progesterone (mid-luteal)	>25 nmol/L to indicate ovulation
17-hydroxyprogesterone	1–20 nmol/L
Inhibin B	5–200 pg/mL
AMH	Low 2.2–15.7 pmol/L
	Satisfactory fertility 15.8–38.6 pmol/L
	Good fertility 28.7–48.5 pmol/L
	>48.5 pmol/L often seen in PCO

* Denotes those tests performed in routine screening of women with amenorrhoea.
FSH, follicle-stimulating hormone; LH, luteinizing hormone; TSH, thyroid-stimulating hormone; TBG, thyroid-binding globulin; SHBG, sex hormone-binding globulin; AMH, anti-Müllerian hormone; PCO, polycystic ovary.

progress of hirsutism, or its response to treatment, by making serial records, either by using a chart or by taking photographs of affected areas of the body.

A measurement of total testosterone (T) is considered adequate for general screening (Table 41.1). It is unnecessary to measure other androgens unless total T is >5 nmol/L (this will depend on the normal range of your local assay). Insulin may be elevated in overweight women and suppresses the production of sex hormone-binding globulin (SHBG) by the liver, resulting in a high free androgen index (FAI) in the presence of a normal total T. The measurement of SHBG is not required in routine practice but is a useful surrogate marker for insulin resistance (IR).

One should be aware of the possibility of Cushing's syndrome in women with stigmata of PCOS and obesity as it is a disease of insidious onset and dire consequences;

additional clues are the presence of central obesity, moon face, plethoric complexion, buffalo hump, proximal myopathy, thin skin, bruising and abdominal striae (which alone are a common finding in obese individuals). Acanthosis nigricans (AN) is a sign of profound insulin resistance and is usually visible as hyperpigmented thickening of the skin folds of the axilla and neck; AN is associated with PCOS and obesity (Fig. 41.1).

> ### Summary box 41.1
>
> A testosterone concentration >5 nmol/L should be investigated to exclude androgen-secreting tumours of the ovary or adrenal gland, Cushing's syndrome and late-onset congenital adrenal hyperplasia (CAH). Whereas CAH often presents at birth with ambiguous genitalia (see Chapter 34, partial 21-hydroxylase deficiency may present in later life, usually in the teenage years, with signs and symptoms similar to PCOS. In such cases, T may be elevated and the diagnosis confirmed by an elevated serum concentration of 17-hydroxyprogesterone (17-OHP); an abnormal ACTH-stimulation test may also be helpful (250 µg ACTH will cause an elevation of 17-OHP, usually between 65–470 nmol/L).
>
> In cases of Cushing's syndrome, a 24-hour urinary-free cortisol will be elevated (>700 nmol/24 hours). The normal serum concentration of cortisol is 140–700 nmol/L at 8 a.m. and less than 140 nmol/L at midnight. A low-dose dexamethasone suppression test (0.5 mg six-hourly for 48 hours) will cause a suppression of serum cortisol by 48 hours. A simpler screening test is an overnight suppression test, using a single midnight dose of dexamethasone 1 mg (2 mg if obese) and measuring the serum cortisol concentration at 8 a.m. when it should be less than 140 nmol/L. If Cushing's syndrome is confirmed, a high-dose dexamethasone suppression test (2 mg six-hourly for 48 hours) should suppress serum cortisol by 48 hours if there is a pituitary ACTH-secreting adenoma (Cushing's disease); failure of suppression suggests an adrenal tumours or ectopic secretion of ACTH – further tests and detailed imaging will then be required.
>
> The measurement of other serum androgen levels can be helpful. Dehydroepiandrosterone sulphate (DHEAS) is primarily a product of the adrenal androgen pathway (normal range <10 µmol/l). If the serum androgen concentrations are elevated, the possibility of an ovarian or adrenal tumour should be excluded by ultrasound or CT scans. The measurement of androstenedione can also be useful in some situations.

Amenorrhoiec women might have hyperprolactinaemia and galactorrhoea. It is important, however, not to examine the breasts before taking blood as the serum prolactin concentration may be falsely elevated as a result of physical examination. Stress may also cause minor

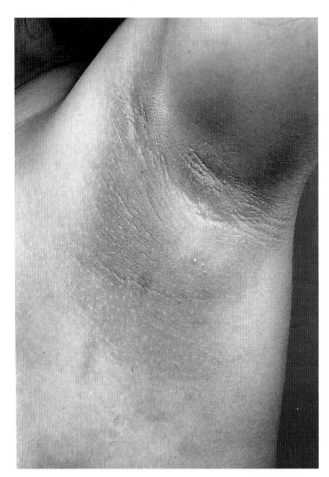

Fig. 41.1 *Acanthosis nigricans*, as seen typically in the skin folds (axilla, neck, elbow, vulva). Reproduced from Balen AH. *Infertility in Practice*, 3rd edn. London: Informa Healthcare, 2008, with permission.

Table 41.2 Classification of secondary amenorrhoea.

Uterine causes	Asherman's syndrome
	Cervical stenosis
Ovarian causes	Polycystic ovary syndrome
	Premature ovarian failure (genetic, autoimmune, infective, radio/chemotherapy)
Hypothalamic causes *(hypogonadotrophic hypogonadism)*	Weight loss
	Exercise
	Chronic illness
	Psychological distress
	Idiopathic
Pituitary causes	Hyperprolactinaemia
	Hypopituitarism
	Sheehan's syndrome
Causes of hypothalamic/pituitary damage *(hypogonadism)*	Tumours (craniopharyngiomas, gliomas, germinomas, dermoid cysts)
	Cranial irradiation
	Head injuries
	Sarcoidosis
	Tuberculosis
	Chronic debilitating illness
Systemic causes	Weight loss
	Endocrine disorders (thyroid disease, Cushing's syndrome, etc.)

elevation of prolactin. If there is suspicion of a pituitary tumour, the patient's visual fields should be checked, as bitemporal hemianopia secondary to pressure on the optic chiasm requires urgent attention.

Thyroid disease is common and the thyroid gland should be palpated and signs of hypothyroidism (dry thin hair, proximal myopathy, myotonia, slow-relaxing reflexes, mental slowness, bradycardia, etc.) or hyperthyroidism (goitre with bruit, tremor, weight loss, tachycardia, hyper-reflexia, exopthalmos, conjunctival oedema, ophthalmoplegia) elicited.

A bimanual examination is inappropriate in a young woman who has never been sexually active, and examination of the external genitalia of an adolescent should be undertaken in the presence of the patient's mother. Furthermore, it may be more appropriate to defer this from the first consultation in order to assure the patient's confidence in future management. A transabdominal ultrasound examination of the pelvis is an excellent non-invasive method for obtaining valuable information in

these patients. Although an examination under anaesthetic is sometimes indicated for cases of intersex with primary amenorrhoea, it is rarely required in cases of secondary amenorrhoea (Table 41.2).

A baseline assessment of the endocrine status should include the measurement of serum prolactin and gonadotrophin concentrations and an assessment of thyroid function. Prolactin levels may be elevated in response to a number of conditions, including stress, a recent breast examination or even having a blood test. The elevation, however, is moderate and transient. A more permanent, but still moderate, elevation (greater than 700 mIU/L) is associated with hypothyroidism and is also a common finding in women with PCOS, where prolactin levels up to 2500 mIU/L have been reported [1]. PCOS may also result in amenorrhoea, which can therefore create diagnostic difficulties, and hence appropriate management, for those women with hyperprolactinaemia and polycystic ovaries. Amenorrhoea in women with PCOS is secondary to acyclical ovarian activity and continuous oestrogen production. A positive response to a progestogen challenge test [e.g. medroxyprogesterone acetate 10–20 mg (depending on body weight) daily for 5 days], which induces a withdrawal bleed, will distinguish patients with PCOS-related hyperprolactinaemia from those with polycystic ovaries and unrelated hyperprolactinaemia, because the latter causes oestrogen deficiency and therefore failure to respond to the progestogen challenge.

A serum prolactin concentration of greater than 1500 mIU/L warrants further investigation. Computed tomography (CT) or magnetic resonance imaging (MRI) of the pituitary fossa may be used to exclude a hypothalamic tumour, a non-functioning pituitary tumour compressing the hypothalamus or a prolactinoma. Serum prolactin concentrations greater than 5000 mIU/L are usually associated with a macroprolactinoma, which by definition is greater than 1 cm in diameter.

The patient's oestrogen status may be assessed clinically by examination of the lower genital tract or by means of a progestogen challenge. Serum measurements of oestradiol are of limited value as they vary considerably, even in a patient with amenorrhoea. If the patient is well oestrogenized, the endometrium will be clearly seen on an ultrasound scan and should be shed on withdrawal of the progestogen.

Serum gonadotrophin measurements help to distinguish between cases of hypothalamic or pituitary failure and gonadal failure. Elevated gonadotrophin concentrations indicate a failure of negative feedback as a result of primary ovarian failure. A serum follicle-stimulating hormone (FSH) concentration of greater than 15 IU/L that is not associated with a preovulatory luteinizing hormone (LH) surge suggests impending ovarian failure. FSH levels of greater than 40 IU/L are suggestive of irreversible ovarian failure. The exact values vary according to individual assays, and so local reference levels should be checked. It is also important to assess serum gonadotrophin levels at baseline, that is during the first 3 days of a menstrual period. In patients with oligo/amenorrhoea, it may be necessary to perform two or more random measurements, although combining an assessment of endocrinology with an ultrasound scan on the same day aids the diagnosis.

An elevated LH concentration, when associated with a raised FSH concentration, is indicative of ovarian failure. However, if LH is elevated alone (and is not attributable to the preovulatory LH surge), this suggests PCOS. This may be confirmed by a pelvic ultrasound scan. Rarely, an elevated LH in a phenotypic female may be due to androgen insensitivity syndrome (AIS), although this condition presents with primary amenorrhoea.

Inhibin B is thought to be the ovarian hormone which has the greatest influence on pituitary secretion of FSH. Previously, it was thought that serum concentrations of inhibin B might provide better quantification of ovarian reserve than serum FSH concentrations. However, it appears that basal FSH concentration and age are better predictors for clinical end-points such as outcome of fertility treatment.

Anti-Müllerian hormone (AMH) is best known as a product of the testes during fetal development that suppresses the development of Müllerian structures. AMH is also produced by the preantral and antral follicles and appears to be a more stable predictor of the ovarian follicle pool as it does not fluctuate through the menstrual cycle. Indeed, it has been reported that higher AMH concentrations are associated with increased numbers of mature oocytes, embryos and clinical pregnancies during *in vitro* fertilization (IVF) treatment. Assays for AMH are now becoming available for routine use and it is this hormone that currently offers the greatest promise for future assessment of ovarian reserve and function. The number of antral follicles in the ovary, as assessed by pelvic ultrasound, also correlates well with ovarian reserve and serum AMH levels. Indeed, it is the number of small antral follicles, 2–6 mm in diameter, that declines significantly with age while there is little change in the larger follicles of 7–10 mm, which is still below the size at which growing follicles have been recruited.

Failure at the level of the hypothalamus or pituitary is reflected by abnormally low levels of serum gonadotrophin concentrations, and gives rise to hypogonadotrophic hypogonadism. Kallmann's syndrome is the clinical finding of hyposmia and/or colour blindness associated with hypogonadotrophic hypogonadism – usually a cause of primary amenorrhoea. It is difficult to distinguish between a hypothalamic and pituitary aetiology as both respond to stimulation with gonadotrophin-releasing hormone (GnRH). CT or MRI should be performed if indicated.

Karyotype and other tests

Women with premature ovarian failure (POF) (under the age of 40 years) may have a chromosomal abnormality [e.g. Turner's syndrome (45X or 46XX/45X mosaic) or other sex chromosome mosaicisms]. A number of genes have also been associated with familial POF, but have not been assessed in routine clinical practice. An autoantibody screen should also be undertaken in women with a premature menopause, although it can be difficult to detect antiovarian antibodies and many will have evidence of other autoantibodies (e.g. thyroid), which then indicates the need for further surveillance.

A history of a recent endometrial curettage or endometritis in a patient with normal genitalia and normal endocrinology, but with absent or only a small withdrawal bleed following a progestogen challenge, is suggestive of Asherman's syndrome. A hysterosalpingogram (HSG) may be helpful and a hysteroscopy will confirm the diagnosis (Fig. 41.2).

Measurement of bone mineral density (BMD) is indicated in amenorrhoeic women who are oestrogen-deficient. Measurements of density are made in the lumbar spine and femoral neck. The vertebral bone is more sensitive to oestrogen deficiency and vertebral fractures tend to occur in a younger age group (50–60 years) than fractures at the femoral neck (70+ years). However,

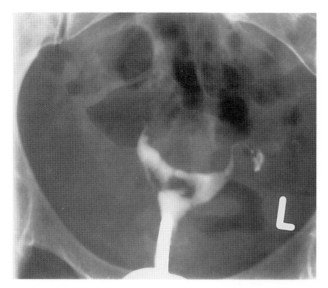

Fig. 41.2 Conventional X-ray hysterosalpingogram demonstrating Asherman's syndrome, with intrauterine synechiae. There is no flow of contrast through the right tube, although thickening of the cornual end of the tube suggests the possibility of tubal spasm. There is flow to the end of the left fallopian tube, although no free spill into the peritoneal cavity. This raises the possibility of sacculated adhesions around the fimbrial end of the tube. Reproduced from Balen AH. *Infertility in Practice*, 3rd edn. London: Informa Healthcare, 2008, with permission.

it should be noted that crush fractures can spuriously increase the measured BMD. An X-ray of the dorsolumbar spine is therefore often complimentary, particularly in patients who have lost height.

Amenorrhoea may also have long-term metabolic and physical consequences. In women with PCOS and prolonged amenorrhoea, there is a risk of endometrial hyperplasia and adenocarcinoma. If on resumption of menstruation there is a history of persistent intermenstrual bleeding, or on ultrasound there is a postmenstrual endometrial thickness of greater than 10 mm, an endometrial biopsy is indicated.

Serum cholesterol measurements are important because of the association of an increased risk of heart disease in women with premature ovarian failure. Women with PCOS [2], although not oestrogen-deficient, may have a subnormal high-density lipoprotein (HDL):total cholesterol ratio. This is as a consequence of the hypersecretion of insulin that occurs in many women with PCOS, which may increase the lifetime risk of heart disease.

Glucose tolerance

Women who are obese, and also many slim women with PCOS, will have insulin resistance and elevated serum concentrations of insulin (usually <30 mIU/L fasting). A 75 g oral glucose tolerance test (GTT) should be performed in women with PCOS and a BMI >30 kg/m^2, with an

Table 41.3 Definitions of glucose tolerance after a 75 g glucose tolerance test (GTT).

	Diabetes mellitus	Impaired glucose tolerance (IGT)	Impaired fasting glycaemia
Fasting glucose (mmol/L)	≥7.0	<7.0	≥6.1 and <7.0
2-hour glucose (mmol/L)	≥11.1	≥7.8 and ≤11.1	<7.8

assessment of the fasting and 2-hour glucose concentration (Table 41.3). It has been suggested that South Asian women should have an assessment of glucose tolerance if their BMI is greater than 25 kg/m^2 because of the greater risk of insulin resistance at a lower BMI than seen in the white population.

Polycystic ovary syndrome

The PCOS is a heterogeneous collection of signs and symptoms that, gathered together, form a spectrum of a disorder with a mild presentation in some but a severe disturbance of reproductive, endocrine and metabolic function in others. The pathophysiology of PCOS appears to be multifactorial and polygenic. The definition of the syndrome has been much debated. Key features include menstrual cycle disturbance, hyperandrogenism and obesity. There are many extraovarian aspects to the pathophysiology of PCOS, yet ovarian dysfunction is central. The joint ESHRE/ASRM (European Society for Human Reproduction and Embryology/American Society for Reproductive Medicine) consensus defined PCOS as requiring the presence of two out of the following three criteria:

1 oligo- and/or anovulation (that is oligomenorrhoea or amenorrhoea);

2 hyperandrogenism (clinical features and/or biochemical elevation of testosterone); and/or

3 polycystic ovaries assessed by ultrasound [3].

Other aetiologies of hyperandrogenism and menstrual cycle disturbance should be excluded by appropriate investigations, as described within this chapter. The morphology of the polycystic ovary (PCO) has been redefined as an ovary with 12 or more follicles measuring 2–9 mm in diameter and/or increased ovarian volume (>10 cm^3) [4].

There is considerable heterogeneity of symptoms and signs among women with PCOS and for an individual these may change over time [1]. PCOS is familial, and various aspects of the syndrome may be differentially inherited. Polycystic ovaries can exist without clinical

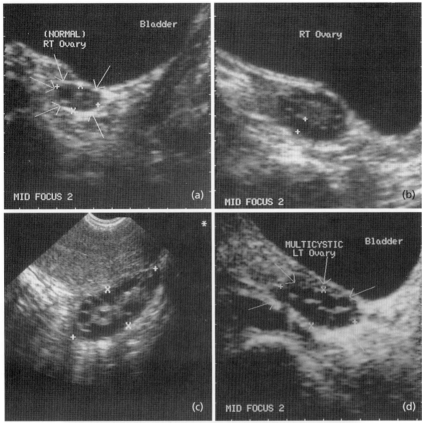

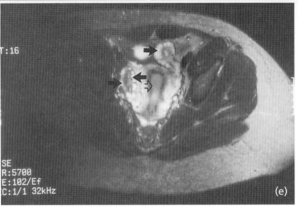

Fig. 41.3 (a) Transabdominal ultrasound scan of a normal ovary. (b) Transabdominal ultrasound scan of a polycystic ovary. (c) Transvaginal ultrasound scan of a polycystic ovary. (d) Transabdominal ultrasound scan of a multicystic ovary. (e) Magnetic resonance imaging (MRI) of a pelvis, demonstrating two polycystic ovaries (closed arrows) and a hyperplastic endometrium (open arrow). Reproduced from Balen AH. *Infertility in Practice*, 3rd edn. London: Informa Healthcare, 2008, with permission.

signs of the syndrome, which may then become expressed in certain circumstances. There are a number of factors that affect expression of PCOS, for example a gain in weight is associated with a worsening of symptoms while weight loss may ameliorate the endocrine and metabolic profile and symptomatology.

Genetic studies have identified a link between PCOS and disordered insulin metabolism, and indicate that the syndrome may be the presentation of a complex genetic trait disorder. The features of obesity, hyperinsulinaemia and hyperandrogenaemia, which are commonly seen in PCOS, are also known to be factors that confer an increased

risk of cardiovascular disease and non-insulin-dependent diabetes mellitus (NIDDM) [5]. There are studies indicating that women with PCOS have an increased risk for these diseases, which pose long-term risks for health, and this evidence has prompted debate as to the need for screening women for PCOS [6] (Fig. 41.3).

Polycystic ovaries are commonly detected by ultrasound or other forms of pelvic imaging, with estimates of the prevalence in the general population being in the order of 20–33% [7]. Although the ultrasound criteria for the diagnosis of polycystic ovaries have not, until now, been universally agreed, the characteristic features are accepted as being an increase in the number of follicles and the amount of stroma compared with normal ovaries, resulting in an increase in ovarian volume. The 'cysts' are not cysts in the sense that they do contain oocytes and indeed are follicles whose development has been arrested. The actual number of cysts may be of less relevance than the volume of ovarian stroma or of the ovary itself, which has been shown to closely correlate with serum testosterone concentrations.

At the ESHRE/ASRM consensus meeting, a refined definition of the PCOS was agreed, encompassing a description of the morphology of the PCO. According to the available literature, the criteria fulfilling sufficient specificity and sensitivity to define the PCO are the presence of 12 or more follicles measuring 2–9 mm in diameter and/or increased ovarian volume ($>10\,cm^3$) [4]. If there is a follicle greater than 10 mm in diameter, the scan should be repeated at a time of ovarian quiescence in order to calculate volume and area. The presence of a single PCO is sufficient to provide the diagnosis. The distribution of the follicles and the description of the stroma are not required in the diagnosis. Increased stromal echogenicity and/or stromal volume are specific to PCO, but it has been shown that the measurement of the ovarian volume (or area) is a good surrogate for the quantification of the stroma in clinical practice. A woman having PCO in the absence of an ovulation disorder or hyperandrogenism ('asymptomatic PCO') should not be considered as having PCOS, although she may develop symptoms over time, for example if she gains weight.

Genetics of polycystic ovary syndrome

Polycystic ovary syndrome has long been noted to have a familial component. Genetic analysis has been hampered by the lack of a universal definition for PCOS. Most of the criteria used for diagnosing PCOS are continuous traits, such as degree of hirsutism, level of circulating androgens, extent of menstrual irregularity, and ovarian volume and morphology. To perform genetic analyses, these continuous variables have to be transformed into nominal variables. Family studies have revealed that about 50% of first-degree relatives have PCOS, suggesting a dominant mode of inheritance [8]. Commonly, first-degree male relatives appear more likely to have the metabolic syndrome. As hyperandrogenism is a key feature of PCOS, it is logical to explore the critical steps in steroidogenesis and potential enzyme dysfunction. Some studies have found an abnormality with the cholesterol side-chain cleavage gene (*CYP11a*), which is a rate limiting step in steroidogenesis. It has also been hypothesized that polymorphisms in the insulin receptor (*INSR*) gene that induce mild changes in insulin receptor function may contribute to the development of PCOS, as it is unlikely that a major mutation is present given the wide variability of insulin resistance in women with PCOS.

Further discussion of this complex area is beyond the scope of this chapter and much research is being performed to provide a more detailed account of the various genetic abnormalities that may be involved in the pathogenesis of PCOS.

The pathophysiology of polycystic ovary syndrome

Hypersecretion of androgens by the stromal theca cells of the PCO leads to the cardinal clinical manifestation of the syndrome, hyperandrogenism, and is also one of the mechanisms whereby follicular growth is inhibited with the resultant excess of immature follicles. Hypersecretion of luteinizing hormone (LH) by the pituitary – a result of both disordered ovarian–pituitary feedback and exaggerated pulses of GnRH from the hypothalamus – stimulates testosterone secretion by the ovary. Furthermore, insulin is a potent stimulus for androgen secretion by the ovary, which, by way of a different receptor for insulin, does not exhibit insulin resistance. Insulin therefore amplifies the effect of LH, and additionally magnifies the degree of hyperandrogenism by suppressing liver production of the main carrier protein, sex hormone-binding globulin (SHBG), thus elevating the 'free androgen index'. It is a combination of genetic abnormalities combined with environmental factors, such as nutrition and body weight, which then affect expression of the syndrome.

Racial differences in expression of polycystic ovary syndrome

The highest reported prevalence of PCOS has been 52% among South Asian immigrants in Britain, of whom 49.1% had menstrual irregularity [9]. Rodin *et al.* [9] demonstrated that South Asian women with PCOS had a comparable degree of insulin resistance to controls with established type 2 diabetes mellitus. Insulin resistance and hyperinsulinaemia are common antecedents of type 2 diabetes, with a high prevalence in South Asian people. Type 2 diabetes also has a familial basis, inherited as a complex genetic trait that interacts with environmental factors, chiefly nutrition, commencing during fetal life. We have found that South Asian people with anovulatory PCOS have greater insulin resistance and more severe symptoms of the syndrome than anovulatory white people with PCOS [10]. Furthermore, we have found that women from South Asia living in the UK appear to express symptoms at an earlier age than their white British counterparts (Table 41.4).

Heterogeneity of polycystic ovary syndrome

The findings of a large series of more than 1700 women with PCOs detected by ultrasound scan are summarized in Table 41.5 [1]. All patients had at least one symptom of PCOS. Thirty eight per cent of the women were overweight (BMI $>25\,kg/m^2$) and obesity was significantly

Table 41.4 Signs and symptoms of polycystic ovary syndrome.

Symptoms
Hyperandrogenism (acne, hirsutism, alopecia – *not* virilization)
Menstrual disturbance
Infertility
Obesity
Sometimes: asymptomatic, with polycystic ovaries on ultrasound
    scan

Serum endocrinology
↑ Fasting insulin (not routinely measured; insulin resistance or
    impaired glucose tolerance assessed by GTT)
↑ Androgens (testosterone and androstenedione)
↑ or normal luteinizing hormone (LH), normal follicle-stimulating
    hormone (FSH)
↓ Sex hormone binding globulin (SHBG), results in elevated 'free
    androgen index'
↑ Oestradiol, oestrone (neither measured routinely as very wide
    range of values)
↑ Prolactin

Possible late sequelae
Diabetes mellitus
Dyslipidaemia
Hypertension, cardiovascular disease
Endometrial carcinoma
Breast cancer (?)

Table 41.5 Characteristics of 1741 women with ultrasound-detected polycystic ovaries. Mean and 5–95 percentiles (*normal range).

Age (years)	31.5 (14–50)
Ovarian volume (cm^3)	11.7 (4.6–22.3)
Uterine area (cm^2)	27.5 (15.2–46.3)
Endometrium (mm)	7.5 (4.0–13.0)
BMI (kg/m^2) (19–25)*	25.4 (19.0–38.6)
FSH IU/L (1–10)*	4.5 (1.4–7.5)
LH IU/L (1–10)*	10.9 (2.0 –27.0)
Testosterone nmol/L (0.5–2.5)*	2.6 (1.1–4.8)
Prolactin (<350 mIU/L)*	342 (87–917)

associated with an increased risk of hirsutism, menstrual cycle disturbance and an elevated serum testosterone concentration. Obesity was also associated with an increased rate of infertility and menstrual cycle disturbance. Twenty six per cent of patients with primary infertility and 14% of patients with secondary infertility had a BMI of more than 30 kg/m^2.

Approximately 30% of the patients had a regular menstrual cycle, 50% had oligomenorrhoea and 20% had amenorrhoea. A rising serum concentration of testosterone was associated with an increased risk of hirsutism, infertility and cycle disturbance. The rates of infertility and menstrual cycle disturbance also rose with increasing

serum LH concentrations to greater than 10 IU/L. The serum LH concentration of those with primary infertility was significantly higher than that of women with secondary infertility, and both were higher than the LH concentration of those with proven fertility. Ovarian morphology appears to be the most sensitive marker of the PCOS compared with the classical endocrine features of raised serum LH and testosterone, which were found in only 40% and 30% of patients, respectively, in this series [1]. It is generally the slim women with PCOS who have a high LH level as the main driver for androgen excess whereas in obese women it is insulin that additionally stimulates the ovaries to overproduce androgens.

Health consequences of polycystic ovary syndrome

Obesity and metabolic abnormalities are recognized risk factors for the development of ischaemic heart disease (IHD) in the general population, and these are also recognized features of PCOS. The question is whether women with PCOS are at an increased risk of IHD, and whether this will occur at an earlier age than women with normal ovaries. The basis for the idea that women with PCOS are at a greater risk for cardiovascular disease is that these women are more insulin resistant than weight-matched controls and that the metabolic disturbances associated with insulin resistance are known to increase cardiovascular risk in other populations. Insulin resistance is defined as a diminution in the biological responses to a given level of insulin. In the presence of an adequate pancreatic reserve, normal circulating glucose levels are maintained at higher serum insulin concentrations. In the general population, cardiovascular risk factors include insulin resistance, obesity, glucose intolerance, hypertension and dyslipidaemia.

There have been a large number of studies demonstrating the presence of insulin resistance and corresponding hyperinsulinaemia in both obese and non-obese women with PCOS [5]. Obese women with PCOS have consistently been shown to be more insulin resistant than weight-matched controls. It appears that obesity and PCOS have an additive effect on the degree and severity of the insulin resistance and subsequent hyperinsulinaemia in this group of women. The insulin resistance causes compensatory hypersecretion of insulin, particularly in response to glucose, so euglycaemia is usually maintained at the expense of hyperinsulinaemia. Insulin resistance is restricted to the extrasplanchnic actions of insulin on glucose dispersal. The liver is not affected (hence the fall in SHBG and HDL), neither is the ovary (hence the menstrual problems and hypersecretion of androgens) nor the skin, hence the development of acanthosis nigricans. Women with PCOS who are oligomenorrhoeic are more likely to be insulin resistant than those with regular cycles, irrespective of their BMI, with the intermenstrual interval correlating with the degree of insulin resistance [2].

Women with PCOS have a greater truncal abdominal fat distribution as demonstrated by a higher waist:hip ratio. The central distribution of fat is independent of BMI and associated with higher plasma insulin and triglyceride concentrations and reduced HDL cholesterol concentrations. From a practical point of view, if the measurement of waist circumference is greater than 80 cm, there will be excess visceral fat and an increased risk of metabolic problems.

Thus, there is evidence that insulin resistance, central obesity and hyperandrogenaemia have an adverse effect on lipid metabolism, yet these are surrogate risk factors for cardiovascular disease. However, Pierpoint *et al.* [11] reported the mortality rate in 1028 women diagnosed as having PCOS between 1930 and 1979. All the women were older than 45 years and 770 women had been treated by wedge resection of the ovaries. A total of 786 women were traced; the mean age at diagnosis was 26.4 years and the average duration of follow-up was 30 years. There were 59 deaths, of which 15 were from circulatory disease. Of these 15 deaths, 13 were from ischaemic heart disease. There were six deaths from diabetes as an underlying or contributory cause compared with the expected 1.7 deaths. The standard mortality rate both overall and for cardiovascular disease was not higher in the women with PCOS than the national mortality rates in women, although the observed proportion of women with diabetes as a contributory or underlying factor leading to death was significantly higher than expected [odds ratio 3.6, 95% confidence interval (CI) 1.5–8.4]. Thus, despite surrogate markers for cardiovascular disease, no increased rate of death from CVS disease could be demonstrated in this study.

Polycystic ovary syndrome in younger women

The majority of studies that have identified the risk factors of obesity and insulin resistance in women with PCOS have investigated adult populations, commonly including women who have presented to specialist endocrine or reproductive clinics. However, PCOS has been identified in much younger populations [7], in which women with increasing symptoms of PCOS were found to be more insulin resistant. These data emphasize the need for long-term prospective studies of young women with PCOS in order to clarify the natural history and to determine which women will be at risk of diabetes and cardiovascular disease later in life. A study of women with PCOS and a mean age of 39 years followed over a period of 6 years found that 9% of those with normal glucose tolerance developed impaired glucose tolerance (IGT) and 8% developed NIDDM [12], while 54% of women with IGT at the start of the study had NIDDM at follow-up. The

risks of disease progression, not surprisingly, were greatest in those who were overweight.

Endometrial cancer

Endometrial adenocarcinoma is the second most common female genital malignancy, but only 4% of cases occur in women aged under 40 years. The risk of developing endometrial cancer has been shown to be adversely influenced by a number of factors, including obesity, long-term use of unopposed oestrogens, nulliparity and infertility. Women with endometrial carcinoma have had fewer births than controls, and it has also been demonstrated that infertility *per se* gives a relative risk of 2 [13]. Hypertension and type 2 diabetes mellitus have long been linked to endometrial cancer – conditions that are now known also to be associated with PCOS. The true risk of endometrial carcinoma in women with clearly defined PCOS, however, is difficult to ascertain [14].

Endometrial hyperplasia may be a precursor to adenocarcinoma, although the rate of progression is difficult to predict. Although the degree of risk has not been clearly defined, it is generally accepted that for women with PCOS who experience amenorrhoea or oligomenorrhoea, the induction of artificial withdrawal bleeds to prevent endometrial hyperplasia is prudent management [6]. Indeed, we consider it important that women with PCOS shed their endometrium at least every 3 months. For those with oligo-/amenorrhoea who do not wish to use cyclical hormone therapy, we recommend an ultrasound scan to measure endometrial thickness and morphology every 6–12 months (depending upon menstrual history). An endometrial thickness greater than 10 mm in an amenorrhoiec woman warrants an artificially induced bleed, which should be followed by a repeat ultrasound scan and endometrial biopsy if the endometrium has not been shed. Another option is to consider a progestogen-secreting intrauterine system, such as the Mirena® (Bayer Pharma, Newburg, UK).

Breast cancer

Obesity, hyperandrogenism and infertility occur frequently in PCOS and are features known to be associated with the development of breast cancer. However, studies examining the relationship between PCOS and breast carcinoma have not always identified a significantly increased risk. The study by Coulam *et al.* [15] calculated a relative risk of 1.5 (95% CI 0.75–2.55) for breast cancer in their group of women with chronic anovulation, which was not statistically significant. After stratification by age, however, the relative risk was found to be 3.6 (95% CI 1.2–8.3) in the postmenopausal age group. Pierpoint *et al.* [11] assessed mortality from the national registry of deaths and standardized mortality rates (SMR) calculated for patients with PCOS compared with the normal population. The average follow-up period was 30 years. The

SMR for all neoplasms was 0.91 (95% CI 0.60–1.32) and for breast cancer was 1.48 (95% CI 0.79–2.54). In fact, breast cancer was the leading cause of death in this cohort.

Ovarian cancer

In recent years there has been much debate about the risk of ovarian cancer in women with infertility, particularly in relation to the use of drugs to induce superovulation for assisted conception procedures. Inherently the risk of ovarian cancer appears to be increased in women who have multiple ovulations – that is those who are nulliparous (possibly because of infertility) with an early menarche and late menopause. Thus, it may be that inducing multiple ovulations in women with infertility will increase their risk – a notion that is by no means proven. Women with PCOS who are oligo-/anovulatory might therefore be expected to be at low risk of developing ovarian cancer if it is lifetime number of ovulations rather than pregnancies that is critical. Ovulation induction to correct anovulatory infertility aims to induce unifollicular ovulation, and so in theory should raise the risk of a woman with PCOS to that of a woman with normal ovulation. The PCO, however, is notoriously sensitive to stimulation and it is only in recent years with the development of high-resolution transvaginal ultrasonography that the rate of unifollicular ovulation has attained acceptable levels. There are a few studies which have addressed the possibility of an association between PCOs and ovarian cancer. The results are conflicting and the ability to generalize is limited owing to problems with the study designs. In the large UK study by Pierpoint *et al.* [11], the standardized mortality rate for ovarian cancer was 0.39 (95% CI 0.01–2.17).

Management of the polycystic ovary syndrome

Obesity

The clinical management of a women with PCOS should be focused on her individual problems. Obesity worsens both symptomatology and the endocrine profile and so obese women (BMI $>30 \text{kg/m}^2$) should therefore be encouraged to lose weight. Weight loss improves the endocrine profile, the likelihood of ovulation and a healthy pregnancy. Much has been written about diet and PCOS. The right diet for an individual is one that is practical, sustainable and compatible with her lifestyle. It is sensible to keep carbohydrate content down and to avoid fatty foods. It is often helpful to refer to a dietitian. Antiobesity drugs such as Orlistat® may help with weight loss. Bariatric surgery (either gastric banding or gastric bypass procedures) are also very effective for women with a BMI of $>35 \text{kg/m}^2$, although it is inadvisable to conceive immediately after surgery until metabolism has stabilized after the initial rapid loss of weight [16].

Menstrual irregularity

Amenorrhoeic women with PCOS are not oestrogen deficient and are not at risk of osteoporosis. Indeed, they are oestrogen replete and at risk of endometrial hyperplasia (see above). The easiest way to control the menstrual cycle is the use of a low-dose combined oral contraceptive preparation. This will result in an artificial cycle and regular shedding of the endometrium. An alternative is a progestogen [such as medroxyprogesterone acetate (Provera®)] for 12 days every 1–3 months to induce a withdrawal bleed, or the continuous provision of progesterone into the uterine cavity by Mirena. It is important once again to encourage weight loss.

Hyperandrogenism and hirsutism

The bioavailability of testosterone is affected by the serum concentration of SHBG. High levels of insulin lower the production of SHBG and so increase the free fraction of androgen. Elevated serum androgen concentrations stimulate peripheral androgen receptors, resulting in an increase in 5α reductase activity, directly increasing the conversion of testosterone to the more potent metabolite, dihydrotestosterone. Women with PCOS do not become virilized (that is, they do not develop deepening of the voice, increased muscle mass, breast atrophy or clitoromegaly). A total testosterone level of greater than 5 nmol/L or rapid onset of signs of hyperandrogenism requires further investigation. Late-onset congenital adrenal hyperplasia (CAH) is not common in the UK but is more prevalent in certain ethnic groups (e.g. Mediterranean, South American and some Jewish populations).

Hirsutism is characterized by terminal hair growth in a male pattern of distribution, including the chin, upper lip, chest, upper and lower back, upper and lower abdomen, upper arm, thigh and buttocks. A standardized scoring system, such as the modified Ferriman and Gallwey score, may be used to evaluate the degree of hirsutism before and during treatments (Fig. 41.4). Many women attend having already tried cosmetic techniques and so it may be difficult to obtain a baseline assessment.

Drug therapies may take 6–9 months or longer before any improvement of hirsutism is perceived. Physical treatments including electrolysis, waxing and bleaching may be helpful while waiting for medical treatments to work. Electrolysis is time-consuming, painful and expensive, and should be performed by an expert practitioner. Regrowth is not uncommon and there is no really permanent cosmetic treatment. Laser and photothermolysis techniques are more expensive but may have a longer duration of effect. Comparative studies, however, have not been performed. Repeated treatments are required for a near-permanent effect because only hair follicles in the growing phase are obliterated at each treatment. Hair growth occurs in three cycles, so 6–9 months of regular

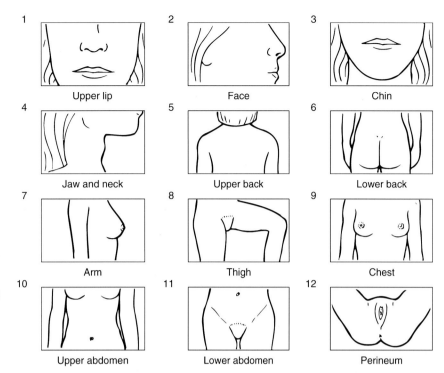

Fig. 41.4 The Ferriman–Gallwey Hirsutism Scoring System. The chart is used both to provide an initial score, with a scale of 0–3 at each of 12 points, depending on severity, and for the monitoring of progress with therapy. Reproduced from Balen AH, Jacobs HS. *Infertility in Practice*, 2nd edn. Churchill Livingstone, 2003, with permission.

treatments are typical. The topical use of eflornithine may be effective. It works by inhibiting the enzyme ornithine decarboxylase in hair follicles and may be a useful therapy for those who wish to avoid hormonal treatments, but may also be used in conjunction with hormonal therapy. Eflornithine may cause some thinning of the skin and so high factor sun block is recommended when exposed to the sun.

Medical regimens should stop further progression of hirsutism and decrease the rate of hair growth. Adequate contraception is important in women of reproductive age as transplacental passage of antiandrogens may disturb the genital development of a male fetus. First-line therapy has traditionally been the preparation Dianette®, which contains ethinyloestradiol (30 μg) in combination with cyproterone acetate (2 mg). The addition of higher doses of the synthetic progestogen, cyproterone acetate (CPA, 50–100 mg), do not appear to confer additional benefit [17], but are sometimes prescribed for the first 10 days of each 21-day cycle for women who are particularly resistant to treatment with Dianette alone. The effect on acne and seborrhoea is usually evident within a couple of months. Cyproterone acetate can rarely cause liver damage, and liver function should be checked regularly (after 6 months and then annually). Once symptom control has been obtained, it is advisable to switch to a combined oral contraceptive pill containing a lower dose of ethinyl oestradiol because of concerns about the increased risk of thrombo-embolism with Dianette.

Spironolactone is a weak diuretic with antiandrogenic properties that may be used in women in whom the combined oral contraceptive pill is contraindicated at a daily dose of 25–100 mg. Drosperinone is a derivative of spironolactone and is contained in the combined oral contraceptive pill Yasmin®, which may also be beneficial for women with PCOS.

Other antiandrogens such as ketoconazole, finasteride and flutamide have been tried, but are not widely used in the UK for the treatment of hirsutism in women owing to their adverse side effects. Furthermore, they are no more effective than cyproterone acetate.

Infertility

Various factors influence ovarian function, and fertility is adversely affected by an individual being overweight or having elevated serum concentrations of LH. Strategies to induce ovulation include weight loss, oral antioestrogens (principally clomifene citrate [CC] or tamoxifen), parenteral gonadotrophin therapy and laparoscopic ovarian surgery. Clomifene is the traditional first-line therapy and can be continued for 6–12 cycles of treatment if the patient is ovulating with normal endocrinology. For those who do not ovulate, the options include daily injections of either recombinant follicle-stimulating hormone (FSH), human menopausal gonadotrophins (hMGs, which contain both FSH and LH activity) or laparoscopic ovarian diathermy (LOD) [18]. Women with PCOS are at risk of ovarian hyperstimulation syndrome (OHSS) and multiple pregnancy, and so ovulation induction has to be carefully monitored with serial ultrasound scans.

Improvement in lifestyle with a combination of exercise and diet to achieve weight reduction is important to improve the prospects of both spontaneous and drug-induced ovulation. In addition, overweight women with PCOS are at increased risk of obstetric complications, gestational diabetes mellitus and pre-eclampsia, and their fetuses are at increased risk of congenital malformations and miscarriage [19].

Ovulation can be induced with the antioestrogen clomifene citrate (50–100 mg) taken from days 2–6 of a natural or artificially induced bleed. While clomifene is successful in inducing ovulation in over 80% of women, pregnancy only occurs in about 40%. CC should only be prescribed in a setting where ultrasound monitoring is available (and performed) in order to minimize the 10% risk of multiple pregnancy and to ensure that ovulation is taking place [20,21]. A daily dose of more than 100 mg rarely confers any benefit and can cause thickening of the cervical mucus, which can impede passage of sperm through the cervix. Once an ovulatory dose has been reached, the cumulative conception rate continues to increase for up to 10–12 cycles [20].

The therapeutic options for patients with anovulatory infertility who are resistant to antioestrogens are either parenteral gonadotrophin therapy or laparoscopic ovarian diathermy. Because the PCO is very sensitive to stimulation by exogenous hormones, it is extremely important to start with very low doses of gonadotrophins and follicular development must be carefully monitored by ultrasound scans. The advent of transvaginal ultrasonography has enabled the multiple pregnancy rate to be reduced to less than 5% because of its higher resolution and clearer view of the developing follicles. Cumulative conception and livebirth rates after 6 months may be 62% and 54%, respectively, and after 12 months 73% and 62%, respectively [21] (Fig. 41.5). Close monitoring should enable treatment to be suspended if more than two mature follicles develop, as the risk of multiple pregnancy increases (Fig. 41.6).

Women with the PCOS are also at increased risk of developing the ovarian hyperstimulation syndrome (OHSS). This occurs if too many follicles (>10 mm) are stimulated and results in abdominal distension, discomfort, nausea, vomiting and sometimes difficulty in breathing. The mechanism for OHSS is thought to be secondary to activation of the ovarian renin–angiotensin pathway and excessive secretion of vascular epidermal growth factor (VEGF). The ascites, pleural and pericardial effusions exacerbate this serious condition and the resultant haemoconcentration can lead to thromboembolism. The situation worsens if a pregnancy has resulted from the treatment as human chorionic gonadotrophin from the placenta further stimulates the ovaries. Hospitaliza-

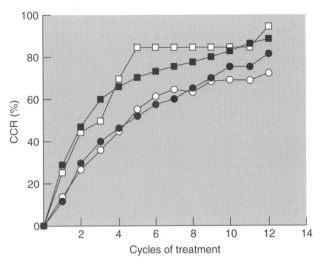

Fig. 41.5 Cumulative conception rates over successive cycles in normal women (triangle) and after ovulation induction in 103 women with anovulatory polycystic ovary syndrome (circle), 77 women with hypogonadotrophic hypogonadism (diamond) and 20 patients with weight-related amenorrhoea (square). While patients with weight-related amenorrhoea conceive readily after ovulation induction we now believe that their management should be weight gain before conception (see text). From Balen *et al.*, 1994 [21].

tion is sometimes necessary in order for intravenous fluids and heparin to be given to prevent dehydration and thromboembolism. Although the OHSS is rare, it is potentially fatal and should be avoidable with appropriate monitoring of gonadotrophin therapy.

Ovarian diathermy is free of the risks of multiple pregnancy and ovarian hyperstimulation and does not require intensive ultrasound monitoring. Laparoscopic ovarian diathermy has taken the place of wedge resection of the ovaries (which resulted in extensive periovarian and tubal adhesions) and carries a reduced risk of multiple pregnancy compared with gonadotrophin therapy in the treatment of clomifene-insensitive PCOS. Pregnancy rates are greater with 6 months of gonadotrophin therapy compared with 6 months after laparoscopic ovarian diathermy [22].

Insulin-sensitizing agents and metformin

A number of pharmacological agents have been used to amplify the physiological effect of weight loss, notably metformin. This biguanide inhibits the production of hepatic glucose and enhances the sensitivity of peripheral tissue to insulin, thereby decreasing insulin secretion. It has been shown that metformin may ameliorate hyperandrogenism and abnormalities of gonadotrophin secretion in some women with PCOS, and therefore it was suggested that it might restore menstrual cyclicity and fertility. The insulin-sensitizing agent troglitazone also appeared to significantly improve the metabolic and

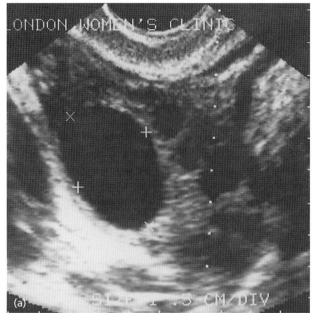

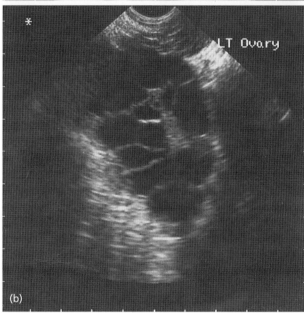

Fig. 41.6 (a) Transvaginal ultrasound scan of unifollicular development in a polycystic ovary and (b) an overstimulated polycystic ovary. Reproduced from Balen AH. *Infertility in Practice*, 3rd edn. London: Informa Healthcare, 2008, with permission.

reproductive abnormalities in PCOS, although it was withdrawn because of reports of deaths from hepatotoxicity, and other thiazolidinediones such as rosiglitazone and pyoglitazone are not advocated for women trying to conceive.

Most of the initial studies of metformin in the management of PCOS were observational. Metformin appears to be less effective in those who are significantly obese (BMI >35 kg/m²). The largest appropriately powered prospec-

---

Summary box 41.2

- PCOS is the commonest endocrine disorder in women (prevalence 15–20%).
- PCOS runs in families and affects approximately 50% of first-degree relatives.
- PCOS is a heterogeneous condition. Diagnosis is made by two out of the following three criteria: (i) oligo- and/or anovulation, (ii) hyperandrogenism (clinical and/or biochemical) or (iii) polycystic ovaries, with the exclusion of other aetiologies of menstrual irregularity and androgen excess.
- Management is symptom-orientated.
- If obese, weight loss improves symptoms and endocrinology and should be encouraged. A glucose tolerance test should be performed if the BMI is >30 kg/m² (or >25 kg/m² if Asian). Dietary advice and exercise are essential components of a weight-reducing programme. Antiobesity drugs or surgery may be indicated.
- Menstrual cycle control may be achieved by using cyclical oral contraceptives or progestogens.
- Ovulation induction may be difficult and require progression through various treatments which should be monitored carefully to prevent multiple pregnancy.
- Hyperandrogenism is usually managed with Dianette®, containing ethinyloestradiol in combination with cyproterone acetate, or Yasmin®, which contains drosperinone. Alternatives include spironolactone, and reliable contraception is required.
- There is no place for insulin-sensitizing agents (e.g. metformin) in the absence of impaired glucose tolerance or type 2 diabetes.

---

tive randomized double-blind placebo-controlled study set out to evaluate the combined effects of lifestyle modification and metformin in 143 obese anovulatory women with a mean BMI of 38 kg/m² [23]. All subjects had an individualized assessment by a dietitian in order to set a realistic goal that could be sustained with an average reduction of energy intake of 500 kcal per day. As a result, both the metformin-treated and placebo groups managed to lose weight, but the amount of weight reduction did not differ between the two groups. An increase in menstrual cyclicity was observed in those who lost weight but again did not differ between the two arms of the study.

Two large randomized controlled trials also concluded that as first-line therapy for the treatment of anovulatory infertile women with PCOS, metformin alone was significantly less effective than CC alone, and that the addition of metformin to CC produced no significant benefit [24,25]. The recent Cochrane review has also concluded no benefit of metformin in achieving an increased rate of livebirth either alone or in combination [26], and so the use of metformin is only recommended when there is impaired glucose tolerance or type 2 diabetes [18].

Secondary amenorrhoea

Cessation of menstruation for six consecutive months in a women who has previously had regular periods is the usual criteria for investigation. However, some authorities consider 3 or 4 months of amenorrhoea to be pathological, but this is the debate between the definition of amenorrhoea and oligomenorrhoea. Women with secondary amenorrhoea must have a patent lower genital tract, an endometrium that is responsive to ovarian hormone stimulation and ovaries that have responded to pituitary gonadotrophins.

Secondary amenorrhoea is best classified according to its aetiological site of origin and can be subdivided into disorders of the hypothalamic–pituitary–ovarian–uterine axis and generalized systemic disease. The principal causes of secondary amenorrhoea are outlined in Table 41.2. The frequency with which these conditions present, on the other hand, can be seen in Table 41.6.

Management of secondary amenorrhoea

Genital tract abnormalities

Asherman's syndrome

Asherman's syndrome is a condition in which intrauterine adhesions prevent normal growth of the endometrium [27]. This may be the result of an over-vigorous endometrial curettage affecting the basalis layer of the endometrium or adhesions that may follow an episode of endometritis. It is thought that oestrogen deficiency increases the risk of adhesion formation in breast-feeding women who require a puerperial currettage for retained placental tissue. Typically, amenorrhoea is not absolute, and it may be possible to induce a withdrawal bleed using a combined oestrogen/progestogen preparation. Intrauterine adhesions may be seen on an HSG (Fig. 41.2). Alternatively, hysteroscopic inspection of the uterine cavity will confirm the diagnosis and enable treatment by adhesiolysis. The adhesions bridge the anterior and posterior walls of the uterine cavity and are usually avascular, although may contain vessels, muscle and even endometrium. Following surgery, a 3-month course of cyclical progesterone/oestrogen should be given. Some clinicians insert a foley catheter into the uterine cavity for 7–10 days postoperatively or an intrauterine contraceptive device for 2–3 months in order to prevent recurrence of adhesions.

In a series of 292 infertile women who were thought to have intrauterine adhesions, as detected by HSG, 46%

Table 41.6 The aetiology of secondary amenorrhoea in 570 patients attending an endocrine clinic [47].

Polycystic ovary syndrome	37%
Premature ovarian failure	24%
Hyperprolactinaemia	17%
Weight related amenorrhoea	10%
Hypogonadotrophic hypogonadism	6%
Hypopituitarism	4%
Exercise-related amenorrhoea	3%

conceived without treatment but only 53% delivered a live infant, and 13% had placenta accreta (Schenker and Margalioth, 1992 [28]). It has been suggested that the pregnancy rates after hysteroscopic treatment of intrauterine adhesions depend upon the degree of the initial problem (Valle and Sciarra, 1988 [29]), being 93% for mild and 57% for severe disease. The outcome of the pregnancy would appear to depend upon the post-treatment contour of the uterine cavity.

Cervical stenosis
Cervical stenosis is an occasional cause of secondary amenorrhoea. It was relatively common following a traditional cone biopsy for the treatment of cervical intraepithelial neoplasia. However, modern procedures, such as laser or loop diathermy, have less postoperative cervical complications. It still occasionally occurs following curettage of the uterus which inadvertently damages the endocervix. Treatment for cervical stenosis consists of careful cervical dilatation.

Ovarian causes of secondary amenorrhoea

Polycystic ovary syndrome (see above)

Premature ovarian failure
Ovarian failure by definition is the cessation of periods accompanied by a raised gonadotrophin level prior to the age of 40 years. It may occur at any age. The exact incidence of this condition is unknown as many cases go unrecognized, but estimates vary at between 1% and 5% of the female population. Studies of amenorrhoiec women report the incidence of premature ovarian failure to be between 10% and 36%.

Chromosomal abnormalities have been found in 70% of patients with primary amenorrhoea and in 2–5% of women with secondary amenorrhoea due to premature ovarian failure [30]. Ovarian failure occurring before puberty is usually due to a chromosomal abnormality or a childhood malignancy that required chemotherapy or radiotherapy. Adolescents who lose ovarian function soon after menarche are often found to have a Turner's mosaic (46XX/45X) or an X-chromosome trisomy (47XXX). There are some genetic anomalies that run in families with POF, although these are not assessed in routine clinical practice.

Overall, the most common cause of premature ovarian failure is autoimmune disease, with infection, previous surgery, and chemo- and radiotherapy also contributing to the aetiology. Ovarian autoantibodies can be measured and have been found in up to 69% of women with POF. However, the assay is expensive and not readily available in most units. It is therefore important to consider other autoimmune disorders and screen for autoantibodies to the thyroid gland, gastric mucosa parietal cells and adrenal gland if there is any clinical indication.

Before the absolute cessation of periods of true POF, some women experience an intermittent return to menses, interspersed between variable periods of amenorrhoea. Gonadotrophin levels usually remain moderately elevated during these spontaneous cycles, with plasma FSH levels of 15–20 IU/L. This occult ovarian failure, or resistant ovary syndrome, is associated with the presence of primordial follicles on ovarian biopsy (which incidentally is not a procedure that should be performed to make the diagnosis). Pregnancies are sometimes achieved, although the ovaries are usually resistant to exogenous gonadotrophins as they are to endogenous hormones. It is probable that reports of pregnancy in women with POF represent cases of fluctuating ovarian function rather than successes of treatment [31].

It is, however, possible to achieve pregnancy by oocyte donation, as part of *in vitro* fertilization (IVF) treatment. For women who are predicted to develop ovarian failure as a result of sterilizing chemotherapy for malignancy, it is now possible to cryopreserve oocytes collected during an IVF-stimulation protocol, which are frozen either as oocytes or as fertilized oocytes (embryos) if the patient has a partner. An alternative approach is the surgical removal of a whole ovary and transplantation of cryopreserved ovarian tissue once the cancer treatment is completed. Live births have been achieved by all these methods, although the technology for oocyte cryopreservation is less efficient than for embryo cryopreservation and ovarian tissue freezing is still in its infancy.

The diagnosis and consequences of POF require careful counselling of the patient. It may be particularly difficult for a young women to accept the need to take oestrogen preparations that are clearly labelled as being intended for older postmenopausal women while at the same time having to come to terms with the inability to conceive naturally. The short- and long-term consequences of ovarian failure and oestrogen deficiency are similar to those occurring in the fifth and sixth decade. However, the duration of the problem is much longer and therefore HRT is advisable in order to reduce the consequences of oestrogen deficiency in the long term.

Younger women with premature loss of ovarian function have an increased risk of osteoporosis. A series of 200 amenorrhoeic women between the ages of 16 and 40 years demonstrated a mean reduction in bone mineral density of 15% compared with a control group and after correction for body weight, smoking and exercise [32]. The degree of bone loss was correlated with the duration of the amenorrhoea and the severity of the oestrogen deficiency rather than the underlying diagnosis, and was worse in patients with primary amenorrhoea than in those with secondary amenorrhoea. A return to normal oestrogen status may improve bone mass density, but bone mineral density is unlikely to improve by more than 5–10% and it probably does not return to its normal value. However, it is not certain if the radiological improvement seen will actually reduce the risk of fracture, as remineralization is not equivalent to the re-strengthening of bone. Early diagnosis and early correction of oestrogen status is therefore important.

Women with POF may have an increased risk of cardiovascular disease. Oestrogens have been shown to have beneficial effects on cardiovascular status in women. They increase the levels of cardioprotective high-density lipoprotein but also total triglyceride levels, while decreasing total cholesterol and low-density lipoprotein levels. The overall effect is of cardiovascular protection.

The HRT preparations prescribed for menopausal women are also preferred for young women. The reason for this is that even modern low-dose combined oral contraceptive (COC) preparations contain at least twice the amount of oestrogen that is recommended for HRT in order to achieve a contraceptive suppressive effect on the hypothalamic–pituitary axis. HRT also contains 'natural' oestrogens (oestradiol) rather than the synthetic ethinyloestradiol that is found in most COCs.

Pituitary causes of secondary amenorrhoea

Hyperprolactinaemia is the commonest pituitary cause of amenorrhoea. There are many causes of a mildly elevated serum prolactin concentration, including stress, and a recent physical or breast examination. If the prolactin concentration is greater than 1000 mIU/L then the test should be repeated and if still elevated it is necessary to image the pituitary fossa (CT or MRI scan). Hyperprolactinaemia may result from a prolactin-secreting pituitary adenoma or from a non-functioning 'disconnection' tumour in the region of the hypothalamus or pituitary, which disrupts the inhibitory influence of dopamine on prolactin secretion. Large non-functioning tumours are usually associated with serum prolactin concentrations of <3000 mIU/L, while prolactin-secreting macroadenomas usually result in concentrations of 8000 mIU/L or more. Other causes include hypothyroidism, PCOS (up to 2500 mIU/L) and several drugs (e.g.

the dopaminergic antagonist phenothiazines, domperidone and metoclopramide).

In women with amenorrhoea associated with hyperprolactinaemia, the main symptoms are usually those of oestrogen deficiency. In contrast, when hyperprolactinaemia is associated with PCOS, the syndrome is characterized by adequate oestrogenization, PCOs on ultrasound scan and a withdrawal bleed in response to a progestogen challenge test. Galactorrhoea may be found in up to one-third of patients with hyperprolactinaemia, although its appearance is correlated neither with prolactin levels nor with the presence of a tumour. Approximately 5% of patients present with visual field defects.

A prolactin-secreting pituitary microadenoma is usually associated with a moderately elevated prolactin (1500–4000 mIU/L) and is unlikely to result in abnormalities on a lateral skull X-ray. On the other hand, a macroadenoma, associated with a prolactin greater than 5000–8000 IU/L and by definition greater than 1 cm diameter, may cause typical radiological changes – that is, an asymmetrically enlarged pituitary fossa with a double contour to its floor and erosion of the clinoid processes. Skull X-rays are rarely performed these days as CT and MRI scans now allow detailed examination of the extent of the tumour and, in particular, identification of suprasellar extension and compression of the optic chiasma or invasion of the cavernous sinuses. Prolactin is an excellent tumour marker, and so the higher the serum concentration the larger the size of the tumour expected on the MRI scan. In contrast, a large tumour on the scan with only a moderately elevated serum prolactin concentration (2000–3000 mIU/L) suggests a non-functioning tumour with 'disconnection' from the hypothalamus (Fig. 41.7).

The management of hyperprolactinaemia centres around the use of a dopamine agonist, of which bromocriptine is the most widely used. Of course, if the hyperprolactinaemia is drug induced, stopping the relevant preparation should be commended. This may not, however, be appropriate if the cause is a psychotropic medication, for example a phenothiazine being used to treat schizophrenia. In these cases it is reasonable to continue the drug and prescribe a low-dose combined oral contraceptive preparation in order to counteract the symptoms of oestrogen deficiency. Serum prolactin concentrations must then be carefully monitored to ensure that they do not rise further.

Most patients show a fall in prolactin levels within a few days of commencing bromocriptine therapy and a reduction of tumour volume within 6 weeks. Side effects can be troublesome (nausea, vomiting, headache, postural hypotension) and are minimized by commencing the therapy at night for the first 3 days of treatment and taking the tablets in the middle of a mouthful of food. Longer term side effects include Raynaud's phenomenon,

Table 41.7 Drug therapy for hyperprolactinaemia.

Bromocriptine	2.5–20 mg daily, divided doses	Maintenance usually 5–7.5 mg/day
Cabergoline	0.25–1 mg twice weekly	Maintenance usually 1 mg/week
Quinagolide	75–150 mcg daily, at night	

constipation and psychiatric changes – especially aggression, which can occur at the start of treatment.

Bromocriptine should be commenced at a dose of 1.25 mg at night and increased gradually every 5 days to 2.5 mg at night, and then 1.25 mg in the morning with 2.5 mg at night until the daily dose is 7.5 mg (in two or three divided doses). The maintenance dose should be the lowest that reduces prolactin to normal levels and is often lower than that needed initially to initiate a response (Table 41.7).

Longer acting preparations (e.g. twice-weekly cabergoline) may be prescribed to those patients who develop unacceptable side effects. Cabergoline generally appears to be better tolerated and more efficacious than bromocriptine but is currently not recommended for women trying to conceive as the safety data for pregnancy are not available, even though there is unlikely to be a problem with teratogenicity on the data available so far. If a woman is not wishing to conceive, then cabergoline should be prescribed and then switched to bromocriptine when (or if) she wishes to try for a pregnancy.

Surgery, in the form of a trans-sphenoidal adenectomy, is reserved for cases of drug resistance and failure to shrink a macroadenoma or if there are intolerable side effects of the drugs (the most common indication). Non-functioning tumours should be removed surgically and are usually detected by a combination of imaging and a serum prolactin concentration of <3000 mIU/L. When the prolactin level is between 3000 and 8000 mIU/L, a trial of bromocriptine is warranted, and if the prolactin level falls it can be assumed that the tumour is a prolactin-secreting macroadenoma. Operative treatment is also required if there is suprasellar extension of the tumour that has not regressed during treatment with bromocriptine and a pregnancy is desired. With the present day skills of neurosurgeons in transsphenoidal surgery, it is seldom necessary to resort to pituitary irradiation, which offers no advantages, and long-term surveillance is required to detect consequent hypopituitarism (which is immediately apparent if it occurs after surgery).

Women with a microprolactinoma who wish to conceive can be reassured that they may stop bromocriptine when pregnancy is diagnosed and require no further monitoring, as the likelihood of significant tumour expansion is very small (less than 2%). On the other hand, if a

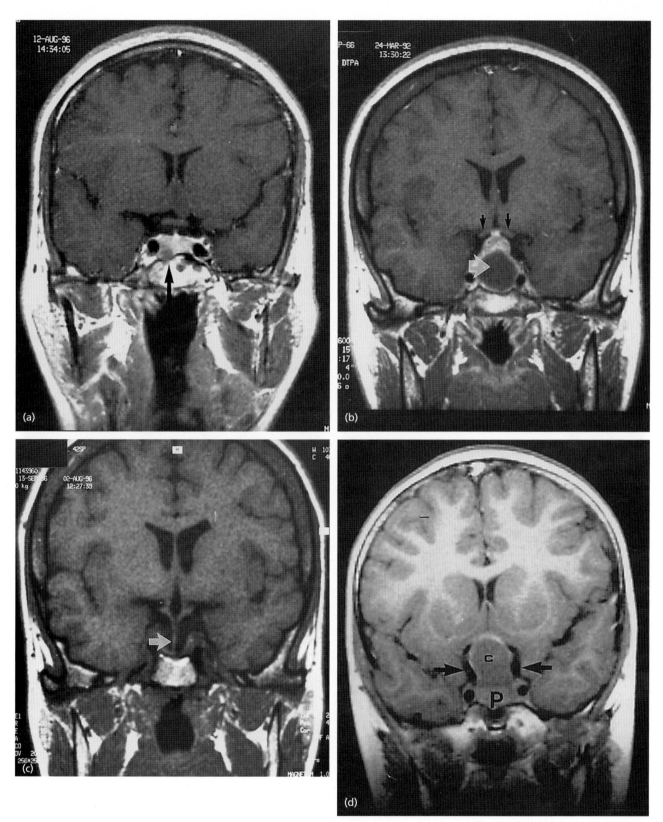

Fig. 41.7 (a) Pituitary microadenoma. Cranial magnetic resonance imaging (MRI). A coronal section T1-weighted spin echo sequence after i.v. gadolinium. The normal pituitary gland is hyperintense (bright) while the tumour is seen as a 4mm area of non-enhancement (grey) in the right lobe of the pituitary, encroaching up to the right cavernous sinus. It is eroding the right side of the sella floor (arrow). Pituitary macroadenoma. MRI scans of a pituitary macroadenoma before and after bromocriptine therapy: (b) T1-weighted image post gadolinium enhancement demonstrating a macroadenoma with a large central cystic component (large arrow). There is suprasellar extension with compression of the optic chiasm (small arrows).

(c) After therapy the tumour has almost completely resolved and there is tethering of the optic chiasm (arrow) to the floor of the sella. (d) Craniopharyngioma. Cranial MRI: coronal T1-weighted section after gadolinium enhancement. The tumour signal intensity on the T1 image and only part of the periphery of the tumour enhances. The carotid arteries have a low signal intensity (black arrows) due to the rapid flow within them and are deviated laterally and superiorly by the mass (C), which arises out of the pituitary fossa (P). Reproduced from Balen AH. *Infertility in Practice*, 3rd edn. London: Informa Healthcare, 2008, with permission.

patient with a macroprolactinoma is not treated with bromocriptine, the tumour has a 25% risk of expanding during pregnancy. This risk is probably also present if the tumour has been treated but has not shrunk, as assessed by CT or MRI scan. The first-line approach to treatment of macroprolactinomas is therefore with bromocriptine combined with barrier methods of contraception. In cases with suprasellar expansion, a follow-up CT (or MRI) scan should be performed after 3 months of treatment to ensure tumour regression before it is safe to embark upon pregnancy. Bromocriptine can be discontinued during pregnancy, although an MRI scan should be performed if symptoms suggestive of tumour re-expansion occur, and it is necessary to recommence bromocriptine therapy if there is continuing suprasellar expansion. These patients also require expert assessment of their visual fields during pregnancy.

If the serum prolactin is found to be elevated and the patient has a regular menstrual cycle, no treatment is necessary unless the cycle is anovulatory and fertility is desired. Amenorrhoea is the 'bioassay' of prolactin excess and should be corrected for its sequelae, rather than for the serum level of prolactin.

Hypothalamic causes of secondary amenorrhoea

Hypothalamic causes of amenorrhoea may be either primary or secondary. Primary hypothalamic lesions include craniopharyngiomas, germinomas, gliomas and dermoid cysts. These hypothalamic lesions either disrupt the normal pathway of prolactin inhibitory factor (dopamine), thus causing hyperprolactinaemia, or compress and/or destroy hypothalamic and pituitary tissue. Treatment is usually surgical, with additional radiotherapy if required. HRT is required to mimic ovarian function, and if the pituitary gland is damaged either by the lesion or by the treatment, replacement thyroid and adrenal hormones are required.

Secondary hypogonadotrophic hypogonadism (HH) may result from systemic conditions including sarcoidosis and tuberculosis as well as following head injury or cranial irradiation. Sheehan's syndrome, the result of profound and prolonged hypotension on the sensitive pituitary gland, enlarged by pregnancy, may also be a cause of HH in someone with a history of a major obstetric haemorrhage [33]. It is essential to assess the pituitary function fully in all these patients and then instigate the appropriate replacement therapy. Ovulation may be induced with pulsatile subcutaneous GnRH or human menopausal gonadotrophins (hMG). The administration of pulsatile GnRH provides the most 'physiological' correction of infertility caused by HH and will result in unifollicular ovulation, while hMG therapy requires close monitoring to prevent multiple pregnancy. Purified or recombinant FSH preparations are not suitable for women with HH (or pituitary hypogonadism) as these patients have absent endogenous production of LH, and so while follicular growth may occur, oestrogen biosynthesis is impaired [34]. Thus, hMG, which contains FSH and LH activity, is necessary for these patients.

Systemic disorders causing secondary amenorrhoea

Chronic disease may result in menstrual disorders as a consequence of the general disease state, weight loss or by the effect of the disease process on the hypothalamic–pituitary axis. Furthermore, a chronic disease that leads to immobility, such as chronic obstructive airway disease, may increase the risk of amenorrhoea-associated osteoporosis.

Some diseases affect gonadal function directly. Women with chronic renal failure have a discordantly elevated LH, possibly as a consequence of impaired clearance. Prolactin is also elevated in these women owing to failure of the normal inhibition by dopamine. Liver disease affects the level of circulating sex hormone-binding globulin and thus hormone levels, thereby disrupting the normal feedback mechanisms. Metabolism of various hormones including testosterone are also liver-dependent; both menstruation and fertility return after liver transplantation (Cundy *et al* 1990 [35]).

Endocrine disorders such as thyrotoxicosis and Cushing's syndrome are commonly associated with gonadal dysfunction. Autoimmune endocrinopathies may be associated with POF because of ovarian antibodies. Diabetes mellitus may result in functional hypothalamic–pituitary amenorrhoea.

Management of these patients should concentrate on the underlying systemic problem and on preventing complications of oestrogen deficiency. If fertility is required, it is desirable to achieve maximal health and where possible to discontinue teratogenic drugs.

Weight-related amenorrhoea

Weight can have profound effects on gonadotrophin regulation and release. Weight and eating disorders are also common in women. A regular menstrual cycle will not occur if the BMI is $<19 \text{kg/m}^2$. Fat appears to be critical to a normally functioning hypothalamic–pituitary–gonadal axis. It is estimated that at least 22% of body weight should be fat in order to maintain ovulatory cycles [36]. This level enables the extraovarian aromatization of androgens to oestrogens and maintains appropriate feedback control of the hypothalamic–pituitary–ovarian (HPO) axis. Therefore, girls who are significantly underweight prior to puberty may have primary amenorrhoea, while those who are significantly underweight after puberty will have secondary amenorrhoea. The clinical presentation depends upon the severity of the nutritional insult and its age of onset. To cause amenorrhoea, the loss must be 10–15% of the women's normal weight for height. Weight loss may be due to a number of causes including self-induced abstinence, starvation, illness and exercise.

Whatever the precipitating cause, the net result is impairment of gonadotrophin secretion. In severe weight loss, oestrogen may be catabolized to the antioestrogen 2-hydroxy-oestrone rather than to the usual oestradiol, which may further suppress gonadotrophin secretion. This pathway is enhanced by cigarette smoking. Weight-related gonadotrophin deficiency is more pronounced with LH than FSH [37]. This and the reduction in pulsatility of gonadotrophin secretion may result in a 'multicystic' pattern in the ovary. This appearance is typical of normal puberty and is seen when there are several cysts (about 5–10 mm in diameter together with a stroma of normal density.

Anorexia nervosa is at the extreme end of a spectrum of eating disorders and is invariably accompanied by menstrual disturbance, and indeed may account for between 15% and 35% of patients with amenorrhoea. Women with anorexia nervosa should be managed in collaboration with a psychiatrist, and it is essential to encourage weight gain as the main therapy.

An artificial cycle may be induced with the combined oral contraceptive pill. However, this may corroborate in the denial of weight loss being the underlying problem. Similarly, while it is possible to induce ovulation with GnRH or exogenous gonadotrophins, treatment of infertility in the significantly underweight patient is associated with a notable increase in intrauterine growth retardation and neonatal problems. Furthermore, since three-quarters of the cell divisions that occur during pregnancy do so during the first trimester, it is essential that nutritional status is optimized before conception. Low birth weight is also now being related to an increased risk of cardiovascular disease, obstructive lung disease and schizophrenia in adult life [38].

Weight-related amenorrhoea may also have profound long-term effects on bone mineral density. The age of onset of anorexia nervosa is also important, as prolonged amenorrhoea before the normal age at which peak bone mass is obtained (approximately 25 years) increases the likelihood of severe osteoporosis.

Worldwide involuntary starvation is the commonest cause of reduced reproductive ability, resulting in delayed pubertal growth and menarche in adolescents [39] and infertility in adults. Acute malnutrition, as seen in famine conditions and during and after the Second World War, has profound effects on fertility and fecundity [40]. Ovulatory function usually returns quickly on restoration of adequate nutrition. The chronic malnutrition common in developing countries has fewer profound effects on fertility but is associated with small and premature babies.

Psychological stress

Studies have failed to demonstrate a link between stressful life events and amenorrhoea of greater than 2 months (Bachmann *et al.*, 1982 [41]). However, stress may lead to physical debility such as weight loss, which may then cause menstrual disturbance.

Exercise-related amenorrhoea

Menstrual disturbance is common in athletes undergoing intensive training. Between 10% and 20% have oligomenorrhoea or amenorrhoea, compared with 5% in the general population [42]. Amenorrhoea is more common in athletes under the age of 30 years and is particularly common in women involved in the endurance events (such as long-distance running). Up to 50% of competitive runners training 80 miles per week may be amenorrhoeic [43].

The main aetiological factors are weight and percentage body fat content, but other factors have also been postulated. Physiological changes are consistent with those associated with starvation and chronic illness.

Ballet dancers provide an interesting subgroup of sportswomen, because their training begins at an early age. They have been found to have a significant delay in menarche (starting at the age of 15.4 years compared with 12.5 years in non-ballet dancers) and a retardation in pubertal development which parallels the intensity of their training [44]. Menstrual irregularities are common, and up to 44% have secondary amenorrhoea [45]. In a survey of 75 dancers, 61% were found to have stress fractures and 24% had scoliosis; the risk of these pathological features was increased if menarche was delayed or if there were prolonged periods of amenorrhoea [45]. These findings may be explained by delayed pubertal maturation resulting in attainment of a greater than expected height and a predisposition to scoliosis, as oestrogen is required for epiphyseal closure.

Exercise-induced amenorrhoea has the potential to cause severe long-term morbidity, particularly with regard to osteoporosis. Studies on young ballet dancers have shown that the amount of exercise undertaken by these dancers does not compensate for these osteoporotic changes [45]. Oestrogen is also important in the formation of collagen, and soft-tissue injuries are also common in dancers [46]. Whereas moderate exercise has been found to reduce the incidence of postmenopausal osteoporosis, young athletes may be placing themselves at risk at an age when the attainment of peak bone mass is important for long-term skeletal strength. Appropriate advice should be given, particularly regarding diet, and the use of a cyclical oestrogen–progestogen preparation should be considered.

Iatrogenic causes of amenorrhoea

There are many iatrogenic causes of amenorrhoea, which may be either temporary or permanent. These include malignant conditions that require either radiation to the abdomen/pelvis or chemotherapy. Both of these treatments may result in permanent gonadal damage – the amount of damage being directly related to the age of the patient, the cumulative dose and the patient's previous menstrual status.

Gynaecological procedures such as oophorectomy, hysterectomy and endometrial resection inevitably result in amenorrhoea. Hormone replacement should be prescribed for these patients where appropriate. Hormone therapy itself can be used to deliberately disrupt the menstrual cycle. However, iatrogenic causes of ovarian quiescence have the same consequences of oestrogen deficiency due to any other aetiology. Thus, the use of GnRH analogues in the treatment of oestrogen-dependent conditions (e.g. precocious puberty, endometriosis, uterine fibroids) results in a significant decrease in bone mineral density in as little as 6 months. However, the demineralization is reversible with the cessation of therapy, especially for the treatment of benign conditions in young women who are in the process of achieving their peak bone mass. The concurrent use of an androgenic progestogen or oestrogen 'add-back' therapy may protect against bone loss.

References

1 Balen AH, Conway GS, Kaltsas G *et al.* Polycystic ovary syndrome: The spectrum of the disorder in 1741 patients. *Hum Reprod* 1995;10:2107–2111.

2 Conway GS, Agrawal R, Betteridge DJ, Jacobs HS. Risk factors for coronary artery disease in lean and obese women with the polycystic ovary syndrome. *Clin Endocrinol* 1992;37:119–125.

3 The Rotterdam ESHRE/ASRM-sponsored PCOS Consensus Workshop Group; Fauser B, Tarlatzis B *et al.* Revised 2003 consensus on diagnostic criteria and long-term health risks related to polycystic ovary syndrome (PCOS). *Hum Reprod* 2004;19:41–47.

4 Balen AH, Laven JSE, Tan SL, Dewailly D. Ultrasound assessment of the polycystic ovary: international consensus definitions. *Hum Reprod* 2003;9:505–514.

5 Rajkowha M, Glass MR, Rutherford AJ, Michelmore K, Balen AH. Polycystic ovary syndrome: a risk factor for cardiovascular disease? *Br J Obstet Gynaecol* 2000;107:11–18.

6 RCOG. *Long-term Consequences of Polycystic Ovary Syndrome.* RCOG Guideline Number 33,2003.

7 Michelmore KF, Balen AH, Dunger DB, Vessey MP. Polycystic ovaries and associated clinical and biochemical features in young women. *Clin Endocrinol Oxf* 1999;51:779–786.

8 Legro RS. Polycystic ovary syndrome, phenotype and genotype. *Endocrinol Metabol Clin North Am* 1999;28:379–396.

9 Rodin DA, Bano G, Bland JM, Taylor K, Nussey SS. Polycystic ovaries and associated metabolic abnormalities in Indian subcontinent Asian women. *Clin Endocrinol* 1998;49:91–99.

10 Wijeyaratne CN, Balen AH, Barth J, Belchetz PE. Clinical manifestations and insulin resistance (IR) in polycystic ovary syndrome (PCOS) among South Asians and Caucasians: is there a difference? *Clin Endocrinol* 2002;57:343–350.

11 Pierpoint T, McKeigue PM, Isaacs AJ, Wild SH, Jacobs HS. Mortality of women with polycystic ovary syndrome at long-term follow-up. *J Clin Epidemiol* 1998;51:581–586.

12 Norman RJ, Masters L, Milner CR, Wang JX, Davies MJ. Relative risk of conversion from normoglycaemia to impaired glucose tolerance or non-insulin dependent diabetes mellitus in polycystic ovary syndrome. *Hum Reprod* 2001;16:1995–1998.

13 MacMahon B. Risk factors for endometrial cancer. *Gynecol Oncol* 1974;2:122–129.

14 Balen AH. Polycystic ovary syndrome and cancer. *Hum Reprod* 2001;7:522–525.

15 Coulam CB, Annegers JF, Kranz JS. Chronic anovulation syndrome and associated neoplasia. *Obstet Gynecol* 1983;61:403–407.

16 Scholtz S, Le Roux C, Balen AH. *The Role of Bariatric Surgery in the Management of Female Fertility.* RCOG SAC Paper, 2009.

17 Barth JH, Cherry CA, Wojnarowska F, Dawber RPR. Cyproterone acetate for severe hirsutism: results of a double-blind dose-ranging study. *Clin Endocrinol* 1991;35:5–10.

18 The Thessaloniki ESHRE/ASRM-sponsored PCOS Consensus Workshop Group, Thessaloniki, Greece; Tarlatzis BC, Fauser JM, Chang J *et al.* Consensus on infertility treatment related to polycystic ovary syndrome. *Hum Reprod* 2008;23:462–477.

19 Balen AH, Anderson R. Impact of obesity on female reproductive health: British Fertility Society, Policy and Practice Guidelines. *Hum Fertil* 2007;10:195–206.

20 Kousta E, White DM, Franks S. Modern use of clomifene citrate in induction of ovulation. *Hum Reprod* 1997;3:359–365.

21 Balen AH, Braat DDM, West C, Patel A, Jacobs HS. Cumulative conception and live birth rates after the treatment of anovulatory infertility. *Hum Reprod* 1994;9:1563–1570.

22 Bayram N, van Wely M, Kaaijk EM, Bossuyt PMM, van der Veen F. Using an electrocautery strategy or recombinant FSH to induce ovulation in polycystic ovary syndrome: a randomized controlled trial. *BMJ* 2004;328:192–195.

23 Tang T, Glanville J, Hayden CJ, White D, Barth JH, Balen AH. Combined life-style modification and metformin in obese patients with polycystic ovary syndrome (PCOS). A randomized, placebo-controlled, double-blind multi-centre study. *Human Reprod* 2006;21:80–89.

24 Moll E, Bossuyt PM, Korevaar JC, Lambalk CB, van der Veen F. Effect of clomifene citrate plus metformin and clomifene citrateplus placebo on induction of ovulation in women with newly diagnosed polycystic ovary syndrome: randomized double blind clinical trial. *BMJ* 2006;332:1485.

25 Legro RS, Barnhart HX, Schlaff WD *et al.* Cooperative Multicenter Reproductive Medicine Network. Clomiphene, metformin, or both for infertility in the polycystic ovary syndrome. *N Engl J Med.* 2007;356:551–628.

26 Tang T, Lord JM, Norman RJ, Yasmin E, Balen AH. Insulin-sensitizing drugs (metformin, rosiglitazone, pioglitazone, D-chiro-inositol) for women with polycystic ovary syndrome, oligo-amenorrhoea and subfertility. *Cochrane Database Syst Rev* 2009; DOI:10.1002/14651858.CD003053.pub2.

27 Asherman JG. Traumatic intrauterine adhesions. *J Obstet Gynaecol Brit Empire* 1950;57:892–896.

28 Schenker JG, Margalioth EJ. Intravterine adhesions: an updated appraisal. *Fertil Steril* 1992;37:593–610.

29 Valle RF, Sciarra JJ. Intrauterine adhesions: hysteroscopic diagnosis, classification, treatment and reproduction outcome. *Am J Obstet Gynecol* 1988;158:1459–1470.

30 Hague WM, Tan SL, Adams J, Jacobs HS. Hypergonadotrophic amenorrhoea – aetiology and outcome in 93 young women. *Int J Gynaecol Obstet* 1987;25:121–125.

31 Check JH, Nowroozi K, Chase JS, Nazari A, Shapse D, Vaze M. Ovulation induction and pregnancies in 100 consecutive women with hypergonadotrophic amenorrhoea. *Fertil Steril* 1990;53:811–816.

32 Davies MC, Hall M, Davies HS. Bone mineral density in young women with amenorrhoea. *Br Med J* 1990;301:790–793.

33 Sheehan HL. Simmond's disease due to post-partum necrosis of the anterior pituitary. *Q J Med* 1939;8:277.

34 Shoham Z, Balen AH, Patel A, Jacobs HS. Results of ovulation induction using human menopausal gonadotropin or purified follicle-stimulating hormone in hypogonadotropic hypogonadism patients. *Fertil Steril* 1991;56:1048–1053.

35 Cundy TF, O'Grady JG, Williams R. Recovery of menstruation and pregnancy after liver transplantation. *Gut* 1990;31:337–338.

36 Frisch RE. Fatness of girls from menarche to age 18 years, with a nomogram. *Hum Biol* 1976;48:353–359.

37 Warren MP, Vande Wiele RL. Clinical and metabolic features of anorexia nervosa. *Am J Obstet Gynecol* 1973;117:435–449.

38 Barker DJP. The fetal and infant origins of adult disease. *Br Med J* 1990;301:111.

39 Kulin HE, Bwibo N, Mutie D, Santner SJ. The effect of chronic childhood malnutrition on pubertal growth and development. *Am J Clin Nutrition* 1982;36:527–536.

40 Van der Spuy ZM, Steer PJ, McCusker M, Steele SJ, Jacobs HS. Outcome of pregnancy in underweight women after spontaneous and induced ovulation. *Br Med J* 1988;296:962–965.

41 Bachmann G, Kemmann E. Prevalence of oligomenorrhea and amenorrhea in a college population. *Am J Obstet Gynecol* 1982;144:98–102.

42 Schwartz B, Cumming DC, Riordan E, Selye M, Yen SSC, Rebar RW. Exercise-associated amenorrhoea: A distinct entity? *Am J Obstet Gynecol* 1981;141:662–670.

43 Cumming DC, Rebar RW. Exercise and reproductive function in women. *Am J Indust Med* 1983;4:113–125.

44 Warren MP: The effects of exercise on pubertal progression and reproductive function in girls. *J Clin Endocrinol Metab* 1980;51:1150–1157.

45 Warren MP, Brooks-Gunn J, Hamilton LH, Warren LF, Hamilton WG. Scoliosis and fractures in young ballet dancers. *N Engl J Med* 1986;314:1348–1353.

46 Bowling A. Injuries to dancers: prevalence, treatment and perception of causes. *Br Med J* 1989;298:731–734.

47 Balen AH, Tan SL, Jacobs HS. Hypersecretion of luteinizing hormone – A significant cause of infertility and miscarriage. *Br J Obstet Gynaecol* 1993;100:1082–1089.

Further reading

Balen A, Franks S, Homburg R, eds. *Polycystic Ovary Syndrome*. London: RCOG Press, 2010.

Balen A, Franks S, Homburg R, Kehoe S. Current Management of Polycystic Ovary Syndrome. Proceedings of 59th RCOG Study Group. London: RCOG Press.

Balen AH. *Reproductive Endocrinology for the MRCOG and Beyond*, 2nd edn. London: RCOG Press, 2007.

Balen AH. *Infertility in Practice*, 3rd edn. London: Informa Healthcare, 2008.

Chapter 42
Menstrual Problems: Heavy Menstrual Bleeding and Primary Dysmenorrhoea

Andrew W. Horne and Hilary O.D. Critchley
MRC Centre for Reproductive Health, University of Edinburgh, The Queen's Medical Research Institute, Edinburgh, UK

Heavy menstrual bleeding

Definition

There is confusion over the various terminologies used for abnormalities of menstrual blood loss. Heavy menstrual bleeding (HMB) is now a preferred description as it is simple and easily translatable into other languages [1–3]. HMB is defined as excessive menstrual blood loss (over several consecutive cycles) that has a major effect on a woman's quality of life. The objective definition of HMB (defined as a blood loss of greater than 80 mL per menstruation) is no longer used except for research purposes [4,5]. It is also important in clinical practice to distinguish between regular and abnormal bleeding, such as intermenstrual and post-coital bleeding.

> ### Summary box 42.1
>
> - 'Heavy menstrual bleeding (HMB)' replaces 'menorrhagia'.
> - 'Bleeding of endometrial origin' replaces 'dysfunctional uterine bleeding'.
> - Distinguish between 'regular' and 'abnormal' bleeding.

Prevalence and impact

Heavy menstrual bleeding affects one in three women of reproductive age [5,6]. The complaint of HMB results in significant morbidity. In the UK, ~1.5 million women per year consult their general practitioner with menstrual complaints. Annual treatment costs exceed £65m, an estimated 3.5 million work-days are lost annually [7] and current medical therapy may be associated with undesirable side effects. As many as one in five women discontinue use of progestin therapies (systemic and locally delivered) for HMB on account of unscheduled bleeding [8]. Surgery is favoured by many women with severe symptoms [9] and HMB is a leading indication for hysterectomy [10]. In the UK, regional differences in surgical rates for HMB have persisted despite changes in practice and improved evidence, suggesting that there is still scope for improving the management of HMB within health services [11].

Causes of heavy menstrual bleeding

Fibroids

Submucosal and intramural fibroids are the subtype most commonly associated with HMB, but the exact number of cases of HMB resulting from fibroids is not known. About 50% of fibroids cause no symptoms. Furthermore, the mechanisms involved in fibroid-associated HMB are yet to be determined. Bleeding from a fibroid itself is relatively rare, although there may be bleeding from the surrounding rich vasculature. Alternatively, differential expression of angiogenic factors and growth factors between leiomyoma cells and normal myometrium has been proposed to explain fibroid-associated bleeding [12].

Polyps

Polyps are common and frequently asymptomatic and their exact cause remains unknown. Polyps may cause unpredictable intermenstrual bleeding as well as being associated with an increased volume of bleeding with fibroid polyps [13,14].

Coagulopathy

As many as 10–20% of women with HMB will have a systemic disorder of haemostasis [15]. These disorders may be inherited or acquired and the severity of the disorder varies (majority mild to moderate). The overall clinical impact is unknown. The most common inherited disorder is von Willebrand's disease, found in 13% of women with HMB [16,17]. This aetiology should be considered in women who fail to respond to medical management or women who present at a young age. Acquired conditions include severe thrombocytopenia, thrombocytopathies, such as Glanzmann disease [18], and other rare bleeding/factor deficiencies.

Malignancy

Both endometrial and cervical carcinoma are potential causes of intermenstrual and post-coital bleeding, and rarely HMB. Sarcomas of myometrial origin, such as leiomyosarcoma, are rare (~2 in 1000 women with fibroids) but not infrequently present with abnormal bleeding [19]. The most relevant premalignant condition that may cause abnormal bleeding is endometrial hyperplasia [20,21].

Thyroid disease

Untreated hypothyroidism causes anovulation that typically manifests as amenorrhoea, but this endocrine state may also be associated with HMB [22,23]. Thyroid evaluation should be considered in the patient who presents with HMB and symptoms of thyroid dysfunction.

Pelvic infection

Data do exist to support an association between chronic endometrial infection and abnormal uterine bleeding, both intermenstrual and heavy bleeding [14,24]. *Chlamydia trachomatis* has been proposed as a cause of HMB [24], and the prevalence of *C. trachomatis* in women with abnormal uterine bleeding (AUB) may be underestimated. This is confounded by the fact that 85% cases of chlamydial infection are asymptomatic. Further research is required to determine whether all women with HMB should be screened for *C. trachomatis*.

Arteriovenous malformations

An arteriovenous malformation (AVM) is a congenital or acquired localized collection of abnormally connected arteries and veins. When they occur in the uterus, they have been associated with episodes of acute excessive bleeding [25]. Congenital AVM are rare, as are acquired AVM, which may occur following uterine curettage after pregnancy [26]. These vascular lesions of the uterus pose difficult management decisions and may present with heavy uterine bleeding following early pregnancy loss (EPL). Colour Doppler imaging is a useful diagnostic modality if an arteriovenous malformation is suspected. In cases associated with an EPL (likely due to subinvolution of the placental bed), the uterine lesion resolves once the human chorionic gonadotrophin (HCG)level has returned to normal. Acute heavy bleeding from an AVM may be required to be managed with therapeutic uterine artery embolization.

Iatrogenic

Iatrogenic causes include the use of anticoagulants in women with thromboembolic disease, pharmacological drugs known to impact on ovulation by prolactin-related disruption of the hypothalamic–pituitary–ovarian (HPO) axis (e.g. tricyclic antidepressants and phenothiazines) and copper intrauterine contraceptive devices (the effect is thought to be due to a local inflammatory process).

Bleeding of endometrial origin

In the majority of cases of HMB, it is probable that the precise cause of heavy bleeding lies at the level of the endometrium itself. This has previously been termed 'dysfunctional uterine bleeding' (DUB) and is a diagnosis of exclusion. However, the exact endometrial mechanisms leading to HMB remain undefined and an area of active research enquiry. Containment of menstrual blood loss is controlled in a major part by vasoconstriction [27,28]. In the absence of pregnancy, with luteal regression, the withdrawal of sex steroids (progesterone and oestrogen) results in vasoconstriction of the spiral arterioles. Factors regulating vascular tone thus play an important role and include prostaglandins, endothelins and nitric oxide. Aberrant expression of local regulators of vascular tone have been implicated in the problem of HMB. For example, reduced endometrial expression of the vasoconstrictor endothelin has been described in women with HMB [29]. Disturbance in prostaglandin synthesis/pathways is also implicated in the problem of HMB [30–33]. Early research in this area demonstrated increased levels of total prostaglandins (PG) in the endometrium of women with HMB [31]. Administration of COX-inhibitors is a first-line treatment during menses for women with HMB [5]. Endometrial haemostasis differs from haemostasis elsewhere in the body. Platelets in the endometrial cavity are deactivated. The endometrium is a rich source of plasminogen activators (uPA and tPA) but coagulation is rapidly reversed by marked fibrinolysis. Since menstrual loss is mainly controlled by vasoconstriction, there is a lesser need for coagulation. Women with HMB are reported to exhibit increased endometrial fibrinolytic activity [34]. Antifibrinolytics commonly prescribed for complaint of HMB reduce blood loss by 40–50% [35].

 Summary box 42.2

Causes of HMB:
- In most women, no cause for HMB is found.
- Coagulopathies may account for 10–20% of cases of HMB.
- Malignancy should always be excluded.
- Remember iatrogenic causes.

Clinical evaluation

History

The primary aim of the history is to determine the full impact that the bleeding is having on the woman's quality of life, and a menstrual diary is often helpful to determine the amount and timing of the bleeding [36]; flooding and clots indicate significant loss. An accurate history may also indicate the cause of the bleeding. Intermenstrual bleeding and postcoital bleeding are suggestive of an anatomical cause, whereas pressure symptoms, including bowel and urinary symptoms, can indicate the presence of a large fibroid. A coagulation disorder may be implicated in the complaint of HMB and a structured history to elicit such is valuable [14,37]. It is likely if there is a history of excessive bleeding since menarche, postpartum haemorrhage, surgery-related bleeding or bleeding associated with dental work, or a history of two or more of the following: bruising greater than 5 cm, epistaxis once a month, frequent bleeding or a family history of bleeding symptoms.

A sexual, smear and contraceptive history are essential and should include questioning about the woman's desire for future pregnancy as this will affect future symptom management.

Examination

A general evaluation of the patient should be performed to exclude signs of anaemia, evidence of systemic coagulopathy (bruising, petechiae) and thyroid disease (goitre). An abdominal examination should be performed to reveal a pelvic mass (fibroid); a speculum examination should be performed to assess the vulva, vagina and cervix (this may reveal sources of bleeding, such as a tumour, or a discharge suggesting infection); and a bimanual examination should be performed to elicit uterine enlargement.

Investigations

A full blood count is indicated in all women with HMB. If the history and examination strongly suggest cyclical HMB without the presence of pathology in a woman under 45 years old, it is appropriate to implement first-line medical treatment without further investigation [5]. In older women, and in younger women in whom medical treatment has failed, further investigation is warranted (see Table 42.1).

Histological assessment of the endometrium

The authors of a recent study reviewed the histology reports of all women aged 30–50 years who presented to a large UK hospital with unscheduled uterine bleeding between 1998 and 2007 [38]. They categorized the patients according to age and the type of unscheduled bleeding that they presented with, i.e. cyclical HMB or irregular bleeding. Their data demonstrate categorically that the age cut-off of 45 years has the highest sensitivity in detecting the maximum proportion of all types of endometrial

Table 42.1 Investigations of patients complaining of heavy menstrual bleeding (HMB).

Investigation	Indication
Full blood count	All women with HMB
Coagulation screen	If a focused/structured history is suggestive of a coagulation disorder
Thyroid function tests	Only from women with other symptoms of thyroid disease
Endocervical/high vaginal swabs	If history suggestive of risk of infection
Colposcopic examination	Suspicion of cervical malignancy
Histological assessment of the endometrium	Symptomatic women >45 years old, younger women when medical treatment has failed and all women prior to surgical intervention
Evaluation of the uterine cavity (pelvic ultrasound, including saline infusion sonography, and outpatient hysteroscopy)	Intermenstrual or postcoital bleeding, irregular HMB, suspected structural pathology or when medical management has failed

hyperplasia and carcinoma, while having a reasonably high specificity so as to avoid false negatives. Reassuringly, these data support the guidelines produced in the UK by the National Institute of Clinical Excellence (NICE) [5].

Evaluation of the uterine cavity

Blind sampling methodologies (outpatient endometrial biopsy) are reasonable screening techniques but they are ineffective at diagnosing focal lesions. Published research has provided the clinician with high-quality data regarding the accuracy of pelvic ultrasound and outpatient hysteroscopy in the diagnosis of structural lesions endometrial disease [36,39]. Despite this, controversy remains regarding the clinical utility of these uterine imaging modalities. Furthermore, magnetic resonance imaging (MRI) is now being used in specific clinical scenarios in the evaluation of HMB [40]. It is non-invasive, differentiates uterine anatomy in response to exogenous hormones or the normal menstrual cycle, and reliably localizes pelvic pathology and size of lesions. When uterine conservation is desired in women with fibroids and ultrasound is unsuccessful in determining depth of myometrial involvement of a fibroid, MRI should be considered. The precision of MRI in the localization of submucosal fibroids can obviate the need for hysterectomy and permit hysteroscopic resection of the fibroids. MRI is also of value in determining the role of embolization as a treatment option. However, future research needs to be directed towards providing effectiveness and cost-effectiveness data (MRI is expensive) in order to resolve the ongoing debate and guide best clinical practice.

Summary box 42.3

Evaluation of patient with HMB:
- Objective definition of HMB is no longer used in clinical practice.
- Determine impact of HMB on quality of life.
- Perform structured history to determine coagulation disorder.
- Full blood count should be performed in all patients.
- Controversy remains over clinical utility of imaging modalities.
- Endometrial histology is only warranted in women >45 years, younger women when medical treatment has failed and all women prior to surgical intervention.

Management of heavy menstrual bleeding

For some women, the demonstration that their blood loss is in fact 'normal' may be sufficient to reassure them and make further treatment unnecessary. However, when treatment is advised by the healthcare professional, women with HMB should be given information about treatment options [5] and given adequate time and support in the decision-making process. A care pathway for HMB is shown in Fig. 42.1 (adapted from NICE, 2007) [5].

Non-hormonal treatments

If a woman is wishing to conceive, hormonal treatments and most surgical interventions are unacceptable.

Antifibrinolytics

Antifibrinolytics, such as tranexamic acid, reduce blood loss by up to 50% by inhibiting endometrial fibrinolysis [41–43]. Side effects are rare but include gastrointestinal symptoms.

Prostaglandin synthetase inhibitors

Prostaglandin synthetase inhibitors, such as non-steroidal anti-inflammatories (NSAIDs), inhibit endometrial prostaglandin production, leading to a reduction in menstrual blood loss. Mefenamic acid is the most frequently used agent and reduces blood loss by approximately 25% [44–46]. The drug is taken during menstruation and has the

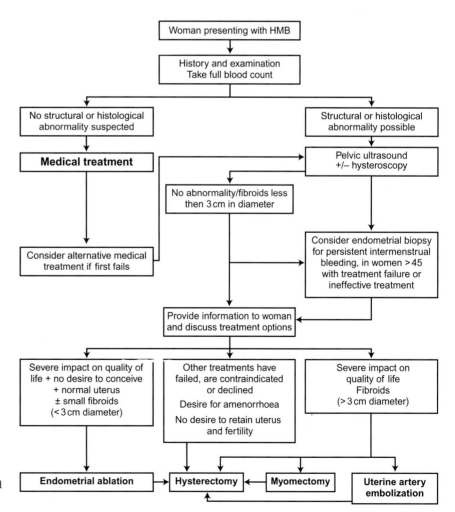

Fig. 42.1 Suggested care pathway for heavy menstrual bleeding (HMB) (adapted from NICE Guideline 44, 2007).

advantage of containing analgesic properties. However, NSAIDs are associated with gastrointestinal side effects. There have also been isolated reports of NSAID-associated reversible female infertility [47], and the probable mechanism is ovulatory failure due to non-rupture of mature follicles. If a woman presents with infertility and is found to be taking a NSAID for HMB, this potential cause should be considered.

Hormonal treatments

Combined oral contraceptive pill

From clinical experience, the combined oral contraceptive pill (COCP) is generally considered to be effective in the management of HMB. Furthermore, as amenorrhoea becomes more acceptable, many women use the COCP continuously for periods of between 3 and 6 months to avoid menstruation altogether [48,49]. However, there are limited studies to support the effectiveness of the COCP (taken either cyclically or continuously) in the management of HMB. Evidence from one randomized controlled trial (RCT) of the COCP (ethinyl oestradiol 30 mcg and levonorgestrel 150 mcg for 21 days) found a reduction in blood loss of 43% [50]. There are no available RCT data to date on other COCP preparations. Risks of COCP treatment include thromboembolic disease and migraine (increased in the older woman, particularly if she is a smoker).

Levonorgestrel-releasing intrauterine system

The levonorgestrel-releasing intrauterine system (LNG-IUS) is an excellent alternative to surgery for women with HMB who also seek reliable long-acting reversible contraception [5,51]. An estimated 9.8 million women worldwide use the LNG-IUS. This usage will be mainly for contraception, but the added health benefits of reduced menstrual bleeding and less anaemia make this an attractive option to many women worldwide. The uptake of LNG-IUS has undoubtedly been further increased because the low dose of LNG released into the uterine cavity leads to endometrial atrophy, so that for many women its use is associated with little or no vaginal bleeding. RCTs show that the LNG-IUS, or Mirena®, will reduce menstrual loss by up to 96% after 1 year but that the full benefit may not be seen for 6 months [52,53]. As its action is local, progestogen-related side effects are much less than with oral agents. Women should be fully counselled that they are likely to experience unscheduled spotting/bleeding during the initial months of use [54, 55]. In a UK study, 10.5% of new users of LNG-IUS ceased use by the end of the first year owing to bleeding problems, and this accounted for much of the total 5-year cumulative discontinuation rate for bleeding problems (16.7%) [56]. To date, effective interventions to prophylactically ameliorate unscheduled bleeding in women using the LNG-IUS

remain elusive [55]. The LNG-IUS may be inserted in the outpatient setting and requires change every 5 years.

Oral progestogens

Oral progestogens are helpful in the management of women with irregular (anovulatory) HMB at the extremes of reproductive life. Cyclical administration of progestogens in ovulatory women is of no benefit [45,57]. Only norethisterone acetate (5 mg, three times daily), if prescribed for 21 days, is effective for treatment of ovulatory HMB [58].

Injected/depot progestogens

There is no published evidence relating to the use of injected progestogens for the treatment of HMB. Nevertheless, it is well recognized that amenorrhoea occurs in many women when injected progestogens are used for contraception, and they are commonly used for the treatment of HMB.

Gonadotrophin-releasing hormone analogues

Limited use of gonadotrophin-releasing hormone (GnRH) analogues (GnRHa) may be considered when all other management options have been explored [59]. GnRHa act by downregulating the HPO axis and induce ovarian suppression, leading to amenorrhoea. Unfortunately, their beneficial effect does not continue after stopping treatment and their adverse effect on bone density limit their use beyond 6 months. If used for over 6 months, the addition of 'add-back' hormone replacement therapy (HRT) is recommended.

Danazol, ethamsylate and gestrinone are no longer recommended for routine use in the treatment of HMB owing to their unacceptable side effects. Selective progesterone receptor modulators are a group of novel compounds, which thus far have been shown to reduce menstrual bleeding without the unwanted effect of unscheduled bleeding episodes [60,61]. Further research is needed into the efficacy and safety of these drugs, which appear to have great potential in reducing menstrual blood loss.

Summary box 42.4

Medical treatments for HMB:
- Antifibrinolytics and prostaglandin synthetase inhibitors are appropriate first-line treatments.
- The COCP is considered effective.
- The levonorgestrel-releasing intrauterine system is an excellent long-term alternative to surgery.

Surgical treatments

It is unclear whether operative interventions should be used as the initial treatment for HMB or whether medical intervention should always be tried first. Typically, surgical management is only considered in women who have completed their family, with the exception of polypectomy and myomectomy where fertility can be retained. The number of hysterectomies performed for HMB is only one-third that of a decade ago [62]. This reduction in hysterectomy rates is considered to reflect not only the introduction of successful treatment options, such as the LNG-IUS, but also the increased management in primary care of menstrual bleeding complaints. Dilatation and curettage should not be used as a therapeutic treatment in any clinical situation.

Polypectomy

Endocervical polyps can be avulsed in the outpatient setting. Endometrial polyps can be removed blindly under general anaesthetic, or by hysteroscopic resection either under general anaesthetic or in the outpatient setting. There is evidence that hysteroscopically directed polypectomy is associated with reduced recurrence [63] but there is no evidence for reduction of bleeding.

Endometrial ablation

Endometrial ablation is the targeted destruction of the endometrium and some of the underlying myometrium. The technique is suitable for women who have completed their family and in whom all organic and structural causes of HMB have been excluded (fibroids <4 cm are an exception). First-generation techniques include hysteroscopic transcervical resection of the endometrium, using an electrical diathermy loop, and roller-ball ablation. These techniques offer treatment for uterine cavities with submucous fibroids. Simpler, quicker second-generation alternatives have subsequently been developed for smoother, smaller cavities. These include fluid-filled thermal balloon endometrial ablation (Thermachoice™), microwave ablation (Microsulis™) and impedance-controlled endometrial ablation (Novasure™). Overall, the existing evidence suggests that success rates and complication profiles of newer techniques of ablation compare favourably with first-generation hysteroscopic techniques [64]. All can be performed as day-care procedures, either under general anaesthetic or under local anaesthetic in the outpatient setting. Women who undergo this procedure should be advised to use long-term effective contraception. The rationale for this is the lack of knowledge about the effects of endometrial ablation on future reproductive potential. It is also recommended that pre-ablation endometrial histology is obtained and that a hysteroscopy is performed before (following cervical dilatation) and after each treatment to exclude uterine perforation. Postoperatively, patients may complain of transient crampy abdominal pain and a watery brown discharge for between 3 and 4 weeks. Prophylactic antibiotic therapy is often used to reduce the risk of endometritis. Patients must be coun-

selled before the procedure about the potential complications, which may include device failures at time of procedure, endometritis, haematometra, fluid overload due to absorption of distension medium (resection only), perforation and intra-abdominal injury (including visceral burns). Endometrial thinning agents (e.g. GnRH analogues) are not usually indicated for the newer ablative techniques but can be employed at the operator's preference for endometrial resection. As a general rule, of all women undergoing endometrial ablation with a second-generation technique, 40–50% will become amenorrhoeic, 40–60% will have markedly reduced menstrual loss and 20% will have no difference in their bleeding. When the effects of the LNG-IUS and endometrial ablation in reducing HMB are compared, a meta-analysis of six randomized clinical trials reported that the efficacy of the LNG-IUS in the management of HMB appeared to have similar therapeutic effects to that of endometrial ablation up to 2 years after treatment [65]. Nonetheless, it is clear from longer-term trials that while most women are initially satisfied, many subsequently choose or require repeat endometrial ablation (technique dependent) or hysterectomy [66].

Myomectomy

Myomectomy is the surgical removal of fibroids from the uterine wall with conservation of the uterus [67]. In woman with multiple fibroids or a significantly enlarged uterus, the abdominal approach is most appropriate. However, advances in surgical instruments and techniques are expanding the role of the laparoscopic myomectomy in well-selected individuals. If the fibroid protrudes into the uterine cavity, it may be removed hysteroscopically. GnRH analogue therapy is often used for three months prior to surgical intervention in an attempt to reduce the vascularity of the fibroids. Immediate complications usually relate to excessive blood loss and a blood transfusion may be required intra- or postoperatively. Difficulty achieving haemostasis occurs more frequently than at hysterectomy and progression to hysterectomy to control blood loss is not uncommon. Patients should therefore be carefully counselled preoperatively about this risk. Intermediate postoperative risks include infection and further bleeding. Pregnancy following myomectomy appears to be safe, with a very low risk of uterine rupture with a vaginal delivery [68].

Uterine artery embolization

Uterine artery embolization (UAE) is a well-established technique for the treatment of fibroids [69]. The procedure is carried out by an interventional radiologist, usually under local anaesthetic with or without sedation. The femoral artery is canalized on one or both sides and fed into the iliac and then the uterine artery. Angiography is carried out to confirm the correct position before introduction of the embolic agent. Blockage of both uterine arteries results in fibroids becoming avascular and shrinking. As the normal myometrium subsequently derives its blood supply from the vaginal and ovarian vasculature, UAE is thought to have no permanent effect on the rest of the uterus. The procedure requires only a short hospital stay and may be done as a day case in selected women. Post UAE, a mean reduction of fibroid volume of 30–46% has been reported and symptomatic improvement has been reported in up to 85% of women [70]. However, there is no evidence of benefit of UAE compared with surgery (hysterectomy/myomectomy) for satisfaction [69]. In the immediate postoperative period, patients may experience ischaemic pain (usually responsive to simple analgesics) and infection is not uncommon. Occasionally, the rapid change in uterine size can result in passage of the fibroid vaginally following UAE. Rarely, subserosal fibroids can be adherent to the bowel and UAE can lead to bowel necrosis and peritonitis. Although there is a theoretical risk of premature ovarian failure after UAE, a recent study has shown that there is no evidence of a deterioration in ovarian function after 1 year [71]. This procedure is not currently recommended for women who wish to maintain their fertility. A small risk of sepsis after the procedure is acknowledged, even several months later. There appears to be a significant re-intervention rate and, although recovery time is quick, cost-effectiveness may be lost by 5 years owing to the re-intervention rate (Moss *et al.* [72]).

Hysterectomy

Hysterectomy should only be considered in the treatment of HMB when a woman has completed her family and when medical and less-invasive surgical options have failed or are inappropriate. Hysterectomy is an established, effective treatment for HMB that induces amenorrhoea, but this must be balanced against its potential morbidity and mortality. The UK NICE guidelines for HMB [5] advise that the hysterectomy route for HMB should be considered in the following order: vaginal, abdominal and laparoscopic. However, individual patient characteristics and surgical expertise are important determinants.

Vaginal hysterectomy

Vaginal hysterectomy is appropriate for women with HMB with a small uterus. Advantages of the vaginal route include the obvious absence of an abdominal wound and minimal disturbance of the intestines. This results in less postoperative pain, earlier mobilization and earlier discharge from hospital [73].

Abdominal hysterectomy

An abdominal approach is necessary/indicated in women with a uterine size greater than the equivalent of 12 weeks of pregnancy; endometriosis or history of pelvic inflammatory disease; a history of previous Caesarean section; or a long vagina and/or narrow pubic arch, making the vaginal approach technically difficult. An abdominal hysterectomy involves removal of the uterus and/or cervix (subtotal and total, respectively) through an abdominal incision under general anaesthetic. A subtotal abdominal hysterectomy may be performed according to patient preference or if the surgery is technically difficult owing to adhesions or endometriosis. Although a subtotal is associated with decreased morbidity, patients must be warned of a 15% incidence of residual bleeding from the cervix. In young patients with HMB, the ovaries are usually conserved, but a bilateral salpingo-oophrectomy may be carried out simultaneously after detailed discussion with the patient, with particular attention to family history. In this situation, patients must be counselled about the need for HRT.

Laparoscopic hysterectomy

The proportion of hysterectomies performed laparoscopically has gradually increased and, although the procedure takes longer, proponents have emphasized several advantages. These include the opportunity to diagnose and treat other pelvic diseases (such as endometriosis), to carry out adnexal surgery, the ability to secure thorough intraperitoneal haemostasis at the end of the procedure and a rapid recovery time. Laparoscopic hysterectomy should be used as a general term, whereas operative laparoscopy before hysterectomy, laparoscopically assisted vaginal hysterectomy (with or without laparoscopic uterine vessel ligation), and laparoscopic total and subtotal hysterectomy should be used to describe the types of laparoscopic hysterectomy. In laparoscopically assisted vaginal hysterectomy (LAVH), the procedure is done partly laparoscopically and partly vaginally, but the laparoscopic component does not involve uterine vessel ligation. In uterine vessel ligation laparoscopic hysterectomy, although the uterine vessels are ligated laparoscopically, part of the operation is done vaginally. In total laparoscopic hysterectomy, the entire operation, including suturing of the vaginal vault, is done laparoscopically. These methods of hysterectomy require more specific surgical training than that required for the vaginal and abdominal methods. A full description of all these techniques is outwith the scope of this book.

Complications of hysterectomy

A prospective observational study of >10 000 hysterectomies in Finland revealed an overall complication rate of 17.2% for abdominal, 23.3% for vaginal and 19% for laparoscopic hysterectomy [74]. Mortality is a recognized complication of hysterectomy. The risk of death for the abdominal approach is estimated as one in every 4000 procedures. Serious risks include damage to the bladder and/or ureters (7/1000), damage to the bowel (0.4/1000), major haemorrhage (15/1000), infection/pelvic abscess (2/1000) and thromboembolism (4/1000), and long-term increased risk of prolapse and urinary incontinence. Notwithstanding these complications, patient satisfaction following hysterectomy for HMB is as high as 95% [75].

> **Summary box 42.5**
>
> Surgical treatments for HMB:
> - Endometrial ablation is safe and effective but may not have longer-term benefits.
> - Uterine artery embolization also has a significant re-intervention rate.
> - Hysterectomy should only be considered when a woman has completed her family and when medical and less invasive surgical options have been considered.

Severe acute heavy menstrual bleeding

Severe acute HMB can occur as a result of a coagulopathy (most commonly von Willebrand's disease), prolapsed fibroids, AVMs (see earlier section) or anticoagulants. Initial management is based on haemodynamic stability. One reported regimen is ethinyl oestradiol 30 µg/norgestrel 0.3 mg four times daily for 4 days, followed by three times daily for 3 days, followed by two times daily for 2 days, followed by once daily for 3 weeks [76]. Two further regimens [multidose oral contraceptive pill and multidose medroxyprogesterone acetate (MPA)] that have been reported to be effective and reasonably well tolerated (RCT, albeit limited by sample size) [77] are norethindrone 1 mg/ethinyl oestradiol 35 µg given three times daily for 1 week, then daily for 3 weeks, and MPA 20 mg orally three times daily for 1 week and then daily for 3 weeks. Cessation of bleeding was achieved by 10–14 days in 88% and 76% patients, respectively, with the median time to cessation of bleeding being 3 days. Once the patient is clinically stable, an investigation into the cause of bleeding should be performed.

Dysmenorrhoea

The prevalence of dysmenorrhoea (painful menstrual cramps of uterine origin) is difficult to determine because of different definitions of the condition – estimates vary from 45% to 95% [78]. Despite the substantial effect on quality of life and general well-being, few women with dysmenorrhoea seek treatment as they believe it will not help. Primary dysmenorrhoea is thought to be due to prostaglandin production in the myometrium during menstruation, triggering myometrial contractions and increasing uterine tone. This results in decreased blood flow and subsequent pain. Secondary dysmenorrhoea

and deep dyspareunia may be due to endometriosis, adenomyosis, fibroids or adhesions. Primary dysmenorrhoea is commoner in women under the age of 30 years, and secondary dysmenorrhoea usually occurs in women between the ages of 30 and 45 years old. Pain occurring with onset of menstruation is indicative of primary dysmenorrhoea. Pain preceding periods and relieved by menstruation is more likely to be due to secondary dysmenorrhoea. Primary dysmenorrhoea will usually respond to treatment with non-steroidal anti-inflammatory analgesics. These limit the production of prostaglandins and reduce myometrial contractility. Alternatively, the COCP can be used to alleviate symptoms. For women seeking alternative therapies, heat, thiamine, magnesium, and vitamin E may be effective [78]. The management of identified causes of secondary dysmenorrhoea are addressed in the relevant pathology sections.

Acknowledgements

We thank Dr Sue Milne, Dr Christine West and Dr Paul Dewart for helpful comments on chapter content; Ronnie Grant and Sheila Milne for help with chapter preparation. Dr Andrew Horne is supported by an MRC Clinician Scientist Fellowship.

References

1 Fraser IS, Critchley HO, Munro MG *et al.* A process designed to lead to international agreement on terminologies and definitions used to describe abnormalities of menstrual bleeding. *Fertil Steril* 2007;87:466–476.

2 Fraser IS, Critchley HO, Munro MG *et al.* Can we achieve international agreement on terminologies and definitions used to describe abnormalities of menstrual bleeding? *Hum Reprod* 2007;22:635–643.

3 Woolcock JG, Critchley HO, Munro MG *et al.* Review of the confusion in current and historical terminology and definitions for disturbances of menstrual bleeding. *Fertil Steril* 2008;90: 2269–2280.

4 Warner PE, Critchley HO, Lumsden MA *et al.* Menorrhagia II: is the 80-mL blood loss criterion useful in management of complaint of menorrhagia? *Am J Obstet Gynecol* 2004;190: 1224–1229.

5 NICE. Clinical Guideline 44; Heavy menstrual bleeding, 2007. Available at: http://www.nice.org.uk/nicemedia/pdf/CG44FullGuideline.pdf.

6 Kennedy AD, Sculpher MJ, Coulter A *et al.* A multicentre randomized controlled trial assessing the costs and benefits of using structured information and analysis of women's preferences in the management of menorrhagia. *Health Technol Assess* 2003;7:1–76.

7 Weeks AD, Duffy SR, Walker JJ. A double-blind randomized trial of leuprorelin acetate prior to hysterectomy for dysfunctional uterine bleeding. *BJOG* 2000;107:323–328.

8 Abdel-Aleem H, d'Arcangues C, Vogelsong KM *et al.* Treatment of vaginal bleeding irregularities induced by progestin only contraceptives. *Cochrane Database Syst Rev* 2007;CD003449.

9 Coulter A, Peto V, Doll H. Patients' preferences and general practitioners' decisions in the treatment of menstrual disorders. *Fam Pract* 1994;11:67–74.

10 Marjoribanks J, Lethaby A, Farquhar C. Surgery versus medical therapy for heavy menstrual bleeding. *Cochrane Database Syst Rev* 2006;CD003855.

11 Cromwell DA, Mahmood TA, Templeton A *et al.* Surgery for menorrhagia within English regions: variation in rates of endometrial ablation and hysterectomy. *BJOG* 2009;116: 1373–1379.

12 Stewart EA, Nowak RA. Leiomyoma-related bleeding: a classic hypothesis updated for the molecular era. *Hum Reprod Update* 1996;2:295–306.

13 Van Bogaert LJ. Clinicopathologic findings in endometrial polyps. *Obstet Gynecol* 1988;71:771–773.

14 Munro MG. *Abnormal Uterine Bleeding*. Cambridge: Cambridge University Press, 2010; pp. 40–41, 54, 59.

15 Kadir RA, Economides DL, Sabin CA, Owens D, Lee CA. Frequency of inherited bleeding disorders in women with menorrhagia. *Lancet* 1998;351:485–489.

16 Shankar M, Lee CA, Sabin CA *et al.* von Willebrand disease in women with menorrhagia: a systematic review. *BJOG* 2004;111:734–740.

17 Munro MG, Lukes AS. Abnormal uterine bleeding and underlying hemostatic disorders: report of a consensus process. *Fertil Steril* 2005;84:1335–1337.

18 Vijapurkar M, Mota L, Shetty S *et al.* Menorrhagia and reproductive health in rare bleeding disorders: a study from the Indian subcontinent. *Haemophilia* 2009;15:199–202.

19 Parker WH, Fu YS, Berek JS. Uterine sarcoma in patients operated on for presumed leiomyoma and rapidly growing leiomyoma. *Obstet Gynecol* 1994;83:414–418.

20 Gultekin M, Diribas K, Dursun P *et al.* Current management of endometrial hyperplasia and endometrial intraepithelial neoplasia (EIN). *Eur J Gynaecol Oncol* 2009;30:396–401.

21 Lacey JV, Jr., Chia VM. Endometrial hyperplasia and the risk of progression to carcinoma. *Maturitas* 2009;63:39–44.

22 Weeks AD. Menorrhagia and hypothyroidism. Evidence supports association between hypothyroidism and menorrhagia. *BMJ* 2000;320:649.

23 Moragianni VA, Somkuti SG. Profound hypothyroidism-induced acute menorrhagia resulting in life-threatening anaemia. *Obstet Gynecol* 2007;110:515–517.

24 Toth M, Patton DL, Esquenazi B *et al.* Association between Chlamydia trachomatis and abnormal uterine bleeding. *Am J Reprod Immunol* 2007;57:361–366.

25 O'Brien P, Neyastani A, Buckley AR *et al.* Uterine arteriovenous malformations: from diagnosis to treatment. *J Ultrasound Med* 2006;25:1387–1392; quiz 1394–1385.

26 Darlow KL, Horne AW, Critchley HO *et al.* Management of vascular uterine lesions associated with persistent low-level human chorionic gonadotropin. *J Fam Plann Reprod Health Care* 2008;34:118–120.

27 Markee JE. Menstruation in intraocular transplants in the rhesus monkey. *Contr Embryol Carnegie Instn* 1940;28:219–308.

28 Smith SK. Angiogenesis and implantation. *Hum Reprod* 2000;15(Suppl 6):59–66.

29 Marsh MM, Malakooti N, Taylor NH *et al.* Endothelin and neutral endopeptidase in the endometrium of women with menorrhagia. *Hum Reprod* 1997;12:2036–2040.

30 Willman EA, Collins WP, Clayton SG. Studies in the involvement of prostaglandins in uterine symptomatology and pathology. *Br J Obstet Gynaecol* 1976;83:337–341.

31 Smith SK, Abel MH, Kelly RW *et al.* Prostaglandin synthesis in the endometrium of women with ovular dysfunctional uterine bleeding. *Br J Obstet Gynaecol* 1981;88:434–442.

32 Adelantado JM, Rees MC, Lopez Bernal A *et al.* Increased uterine prostaglandin E receptors in menorrhagic women. *Br J Obstet Gynaecol* 1988;95:162–165.

33 Smith OP, Jabbour HN, Critchley HO. Cyclooxygenase enzyme expression and E series prostaglandin receptor signalling are enhanced in heavy menstruation. *Hum Reprod* 2007;22: 1450–1456.

34 Gleeson N, Devitt M, Sheppard BL *et al.* Endometrial fibrinolytic enzymes in women with normal menstruation and dysfunctional uterine bleeding. *Br J Obstet Gynaecol* 1993;100: 768–771.

35 Preston JT, Cameron IT, Adams EJ *et al.* Comparative study of tranexamic acid and norethisterone in the treatment of ovulatory menorrhagia. *Br J Obstet Gynaecol* 1995;102: 401–406.

36 Critchley HO, Warner P, Lee AJ *et al.* Evaluation of abnormal uterine bleeding: comparison of three outpatient procedures within cohorts defined by age and menopausal status. *Health Technol Assess* 2004;8:iii–iv,1–139.

37 Kadir RA, Economides DL, Sabin CA *et al.* Frequency of inherited bleeding disorders in women with menorrhagia. *Lancet* 1998;351:485–489.

38 Iram S, Musonda P, Ewies AA. Premenopausal bleeding: When should the endometrium be investigated?–A retrospective noncomparative study of 3006 women. *Eur J Obstet Gynecol Reprod Biol* 2010;148:86–89.

39 Clark TJ. Outpatient hysteroscopy and ultrasonography in the management of endometrial disease. *Curr Opin Obstet Gynecol* 2004;16:305–311.

40 Bradley LD, Falcone T, Magen AB. Radiographic imaging techniques for the diagnosis of abnormal uterine bleeding. *Obstet Gynecol Clin North Am* 2000;27:245–276.

41 Lethaby A, Farquhar C, Cooke I. Antifibrinolytics for heavy menstrual bleeding. *Cochrane Database Syst Rev* 2000;CD000249.

42 Andersch B, Milsom I, Rybo G. An objective evaluation of flurbiprofen and tranexamic acid in the treatment of idiopathic menorrhagia. *Acta Obstet Gynecol Scand* 1988;67:645–648.

43 Gleeson NC, Buggy F, Sheppard BL *et al.* The effect of tranexamic acid on measured menstrual loss and endometrial fibrinolytic enzymes in dysfunctional uterine bleeding. *Acta Obstet Gynecol Scand* 1994;73:274–277.

44 Lethaby A, Augood C, Duckitt K *et al.* Nonsteroidal anti-inflammatory drugs for heavy menstrual bleeding. *Cochrane Database Syst Rev* 2007;CD000400.

45 Cameron IT, Haining R, Lumsden MA *et al.* The effects of mefenamic acid and norethisterone on measured menstrual blood loss. *Obstet Gynecol* 1990;76:85–88.

46 van Eijkeren MA, Christiaens GC, Geuze HJ *et al.* Effects of mefenamic acid on menstrual hemostasis in essential menorrhagia. *Am J Obstet Gynecol* 1992;166:1419–1428.

47 Gaytan M, Morales C, Bellido C *et al.* Non-steroidal anti-inflammatory drugs (NSAIDs) and ovulation: lessons from morphology. *Histol Histopathol* 2006;21:541–556.

48 Loudon NB, Foxwell M, Potts DM *et al.* Acceptability of an oral contraceptive that reduces the frequency of menstruation: the tri-cycle pill regimen. *Br Med J* 1977;2:487–490.

49 Glasier AF, Smith KB, van der Spuy ZM *et al.* Amenorrhoea associated with contraception-an international study on acceptability. *Contraception* 2003;67:1–8.

50 Fraser IS, McCarron G. Randomised trial of 2 hormonal and 2 prostaglandin-inhibiting agents in women with a complaint of menorrhagia. *Aust N Z J Obstet Gynaecol* 1991;31:66–70.

51 Hurskainen R, Teperi J, Rissanen P *et al.* Clinical outcomes and costs with the levonorgestrel-releasing intrauterine system or hysterectomy for treatment of menorrhagia: randomised trial 5-year follow-up. *JAMA* 2004;291:1456–1463.

52 Milsom I, Andersson K, Andersch B *et al.* A comparison of flurbiprofen, tranexamic acid, and a levonorgestrel-releasing intrauterine contraceptive device in the treatment of idiopathic menorrhagia. *Am J Obstet Gynecol* 1991;164:879–883.

53 Lethaby AE, Cooke I, Rees M. Progesterone or progestogen-releasing intrauterine systems for heavy menstrual bleeding. *Cochrane Database Syst Rev* 2005;CD002126.

54 Backman T, Huhtala S, Blom T *et al.* Length of use and symptoms associated with premature removal of the levonorgestrel intrauterine system: a nation-wide study of 17,360 users. *BJOG* 2000;107:335–339.

55 Warner P, Guttinger A, Glasier AF *et al.* Randomised placebo-controlled trial of CDB-2914 in new users of a levonorgestrel-releasing intrauterine system shows only short-lived amelioration of unscheduled bleeding. *Hum Reprod* 2010;25:345–353.

56 Cox M, Tripp J, Blacksell S. Clinical performance of the levonorgestrel intrauterine system in routine use by the UK Family Planning and Reproductive Health Research Network: 5-year report. *J Fam Plann Reprod Health Care* 2002;28:73–77.

57 Higham JM, Shaw RW. A comparative study of danazol, a regimen of decreasing doses of danazol, and norethindrone in the treatment of objectively proven unexplained menorrhagia. *Am J Obstet Gynecol* 1993;169:1134–1139.

58 Irvine GA, Campbell-Brown MB, Lumsden MA *et al.* Randomized comparative trial of the levonorgestrel intrauterine system and norethisterone for treatment of idiopathic menorrhagia. *Br J Obstet Gynaecol* 1998;105:592–598.

59 Thomas EJ. Add-back therapy for long-term use in dysfunctional uterine bleeding and uterine fibroids. *Br J Obstet Gynaecol* 1996;103(Suppl 14):18–21.

60 Wilkens J, Chwalisz K, Han C *et al.* Effects of the selective progesterone receptor modulator asoprisnil on uterine artery blood flow, ovarian activity, and clinical symptoms in patients with uterine leiomyomata scheduled for hysterectomy. *J Clin Endocrinol Metab* 2008;93:4664–4671.

61 Wilkens J, Critchley H. Progesterone receptor modulators in gynaecological practice. *J Fam Plann Reprod Health Care* 2010;36:87–92.

62 Reid PC, Mukri F. Trends in number of hysterectomies performed in England for menorrhagia: examination of health episode statistics, 1989 to 2002–3. *BMJ* 2005;330:938–939.

63 Preutthipan S, Herabutya Y. Hysteroscopic polypectomy in 240 premenopausal and postmenopausal women. *Fertil Steril* 2005;83:705–709.

64 Lethaby A, Hickey M, Garry R *et al.* Endometrial resection/ablation techniques for heavy menstrual bleeding. *Cochrane Database Syst Rev* 2009;CD001501.

65 Kaunitz AM, Meredith S, Inki P *et al.* Levonorgestrel-releasing intrauterine system and endometrial ablation in heavy menstrual bleeding: a systematic review and meta-analysis. *Obstet Gynecol* 2009;113:1104–1116.

66 McGurgan P, O'Donovan P. Second-generation endometrial ablation: an overview. *Best Pract Res Clin Obstet Gynaecol* 2007;21:931–945.

67 Luciano AA. Myomectomy. *Clin Obstet Gynecol* 2009;52:362–371.

68 Campo S, Campo V, Gambadauro P. Reproductive outcome before and after laparoscopic or abdominal myomectomy for subserous or intramural myomas. *Eur J Obstet Gynecol Reprod Biol* 2003;110:215–219.

69 Edwards RD, Moss JG, Lumsden MA *et al.* Uterine-artery embolisation versus surgery for symptomatic uterine fibroids. *N Engl J Med* 2007;356,360–370.

70 Gupta JK, Sinha AS, Lumsden MA *et al.* Uterine artery embolisation for symptomatic uterine fibroids. *Cochrane Database Syst Rev* 2006;CD005073.

71 Rashid S, Khaund A, Murray LS *et al.* The effects of uterine artery embolization and surgical treatment on ovarian function in women with uterine fibroids. *BJOG* 2010;117:985–989.

72 Moss JG, Cooper KG, Khaund A *et al.* Randomised comparison of uterine artery embolisation (UAE) with surgical treatment in patients with symptomatic uterine fibroids (REST trial): 5-year results. *BJOG* 2011;118:936–944.

73 Garry R, Fountain J, Brown J *et al.* EVALUATE hysterectomy trial: a multicentre randomized trial comparing abdominal, vaginal and laparoscopic methods of hysterectomy. *Health Technol Assess* 2004;8:1–154.

74 Makinen J, Johansson J, Tomas C *et al.* Morbidity of 10,110 hysterectomies by type of approach. *Hum Reprod* 2001;16:1473–1478.

75 Crosignani PG, Vercellini P, Apolone G *et al.* Endometrial resection versus vaginal hysterectomy for menorrhagia: long-term clinical and quality-of-life outcomes. *Am J Obstet Gynecol* 1997;177:95–101.

76 Ely JW, Kennedy CM, Clark EC *et al.* Abnormal uterine bleeding: a management algorithm. *J Am Board Fam Med* 2006;19:590–602.

77 Munro MG, Mainor N, Basu R *et al.* Oral medroxyprogesterone acetate and combination oral contraceptives for acute uterine bleeding: a randomised controlled trial. *Obstet Gynecol* 2006;108:924–929.

78 Proctor M, Farquhar C. Diagnosis and management of dysmenorrhoea. *BMJ* 2006;332:1134–1138.

Chapter 43
Premenstrual Syndrome

P.M. Shaughn O'Brien
Keele University School of Medicine, Stoke on Trent, UK

Introduction

Premenstrual symptoms occur in most women and there may have been evolutionary benefit to this. Social behaviour resulting in intercourse would have occurred more frequently at the time of ovulation and less frequently once ovulation had passed. As the female becomes less receptive and possibly aggressive to males during the non-fertile premenstrual phase, the males would seek more receptive ovulating females leading to an increase in the population. This is pure conjecture of course – but that is the nature of evolutionary theory. As with all biological parameters there are extremes so that some women have minimal or no symptoms (5–9%) while a similar number have such severe symptoms that there is major impairment of their lives, that of their families, their interpersonal relationships and normal day-to-day functioning. This extreme is premenstrual syndrome (PMS).

Definitions

The terminology used for premenstrual disorders is complex. Premenstrual tension was the term originally used, but it has now become the usual lay term; PMS is the medical term most often used in the UK. Premenstrual dysphoric disorder (PMDD) is the extreme, predominantly psychological end of the PMS spectrum estimated to occur in 3–5% of women [1] (Table 43.1). It is the term used increasingly by psychiatrists in the USA, but strictly speaking only for research purposes. It should be noted that much recent research into aetiology and treatment has been undertaken on women who fulfil the criteria for PMDD, particularly for clinical trials on selective serotonin reuptake inhibitors (SSRIs). Women designated as having PMDD will also fulfil criteria for PMS but not necessarily vice versa. The term PMDD may become more established in Europe but as yet it is far from universally accepted.

Premenstrual syndrome is defined in the Tenth Revision of the International Classification of Disease (ICD-10): a woman is considered to have PMS if she complains of recurrent psychological or somatic symptoms (or both) occurring specifically during the luteal phase of the menstrual cycle and which resolve in the follicular phase at least by the end of menstruation [2]. PMDD is more specific with regard to symptoms and (reflecting the introduction of the term by psychiatrists) pays little attention to physical symptoms (Table 43.1).

Because the ICD-10 definition makes no reference to impairment, it is probably too liberal to be of practical use clinically or for research purposes. The Diagnostic and Statistical Manual of Mental Disorders – 4th edn (DSM-IV) classification is too restrictive for clinical use and may have the detrimental effect of under-recognizing patients who are severely debilitated.

Symptoms

A wide range of PMS symptoms has been described, but it is their timing and impact that are most important, more so than their specific character [3].

Depression, irritability, anxiety, tension, aggression, inability to cope and feeling out of control are typical psychological symptoms. Bloatedness, mastalgia and headache are classical physical symptoms.

Because most normal women have some degree of symptomatology in the days leading up to menstruation, it is considered that it is the impact of symptoms, namely that they significantly disrupt normal functioning, that distinguishes those women with PMS from those with no more than normal physiological symptoms.

Essentially, symptoms of PMS are non-specific, must cause significant impairment and the symptoms (and the impairment) must resolve by the end of menstruation.

Dewhurst's Textbook of Obstetrics & Gynaecology, Eighth Edition. Edited by D. Keith Edmonds.
© 2012 John Wiley and Sons, Ltd. Published 2012 by John Wiley and Sons, Ltd.

Table 43.1 *Diagnostic and Statistical Manual of Mental Disorders – 4th edn (DSM-IV) research diagnostic criteria for premenstrual dysphoric disorder (PMDD) (1994).*

A	In most menstrual cycles, five (or more) of the following symptoms are present, with at least one of the symptoms being either (1), (2), (3) or (4)
1	Markedly depressed mood, feelings of hopelessness or self-deprecating thoughts
2	Marked anxiety, tension, feeling of being 'keyed up' or 'on edge'
3	Marked affective lability (e.g. feeling suddenly sad or tearful or increased sensitivity to rejection)
4	Persistent and marked anger or irritability or increased interpersonal conflicts
5	Subjective sense of difficulty in concentrating
6	Decreased interest in usual activities (e.g., work, school, friends, hobbies)
7	Lethargy, easy fatigability or marked lack of energy
8	Marked change in appetite, overeating or specific food cravings
9	Hypersomnia or insomnia
10	A sense of being overwhelmed or out of control
11	Other physical symptoms, such as breast tenderness or swelling, headaches, joint or muscle pain, a sensation of 'bloating', weight gain
B	Interference with work, school or social relationships
C	Symptoms of PMDD must be present for most of the time during the last week of the luteal phase (premenses) and absent during the week after menses
D	The disturbance cannot merely be an exacerbation of the symptoms of another disorder
E	Confirmation by prospective daily ratings for two consecutive menstrual cycles

Diagnosis

There are no objective tests (physical, biochemical, endocrine or imaging) to assist the diagnosis of PMS and so the use of prospectively completed symptom charts is essential (Fig. 43.1). Retrospective reporting of symptoms is inaccurate, but also significant numbers of women who present to a PMS clinic have separate underlying problems such as perimenopause, thyroid disorder, migraine, chronic fatigue syndrome, irritable bowel syndrome, seizures, anaemia, endometriosis, drug or alcohol abuse and menstrual disorders as well as psychiatric disorders such as depression, bipolar illness, panic disorder, personality disorder and anxiety disorder.

The confirmation of luteal-phase timing with the relief of symptoms by the end of menstruation is diagnostic providing the symptoms are of such severity to impact on the patient's normal functioning. It is also important to identify patients who have a premenstrual exacerbation (PME) of an underlying psychological, physical or medical disorder. For example, there are many documented cases of premenstrual suicide, asthma and epilepsy.

Many validated assessment instruments are available – they are all paper-based self-assessment scales and are not objective. Most researchers and clinicians opt for the Daily Record of Severity of Problems (DRSP) form (Fig. 43.1), which was recommended in the (downloadable) Royal College of Obstetricians and Gynaecologists (RCOG) Green Top guideline no. 48 in 2007 [4]. Such charts are invaluable. They enable the clinician to characterize instantly the pattern of premenstrual symptoms, their absence during the follicular phase and the degree of impairment caused. Despite the guideline's recommendation that the DRSP charts be administered for 2 months prospectively in order to establish the diagnosis before initiating treatment, less than 10% of clinical directors report that this strategy had been adopted in their gynaecology/PMS clinics (O'Brien and Samad, unpublished national survey data) (Fig. 43.2).

Gonadotrophin-releasing hormone agonists in diagnosis

The use of the so-called 'GnRH (gonadotrophin-releasing hormone) analogue test' may be of benefit in clarifying the diagnosis where there is a mixed picture. Although there are several studies to demonstrate that this group of drugs successfully eradicates symptoms in well-defined patients, it has never been proven scientifically as a clinical test nor indeed even assessed as such. It is used extensively by gynaecologists (off licence and with due discussion with the patient) for the purposes of removing the ovarian cycle to determine which of a patient's symptoms are clearly related to the menstrual cycle and which (i.e. those which persist despite suppression of the cycle) are not. It is also a valuable way of demonstrating whether symptoms or medical problems such as premenstrual migraine, asthma and epilepsy are truly related to the cycle or are independent. This can be illustrated by the following commonly encountered clinical problem. If a woman is to be considered for hysterectomy for a gynaecological indication such as HMB due to fibroids, symptom information gathered during GnRH therapy

DAILY RECORD OF SEVERITY OF PROBLEMS

Please print and use as many sheets as you need for at least two FULL months of ratings

Name or Initials _____ T F _____

Month/Year _____ N O V E M B E R _____

Each evening note the degree to which you experienced each of the problems listed below. Put an "x" in the box which corresponds to the severity: **1** - not at all, **2** - minimal, **3** - mild, **4** - moderate, **5** - severe, **6** - extreme.

Enter day (Monday="M", Thursday="R", etc) >	T	W	T	F	S	S	M	T	W	T	F	S	S	M	T	W	T	F	S	S	M	T	W	T	F	S	S	M	T	W	T
Note spotting by entering "S" >																			S	S	S					S	S	S			
Note menses by entering "M" >																									M	M	M				
Begin rating on correct calendar day >	1	2	3	4	5	6	7	8	9	10	11	12	13	14	15	16	17	18	19	20	21	22	23	24	25	26	27	28	29	30	31

The chart contains the following numbered problem items rated on a 1–6 severity scale:

1. Felt depress, sad, "down", or "blue" or felt hopeless; or felt worthless or guilty
2. Felt anxious, tense, "keyed up" or "on edge"
3. Had mood swings (i.e. suddenly feeling sad or tearful) or was sensitive to rejection or feelings were easily hurt
4. Felt angry, or irritable
5. Had less interest in usual activities (work, school, friends, hobbies)
6. Had difficulty concentrating
7. Felt lethargic, tired, or fatigued; or had lack of energy
8. Had increased appetite or overate; or had cravings for specific foods
9. Slept more, took naps, found it hard to get up when intended; or had trouble getting to sleep or staying asleep
10. Felt overwhelmed or unable to cope; or felt out of control
11. Had breast tenderness, breast swelling, bloated sensation, weight gain, joint or muscle pain, or other physical symptoms (J O I N T P A I N)

At work, school, home or in daily routine, at least one of the problems noted above caused reduction of productivity or inefficiency

At least one of the problems noted above caused avoidance or or less participation in hobbies or social activities

At least one of the problems noted above interfered with relationships with others

Fig. 43.1 Daily Record of Severity of Problems (DRSP) chart prospectively completed by a patient suffering from moderately severe premenstrual syndrome (PMS) demonstrating (a) the cyclicity of symptoms, (b) occurrence premenstrually, (c) absence of symptoms in the follicular phase and (d) impairment.

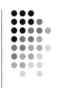

National Audit

Does any formal evaluation take place for PMS patients

before treatment is initiated?

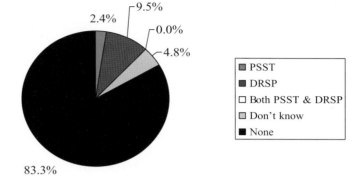

Fig. 43.2 National survey of Clinical Directors. Implementation of RCOG Guidance on Diagnosis. DRSP, Daily Record of Severity of Problems; PSST, Premenstrual Symptom Screening Tool.

may help the patient make the decision about whether to conserve or retain her ovaries. If her PMS (or other significant premenstrual symptom) is severe and is eradicated by GnRH, it is likely (though not guaranteed) that she would also benefit from removal of ovaries when the hysterectomy is being undertaken. This information would be invaluable in the final preoperative counselling.

Aetiology

Premenstrual syndrome is not due to a single factor but its basis is multifactorial, with genetic, environmental and underlying psychological influences being important. This is of course true for all mood disorders but in PMS the ovarian cycle comes into play, with ovulation being almost certainly the key factor.

Ovulation and progesterone

The principal cause of PMS is uncertain. There is evidence to suggest that the cyclical endogenous progesterone produced in the luteal phase of the cycle after ovulation is the key provoking factor. Women with PMS appear to be unusually 'sensitive' to the normal levels of progesterone [5]; differences have not been demonstrated in progesterone levels between women with and without PMS [6]. It has been hypothesized that the mechanism of this increased sensitivity is related to a neurochemical factor, and most evidence points to a dysregulation of serotonin metabolism [5].

Throughout reproductive life, progesterone production seems to be linked to women's psychological health. Progesterone and metabolites, such as allopregnanolone, are produced by the ovary and the adrenals, and also *de novo* in the brain. These hormones are effectively neurosteroids that readily cross the blood–brain barrier. Progesterone has known mood-altering and sedative effects when administered. It is well known that women have no PMS symptoms before puberty, during pregnancy or after the menopause – these are times where ovarian hormone cycling has not begun or ceases temporarily or permanently. Not surprisingly, if the assumptions made above are true, PMS-like symptoms can also be reintroduced by the administration of oestrogen/progestogen hormone replacement therapy (HRT) and this is frequently seen in clinical practice.

Suppression of the ovarian endocrine cycle with danazol by administration of analogues of GnRH or following bilateral oophorectomy results in the elimination of PMS symptoms. Therefore, the hypothesis that ovarian steroids, particularly ovulatory progesterones, have a role in the pathophysiology of the syndrome is intuitively obvious.

Research, none of which is recent, into PMS has generated data which could support theories of progesterone deficiency, oestrogen/progesterone imbalance or progesterone excess. However, the consensus is that ovarian steroid concentrations in blood do not differ in these women. Interactions of fluctuating levels of ovarian steroids or their metabolites with neurotransmitter systems or receptor imbalances in the brain are directly relevant to the pathogenesis of PMS [7]. This is believed to render women more sensitive to physiological levels of progesterone.

Summary box 43.2

Aetiology of PMS is uncertain, although ovulation is almost certainly the trigger in women who are sensitive to endogenous progesterone following ovulation and exogenous progestogen used therapeutically. It is likely that this sensitivity is related to an abnormality of neurotransmitter function. This has yet to be determined, but research evidence points to the serotonergic system.

Neurotransmitters

Oestrogen has clear effects on several neurotransmitters, including serotonin, acetylcholine, noradrenaline, γ-aminobutyric acid (GABA) and dopamine. It cumulatively acts as an agonist on serotonergic function by increasing the number of serotonin receptors, serotonin (5-HT) postsynaptic responsiveness, and neurotransmitter transport and uptake. It also increases serotonin synthesis and boosts the levels of the metabolite 5-hydroxy indole acetic acid (5-HIAA). It is well known that the serotonergic system plays a substantial role in regulating mood, sleep, sexual activity, appetite and cognitive ability. Serotonin dysregulation is a major component in the development of depression. Our knowledge of the role of serotonin in depression has been extended into PMS research [5], and several studies have demonstrated altered 5-HT metabolism in these patients. Blood levels and platelet uptake of 5-HT have been found to be low in patients with PMDD, and acute depletion of tryptophan, the precursor of serotonin, aggravates symptoms of PMS and PMDD. This hypothesis is supported indirectly by the observation that serotonin-receptor concentrations vary with changes in the oestrogen and progesterone level and because the well-known selective serotonin reuptake inhibitors (SSRIs) fluoxetine, paroxetine, citalopram and sertraline have been shown to be extremely efficacious in treating severe PMS and PMDD [7]. This gives additional, albeit indirect, support to the theory of involvement of serotonin in the aetiology of PMS.

Low activity of GABA has been reported in patients with depression, PMDD and PMS. Oestrogen increases binding of GABA agonists and the upregulation of GABA receptors. In addition to the effect of SSRIs on the serotonergic system, they have been shown to enhance GABA function, hence improving depressive symptoms. The GABA receptor is one of the principal receptors involved in the mechanism of action of alcohol and diazepam. Investigations of the metabolites of progesterone have shown that women with PMS had lower levels of allopregnanolone in the luteal phase [8]. This provides another plausible theory, as allopregnanolone has GABA-ergic activities and its deficiency can induce symptoms similar to those experienced in PMS (Fig. 43.2).

Vitamin B6 (pyridoxine) is a cofactor in the final step of the synthesis of serotonin and dopamine from dietary tryptophan. However, no data have yet demonstrated consistent abnormalities either of brain amine synthesis or deficiency of cofactors such as vitamin B6, and supplementation studies have shown that it is probably ineffective as a method of treatment.

Treatment

 Summary box 43.3

Treatment can be achieved effectively either by suppressing or removing ovulation or by modulating central nervous function with psychological interventions or psychotropic drugs.
The SSRIs are particularly useful.

Non-medical therapies

Claims, mainly unsubstantiated, have been made for the supplementation of calcium, vitamin E, magnesium, dietary change, vitamin B6, evening primrose oil, exercise, yoga, acupuncture, psychotherapy and many more. There is very little evidence that any of these treatments for PMS are effective, with the exception of exercise and cognitive behavioural therapy, and very limited evidence for the effects of calcium and magnesium. It is important to realise that the placebo effect for any treatment method is associated with a very high placebo response, so many therapies appear on the face of it to be effective. On the other hand, because of this placebo effect, therapeutic research requires the recruitment of such large numbers of patients to reach the power to demonstrate statistical superiority that many studies are almost impossible to undertake where the additional therapeutic affect over and above that of the placebo is only marginal.

Medical therapies

The management of PMS has, over the past few years, become increasingly easy to undertake, if somewhat more invasive. First, it should be stated that there is overwhelming evidence that progesterone pessaries and oral progestogens are ineffective [9]. Ironically, these are the only drugs in the UK that have a pharmaceutical licence for the management of PMS. All known effective therapies are unlicensed.

Our proposed aetiology of PMS suggests that normal postovulatory progesterone gives rise to symptoms in women who have increased sensitivity to endogenous progesterone and this sensitivity is considered to be due to a neurotransmitter dysregulation such as serotonin 'deficiency'. If this is so, then, broadly speaking, treatment should be achievable either by suppressing ovulation or by enhancing serotonin levels in the central nervous system to 'reduce the sensitivity to progesterone'. The first of these is achieved pharmacologically or by surgical intervention, the latter by elevating serotonin levels using drugs such as the SSRIs. Although theoretical, treatment based on this notion is very useful practically.

Psychotropics – selective serotonin reuptake inhibitors

Elevating serotonin levels can readily be achieved by the use of SSRIs [7]. Such treatment is clearly beneficial, although none of these drugs has a pharmaceutical licence for the management of either PMS or PMDD. Fluoxetine 20 mg daily is usually sufficient to improve symptoms in most women. Side effects such as loss of libido may be partially avoided by administering the drug during the luteal phase only. The effect of the SSRIs is more instantaneous for PMS symptoms than it is for the treatment of symptoms of depression. While SSRIs are not licensed in the UK or Europe for PMS, in the USA fluoxetine and indeed most other SSRIs are licensed for PMDD.

Ovarian cycle suppression

Suppression of the ovarian cycle can be achieved with oestrogen [10], danazol [11], GnRH agonist analogues [12] or bilateral oophorectomy [13].

Summary box 43.4

The few drugs that are licensed to manage PMS are ineffective – those that are effective must be used off licence and patients should be made aware of this.

Surgery

Bilateral oophorectomy

Bilateral oophorectomy (usually with hysterectomy) is almost always too invasive for the majority of patients with PMS and, even though it is the only certain cure [13], its use is rarely justifiable other than as a last resort measure for the most severely affected women – those who have failed to respond to other measures. When removal of the ovaries and uterus is considered appropriate, oestrogen replacement can follow without the need to consider endometrial protection using progestogen, which inevitably would restimulate the PMS symptoms. We should note here that in those studies which appear to have described (retrospectively) increased morbidity and mortality in later life if ovaries are removed are methodologically flawed. Women whose ovaries were conserved were compared with those having hysterectomy or bilateral oophorectomy but without any subsequent oestrogen replacement. No gynaecologist would withhold oestrogen replacement in such women and, while such studies are not yet available, it would be anticipated that outcomes following oophorectromy plus oestrogen therapy would actually be far more favourable. It should be added that the studies described general gynaecological patients and not those undergoing surgery for PMS.

Any treatment technique where the uterus is retained and oestrogen replacement is given will require the administration of progestogen in order to protect the patient from the risk of endometrial cancer in the residual endometrium. Systemic progestogen will then almost certainly cause the reappearance of PMS symptoms in most women. Hence, if the ovaries are to be removed for PMS, then in most cases subsequent management is made simpler and more effective by removing the uterus at the same time. Laparoscopic bilateral oophorectomy has its attractions as it is less invasive, but the subsequent management difficulties posed by the presence of the endometrium are not inconsiderable. Whether it is preferable to use a Mirena® intrauterine system (IUS) (see below) or to remove the uterus is probably more dependent on patient choice as there is no evidence to influence the decision either way

There is no logic in recommending endometrial ablation for PMS because cyclical ovarian function will continue along with the resulting PMS symptoms. Where claims are made for the beneficial effects of ablation, these are based on studies designed to evaluate the treatment of heavy periods and they are not valid for interpretation in terms of PMS treatment.

Danazol

When danazol is given orally, even at doses of 200 mg, it is particularly effective for most symptoms of PMS. Its use has been very much limited by anxieties related to the risk of masculinization. Attempts to reduce side effects by prescribing it for use in the luteal phase only (presumably through its direct effect on target tissue rather than ovulation suppression) have shown it be ineffective for nearly all symptoms of PMS with the exception of cyclical mastalgia [11].

Gonadotrophin-releasing hormone agonist analogues (and add-back therapy)

Gonadotrophin-releasing hormone agonist analogues are extremely effective [12]. These are best administered as injected depot preparations (goserelin or leuprorelin) as, unlike nasal preparations, compliance is virtually guaranteed. These drugs are agonist analogues and so omission of a nasal dose (or indeed late administration of depot preparations) can result in incomplete suppression and even re-stimulation of cycles.

Treatment without add-back treatment will almost always be successful for PMS, but confusion can arise owing to the development of new symptoms usually associated with the menopause. With continuous add-back therapy (particularly tibolone), the analogues remain equally effective for the PMS while eliminating menopause symptoms. [12]. It is difficult to know whether long-term use of this combination is justified either medically or economically. It is probably reasonable to use it in those women approaching the menopause and medium term in younger women. In those who do receive longer-term therapy, it is considered advisable to monitor bone density at 2-yearly intervals as is recommended for patients being treated for endometriosis with long-term GnRHa and add-back.

Oestrogen

Suppression of ovulation using oestrogen has significant advantages over oophorectomy and GnRHa in that these latter approaches still require the addition of oestrogen to prevent the hypo-oestrogenic effects resulting from the primary treatment approach. Its disadvantage is that in those women who retain their uterus and endometrium, it is necessary to protect from endometrial cancer using potentially 'PMS-inducing' progestogens.

Oestrogen can be given in several ways, including via the combined oral contraceptive pill, conventional cyclical or continuous HRT, and oestradiol patches or implants. Standard preparations of HRT, be they cyclical, continuous combined or tibolone, are of insufficient dose to suppress ovulation and they would inevitably fail to improve symptoms and increase the incidence of abnormal uterine bleeding.

While the use of conventional combined oral contraception certainly suppresses ovulation, the progestogen component introduces a new progestogen cycle. This may be the reason why oral contraceptive therapy has in the main proven to be ineffective in several well-conducted trials. The use of continuous combined oral contraceptive therapy would appear to be a more logical approach, but clinical anecdotes are contradictory and there have been no therapeutic studies of continuous combined, back-to-back or tricycling regimens. Relatively recently, oral contraceptives containing a newer progestogen, drospirenone, have been introduced. Drospirenone is derived from spironolactone and thus has antiandrogenic and antialdosterone properties which may antagonize or at least avoid restimulation of the PMS-like symptoms. Early studies are encouraging but not definitive.

Transdermal oestradiol (as patches or implants) suppresses the ovarian cycle effectively without inducing the negative consequences of surgically induced premature menopause or 'medical oophorectomy' [10]. Consequently, they reliably treat PMS symptoms. In the presence of an intact uterus, it remains necessary to prevent endometrial hyperplasia and cancer – this, as has already been discussed, reintroduces 'PMS' [14].

While the possibility of giving oestrogen alone and regularly checking the endometrium with scans or endometrial sampling is feasible, the risk will remain and additionally the likelihood that patients will have troublesome bleeding is very considerable.

Other unresearched and potential alternatives to avoid restimulation of PMS symptoms exist, including:
- administering cyclical progesterone combined with simultaneous SSRI;
- the use of less androgenic progestogens; and
- administration of the progesterone at less frequent intervals.

Probably the most realistic and effective method to achieve endometrial protection without reintroducing PMS would be to administer the progestogen into the uterine cavity using the levonorgestrel intrauterine system (LNG IUS Mirena) where it will act directly on the endometrium. With this approach, oestrogen suppresses ovulation and avoids menopausal symptoms. The intrauterine progestogen provides endometrial protection without achieving systemic levels that would act on the central nervous system to reintroduce PMS symptoms. This combination could have the added benefit of improving any menstrual problem and would provide effective contraception. There is only limited evidence to support the use of this combination. There is, however, good evidence to demonstrate that oestrogen in sufficient doses achieves ovarian suppression and elimination of PMS symptoms – there is good evidence that the LNG IUS can prevent and even reverse established endometrial hyperplasia. There is an enormous amount of clinical anecdotal experience to suggest that the combination is effective. Large-scale studies are required to demonstrate this efficacy as it has the ability to achieve all that hysterectomy and bilateral oophorectomy plus oestrogen achieves but without major surgery.

If general practitioners or gynaecologists should use this approach, it is important that they and their patients are aware that, as well as the LNG IUS-induced bleeding in the months following its insertion, there can be initial absorption of the LNG into the circulation, and thus bringing back PMS symptoms in the early months. Both are transient in most patients. Finally, the author has shown (unpublished data) that in a significant number of women who have received pretreatment with GnRH suppression before insertion of LNG IUS during the third month (when presumably the endometrium is thinned and avascular), both bleeding and PMS are minimized. As yet, this requires formal evaluation in research studies (Fig. 43.3).

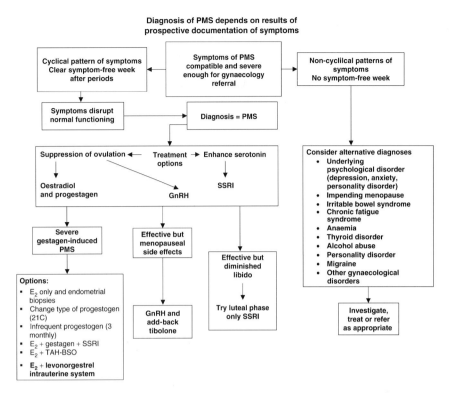

Fig. 43.3 Algorithm for the diagnosis and management of premenstrual syndrome (PMS).

 Summary box 43.5

In general, the more effective a treatment method is, the more invasive it is. Paradoxically, then, the worse the symptoms are, the easier it is to treat them as the more invasive treatment methods can be justified – assuming, of course, that the diagnosis is sound.

Conclusion

Suppression of the ovarian cycle eliminates PMS effectively. This can most precisely be achieved by GnRHa with add-back tibolone. The scope for long-term therapy using this approach is limited, and if it is required (rarely) it is prudent to monitor bone mineral density. Bilateral oophorectomy with hysterectomy is a last resort for all but a few well-selected women. Oestrogen suppresses ovulation reliably and eliminates PMS without generating menopausal side effects. Intrauterine progestogen (LNG IUS) can be used to protect the endometrium and avoid re-stimulation of premenstrual symptoms; it also reduces periods and provides contraception. There can be initial bleeding and re-stimulation of symptoms in the first months. The oral contraceptive pill appears to have extremely limited efficacy using conventional pills. Newer drospirenone-containing OCs have the potential to sup-

press ovulation without re-introducing PMS. SSRIs are the simplest and most effective non-hormonal approach to treatment. Some consider that they should be used as first-line medical therapy, although many patients consider this form of therapy to be stigmatizing.

St John's Wort and agnus castus have been shown to be effective when used in depression. They could be tried as a self-help measure in PMS as there is limited evidence for their efficacy – there are known interactions if taken at the same time as SSRIs. There is limited evidence to demonstrate that exercise and cognitive behavioural therapy are effective, but access to clinical psychology services and lifestyle intervention programmes within the National Health Service are extremely limited in the UK.

Other non-medical treatments are of doubtful efficacy but are usually harmless. They can be tried before resorting to medical therapy when there are no risks other than the inevitable delay in initiating a known effective therapy. The majority of patients can be treated simply in community-based practices by general practitioners or by self-help. Patient groups such as the National Association for PMS are very useful for this approach (NAPS, www.pms.org.uk). Correct diagnosis is all important, and those patients without a symptom-free week probably have a continuous underlying psychological disorder. They should be referred back to the general practitioner or, in severe cases, referred on to a psychiatrist. Suicidal ideation and attempts call for urgent referral to doctors with the specific skills to manage these problems.

Only the most severely affected patients with clear-cut PMS requiring medical or surgical intervention should be referred for secondary gynaecological management. Gynaecologists, preferably those with an interest, understanding and expertise in the area, should be asked to manage PMS patients only when symptoms are severe enough to justify such endocrine or surgical intervention.

References

1 American Psychiatric Association. *Diagnostic and Statistical Manual of Mental Disorders: DSM-IV, 4th edn.* Washington, DC: American Psychiatric Association, 1994.

2 World Health Organization. *Mental, Behavioural and Developmental Disorders.* Geneva: WHO, 1996.

3 Ismail KMK, Crome I, O'Brien PMS. *Psychological Disorders in Obstetrics and Gynaecology for the MRCOG and Beyond.* London: RCOG Press, 2006, pp. 29–40.

4 RCOG Green Top Guideline No 48, Management of Premenstrual Syndrome. RCOG Press. Available at: http://www.rcog.org.uk/womens-health/clinical-guidance/management-premenstrual-syndrome-green-top-48.

5 Rapkin AJ. The role of serotonin in premenstrual syndrome. *Clin Obstet Gynecol* 1992;35:629–636.

6 Backstrom T, Andreen L, Birzniece V *et al.* The role of hormones and hormonal treatments in the premenstrual syndrome. *CNS Drugs* 2003;17:325–342.

7 Dimmock P, Wyatt K, Jones P, O' Brien PMS. Efficacy of selective serotonin re-uptake inhibitors in premenstrual syndrome: a systematic review. *Lancet* 2000;356:1131–1136.

8 Rapkin AJ, Morgan M, Goldman L *et al.* Progesterone metabolite allopregnanolone in women with premenstrual syndrome. *Obstet Gynecol* 1997;90:709–714.

9 Wyatt K, Dimmock P, Jones P, Obhrai M, O'Brien PMS. Efficacy of progesterone and progestogens in management of premenstrual syndrome: systematic review. *BMJ* 2001;323:776–780.

10 Watson NR, Studd JW, Savvas M *et al.* Treatment of severe premenstrual syndrome with oestradiol patches and cyclical oral norethisterone. *Lancet* 1989;2:730–732.

11 O' Brien PMS, Abukhalil IEH. Randomized controlled trial of the management of premenstrual syndrome and premenstrual mastalgia using luteal phase only danazol. *Am J Obstet Gynecol* 1999;180:18–23.

12 Wyatt KM, Dimmock PW, Ismail KMK *et al.* The effectiveness of GnRHa with or without 'addback' therapy in treating premenstrual syndrome: a meta analysis. *BJOG* 2004;111:585–593.

13 Casson P, Hahn PM, Van Vugt DA *et al.* Lasting response to ovariectomy in severe intractable premenstrual syndrome. *Am J Obstet Gynecol* 1990;162:99–105.

14 Hammarback S, Backstrom T, Holst J *et al.* Cyclical mood changes as in the premenstrual tension syndrome during sequential oestrogen-progestogen postmenopausal replacement treatment. *Acta Obstet Gynecol Scand* 1985;64:393–397.

Chapter 44
Menopause and the Postmenopausal Woman

Nick Panay
Queen Charlotte's & Chelsea Hospital; Chelsea and Westminster Hospital; West London Menopause & PMS Centre, London, UK

Introduction

The diagnosis of menopause, from the Greek 'menos' (month) and 'pausis' (cessation), is defined as the last menstrual period after a minimum of 1 year's amenorrhoea. However, it is becoming increasingly recognized that the physiological changes which result in the final menstrual period (FMP) start many years before the cessation of periods. This episode of dynamic neuroendocrine change occurs as a result of a progressive reduction ovarian reserve and can be associated with various distressing physical and psychological symptoms in the last decade of a woman's reproductive lifespan. It culminates in 'the climacteric', from the Greek 'klimax' (ladder), i.e. the climb to the menopause.

The population continues to age such that an ever-growing population continues to suffer the short- and long-term sequelae of the menopause. Even though our understanding of hormonal and complementary therapies has evolved, women and their clinicians continue to be concerned about the purported risks. As a result, newly symptomatic menopausal women remain confused as to how to manage their symptoms. Also, symptomatic women who discontinued therapy owing to fears generated by ill-conceived and misreported trials remain too scared to recommence therapy.

The aim of this chapter is to bring the reader up to date with the state of the art of postreproductive medicine. New data are discussed, including the prediction and diagnosis of menopause, causes of menopausal flushing, e.g. the concept of the thermoneutral zone, and new treatment regimens such as ultra low-dose hormone replacement therapy (HRT), body-identical HRT, highly selective therapies and alternatives to HRT, both complementary and pharmacological.

Premature ovarian failure/dysfunction

Premature ovarian failure is said to have occurred when menstruation ceases before the age of 40 years and early menopause before the age of 45 years. The author prefers the term premature ovarian dysfunction to signify that the transition into menopause can be lengthy and occasionally may even reverse itself [1]. Although there are many causes of early ovarian failure, the majority are idiopathic. The main identified genetic causes are Turner's syndrome and fragile X. The proportion of women with iatrogenic premature ovarian failure is growing as increasing numbers of women survive leukaemias, lymphomas and gynaecological cancers as a result of improved surgical techniques, radiotherapy and chemotherapeutic regimens. Work is ongoing to build a global database of patients with premature ovarian failure to develop a clearer understanding on what causes the disorder and how best it should be treated [2,3].

Consequences of the menopause

Aetiology of hot flushes and sweats – the latest theory

It is generally accepted that oestrogen plays an integral role in the genesis of vasomotor symptoms, but the precise aetiology remains unknown. The latest theory, proposed by Robert Freeman, seems the most plausible to date [4,5]. In the asymptomatic woman, there is a thermoneutral zone (about 0.4°C) within which fluctuations of core body temperature do not trigger compensatory autonomic mechanisms such as flushing or sweating. In the symptomatic woman, the thermoneutral zone is considerably reduced, so that even minor fluctuations in core

Dewhurst's Textbook of Obstetrics & Gynaecology, Eighth Edition. Edited by D. Keith Edmonds.
© 2012 John Wiley and Sons, Ltd. Published 2012 by John Wiley and Sons, Ltd.

body temperature reach the limits of the zone and initiate a thermoregulatory response. The narrowing of the zone may be due to elevated central noradrenergic activation and is probably precipitated by changes in oestrogen. Obese women are relatively protected from vasomotor symptoms owing to their production of oestrone and low sex hormone-binding globulin levels, which leaves more unbound free, active hormone.

Other early symptoms

Other typical immediate menopausal symptoms include insomnia, anxiety, irritability, memory loss, tiredness and poor concentration. Falling oestrogen levels are thought to lead to similar falls in neurotransmitter levels such as serotonin, which trigger mood symptoms. Women who have suffered from postnatal depression and premenstrual syndrome (PMS) appear to be particularly predisposed to depression in the perimenopause [6]. The menopause transition can also be associated with a significant reduction in sexuality and libido.

Intermediate symptoms

Oestrogen deficiency leads to the rapid loss of collagen, which contributes to the generalized atrophy that occurs after the menopause. In the genital tract, this is manifested by dyspareunia and vaginal bleeding from fragile atrophic skin. In the lower urinary tract, atrophy of the urethral epithelium occurs with decreased sensitivity of urethral smooth muscle and a decreased amount of collagen in periurethral collagen. All this results in dysuria, urgency and frequency, commonly termed the urethral syndrome. A recent position statement from the International Menopause Society [7] emphasizes the importance of enquiring about urogenital symptoms, the history of which might not be readily volunteered by the menopausal patient.

Long term: osteoporosis

Osteoporosis is a disorder of the bone matrix resulting in a reduction of bone strength to the extent that there is a significant increased risk of fracture. These fractures cause considerable morbidity in the elderly, requiring prolonged hospital care and difficulties in remobilization. Osteoporosis is predominantly a disease of women, who achieve a lower peak bone mass than men and are then subjected to an accelerated loss of bone density following the menopause. Women lose 50% of their skeleton by the age of 70 years, but men only lose 25% by the age of 90 years. Recent work has shown that loss of height occurs not only due to vertebral fractures but also loss of the intervertebral disc space as a result of deterioration and loss of collagen [8].

Cardiovascular

Women are protected against cardiovascular disease before the menopause, after which the incidence rapidly increases, reaching a similar frequency to men by the age of 70 years.

As oestrogen levels begin to fall, the somatotrophic axis becomes less active, leading to insulin resistance and a rise in central adiposity. This in turn leads to the change in body shape from the female gynaecoid shape to the male android shape, itself an independent risk factor for coronary heart disease [9]. There are a number of factors involved in perimenopausal weight gain including genetic predisposition, socioeconomic influences, reduction in caloric need and expenditure, reduced lean body mass and a reduction in resting basal metabolic rate. Preliminary work suggests that these changes can be ameliorated by the use of insulin-sensitizing agents, the value of which is being assessed in clinical trials.

Lipids and lipoproteins

The protective effect of oestrogen in premenopausal women is also thought to be mediated by an increase in high-density lipoprotein (HDL) and a decrease in low-density lipoprotein (LDL), nitric oxide-mediated vasodilatation leading to increased myocardial blood flow, an antioxidant effect on endothelial cells and a direct effect on the aorta decreasing atheroma. Cross-sectional and prospective observational studies have shown that women going through the menopause transition have elevation of cholesterol, triglyceride and LDL levels, a reduction in HDL2 levels and a rise in insulin resistance.

Central nervous system

Oestrogen appears to have a direct effect on the vasculature of the central nervous system and promotes neuronal growth and neurotransmission. Studies have demonstrated that oestrogen may improve cerebral perfusion and cognition in women below the age of 60 years. In the long term, this may prevent diseases with a vascular aetiology such as vascular dementia and Alzheimer's as the vasculature is clearly involved in this. The failure to show benefit for dementia in older populations, and possibly an increased risk with HRT in some studies, may reflect the predominance of the prothrombotic effect of oestrogen in this age group.

Prediction of menopause

Until recently, early follicular-phase follicle-stimulating hormone (FSH) levels were used to predict ovarian reserve with a level of >10 IU/L indicating reduced reserve and >40 IU/L regarded as being diagnostic of the menopause. However, this test can be misleading; levels vary according to the timing of the sample and often change in subsequent cycles depending on ovarian activity. The most accurate predictors of ovarian reserve currently available appear to be measurement of anti-Müllerian hormone (AMH) production by the primordial and pre-antral follicles and estimation of antral follicle count on ultrasonographic estimation [10]. AMH is independent of the day of cycle and its predictive value of ovarian reserve is claimed to last for up to 2 years from when the sample was taken.

Two recent studies have suggested that the timing of the menopause transition can be predicted. In the first study, 300 archival follicular-phase specimens were analysed from 50 women from the Michigan Bone Health and Metabolism Study which had been taken on six annual visits from 1993. Each woman had a documented FMP. As AMH levels declined to undetectable, this was highly associated with a time point 5 years prior to FMP (*P* < 0.0001). Baseline AMH levels also correlated with the age at FMP (*P* < 0.035) [11]. Another group reported similar findings [12], and at a recent meeting (ESHRE, 2010) claimed that menopause could actually be predicted from a younger age, thus allowing women to make choices regarding family planning and allowing the possibility of the institution of primary prevention measures.

Summary box 44.1

Menopause diagnosis:
- The average age of menopause is 51 years.
- Premature ovarian failure (also known as premature ovarian insufficiency) is diagnosed when menopause occurs before 40 years of age.
- The climacteric defines the period (often symptomatic) around the menopause transition.
- Menopause is diagnosed retrospectively when the last menstrual period has occurred 1 year earlier.
- Elevated FSH/LH levels may predict the menopause – more data are required.

Patient assessment and ongoing monitoring

The diagnosis of natural menopause can usually be made from the characteristic history of the vasomotor symptoms of hot flushes and night sweats and prolonged episodes of amenorrhoea. Measurement of plasma hormone levels [oestradiol, FSH, lutinizing hormone (LH)] in women in their late 40s onwards with classical symptoms are not essential as they do not change clinical management. However, in the young patient or in a woman after hysterectomy, where the diagnosis is more difficult and the metabolic implications may be more serious, measurement of FSH levels may be helpful, in which case repeated measurements of 15 IU/L or above may be regarded as climacteric. Women diagnosed with spontaneous premature ovarian dysfunction should, in addition to hormonal investigations, also have an autoantibody screen, karyotype and fragile X genetic analysis performed, although the aetiology is usually idiopathic.

After the diagnosis has been established, investigations should be no more than the annual screening which is

normally applicable to middle-aged women. This should include assessment of weight, blood pressure and routine cervical cytology. A recent consensus between menopause experts and cardiologists has highlighted the important role that gynaecologists can play in cardiovascular screening [13]. Fasting lipid profile and insulin resistance estimations are recommended in women with risk factors, e.g. increased waist circumference or personal/family history of diabetes/cardiovascular disease. In women with persistent symptoms or with side effects on HRT, it might be of benefit to perform hormone assays, e.g. oestradiol levels to determine the degree of response to therapy as adjustment of the dose might be required.

Although advice should be given to women about being aware of changes in their breasts and perineum, routine breast palpation and pelvic examination is unnecessary; these need only be performed if clinically indicated. Mammography should be performed as part of the national screening programme every 3 years unless more frequent examinations are clinically indicated. However, if a woman chooses to use HRT beyond the current age of breast screening cessation (70 years), mammographic screening should also continue. In women over 45 years of age, it is best to arrange screening before starting oestrogen therapy to identify patients with subclinical disease. Ultrasound examination of the pelvis and/or endometrial biopsy are not a necessary prerequisite to treatment with HRT unless there is undiagnosed bleeding.

The gold standard measurement of osteoporosis risk is still dual energy X-ray absorptiometry (DEXA) measurement of the lumbar spine and hip; some units are now using computerized tomography to perform this assessment. Markers of bone formation and breakdown can be useful in that changes occur more rapidly than with bone density, but their use is largely confined to research. The Royal College of Physicians still advises that DEXAs are performed no more frequently than every 2 years because changes in bone mineral density are so small that they often do not exceed the margin of error of the equipment and assessor. The World Health Organization (WHO) has recently advised that the decision to treat osteoporosis is made by taking into account not only the bone mineral density, but also age and body mass index [14]. The formula for calculating the probability of fracture (FRAX) is available online (http://www.shef.ac.uk/FRAX).

Interventions

Lifestyle measures
Common sense dictates that every woman should be encouraged to take plenty of regular exercise in addition to having a well-balanced diet, rich in isoflavones, and to avoid smoking. Data suggest that women who are more active tend to suffer less from the symptoms of the

menopause. Women who take regular weight-bearing exercise have higher bone mineral densities than sedentary controls. There is also evidence for reduction in bone loss by the daily use of calcium (approximately 1500 mg elemental calcium) and vitamin D (4–600 IU) supplements. However, recent data have shown that excessive calcium intake can lead to significant adverse events such as myocardial infarction [15]. A reduction of alcohol and caffeine intake can also reduce the severity and frequency of vasomotor symptoms.

Hormone replacement therapy

Summary box 44.2

HRT:
- The primary indication for HRT is relief of menopause symptoms.
- A window of opportunity exists for initiation of treatment with HRT (below the age of 60 years) during which there may be primary prevention opportunities.
- Women with premature ovarian failure need adequate hormonal support at least until the average age of the menopause.
- Based on current data, low dose, transdermal, body identical hormones optimise benefits and minimise side effects and risks.

Oestrogen

Dose

There is now consensus that the minimum effective dose of oestradiol should be prescribed and increased if required to alleviate symptoms. Although there is no direct evidence that higher doses of exogenous oestrogen are associated with increased risk of breast cancer or heart disease, there are dose–response effects with venous thromboembolism and stroke. Importantly, lower doses of oestrogen are less likely to cause breast tenderness and bleeding problems (less endometrial stimulation), which will encourage continuation of therapy.

The recommended starting doses of currently available systemic oestrogen are as follows:
- 0.3 mg of oral conjugated equine oestrogens;
- 1 mg of oral micronized oestradiol or oestradiol valerate;
- 25–50 mcg transdermal oestradiol;
- two (0.5 mg) metered doses of oestradiol gel; and
- 25–50 mg of implanted oestradiol.

Recent data suggest that the benefits of a 1 mg dose of oestradiol for symptoms and bone protection can be achieved with a 0.5 mg dose [16]. Side effects such as bleeding problems are minimized by this dosage and metabolic impact is neutralized [17]. It appears that a

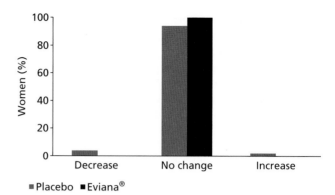

Fig. 44.1 Mammographic density. Percentage scale showing the change in breast density from baseline to week 24. Adapted from [18].

neutral effect on breast symptoms and mammographic density is possible at these low doses (Fig. 44.1) [18]. Exceptions to this 'low dose rule' are women who suffer premature ovarian failure and need higher doses of oestrogen to reproduce the physiological hormone levels which would have been present if the ovaries had not failed early. Sadly, very little work has been carried out to determine what the optimum route of administration or dosage is in this group of young women.

Route of administration

If we adhere to the principle that we should try to reproduce the most physiological state possible with a 2:1 oestradiol:oestrone ratio, then we should avoid the oral route altogether. Oral oestradiol preparations are partially metabolized to oestrone by hepatic first-pass metabolism and therefore do not fully restore this ratio. There are now observational and case–control data showing that the thromboembolic risk is neutralized by avoidance of first-pass stimulation of coagulation factors, even in women who are obese and thrombophilic [19].

There are twice-weekly or once-weekly transdermal systems containing both oestrogen and progestogen which can be used either sequentially or as continuous combined HRT. The hormone is adsorbed onto the adhesive matrix, which avoids the skin reactions caused by the old alcohol reservoir patches. Oestradiol is also available as a low-volume daily transdermal gel and work is ongoing to produce an oral tab/wafer which maintains the ease of oral administration while absorption avoids first-pass metabolism.

Local (vaginal) oestrogen

Creams, tablets and rings containing oestriol and oestradiol do not produce endometrial hyperplasia according to endometrial biopsy data following 1 year of usage. These preparations provide effective relief of local symptoms without any significant endometrial effects and can be used without progestogenic opposition. The

International Menopause Society has recently highlighted the under-utilization of these preparations, which can be of benefit even in women on pre-existing systemic therapy [7].

The regulatory authorities in the UK (Medicines and Healthcare Products Regulatory Agency) have recently granted an 'indefinite use' licence to 25 μg vaginal tablets. A recently developed 10 μg oestradiol vaginal tablet will soon be licensed with the aim of providing the minimum effective dose for relief of urogenital symptoms – a year of use will expose the user to only 1.4 mg of oestradiol in total with no endometrial effects [20].

Options for local vaginal oestrogen are as follows:
- 0.01% oestriol cream and pessaries;
- 0.1% oestriol cream;
- 25 mcg/24 h oestradiol vaginal tablets;
- 7.5 mcg/24 h oestradiol-releasing silicone ring; and
- conjugated equine oestrogen cream.[1]

Summary box 44.3

Vaginal preparations:
- Vaginal atrophy occurs in up to 50% of postmenopausal women.
- Distressing symptoms often occur, e.g. vaginal dryness, pain at intercourse, urinary symptoms.
- Non-hormonal options include lubricants and moisturisers.
- Vaginal oestrogen, e.g. tablets, creams, rings, are highly effective in alleviating symptoms.
- Progestogenic opposition is not required with low-dose vaginal oestrogen.

Progestogens/progesterone

Regimens

Women commencing oestrogen should use progestogen to avoid endometrial hyperplasia and carcinoma. If the last menstrual period occurred less than 1 year prior to starting HRT, a sequential combined regimen should be started, i.e. continuous oestrogen with progestogen for 12–14 days per month. A progestogen challenge should be considered after 3–6 months of oestrogen alone in women who have had a subtotal hysterectomy to test for residual endometrium. Low-dose continuous progestogen should also be used after endometrial ablation and pelvic radiotherapy in case any endometrium remains.

The typical dosages of the more commonly used progestogens are shown in Table 44.1.

---

[1]This can cause endometrial hyperplasia; it requires progestogenic opposition after 3 months.

Table 44.1 Minimum doses of progestogen given orally in hormone replacement therapy (HRT) as endometrial protection.

Progestogen type	Sequential combined daily dosage	Continuous combined daily dosage
Testosterone-derived progestogens		
Norethisterone	5 mg	0.1 mg
Levonorgestrel	75 μg	n/a
Levonorgestrel (IUS)	n/a	20 μg (12 and 16 μg in development)
Norgestrel	150 μg	50 μg
Progesterone-derived progestogens		
Cyproterone	2 mg	1 mg
Medroxyprogesterone acetate	5 mg	2.5 mg
Micronized progesterone	200 mg	100 mg
Cyclogest pessaries	400 mg	200 mg
Crinone gel (8%)	Alternate days/12 days per cycle	Twice weekly
Spironolactone-derived progestogens		
Drospirenone	n/a	2 mg

IUS, intrauterine system.

Bleeding problems

If bleeding is heavy or erratic, the dose of progestogen can be doubled or its duration can be increased to 21 days. Persistent bleeding problems beyond 6 months warrant investigation with ultrasound scan and/or endometrial biopsy. After 1 year of therapy (2 years in premature ovarian failure), women can switch to a continuous combined regimen which aims to give a bleed-free HRT regimen, which will also minimize the risk of endometrial hyperplasia. Alternatively, women can be switched to the tissue-selective agent tibolone. With both of these regimens there may be some erratic bleeding to begin with, but 90% of those that persist with this regimens will eventually be completely bleed free. If starting HRT *de novo*, a bleed-free regimen can be used from the outset if the last menstrual period was over a year ago.

Progestogenic side effects

It is vital that compliance is maximized if patients are to receive the full benefits from HRT [21]. One of the main factors for reduced compliance is that of progestogen intolerance. Progestogens have a variety of effects apart from the one for which their use was intended, that of secretory transformation of the endometrium. Symptoms of fluid retention are produced by the sodium-retaining effect of the renin–aldosterone system, which is triggered by stimulation of the mineralocorticoid receptor.

Androgenic side effects such as acne and hirsuitism are a problem of the testosterone-derived progestogen due to stimulation of the androgen receptors. Mood swings and PMS-like side effects result from stimulation of the central nervous system progesterone receptors.

Minimizing progestogen side effects

The dose can be halved and duration of progestogen can be reduced to 7–10 days. However, this may result in bleeding problems and hyperplasia in a few cases (5–10%), so there should be a low threshold for performing ultrasound scans and endometrial sampling in these women. Natural progesterone has fewer side effects owing to progesterone receptor specificity and is now available in an oral micronized form, vaginal pessaries and gel (see Table 44.1). Recent evidence suggests that HRT regimens containing natural progesterone can minimize the metabolic impact and reduce the risk of thromboembolism [22]. The levonorgestrel intrauterine system, which has a 4-year licence in the UK for progestogenic opposition (5 years in other countries), also minimizes systemic progestogenic side effects by releasing the progestogen directly into the endometrium with low systemic levels. Drospirenone, a spironolactone analogue, has recently been incorporated with low-dose oestrogen in a continuous combined formulation. It is not only progesterone receptor-specific but also has antiandrogenic and antimineralocorticoid properties, the former making it useful for hirsuitism and the latter for fluid retention. Also, it may have blood pressure lowering effects [23].

Bio/body-identical hormone replacement therapy

Bioidentical hormones are precise duplicates of oestradiol, progesterone and testosterone as synthesized by the human ovary. They are manufactured from plant sources in the laboratory and are available from pharmaceutical companies as micronized oral tablets, transdermal patches, implants and gels. Regulated bioidentical products must not be confused with unregulated products from compounding pharmacists. In order to avoid confusion, the author proposes that regulated products should be referred to as 'body' rather than 'bio' identical [24]. The published data thus far suggest that differential effects can be achieved by the use of body-identical hormones in comparison with synthetic non-body-identical HRT. The E3N cohort study established in 1990 with 98 995 women from a health insurance scheme covering French teachers is part of the European Prospective Investigation into Cancer and Nutrition (EPIC). Oestrogen–progesterone combination HRT was found to be associated with a significantly lower relative risk (neutral for 'ever use' of HRT) than for other types of combined HRT (recurrence rates 1.7–2.0) (Fig. 44.2) [25]. Further data from larger studies on major breast end points are required to confirm this effect.

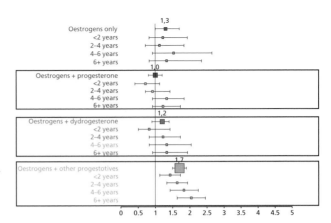

Fig. 44.2 Results showing the risk of invasive breast cancer. Adapted from [25].

Androgens

Women with distressing low sexual desire and tiredness should be counselled that androgen supplementation is an option. Until recently, only 100 mg implanted testosterone pellets were licensed for female testosterone replacement. The realization that there was an unfilled niche in the market for other female androgenic options led to the development of the 300 mcg per day testosterone transdermal system to treat hyposexual desire disorder (HSDD). HSDD is the American Psychiatric Association's definition of distressing low sexual desire. The current licence for this product in Europe is in surgically menopausal women on concomitant oestrogen, but it is expected that licences will be granted for naturally menopausal women and women using testosterone without oestrogen [26,27]. Unlicensed options include testosterone gel, which comes in 50 mg, 5 mL sachets or tubes at a dose of 0.5–1.0 mL/day. In the author's clinical experience, if the free androgen index is kept within the physiological range, there are rarely any side effects such as hirsuitism and acne. The Food and Drug Administration in the USA has requested a 5-year study (currently ongoing) on cardiovascular and breast safety before considering a licence for testosterone in women; no significant problems have been found in previous shorter studies.

Dehydroepiandrosterone (DHEA) is a weak androgenic steroid produced by the adrenal gland. It is mostly produced in a sulphated form (DHEAS) which may be converted to DHEA in many tissues. Blood levels of DHEA drop dramatically with age. This had led to suggestions that the effects of ageing can be counteracted by DHEA 'replacement therapy'. DHEA is increasingly being used in the USA, where it is classed as a food supplement, for its supposed anti-ageing effects. Some studies have shown benefits on the skeleton, cognition, well-being, libido and the vagina; these data require confirmation [28].

Risks of hormone replacement therapy

The Women's Health Initiative (WHI) [29] and Million Women Study (MWS) [30] both demonstrated an excess risk of cardiovascular disease, stroke and breast cancer in women using combined oestrogen and progestogen HRT. However, these studies were heavily criticized owing to their design, particularly the WHI study where the average age of recruitment was 63 years with an excess of obesity, hypertension and pre-existing cardiovascular disease leading to prothrombotic problems. In contrast, a recent subanalysis of the WHI [31] has shown that the cardiovascular risks were confined to the oldest age group (Fig. 44.3). Women in the youngest cohort (typically seen in our clinics with menopausal symptoms) had a trend towards improvement of cardiovascular risk and significant reduction in all cause mortality. Guidance issued by the International Menopause Society (IMS) has emphasized that in the WHI study, the risks of breast cancer did not become significant until 7 years of usage (approximately 1 extra case per 1000 women per annum): they stated that for women in the normal menopause transition, the benefits of HRT far outweigh the risks and may even confer cardiovascular benefits [32]. In addition, the IMS guidance emphasized the neutral impact of oestrogen alone on the breast. Research is currently being con-

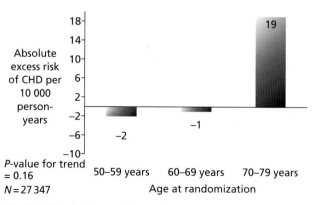

Fig. 44.3 The absolute risk by age of patients taking hormone replacement therapy developing coronary heart disease (CHD). Adapted from [31].

ducted in two studies (ELITE and KEEPS) [33] using lower-dose body-identical HRT in younger populations looking at surrogate markers of cardiovascular disease, e.g. intima media thickness and coronary calcium scores. The aim is to prove that use of modern preparations in the appropriate women can confer benefits rather than risks.

Contraindications to hormone replacement therapy

Hormone replacement therapy is contraindicated in women with a history of cardiovascular disease and stroke. Data from one pilot study suggest that there can be beneficial effects, but this requires confirmation. Although also contraindicated in venous thromboembolic disease, there is some evidence that transdermal preparations are safer by avoiding first-pass metabolism [19].

Natural oestrogens, when given to normotensive or hypertensive women, do not cause an elevation in blood pressure, and when given in combination with oral natural progesterone or drospirenone may actually lower blood pressure [23]. There is therefore little justification for withholding HRT from controlled hypertensive women.

Treatment of patients with a history of endometrial cancer is controversial, but there are reports of oestrogen use without any detrimental effects in stage I–III disease. Squamous cervical cancer is not oestrogen sensitive. There are no adverse data in ovarian cancer survivors, although there may be a very small increased risk of ovarian cancer with long-term unopposed oestrogen use in healthy women. There are no data for adenocarcinoma of the cervix, vaginal or vulval cancer.

Women seeking HRT with a history of severe endometriosis should be given continuous combined therapy even after hysterectomy to prevent recurrence of the endometriosis.

Breast cancer must be regarded as the principal contraindication to oestrogen treatment, but high-risk women with a strong family history of breast malignancy or those with benign breast disease should not necessarily be denied treatment. It is unclear what the precise risk of breast cancer recurrence is with HRT use. A large randomized placebo-controlled study (LIBERATE) in survivors of breast cancer using tibolone recently demonstrated a marginal increase in recurrence rates (1.4) [34].

Duration of therapy

It is recognized that symptoms often return when HRT is ceased, even after many years of use. If the underpinning principle of HRT is that it should be used to improve and maintain a good quality of life, in women in whom this principle is maintained it is difficult to argue that they should have arbitrary deadlines imposed on them.

Although breast cancer risks appear to be duration-dependent, evidence suggests that overall mortality is actually reduced in women commencing HRT before the age of 60 years [35]. Thus, duration of therapy requires careful judgement of benefits and risks on an individual basis. If therapy is to be discontinued, the dose should be reduced in a stepwise fashion over a minimum of 6 months to reduce the risk of immediate severe symptom resurgence.

Official prescribing advice

It is still recommended by the regulatory authorities that HRT be used merely for symptom relief in the short term at the lowest effective dose and alternatives should be considered in the long term for prevention of osteoporosis. Annual reappraisal of HRT use should be carried out with weighing up of the pros and cons on an individual basis. However, the British, European and International Menopause Societies (see website listed at the end of the chapter) consensus statements advise that prescribing habits need not be changed by the WHI studies. The recent favourable reanalyses of the WHI data and the finding that long-term use of bisphosphonates and other alternatives to HRT have led the National Osteoporosis Society (NOS) to reconsider its position on HRT. Although still in consultation phase, it is likely that the NOS will come into line with the menopause societies that HRT should still be a first-line agent in young women (up to the age of 60 years) requiring osteoporosis prophylaxis (see NOS website listed at the end of the chapter).

Complementary therapies/alternatives to hormone replacement therapy

An integrated approach to the management of vasomotor symptoms should be considered in women wanting to consider alternatives to (or contraindicated to) HRT. An algorithm drawn up by a consensus group of international experts integrating lifestyle, complementary and pharmacological interventions is shown below (Fig. 44.4). Lifestyle changes and supplements such as red clover, soy isoflavones and other alternatives can be incorporated into the routine management of women with vasomotor symptoms [36]. The algorithm is not intended for women

 Summary box 44.5

Future avenues of HRT research:
- The cardiovascular impact of low-dose systemictransdermal oestradiol with modern progestogens/progesterone.
- The impact of body-identical hormones on breast epithelial cell division/breast cancer.
- The benefits and risks of tissue-selective agents (e.g. selective estrogen receptor modulators).
- Effectiveness of local androgens for vaginal symptoms.

with premature menopause or for those with other risk factors such as osteoporosis.

Non-pharmacological alternatives

Gels for vaginal symptoms

Vaginal bioadhesive moisturizers are a more physiological way of replacing vaginal secretions than with lubricant vaginal gels such as K-Y Jelly®. They are hydrophilic and actually rehydrate the vaginal tissues, providing a reasonable alternative for women wishing to avoid vaginal oestrogen [36–38].

Pharmacological alternatives

Alpha-2 agonists

Clonidine, a centrally active α2 agonist, has been one of the most popular alternative preparations for the treatment of vasomotor symptoms. A recent meta-analysis of the few randomized controlled trials has shown a marginal benefit of clonidine over placebo [38].

Selective serotonin reuptake inhibitors/noradrenaline reuptake inhibitors

A significant amount of evidence exists for the efficacy of SSRIs and selective noradrenaline reuptake inhibitors (SNRIs) in the treatment of vasomotor symptoms. Although there are some data for SSRIs, such as fluoxetine and paroxetine, the most convincing data are for the SNRI (venlafaxine) at a dose of 37.5 mg twice daily. The key effect with these preparations appears to be stimulation of the noradrenergic as opposed to the serotonergic pathways, hence the preferential effect of SNRIs [38]. Recent work has focused on desvenlafaxine succinate, a derivative of venlafaxine, as a way of maintaining the benefits of the parent molecule but minimizing side effects.

Gabapentin

Recent work with the antiepileptic drug gabapentin has shown efficacy for hot flush reduction compared with placebo. In a recent study using gabapentin at a dose of 900 mg per day, a 45% reduction of hot flush frequency and a 54% reduction of symptom severity was demonstrated [38]. Further work is being conducted to confirm the efficacy and safety of this preparation, but for the moment its use is restricted to specialist centres. Its use is limited by side effects such as drowsiness and somnolence, particularly at high doses.

Complementary therapies: phytoestrogens

The role of phytoestrogens has stimulated considerable interest since populations consuming a diet high in isoflavones such as the Japanese appear to have lower rates of menopausal vasomotor symptoms, cardiovascular

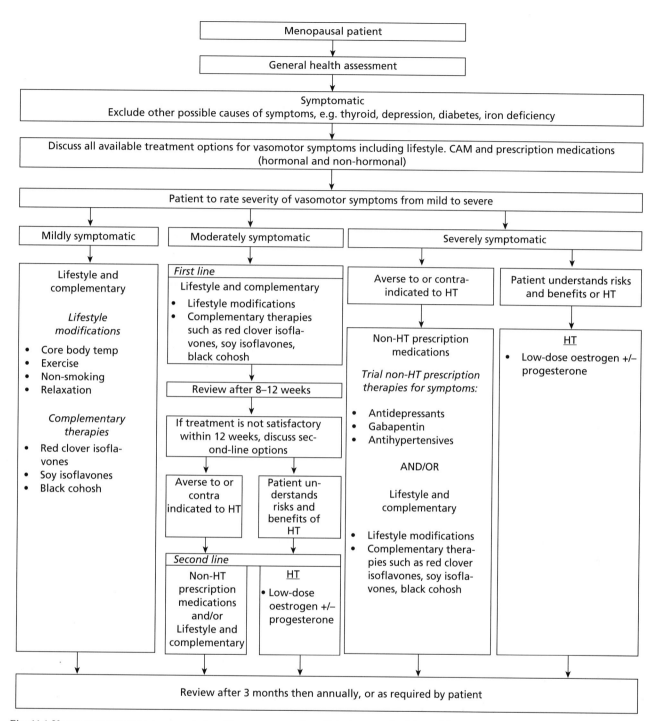

Fig. 44.4 Vasomotor symptom treatment algorithm: a conservative clinical approach. Adapted from reference 36. HT, hormone therapy.

disease, osteoporosis, and breast, colon, endometrial and ovarian cancers. The normal Japanese diet contains 200 mg of phytoestrogens per day in comparison to the average Western diet, which contains less than 1 mg. However, epidemiological studies need to be supported by data with analyses of the isoflavone content of foods and measures of their bioavailability.

Data from some of the better-researched phytoestrogen-containing preparations appear to demonstrate some benefits, not only for symptom relief but also on the skel-eton and cardiovascular system. Efficacy for vasomotor symptom relief is lower than with traditional HRT (maximally 60–70% symptom reduction compared with 90–100% with traditional HRT). Beneficial effects have been shown on cardiovascular risk markers such as lipids and arterial compliance and on bone markers/density, with possible SERM (selective oestrogen receptor modulator)-type effects [39]. There are as yet no hard data on major outcome measures such as coronary heart disease and fractures. Laboratory data suggest avoidance of stimulation of oestrogen receptors in the endometrium and breast and safety in observed populations [40], but, once again, sufficiently powered randomized controlled trial data on endometrial and breast cancer incidence are absent. Studies such as PHYTOS and PHYTOPREVENT are currently running in the European Union examining the role of phytoestrogens in osteoporosis, metabolism and cancer (see websites listed at the end of the chapter).

Future research

In the future, targeted agents able to switch on receptors in tissues where this is desirable and avoid receptors in tissues such as the breast and endometrium will undoubtedly succeed traditional HRT, which produces more a generalized effect. There are problems with all the currently available tissue-selective agents. The only SERM (selective oestrogen receptor modulator) currently licensed in the UK, raloxifene, while being agonistic in the bone and cardiovascular system and antagonistic in the endometrium and breast, unfortunately does not relieve and may precipitate vasomotor symptoms. ANGELS (activators of non-genomic oestrogen-like signalling) look promising in that they avoid stimulating the genomic pathways by targeting non-genomic stimulation of selected tissues, e.g. osteoblasts. There are good laboratory bone data in rats while avoiding mammary cell stimulation but there is still along way to go before these compounds are trialled in the clinical situation. Realistically, we are probably at least 10 years away from the ideal tissue-selective agent, but this is undoubtedly the holy grail in terms of menopause therapy. In the meantime, a compound is close to being licensed which appears to maintain the benefits of SERMS but also harnesses the effect of oestrogen on vasomotor symptoms. This TSEC (tissue-selective oestrogen complex), a combination of the SERM bazedoxifene and conjugated equine oestrogens, has already been shown in phase III clinical trials to relieve vasomotor symptoms while avoiding endometrial stimulation, without the need for progestogen [41].

Conclusions

Scientists strive to develop the ultimate menopause therapy which truly has all the benefits without any side effects and risks. In the meantime, clinicians should aim to provide the best evidence-based advice possible in order to allow women to make an informed choice as to how to maintain their health during the menopause transition and beyond. The overzealous reporting of recent clinical trials has made it imperative that health professionals involved in this area, and their patients, can access well-balanced evidence-based information. We are now beginning to understand how we can optimize therapy in order to alleviate distressing menopausal symptoms while avoiding side effects and risks. Effective management of the menopause is taking on ever-increasing importance in view of our ageing population. In the author's opinion, current best practice should involve the following:

1 Discussion of lifestyle measures, HRT and alternatives should take place from the outset.

2 Management should be individualized, taking into account risks and benefits.

3 The main indication for use of HRT should be for symptom relief rather than for prevention of long-term problems.

4 Low-dose HRT should usually be commenced and increased if necessary to achieve effective symptom relief, except in premature ovarian failure where higher doses are physiological.

5 Androgen therapy should be offered to women with persistent low libido and energy levels.

6 Rigid cut-offs in duration of therapy should be avoided with regular reappraisal (at least annual) of the benefits and risks for each individual.

7 Delivery of services should be from a multidisciplinary team if possible with close liaison with allied specialties and experts.

References

1 Kalu E, Panay N. Spontaneous premature ovarian failure: management challenges. *Gynecol Endocrinol* 2008;24:273–279.

2 Panay N, Fenton A. Premature ovarian failure: A growing concern. *Climacteric* 2008;11:1–3.

3 Maclaran K, Horner E, Panay N. Premature ovarian failure: long-term sequelae. *Menopause Int* 2010;16:38–41.

4 Freedman RR. Pathophysiology and treatment of hot flashes. *Semin Reprod Med* 2005;23:117–125.

5 Sturdee D. The menopausal hot flush – anything new? *Maturitas* 2008;60:42–49.

6 Panay N, Studd JWW. The psychotherapeutic effects of estrogens. *Gynaecol Endocrinol* 1998;12:353–365.

7 Sturdee D, Panay N. Recommendations for the management of postmenopausal vaginal atrophy. *Climacteric* 2010;13:1–15.

8 Calleja-Agius J, Muscat-Baron Y, Brincat MP. Estrogens and the intevertebral disc. *Menopause Int* 2009;15:127–130.

9 Lejsková M, Alušík S, Suchánek M, Zecová S, Pitha J. Menopause: clustering of metabolic syndrome components and population changes in insulin resistance. *Climacteric* 2011;14:83–91.

10 Nardo LG, Christodoulou D, Gould D, Roberts SA, Fitzgerald CT, Laing I. Anti-Müllerian hormone levels and antral follicle count in women enrolled in *in vitro* fertilisation cycles: Relationship to lifestyle factors, chronological age and reproductive history. *Gynecol Endocrinol* 2007;24:1–8.

11 Sowers M, McConnell D, Gast K *et al.* Anti-mullerian hormone and inhibin B in the definition of ovarian ageing and the menopause transition. *J Clin Endocrinol Metab* 2008;93:3478–3483.

12 Tehrani FR, Solaymani-Dodaran M, Azizi F. A single test of anti-mullerian hormone in late reproductive-aged women is a good predictor of menopause. *Menopause* 2009;16:797–802.

13 International Menopause Society Consensus Statement. Ageing, menopause, cardiovascular disease and HRT. *Climacteric* 2009;12:368–377.

14 van Geel TA, van den Bergh JP, Dinant GJ, Geusens PP. Individualising fracture risk prediction. *Maturitas* 2010;65: 143–148.

15 Bolland MJ, Avenell A, Baron JA et al. Effect of calcium supplements on risk of myocardial infarction and cardiovascular events: meta-analysis. *BMJ* 2010;341:c3691.

16 Panay N, Ylikorkala O, Archer DF, Rakov V, Gut R, Lang E. Ultra low-dose estradiol and norethisterone acetate: Effective menopausal symptom relief. *Climacteric* 2007;10:120–131.

17 Sturdee DW, Archer DF, Rakov V, Lang E; CHOICE Study Investigators. Ultra-low-dose continuous combined estradiol and norethisterone acetate: improved bleeding profile in postmenopausal women. *Climacteric* 2008;11:63–73.

18 Lundström E, Bygdeson M, Svane G, Azavedo E, von Schoultz B. Neutral effect of ultra-low-dose continuous combined estradiol and norethisterone acetate on mammographic breast density. *Climacteric* 2007;10:249–256.

19 Scarabin PY, Olger E, Plu–Bureau G. Differential association of oral and transdermal oestrogen replacement therapy with venous thromboembolism risk. *Lancet* 2003;362:428–432.

20 Ulrich LS, Naessen T, Elia D, Goldstein JA, Eugster-Hausmann M; VAG-1748 trial investigators. Endometrial safety of ultra-low-dose Vagifem 10 microg in postmenopausal women with vaginal atrophy. *Climacteric* 2010;13:228–237.

21 Panay N, Studd JWW. Progestogen intolerance and compliance with hormone replacement therapy in menopausal women. *Hum Reprod Update* 1997;3:159–171.

22 Canonico M, Oger E, Plu-Bureau G et al.; Oestrogen and Thromboembolism Risk (ESTHER) Study Group. Hormone therapy and venous thromboembolism among postmenopausal women: impact of the route of oestrogen administration and progestogens: the ESTHER study. *Circulation* 2007;115:840–845.

23 White WB, Hanes V, Chauhan V, Pitt B. Effects of a new hormone therapy, drospirenone and 17-beta-estradiol, in postmenopausal women with hypertension. *Hypertension* 2006;48: 246–253.

24 Panay N, Fenton A. Bioidentical hormones: what is all the hype about? *Climacteric* 2010;13:1–3.

25 Fournier A, Fabre A, Mesrine S, Boutron-Ruault MC, Berrino F, Clavel-Chapelon F. Use of different postmenopausal hormone therapies and risk of histology- and hormone receptor-defined invasive breast cancer. *J Clin Oncol* 2008;26:1260–1268.

26 Davis SR, Moreau M, Kroll R et al. Testosterone for low libido in postmenopausal women not taking oestrogen. *N Engl J Med* 2008;359:2005–2017.

27 Panay N, Al-Azzawi F, Bouchard C et al. Testosterone treatment of HSDD in naturally menopausal women: the ADORE study. *Climacteric* 2010;13:121–131.

28 Rees M, Panay N. *The Use of alternatives to HRT for the Management of Menopause Symptoms*. RCOG Scientific Advisory Committee 2006; Opinion Paper 6 (in revision for 2010). Available at: www.rcog.org.uk.

29 Writing Group for the Women's Health Initiative Investigators. Risks and benefits of oestrogen plus progestin in healthy postmenopausal women: principal results From Women's Health Initiative randomised controlled trial. *JAMA* 2002;288:321–333.

30 Million Women Study Collaborators. Breast cancer and HRT in the Million Women Study. *Lancet* 2003;362:419–427.

31 Rossouw JE, Prentice RL, Manson JE et al. Postmenopausal hormone therapy and risk of cardiovascular disease by age and years since menopause. *JAMA* 2007;297:1465–1477.

32 Pines A, Sturdee DW, Birkhauser MH, Schneider HP, Gambacciani M, Panay N. IMS updated recommendations on postmenopausal HRT. *Climacteric* 2007;10:181–194.

33 Harman SM, Brinton EA, Cedars M et al. KEEPS: The Kronos Early Oestrogen Prevention Study. *Climacteric* 2005;8:3–12.

34 Kenemans P, Bundred NJ, Foidart JM et al. Safety and efficacy of tibolone in breast-cancer patients with vasomotor symptoms: a double-blind, randomized, non-inferiority trial. *Lancet Oncol* 2009;10:135–146.

35 Salpeter SR, Walsh JM, Greyber E, Ormiston TM, Salpeter EE. Mortality associated with HRT in younger and older women: a meta-analysis. *J Gen Intern Med* 2004;19:791–804.

36 Panay N. Integrating phytoestrogens with prescription medicines – A conservative clinical approach to vasomotor symptom management. *Maturitas* 2007;57:90–94.

37 Panay N, Fenton A. Complementary therapies for managing the menopause: has there been any progress? *Climacteric* 2010; 13:201–202.

38 Nelson HD, Vesco KK, Haney et al. Non-hormonal therapies for menopausal hot flashes: systematic review and meta – analysis. *JAMA* 2006;295:2057–2071.

39 Somjen D, Katzburg S, Livne E, Yoles I. 'DT56a (Femarelle/Tofupill) stimulates bone formation in female rats'. *BJOG* 2005; 112:981–985.

40 Powles TJ, Howell A, Evans DG et al. Red clover isoflavones are safe and well tolerated in women with a family history of breast cancer. *Menopause Int* 2008;14:6–12.

41 Pickar JH, Macneil T, Ohleth K. SERMs: Progress and future perspectives. *Maturitas* 2010;67:129–138.

Further reading

Panay N. *Climacteric – The Journal of the International Menopause Society*. Informa Press.

Studd J. *Menopause International – The Journal of the British Menopause Society*. RSM Press.

Rees M. *Maturitas – The Journal of the European Menopause Society*. Elsevier Press.

Rees M, Stevenson J, Hope S, Rozenberg S, Palacios S. (eds) *Management of the Menopause: The Handbook*, 5th edn. London: RSM Press, 2009.

Singer D, Hunter M (eds) *Premature Menopause: A Multidisciplinary Approach*. London: Wiley Blackwell.

Useful websites

Top recommendations

www.the-bms.org (British Menopause Society site – see consensus statements)

www.imsociety.org (International Menopause Society – see consensus statements)

http://emas.obgyn.net (European Menopause Society)

Other

www.mhra.gov.uk (The Medical and Healthcare Products Regulatory Agency)

www.shef.ac.uk/FRAX/ (WHO osteoporosis fracture risk calculator)

www.nos.org.uk (National Osteoporosis Society – professionals and patients)

www.menopause.org (North American Menopause Society)

www.emea.eu.int (European Medicines Agency)

http://nccam.nih.gov/health/alerts/menopause/ (National Centre for Complementary and Alternative Medicine. Alternative therapies for managing menopausal symptoms.)

www.phytohealth.org (The PHYTOHEALTH Network)

http://dietary-supplements.info.nih.gov (The NIH Office of Dietary Supplements)

www.whi.org (Women's Health Initiative Website)

www.rcplondon.ac.uk/pubs/wp_osteo_update.htm (Royal College of Physicians Guidelines on Osteoporosis)

http://ec.europa.eu/research/endocrine/pdf/qlk1-ct2000–00431-year1.pdf (PHYTOS)

www.ist-world.org/ProjectDetails.aspx?ProjectId=2f26ce134aca48e78b08fbfc9c8e2cbd (PHYTOPREVENT)

Patient information and contacts

www.menopausematters.co.uk (very informative menopause website)

www.pms.org.uk (Premenstrual Syndrome website)

www.nos.org.uk (National Osteoporosis Society – professionals and patients)

www.womens-health-concern.org/(Women's Health Group – including 'ask the experts')

Part 11
Inability to Conceive

Chapter 45
Infertility

Mark Hamilton

Department of Obstetrics and Gynaecology, University of Aberdeen, Aberdeen Maternity Hospital, Aberdeen, UK

Infertility

This chapter provides an overview of the clinical problem of infertility as it presents to gynaecologists in practice. The epidemiology of infertility is discussed, leading to a description of the assessment of infertile couples. A critique of the place of secondary investigations under the broad headings of male factor infertility, disorders of ovulation, tubal factor infertility, endometriosis and uterine factors, and unexplained infertility is provided. Some remarks on treatment options are provided. Insights that assisted conception techniques bring to our understanding of the pathogenesis of infertility are briefly examined. Integration of services to enable efficient evidence-based management of individuals who are infertile is emphasized throughout.

Epidemiology

A common definition employed in describing infertility is the inability of a couple to conceive following 12–24 months of exposure to pregnancy. In the general population, about 85% of couples have achieved conception within a year of trying and by the time 2 years has elapsed, some 92% will have conceived [1]. In practical terms, the failure to achieve pregnancy causes enormous distress to those affected. For people with fertility problems, using a definition of a year to describe infertility is usual and most will have sought medical advice or assistance by that time. While natural fertility rates decline as women become older, in an ultimately fertile group of women it is not certain that monthly fecundability (percentage chance of conception) is any less than in younger women. It is sensible to consider specialist referral of women over the age of 35 years in advance of 1 year, although in many instances conception will occur naturally in these cases.

Estimates of the prevalence of infertility in the population are influenced by the duration of infertility used in the definition and the population studied, e.g. primary care [2] or hospital clinics [3]. Community-based data which would give an accurate reflection of prevalence within the general population are limited. It is not surprising, therefore, that existing studies suggest a range of lifetime prevalence of infertility extending from 6.6% to 32.6%. One population-based study in the north-east of Scotland [4], which took account also of conceptions resulting in miscarriage and ectopic pregnancy, found a prevalence of 14% using a 2-year definition.

Factors that could influence trends in the prevalence of infertility include the incidence of sexually transmitted infections (STIs) such as *Chlamydia trachomatis* in the young [5]. In addition, there have been suggestions that environmental factors may affect male fertility [6], and one should wonder about the possible effects on female fertility of delayed childbearing as determined by changes in lifestyle and working patterns. Despite these concerns, when the population-based study was repeated [7], the observed prevalence of infertility had not increased in north-east Scotland in the succeeding 20 years.

The promotion of safe sexual practices limiting exposure to the risk of STIs is clearly important in the prevention of infertility. Rubella immunization programmes should be in place for teenage girls. Education of the public about the known decline in fertility with age is important. The need to make certain lifestyle adjustments such as stopping smoking and reducing alcohol consumption as well as achieving optimal weight should be promoted [8].

The requirement to take account of future reproductive needs in women is essential where abdominal or pelvic surgery is carried out, and careful technique should be employed to minimize the risk of pelvic adhesions. Where uterine instrumentation is considered, particularly in women under the age of 25 years, the prevention of *Chlamydia* infection is receiving appropriate attention [5]. Screening tests to detect the organism in first-void urine

Dewhurst's Textbook of Obstetrics & Gynaecology, Eighth Edition. Edited by D. Keith Edmonds.
© 2012 John Wiley and Sons, Ltd. Published 2012 by John Wiley and Sons, Ltd.

Table 45.1 Diagnostic categories and distribution of couples with primary and secondary infertility.

Diagnostic category	Infertility	
	Primary (%)	Secondary (%)
Male factor	25	20
Disorders of ovulation	20	15
Tubal factor	15	40
Endometriosis	10	5
Unexplained	30	20

samples or cervical swabs using nucleic acid amplification techniques should routinely be available and antibiotic treatment given for identified cases and potential contacts. Good lines of communication to sexual health and genitourinary medicine services will facilitate swift management.

The management of people with infertility problems is largely dictated by the major diagnostic category into which they fit. Typical figures are shown in Table 45.1.

Diagnostic categories in most studies include male factors, disorders of ovulation, tubal factors, endometriosis and unexplained infertility. The distribution of causes, when analysed, will be affected by whether the female has been pregnant in the past: secondary infertility. This has an association with an increased risk of tubal factor infertility as compared with those couples with primary infertility, i.e. where there has not been a pregnancy in the past. The possibility that male factors may contribute to a couple's infertility should not be ignored even in cases where the man has fathered a pregnancy in the past. It should be borne in mind that more than one factor may contribute to a couple's infertility and each may require simultaneous management, e.g. ovulation induction for a woman who is not ovulating in combination with donor insemination. Decisions to initiate active treatment will be influenced by the age of the female, the duration of infertility and whether or not there has been a pregnancy in the past. Initiating intrusive and potentially harmful treatment should take account of natural expectations of pregnancy. In many instances expectant management will be appropriate.

Initial assessment

The point at which any couple might seek assistance will be influenced by a number of factors, not least the degree of anxiety which couples feel in confronting seemingly relentless monthly disappointments. It should be borne

in mind that libido and consequently coital frequency may be influenced by the experience of infertility and thus affect prognosis. While there is some evidence that sperm parameters may be adversely affected by very frequent ejaculation, the evidence suggests that fertility potential is unaffected. Bearing in mind that sperm survival can be expected for up to 7 days within the female reproductive tract, couples should be advised to have intercourse every 2–3 days to optimize the chance of conception. The use of temperature charts or luteinizing hormone (LH) prediction kits to time intercourse should be discouraged.

It may be apparent to individuals that they may be at risk of a fertility problem and advice should be sought at an early stage. For example, the male may have had a vasectomy or undergone testicular surgery in childhood, e.g. orchidopexy; either partner may be a survivor of childhood cancer and have undergone chemotherapy; or the female may be aware of an association of absent or irregular periods with infertility.

All people seeking advice about fertility should have prompt access to an integrated multidisciplinary service which by definition must include the general practitioner (GP), whose role is of fundamental importance [9]. Infertility, its investigation and treatment can threaten domestic stability and it is often the GP, through longstanding knowledge of the couple and their families, who may be in the best position to provide support for those struggling to come to terms with continued disappointment. Once a referral is made to a specialist clinic, increasing the demands on couples' time, the intrusive nature of some of the investigations may add to the stress of the situation.

Preliminary assessment of the infertile couple

Points requiring particular attention in the history and examination of the female and male are shown in Tables 45.2 and 45.3.

Appropriate initial investigations

Should couples present in advance of a year's duration of infertility, then it may be unnecessary to pursue vigorous investigation unless there is something obvious in either the history or the examination. It is advisable to ensure that the female is immune to rubella and that she is taking an appropriate dose of folic acid supplementation to reduce the chance of the fetus developing a neural tube defect.

Merely providing the couple with an outline of their excellent fertility potential over the next year may be all that is required, but more urgency may be required where the female partner is over 35 years of age.

Table 45.2 The initial assessment of female infertility: history and examination.

Area of investigation	History	Area of investigation	Examination
Infertility	Duration of infertility Length and type of contraceptive use Fertility in previous relationships as well as in present liaison Previous investigation and treatment Fertility subsequently, if known, in any former partners Previous fertility investigations and treatment	General	Height, weight, BMI Fat and hair distribution (Ferriman–Gallwey score to quantify hirsutism) Note presence or absence of acne and galactorrhoea
Medical	Menstrual history: menarche, cyclicity, pain, bouts of amenorrhoea, menorrhagia, intermenstrual bleeding Number of previous pregnancies including abortions, miscarriages and ectopic pregnancies Any associated sepsis Time to initiate previous pregnancies Drug history and present, e.g. agents which cause hyperprolactinaemia, past cytotoxic treatment or radiotherapy	Abdominal	Check for abdominal masses or tenderness
Surgical	Previous abdominal or pelvic surgery, in particular gynaecological procedures	Pelvis	Assess state of hymen Assess normality of clitoris and labia Assess vagina, looking for such problems as infection or vaginal septa, endometriotic deposits Check for presence of cervical polyps Assess accessibility of the cervix for insemination Record uterine size, position, mobility and tenderness Perform cervical smear if appropriate
Occupational	Work patterns including separation from partner		
Sexual	Coital frequency and timing, including knowledge of the fertile period Dyspareunia Postcoital bleeding		

Table 45.3 The initial assessment of male infertility: history and examination.

Area of investigation	History	Area of investigation	Examination
Infertility	Duration of infertility Fertility in previous relationships as well as in present liaison Fertility subsequently, if known, in any former partners Previous fertility investigations and treatment	General	Height, weight, body mass index Fat and hair distribution Evidence of hypoandrogenism or gynaecomastia
Medical	Sexually transmitted infection Epididymitis Mumps orchitis Testicular maldescent Chronic disease Drug/alcohol abuse Recent febrile illness Recurrent urinary tract infection	Groin	Exclude inguinal hernia (patient in upright position) Check for inguinal mass, e.g. ectopic testicle

(Continued)

Table 45.3 (*Continued*)

Area of investigation	History	Area of investigation	Examination
Surgical	Herniorrhaphy Testicular injury Torsion Orchidopexy Vasectomy and/or reversal	Genitalia	Note site of testicles in the scrotum and measure volume using an orchidometer Palpate epididymis for nodularity or tenderness Check presence and normality of the vasa deferentia Check for the presence of a varicocele Examine penis for any structural abnormality, e.g. hypospadias
Occupational	Toxic substance exposure including chemicals, radiation Time away from home through work		
Sexual	Onset of puberty Coital habits Premature ejaculation Libido/impotence Use and knowledge of the fertile period		

An explanation of the steps in the process of investigation should be given to the couple at the outset. Three simple questions require to be answered:

1 Are sperm available, i.e. is there evidence of normal spermatogenesis and ejaculatory competence?
2 Are eggs available, i.e. is the woman ovulating?
3 Can the gametes meet, i.e. is there a pelvic problem in the female impairing normal gamete/embryo transport and is coital function adequate?

Summary box 45.1

- Fifteen per cent of couples have difficulty conceiving.
- Female age, duration of infertility and history of a previous pregnancy are the most important prognostic factors.
- Couples should normally be referred for investigation if the duration of infertility exceeds a year.

Male factor infertility

Semen analysis remains the cornerstone of assessment. Clear instructions on the provision of samples should be given – a period of abstinence of at least 3 days but no longer than 1 week is desirable, and the sample should be kept at body temperature in transportation and should arrive at the laboratory if being provided off site within 1 hour of production. In most instances a single sample will suffice if the result is normal. If an abnormality is found then the sample should be repeated, usually after

Table 45.4 Laboratory reference range for semen characteristics.

Semen parameter	Lower reference limit (fifth centiles + 95% confidence intervals)
Semen volume (mL)	1.5 (1.4–1.7)
Total sperm number ($\times 10^6$ per ejaculate)	39 (33–46)
Sperm concentration ($\times 10^6$ per mL)	15 (12–16)
Total motility: progressive + non-progressive (%)	40 (38–42)
Progressive motility (%)	32 (31–34)
Sperm morphology (normal forms, %)	4 (3.0–4.0)

From reference 10.

1 month, although resolution of any transient insult leading to defects in sperm production may not be apparent for up to 3 months.

What constitutes a normal result is a matter of debate. Large laboratories may have their own local population-based normal ranges, but in the absence of local information the World Health Organization (WHO) values for definition of normality can be applied. These have recently been updated [10] (Table 45.4). Such definitions of normality as predictors of pregnancy are poor. More complex tests of sperm function, including their potential for movement, cervical mucus penetration, capacitation, zona recognition, the acrosome reaction and sperm–oocyte fusion, have been developed [11].

In practice, such additional complex tests of sperm function are rarely required. Particular debate has centred on the use of the postcoital test (PCT). The test is intrusive in so far as the couple is asked to have intercourse at a prescribed time and then the female attends the clinic for a sample of mucus to be obtained from the cervix. The investigator examines the specimen to determine if there are motile sperm visible under light microscopy. In theory, the test could give an indication that intercourse has taken place, that timing is correct, that the mucus is receptive and that sperm numbers and motility are adequate. In critically evaluating the usefulness of the PCT in clinical practice, many would argue that it lacks predictive power in its ability to identify those who will conceive naturally from those who will not [12]. Furthermore, there is no standardization of the methodology of the test, e.g. timing of intercourse in relation to ovulation, timing of examination of sampled mucus relative to intercourse, and what sperm numbers and motility levels within examined mucus are normal [1]. One study [13] found the PCT to be useful in predicting spontaneous conception in couples with otherwise unexplained infertility of a short duration (<3 years). A study which examined whether intrauterine insemination improved the chance of conception where a PCT was negative, however, only showed a marginal effect [14].

Endocrine investigation in the male will include the measurement of serum follicle-stimulating hormone (FSH), prolactin and testosterone but is only indicated in particular circumstances. If there is azoospermia (no sperm in the ejaculate) or severe oligozoospermia (sperm density <1 M/mL), then a high FSH level may indicate testicular failure. In these circumstances a karyotype should be performed. Conditions such as Klinefelter's syndrome (47XXY) may be found. If the FSH is normal, then this may indicate an obstructive cause and surgical sperm retrieval may be possible. If the vas is impalpable on examination, screening for cystic fibrosis (CF) gene mutations should be performed because of the association with congenital absence of the vas deferens. If there is a suspicion of hypogonadism, then measurement of testosterone and prolactin is important. Men with impotence may have high prolactin levels and, if found, magnetic resonance imaging (MRI) of the pituitary gland to exclude a tumour should be performed. It should be remembered that certain drugs may cause high prolactin levels. Occasionally, some men may experience orgasm but fail to ejaculate. Retrograde ejaculation should be considered and it may be possible to identify sperm in a post-ejaculation first-void specimen of urine. A history of diabetes or previous prostatic surgery may be implicated. Nowadays, it is rare for a testicular biopsy to be required in the investigation of male infertility, although in onward fertility care a biopsy may be required to obtain sperm for use in assisted reproduction.

There are few conditions in male infertility that are easily reversible. Hypogonadotrophic hypogonadism (low FSH, low testosterone) may be reversible with exogenous gonadotrophins, although treatment may take several months. If there is erectile dysfunction, as might occur after spinal cord injury, then it may be possible to achieve ejaculation through the use of vibrators or electro-ejaculation. Samples obtained in this way may be suitable for artificial insemination, but if the quality is poor, *in vitro* fertilization (IVF) may be necessary. On occasion, the use of phosphodiesterase type-5 inhibitors, such as sildenafil, may help men struggling with impotence. Sometimes intracavernosal injection of prostaglandin E1 (alprostadil) may be helpful. Current evidence would suggest that treatment of a varicocele in an infertile man is unlikely to improve the sperm count and should be reserved for those with symptoms.

If the semen analysis reveals significant agglutination of sperm, then antisperm antibodies may be present. In these circumstances, IVF may be necessary when intracytoplasmic sperm injection (ICSI) will usually be used to maximize the chance of successful fertilization. If a man has previously had a vasectomy, then in skilled hands good results can be obtained for vasectomy reversal. Alternatively, IVF may be required.

Empirical treatment in the face of a moderately impaired sperm count has little to commend it. The use of gonadotrophins, antioestrogens (e.g. clomifene), androgens, bromocriptine, kallikrein, antioxidants, mast cell blockers and alpha blockers have been studied with no convincing evidence of benefit. Assisted reproduction encompassing intrauterine insemination and IVF techniques are more successful and are discussed in Chapter. In some men with primary testicular failure, e.g. azoospermia associated with Klinefelter's syndrome, the only option will be the use of donor sperm. This will inevitably raise complex ethical questions for couples.

 Summary box 45.2

- Semen parameters alone are not strong predictors for chance of future conception.
- Tests of sperm function have a limited role in investigation.
- Genetic investigation will be required in cases of severe oligozoopermis or azoospermia.
- Endocrine investigation may be helpful in cases of suspected hyperandrogenism.
- Varicocele is unproven as a cause of male infertility.
- The postcoital test is of little use in the evaluation of the infertile male.

Disorders of ovulation

Disturbances in ovulation are the principal factor in about 20% of couples presenting with fertility difficulties to clinics. In women who have regular monthly menstrual cycle (21–42 days), it is most likely that ovulation occurs normally. The release of the oocyte is usually inferred through indirect methods, most often the measurement of progesterone (P_4) in the putative luteal phase of the cycle. Serum P_4 levels in excess of 30 nmol/L 7 days after ovulation are usually taken as indicative of satisfactory ovulation, although lower levels are not incompatible with egg release and corpus luteum formation [15,16]. It is important to relate P_4 levels to the timing of subsequent menstruation. Samples will typically be checked on day 21 of a 28-day cycle. Serial checks will be required if the cycle is longer than this or is variable in length. Shorter cycle length will require an assessment earlier than day 21. Urinary kits are available to detect LH and can be helpful in treatment cycles where the timing of artificial insemination is critical. Their use in detecting ovulation in routine investigation is not encouraged.

Clinical signs, in addition to regular menstruation, which would suggest that ovulation is occurring include the presence of mittelschmerz (mid-cycle abdominal discomfort) or mid-cycle spotting induced through a transient fall in E_2 coincidental to the LH surge. The production of mid-cycle mucus is oestrogen-dependent, and a change in consistency and stretchability (spinnbarkeit) occurs under the influence of P_4. This is used in natural family planning techniques as a contraceptive method, but conversely may occasionally have a place in timing intercourse or artificial insemination in promoting fertility. Under the influence of progesterone, basal body temperature (BBT) may rise by 0.5–1.0°C after ovulation. While for some the finding of such a rise through serial measurement taken each morning through the periovulatory phase of the cycle is reassuring, the correlation with serum P_4 levels is poor and often couples find the confusion and uncertainty this brings to be stressful.

If there is a history of irregular periods or amenorrhoea, especially if associated with galactorrhoea, hirsutism or obesity, then additional endocrine investigations will be required. These would include the measurement of FSH, LH, thyroid-stimulating hormone (TSH) and prolactin, timing sampling to coincide with the early follicular phase of the cycle if the woman is having periods. If significant hirsutism or acne is present, then the measurement of testosterone, sex hormone-binding globulin and adrenal androgens including androstenedione, dehydroepiandrosterone, dehydroepiandrosterone sulphate and 17-hydroxy progesterone should be performed.

Ovarian ultrasound to track follicular development, rupture and corpus luteum formation may be useful in ovulation-induction treatment cycles but is time consum-

Table 45.5 The World Health Organization classification of ovulatory disorders.

Group	Type of disorder	%	Biochemical characteristics
I	Hypothalamic pituitary failure (hypothalamic amenorrhoea or hypogonadotrophic hypogonadism)	10	Low basal gonadotrophins, normal prolactin, low oestrogen
II	Hypothalamic pituitary dysfunction	85	Gonadotrophins and oestrogen levels in the normal range
III	Ovarian failure	4–5	High gonadotrophins, low oestrogen

ing and intrusive, and thus rarely used in the routine investigation of ovulation. Early follicular phase scanning is, however, helpful in assessing ovarian morphology. A diagnosis of the polycystic ovary is made if there are at least 12 follicles 2–9 mm in diameter and/or the ovarian volume is greater than 10 cm^3. Assessment of endometrial thickness within the uterus may be a useful indicator of the level of oestrogen exposure in women presenting with amenorrhoea, which can be of assistance in reaching a diagnosis.

The WHO classification of ovulatory dysfunction (Table 45.5) is a helpful system of categorizing disorders of ovulation based on the pathogenesis of the disorder. WHO type I ovulatory dysfunction may be due to a failure of the hypothalamus to produce gonadotrophin-releasing hormone (GnRH), which regulates the production of gonadotrophins by the pituitary gland. Typically, FSH and LH levels are low (<5 IU/L). Oestrogen levels are also low, and an ultrasound scan of the uterus will show a thin or absent endometrial stripe. The patient fails to menstruate after exposure to a short course of progestogen treatment.

A similar situation may arise in cases of hyperprolactinaemia, which may be associated with galactorrhoea as well as amenorrhoea. Normal pulsatile release of GnRH from the hypothalamus is compromised and follicular growth ceases with resultant amenorrhoea. This may also occur in some instances of hypothyroidism where high levels of thyrotropin-releasing hormone (TRH) can alter dopamine-mediated regulation of the anterior pituitary and cause hyperprolactinaemia. If hyperprolactinaemia is found, then pituitary imaging by MRI may identify a microadenoma or occasionally a larger pituitary tumour. Some drugs that block the effect of dopamine, e.g. phenothiazines, certain antipsychotics, metoclopramide and others, can cause hyperprolactinaemia.

Acquired GnRH deficiency may also arise in association with weight loss, as seen in anorexia nervosa, and in individuals who take excessive exercise. Kallmann's syndrome presents as hypothalamic amenorrhoea associated with anosmia, and results from a congenital absence of GnRH-releasing neurones in the hypothalamus. The syndrome is characterized by a lack of gonadotrophin secretion from the anterior pituitary and consequent hypogonadism. Pituitary failure may arise as a result of necrosis or thrombosis secondary to tumour formation. Rarely, massive obstetric haemorrhage and prolonged hypotension can lead to pituitary infarction (Sheehan's syndrome).

The commonest ovulation disturbances (WHO type II) are associated with disordered hypothalamic–pituitary–ovarian function. Women with this dysfunction will have oestrogen levels in the normal range and many are overweight, presenting with infrequent or absent periods. A common finding is the presence of polycystic ovaries on ultrasound, seen in up to 90% of such cases. In contrast to WHO type I patients, these women will usually menstruate after exposure to a short course of progestogen treatment. Ultrasound scanning should be timed to coincide with either a natural or progestogen-induced menstrual period. Where there is clinical or biochemical evidence of hyperandrogenism, then this together with menstrual irregularity and ovarian morphology should be taken into account in reaching a diagnosis of polycystic ovarian syndrome (PCOS). A consensus view on standardized criteria for the diagnosis of PCOS has helped in establishing a uniform approach and facilitated easier comparison of clinical and research experience in different centres [17]. It was agreed that the presence of any two of the following triad are sufficient to make the diagnosis:

1 oligo- and/or anovulation;
2 polycystic ovaries on ultrasound; and/or
3 clinical and/or biochemical hyperandrogenism.

About 10–20% of patients with PCOS have an associated elevation in PRL, but this is usually mild and not of clinical consequence. On occasions, ovulatory failure may result from 21-hydroxylase deficiency in the adrenal gland, leading to elevated serum levels of 17-hydroxy progesterone, an androgenic steroid precursor of cortisol. High androgens disturb normal follicular growth and patients may present with irregular or absent periods associated with signs of androgen excess including hirsutism, acne and enlargement of the clitoris. Other causes of hyperandrogenism such as adrenal tumours and Cushing's syndrome may need to be considered where adrenal androgen levels are found to be high.

Insulin resistance has been well described in women with PCOS and it has been estimated that they have a three to seven times greater risk in later life of developing type 2 diabetes, for which regular screening may therefore be appropriate. Amenorrhoea in PCOS may also be associated with an increased lifetime risk of endometrial cancer. Progestogen-induced menstruation should thus be facilitated three or four times per year, particularly if increased endometrial thickness is seen on ultrasound.

In patients presenting with amenorrhoea and where initial biochemical screening and physical examination lead one to suspect ovarian failure (WHO type III), then the presence of a genetic disorder such as Turner's syndrome (45XO) or Turner mosaic (45XO/46XX) should be considered and a karyotype performed. Occasionally, deletions in one of the X chromosomes or defects in the fragile X gene may lead to ovarian failure, but agenesis of the ovaries (associated with primary amenorrhoea) and premature ovarian failure (presenting as secondary amenorrhoea before the age of 40 years) is sometimes found in the presence of a normal karyotype. Acquired ovarian failure may occur as a result of previous medical treatment such as chemotherapy or radiotherapy for cancer. Autoimmune ovarian failure should be considered, and screening for antiovarian antibodies may be useful in reaching a diagnosis. If the result is positive, then screening for other autoimmune disorders including hypothyroidism, adrenal insufficiency (Addison's disease), diabetes mellitus and pernicious anaemia should be considered.

The treatment of infertility associated with disturbed ovulation depends on the diagnosis. Ovulation induction requires care in choice of treatment modality and in monitoring ever mindful of the risks of multiple pregnancies.

The commonest group requiring treatment includes women with PCOS (WHO type II). Many are overweight and have associated insulin resistance. A reduction in body weight by 5–10% may restore ovulation in some and will maximize the likelihood of a response to ovulation induction agents. Insulin-sensitizing agents such as metformin have a limited effect on ovulation rates and any improvement usually is associated with weight loss. Lifestyle measures are thus an important element in management and care in diet and attention to exercise should be emphasized to patients.

Antioestrogen treatment (e.g. clomifene) is the commonest form of therapy. A 50 mg/day regime from days 2–6 of the cycle is the usual starting dose. Ultrasound monitoring for multiple follicular development is recommended in the first cycle. If an exuberant response is seen, then a 25 mg dose should be used. In women who do not respond to the initial dose, then the dose may be increased in 50 mg increments in subsequent cycles to a maximum of 150 mg/day. Ovulation will be achieved in at least 80% of women, with pregnancy rates in excess of 20–25% per cycle. Multiple pregnancy rates should be no higher than 5%. Usually a maximum of 12 treatment cycles will be offered.

In women who fail to conceive with clomifene, gonado-trophin therapy may be employed. A low-dose step-up regime is most often used, starting at 37.5IU/day of FSH. Ideally, monofollicular development will ensue. The dose of FSH should be increased in 37.5IU increments and 75% of women will respond by 75IU/day dose levels. Human chorionic gonadotrophin (hCG) is used to trigger ovulation when an adequate response is seen. Monitoring entails attendance for regular ovarian ultrasound assessments and thus the treatment is quite intrusive and should be carried out only in centres with access to monitoring facilities. If more than two mature follicles develop, the risk of multiple pregnancy is unacceptable and the ovulatory dose of hCG should be withheld. Patients who embark on gonadotrophin treatment because they failed to ovulate on clomifene have higher pregnancy rates than those who fail to conceive with clomifene despite ovulation.

Laparoscopic ovarian diathermy can also be used in women with PCOS-associated anovulation. The duration of effect is variable, but in some women ovulation may be restored and improved responsiveness to pharmacological ovulation induction may occur. Aromatase inhibitors such as letrozole have also been used in women resistant to clomifene treatment. Ovulation rates of 75% have been described using a dose of 2.5mg per day from days 3–7 of the cycle [18].

In women with WHO type I-associated anovulation, clomifene is less successful. Many are underweight and for them achieving a body mass index (BMI) of >20kg/m^2 may be effective treatment. For them, gonadotrophin treatment should be considered or alternatively pulsatile GnRH. In women with hyperprolactinaemia, dopamine agonists, for example bromocriptine or cabergoline, are effective. Should ovulation induction treatment be unsuccessful, IVF should be considered.

Ovulation induction also carries the risk of ovarian hyperstimulation syndrome. This occurs much less frequently than with ovarian stimulation in IVF but is a dangerous condition if not managed appropriately. Women who develop an excessive number of follicles are most at risk of the condition and the ovulatory dose of hCG should be withheld when this occurs.

Summary box 45.3

- Progesterone testing should be timed according to menstrual cycle length.
- Other endocrine investigations should be reserved for women with irregular cycles and/or signs of androgen excess.
- Clomifene is an effective and safe first-line agent in 90% of cases of ovulatory problems.
- Multiple pregnancy risks should be carefully considered in delivering treatment.

Tubal factor infertility

Tubal pathology is a contributory factor in 15–30% of women presenting with infertility. Normal tubal function should permit gamete transport and fertilization and the subsequent passage of the embryo to the uterus such that implantation can take place at the appropriate stage in the menstrual cycle. The most common cause of tubal factor infertility is past pelvic infection through an STI, for example *Chlamydia trachomatis*, although previous pregnancy, both successful and failed, or history of pelvic surgery or endometriosis can be implicated. Occasionally, a Müllerian developmental anomaly may be involved.

The following tests of pelvic anatomy are commonly performed in the diagnostic workup of women with infertility:
1 X-ray hysterosalpingography;
2 laparoscopy; and
3 hysterosalpingo-contrast sonography (HyCoSy).

If the duration of infertility is short (<1 year) and the history and examination findings do not suggest that a tubal factor is likely, then the examination of the pelvis may be deferred until nearly 18 months duration of infertility. However, if there is a positive feature in the history, if the pelvic findings on bimanual examination are abnormal or if a screening test for *Chlamydia* is positive, then an assessment should be arranged without delay.

X-ray hysterosalpingography

This is an outpatient examination and involves the instillation of either a water- or oil-soluble contrast medium through a cannula attached to the cervix. The fluid, being radio-opaque, can be visualized under X-ray screening conditions. An assessment is made of the normality of the uterine cavity. Passage of dye to the side of the uterus permits an assessment of tubal anatomy. Unimpaired passage of dye throughout tubal length and dispersal into the peritoneal cavity is suggestive of normal anatomy. If there is impaired flow or localization of spill distally, then one should be suspicious of peritubal adhesions. The finding of a hydrosalpinx will be indicative of severe tubal damage. It is important, particularly in women under the age of 25 years, to consider the need for antibiotic prophylaxis since *Chlamydia* infection could be reactivated in susceptible women. Azithromycin or doxycycline is usually used.

A hysterosalpingography (HSG) should not be carried out if the patient is menstruating. In addition, women should be advised to avoid conception in the cycle in which the procedure is carried out. If unprotected intercourse has occurred, then the examination should be deferred.

The contrast medium used in an HSG may contain iodine, and the possibility of allergic reactions should be borne in mind. Significant extravasation of oil-soluble contrast media within the pelvis may lead to lipogranuloma formation. There is some evidence that the use of an oil-soluble contrast medium (lipiodol) may enhance the chance of pregnancy in unexplained infertility [19] although it has not gained widespread popularity as a therapeutic choice.

A meta-analysis evaluating HSG assessment of tubal patency using laparoscopy as the gold standard showed a 65% sensitivity rate and 83% specificity rate [20,21]. One would deduce from this that although the HSG is of limited value in detecting tubal blockage because of its low sensitivity, its high specificity makes it a better test for identification of tubal patency.

Laparoscopy and dye hydrotubation

It is generally accepted that laparoscopy and dye hydrotubation is the gold standard of tubal assessment. In this procedure, which, like HSG, should avoid the time of menstruation and any chance of pregnancy, a coloured dye is injected through the cervix while carrying out a laparoscopic inspection of the pelvis. Failure of dye to pass through the tube is indicative of blockage.

Direct visualization of the pelvis permits identification of adhesions, fibroids, endometriosis, ovarian cysts and other pathology which may be relevant to infertility and would be missed at HSG. The likelihood of finding tubal disease is increased if the patient has a positive *Chlamydia* screening test [22]. Immediate treatment of pathology is also possible at laparoscopy, which may be particularly relevant where endometriosis is found.

The procedure should be carried out in a systematic fashion and a written record, together with photographs if possible, made of the findings. The use of a diagram such as that produced by the American Society for Reproductive Medicine (ASRM) [23] to record findings is often helpful in explaining to patients what has been seen and done as well as providing a formal record of the findings, particularly if endometriosis is found.

General anaesthesia carries with it a small risk of reaction to the drugs used, and in addition the introduction of laparoscopic instruments presents a risk of injury to intra-abdominal structures such as the bowel, bladder and blood vessels. Patients who have undergone previous abdominal surgery, in particular those with a mid-line incision, are particularly at risk. The technique used in the introduction of instruments may need to be adapted to take account of this increased hazard. Alternatively, an HSG may be preferred.

Hysterosalpingo-contrast sonography

In the last two decades, HyCoSy has attracted some interest as an additional method for assessing tubal patency [24]. Carried out as an outpatient or office procedure, a small balloon catheter is inserted in to the uterine cavity through the cervix. A vaginal scan is performed while a suspension of an ultrasound contrast agent (Echovist) is injected through the catheter. Usually, only 2–5 mL of fluid will be required. The media contain galactose granules and if flow is seen through the length of the tube it is likely to be patent. Hydrosalpinges can also be identified. Saline alone can be used if inspection of the uterine cavity only is required and good imaging of endometrial polyps can be obtained. The technique requires considerable ultrasound skills and occasionally some patients find the instillation of the fluid uncomfortable. There is no evidence of therapeutic benefit through flushing with the media used in HyCoSy [25].

Hysteroscopy

Hysteroscopic examination of the uterine cavity may be performed as an outpatient procedure, although if a laparoscopic assessment is being carried out then it is a simple affair to combine the two procedures. Uterine malformations, fibroids, endometrial polyps, adhesions and other conditions may be identified and treated using this technique, although it is controversial whether some of these findings contribute to infertility to any great degree.

Evaluation of diagnostic tests of tubal factor infertility

A meta-analysis evaluating HSG assessment of tubal patency using laparoscopy as the gold standard showed a 65% sensitivity rate and 83% specificity rate [20,21]. One would deduce from this that although the HSG is of limited value in detecting tubal blockage because of its low sensitivity, its high specificity makes it a better test for identification of tubal patency. The negative predictive value (94%) of the test as a predictor of tubal patency is also high, suggesting that the finding of normal tubes at HSG is likely to be correct. However, a low positive predictive value of 38% of the test would suggest that HSG is not a reliable indicator of tubal occlusion and that it would be wise in the circumstances of an abnormal HSG result to consider a laparoscopic assessment to confirm or refute the findings [8].

HyCoSy also performs fairly well in detecting normality and hydrosalpinx formation, but, similar to HSG, performs less well in its reliability in identifying tubal blockage [24].

Endoscopic assessment of the tubal lumen to study mucosal appearance has not proved to be helpful in routine work-up of infertility. Falloposcopy achieves access to the tube per vaginam [26]. Salpingoscopy can be performed at laparoscopy or laparotomy where the tube is cannulated through the fimbria [27]. Initially thought to be of potential use in selecting patients with healthy tubal epithelium who might be suitable for tubal surgery, neither of the techniques has gained much popularity and they are rarely used.

A number of factors should be considered when considering appropriate management of tubal factor infertility:

- Female age – fecundity diminishes markedly over the age of 40 years.
- Extent of disease – surgery is less likely to be successful with more severe disease. The presence of a hydrosalpinx may affect IVF outcome and removal should be considered. Microsurgical techniques of sterilization reversal have high success rates in women below the age of 40 year.
- Site of disease – proximal disease may be amenable to tubal recanalization by selective salpingography. Isolated distal disease may be treated with salpingostomy. Peritubal adhesions can be treated with adhesiolysis.
- Presence of other fertility factors – these may identify individuals most suited to IVF.
- Surgical expertise – the skill of the surgeon is an important determinant of success.
- Future pregnancy – ectopic pregnancy is a risk following tubal surgery. IVF may diminish but does not abolish the risk.

Endometriosis, fibroids and uterine factors

Endometriosis is a debilitating condition which has associations with infertility, particularly where there is anatomical distortion of the pelvis. Women who are susceptible to the condition may have genetic, immunological, hormonal or environmental factors contributing to the problem [28]. A family history of the condition should alert the gynaecologist to the possibility, particularly if the common symptoms of dysmenorrhoea and chronic pelvic pain are present. Pelvic examination may reveal a fixed, tender retroverted uterus and on occasions there may be endometriotic nodules presenting the vault of the vagina or the rectovaginal septum. A combined rectal and vaginal examination may be helpful if this is suspected. Laparoscopic visualization of endometriotic lesions is the cornerstone of diagnosis, although a histological confirmation of an excised lesion is strictly necessary to be absolutely certain. The accuracy of the diagnosis therefore depends on the degree of skill and vigilance of the surgeon. If endometriosis is found at laparoscopy, it is helpful to stage the disease by reference to the ASRM guidelines [23]. There is some evidence that women with mild endometriosis have reduced fertility [29] and that treatment, for example with diathermy, may improve the natural chances of conception in minimal/mild disease [30]. A suspicion of endometriosis may be raised if vaginal ultrasound examination of the pelvis is painful or a cyst with a hazy 'ground glass' appearance is seen in the ovary, suggestive of an endometrioma. MRI of the uterus may be helpful if one suspects adenomyosis. Biochemical assay of CA-125, if raised, may be suggestive of endometriosis although this is non-specific. Women with Müllerian abnormalities promoting retrograde menstruation are at greater risk of developing endometriosis.

Medical options in the management of endometriosis include the use of continuous combined oral contraceptive preparations, progestogens, danazol, gestrinone and GnRH analogues. The suppression of ovulation addresses the oestrogen-associated pathogenesis of the condition. However, there is little evidence to suggest that medical treatment enhances fertility rates.

In addition, surgery may be helpful in cases of advanced disease, particularly if there is significant pain or large ovarian cysts. Bowel involvement may require the input of colorectal surgeons. Laparoscopic or open surgical approaches may be used dependent on the skill of the surgical team.

Fibroids are among the commonest benign tumours in women, with a reported prevalence of 3–8% in unselected women of reproductive age [31], although they occur with higher frequency in older women and in certain ethnic populations. Fibroids are often asymptomatic but an association with infertility is possible [32], particularly where the tumour impinges on the cavity of the uterus [33,34]. Abdominal palpation and vaginal examination may reveal a mass arising from the pelvis. Ultrasound examination is usually performed to confirm the diagnosis. If the relationship between the fibroid and the uterine cavity is unclear from an initial ultrasound assessment, then hysterosalpingo contrast sonography or a HSG may be useful to distinguish submucosal from intramural lesions. Hysteroscopic evaluation of the degree of myometrial penetration by the fibroid is essential if surgical excision is contemplated [35]. Laparoscopic or open myomectomy can be carried out, although there is a risk of postoperative adhesions which may compromise fertility. Uncontrolled haemorrhage may lead to hysterectomy. Preoperative shrinkage of the fibroid with GnRH analogue therapy may be associated with a reduction in bleeding. Discrimination between adenomyosis and fibroids may be facilitated with the use of ultrasound where the absence of a tumour capsule and lacunae within the lesion may suggestive of the former. MRI scanning can also be of help.

Undiagnosed uterine pathology as a cause of infertility, recurrent implantation failure (RIF) or recurrent miscarriage is an attractive concept. However, the evidence that disturbed endometrial receptivity is important in infertility is mixed. Endometrial assessment by timed sampling and histological dating is the most described method of assessing the normality of endometrial development. It is dependent on accurate timing of sampling endometrium relevant to the LH surge [36] and in routine practice has largely been abandoned, as has the concept of luteal-phase deficiency as a major cause of infertility. Ultrasound-measured endometrial thickness is a poor predictor of implantation potential in IVF [37], particularly where high-quality embryos are available. Disturbances in cytokine expression and action have been postulated as a cause of RIF, but analysis of these factors remains a research rather than a clinical tool. The role that immunological causes and thrombophilia may have in infertility is also uncertain. Some early studies suggested an association between antiphospholipid syndrome and RIF, but this has not been confirmed in larger prospective studies. The role that natural killer cells may play in RIF is disputed [38]. For the moment there is no convincing evidence for an association. An association between hereditary thrombophilia and RIF has also been described in some, but not all, studies and screening for these disorders is still controversial.

 Summary box 45.5

- Before undergoing uterine instrumentation, women who are at risk should be screened for *Chlamydia trachomatis* infection.
- Affected women and their partners should be referred to genitourinary medicine services for treatment.
- Surgery may be effective in appropriately selected women.
- Myomectomy should be considered for fibroids if there is significant distortion of the uterine cavity, although the risks of surgery should be discussed.
- Medical management of endometriosis does not enhance fertility.

Unexplained infertility

Despite our use of investigation of pathways as outlined above, it is debatable whether the basic tests of semen quality, ovulation and tubal patency are in any way accurate in predicting live birth [39]. From the above discussion it will also be clear that there is an ongoing, and relevant, debate concerning the existence of subtle disturbances in reproductive function in the female and their impact on fertility. While endometrial function is undoubtedly important in the genesis of conception, a number of other elements in the path to establishment of pregnancy have been considered as causes of infertility. Few are amenable to simple investigation. Possibilities are listed in Table 45.6.

Unexplained infertility presents a frustrating diagnosis for both clinician and patient. The range and accuracy of the tests which are used to investigate the infertile will influence the chance of a 'diagnostic label' being attached to the problem [40]. Whether such a label is helpful in forming a prognosis or formulating a treatment plan is

Table 45.6 Putative causes of unexplained infertility.

Endocrine factors	Abnormal follicle growth
	Suboptimal progesterone secretion (luteal phase deficiency)
	Luteinized unruptured follicle syndrome
	Hypersecretion of luteinizing hormone
	Ovulatory hyperprolactinaemia
Ovarian factors	Zona pellucida antibodies
	Diminished ovarian reserve (ovarian ageing)
Uterine/endometrial factors	Congenital uterine abnormalities
	Submucous fibroids
	Abnormal uterine perfusion
	Altered cytokine expression and action
	Disturbed T-cell and natural killer cell function
Tubal factors	Disturbed tubal function, i.e. peristalsis, cilia
	Suboptimal metabolic support of gametes and embryos
	Altered immune activity
Peritoneal factors	Mild endometriosis
	Occult infection
	Altered immune activity
Genetic factors	Gamete and embryo aneuploidy
	Poor embryo morphology, cleavage and blastocyst formation
Sperm cervical mucus interaction	Altered cervical mucus production
	Anti-sperm antibodies
Psychogenic factors	Inadequate coital function

debatable [41]. In some instances the finding of 'abnormality' occurs with similar frequency in both those who ultimately conceive naturally and those who remain infertile [42]. In recent times, the age profile of patients attending fertility clinics has changed as many women, for a variety of reasons, are now delaying childbearing. For many, age alone is a major factor in determining prognosis and age may also influence the probability of a diagnosis of unexplained infertility being made. It has been estimated that the chance of reaching a diagnosis of unexplained infertility is doubled if the female is >35 years of age as compared with females <30 years old [43]. As discussed below, diminished ovarian reserve may, in theory, be a missed cause of infertility in otherwise unexplained infertility. For most clinics, female age together with parity and the duration of infertility will be the three factors having the greatest bearing on prognosis.

A move to empirical treatment should take account of evidence of effectiveness. Expectant management is appropriate if the duration of infertility is less than 3 years, although in women >35 years of age there may be a case for earlier treatment. Clomifene has often been used but current evidence suggests it may not be effective. Timed intrauterine insemination is sometimes considered, but unless there are sexual difficulties it is unlikely to be helpful. If combined with superovulation, there may be an increased chance of pregnancy but multiple pregnancy risks will be greater [44].

Insights from assisted conception

The population using assisted conception will usually include those who have prolonged infertility and, as such, is arguably not truly representative of the general population with infertility. However, outcomes in those who access IVF treatment, although under very different conditions, may give some insight into what may be occurring in natural attempts to conceive and afford help to couples in coming to terms with their infertility. Occasionally, poor fertilization outcomes may unmask functional problems to do with sperm or egg quality. Failed fertilization may be due to hardening of the zona pellucida, which is associated with ageing of the oocyte. Embryo quality as judged by morphology and cleavage patterns may be consistently suboptimal. The association with such findings and aneuploidy in embryos is well established. Women who fail to respond well to ovarian stimulation may have a qualitative or quantitative disturbance in follicular physiology. Tests of ovarian reserve to predict outcome have been widely used in those who are embarking on IVF treatment. Measures of early follicular-phase FSH, anti-Müllerian hormone (AMH), inhibin-B and ovarian ultrasound observed antral follicle count (AFC) are the most popular. Dynamic tests of ovarian reserve have also been described using clomifene or exogenous gonadotrophin stimulation. The predictive power of all these tests relevant to a number of end-points including eggs retrieved and clinical pregnancy, save at the extremes of range, is, however, poor. For the moment they should be regarded as unsuited for routine evaluation of the infertile female [45]. This will be discussed in greater detail elsewhere.

Conclusion

Infertility is a major public health problem, causing significant distress to those directly involved as well as to family and friends. The preliminary assessment of the availability of eggs and sperm, together with a determination that the gametes can meet, should provide a diagnosis for the majority of couples. A prognosis, usually favourable, should be able to be provided and, where necessary, treatment initiated within a relatively short time.

References

1 Evers JLH. Female subfertility. *Lancet* 2002;360:151–159.
2 Snick HKA, Snick TS, Evers JLH, Collins JA. The spontaneous pregnancy prognosis is untreated subfertile couples: the Walcheren primary care study. *Hum Reprod* 1997;12: 1582–1588.
3 Hull MGR, Glazener CMA, Kelly NJ *et al.* Population study of causes, treatment and outcome of infertility. *BMJ* 1985;291:1693–1697.
4 Templeton A, Fraser C, Thompson B. The epidemiology of infertility in Aberdeen. *BMJ* 1990;301:148–152.
5 Macmillan S, Templeton A. Screening for *Chlamydia trachomatis* in subfertile women. *Hum Reprod* 1999;12:3009–3012.
6 Oliva A, Spira A, Multigner L. Contribution of environmental factors to the risk of male infertility. *Hum Reprod* 2001;16: 1768–1776.
7 Bhattacharya S, Porter M, Raja EA *et al.* The epidemiology of infertility in the North East of Scotland. *Hum Reprod* 2009;24: 3096–3107.
8 NICE: National Collaborating Centre for Women's and Children's Health for the National Institute of Clinical Excellence. *Fertility: Assessment and Treatment for People with Fertility Problems.* London: RCOG Press, 2004.
9 Hamilton MPR. The initial assessment of the infertile couple. *Curr Obstet Gynaecol* 1992;2:2–7.
10 World Health Organization. *WHO Laboratory Manual for the Examination and Processing of Human Semen*, 5th edn. Geneva: WHO, 2010.
11 Aitken RJ. Sperm function tests and fertility. *Int J Androl* 2006;29:69–75.
12 Oei SG, Helmerhorst FM, Keirse MJNC. When is the post-coital test normal? A critical appraisal. *Hum Reprod* 1995;10: 1711–1714.
13 Glazener CMA, Ford WCL, Hull MGR. The prognostic power of the post-coital test for natural conception depends on the duration of infertility. *Hum Reprod* 2000;15:1953–1957.
14 Mol BW. Diagnostic potential of the post-coital test. In: Heineman MJ (ed) *Evidence Based Reproductive Medicine in Clinical Practice.* Birmingham: American Society for Reproductive Medicine, 2001: 73–82.
15 Hull MG, Savage PE, Bromham DR, Ismail AA, Morris AF. The value of a single serum progesterone measurement in the mid-luteal phase as a criterion of a potentially fertile cycle ('ovulation') derived from treated and untreated conception cycles. *Fertil Steril* 1982;37:355–360.
16 Wathen NC, Perry L, Lilford RJ, Chard T. Interpretation of single progesterone measurement in diagnosis of anovulation and defective luteal phase: observations on analysis of the normal range. *BMJ* 1984;288:7–9.
17 The Rotterdam ESHRE/ASRM-sponsored PCOS Consensus Workshop Group. Revised 2003 Consensus on diagnostic criteria and long-term health risks related to polycystic ovary syndrome (PCOS). *Hum Reprod* 2004;19:41–47.
18 Mitwally MF, Casper RF. Use of an aromatase inhibitor for induction of ovulation in patients with an inadequate response to clomiphene citrate. *Fertil Steril* 2001;75:305–309.
19 Johnson NP, Farquhar CM, Hadden WE, Suckling J, Yu Y, Sadler L. The FLUSH trial – Flushing with Lipiodol for Unexplained (and endometriosis-related) Subfertility by

Hysterosaplingograpgy: a randomised trial. *Hum Reprod* 2004;19:2043–2051.

20 Swart P, Mol BWJ, van der Veen F, van Beurden M, Redekop WK, Bossuyt PMM. The accuracy of hysterosalpingography in the diagnosis of tubal pathology, a meta-analysis. *Fertil Steril* 1995;64:486–491.

21 Mol BWJ, Swart P, Bossuyt PMM, van Beurden M, van der Veen F. Reproducibility of the interpretation of hysterosalpingography in the diagnosis of tubal pathology *Hum Reprod* 1996;11:1204–1208.

22 Coppus SFPJ, Opmeer BC, Logan S, van der Veen F, Bhattacharya S, Mol BWJ. The predictive value of medical history taking and Chlamydia IgG ELISA antibody testing (CAT) in the selection of subfertile women for diagnostic laparoscopy: a clinical prediction model approach. *Hum Reprod* 2007;22:1353–1358.

23 American Society for Reproductive Medicine. Revised American Society for Reproductive Medicine: classification of endometriosis. *Fertil Steril* 1996;67:817–821.

24 Hamilton JA, Larson AJ, Lower AM, Hasnain S, Grudzinskas JG. Evaluation of the performance of hysterosalpingo contrast sonography in 500 consecutive, unselected, infertile women. *Hum Reprod* 1998;13:1519–1526.

25 Lindborg L, Thorburn J, Bergh C, Strandell A. Influence of HyCoSy on spontaneous pregnancy: a randomized controlled trial. *Hum Reprod* 2009;24:1075–1079.

26 Rimbach S, Bastert G, Wallwiener D. Technical results of falloposcopy for fertility diagnosis in a large multicentre study. *Hum Reprod* 2001;16:925–930.

27 de Bruyne F, Hucke J, Willers R. The prognostic value of salpingoscopy. *Hum Reprod* 1997;12:266–271.

28 Crosignagni PG, Olive D, Bergqvist A, Luciano A. Advances in the management of endometriosis: an update for clinicians. *Hum Reprod Update* 2006;12:179–189.

29 Akande VA, Hunt LP, Cahill D, Jenkins JM. Difference in time to natural conception between women with unexplained infertility and infertile women with minor endometriosis. *Hum Reprod* 2004;19:96–103.

30 Marcoux S, Maheux R, Berube S. Laparoscopic surgery in infertile women with minimal or mild endometriosis. *N Engl J Med* 1997;337:217–222.

31 Borgfeldt C, Andolf E. Transvaginal ultrasonographic findings in the uterus and the endometrium: low prevalence of leiomyoma in a random sample of women age 25–40 years. *Acta Obstet Gynecol Scand* 2000;79:202–207.

32 Somigliana E, Vercellini P, Daguati R, Pasin R, de Giorgi O, Crosignani PG. Fibroids and female reproduction: a critical analysis of the evidence. *Hum Reprod Update* 2007;13:465–476.

33 Khalaf Y, Ross C, El-Toukhy T, Hart R, Seed P, Braude P. The effect of small intramural uterine fibroids on the cumulative outcome of assisted conception. *Hum Reprod* 2006;21: 2640–2644.

34 Klatsky PC, Lane DE, Ryan IP, Fujimoto VY. The effect of fibroids without cavity involvement on ART outcomes independent of ovarian age. *Hum Reprod* 2007;22:521–526.

35 Di Spiezio Sardo A, Mazzon I, Bramante S et al. Hysteroscopic myomectomy: a comprehensive review of surgical techniques. *Hum Reprod Update* 2008;14:101–119.

36 Li TC, Tuckerman EM, Laird SM. Endometrial factors in recurrent miscarriage. *Hum Reprod Update* 2002;8:43–52.

37 Margalioth EJ, Ben-Chetrit A, Gal M, Eldar-Geva T. Investigation and treatment of repeated implantation failure after IVF-ET. *Hum Reprod* 2006;21:3036–3043.

38 Rai R, Sacks G, Trew G. Natural killer cells and reproductive failure – theory, practice and prejudice. *Hum Reprod* 2005;20:1123–1126.

39 Taylor PJ, Collins JA. *Unexplained Infertility*. Oxford: Oxford University Press, 1992.

40 Gleicher N, Barad D. Unexplained infertility: does it really exist? *Hum Reprod* 2006;21:1951–1955.

41 Siristatidis C, Bhattacharya S. Unexplained infertility: does it really exist? Does it matter? *Hum Reprod* 2007;22:2084–2087.

42 Guzick DS, Grefenstette I, Baffone K et al. Infertility evaluation in fertile women: a model for assessing the efficacy of infertility testing. *Hum Reprod* 1994;9:2306–2310.

43 Maheshwari A, Hamilton M, Bhattacharya S. Effect of female age on the diagnostic categories of infertility. *Hum Reprod* 2008;23:538–542.

44 Bhattacharya S, Harrild K, Mollison J et al. Clomifene citrate or unstimulated intrauterine insemination compared with expectant management for unexplained infertility: pragmatic randomized controlled trial. *BMJ* 2008;337:a716.

45 Maheshwari A, Fowler P, Bhattacharya S. Assessment of ovarian reserve – should we perform tests of ovarian reserve routinely? *Hum Reprod* 2006;21:2729–2735.

Chapter 46
Assisted Reproduction

Geoffrey Trew and Stuart Lavery
Hammersmith Hospital, London, UK

Introduction

Assisted conception is the facilitation of natural conception by some form of scientific intervention. It has been available for many years, but one of the first recorded and possibly best known instances of assisted conception was that performed by the eminent surgeon John Hunter, in London in 1785. The husband, in this infertile couple, had hypospadias, and artificial insemination of ejaculated sperm was performed on his wife. This resulted in a successful pregnancy and subsequent birth. This basic assisted conception continued until scientific techniques improved in the middle of the twentieth century. The advent of improved techniques, particularly in the form of ovulation induction and controlled ovarian stimulation, has allowed the successful treatment of the anovulatory female. The purification and use of human menopausal gonadotrophins (hMGs) in the 1960s led to multiple follicular development allowing *in vitro* fertilization (IVF). Over the last 40 years there have been dramatic improvements in the treatment of the infertile female as well as the male. There is now a full panoply of techniques with abbreviations ranging from the more well known such as IUI (intrauterine insemination), IVF, ICSI (intracytoplasmic sperm injection) and PGD (preimplantation genetic diagnosis), through to ones that have now become more esoteric because of their low success rates, such as DOT (direct oocyte transfer), PROST (pronuclear stage transfer) and even DIPI (direct intraperitoneal insemination; Table 46.1). With these advances it is possible to treat the vast majority of subfertile men and women successfully and give them the child they so desire.

Investigations prior to assisted conception

Even though the diagnosis may have been made and the most appropriate form of treatment decided upon, there are a few essential investigations that should be performed prior to any form of assisted conception. These will not only ensure the best results when the assisted conception is performed, but also reduce the chance of any diagnosis being missed before multiple cycles are embarked upon with the subsequent emotional and financial cost to the patient if they are unsuccessful.

> **Summary box 46.1**
>
> Investigations prior to assisted reproduction:
> - Hormone profile: AMH, FSH, E2 (measurement of ovarian reserve), progesterone (check of ovulation)
> - Semen analysis
> - Pelvic ultrasound
> - Evaluation of uterine cavity and fallopian tubes: HSG, laparoscopy and hysteroscopy

Female

Tests of ovarian reserve have been utilized for many years – previously an early follicular phase follicle-stimulating hormone (FSH) level was used and is still the mainstay in most countries. The use of a relatively new blood test, anti-Müllerian hormone (AMH), is now more widespread and gives a more accurate assessment of the ovarian reserve. It has better intra- and intercycle variability and has a better correlation to ovarian response to supraovulation and success rates than any other test. Indeed, it is often used to assess the patient's suitability for techniques such as IVF prior to treatment. A very low level of <3 pmol/L would suggest a live birth rate of <2%, and hence IVF using the patient's own eggs would rarely be successful. Conversely, a high level (>50 pmol/L) would suggest very sensitive ovaries and a higher chance of developing ovarian hyperstimulation syndrome (OHSS) if the dose of FSH is not reduced.

Most forms of assisted conception, excluding egg donation, require normal ovarian reserve to have any significant chance of success. If the patient has irregular periods, then prolactin, thyroid function and, if appropri-

Dewhurst's Textbook of Obstetrics & Gynaecology, Eighth Edition. Edited by D. Keith Edmonds.
© 2012 John Wiley and Sons, Ltd. Published 2012 by John Wiley and Sons, Ltd.

Table 46.1 Assisted contraception abbreviations.

Abbreviation	Definition
IVF	*In vitro* fertilization
IUI	Intrauterine insemination
ICSI	Intracytoplasmic sperm injection
PGD	Preimplantation genetic diagnosis
PGS	Preimplantation genetic screening
DOT	Direct oocyte transfer
PROST	Pronuclear stage transfer
DIPI	Direct intraperitoneal insemination
MESA	Microepididymal sperm aspiration
PESA	Percutaneous epididymal sperm aspiration
TESE	Testicular sperm extraction
GIFT	Gamete intrafallopian transfer

ate, testosterone and sex hormone-binding globulin (SHBG) levels should also be performed.

If the patient is undergoing a licensed form of assisted conception, under the 1990 Human Fertilisation and Embryology Act, then both the male and female partner have to be screened for hepatitis B, hepatitis C and human immunodeficiency virus (HIV). If either partner is positive for these conditions this does not preclude them from being treated, but unless specific embryo cryopreservation facilities are available freezing of surplus embryos cannot be performed because of the theoretical risk of cross-infection between the patients' embryos and unaffected embryos from other patients.

Ultrasound

Virtually all ultrasound scanning in assisted conception is performed transvaginally. The initial scan assesses several areas: (i) the ovarian morphology – if there are underlying polycystic ovaries, they may be hyper-responsive to stimulation with gonadotrophins; (ii) the presence of ovarian cysts – if present, suitable treatment should be arranged; (iii) many centres now also measure the ovarian volumes as well as the antral follicle count as these are also used in the dose calculation of FSH for the stimulation phase of IVF; (iv) the ovaries are assessed for accessibility, not just for the monitoring itself but also if transvaginal oocyte retrieval (TVOR) is planned, to ensure that this can be performed without undue difficulty. Sometimes patients who have abdominal adhesions [from iatrogenic causes, previous pelvic inflammatory disease (PID) or endometriosis] then gentle abdominal pressure can be applied during the screening ultrasound to ensure that the ovary can be moved down to a more accessible position for egg collection; (v) the uterus is also assessed for the presence of abnormalities, such as uterine fibroids, to make sure the endometrium appears normal and there are no other abnormalities; and (vi) the rest of the pelvis

is also screened in a systematic fashion to exclude other pathology.

Uterine cavity and tubal patency

Both the uterine cavity and the fallopian tubes should be examined prior to all forms of assisted conception. For techniques such as IUI, in which either one or both fallopian tubes are required to be patent, it is obvious why both the cavity and the tubes should be checked. Less obviously, the fallopian tubes require inspection for techniques such as IVF, even though they are not required for the actual procedure. Grade A evidence [1] suggests that the presence of hydrosalpinges can significantly reduce the implantation rate due to reflux of the hydrosalpingeal fluid into the uterine cavity (see p. 580). The integrity of the uterine cavity should be evaluated as various forms of pathology ranging from intrauterine adhesions, congenital abnormalities such as large septate uterus, submucous fibroids and intrauterine polyps can all significantly reduce the implantation rate and hence the subsequent live birth rate, from all forms of assisted conception. If a significant problem is noted in the uterine cavity, this should be corrected prior to the assisted conception cycles being performed. The uterine cavity and the fallopian tubes can be investigated by the following means.

Hysterosalpingography

Hysterosalpingography (HSG) has been used for many decades but has a reputation for being painful. With newer techniques, and in particular the advent of suction caps and small balloon catheters, the need for unnecessary trauma is obviated. It allows assessment of both the uterine cavity and the fallopian tubes and it is an extremely useful screening test that can be performed with a high degree of accuracy without the need for a general anaesthetic. It is recommended that chlamydial screening is performed beforehand, preferably as part of the initial work-up of the female partner, and antibiotic cover for the procedure should be used.

Hysterocontrast sonography

There have been several ultrasound techniques developed to try to assess tubal patency, the most commonly used being Echovist®. This is an echogenic fluid instilled inside the uterine cavity and down the fallopian tubes, which can be tracked by ultrasound. This can be a good method for assessing tubal patency, but owing to the high echogenicity of the fluid, it can sometimes miss the uterine cavity lesions such as intrauterine adhesions and subtle distortions by submucous fibroids [2].

Laparoscopy and hysteroscopy

These are commonly performed infertility investigations used particularly if the patient has other presenting complaints, notably pelvic pain.

If a screening test such as hysterosalpingogram has been performed and an intrauterine lesion found, then hysteroscopy would also be performed and, if the diagnosis is confirmed, the lesion is then removed. For example, if there are intrauterine adhesions, these can be divided hysteroscopically, or a submucous fibroid can be resected by transcervical resection of this fibroid.

Male partner

A comprehensive semen analysis should be performed on all males referred for assisted conception to ascertain the most appropriate technique suitable for the patient. Most assisted conception units not only look at the normal World Health Organization (WHO) sperm criteria, but also perform sperm function tests to assess the best way to use the sperm – generally IVF if the parameters are good and ICSI if there is a severe problem. The presence of other problems, such as antisperm antibodies within the ejaculate, are also ascertained and, if present, further samples can be obtained with the patient ejaculating directly into culture medium to try to lessen the impact of these antibodies on sperm function. This can sometimes mean that a sample severely affected by antisperm antibodies deemed suitable only for IVF can sometimes be 'upgraded' to techniques such as IUI if ejaculation into medium is performed.

Important coexistent pathologies

There are several other coexistent pathologies that can significantly reduce the successful outcome of assisted conception or increase the complication rate from it.

Uterine fibroids

Uterine fibroids are commonly picked up by transvaginal scanning of the infertile woman. It has always been difficult to ascertain the causality of these fibroids pertaining to the patient's infertile status. The presence of fibroids does not necessarily mean there is a direct causative link between the fibroids and infertility. On the other hand, there are a number of reported case series where removal of fibroids resulted in subsequent improved conception rates between 30% and 80% [3]. It was previously thought that fibroids only significantly reduced implantation rates if the uterine cavity was distorted. There are two series looking at the effect on implantation in IVF cycles of fibroids in other locations. In the first, Eldar-Geva et al. [4] showed that intramural fibroids significantly reduced implantation rates; this was then confirmed by Hart et al. [5]. Both of these studies confirmed the impact of fibroids that do not distort the uterine cavity, but this appears to be only for fibroids larger than 3 cm. Therefore, any patient who has fibroids larger than 3 cm, and in particular who have recurrent implantation failures, should be considered for myomectomy prior to further assisted conception. Although there does appear to be an impact on the removal of fibroids on implantation rates, Surrey et al.

[3], in a randomized trial, failed to demonstrate improved live birth rates.

Hydrosalpinges

There have been several studies that have shown the adverse effect of hydrosalpinges on IVF outcome. Indeed, three randomized controlled trials were included in the Cochrane review [6] to see if salpingectomy would be useful for patients with hydrosalpinges prior to undergoing IVF. Surgical treatment of these hydrosalpinges versus non-surgical treatment increased the odds of live birth plus ongoing pregnancy [odds ratio (OR) 2.13; 95% confidence interval (CI) 1.24–3.65] and of pregnancy (OR 1.75; 95% CI 1.07–2.86). It has now been shown that removal of these diseased tubes by salpingectomy prior to IVF leads to implantation rates that would be expected in patients unaffected with hydrosalpinges. Whether these hydrosalpinges are removed or blocked in the proximal portion (by clipping or coagulation) will depend on several factors, such as degree of damage and whether the patient has pain associated with the hydrosalpinges. Salpingectomy used to be the routine but more units are now coagulating the proximal portion because of the concern that salpingectomy may compromise ovarian vasculature and reduce subsequent response to stimulation [7]. Most practitioners would individualize the treatment of hydrosalpinges and take all other variable parameters into consideration, ranging from any male factor present through to the degree of tubal disease, as well as the known ovarian function of the patient prior to removing them.

Polycystic ovaries

Polycystic ovaries as seen by ultrasound are an extremely common finding in women of childbearing age and can occur in ~30% of patients. Patients with polycystic ovaries can be more difficult to stimulate with gonadotrophins for either IUI or IVF. Initially there can be a degree of resistance at lower doses, but then a very narrow therapeutic window before the patient hyperstimulates, and this can quite often lead to cycle cancellation. In view of the severe complications resulting from OHSS, one should always start with a low dose and increase in small increments until the appropriate therapeutic window is achieved. Some have advocated the use of laparoscopic ovarian drilling to try to improve this therapeutic window, as well as the precycle treatment of all insulin-sensitizing agents such as metformin. There is now evidence that metformin does not improve the success rate but can improve the safety of the cycle [8].

Endometriotic cysts

Endometriosis is a common coexistent pathology in patients undergoing assisted conception. Whereas there has been no suggestion of improvement in assisted conception cycles by treating peritoneal endometriosis, there can be a benefit to treating large endometriomas prior to IVF. It is thought this may benefit the cycle in several ways including the ovarian response itself and overall number of eggs obtained (particularly in the ovary containing the endometrioma). The second concern with ovarian endometriomas is that these can be inadvertently punctured during TVOR and there is a significant risk of ovarian abscess formation if this occurs. Precycle drainage by needle aspiration can also give a significant rate of ovarian abscesses and this is generally not advised. If the ovarian endometrioma is felt to be a significant size that it may adversely affect the cycle or there is a significant chance of inadvertent needling, then it is better for these to be surgically treated prior to the initiation of the cycle. Prolonged downregulation with gonadotrophin-releasing hormone (GnRH) analogues can shrink the cysts but this may make it more difficult to stimulate the ovaries.

Smoking

Patients should be advised to stop smoking as this significantly reduces the effectiveness of all forms of assisted conception.

Obesity

It is recommended that a patient should have a body mass index (BMI) of between 19 and 30. Outside this range, success rates of assisted conception are reduced. If the BMI is above 30, not only are success rates lower, but miscarriage rates higher and the incidence of complications such as OHSS is also increased.

Types of assisted conception

There are many types of assisted conception available ranging from less invasive procedures such as IUI to the widely known IVF, with or without ICSI. The use of other procedures such as gamete intrafallopian transfer (GIFT) has reduced because of the improving success rates of IVF. Other techniques associated with assisted conception cycles such as preimplantation genetic diagnosis (PGD) and preimplantation genetic screening (PGS) are also performed in a few specialized centres.

Intrauterine insemination

Intrauterine insemination (IUI) consists of a prepared sample of sperm (normally produced by masturbation) being placed into the uterine cavity using a cannula, at the appropriate time of the patient's menstrual cycle. Approximately 2 weeks later a pregnancy test is performed to see if the cycle has been successful.

Protocols

Intrauterine insemination can be performed in a natural cycle with Clomid® alone, with Clomid followed by FSH injection or purely with FSH. If any form of ovulation induction has been used, it is normal practice to use a single human chorionic gonadotrophin (hCG) injection approximately 36 h prior to the insemination to ensure optimal timing with ovulation.

Monitoring

Although for unstimulated cycles it is possible to do urinary luteinizing hormone (LH) monitoring by home dipstick methods, this does not give the best success rates. If any form of ovulation induction has been used, more accurate monitoring is performed. This is normally follicle tracking using transvaginal ultrasound and has the benefit of not only deciding the best time to give the dose of hCG and hence the timing of the insemination, but also ensuring that the ovulation induction is having the desired effect, that is one (or at most two) developing follicle(s) over 18 mm. If there are more than two follicles, this can be detected by the ultrasound; the cycle should be cancelled and the patient advised against having unprotected intercourse due to the increased risk of higher order multiple pregnancies.

Success rates increase from unstimulated IUI through to stimulation with Clomid and FSH. The overall success rate, as with any subfertile couple, depends on multiple factors, most importantly female age and, with IUI, the quality of the sperm. Though IUI can be used for mild male factor problems, it is not recommended for more severe problems. Success rates of around 5% per cycle have been quoted for unstimulated IUI, increasing to 8–10% for stimulation with Clomid and 12–18% per cycle when FSH is used in the protocol. Although success rates of 35% have been quoted in the literature, these tend to be highly selective series and do not necessarily represent a general case mix of patients across a wider age range [9].

Complications

The main complication of IUI occurs when FSH has been used and this is higher order multiple births. Most centres would expect a twinning rate of between 10% and 15% and a triplet rate of less than 1%. If the triplet rate is higher than 1%, and in particular if there are even higher numbers than this, then this is normally due to inadequate monitoring and inadequate numbers of cycles being cancelled when an over-response of the ovaries has been seen.

Although ovarian hyperstimulation can occur, particularly in the protocols where FSH is used, this would normally be mild to moderate, and it is very unusual to get a case of severe hyperstimulation in IUI cycles. If this happens it tends to be when an inappropriate starting dose of FSH has been used and again when inadequate monitoring has been performed.

The patient should also be warned about the possibility of ectopic pregnancies, and most clinics would offer an early ultrasound scan to patients who have had a positive pregnancy test, at between 6 and 7 weeks' gestation.

Advantages

Intrauterine insemination is a relatively simple technique that is cost-effective and can be offered by both secondary and tertiary fertility centres. It is not as invasive as IVF and allows fertilization to occur within the fallopian tubes, and therefore it is generally acceptable to most religious groups.

Disadvantages

The success rates for IUI are lower than those for IVF, and if the cycle fails less information is obtained than would be with an IVF cycle – particularly pertaining to possible egg or subsequent embryo quality. It also requires at least one healthy fallopian tube and reasonable sperm parameters. If monitoring is suboptimal then there can be a significant increase in higher order multiple births with the expected sequelae of these.

Indications

- Unexplained infertility.
- Mild male factor.
- Ejaculatory problems.
- Cervical problems.
- Ovulatory disorders.
- Mild endometriosis.
- To optimize the use of donor sperm.

In vitro fertilization

In vitro fertilization involves surgical removal of the mature oocyte from the ovary and fertilization by sperm in the laboratory. The world's first successful IVF baby was delivered by Patrick Steptoe in 1978 after a number of years collaborating with Robert Edwards. Over the last 25 years, the success rates and types of IVF have greatly improved and at present there are over 2 million babies born throughout the world by this technique.

Indications

- Severe tubal disease – tubal blockages.
- Severe endometriosis.
- Moderate male factor.
- Unexplained infertility.
- Unsuccessful IUI.

Summary box 46.2

Stages of *in vitro* fertilization:
- Pituitary downregulation.
- Ovarian stimulation.
- hCG trigger.
- Oocyte retrieval.
- Fertilization (insemination or ICSI).
- Embryo culture.
- Embryo transfer.
- Luteal support.

Protocols

Initially, simple forms of ovulation induction using Clomid and hMGs were used. Over the last 20 years protocols have been refined and these are now broken down into three main categories:
1. natural cycle;
2. long protocol – agonist cycles; and
3. short protocol – antagonist cycles.

Although there are other short protocols using agonists, these are now less frequently used because of their poorer success rates.

Agonist cycles

Long protocols are still at present the most widely used protocols throughout the world. They involve the use of a GnRH agonist that can be taken nasally on a daily basis (e.g. buserelin, nafarelin) or daily subcutaneous injection (e.g. buserelin, leuprorelin) or in a depot preparation (goserelin, leuprorelin). The agonist is given continuously and initially increases the production of gonadotrophins (FSH and LH) from the pituitary gland. If this continuous administration is maintained then the so-called downregulation effect on the GnRH receptors is achieved. This causes a reduction in LH and FSH levels and with this a reduction in stimulation of the ovary. As a result, folliculogenesis is suppressed and blood oestradiol levels fall to menopausal levels within 3 weeks. As long as the agonists are continued then the ovary is suppressed unless exogenous gonadotrophins are given.

The start of agonist administration can be on either day 2 of the preceding menstrual cycle or, more commonly, day 21.

The rationale behind using these long protocols is to create a temporary menopause from which the ovaries can then be stimulated by the daily use of FSH/hMG injections.

In a mid-luteal start (normally around day 21), the patient is reviewed when her period starts (approximately 7–10 days after the agonist is initiated). A scan and often a blood oestradiol level are performed to ensure that the patient is adequately suppressed. If this is the case, then exogenous gonadotrophins are started the following day and continued until an adequate ovarian response is gained.

Early follicular, or day 2, can also be used and the patient brought back for her scan and blood test, on average 2 weeks later, to see if she is suppressed. As in the luteal start, if adequate suppression is obtained, then exogenous gonadotrophins are started and then continued until satisfactory ovarian response is obtained.

Antagonist protocols

Antagonists (ganirelix and cetrorelix) have been in use for the last 5 years. The antagonist has an almost immediate effect on the pituitary and, unlike agonists, does not need several days to achieve menopausal levels of the pituitary derived gonadotrophins. Therefore, the patient is prevented from having a premature LH surge and ovulating within an hour of the start of the antagonist. A daily dose of 0.25 mg is normally given and there is also a 3 mg dose of Cetrorelix, which can last for several days. The drugs are given subcutaneously and are started either on a fixed day of FSH stimulation (normally on the fifth day) or when the lead follicle is a certain size by ultrasound monitoring (normally 14 mm). The antagonists are continued alongside the gonadotrophin stimulation until an adequate response is achieved and then stopped prior to the hCG injection.

The benefits of antagonists over agonists are:
- no menopausal side-effects;
- no cyst formation from the initial gonadotrophin surge;
- shorter cycle duration; and
- less gonadotrophin required in each cycle, and thus lower drug costs.

Monitoring

It is essential that adequate monitoring is performed during stimulation of the ovaries with exogenous gonadotrophins. Serial transvaginal ultrasounds to assess the follicular growth should be used. A decreasing number of units continue to use serial oestradiol levels to add to the information obtained from the ultrasound. The use of serial oestradiol can be useful in some patient groups, particularly if an under- or over-response is anticipated. An under-response can sometimes be anticipated in the older patient or the patient with previously raised FSH levels. An over-response can sometimes be anticipated if there has been a previous over-response or if the patient has a polycystic ovarian morphology on her initial diagnostic ultrasound. There seems to be no value in routine oestradiol monitoring.

Monitoring during the stimulatory phase allows the dose to be increased or decreased, if appropriate, as well as to allow timing of the hCG injection.

Human chorionic gonadotrophin injection

This is used to induce final maturation of the oocytes prior to the oocyte retrieval. Generally, 10 000 units of urinary hCG is used, although in patients with an over-response this can be decreased to 5000 units. If recombinant hCG is used, the usual dose is 150 µg given subcutaneously in a prefilled pen.

Human chorionic gonadotrophin should be given when either one or two lead follicles have reached 18 mm. The injection is normally given around midnight to allow for oocyte retrieval approximately 34 h later prior to physiological ovulation occurring. If the hCG injection is incorrectly administered then very few or no eggs will be obtained at the egg collection itself.

Oocyte retrieval

Originally, this was done laparoscopically, but with the advent of real-time ultrasound this allowed a less invasive oocyte retrieval by ultrasound-directed needling of the ovaries. Smaller and better quality ultrasound probes, particularly with the advent of transvaginal scanning, has allowed both the monitoring of the ovary during stimulation and the actual retrieval itself to be done transvaginally. Virtually all oocyte retrievals are performed by this transvaginal ultrasound-directed route. The laparoscopic route is still occasionally used if the ovaries are inaccessible transvaginally. This can occur in frozen pelvises or when the ovaries have been moved out of the pelvis prior to pelvic irradiation.

Transvaginal egg (oocyte) retrievals (TVORs) can be performed under general anaesthesia or, more commonly these days, local anaesthesia and some form of intravenous sedation. The procedure generally takes 20–30 min, depending on how many follicles are present. A single-use disposable needle is inserted under ultrasound control directly into the follicles of one ovary and the fluid aspirated and given directly to the embryologist. If the egg is not found after all the fluid has been aspirated, then the follicle is flushed and reaspirated to try to find the egg, as well as using gentle needle agitation (Fig. 46.1). After all the follicles have been exhausted from one ovary, the needle is then withdrawn and reinserted under ultrasound control into the other ovary, and the process repeated. After the ultrasound probe is removed, the vaginal vault is checked for bleeding and although usually not a problem, occasionally an absorbable suture has to be inserted under direct vision for a specific bleeding point. Most patients go home a few hours after the procedure has finished.

Embryo transfer

Eggs are fertilized either by routine insemination with a concentration of approximately 100 000 normally motile sperm per millilitre or by ICSI (see p. 586). They are incubated in a commercially prepared culture medium under strict laboratory conditions. The temperature is carefully controlled within the incubators, as are the gas content, humidity and pH.

Traditionally, most embryos are transferred at day 2 following egg collection. There is increasing evidence that, at the blastocyst stage, if embryos are left in extended culture conditions and transferred on day 5, higher pregnancy rates can be achieved [10]. Approximately 55–60% of all mature eggs fertilize normally and these are graded by the embryologist on day 2 (Fig. 46.2). At present, the guidelines in the UK from the Human Fertilisation and Embryology Authority (HFEA) state that only two embryos should be transferred in people under the age of 40, unless exceptional circumstances are present, but over the age of 40 three embryos can be transferred. In other

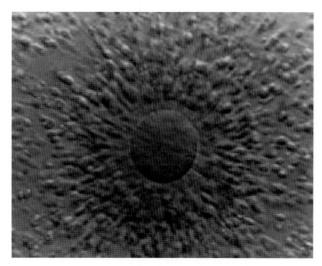

Fig. 46.1 Human oocyte with cumulus cells.

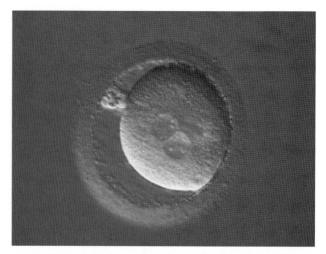

Fig. 46.2 Human embryo 2 pronuclear (PN) stage day 1 – normal fertilization.

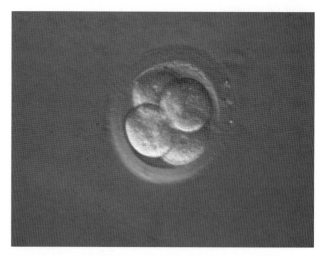

Fig. 46.3 Four cell stage – day 2.

countries, there is less regulation; in the USA, it would not be unusual for between three and five embryos to be transferred, depending on the age of the patient. On the other hand, in some Scandinavian countries, if the patient is aged ≥35 years, then she is moving towards elective single embryo transfer to reduce the incidence of twins or triplets. Although this would have a slight decrease in success rates, the other normal embryos are frozen and, hence, if a cycle is unsuccessful the patient can undergo repeated single embryo transfers from frozen embryo replacement cycles. Evidence from elective single embryo transfer programmes in Scandinavia and Belgium have shown that twin rates can be virtually eliminated while maintaining acceptable overall pregnancy rates [11]. Regulatory bodies in the UK are now encouraging the use of elective single embryo transfer in selected patients (usually women older than 36 years of age in their first treatment cycle).

The benefits of a day 2 transfer are that a single-stage culture medium can be used and that the majority of normal embryos survive to this stage. After two or three embryos have been replaced, there may be surplus embryos of a satisfactory quality that are suitable for cryopreservation. The potential downside of a day 2 transfer is that in a normal menstrual cycle the day 2 embryo is still in the fallopian tube and not in the uterine cavity, and so the environment for embryo development is not ideal. The grading system utilized by the embryologist is not totally accurate, and therefore it can sometimes be difficult to judge the best two embryos – out of potentially six or seven – to transfer fresh. The benefit of a day 5, or blastocyst, transfer is that the embryo has been replaced when it would physiologically be in the uterine cavity – this may have some benefits regarding certain growth factors that can improve embryo development. Blastocyst transfer also allows better selection of the embryos as the majority of abnormal embryos perish

between day 2 and day 5 (Figs 46.3–46.6). However, even in the best cycles there are quite often only two, or sometimes three, blastocysts left after 5 days of culture. The downside of blastocyst transfer is that it requires a two-stage culture medium as the blastocyst metabolic requirements change after day 2 and that there are generally fewer embryos remaining that would be suitable for freezing. The other potential downside is that all of the embryos may perish before day 5 and hence the patient may have nothing to transfer at all. It is for this reason that the majority of centres will perform a blastocyst transfer only if the patient has sufficient numbers of good-quality embryos. Embryo transfer is performed without any anaesthetic. A Cusco's speculum is generally used to visualize the cervix, which is cleaned carefully, and a sterile, single-use embryo transfer catheter is carefully inserted through the cervical canal. Where in the uterine cavity the embryos should be placed is a topic of great debate, but it is not uncommon for them to be

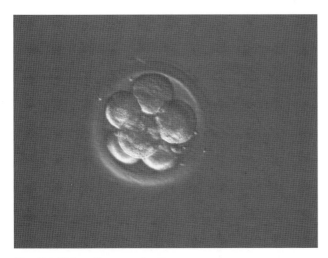

Fig. 46.4 Eight cell stage – day 3.

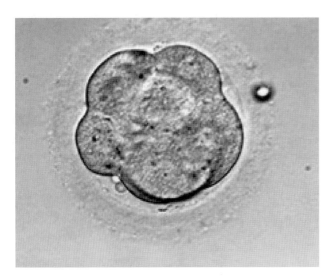

Fig. 46.5 Morula – day 4.

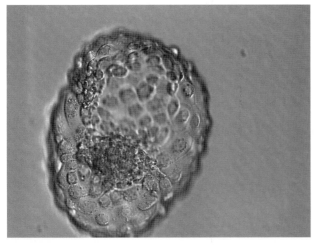

Fig. 46.6 Blastocyst – day 5.

placed in the mid-cavity portion and generally for insertion of the catheter to be stopped before the fundus because it could potentially cause some slight trauma and bleeding. Evidence suggests that embryo transfer should be performed under ultrasound guidance as this allows more accurate placement of the embryos in the uterine cavity and has been shown to significantly improve success rates [12]. After the outer sheath has been inserted in the correct location, an inner catheter containing the embryos is inserted. When it is in the correct position, a very small aliquot of fluid is used to emit the embryos from the end of the catheter. The inner catheter is then removed and handed back to the embryologists to confirm that no embryos have been retained in the inner catheter. If the catheter is empty, then the outer sheath is gently withdrawn and the speculum removed.

Although there is no evidence that the embryos can 'fall out', not surprisingly many patients are very cautious at this stage and quite often are allowed to rest in a supine position for any time up to 2 hours before leaving the hospital. There has been no evidence that leaving patients in a supine position increases pregnancy rates, but it may help the patients psychologically.

Luteal phase support

With modern assisted conception, utilizing either agonist or antagonist protocols, some form of luteal phase support (LPS) is generally thought necessary. Although natural-cycle IVF does not need this, superovulation may impair normal corpus luteal function, and the use of LPS has been shown to improve success rates [13]. The use of LPS with antagonist cycles is more debatable, but pregnancy rates without it are generally thought to be significantly lower [14]. LPS is broadly divided into two types – the use of luteotropic preparations, such as hCG, and the use of progestogens or progesterone. hCG is given by a subcutaneous injection in small aliquots that stimulates the patient's own ovaries to produce more progesterone. It has been shown to be as efficacious as progesterone, but it does require an injection and also increases the risk of ovarian hyperstimulation syndrome in some patients.

The use of progesterone is more common and it can be given as tablets, injections, a vaginal gel or vaginal pessaries/rectal suppositories. Intravaginal or rectal use of progesterone achieves extremely good tissue levels very rapidly. LPS should be given for a minimum of 2 weeks, but some clinics routinely offer it up to 12 weeks or even later. However, there is no evidence that continuing it beyond 2 weeks significantly improves pregnancy rates. The minimum dose required is 200 mg per day, but the most commonly prescribed dose is 400–800 mg a day.

Pregnancy test

The wait between the embryos being replaced and the pregnancy test is the most psychologically stressful time for the majority of patients. Some patients start bleeding prior to the pregnancy test, although it is not unusual for the progesterone to delay this bleeding even if they are not pregnant. Generally, pregnancy tests are performed around 12 days after the embryo transfer and can be performed either at home with a urinary pregnancy test or at the clinic with a serum pregnancy test. A home pregnancy test is obviously more convenient, and the newly available kits have excellent sensitivity. If the pregnancy test is positive and in the normal range, then it is usual to offer the patient a transvaginal scan 2–3 weeks later to ensure that the pregnancy is intrauterine and also to assess its viability. If the initial hCG level is low, then this is often repeated 48h later to assess the rise, and, if it is suboptimal, then the possibility of an ectopic pregnancy or miscarriage has to be considered.

Results

In 2007 around 1.5% of all births and 1.8% of all babies in the UK were a result of IVF or donor insemination. The latest trends in assisted conception treatment in the UK are demonstrated in Table 46.2. It can be seen that over the most recent 3 years of available data, the number of treatment cycles and patients treated continues to increase. At the same time, pregnancy rates are improving while multiple pregnancy rates are not showing the same rate of increase. The most important factor influencing pregnancy success by IVF is female age (see Table 46.3, which shows the most recent data from the HFEA for treatment in the UK). Male age, in comparison, has very little impact. The two adverse factors that patients can influence themselves are smoking and obesity (see National Institute for Health and Clinical Excellence guidelines; futher reading).

Intracytoplasmic sperm injection

Intracytoplasmic sperm injection is when an individual, morphologically normal, sperm is immobilized by 'striking' the tail injected into a mature oocyte that has had its surrounded cumulus and corona cells removed. An inverted microscope with a heated stage and micromanipulating equipment (Fig. 46.7) are used. The oocyte is carefully positioned using a holding pipette under gentle suction. A very sharp glass injecting pipette is slowly inserted to rupture the oolemma and the immobilized sperm is injected into the oocyte with a very small volume of the medium. The injecting pipette is then carefully removed and the oocyte incubated under the usual stringent laboratory conditions.

Indications
- Severe male factor infertility including azoospermia and subsequent surgical sperm retrieval by, for example, microepididymal sperm aspiration (MESA), testicular sperm extraction (TESE) or percutaneous epididymal sperm aspiration (PESA).
- Severe oligoasthenoteratozoospermia.
- Poor or total non-fertilization from previous IVF cycles.
- Preimplantation genetic diagnosis cycles.

Most IVF units would have approximately 40–60% of their total IVF cycles using ICSI. Studies have been performed to determine if ICSI with normal sperm improves pregnancy rates, but there is no evidence for this strategy [15].

Results

Pregnancy rates of 36.5% per transfer are reported [16] with live birth rates of 30.4% per transfer in over 28 800 cycles.

Table 46.2 Latest trends in *in vitro* fertilization in the UK.

	2005	2006	2007	% change 2006–2007
Number of IVF cycles	41 932	44 275	46 829	Up 5.8%
Number of patients	32 626	34 855	36 861	Up 5.8%
Number of babies born	11 262 babies from 9058 births	12 596 babies from 10 242 births	13 672 babies from 11 091 births	Babies up 8.5% Births up 8.3%
Live birth rate/cycle started	21.6%	23.1%	23.7%	Up 0.6%
Multiple birth rate	24%	22.7%	23%	Up 0.3%

Table 46.3 *In vitro* fertilization success rates by age in the UK for 2007 using fresh and frozen embryos.

	Number of patients	Number of births	LBR < 35	LBR 35–37	LBR 38–39	LBR 40–42	LBR 43–44	LBR > 44
Fresh	30 435	9011	32.3%	27.7%	19.2%	11.9%	3.4%	3.1%
Frozen	7489	1534	20.4%	19%	16.3%	12.5%	10.8%	12.5%

LBR, live birth rate/cycle started.

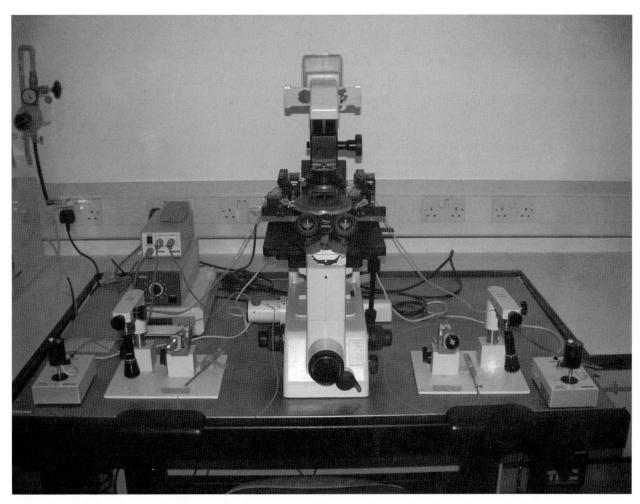

Fig. 46.7 Intracytoplasmic sperm injection micromanipulator.

Safety

Intracytoplasmic sperm injection has been in clinical use since the early 1990s, and results of the follow-up studies are generally reassuring. The current recommendations are that any male who has sperm parameters that require ICSI should be offered screening for karyotype. Some centres also advocate the use of Y chromosome microdeletion screening, although this is not routinely offered. Cystic fibrosis screening is essential in cases of azoospermia, particularly if it is related to the condition of congenital bilateral absence of the vas deferens, as a significant proportion of these patients will be carriers of the cystic fibrosis mutations. Being a carrier does not preclude them being treated as a couple, but the female partner is then offered screening, and if she is also found to be a carrier, then the couple should be referred for consideration of IVF – ICSI with PGD.

If all the above results are normal, then the patients should be counselled carefully that there is a slight increase in genetic abnormalities of the offspring. Most of these abnormalities are thought to be minor and the major congenital malformation rate is thought to be similar to that of the general population.

Gamete intrafallopian tube transfer

Gamete intrafallopian tube transfer was first used around 1984. and here the eggs are collected laparoscopically, identified by the embryologist and then placed back in the fallopian tube, again laparoscopically, with a small aliquot of specially prepared highly motile sperm. The use of GIFT reached a peak in the early 1990s and has diminished thereafter.

Advantages

Gamete intrafallopian tube transfer was initially developed to increase the availability of assisted conception because of the scarcity of suitable laboratory facilities and embryological skills. As the eggs did not have to be cultured outside the body, few of the usual laboratory facilities were needed. It appears to be very physiologically sound as both the egg and sperm are in the appropriate environment at the appropriate time. The embryo travels physiologically down into the uterine cavity, and hence there is no disruption of the endometrial environment, as there would be with normal embryo transfer from IVF.

Disadvantages

Gamete intrafallopian tube transfer is more invasive than IVF because a laparoscope is used to replace the embryos and sperm through the fimbrial end of the fallopian tube. The eggs are generally collected by transvaginal egg collection as it has been shown that more eggs are obtained by this route. As part of good clinical practice, only a limited number of eggs are replaced, even though it is not known whether these will fertilize normally by the sperm that is added. Therefore, less information is obtained than with an IVF cycle. At least one fallopian tube should be healthy. Normal sperm parameters are also optimal, although GIFT can be used in cases of mild male factor disease.

The place of GIFT in today's society is often debated and its routine use is now very limited. Most European centres would use it only in cases where IVF is not allowed for religious reasons. As conception occurs within the body, GIFT is often acceptable even though IVF is not. In some cases of totally unexplained infertility, where there has been repeated IUI and IVF failures, GIFT may also have a small place.

Success rates

Success rates vary enormously depending on patient selection, but in appropriate circumstances they can be 30% live birth per transfer [14]. Apart from a few enthusiasts, the use of GIFT in most large clinics accounts for less than 0.5% of all their assisted reproductive technology (ART) cycles.

Frozen embryo replacement cycle (FERC)

The first pregnancy resulting from a frozen human embryo was in 1985 and since then the use of frozen cycles has increased dramatically. Freezing surplus morphologically normal embryos allows the use of those embryos which otherwise may have been wasted. Normally embryos are frozen on day 2 after the selected ones have been replaced fresh, but can be frozen any time from day 1 through to day 5 if excess blastocysts are obtained. The use of day 1 freezing is normally confined to elective freezing of all embryos when there is a high risk of ovarian hyperstimulation syndrome occurring. At day 2 any morphologically normal embryos of suitable quality are selected and, through specific cryopreservation protocols, are frozen and stored in liquid nitrogen in specially monitored tanks. The success rates of day 1 and day 2 embryos are cited as 20.4% live birth rate per transfer [16]. The success rates of frozen blastocyst cycles are still suboptimal, although work is ongoing at present to improve the cryoprotectants used as well as the actual programmes for preservation.

Transfer of frozen embryos

There are two main ways to transfer frozen embryos: first, replace them in a spontaneous menstrual cycle or, second, suppress the patient's own menstrual cycle with GnRH agonists and then supplement with oestrogen to thicken the endometrium prior to embryo replacement.

Natural cycle

The patient has to have regular menstrual cycles for this to be a feasible option. The patient's cycle is monitored by serial ultrasound scan as well as hormone profiling, including oestradiol and LH measurement. As long as there are no adverse factors noted on these measurements, the embryos are thawed and replaced approximately 3 days after the LH surge has been detected. Approximately two-thirds of all frozen embryos survive the thaw process, and, depending on the age of the patient, two or three embryos are replaced. No luteal phase support is required as the ovaries are not downregulated, and sufficient natural progesterone is produced from the patient's own corpus luteum.

Suppressed cycles

The majority of FERCs are with suppressed cycles as these give better control and results. A GnRH agonist is used to suppress the patient's menstrual cycle and is normally started on day 21. If the patient is menopausal then this is not required and only oestrogen supplementation is used. After adequate suppression has been achieved then hormone supplementation in the form of oestrogen is used. This is generally an increasing regime with either tablets or patches until sufficient endometrial thickness has been achieved (preferably around 9 mm). The embryos are replaced in a similar fashion to IVF and, owing to ovarian suppression, LPS is required. If the patient is pregnant this is continued up to approximately 12 weeks of pregnancy.

Virtually all IVF units should have a frozen embryo replacement programme and it is generally accepted not only as a safe and effective means of treatment but also one that is cost beneficial, maximizing the use of the patient's fresh cycle.

Egg donation

Oocyte donation involves a donor oocyte obtained from a fresh IVF cycle from a suitable screened donor, which is fertilized with the recipient's partner's sperm. The fertilized embryo is re-placed into the recipient. The first successful pregnancy from an egg donation cycle was in 1983.

Procedure

Unfertilized mature oocytes are obtained from a donor who should be younger than 37 years old, healthy and preferably of known fertility. The donor is screened for hepatitis B, hepatitis C and HIV as well as for appropriate genetic diseases. It is generally recommended that both the donor and recipient undergo counselling with regard to the implications of egg donation and the possible outcome. A routine IVF cycle is then performed and, depending on the sperm parameters of the male partner of the recipient, the eggs are fertilized either routinely or with ICSI. The resultant embryos can be replaced fresh or in a frozen cycle.

The recipient is prepared in a similar way to FERCs – if the menstrual cycle is regular the embryos can be replaced in a natural cycle (although this is unusual as recipients rarely have normal menstrual cycles). More often than not, they are replaced as in a suppressed FERC with the use of oestrogen to get an optimum endometrium for implantation.

Indications
- Ovarian failure – either premature or physiological.
- Patients with very poor ovarian function where previous IVF has repeatedly failed.
- Patients over the age of 45 and with severe male factor disease necessitating ICSI.
- Patients with hereditary genetic disease where using the patient's own gametes is not advisable.

Benefits
The recipient adopts the success rate corresponding to the age of the donor. Therefore, success rates with egg donation are generally high. Any resultant offspring have the aneuploidy rates of the age of the donor as well. Therefore, for a patient who is over the age of 40, the success rates are far greater and the risk of genetic disease, such as Down's syndrome, significantly lower.

Problems
The main problem with oocyte donation is obtaining eggs. In the UK it is illegal at present to pay donors for their eggs and they are only allowed to be compensated minimally for their time and inconvenience. Since 1 April 2005 anonymity for donors has also been repealed and any resultant offspring can trace his or her genetic mother from the age of 18. Not surprisingly, there is therefore a paucity of suitable egg donors in the UK and most programmes at present rely on altruistic donors brought in by the recipients themselves. These are generally either family members or friends.

Egg share programmes can be used, where a person requiring IVF for personal reasons agrees to donate half her eggs to an unknown recipient in lieu of having a reduced cost for her own IVF cycle. The use of egg share programmes has diminished since 1 April 2005, again because of this lack of anonymity to the donor.

Elsewhere in the world, particularly in the USA, donors are paid, so there tends not to be a lack of donors, but cycle costs are considerably higher. There is now a considerable amount of fertility tourism, whereby couples travel to overseas clinics to bypass their own country's regulatory authorities. This is particularly popular in patients requiring anonymous egg donors.

Surrogacy
Surrogacy is used when a patient's uterus is either absent or unable to maintain a pregnancy, and a surrogate or host uterus is used to carry the pregnancy. Generally this procedure is used when a young patient has lost her uterus to cancer or to uncontrollable bleeding, for example from postpartum haemorrhage or following a difficult myomectomy, or in patients with congenital absence of the uterus. The patient's own eggs are obtained as in an IVF cycle, fertilized by her partner's sperm and the resultant embryos replaced within the surrogate. Counselling is obligatory for both the patients and the surrogate. Generally, surrogates are women who have already had children themselves and are recruited either by the patients or through an organization such as COTS (Childlessness Overcome Through Surrogacy). Surrogacy is legal in the UK and the surrogate can be compensated for time lost away from employment during the pregnancy. However, the child's legal mother is the woman who delivers the child and therefore the patient and the husband have to undergo formal adoption procedures to become the legal parents of their genetic offspring which the surrogate has delivered. The laws governing surrogacy vary widely from country to country.

Egg freezing
Egg freezing involves eggs being obtained from an IVF cycle, but instead of being fertilized with sperm they are left unfertilized and frozen for future use. Unfortunately, unfertilized eggs do not survive the freeze–thaw process anywhere near as well as an embryo owing to the large size of the unfertilized eggs and their high water content. This causes problems during the freezing process as ice crystals can form within the egg, disrupting the delicate structures and resulting in its demise when thawed. (Once an oocyte is fertilized the resultant cells are considerably smaller and therefore the problem of ice formation within these cells is significantly lower.) Success rates of egg freezing programmes using conventional slow freezing techniques are associated with low pregnancy rates of under 10% per transfer. As a result, such treatment is usually recommended only for young patients with cancer facing treatments such as chemotherapy, radiotherapy or sterilizing surgery. Recently, an alternative approach to cryopreservation called vitrification has been attempted. Although still relatively new, improvements in freeze–thaw rates are encouraging and pregnancy rates of up to 35% per transfer have been reported [17]. This new technology may justify an expansion of the indications of egg storage from fertility preservation in oncology patients who have no partner to the so-called 'social' egg freezing, which may be popular with professional

women trying to delay the impact of age-related decreases in ovarian function and egg quality.

Preimplantation genetic diagnosis

Preimplantation genetic diagnosis is a form of very early prenatal diagnosis. It combines the techniques of assisted conception with molecular and cytogenetics to detect genetic disease in embryos at the preimplantation stage. It allows couples who carry serious genetic disorders to have embryos free of these diseases transferred into the uterus. This prevents the need for invasive prenatal diagnosis and the difficult decision on whether to terminate an affected pregnancy. The technique was pioneered at the Hammersmith Hospital in the early 1990s [18], and can now be applied to almost all hereditary conditions where the mutation is known.

Indications
• Single-gene defects such as cystic fibrosis, thalassaemia or sickle cell disease.
• Chromosomal rearrangements such as translocations.
• human leukocyte antigen (HLA) matching for donor sibling stem cell transplantation.

Procedure
The embryos are obtained as with any routine IVF procedure, although generally ICSI is now used to minimize the potential for genetic contamination. Biopsy may be of the polar body (at the MII oocyte phase), the blastocyst on day 5 or, more commonly, at the cleavage stage of development. The zona pellucida of the embryo is then opened using either acid-tyrodes or special lasers, and one or two blastomeres are gently teased out of the embryo for the specific test itself. If it is a specific single-gene defect, the embryos are tested by polymerase chain reaction (PCR). Chromosomal rearrangements are usually detected by fluorescent *in situ* hybridization (FISH). Unaffected embryos are then transferred to the uterus.

Preimplantation genetic screening

Chromosomal aneuploidy in human embryos is one of the commonest reasons for failure of implantation following IVF. These aneuploidies may be age-related aneuploidies in the egg (meiotic) or related to early cell division in the embryo (post zygotic). Preimplantation genetic screening is the use of PGD techniques to detect these aneuploidies in an attempt to ameliorate the impact of female age on IVF. Initial indications for the technique were advanced maternal age, recurrent IVF failure at the stage of implantation, previous aneuploid pregnancies and recurrent miscarriage. The technique originally used multicolour FISH and was controversial because of its attractive self-evident hypothesis, but it lacked a robust evidence base. Eventually, following prospective randomized controlled trials, it was shown to be ineffective.

Advances such as whole genome amplification, comparative genomic hybridization and microarray analysis have led to a renewed interest in PGS, and these novel exciting approaches are currently under evaluation.

Surgical sperm retrieval

In cases where there is either azoospermia or necrozoospermia, surgical sperm retrieval can be performed to obtain sperm directly from either the epididymus (MESA) or directly from the testis (TESE or PESA). A biopsy should always be taken from each testis and sent to histopathology, as carcinoma *in situ* can be found in approximately 1% of subfertile men.

These techniques can be performed under either local anaesthetic or a light general anaesthetic. The patient should be screened for cystic fibrosis and karyotyping prior to the procedure. There are major chromosomal abnormalities in just over 2% of infertile men, which is three times the normal incidence. In the case of azoospermia, this increases to over 15%. If semen results are in the normal range, then chromosomal abnormalities are significantly lower. An FSH level is also beneficial as, if this is in the normal range, the chances of obtaining usable spermatozoa are much higher (around 90% if the testicular volumes are normal) whereas if the FSH is markedly raised then the chances are significantly lower (less than 10% if the testicular volumes are reduced).

Any sperm obtained through these techniques is then cryopreserved for future use. The sperm can be used fresh if the operation is timed to coincide with oocyte retrieval. ICSI has to be used in all cases of surgical sperm retrieval as there is inadequate motile sperm for normal fertilization.

Donor sperm

If there is no usable sperm obtained from either surgical sperm retrieval or ejaculation, then the use of donor sperm may be considered. Donor sperm is obtained by masturbation from healthy screened donors. All donor sperm in the UK must be stored for 6 months, and then the donor screened again. Sperm can then be released for use only after both sets of screening have been found to be negative.

Indications
• Azoospermia.
• Carriers of severe genetic disease.
• Lesbian/single women.

Use
Donor sperm used to be inseminated around the cervix using an unprepared specimen around what was thought to be the fertile time. Now, a prepared sample of sperm is used and inseminated directly into the uterine cavity as part of an IUI programme. The patient has the usual

screening tests including a test of tubal patency, and then, provided the menstrual cycle is regular, the cycle is monitored and at the appropriate time, around ovulation, the prepared sample is inseminated directly into the cavity. If the patient has irregular cycles or unstimulated IUI has been unsuccessful, then stimulated IUI can be performed and success rates are generally higher. If the fallopian tubes are severely damaged or blocked, then the donor sperm has to be utilized with techniques such as IVF. Success rates are almost entirely dependent on the age of the patient.

Complications of assisted conception

Multiple births

The most common complication of assisted conception is that of multiple births. Cumulative analysis of IVF over 20 years reveals that approximately 24% of patients will have twins when two or three embryos are transferred. Triplet rates vary depending on the percentage of embryo transfers that are three embryos or more. In the UK a maximum of three embryos can be transferred, but only under exceptional circumstances or if the patient is aged 40 years or older. The majority of embryo transfers in the UK at present are two embryo transfers. The issue is the incidence of preterm birth and cerebral palsy and, with a twin pregnancy, the risk of cerebral palsy is up to eight times greater than that of a singleton pregnancy. In triplet pregnancies, the rate can be as high as 47 times greater. The offspring also are at risk of all the other multiple sequelae of prematurity [19].

To reduce the rate of multiple births, the HFEA has made strong recommendations towards elective single embryo transfers. As clinical and laboratory techniques improve, this should maintain acceptable pregnancy rates and reduce the twin rate to monozygotic twins only. Indeed, in some Scandinavian countries, if the patient is aged 35 or younger then elective single embryo transfer is mandatory. One embryo is transferred fresh and all the other embryos are frozen, and then the patient undergoes repeated single embryo transfer. Although there is increasing evidence to support the advocacy of elective single embryo transfer, it remains difficult to persuade patients that this is desirable as many patients see a twin pregnancy as a desirable outcome.

Summary box 46.3

Complications of assisted reproduction:
- Multiple pregnancy.
- Ovarian hyperstimulation syndrome (OHSS).
- Ectopic pregnancy.
- Complications of ocyte retrieval: haemorrhage, infection.

Ovarian hyperstimulation syndrome

Ovarian hyperstimulation syndrome is an iatrogenic condition that can occur in any IVF cycle, but usually is only mild to moderate. It is characterized by an excessive ovarian response resulting in multiple follicular growth and large numbers of eggs collected. Severe OHHS can be life-threatening and is associated with intravascular fluid depletion and thrombosis, ascites and pleural effusion. It generally occurs in specific at-risk groups, in particular in young patients who have polycystic ovaries. In these situations the starting dose of gonadotrophins should be lowered to take account of the increased sensitivity of the polycystic ovaries. Even in the best centres with adequate monitoring there can be a surprisingly brisk ovarian response and the ovaries can hyperstimulate. In these situations several options are available. The cycle can be abandoned and then restarted at a lower dose or the eggs collected, fertilized and then all the embryos electively frozen as severe hyperstimulation tends to be most severe in patients who become pregnant from a fresh transfer. Lastly, if the risks have been fully considered and thought still acceptable, then the embryos can be transferred and the patient very carefully monitored. If OHHS results, admission to hospital is essential for monitoring fluid balance and plasma protein levels. Human albumin solution may be given if hypoproteinaemia develops. If ascites is present, it can be drained on a daily basis, limited to 1 litre per day in multiple aliquots as this gives symptomatic relief and increases urinary output, but avoids abrupt hypoproteinaemia. If the patient develops pleural effusions, these also can be tapped, although draining the ascites helps these as well. Owing to the increased risk of thromboembolism, patients should also be given thromboprophylaxis in the form of antithrombotic stockings and low-molecular-weight heparin daily. Generally the condition is self-limiting, but the patient should be kept in hospital and closely monitored until the OHSS has resolved. The condition does not appear to adversely affect the fetus and the subsequent pregnancy is usually uneventful. In rare occasions where the situation is deteriorating and the patient's life is at risk, the pregnancy may need to be terminated.

Ectopic pregnancies

Ectopic pregnancies can occur with any of the assisted reproductive techniques. This is not only in patients with tubal disease – any patient undergoing any form of assisted conception is at greater risk. In IVF programmes the generally accepted rate is between 2% and 5%, even though the embryos are transferred directly into the uterine cavity. This may be due to post embryo transfer uterine contractions that force the embryos into the fallopian tubes, only for them to return to the uterine cavity in the majority. Unfortunately, some embryos remain in the tube and develop into an ectopic pregnancy. Patients who successfully become pregnant following assisted conception should always be offered an early scan to ensure that the pregnancy is intrauterine. If the pregnancy is found to be extrauterine, then the full range of treatment options should be discussed with the patient. With the increasing amount of salpingectomies performed for hydrosalpinges, it is hoped that the incidence of ectopic pregnancies with IVF will reduce.

Transvaginal oocyte retrieval complications

There are always accepted risks of complications from ultrasound-guided oocyte retrievals, and these can range from infection of the ovaries causing ovarian abscess to damage to the bowel. These are generally quoted at 1% or less, and all patients should be counselled about them prior to starting their treatment [20].

References

1 Strandell A, Bourne T, Bergh C, Granberg S, Asztely M, Thorburn J. The assessment of endometrial pathology and tubal patency: a comparison between the use of ultrasonography and X-ray hysterosalpingography for the investigation of infertility patients. *Ultrasound Obstet Gynecol* 1999;14: 200–204.

2 Strandell A, Lindhard A, Waldenstrom U, Thorburn J. Hydrosalpinx and IVF outcome: cumulative results after salpingectomy in a randomised controlled trial. *Hum Reprod* 2001; 16:2403–2410.

3 Surrey ES, Minjarez DA, Stevens JM, Schoolcraft WB. Effect of myomectomy on the outcome of assisted reproductive technologies. *Fertil Steril* 2005;83:1473–1479.

4 Eldar-Geva T, Meagher S, Healy DL, MacLachlan V, Breheny S, Wood C. Effect of intramural, subserosal and submucosal intrauterine fibroids on the outcome of assisted reproductive technology treatment. *Fertil Steril* 1998;70:687–691.

5 Hart R, Khalaf Y, Yeong CT, Seed P, Taylor A, Braude P. A post prospective control study on the effect of intramural fibroids on the outcome of assisted conception. *Hum Reprod* 2001;60: 2411–2417.

6 Johnson NP, Mak W, Sowter MC. Surgical treatment for tubal disease in women due to undergo *in vitro* fertilisation. *Cochrane Database Syst Rev* 2004;3:CD002125.

7 Gelbaya TA, Nardo LG, Fitzgerald CT, Horne G, Brison DR, Lieberman BA. Ovarian response to gonadotropins after laparoscopic salpingectomy or the division of fallopian tubes for hydrosalpinges. *Fertil Steril* 2006;85:1464–1468.

8 Swanton A, Lighten A, Granne I *et al.* Do women with ovaries of polycystic morphology without any other features of PCOS benefit from short-term metformin co-treatment during IVF? A double-blind, placebo-controlled, randomized trial. *Hum Reprod* 2011;26:2178–2184.

9 Cohlen BJ, Vandekerckhove P, te Velde ER, Habbma JD. Timed intercourse versus intra-uterine insemination with or without ovarian hyperstimulation for subfertility in men. *Cochrane Database Syst Rev* 2000;2:CD000360.

10 Blake DA, Farquhar CM, Johnson N, Proctor M. Cleavage stage versus blastocyst stage embryo transfer in assisted conception. *Cochrane Database Syst Rev* 2007;4:CD002118.

11 Pandian Z, Bhattacharya S, Ozturk O, Serour G, Templeton A. Number of embryos for transfer following in-vitro fertilisation or intra-cytoplasmic sperm injection. *Cochrane Database Syst Rev* 2009;15:CD003416.

12 Buckett WM. A meta-analysis of ultrasound-guided versus clinical touch embryo transfer. *Fertil Steril* 2003;80:1037–1041.

13 Nosarka S, Kruger T, Siebert I, Grove D. Luteal phase support in IVF: meta-analysis of randomised trials. *Gynecol Obstet Invest* 2005;60:67–74.

14 Daya S, Gunby J. Luteal phase support in assisted reproduction cycles. *Cochrane Database Syst Rev* 2004;3:CD004830.

15 Devroey P. Clinical application of new micromanipulative technologies to treat the male. *Hum Reprod* 1998;13(Suppl 3): 112–122.

16 Society for Assisted Reproductive Technologies. Assisted reproductive technologies in the United States: 2000 results. *Fertil Steril* 2004;81:1207–1220.

17 Ubaldi F, Anniballo R, Romano S *et al.* Cumulative ongoing pregnancy rate achieved with oocyte vitrification and cleavage stage transfer without embryo selection in a standard infertility program. *Hum Reprod* 2010;25:1199–1205.

18 Handyside AH, Kontogianni EH, Hardy K, Winston RM. Pregnancies from biopsied human preimplantation embryos sexed by Y-specific DNA amplification. *Nature* 1990;344 (6268):768–770.

19 Pharoah PO. Risk of cerebral palsy in multiple pregnancies. *Obstet Gynecol Clin North Am* 2005;32:55–67.

20 El-Shawarby S, Margara R, Trew G, Lavery S. A review of complications following transvaginal oocyte retrieval for in-vitro fertilisation. *Hum Fertil (Camb)* 2004;7:127–133.

Further reading

Brinsden P (ed.) *A Textbook of In Vitro Fertilisation and Assisted Reproduction: the Bourn Hall Guide to Clinical and Laboratory Practice*, 2nd edn. London: Parthenon Publishing, 1999.

Gardner DK, Weissman A, Howles CM, Shoham Z (eds) *Textbook of Assisted Reproductive Techniques – Laboratory and Clinical Perspectives*. London: Taylor & Francis, 2004.

Report on Fertility Clinical Guidelines at www.nice.org.uk

Human Fertilisation and Embryology Authority website: www.hfea.gov.uk

Part 12
Pelvic Pain

Chapter 47
Pelvic Infection

Jonathan D.C. Ross
Whittall Street Clinic, Birmingham, UK

Summary box 47.1

Overview of pelvic infection:
- Pelvic inflammatory disease (PID) is a common and often asymptomatic problem in young women.
- Confirmation with a microbiological diagnosis is often not possible.
- Antibiotics are very effective in controlling symptoms when present.
- Surgical intervention is seldom required.
- A single episode of PID treated early with appropriate antibiotics is associated with well-preserved fertility.

Pelvic infection is common and usually results from sexually transmitted pathogens ascending from the lower to upper genital tract. Infection can also occur following pelvic surgery, in the puerperium and after instrumenting the uterus.

Epidemiology and risk factors

How common is pelvic inflammatory disease?

Pelvic inflammatory disease (PID) is a major cause of morbidity in young women, and it is becoming more common. About 2% of young women in the UK give a history of PID when asked, and about 1 in 50 consultations made by young women with general practitioners relate to PID [1]. The number of women in the UK diagnosed with *Chlamydia* infection, which is a major cause of PID, is increasing and this is reflected in a rising prevalence of PID.

Who gets pelvic inflammatory disease?

The risk factors for PID strongly reflect those of any sexually transmitted infection – young age, multiple sexual partners, lack of condom use, lower socioeconomic status and black Caribbean/black African ethnicity. What is less certain is why some women with lower genital tract infection go on to develop upper genital tract disease – what factors encourage infection to spread from the vagina or cervix to the endometrium and fallopian tubes?

Cervical mucus provides an important barrier to ascending infection. Young women with anovulatory cycles have thinner cervical mucus and this, combined with higher rates of cervical ectopy and riskier sexual behaviour, may account for their high rates of PID. The ability of the immune response to control and contain infection will also determine the risk of upper genital tract involvement. Part of that immune response is genetically determined and an increased risk of PID is observed in women of human leukocyte antigen (HLA) subtype A31, while women with HLA DQA 0501 and DQB 0402 have lower rates of infertility following a diagnosis of PID. Polymorphisms in TCR4 and CCR5 antigen receptors, and variable expression of interleukin 10 (IL-10), may also have a role. It is possible that certain strains of bacteria are more likely to cause PID than others, but the evidence for this is limited (e.g. serogroup A strain of *Neisseria gonorrhoeae*, serovar F strain of *Chlamydia trachomatis*).

Differences in behaviour have been linked to the risk of PID. A clear association can be seen between vaginal douching and PID but more recent longitudinal studies suggest that douching does not cause PID; rather, it would appear that the vaginal discharge and menstrual irregularities associated with PID may themselves lead to more douching [2]. Women who smoke are at higher risk of PID but it is unclear whether this is a marker for high-risk sexual behaviour or a direct effect of smoking itself on immune surveillance.

Many women with PID also have bacterial vaginosis with an overgrowth of the normal commensal bacteria in the vagina and loss of vaginal lactobacilli. These same vaginal commensual bacteria are often isolated from the upper genital tract raising the possibility that bacterial vaginosis may lead to PID. Longitudinal studies do not

Dewhurst's Textbook of Obstetrics & Gynaecology, Eighth Edition. Edited by D. Keith Edmonds.
© 2012 John Wiley and Sons, Ltd. Published 2012 by John Wiley and Sons, Ltd.

Table 47.1 Organisms associated with pelvic inflammatory disease.

Aerobic/facultative anaerobic	Anaerobic	Viruses
Neisseria gonorrhoeae	Bacteroides sp.	Herpes simplex
Chlamydia trachomatis	Peptostreptococcus sp.	Echovirus
Ureaplasma urealyticum	Clostridium bifermentans	Coxsackie
Mycoplasma genitalium	Fusobacterium sp.	Respiratory syncytial virus
Gardnerella vaginalis		
Streptococcus pyogenes		
Coagulase-negative Staphylococci		
Escherichia coli		
Haemophilus influenzae		
Mycoplasma hominis		
Streptococcus pneumoniae		
Mycobacterium tuberculosis		

support a direct causal association, although women who catch gonorrhoea or chlamydia are at higher risk of PID if they also have pre-existing bacterial vaginosis, suggesting some synergy between the different infections [3].

The cost of treating pelvic inflammatory disease

The psychological and fiscal costs of PID are substantial. The uncertainty of the diagnosis and difficulty in predicting the subsequent risk of infertility, chronic pelvic pain or ectopic pregnancy add to the anxiety associated with PID, and are in addition to the feelings of blame, guilt and isolation that the diagnosis of a sexually transmitted infection may instil. Most of the monetary costs of PID arise from surgical interventions to diagnose and treat the consequences of tubal damage, and have been estimated at between £650 and £2000 per case [4]. These costs will rise substantially with improved availability of infertility treatments in the future.

Microbiology

Pelvic inflammatory disease is a polymicrobial infection. *N. gonorrhoeae* and *Chlamydia* are the most frequently recognized pathogens but a wide variety of other bacteria

and viruses can also be isolated from the fallopian tubes of women with PID (Table 47.1).

Neisseria gonorrhoeae

Neisseria gonorrhoeae is a Gram-negative diplococcus, therefore when a sample of cervical discharge is spread and fixed on a slide the bacteria can be seen on microscopy as pairs of red kidney-shaped organisms, mostly sitting within polymorphs. Gonorrhoea causes about 5% of PID in the UK [5,6].

N. gonorrhoeae initially infects the cervix but ascends to the upper genital tract in 10–20% of untreated cases. Around half of women with gonorrhoea are asymptomatic, but when symptoms are present the vaginal discharge tends to be thick and purulent. Although isolating gonorrhoea from the cervix supports a diagnosis of PID, its absence in the lower genital tract cannot exclude infection in the fallopian tubes or ovaries.

Chlamydia trachomatis

Chlamydia trachomatis is an unusual bacterium as it requires a host cell to grow (obligate intracellular organism), behaving in some ways more like a virus. To detect the organism, therefore, the optimal specimen needs to contain cells and should be collected by gently rubbing against the endocervix with a swab. The use of sensitive nucleic acid amplification tests (NAAT) also allows the use of other more accessible samples to detect chlamydia, e.g. vulval swabs (which the patient can take herself after appropriate instruction) or first-pass urine. Light microscopy is not useful since *C. trachomatis* is too small to be seen.

Chlamydia, like gonorrhoea, initially infects the cervix and sometimes also the urethra. It is the commonest identified cause of PID in the UK, accounting for 30% of cases [5] and causes a more chronic low-grade infection than gonorrhoea. Over two-thirds of women with chlamydial infection are asymptomatic.

Mycoplasma genitalium

Evidence for the role of *Mycoplasma genitalium* in PID is growing. It has been isolated from the cervix, endometrium and, in a single case, from the fallopian tubes of women with PID [7]. Tubal factor infertility is strongly associated with past infection with *M. genitalium*, and inoculation of the lower genital tract with mycoplasma causes PID in female monkeys [8]. Testing for *M. genitalium* is expensive and not routinely available.

Anaerobes

Anaerobic bacteria are of particular importance in women with severe PID, and can often be isolated from tubo-ovarian abscesses. Their role in mild to moderate PID is less clear. *Bacteroides* spp. *fragilis, peptostreptococcus* and *peptococcus* can all be isolated from the genital tract of women with PID and the production of mucinases and sialidases by anaerobic bacteria may break down cervical mucus, thus facilitating the passage of other bacteria into the upper genital tract.

Actinomyces

Actinomyces israeli is occasionally detected in women with an intrauterine contraceptive device (IUCD) *in situ*. If there are no symptoms of vaginal discharge, intermenstrual bleeding or pelvic pain then the woman should be advised that neither treatment nor removal of the IUCD is required, but she should be reviewed in 6 months or earlier if symptoms develop. If symptoms are present then at least 2 weeks' therapy with a penicillin, tetracycline or macrolide antibiotic is indicated and the IUCD should be removed.

Mycobacterium tuberculosis

Tuberculous PID is largely limited to patients from developing countries. Pelvic infection usually occurs secondary to haematogenous spread from an extragenital source, but occasionally *Mycobacterium tuberculosis* can be transmitted sexually [9]. Usually it is not possible to detect the organism in the lower genital tract and samples should be obtained by uterine curettage or from the fallopian tubes at laparoscopy to be sent for culture or nucleic acid testing. Standard quadruple antituberculous therapy with isoniazid, rifampicin, ethambutol and pyrazinamide is effective but surgical intervention may be required for extensive disease.

Viruses

A number of viruses have been isolated from the upper genital tract in women with PID (Table 47.1) but their role in pathogenesis is unclear.

Clinical presentation

Clinical features

The clinical diagnosis of PID is based on the presence of lower abdominal pain, usually bilateral, combined with either adnexal tenderness or cervical excitation on vaginal examination (Fig. 47.1). A comprehensive medical history and examination including an accurate menstrual and sexual history may help to reach a diagnosis. A pelvic examination is essential and a speculum examination is necessary both to enable appropriate swabs to be taken and also to exclude foreign bodies in the vagina such as retained tampons. The poor specificity and associated low positive predictive value of this approach (65–90%) is

Essential features
Lower abdominal pain (usually bilateral)
or
Adnexal tenderness
or
Cervical motion tenderness

Supporting features
Intermenstrual/abnormal bleeding
Postcoital bleeding
Increased/abnormal vaginal discharge
Deep dyspareunia
Vaginal discharge
Fever
Nausea/vomiting
Right upper abdominal pain and tenderness
Generalized peritonitis

Fig. 47.1 Diagnosing pelvic infection.

justified because a delay in antibiotic therapy of even a few days may increase the risk of impaired fertility [10]. The risks of giving antibiotics to a woman who turns out not to have PID are low, although important differential diagnoses first need to be excluded.

Other clinical features can support a diagnosis of PID but are not essential before starting empirical therapy:
• intermenstrual or postcoital bleeding – resulting from endometritis and cervicitis;
• deep dyspareunia;
• abnormal vaginal discharge – indicating lower genital tract infection;
• fever – non-specific and usually only present in moderate to severe PID; and
• nausea/vomiting – may occur in severe PID but is more commonly associated with appendicitis.

Pelvic inflammatory disease caused by gonorrhoea presents more acutely and is more severe compared with chlamydial PID [11]. It is worth remembering that for every woman presenting with clinical features of PID there are two others who are asymptomatic.

Fitz-Hugh–Curtis syndrome

Inflammation and infection of the liver capsule (perihepatitis) affects 10–20% of women with gonococcal or chlamydial PID and occasionally dominates the clinical presentation. Patients complain of right upper abdominal pain and have tenderness at the liver edge, occasionally accompanied by a hepatic friction rub.

Differential diagnosis

The main differential diagnoses are given in Table 47.2. The features that classically lead towards a diagnosis of PID are the typical 'G string' distribution of the pain and bilateral tenderness on pelvic examination. In

Table 47.2 Differential diagnosis of pelvic inflammatory disease.

Differential diagnosis	Significant features
Ectopic pregnancy	Menstrual history, initially unilateral pain
Ovarian cyst rupture/torsion	Initially unilateral pain, often mid-cycle
Appendicitis	Gastrointestinal symptoms, right-sided pain
Irritable bowel syndrome	Central or left-sided pain, no cervical excitation
Inflammatory bowel disease, e.g. Crohn's, ulcerative colitis, diverticular disease	Colicky central or left-sided abdominal pain, bowel symptoms
Urinary tract infection	Urinary symptoms ± loin pain (chlamydial infections can also present with urinary symptoms)
Bowel torsion	Central pain
Psychosomatic pain	Usually inconsistent symptoms

bowel-related disorders the pain tends to be higher in the abdomen and more central or to the left. Other conditions tend to give unilateral pain, at least at their onset. The main diagnoses to exclude are ectopic pregnancy and causes of an acute abdomen which may require surgical intervention, such as appendicitis and an ovarian 'accident' (e.g. torsion or persistent bleeding from a ruptured cyst). If the diagnosis is not clear then empirical treatment with antibiotics should be commenced, but the patient kept under close observation to ensure that an alternative diagnosis has not been missed.

Investigation

Summary box 47.2

Before diagnosing pelvic inflammatory disease:
• Perform a pregnancy test to help exclude ectopic pregnancy.
• Screen for sexually transmitted infections.

Rather like signs and symptoms, the investigations available to diagnose acute PID lack accuracy. Blood tests such as a white cell count, erythrocyte sedimentation rate and C reactive protein are all relatively non-specific. They may be elevated in PID but in mild cases can be normal. In particular, a leukocytosis is often not seen in non-pyogenic infections.

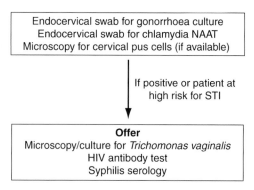

Fig. 47.2 Microbiological investigation of women with pelvic infection.

A pregnancy test, preferably measuring serum beta hCG, is mandatory to exclude an ectopic pregnancy and also the possibility of an ovarian accident associated with a very early intrauterine pregnancy. This should always be performed before commencing empirical antibiotic treatment. In most hospitals this is available as an emergency investigation. If it is not, a simple urinary pregnancy test is almost as accurate.

Microbiological tests

The following microbiology tests should be offered to all women presenting with possible PID (Fig. 47.2):
• endocervical swab for *N. gonorrhoeae* culture – this should be placed in transport medium (either Stuart or Amies) and arrive at the laboratory preferably within 6 h but certainly within 24 h, otherwise viability is rapidly lost. Nucleic acid amplification tests (NAATs) for *N. gonorrhoeae* have greater sensitivity than culture and can be used as an alternative, but confirmation of a positive NAAT is required because of the risk of false-positive results; and
• endocervical swab for *Chlamydia* NAAT – the alternative enzyme-linked immunosorbent assays (EIA) test lack sensitivity.

The detection of gonorrhoea or chlamydia at the cervix greatly increases the likelihood of PID as the cause of lower abdominal pain, but many women with PID also have a negative infection screen from the lower genital tract.

A lack of polymorphs on a Gram-stained smear of cervical discharge makes PID unlikely but their presence is non-specific, i.e. the absence of polymorphs has a good negative predictive value but their presence has a poor positive predictive value for PID [12].

Screening for other sexually transmitted infections should be offered to women who test positive for gonorrhoea or chlamydia, and to those who are at higher risk of infection, e.g. two or more partners within the past year, lack of condom use or previous history of a sexually transmitted infection. An appropriate screen would include:

- microscopy and/or culture for *T. vaginalis* – the sample should be taken from the posterior fornix and transported in Amies or Stuart media arriving at the laboratory within 6 h;
- HIV antibody test; and
- syphilis serology.

If laparoscopy or laparotomy is performed then specimens from the fallopian tube should also be sent requesting bacterial culture, including gonorrhoea. *Chlamydia* nucleic acid amplification tests are not licensed for use for fallopian tube samples and therefore require cautious interpretation. Chlamydial culture can be also performed on this sample but is less sensitive, requires specific transport media and is not widely available.

Radiology investigations

Transvaginal ultrasound of the pelvis may be useful where there is diagnostic difficulty. There are no features, however, that are pathognomonic of acute PID. Free fluid in the pouch of Douglas is a common normal finding and is therefore not helpful. Scanning may help to exclude ectopic pregnancy, ovarian cysts or appendicitis and can also identify dilated fallopian tubes or a tubal abscess. Work with power Doppler has suggested that inflamed and dilated tubes and tubal ovarian masses can be diagnosed reasonably accurately. This investigation, however, requires considerable expertise and may not be readily available in an emergency setting. It therefore has very little benefit to the routine diagnosis of PID.

Magnetic resonance imaging can assist in making the diagnosis where there is difficulty, but it is also not widely available and has not entered routine management. Computed tomography (CT) scanning in acute PID may show obscuring of the pelvic fascial planes, thickening of the uterosacral ligaments and accumulation of fluid in the tubes and endometrial canal. In the upper abdomen it can provide evidence of perihepatitis. Enhancement of the hepatic and splenic capsules on abdominal CT scan has been suggested as characteristic of Fitz-Hugh–Curtis syndrome but is of little value as a routine investigation.

Surgical investigation

For many years the definitive diagnostic procedure for PID was considered to be laparoscopy and it probably remains more sensitive than any other investigation currently available. In many cases there will be clear evidence of dilated, hyperaemic tubes with an inflammatory, fibrinous exudate covering the tubes and the fundus of the uterus. In mild cases, however, intraluminal inflam-mation of the tubes may be missed and significant inter- and intra-observer variation in interpreting the appearance of salpingitis at laparoscopy has been reported [13]. It does enable swabs to be taken from the fimbrial ends of the tubes, which may be more accurate than endocervical swabs, but the principal benefit of laparoscopy is to exclude other diagnoses. As an invasive procedure it should be reserved for those cases where there is an element of doubt as to the diagnosis of acute PID or in cases where the patient fails to respond to antibiotics within 48–72 h.

There is no evidence to support the routine use of hysteroscopy or endometrial biopsy in the routine diagnosis of acute PID. More invasive endoscopic techniques, such as fallaposcopy, may be potentially dangerous and have no place in management.

Histology and pathology

The spread of infection from the cervix to the endometrium leads to an acute, predominately polymorph-mediated endometritis [14]. Transcervical suction biopsy of the endometrium allows assessment of the endometrial inflammation, which correlates well with salpingitis [14]. Unfortunately, the usefulness of this approach to diagnose PID is limited by the risk of introducing infection during the procedure, the time delay in fixing and staining the sample, and the uncertain significance of isolated endometritis.

The inflammatory response seen in the fallopian tubes depends on the underlying pathogen. Gonorrhoea infects the non-ciliated epithelial cells but production of tumour necrosis factor and gamma interferon soon lead to collateral damage to the surrounding tissue and invasion of the submucosa. The tissue damage associated with *Chlamydia* is mediated primarily by the immune response to the infection occurring as a result of a delayed type hypersensitivity reaction to a chlamydial heat shock protein. This is characterized by a low-grade lymphocytic response compared with the acute neutrophil response of gonococcal salpingitis.

Recurrent infection with *Chlamydia* causes further immune stimulation possibly mediated by a cross-reaction between chlamydial and human heat shock protein 60 [15]. This exaggerated immune response following re-exposure to *Chlamydia* may explain the exponential increase in the risk of tubal damage that occurs with repeated infection.

Severe inflammation is associated with tubal occlusion and the production of a tubo-ovarian abscess or hydrosalpinx. Healing following acute inflammation may produce chronic fibrosis with associated damage to the ciliated epithelium, tubal blockage and/or pelvic adhesions. Histologically, this chronic damage produces lymphoid follicles and a mononuclear cell infiltrate.

Treatment

Summary box 47.3

Treating pelvic infection:
- Start appropriate antibiotics promptly after making a clinical diagnosis.
- Arrange for the patient's partner to be screened for sexually transmitted infection and receive empirical antibiotics.
- Ensure that the patient and her partner are treated concurrently.
- Provide information about future use of condoms.
- Discuss the implications of a diagnosis of PID on future fertility.

Patients who are systemically unwell should be advised to rest and should be prescribed adequate analgesia. Regular review to assess progress is required. If no improvement is observed after 3 days of antibiotic therapy then alternative diagnoses should be considered. Most patients can be managed as outpatients, but those with severe symptoms, such as an acute abdomen, will require inpatient care. If the diagnosis is in doubt or if intravenous antibiotics are considered to be necessary then the patient should be admitted to hospital.

Antimicrobials

Broad-spectrum antibiotic cover to include gonorrhoea, chlamydia and anaerobes is required. The optimal choice of antibiotics may be affected by knowledge of local bacterial resistance patterns, severity of disease, cost and patient convenience. Parenteral therapy should be continued until 24h after clinical improvement and then switched to oral.

Randomized controlled trial evidence is available to support the use of the antibiotic regimens in Table 47.3 for outpatients and Table 47.4 for inpatients.

Quinolone resistance in gonorrhoea is common in many areas of the world and is rising in the UK. Ofloxacin or moxifloxacin should therefore be avoided if there is clinical suspicion of gonococcal PID as a result of, for example, clinically severe disease, a history of a partner with gonorrhoea or sexual contact abroad. Oral metronidazole can be discontinued in those with mild to moderate PID if the patient is unable to tolerate it.

Management of partners

Pelvic inflammatory disease is usually secondary to a sexually acquired infection so, unless the male partner(s) are identified and either screened for infection or treated empirically, the woman with PID is at high risk of a recurrence. Current male partners should be offered screening for gonorrhoea and chlamydia, and attempts made to contact other partners within the past 6 months, although

Table 47.3 Outpatient antibiotic regimens.

Regimen 1*	Regimen 2*	Regimen 3*
Ofloxacin 400 mg BD *plus* metronidazole 400 mg BD	Moxifloxacin 400 mg OD	Ceftriaxone 500 mg i.m. immediately *plus* doxycycline 100 mg BD *plus* metronidazole 400 mg BD

* To complete 14 days of therapy.
BD, twice daily; i.m., intramuscularly; OD, once daily.

Table 47.4 Inpatient antibiotic regimens.

Regimen 1	i.v. ceftriaxone 2 g daily *plus* i.v. or oral doxycycline 100 mg BD *followed by** oral doxycycline 100 mg BD *plus* metronidazole 400 mg BD
Regimen 2	i.v. clindamycin 900 mg TID *plus* i.v. gentamycin 2 mg/kg loading dose followed by 1.5 mg/kg TID (a single daily dose may also be used) *followed by** oral doxycycline 100 mg BD *plus* metronidazole 400 mg BD
Regimen 3	i.v. ofloxacin 400 mg BD *plus* i.v. metronidazole 500 mg TID *followed by** oral ofloxacin 400 mg BD *plus* oral metronidazole 400 mg BD
Regimen 4	i.v. ciprofloxacin 200 mg BD *plus* i.v. or oral doxycycline 100 mg BD *plus* i.v. metronidazole 500 mg TID *followed by** oral doxycycline 100 mg BD *plus* metronidazole 400 mg BD

* Parenteral therapy should be continued until 24 h after clinical improvement. Oral therapy to continue to complete 14 days of antibiotics in total.
BD, twice daily; i.m., intramuscularly; i.v., intravenously; QID, four times daily; TID, three times daily.

the exact time period will be influenced by the sexual history. If screening for sexually acquired infections is not possible then antibiotic therapy effective against gonorrhoea and chlamydia should be given empirically to the male partner(s) (see British Association for Sexual Health and HIV guidelines for up-to-date treatment recommendations at www.bashh.org) (Fig. 47.3).

The patient and her partner(s) should be advised to avoid intercourse until she has completed the treatment course.

Summary box 47.4

Follow-up appointment after PID:
- Review response to treatment.
- Ensure that the full course of antibiotics has been taken.
- Check whether the patient's partner has been seen and treated.
- Reinforce advice regarding future condom use.

Test for gonorrhoea and chlamydia
Give empirical therapy for gonorrhoea and chlamydia if testing is not available (see www.bashh.org for current recommended therapies)
Advise to avoid intercourse until index patient and male partner have both completed antibiotic therapy

Fig. 47.3 Management of the male partners of women with pelvic infection.

Surgical intervention

Surgical intervention is rarely required as a treatment for acute PID. Most patients present at an early enough stage of the disease for antibiotic treatment to be fully effective. There may, however, be an indication for laparoscopy or laparotomy to drain a pelvic abscess if this is diagnosed on ultrasound scanning and does not appear to be resolving with conservative antibiotic treatment. In these circumstances most surgeons would prefer to perform a laparotomy, which would allow digital division of all adhesions and access to any loculated areas of abscess formation. The decision whether or not to carry out a salpingo oophorectomy in the presence of a large tubo-ovarian abscess will obviously depend on the patient's age and her reproductive history. In most circumstances, however, if the patient's condition warrants a laparotomy, then removal of the damaged organs may well be the preferred option. If at least one ovary is retained then IVF treatment remains a possibility if the patient wishes to achieve a pregnancy.

In cases of small abscesses or fluid collections in the pouch of Douglas, ultrasound-guided aspiration is less invasive and there is some evidence that it is as effective as laparoscopy or laparotomy. The usual technique is to aspirate the fluid transvaginally using transvaginal scanning. Occasionally, a surgeon may consider draining an abscess in the pouch of Douglas via the rectum, although this may lead to chronic sinus formation.

On the rare occasion when pelvic actinomyces is suspected, surgery should be avoided. The history is likely to be more chronic than in acute PID, there is usually clear clinical evidence of a pelvic mass which does not appear to be an abscess on ultrasound scanning. There is also usually a history of recent use of an intrauterine contraceptive device. If surgery is performed, then there is a significant risk of bowel damage.

Prognosis

The evidence quantifying the frequency of sequelae of PID is complicated by the variable definitions and diagnostic criteria used to identify the index episode of infection.

Chronic pelvic pain

It is generally accepted that episodes of acute PID can lead to symptoms of chronic pelvic pain. The cause of the chronic pelvic pain, however, remains controversial. It may be that damaged tubes act as a nidus for recurrent infections or it may be due to adhesions tethering or encapsulating the pelvic organs. It is even possible that the pain is due to altered behaviour of pelvic nerves damaged by infection. There is also limited evidence as to the incidence of chronic pelvic pain resulting from single or multiple episodes of acute PID. It can be as high as 33% after recurrent episodes [16] and can have a significant effect on a patient's future quality of life [17]. The precautionary use of condoms after an episode of pelvic infection has been found to reduce the risk of chronic pelvic pain developing.

Subfertility and ectopic pregnancy

There is clear, population-based, epidemiological evidence of the relationship between a finding of *Chlamydia trachomatis* specific immunoglobulin G (IgG) antibodies and subsequent tubal subfertility [18].

Some cohort studies have shown a rate of subsequent involuntary infertility of up to 40% after a single episode of PID [19]. There is a relationship between the risk of subfertility and the severity of infection with a relative risk of 5.6 for severe infection compared with mild infection [20].

More recent prospective studies (in clinically mild/moderate disease) have suggested that infertility rates are not significantly increased following a single episode of PID treated appropriately [16]. A delay in antibiotic therapy, however, of even a few days may lead to a large increase in the risk of impaired fertility [10].

There is also clear epidemiological evidence of a relationship between the risk of ectopic pregnancy and a previous episode of PID. In laparoscopically proven cases of PID the risk of an ectopic in the next index pregnancy is six times greater than in controls [20]. The absolute risk of ectopic pregnancy remains low, however, at 0.5–1%, at least in women with mild to moderate disease [16].

Special circumstances

Pregnancy

Pelvic inflammatory disease associated with an intrauterine pregnancy is extremely rare except in cases of septic abortion. Cervicitis is more common and associated with increased fetal and maternal morbidity. Treatment regimes will depend upon the organisms isolated while avoiding those antibiotics that are contraindicated in pregnancy, e.g. tetracycline. Erythromycin and amoxicillin are not known to be harmful in pregnancy. In cases of septic abortion the organisms are more likely to be pyogenic than sexually transmitted. The use of broad-spectrum antibiotics, such as a third-generation cephalosporin together with azithromycin and metronidazole, would comprise a suitable regimen.

Mild endometritis following surgical termination of pregnancy is relatively common (approximately 1–2%) and needs to be treated aggressively to ensure future fertility. If pretreatment screening for sexually transmitted infection has been employed, it is very unusual to find a positive result on repeat swabs. It is, however, prudent to treat with a broad spectrum of antibiotics effective against both *Chlamydia* and anaerobes, e.g. ofloxacin plus metronidazole, or moxifloxacin.

Post pelvic surgery

Pelvic surgery such as hysterectomy is invariably associated with a significant risk of postoperative infection because it is virtually impossible to render the vagina totally aseptic. Prophylactic antibiotics are usually used during surgery, but postoperative pelvic infections, usually secondary to haematoma formation, are not uncommon. Most infections are caused by anaerobes and should be treated with a regime that includes metronidazole or co-amoxiclav.

Pelvic infection and intrauterine contraceptive devices

An IUCD only increases the risk of developing PID in the first few weeks after insertion and, except for subacute infections with *Actinomyces*, there appears to be no evidence of increased risk with the continuing use of an IUCD. Routine screening for chlamydia, gonorrhoea and bacterial vaginosis before insertion will therefore reduce the risk of PID in those women requiring an IUD. The use of progesterone IUDs has been associated with very low rates of PID.

The randomized controlled trial evidence for whether an IUCD should be left *in situ* or removed in women presenting with PID is limited [21,22]. Removal of the IUD should be considered and may be associated with better short-term clinical outcomes [21], but the decision to remove the IUD needs to be balanced against the risk of pregnancy in those who have had otherwise unprotected intercourse in the preceding 7 days. Hormonal emergency contraception may be appropriate for some women in this situation.

Human immunodeficiency virus

Women with HIV may have a more severe clinical presentation of PID, particularly in late-stage HIV disease associated with severe immunosuppression. No alteration in therapy is required although caution is required to check for any interactions between the PID treatment and antiretroviral medication.

Prevention

Chlamydia screening programme

Chlamydia is the commonest identified pathogen causing PID in the UK. Initial infection with *Chlamydia* is usually asymptomatic but, if identified, can be treated simply and cheaply with antibiotics such as doxycycline or azithromycin, and thus preventing the development of PID. Screening young women for chlamydia can be both feasible and cost-effective [23], and a national screening programme is now being rolled out across the UK targeting men and women under the age of 25 (further information is available at www.chlamydiascreening.nhs.uk).

Instrumentation of the uterus

There is a significant risk of introducing infection into the upper genital tract when instrumenting the uterus, particularly in women at high risk of a subclinical cervical *Chlamydia* infection (e.g. those under 25 years old). The most common indications for instrumenting the uterus are therapeutic surgical termination of pregnancy, insertion of an IUCD and investigations for subfertility. It is now considered mandatory to offer either a 'screen and treat' policy or routine prophylaxis for all women undergoing such management. In cases where a 'screen and treat' policy is inappropriate, e.g. insertion of an IUCD for emergency contraception, it is essential to ensure adequate prophylaxis and a single 1 g dose of azithromycin is recommended.

Particular care needs to be taken in patients who are on immunosuppressant treatment (e.g. renal transplant patients) and in those who are immunocompromised because of chemotherapy or HIV.

Contraception

Consistent use of barrier methods has been shown to reduce the risk of recurrent episodes of pelvic infection and also the chronic sequelae of pelvic infection by between 30% and 60%.

All forms of hormonal contraception (e.g. combined oral contraceptive pill [OCP], progesterone-only pill, progesterone injections and implants and Mirena® intrauterine system) have been shown to reduce the incidence of symptomatic PID compared with either the use of a standard IUCD or unprotected intercourse. This is presumed to be due to the protective effect of the progestogens, which decreases the permeability of the cervical mucus both to sperm and pathogens.

It may also have an effect through endometrial suppression or a direct steroidal induced effect on the

Table 47.5 Useful internet sites.

PID Treatment Guidelines – Royal College of Obstetrics and Gynaecologists	www.rcog.org
PID Treatment Guidelines – British Association for Sexual Health and HIV	www.bashh.org
Patient Information Leaflet for PID – Royal College of Obstetrics and Gynaecologists	www.rcog.org
UK Chlamydia Screening Programme – Department of Health	www.dh.gov.uk
Guideline on Screening and Testing for Sexually Transmitted Infections – British Association for Sexual Health and HIV	www.bashh.org
UK Health Protection Agency – UK data on the incidence of sexually transmitted infection and PID	www.hpa.org.uk

inflammatory response in the tubes. The beneficial effect of the OCP may, however, be limited to PID which is symptomatic and caused by *C. trachomatis* [24] and it has been suggested that hormonal contraception may in fact simply be masking infection rather than preventing it [24]. A study that appeared to suggest that injectable progesterone contraception increased the risk of PID was methodologically flawed and hence may not be valid [25]. The true relationship between hormonal contraception and PID therefore still needs to be elucidated.

Further reading

Some useful internet sites are listed in Table 47.5. Other relevant further reading includes:
• Royal College of Obstetrics and Gynaecology guideline on the Management of Acute Pelvic Inflammatory Disease (www.rcog.org.uk);
• PEACH study – one of the largest high-quality PID treatment studies [16];
• *The Prevention of Pelvic Infection* – Allan Templeton [26];
• *Clinical Evidence* – Pelvic Inflammatory Disease (www.clinicalevidence.com); and
• *Chlamydia trachomatis*: summary and conclusions of CMO's Expert Advisory Group (www.dh.gov.uk/).

References

1 Simms I, Rogers P, Charlett A. The rate of diagnosis and demography of pelvic inflammatory disease in general practice: England and Wales. *Int J STD AIDS* 1999;10:448–451.
2 Ness RB, Hillier SL, Richter HE *et al.* Why women douche and why they may or may not stop. *Sex Transm Dis* 2003;30:71–74.
3 Ness RB. Bacterial vaginosis as a cause of PID. British Association for Sexual Health and HIV conference, Bath, 2004.
4 Yeh JM, Hook EW III, Goldie SJ. A refined estimate of the average lifetime cost of pelvic inflammatory disease. *Sex Transm Dis* 2003;30:369–378.
5 Bevan CD, Ridgway GL, Rothermel CD. Efficacy and safety of azithromycin as monotherapy or combined with metronidazole compared with two standard multidrug regimens for the treatment of acute pelvic inflammatory disease. *J Int Med Res* 2003;31:45–54.
6 Eschenbach DA. Acute pelvic inflammatory disease: aetiology, risk factors and pathogenesis. *Clin Obstet Gynecol* 1976;19:147–169.
7 Cohen CR, Manhart LE, Bukusi EA *et al.* Association between *Mycoplasma genitalium* and acute endometritis. *Lancet* 2002;359(9308):765–766.
8 Taylor-Robinson D, Furr PM, Tully JG, Barile MF, Moller BR. Animal models of *Mycoplasma genitalium* urogenital infection. *Isr J Med Sci* 1987;23:561–564.
9 Mardh PA. An overview of infectious agents of salpingitis, their biology, and recent advances in methods of detection. *Am J Obstet Gynecol* 1980;138:933–951.
10 Hillis SD, Joesoef R, Marchbanks PA *et al.* Delayed care of pelvic inflammatory disease as a risk factor for impaired fertility. *Am J Obstet Gynecol* 1993;168:1503–1509.
11 Svensson L, Westrom L, Ripa KT, Mardh PA. Differences in some clinical and laboratory parameters in acute salpingitis related to culture and serological findings. *Am J Obstet Gynecol* 1980;138:1017–1021.
12 Peipert JF, Ness RB, Soper DE, Bass D. Association of lower genital tract inflammation with objective evidence of endometritis. *Infect Dis Obstet Gynecol* 2000;8:83–87.
13 Molander P, Finne P, Sjoberg J, Sellors J, Paavonen J. Observer agreement with laparoscopic diagnosis of pelvic inflammatory disease using photographs. *Obstet Gynecol* 2003;101:875–880.
14 Kiviat NB, Wolner-Hanssen P, Eschenbach DA *et al.* Endometrial histopathology in patients with culture-proved upper genital tract infection and laparoscopically diagnosed acute salpingitis. *Am J Surg Pathol* 1990;14:167–175.
15 Domeika M, Domeika K, Paavonen J, Mardh PA, Witkin SS. Humoral immune response to conserved epitopes of *Chlamydia trachomatis* and human 60-kDa heat-shock protein in women with pelvic inflammatory disease. *J Infect Dis* 1998;177:714–719.
16 Ness RB, Soper DE, Holley RL *et al.* Effectiveness of inpatient and outpatient treatment strategies for women with pelvic inflammatory disease: results from the Pelvic Inflammatory Disease Evaluation and Clinical Health (PEACH) Randomized Trial. *Am J Obstet Gynecol* 2002;186:929–937.
17 Haggerty CL, Schulz R, Ness RB. Lower quality of life among women with chronic pelvic pain after pelvic inflammatory disease. *Obstet Gynecol* 2003;102:934–939.
18 Karinen L, Pouta A, Hartikainen A-K, Bloiga A. Association between *Chlamydia trachomatis* antibodies and subfertility in the Northern Finland Birth Cohort 1966 at the age of 31 years. *Epidemiol Infect* 2004;132:977–984.
19 Pavletic A, Wolner-Hanssen PK, Paavonen JA, Hawes SE, Eschenbach DA. Infertility following pelvic inflammatory disease. *Infect Dis Obstet Gynecol* 1999;7:145–150.
20 Westrom L, Eschenbach D. Pelvic inflammatory disease. In: Holmes KK, Mardh P-A, Sparling PF, Stamm WE, Piot P,

Wasserheit JN, eds. *Sexually Transmitted Diseases*, 3rd edn. New York: McGraw Hill, 1999, pp. 783–810.

21 Altunyurt S, Demir N, Posaci C. A randomized controlled trial of coil removal prior to treatment of pelvic inflammatory disease. *Eur J Obstet Gynecol Reprod Biol* 2003;107:81–84.

22 Soderberg G, Lindgren S. Influence of an intrauterine device on the course of an acute salpingitis. *Contraception* 1981;24: 137–143.

23 Scholes D, Stergachis A, Heidrich FE, Andrilla H, Holmes KK, Stamm WE. Prevention of pelvic inflammatory disease by screening for cervical chlamydial infection. *N Engl J Med* 1996; 334:1362–1366.

24 Washington AE, Gove S, Schachter J, Sweet RL. Oral contraceptives, *Chlamydia trachomatis* infection, and pelvic inflammatory disease. A word of caution about protection. *JAMA* 1985;253: 2246–2250.

25 Morrison CS, Bright P, Wong EL *et al.* Hormonal contraceptive use, cervical ectopy, and the acquisition of cervical infections. *Sex Transm Dis* 2004;31:561–567.

26 Recommendations arising from the 31st Study Group: The Prevention of Pelvic Infection. In: A Templeton, ed. *The Prevention of Pelvic Infection*. London: RCOG Press, 1996, pp. 267–270.

Chapter 48
Chronic Pelvic Pain

R. William Stones

Department of Obstetrics and Gynaecology, Aga Khan University, Nairobi, Kenya

Epidemiology of chronic pelvic pain

Initial reports relied on estimates from hospital series, which are inevitably unrepresentative of the general population. Some population sample survey data are available: a US study reported the responses of women interviewed by telephone [1]. The age range of respondents was 18–50 years. A total of 17 927 households were contacted; 5325 women agreed to participate and of these 925 reported pelvic pain of at least 6 months' duration, including pain within the past 3 months. Having excluded those pregnant or postmenopausal and those with only cycle-related pain, 773 out of 5263 (14.7%) were identified as suffering from chronic pelvic pain (CPP). A British population survey used a postal sample of 2016 women randomly selected from the Oxfordshire Health Authority register of 141 400 women aged 18–49 [2]. Chronic pelvic pain was defined as recurrent pain of at least 6 months' duration, unrelated to periods, intercourse or pregnancy. For the survey, a 'case' was defined as a woman with CPP in the previous 3 months and on this basis the prevalence was 483 out of 2016 (24.0%). In this survey CPP was statistically associated with both dysmenorrhoea and dyspareunia.

Moving from the general population to those seen in general practice, a picture of consulting patterns was obtained using a national database study of UK general practices [3]. Data relating to 284 162 women aged 12–70 who had a general practice contact in 1991 were analysed to identify subsequent contacts over the following 5 years. The monthly prevalence rate was 21.5 per 1000 and the monthly incidence rate was 1.58 per 1000. These prevalence rates are comparable to those for migraine, back pain and asthma in primary care. Older women had higher monthly prevalence rates; for example, the rate was 18.2 per 1000 in the 15–20 year age group and 27.6 per 1000 in women over 60 years of age. This association was thought to be because of persistence of symptoms in older women, the median duration of symptoms being 13.7 months in 13–20 year olds and 20.2 months in women

over the age of 60 years [4]. It is clear that future population-based studies need to include older women.

It is clear that many women with symptoms do not seek care: among 483 women with CPP participating in the Oxfordshire population study discussed above, 195 (40.4%) had not sought a medical consultation, 127 (26.3%) reported a past consultation and 139 (28.8%) reported a recent consultation for pain [5]. The US population-based study discussed above also drew attention to the large numbers of women who have troublesome symptoms but do not seek medical attention: 75% of this sample had not seen a healthcare provider in the previous 3 months. It might be thought that not seeking care would be an indicator of milder symptoms, and, indeed, in the US study those who did seek medical attention had higher pain and lower general health scores than those who did not. However, among those not seeking help questionnaire scores for pain and functional impairment were still substantial, tending to suggest that there are barriers to care seeking, whether organizational or sociocultural.

Summary box 48.1

- Although dysmenorrhoea and dyspareunia often occur as isolated symptoms, they are common in women with CPP.
- In primary care settings, CPP has a similar prevalence to migraine, back pain and asthma.
- Postmenopausal women also report a substantial burden of CPP.

Clinical assessment

For patients presenting with CPP the gynaecological history needs be sufficiently broad as to enable understanding of the impact of symptoms. It is also useful to ascertain at an early stage whether the patient is primarily in search of symptom control, or of diagnosis, advice

Table 48.1 Classification of causes of chronic pelvic pain.

Inflammatory, infective: chronic salpingitis
Inflammatory, non-infective: endometriosis, vulvodynia with
    dermatosis
Mechanical: uterine retroversion, adhesions
Functional: pelvic congestion, irritable bowel syndrome
Neuropathic: post-surgical, dysesthetic vulvodynia, vulval
    vestibulodynia ('vestibulitis')
Musculoskeletal: pelvic floor myalgia, abdominal and pelvic trigger
    points, postural muscle strain

and explanation. Sometimes those with longstanding and disabling symptoms are found to be reluctant to consider symptomatic treatments out of fear that some damaging disease process will be masked and overlooked. Table 48.1 presents a classification of causes of CPP that can be borne in mind while undertaking the clinical assessment.

Pain history

The history needs to include the onset and duration of symptoms, the location and radiation of pain, factors associated with exacerbation and relief, and the relationship of pain to the menstrual cycle. Dysmenorrhoea may be a separate or related symptom. Traditional teaching has emphasized the distinction between primary or spasmodic dysmenorrhoea, with onset of pain at the same time as menstrual flow and symptoms present since menarche, and secondary or congestive dysmenorrhoea where symptoms develop later in reproductive life and pain precedes menstrual flow. The distinction has been used to identify those more or less likely to have specific pathology. However, the intensity of dysmenorrhoea is perhaps a better pointer than the pattern of symptoms to the possibility of specific pathology such as endometriosis: the consequences of missing this diagnosis in young women because pain has been regarded as 'normal' have been emphasized in the literature. Dyspareunia may include pain during intercourse, but for many women a particularly unpleasant symptom is postcoital pain and a specific enquiry about this should be made.

A number of validated pain assessment measures are available for use in research and clinical practice, the most convenient of which are the 10 cm visual analogue scale, the Brief Pain Inventory (BPI), widely used in British pain clinics, and the Short-form McGill Pain Questionnaire. The McGill questionnaire is included in the International Pelvic Pain Society's assessment form, available for downloading at www.pelvicpain.org, and the BPI may be downloaded at www.mdanderson.org, where details of non-English versions may also be obtained. The patient's recall of pain symptoms over the previous month seems

to be adequate and it is probably unnecessary to ask for a daily pain diary: 10 cm visual analogue scales for 'usual' and 'most severe' intensity of pain recalled over the past 4 weeks correlated very well with mean and maximal diary records [6].

Mood and impact on quality of life

It is important to identify coexisting mood disturbance. Although it is unlikely that depression is the cause of CPP, the presence of disturbed mood makes it difficult for patients to engage fully with pain management initiatives and tackle associated lifestyle factors. The absence of laparoscopically visible pathology was not associated with a higher probability of depression [7,8]. In these studies no differences in mood-related symptoms were identified in women with CPP with and without endometriosis. Antidepressant therapy may be indicated to alleviate depression, but sertraline was not effective for relief of pelvic pain in a small but well-conducted randomized trial [9].

With regard to symptom impact, while a validated illness-specific instrument is not currently available, enquiry about the effect of the pain on work, leisure, sleep and sexual relationships is appropriate. This can shed further light on the patient's priorities for treatment. A generic quality of life measure such as the SF-36 may be used for monitoring outcomes but may be too cumbersome for routine clinical use.

Sexual and physical abuse

Child sexual or physical abuse may be an antecedent for CPP but many individuals have suffered such abuse without this or other consequence in later life and the research literature is beset with the problem of appropriate comparison groups. Individual judgement is needed about whether to ask directly about sexual or physical abuse during a gynaecological consultation. Important considerations are the setting and plans for follow-up and support that are available to women following such disclosure. Sometimes such a history may be volunteered by the patient unprompted, especially so during a follow-up consultation when rapport has been established. Some women may even find it easier to raise the subject with an unfamiliar hospital specialist than with a general practitioner with whom they have regular consultations for other matters. It may be useful to incorporate questions on abuse into a self-completion questionnaire, such as that provided by the International Pelvic Pain Society, or in a multidisciplinary clinic to address the topic during a consultation with the nurse or psychologist. We have found it appropriate not to include those items in the package of questionnaires sent to patients for self-completion before the initial consultation.

In a study from a tertiary referral multidisciplinary pain clinic, 40% of those with CPP reported sexual abuse compared with 5 (17%) in each of two comparison groups. In women with pelvic pain, abuse histories were evenly distributed among those with and without identified pelvic pathology such as endometriosis, but somatization scores were higher among those with identified pathology [10]. It has been suggested that the potential link between sexual abuse and pelvic pain might be that abuse is an observable marker for childhood neglect in general [11] and this might explain the association in some studies with physical rather than sexual abuse [12].

Systems review

Many women with chronic abdominal or pelvic pain will turn out to have irritable bowel syndrome (IBS) as their primary problem. These patients do not have good outcomes following (inappropriate) gynaecological referral and investigation [13]. Therefore, it is particularly important that a detailed history is taken of bowel symptoms. The Rome II criteria for the clinical diagnosis of IBS in those with chronic pain include at least two of:

- relief of pain with defecation;
- change in the frequency of stool; and
- change in the appearance or form of stool.

Abdominal bloating in association with acute exacerbations of pain is indicative, but needs to be distinguished from menstrual cycle-related bloating. While dyspareunia is not likely to be due solely to IBS, bowel spasm may account for the experience of those patients who describe an interval between the end of intercourse and the onset of acute pain associated with the urge to defecate and abdominal distension [14].

Bladder symptoms also form an important part of the systems review. Urinary frequency and urgency, but most importantly exacerbation of pain associated with a full bladder, may indicate the presence of interstitial cystitis, a neurogenic inflammatory condition of the bladder associated with chronic pain. As with IBS, it has been suggested that a proportion of cases of CPP seen by gynaecologists are in fact suffering from unrecognized interstitial cystitis on the basis of potassium chloride sensitivity testing [15].

 Summary box 48.2

- The history needs to be sufficiently detailed, with direct questions aiming to elicit symptoms referable to the gastrointestinal and urinary systems.
- The intensity of pain should be documented using a validated tool, taking into account cyclical fluctuations and impairment of function.
- Sexual or physical abuse may be very important antecedents of pain and distress in particular individuals, but the association is not causal and history-taking should be carefully planned.

Physical examination

Observing the patient as she walks may give an indication of a musculoskeletal problem and examination of the back is relevant in those giving a history of pain radiating or originating there. The abdominal examination should focus on distinguishing visceral from abdominal wall tenderness. 'Trigger point' tenderness elicited by palpation with one finger will suggest a nerve entrapment, often involving the ilioinguinal or iliohypogastric nerves. The ilioinguinal nerve runs in relation to abdominal muscle layers, initially superficial to transversus abdominus and deep to internal oblique. It penetrates the belly of the internal oblique muscle to lie deep to the external oblique at a point typically two centimetres medial to the iliac crest, at which point it is susceptible to entrapment. A trigger point is then evident at that site. As well as spontaneous entrapment previous surgery such as appendicectomy or a wide Pfannensteil incision may be responsible. The diagnosis is confirmed after obtaining appropriate consent by infiltration of local anaesthetic such as bupivacaine into the tender area. Interestingly, the duration of relief is often much longer than the action of the local anaesthetic, perhaps because surrounding muscles are made to relax and are no longer pulling on the sensitive area.

'Ovarian point' tenderness has been described as a feature of pelvic congestion syndrome [16] but this sign is problematic in patients with IBS who often have similar abdominal tenderness. A general neurological examination is appropriate to exclude a systemic neuropathy or demyelination and if abnormalities are present a neurology opinion should be sought.

Vaginal examination should commence with a careful inspection of the vulva and introitus, paying particular attention to the presence of erythema, which might suggest primary vulval vestibulitis [17] or evidence of a vulval dermatosis with pain arising from inflammation. More frequently, no erythema is evident but a gentle touch with a cotton-tipped swab in the area just external to the hymeneal ring elicits intense sharp pain, even in patients who do not complain of dyspareunia. This allodynia in the absence of visible erythema probably represents referred sensation from painful areas higher in the pelvis but for some women represents the primary problem and can better be termed 'vestibulodynia' rather than vestibulitis as there is no evidence for an infective aetiology. Vulval varices may indicate incompetence of valves in the pelvic venous circulation; this subgroup of patients may benefit from radiological assessment and treatment such as embolization of the ovarian veins.

Following explanation to and consent from the patient, a gentle one finger digital examination commences with palpation of the pelvic floor muscles. Focal tenderness may be present, indicating a primary musculoskeletal problem that should prompt referral to a pelvic floor physiotherapist for further assessment. As with vestibulodynia, pelvic muscle tenderness may be a residual secondary response to pain from other parts of the pelvis, for example, a previous episode of pelvic infection. Recently, the use of a 'tampon test' has been described in a research setting in order to obtain self report information on pain symptoms in women with vestibulitis/vestibulodynia and vulvodynia. This may prove to be a useful tool for assessing the response to treatment without the need for repeated examination [18].

Further digital examination may reveal nodularity in the pouch of Douglas or restricted uterine mobility suggestive of endometriosis. Adenomyosis may be suggested by a bulky tender uterus. Uterine retroversion should be noted although its relevance to dyspareunia is debatable. Adnexal rather than uterine tenderness may point to pelvic congestion syndrome. In the UK clinic setting pelvic tenderness alone is unlikely to be specific for chronic pelvic inflammatory disease although this diagnosis will be part of the differential among populations where early and appropriate antibiotic treatment for acute pelvic sepsis is less readily available.

Summary box 48.3

- In CPP, the physical examination is highly informative in formulating a diagnosis. The aims are to distinguish neuromuscular (somatic) from visceral tenderness, both in the abdomen and pelvis, and to identify features suggestive of neuropathy such as allodynia.
- In vulval vestibulodynia (or 'vestibulitis') it is usual not to see any signs of inflammation, in contrast to vulval dermatosis.
- Pelvic inflammatory disease should be diagnosed only in presence of supporting evidence and not simply on the basis of pelvic tenderness.

Investigations

Excluding the possibility of ongoing pelvic infection such as *Chlamydia* by taking endocervical swabs, or using the currently available molecular tests in urine or vaginal swab samples is often useful to allay anxiety. Ultrasound examination may be useful in identifying uterine or adnexal pathology and has been shown to be an effective means of providing reassurance [19]. The presence of dilated veins may indicate pelvic congestion [20] but a

power Doppler study suggested that the primary value of sonography was to identify the characteristic multi-cystic ovarian morphology seen in this condition [21] and that venous characteristics were non-specific. Transuterine venography is of limited value in routine clinical practice but is technically simpler than selective catheterization of the ovarian vein. However, where vulval varices are present selective ovarian venous catheterization with a view to embolization provides a combined diagnostic and treatment opportunity. MRI is very helpful in providing a positive diagnosis of adenomyosis but it is not routinely indicated.

Laparoscopy has commonly been undertaken as the primary investigation for CPP. The aims are to give a diagnosis but also to provide 'one-stop' treatment for endometriosis and adhesions where these are identified. This approach is cost-effective for endometriosis treatment, as the expense of a second procedure or hormonal treatment is obviated [22]. The outcomes of this approach are not as good as might be expected: confusion can arise from a 'negative' laparoscopy [23] and where pathology is identified it may be coincidental rather than causal, especially in the case of adhesions. There is a lack of evidence for laparoscopy as a factor improving outcome in hospital referral populations with at least 6 months' history of pain [24,25]. It is therefore sensible to discuss with the patient as a preferred approach deferring laparoscopy and focusing on symptomatic treatment in the first instance.

Pain mapping by laparoscopy under conscious sedation can be a useful procedure, particularly where the site of pain is unilateral, allowing comparison with a 'control' area, to assess the significance of adhesions, to identify unrecognized occult inguinal or femoral hernias and, in the negative sense, to identify individuals with a generalized hyperalgesic chronic pain state for whom further surgical intervention would be hazardous. The role of this procedure remains to be clarified in the overall context of pain assessment and management but reports of experience are now available in the literature [26]. Typical operative technique includes sedation with midazolam and fentanyl, infiltration of puncture sites with bupivicaine, use of a 5-mm laparoscope via a subumbilical puncture together with a fine suprapubic port for a probe. The maximum gas pressure is reduced to around 10 mmHg to minimize discomfort in the upper abdomen. Tenderness at specific sites is recorded on a 0–10 verbal rating scale. In this writer's practice its application has been limited to the small subgroup of patients whose main priority is to obtain a definitive explanation for their problem, rather than symptom relief. Overall, after gaining initial experience following early positive reports, many clinicians no longer consider pain mapping to be useful.

Specific treatments for chronic pelvic pain: evidence from randomized trials

Limited evidence from randomized controlled trials (RCTs) is available to guide treatment decisions in CPP. It is important to be clear whether treatment is directed towards an underlying condition such as adhesions or whether pain itself is the main focus. While hormonal therapy aims to achieve benefit in a non-specific manner by inhibiting ovarian activity, based on the observation that many patients with CPP experience resolution at the time of the menopause, psychological approaches aim to enhance coping skills and reduce pain-associated distress. Many proven treatments for chronic neuropathic pain such as low-dose tricyclic antidepressants and gabapentin are equally relevant in CPP where there are neuropathic features. With regard to specific approaches, systematic review identified 14 RCTs relevant to the management of CPP, the interventions in 12 of which are of practical applicability [27].

Medical therapy

Progestogen [medroxyprogesterone acetate (MPA)] was effective after 4 months' treatment as reflected in pain scores [odds ratio (OR) 2.64; 95% confidence interval (CI) 1.33–5.25; n = 146] and a self-rating scale (OR 6.81; 95% CI 1.83–25.3; n = 44), but benefit was not sustained 9 months after treatment [28,29]. MPA plus psychotherapy was effective in terms of pain scores (OR 3.94; 95% CI 1.2–12.96; n = 43) but not the self-rating scale at the end of treatment. Benefit was not sustained following treatment. Venography scores, symptom and examination scores, mood and sexual function were improved to a greater extent 1 year after treatment with goserelin compared with progestogen [30].

No improvement in pain scores was seen in women taking sertraline compared with placebo. The SF-36 subscale 'health perception' showed a small improvement in the sertraline arm, while the 'role functioning–emotional' subscale showed a large fall in the sertraline arm [9].

Multidisciplinary management

Counselling supported by ultrasound scanning [19] was effective in terms of both pain scores (OR 6.77; 95% CI 2.83–16.19; n = 90) and mood. The use of a multidisciplinary approach [24] led to a positive outcome in a self-rating scale (OR 4.15; 95% CI 1.91–8.99; n = 106) and daily activity but not in pain scores. In British pain clinics, women with CPP rated the intensity of their pain similarly to those with other types of chronic pain. The pattern of interventions used for this group showed less recourse to nerve blocks among those with CPP. Access to clinical psychology input was sadly lacking among all groups of patients [31] (Fig. 48.1).

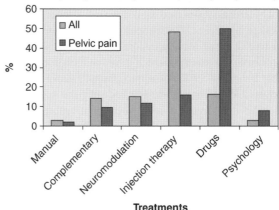

PACS 1998–2001. Treatment modalities used for all pain (N = 40958) and for pelvic pain (N = 472)

Fig. 48.1 Treatments used in UK pain clinics for patients with chronic pain (all causes) and women with CPP (from ref. 30, reproduced with permission).

Surgical treatment

The outcome in women undergoing adhesiolysis was not different to that in women who did not undergo surgery on any outcome measure (OR 1.54; 95% CI 0.81–2.93; n = 148). However, the small subgroup with severe adhesions did show a significant benefit for surgery (OR for self-rating scale 16.59; 95% CI 2.16–127.2; n = 15). Adhesiolysis was performed via laparotomy in one study [32] in contrast with a laparoscopic approach [33]. The latter study also included some men. Thus, there is still uncertainty about the place of adhesiolysis among patients presenting to gynaecologists and the conclusion of this review is that there is 'no evidence of benefit' rather than 'evidence of no benefit'.

Static magnetic therapy

The effects of wearing small magnets as therapy for CPP versus placebo were assessed [34]. No difference was seen following 2 weeks' treatment but some significant differences appeared at 4 weeks as assessed by the Pain Disability Index and the Clinical Global Impression Scale but not the McGill Pain Questionnaire. Analysed in terms of weighted mean differences, the differences were non-significant and there was a substantial dropout rate. It is not clear whether this modality justifies further exploration. A clear mechanistic basis appears to be lacking, but another substantial study did show benefit for magnetic therapy in diabetic neuropathic foot pain, which may indicate some detectable actions of magnetic fields at the neuronal cellular level, such as modifying the abnormal discharge of damaged C fibre afferents [35]. These concepts have been the topic of debate [36].

Photographic reinforcement

Photographic reinforcement after surgery (i.e. showing patients pictures of the findings) does not appear to have any beneficial effect [37]. Unfortunately, the intervention group had a trend for greater pain intensity compared with controls at baseline, which may have confounded a possible beneficial effect of photographic reinforcement. Moreover, 233 women were entered into the trial compared with the target of 450, so the final comparisons were somewhat different to those originally planned. This study is important in demonstrating how a well-intentioned intervention reinforcing patients' knowledge of their condition may not have the intended beneficial impact.

Writing therapy

The aim of this intervention was to allow patients to identify and express through writing the thoughts and feelings associated with their pain, as a means of reducing their impact [38]. The main effects of writing about the stress of pelvic pain were limited: weighted mean differences (95% CI) on the various subcategories of the McGill Pain Questionnaire were: sensory pain 0.07 (−0.31 to 0.45), affective pain −0.12 (−0.42 to 0.18) and evaluation pain −1.16 (−1.96 to −0.36). Women with higher baseline ambivalence about emotional expression appeared to respond more positively to this intervention, thus showing a subgroup that may benefit specifically from this type of psychological approach.

Specific treatments for chronic pelvic pain: other pointers from the literature

A 3-year follow-up study of women with CPP suggested that, as a group, pain intensity and associated measures of psychological distress were improved over time. However, it was not possible to predict individual outcomes based on initial clinical and psychometric assessment. Interestingly, improvement in catastrophizing was strongly associated with improvement in pain intensity, perhaps highlighting the importance of this attitudinal component [39] and emphasizing the scope for supportive psychological interventions, in particular cognitive behaviour therapy. It is helpful to have a cognitive model in mind when discussing potential strategies with the patient [40].

Vulval vestibulitis or vestibulodynia has been treated with topical 5% lidocaine gel, with the aim of desensitizing the cutaneous nociceptors over a period of time. After an initial favourable report [41], comparison has been made with electromyographic biofeedback, and these interventions were found to have similar efficacy over a 4-month course of treatment and follow-up for 1 year.

Lidocaine proved more acceptable with a lower dropout rate [42]. There is a small role for surgical vestibulectomy but this should only be considered in very refractory cases.

While vulvodynia is usually best considered as a type of neuropathic pain and managed with drugs such as amitryptilene, gapapentin or lamotrigine as part of a multidisciplinary pain management programme, an attempt at specific therapy with topical lidocaine or desipramine showed no benefit over placebo in a randomized trial [43]. A specific sub group may benefit from surgical decompression of the pudendal nerve [44]. Nerve conduction studies have not proved to be a conclusive discriminator but these patients should be distinguished from those with 'non-specific' vulvodynia by meeting the Nantes criteria of (i) pain in the anatomical territory of the pudendal nerve; (ii) worsened by sitting; (iii) the patient is not woken at night by the pain; (iv) no objective sensory loss on clinical examination; (v) positive anaesthetic pudendal nerve block [45].

Treatment dilemmas

Women may seek hysterectomy and oophorectomy as a solution to longstanding CPP. The evidence from observational studies is encouraging [46], but this is naturally a treatment of last resort. Where the underlying condition is neuropathic then there is a real possibility of making things worse. It is unclear whether a previous response to gonadotrophin-releasing hormone (GnRH) agonist therapy fully predicts a positive response to oophorectomy, given the complexities of the influences of ovarian hormones on nociception.

There has been a resurgence of interest in pelvic congestion as a cause of CPP owing to increased experience in North America of radiological embolization of pelvic 'varices'. There are issues of case definition and most studies have incomplete clinical documentation [47] but a recent comparative study indicates that this approach may have potential [48]. Radiological appearances of the ovarian veins before and after treatment are shown in Fig. 48.2a and b.

Many women seek complementary or alternative therapies for CPP. At present there is limited research evidence on which to base recommendations for specific treatments. Acupuncture has a place in the management of chronic pain in general, and there is supportive evidence for benefit in dysmenorrhoea [49]. Most importantly, in the author's view, many patients will appreciate a broad consideration of physical conditions, lifestyle factors, psychological stresses and advice on means of dealing with thoughts and feelings as part of a consultation for CPP, whether in 'conventional' or 'complementary' clinic settings.

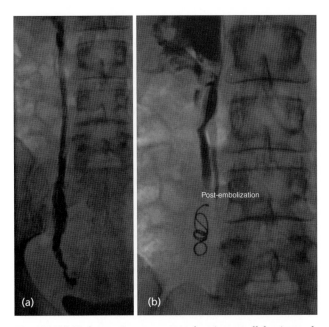

Fig. 48.2 (a) Right ovarian venogram showing parallel veins and venules over the sacral wing. (b) Post-embolization with several distal coils (not shown) and a single mid-vein embolization coil. A local sclerosant 0.5% sodium tetradecyl sulphate (Fibro-Vein™) is mixed with air to form a mousse and injected through the catheter to reflux into small parallel venules and occlude these as well. Images courtesy of Dr Nigel Hacking.

💡 Summary box 48.4

- In clinical practice, RCT evidence is available to guide the recommendation of certain interventions. However, for CPP (as in other types of chronic pain) medical advice should emphasize meeting the patient's goals, the nature of which should not be assumed. Goals may include a need for reassurance as to the absence of dangerous pathology, ability to function including daily activities and sex, or reduction in pain intensity.
- Research strongly supports the use of multidisciplinary approaches to CPP care, and those designing health service delivery models need to take this seriously by removing the barriers to collaborative working, especially relating to provision of cognitive interventions.

Conclusion

To provide useful advice to women with CPP emphasis on careful clinical method is critical: a full history including details of symptoms from all relevant organs, a physical examination that aims to localize tenderness so as to narrow down the diagnostic options and deployment of relevant investigations. Not all patients require laparoscopy, the findings of which can sometimes confuse rather than aid diagnosis through the presence of coincidental findings. There are some therapeutic interventions backed up by randomized trial evidence, but most importantly clinicians need to match their advice to the aspirations and circumstances of each patient.

References

1 Mathias SD, Kuppermann M, Liberman RF, Lipschutz RC, Steege JF. Chronic pelvic pain: prevalence, health-related quality of life, and economic correlates. *Obstet Gynecol* 1996;87:321–327.

2 Zondervan KT, Yudkin PL, Vessey MP *et al.* Chronic pelvic pain in the community – symptoms, investigations, and diagnoses. *Am J Obstet Gynecol* 2001;184:1149–1155.

3 Zondervan KT, Yudkin PL, Vessey MP, Dawes MG, Barlow DH, Kennedy SH. Patterns of diagnosis and referral in women consulting for chronic pelvic pain in UK primary care. *Br J Obstet Gynaecol* 1999;106:1156–1161.

4 Zondervan KT, Yudkin PL, Vessey MP, Dawes MG, Barlow DH, Kennedy SH. Prevalence and incidence of chronic pelvic pain in primary care: evidence from a national general practice database. *Br J Obstet Gynaecol* 1999;106:1149–1155.

5 Zondervan KT, Yudkin PL, Vessey MP *et al.* The community prevalence of chronic pelvic pain in women and associated illness behaviour. *Br J Gen Pract* 2001;51: 541–547.

6 Stones RW, Bradbury L, Anderson D. Randomized placebo controlled trial of lofexidine hydrochloride for chronic pelvic pain in women. *Hum Reprod* 2001;16:1719–1721.

7 Peveler R, Edwards J, Daddow J, Thomas EJ. Psychosocial factors and chronic pelvic pain: a comparison of women with endometriosis and with unexplained pain. *J Psychosom Res* 1995;40:305–315.

8 Waller KG, Shaw RW. Endometriosis, pelvic pain, and psychological functioning. *Fertil Steril* 1995;63:796–800.

9 Engel CC, Walker EA, Engel AL, Bullis J, Armstrong A. A randomized, double-blind crossover trial of sertraline in women with chronic pelvic pain. *J Psychosomatic Res* 1998;44:203–207.

10 Collett BJ, Cordle CJ, Stewart CR, Jagger C. A comparative study of women with chronic pelvic pain, chronic nonpelvic pain and those with no history of pain attending general practitioners. *Br J Obstet Gynaecol* 1998;105:87–92.

11 Fry RPW, Beard RW, Crisp AH, McGuigan S. Sociopsychological factors in women with chronic pelvic pain with and without pelvic venous congestion. *J Psychosom Res* 1997;42:71–85.

12 Rapkin AJ, Kames LD, Darke LL, Stampler FM, Naliboff BD. History of physical and sexual abuse in women with chronic pelvic pain. *Obstet Gynecol* 1990;76:92–96.

13 Prior A, Whorwell PJ. Gynaecological consultation in patients with the irritable bowel syndrome. *Gut* 1989;30:996–998.

14 Whorwell P. The gender influence. *Women & IBS* 1995;2:2–3.

15 Parsons CL, Dell J, Stanford EJ, Bullen M, Kahn BS, Willems JJ. The prevalence of interstitial cystitis in gynecologic patients with pelvic pain, as detected by intravesical potassium sensitivity. *Am J Obstet Gynecol* 2002;187:1395–1400.

16 Beard RW, Reginald PW, Wadsworth J. Clinical features of women with chronic lower abdominal pain and pelvic congestion. *Br J Obstet Gynaecol* 1988;95:153–161.

17 Gibbons JM. Vulvar vestibulitis. In: JF Steage, DA Metzger, BS Levy (eds) *Chronic Pelvic Pain: An Integrated Approach.* Philadelphia: WB Saunders, 1998, pp. 181–187.

18 Foster DC, Kotok MB, Huang LS, Watts A, Oakes D, Howard FM, Stodgell CJ, Dworkin RH. The tampon test for vulvodynia treatment outcomes research: reliability, construct validity, and responsiveness. *Obstet Gynecol* 2009;113:825–832.

19 Ghaly AFF. The psychological and physical benefits of pelvic ultrasonography in patients with chronic pelvic pain and negative laparoscopy. A random allocation trial. *J Obstet Gynaecol* 1994;14:269–271.

20 Stones RW, Rae T, Rogers V, Fry R, Beard RW. Pelvic congestion in women: evaluation with transvaginal ultrasound and observation of venous pharmacology. *Br J Radiol* 1990;63:710–711.

21 Halligan S, Campbell D, Bartram CI *et al.* Transvaginal ultrasound examination of women with and without pelvic venous congestion. *Clin Radiol* 2000;55:954–958.

22 Stones RW, Thomas EJ. Cost-effective medical treatment of endometriosis. In: J Bonnar (ed.) *Recent Advances in Obstetrics and Gynaecology no. 19.* Edinburgh: Churchill Livingstone, 1995, pp. 139–152.

23 Howard FM. The role of laparoscopy in the evaluation of chronic pelvic pain: pitfalls with a negative laparoscopy. *J Am Assoc Gynecol Laparosc* 1996;4:85–94.

24 Peters AA, van Dorst E, Jellis B, van Zuuren E, Hermans J, Trimbos JB. A randomized clinical trial to compare two different approaches in women with chronic pelvic pain. *Obstet Gynecol* 1991;77:740–744.

25 Selfe SA, Matthews Z, Stones RW. Factors influencing outcome in consultations for chronic pelvic pain. *J Womens Health* 1998;7:1041–1048.

26 Howard FM. Pelvic pain. In: EJ Thomas, RW Stones (eds) *Gynaecology Highlights 1998–99.* Oxford: Health Press, 1999, pp. 53–63.

27 Stones W, Cheong Y, Howard FM. Interventions for treating chronic pelvic pain in women. *Cochrane Database Syst Rev* 2005;3:CD000387.

28 Farquhar CM, Rogers V, Franks S, Pearce S, Wadsworth J, Beard RW. A randomized controlled trial of medroxyprogesterone acetate and psychotherapy for the treatment of pelvic congestion. *Br J Obstet Gynaecol* 1989;96:1153–1162.

29 Walton SM, Batra HK. The use of medroxyprogesterone acetate 50 mg in the treatment of painful pelvic conditions: preliminary results from a multicentre trial. *J Obstet Gynaecol* 1992;12(Suppl. 2):S50–S53.

30 Soysal ME, Soysal S, Vicdan K, Ozer S. A randomised controlled trial of goserelin and medroxyprogesterone acetate in the treatment of pelvic congestion. *Hum Reprod* 2001;16:931–939.

31 Stones RW, Price C. Health services for women with chronic pelvic pain. *J Royal Soc Med* 2002;95:531–535.

32 Peters AAW, Trimbos-Kemper GCM, Admiraal C, Trimbos JB. A randomised clinical trial on the benefit of adhesiolysis in patients with intraperitoneal adhesions and chronic pelvic pain. *Br J Obstet Gynaecol* 1992;99:59–62.

33 Swank DJ, Swank-Bordewijk SC, Hop WC *et al.* Laparoscopic adhesiolysis in patients with chronic abdominal pain: a blinded randomised controlled multi-centre trial. *Lancet* 2003; 361(9365):1247–1251.

34 Brown C, Pharm D, Ling F, Wan J, Pills A. Efficacy of static magnetic field therapy in chronic pelvic pain: a double-blind study. *Am J Obstet Gynecol* 2002;187:1581–1587.

35 Weintraub MI, Wolfe GI, Barohn RA *et al.* Static magnetic field therapy for symptomatic diabetic neuropathy: a randomised, double-blind, placebo-controlled trial. *Arch Phys Med Rehab* 2003;84:736–746.

36 Pittler MH, Harlow T, Orton CG. Point/counterpoint. Despite widespread use there is no convincing evidence that static magnets are effective for the relief of pain. *Med Phys* 2008;35:3017–3019.

37 Onwude L, Thornton J, Morley S, Lilleyman J, Currie I, Lilford R. A randomised trial of photographic reinforcement during postoperative counselling after diagnostic laparoscopy for pelvic pain. *Eur J Obstet Gynecol Reprod Biol* 2004;112:89–94.

38 Norman S, Lumley M, Dooley J, Diamond M. For whom does it work? Moderators of the effects of written emotional disclosure in a randomised trial among women with chronic pelvic pain. *Psychosom Med* 2004;66:174–183.

39 Weijenborg PT, Ter Kuile MM, Gopie JP, Spinhoven P. Predictors of outcome in a cohort of women with chronic pelvic pain – a follow-up study. *Eur J Pain* 2009;13:769–775.

40 Weijenborg PT, Ter Kuile MM, Stones W. A cognitive behavioural based assessment of women with chronic pelvic pain. *J Psychosom Obstet Gynaecol* 2009;30:262–268.

41 Zolnoun DA, Hartmann KE, Steege JF. Overnight 5% lidocaine ointment for treatment of vulvar vestibulitis. *Obstet Gynecol* 2003;102:84–87.

42 Danielsson I, Torstensson T, Brodda-Jansen G, Bohm-Starke N. EMG biofeedback versus topical lidocaine gel: a randomised study for the treatment of women with vulvar vestibulitis. *Acta Obstet Gynecol Scand* 2006;85:1360–1367.

43 Foster DC, Kotok MB, Huang LS, Watts A, Oakes D, Howard FM, Poleshuck EL, Stodgell CJ, Dworkin RH. Oral desipramine and topical lidocaine for vulvodynia: a randomised controlled trial. *Obstet Gynecol* 2010;116:583–593.

44 Robert R, Labat JJ, Bensignor M, Glemain P, Deschamps C, Raoul S, Hamel O. Decompression and transposition of the pudendal nerve in pudendal neuralgia: a randomised controlled trial and long-term evaluation. *Eur Urol* 2005;47:403–408.

45 Labat JJ, Riant T, Robert R, Amarenco G, Lefaucheur JP, Rigaud J. Diagnostic criteria for pudendal neuralgia by pudendal nerve entrapment (Nantes criteria). *Neurourol Urodyn* 2008;27:306–310.

46 Beard RW, Kennedy RG, Gangar KF *et al.* Bilateral oophorectomy and hysterectomy in the treatment of intractable pelvic pain associated with pelvic congestion. *Br J Obstet Gynaecol* 1991;98:988–92.

47 Stones RW. Pelvic vascular congestion: half a century later. *Clin Obstet Gynecol* 2003;46:831–836.

48 Chung M-H, Huh C-Y. Comparison of treatments for pelvic congestion syndrome. *Tohoku J Exp Med* 2003;201:131–138.

49 Proctor ML, Smith CA, Farquhar CM, Stones RW. Transcutaneous electrical nerve stimulation and acupuncture for primary dysmenorrhoea. *Cochrane Database Syst Rev* 2002;1:CD002123.

Chapter 49
Endometriosis

Stephen Kennedy[1] and Philippe Koninckx[1,2]
[1]Nuffield Department of Obstetrics and Gynaecology, University of Oxford, Oxford, UK
[2]Department of Obstetrics and Gynaecology, University of Leuven, Leuven, Belgium

Endometriosis has been defined for many years as the presence of endometrial glands and stroma outside the uterus. The most commonly affected sites are the pelvic organs and peritoneum, although other parts of the body such as the lungs are occasionally affected. The disease, as defined, varies from a few superficial, subtle or typical lesions on otherwise normal pelvic organs to solid infiltrating masses and ovarian endometriotic cysts (endometriomas), often with extensive fibrosis and adhesion formation causing marked distortion of pelvic anatomy. Endometriosis should be suspected in women with subfertility, severe dysmenorrhoea, deep dyspareunia and/or chronic pelvic pain. However, many affected women are asymptomatic, in which case the diagnosis is made only when the pelvis is inspected for an unrelated reason, for example sterilization.

Prevalence

The prevalence is estimated to be 8–10% in women in the reproductive years [1], although the precise rate in the general population is unknown because the pelvis has to be inspected at surgery to make a definitive diagnosis. In symptomatic women, the reported rates vary from 2% to 100% (Summary box 49.1) for which several explanations exist: (i) 'subtle' (e.g. small, non-coloured) peritoneal lesions were not recognized before 1985, leading to an apparent increased prevalence since then; (ii) recognition of subtle and deep lesions increases with the surgeon's experience and interest in endometriosis; (iii) the indication for laparoscopy influences how meticulously the pelvis is inspected; (iv) histological confirmation (close to 100% for deep lesions and at best 60% for subtle lesions) is not always obtained or reported, and (v) rarely are the prevalence rates of subtle lesions (very common), typical lesions (20–40%), endometriomas (10–20%) and deep endometriosis (1–2%) assessed separately. Whatever the true prevalence, it remains possible that the most common manifestation – subtle endometriosis – may not be a disease entity at all [2].

💡 Summary box 49.1

Prevalence rates at laparoscopy for different indications

	Number of studies	Number of patients	Number with disease	% with disease (range)	% with Stage I–II disease (range)
Pelvic pain	15	2400	688	24.5 (4.5–62.1)	69.9 (61.0–100)
Infertility	32	14971	2812	19.6 (2.1–78.0)	65.6 (16.3–95.0)
Sterilisation	13	10634	499	4.1 (0.7–43.0)	91.7 (20.0–100)

Eskenazi & Warner *Obstet Gynecol Clin* 1997;24:235

Dewhurst's Textbook of Obstetrics & Gynaecology, Eighth Edition. Edited by D. Keith Edmonds.
© 2012 John Wiley and Sons, Ltd. Published 2012 by John Wiley and Sons, Ltd.

Classification systems

Several systems have been devised to classify disease severity, with varying degrees of prognostic value. The most widely used is one developed by the American Society for Reproductive Medicine [3], in which points are allocated for endometriotic lesions, periovarian adhesions and pouch of Douglas obliteration (Fig. 49.1). The total score is then used to describe the disease as minimal (stage 1), mild (stage 2), moderate (stage 3) or severe (stage 4). Stages 1 and 2 consist mainly of superficial lesions, and stages 3 and 4 of endometriomas. Unfortunately, deep endometriosis, a major cause of pelvic pain and dyspareunia, is typically assigned a low score (stage 1 or 2) because only visible lesions contribute; this partly explains why there is little correlation between the total score and pain severity. Clearly, a more validated method to classify disease severity is needed, which can differentiate between subtle, typical, cystic ovarian and deep endometriosis.

Aetiology

Implantation of viable endometrial cells and metaplasia of coelomic epithelium are reasonable explanations for the occurrence of endometriosis. However, neither theory can account for all aspects of the disease, which could mean that several mechanisms are involved or simply that the theories are inadequate. Both assume that endometriotic tissue consists of 'normal' cells but they fail to explain why development and progression occur only in some women. In contrast, the endometriotic disease theory [4] considers subtle lesions due to intermittent implantation to be a normal, physiological event. If these cells are transformed because of a genetic insult they progress to typical, cystic and deep lesions, consisting of 'abnormal' cells. An alternative explanation is that endometriosis is heterogeneous and not a disease on its own, and the different types, which are considered below, result from different disease processes, each with their own aetiology [5].

American society for Reproductive Medicine revised classification of endometriosis

Patient's name _____   Date _____

Stage I (minimal)	1–5
Stage II (mild)	6–15
Stage III (moderate)	16–40
Stage IV (severe)	>40
Total _____	

Laparoscopy _____ Laparotomy _____ Photography _____
Recommended treatment _____
_____
Prognosis _____

	Endometriosis	<3 cm	1–3 cm	>3 cm
Peritoneum	Superficial	1	2	4
	Deep	2	4	6
Ovary	R Superficial	1	2	6
	Deep	4	10	20
	L Superficial	1	2	4
	Deep	4	16	20
	Posterior culdesac obliteration	Partial — 4		Complete — 40

	Adhesions	<1/3 enclosure	1/3–2/3 enclosure	>2/3 enclosure
Ovary	R Filmy	1	2	4
	Dense	4	8	16
	L Filmy	1	2	4
	Dense	4	8	16
Tube	R Filmy	1	2	4
	Dense	4	8*	16
	L Filmy	1	2	4
	Dense	4	8*	16

*If the fimbriated end of the fallopian tube is completely enclosed change the point assignment to 16.

Denote appearance of superficial implant types as red [(R), red, mid-pink, flamelike, vesicular blobs, clear vesicles], white [(W) specifications, peritoneal defects, yellow-brown], or black [(B) black, hemosiderm deposits, black]. Denote percent of total described as R_____% and B_____%. Total should equal 100%.

Fig. 49.1 American Society for Reproductive Medicine classification system [3].

Peritoneal endometriosis

Peritoneal endometriosis comprises superficial lesions scattered over the peritoneal, serosal and ovarian surfaces. These were described as 'powder-burn' or 'gunshot' deposits until atypical or subtle lesions were recognized, including red implants, polypoid lesions, and serous or clear vesicles. It remains unclear, however, whether these subtle lesions should be considered early disease, or whether they are transient physiological events without any clinical significance. Subtle lesions can readily be explained by Sampson's theory of retrograde menstruation. Menstrual effluent containing viable cells is transported into the peritoneal cavity in a retrograde direction along the fallopian tubes and the refluxed endometrium then implants onto the surface of exposed tissues, principally the peritoneum. The amount of menstrual effluent transported seems important as higher prevalence rates occur in women with increased menstrual exposure due to (i) obstructed outflow associated with Müllerian anomalies and (ii) short menstrual cycles, increased duration of bleeding and decreased parity [1]. However, most women do not develop endometriosis even though retrograde menstruation occurs commonly, for which there are several explanations. The expression of factors such as cell adhesion molecules, proteolytic enzymes and cytokines affecting the adherence, implantation and proliferation of tissue within the peritoneal cavity may differ between women, as may clearance of endometrial cells from the pelvis. Thus, defects in the immunological mechanisms responsible for the clearance of menstrual effluent from the peritoneal cavity may increase the likelihood of endometrial cells implanting. However, it is unclear whether such abnormalities are truly a cause or a result of the disease. Lastly, changes in systemic humoral immunity (altered B-cell function and antibody production) have been implicated, which is interesting as women with endometriosis are reported to have a higher prevalence of autoimmune diseases, e.g. rheumatoid arthritis and systemic lupus erythematosus (SLE).

Cystic ovarian endometriosis (endometriomas)

Several variants on the implantation and metaplasia theories have been proposed to account for ovarian endometriomas. Thus, it has been suggested that superficial lesions on the ovarian cortex become inverted and invaginated, and that endometriomas are derived from functional ovarian cysts or metaplasia of the coelomic epithelium covering the ovary. Endometriomas have features in common with neoplasia such as clonal proliferation, which is consistent with the endometriosis disease theory. They are statistically associated with subtypes of ovarian malignancy, such as endometrioid and clear cell carcinoma. However, it still remains uncertain whether

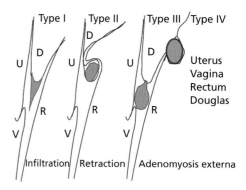

Fig. 49.2 Types of deeply infiltrating endometriosis [7].

such cancers arise from malignant transformation of benign endometriotic tissue.

Deep endometriosis

Several hypotheses explain the aetiology of nodules that extend >5mm beneath the peritoneum and may involve the uterosacral ligaments, vagina, bowel, bladder and ureters. Donnez *et al.* [6] suggested that these are a form of adenomyosis arising in Müllerian rests in the rectovaginal septum. Koninckx and Martin [7] described three macroscopic types [7]. Type I (conical lesions with the largest area exposed to the peritoneal cavity) result from infiltration of superficial disease; they should be considered a form of typical endometriosis (Fig. 49.2). However, type II infiltrating lesions with bowel retracted around and over the nodule and type III lesions, which often occur in an otherwise normal pelvis, are morphologically like adenomyosis with mainly fibromuscular and little glandular tissue. The same applies to infiltrating lesions of the sigmoid (type IV). Type I lesions, like typical ones, can be multifocal, but type II and III are invariably singular: in a series of over 1000 cases, fewer than 50 women had nodules infiltrating both the rectum and sigmoid. Therefore, it has been suggested that deep endometriosis should be redefined as adenomyosis externa on pathological grounds.

Disease risk factors

Risk factors include age, increased peripheral body fat, and greater exposure to menstruation (i.e. short cycles, long duration of flow and reduced parity), whereas smoking, exercise, and oral contraceptive use (current and recent) may be protective [1]. There is no evidence, however, that the natural history of the disease can be influenced by controlling these factors. Genetic predisposition is likely as endometriosis is six to nine times more common in the first-degree relatives of affected women than in controls, and in an analysis of >3000 Australian twin pairs, 51% of the variance of the latent liability to the disease was attributable to additive genetic influences [8]. Disease heritability is also apparent in non-human primates, which develop the disease spontaneously. These data imply that endometriosis is inherited as a complex genetic trait, similar to diabetes or asthma, which means that a number of genes interact with each other to confer disease susceptibility, but the phenotype probably emerges only in the presence of environmental risk factors. A genome-wide linkage study in affected sibling-pair families of European origin has identified a significant susceptibility locus on chromosome 10q26 [9]. More recently, through genome-wide association and replication studies in Japanese cases and controls, significant association has been reported with a single nucleotide polymorphism located in CDKN2BAS on chromosome 9p21, encoding the cyclin-dependent kinase inhibitor 2B antisense RNA [10].

Endometriosis-associated pain symptoms

Severe dysmenorrhoea, deep dyspareunia, chronic pelvic pain, ovulation pain, cyclical or perimenstrual symptoms – often bowel or bladder related, causing dyschezia or dysuria – with or without abnormal bleeding, and chronic fatigue have all been associated with endometriosis. However, the predictive value of any one symptom or set of symptoms is uncertain as each can have other causes, and many affected women are asymptomatic. There is little correlation between disease stage and the type, nature and severity of pain symptoms, suggesting that the current classification systems are inadequate. It is unclear whether subtle lesions cause pain. Typical lesions can cause moderate pain as symptoms are relieved by surgery, but half of the women with such lesions are pain free. Cystic ovarian endometriosis is associated with more severe pain but 10–20% are pain free. Deep endometriosis can be associated with very severe pain, although, again, women sometimes have no pain at all. The suggested causes for the pain include peritoneal inflammation, activation of nociceptors, tissue damage, and nerve irritation/invasion in deep endometriosis. Pain symptoms are usually assessed in clinical trials using a four-point verbal rating scale for three symptoms (dysmenorrhoea, dyspareunia and pelvic pain) and two signs (pelvic tenderness and induration). Increasingly, however, health-related quality of life is also being measured as traditional outcome measures may not adequately assess what the patient considers important. The only patient-generated, disease-specific tool is the Endometriosis Health Profile-30 (EHP-30), a 30-item questionnaire that covers five dimensions: pain, control

and powerlessness, emotional well-being, social support and self image [11].

Endometriosis-associated subfertility

Whether or not endometriosis causes subfertility is also controversial. It is generally accepted that endometriomas cause infertility because severe anatomical distortion must interfere with oocyte pick-up. A causal relationship with Stage I or II disease (particularly subtle lesions) and even deep endometriosis is much less certain. Numerous mechanisms have been proposed, including abnormal folliculogenesis, anovulation, luteal insufficiency, luteinized unruptured follicle syndrome, recurrent miscarriage, decreased sperm survival, altered immunity, intraperitoneal inflammation and endometrial dysfunction. However, all these functional disturbances can occur in subfertile women without endometriosis, which suggests that finding disease during investigation for subfertility may be coincidental.

Diagnosis

History and clinical examination

Making a diagnosis on the basis of symptoms alone is difficult as the presentation is so variable and other conditions such as irritable bowel syndrome and pelvic inflammation mimic the disease. Consequently, there is often a delay of 7 or 8 years between symptom onset and a definitive laparoscopic diagnosis. Finding pelvic tenderness, a fixed retroverted uterus, tender uterosacral ligaments or enlarged ovaries on examination is suggestive of endometriosis, although the findings can be normal. The diagnosis is likely if nodules are found on the uterosacral ligaments or in the pouch of Douglas, and is confirmed if visible lesions are seen in the vagina or on the cervix. Such nodules are most reliably detected when the examination is performed during menstruation [12].

Non-invasive tests

Compared with laparoscopy, transvaginal ultrasound is a useful tool to diagnose and exclude ovarian endometriomas but it has no value for peritoneal disease [13]. Some studies have claimed that magnetic resonance imaging has >90% sensitivity and specificity for endometriomas, but the evidence has not been assessed in a systematic review. CA-125 (cancer antigen 125) measurement has no value as a diagnostic tool for Stage I–II endometriosis [14]. Serum levels are generally elevated in women with deep endometriosis and endometriomas but the test is rarely used because clinical examination and ultrasound usually suffice. Numerous other circulating biomarkers have been studied but none has entered clinical practice [15].

Laparoscopy

Laparoscopy is the gold standard for diagnostic purposes, unless disease is visible in the vagina or elsewhere. Histological confirmation of at least one peritoneal lesion is ideal, and mandatory if deep endometriosis or an endometrioma with a >3 cm diameter is present. The entire pelvis should be inspected systematically, and good practice is to document in detail the type, location and extent of all lesions and adhesions. Ideally, the findings should be recorded. Depending upon the severity of disease found, best practice is to remove/ablate endometriosis at the same time, provided that adequate consent has been obtained.

General treatment issues

Patient participation in the decision-making process is essential as multiple options exist and endometriosis is potentially a chronic problem. Choosing which treatment to have will depend upon a number of factors (Summary box 49.2). Summarizing how these factors influence decision-making is difficult because each patient is different and the decisions are often complex.

Summary box 49.2

Factors influencing choice of treatment:
- Woman's age.
- Fertility status.
- Nature of symptoms.
- Severity of disease.
- Previous treatments.
- Priorities and attitudes.
- Resource implications.
- Costs and side-effect profile.
- Risks of treatment.
- Other subfertility factors.
- Intended duration of treatment.
- Best available evidence.

Treatment aims

The treatment aims should be agreed with the patient (Summary box 49.3). For surgery, the intended benefits and the major risks and complications should be explained and documented on the consent form. When medical treatment is initiated, ideal practice would be to document in the notes, and/or in a letter to the patient, what options were discussed, why the decision to treat was made, as well as the treatment aims and side-effects/risks.

Summary box 49.3

Treatment aims:
- What are you treating (disease, symptoms or both)?
- Why are you treating?

Possible reasons to treat:
- Improve natural fertility.
- Enhance chances of success at assisted reproductive technology.
- Pain relief as an alternative to surgery.
- Pain relief while awaiting surgery.
- Adjunct to surgery.
- Prophylaxis against disease occurrence.
- Symptom recurrence.

Non-hormonal treatment for pain relief

Clinicians and self-help groups recognize that some women control their symptoms with analgesics and/or alternative therapies including Chinese herbal remedies, dietary manipulation, acupuncture and vitamin/mineral supplements. Although these measures can improve quality of life and relieve symptoms, it is inadvisable to make specific recommendations in the absence of evidence to support their effectiveness.

Hormonal treatments

Hormonal treatments have traditionally attempted to mimic pregnancy or the menopause, based upon the clinical impression that the disease regresses during these physiological states, but is never eradicated. The treatments currently available – combined oral contraceptives (COCs), progestagens, danazol, gestrinone, gonadotrophin-releasing hormone (GnRH) agonists and aromatase inhibitors – have been extensively reviewed. Despite different modes of action, they all appear to relieve symptoms even if deep endometriosis or endometriomas are present. Some treatments have been shown to induce atrophy and or decidualization of peritoneal deposits by suppressing ovarian function; however, such lesions often reappear rapidly following therapy. Endometriomas rarely decrease in size and adhesions will be unaffected.

Pain relief

All the hormonal treatments above (with the exception of dydrogesterone given in the luteal phase) relieve endometriosis-associated pain. However, using the total amount of pain (dysmenorrhoea, non-menstrual pain and dyspareunia) as the primary outcome measure inevitably

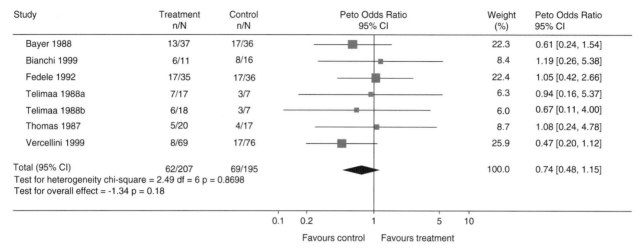

Study	Treatment n/N	Control n/N	Peto Odds Ratio 95% CI	Weight (%)	Peto Odds Ratio 95% CI
Bayer 1988	13/37	17/36		22.3	0.61 [0.24, 1.54]
Bianchi 1999	6/11	8/16		8.4	1.19 [0.26, 5.38]
Fedele 1992	17/35	17/36		22.4	1.05 [0.42, 2.66]
Telimaa 1988a	7/17	3/7		6.3	0.94 [0.16, 5.37]
Telimaa 1988b	6/18	3/7		6.0	0.67 [0.11, 4.00]
Thomas 1987	5/20	4/17		8.7	1.08 [0.24, 4.78]
Vercellini 1999	8/69	17/76		25.9	0.47 [0.20, 1.12]
Total (95% CI)	62/207	69/195		100.0	0.74 [0.48, 1.15]

Test for heterogeneity chi-square = 2.49 df = 6 p = 0.8698
Test for overall effect = -1.34 p = 0.18

0.1   0.2   1   5   10

Favours control   Favours treatment

Fig. 49.3 Cochrane review showing clinical pregnancy rates in studies comparing ovulation suppression and placebo [24].

produces a favourable result as all hormonal treatments abolish menstruation; the effects on non-menstrual pain and dyspareunia are variable. When taken for 6 months, most drugs are equally effective [16–19] but their side-effect and cost profiles differ. These analyses include one randomized controlled trial comparing a combined oral contraceptive (COC) taken conventionally against a gonadotrophin-releasing hormone (GnRH) agonist: the COC was less effective in relieving dysmenorrhoea but there were no significant differences between the treatments in the relief of dyspareunia or non-menstrual pain [20]. It is important to emphasize that a 30% placebo effect is common in endometriosis studies; hence the need for placebo-controlled RCTs.

The duration of GnRH agonist use is limited by the associated loss in bone density – up to 6% in the first 6 months, although the loss is restored almost completely 2 years after stopping treatment. The hypo-oestrogenic symptoms can be alleviated and bone loss prevented, without loss of efficacy, by using 'add-back therapy' in the form of oestrogens, progestagens or tibolone. How long this regimen can safely be continued is unclear, but there is evidence to suggest that bone density can be maintained over 2 years with add-back therapy [21]. However, careful consideration should be given to the use of GnRH agonists with add-back in women who may not have reached their maximum bone density [22]. It has also been suggested that the local release of progestagens may be beneficial: the levonorgestrel intrauterine system (LNG-IUS) has been shown to relieve pain in women with endometriosis, including deep endometriosis and adenomyosis, although experience is limited and long-term studies are needed [23].

Subfertility

Hormonal treatment for subfertility associated with endometriosis does not improve the chances of natural conception [24]. The odds ratio for pregnancy following ovulation suppression versus placebo or no treatment in the meta-analysis was 0.79 (95% CI 0.54–1.14) and 0.80 (95% CI 0.51–1.24), respectively (Fig. 49.3). Clearly treatment can do more harm than good because of the lost opportunity to conceive. In more advanced disease, there is no evidence of an effect on natural conception, but there may be a role for hormonal treatment as an adjunct to assisted conception. A meta-analysis, involving a small number of subjects, has shown that the administration of a GnRH agonist for 3–6 months prior to IVF in women with endometriosis increased the odds of clinical pregnancy fourfold [25]. This strategy can be particularly helpful for a woman who also has severe pain to help relieve her symptoms in the months leading up to IVF treatment.

Surgical treatment

The goal of surgery is to eliminate all visible peritoneal lesions, endometriomas, deep endometriosis and associated adhesions, and to restore normal anatomy. As depth of infiltration is difficult to judge, excision or vaporization is preferable for typical lesions. Excision is the preferred method for endometriomas because recurrence rates following marsupialization and focal treatment are much higher. It is controversial whether conservative discoid resection or resection anastamosis of larger deep lesions should be offered. Laparoscopy should be used as it decreases morbidity and the duration of hospitalization, and therefore cost, compared with laparotomy. Whether laparoscopy also reduces postoperative adhesions is less clear. If local expertise is lacking, then referral to a specialized centre with the necessary expertise to offer all available treatments in a multidisciplinary context, including advanced laparoscopic surgery and laparotomy, is strongly recommended. This particularly applies if deep and/or Stage III or IV endometriosis is suspected or has been diagnosed.

Pain relief

A Cochrane review concluded that laparoscopic surgery results in improved pain outcomes when compared with diagnostic laparoscopy alone [26]; however, there is no evidence that laparoscopic uterine nerve ablation (LUNA) is a necessary component, as LUNA alone has no effect on dysmenorrhoea associated with endometriosis [27]. Few women with severe endometriosis were included in the meta-analysis and no RCTs have been conducted comparing surgery for deep endometriosis or endometriomas against diagnostic laparoscopy for obvious ethical reasons. However, a number of retrospective studies demonstrate that approximately 80% of women with severe symptoms are pain free following surgery for severe disease – a figure that clearly exceeds any likely placebo effect.

Subfertility

A Cochrane review concluded that ablation of lesions plus adhesiolysis in Stage I or II endometriosis enhances fertility significantly better than diagnostic laparoscopy alone with a number needed to treat (NNT) of 12 (95% CI 7–49), i.e. 12 women need to undergo surgery to achieve one additional pregnancy [28]. Two relevant RCTs were identified (Fig. 49.4): the larger showed an increased chance of pregnancy and ongoing pregnancy rate after 20 weeks but the smaller one failed to show benefit. The findings are nevertheless controversial because the patients were seemingly not blinded to whether or not they were treated in the larger study. Moreover, the cumulative pregnancy rate of approximately 30% in the treated group is comparable to previously reported rates in women with typical endometriosis treated expectantly. What cannot be excluded is the possibility that the low cumulative pregnancy rate in the non-treated group arose

because of the awareness that endometriosis was still present.

No RCTs have been conducted to determine whether surgery for Stage III–IV disease improves pregnancy rates, which is not surprising as many of these women also have pain. Nevertheless, cumulative pregnancy rates after surgery for endometriomas are around 60% in most published retrospective studies, although it is unclear to what extent adhesiolysis and ablation of other endometriotic lesions contribute to the effect.

Ovarian endometriomas

Cystectomy for endometriomas is the treatment of choice and is preferable to focal coagulation or laser vaporization with regard to recurrence of cysts and symptoms and subsequent spontaneous pregnancy in women who were previously subfertile [29]. If an endometrioma ≥4 cm in diameter is present before IVF, many authorities recommend cystectomy to confirm the diagnosis histologically, reduce the risk of infection following egg retrieval and improve access to follicles [20]. It had also been suggested that cystectomy might improve the ovarian response to gonadotrophins and thereby pregnancy rates; however, a recent meta-analysis showed no benefit [30]. When the endometrioma is large, the remaining ovarian capsule is so thin that excision and coagulation will almost invariably remove or destroy a large part of the normal ovarian tissue. Therefore, a two-step procedure (marsupialization and rinsing followed by 3 months' GnRH agonist therapy and then repeat surgery) should be considered if fertility is to be conserved; otherwise, an oophorectomy may be performed as it is technically easier. Fertility patients should be counselled about the risks of reduced ovarian function after endometrioma excision and the loss of an ovary. Interestingly, although cystectomy is considered a level 1 laparoscopic procedure by the Royal College of Obstetricians and Gynaecologists, it is technically difficult and demanding surgery for endometriomas because

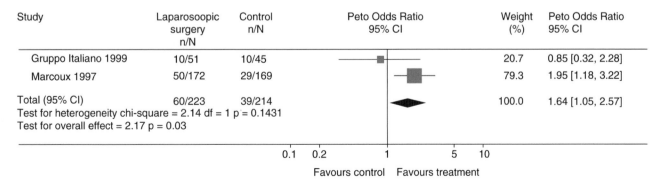

Fig. 49.4 Cochrane review showing ongoing pregnancy or live birth rates in controls and women undergoing laparoscopic surgery [28].

of the risks of damaging the vasculature and surrounding ovarian tissue.

Surgery for deep endometriosis

If there is clinical evidence of deep endometriosis, the possibility of ureteric, bladder and bowel involvement should be considered preoperatively to determine the best management. Surgery needs to be performed as safely as possible and by appropriately trained surgeons because it may be necessary to resect part of the bladder and/or ureter, as well as bowel wall; occasionally, more extensive bowel resection (e.g. the rectum and/or sigmoid) is needed. Clearly, therefore, many gynaecologists will need to seek advice/help from surgeons in other specialties to deal with disease of this severity.

Preoperative assessment is important as it aims to predict as accurately as possible the expected difficulty and which specialities should be available to avoid unnecessary complications and leaving disease behind. The ideal work-up should comprise an IVP to detect ureteric strictures and hydronephrosis and a contrast enema to diagnose extensive narrowing at the level of the rectum or sigmoid (an indication for bowel resection especially at the level of the sigmoid). Preoperative ureteric stenting is mandatory in the presence of hydronephrosis or a bladder nodule close to the ureter. The reliability of ultrasound and magnetic resonance imaging depends greatly on local expertise; unfortunately, there are no data indicating how preoperative imaging should influence the decision to refer to a tertiary centre.

How radical the surgery should be is also controversial. If a general principle of removing all endometriosis is adopted, then bowel resection with 2 cm safety margins should be considered because small endometriotic foci can be found up to 2 cm from a bowel lesion. A conservative discoid resection, however, is preferable for most patients as it is associated with fewer complications. Moreover, a recurrence rate of only 1% casts doubt on the need to remove large segments of bowel. Another important consideration in the decision-making is that the complication rates and long-term morbidity associated with bowel resection are much lower for the sigmoid than for the low rectum.

Postoperative hormonal treatment

The need for postoperative treatment varies with the completeness of the surgical excision; if complete, there is usually little need. Having said that, compared with surgery alone or surgery plus placebo, postoperative hormonal treatment does not produce a significant reduction in pain recurrence at 12 or 24 months, and has no effect on disease recurrence; similarly, it has no effect on pregnancy rates [31]. Prescribing hormone replacement therapy (HRT) after bilateral oophorectomy is advisable in young women but the ideal regimen is unclear. Adding a progestagen after hysterectomy is unnecessary (unless deep endometriosis is left behind) but should theoretically protect against the unopposed action of oestrogen on any residual disease – causing reactivation or, in rare circumstances, malignant transformation. A recently published EMAS (European Menopause and Andropause Society) statement on the subject recommended either form of HRT 'in both hysterectomized and non-hysterectomized women as the risk of recurrence and malignant transformation of residual endometriosis may be reduced' [32]. There is no evidence to justify delaying the start of HRT.

Assisted reproduction

In women with Stage I–II endometriosis and patent fallopian tubes, treatment with intrauterine insemination (IUI) plus ovarian stimulation improves fertility, but it is uncertain whether unstimulated IUI is effective. *In vitro* fertilization (IVF) is appropriate treatment for all disease severities, especially if tubal function is compromised or there are other problems, such as male factor subfertility [22]. However, a systematic review (Fig. 49.5) showed that IVF pregnancy rates are lower in patients with endometriosis than in those with tubal subfertility [33], even though endometriosis does not appear to adversely affect pregnancy rates in some large national databases [e.g. Society for Assisted Reproductive Technology (SART) and Human Fertilisation and Embryology Authority (HFEA)]. A poorly addressed issue is whether surgery should be considered before IVF in women with endometriomas to prevent complications (see section Ovarian endometriomas). In the case of deep endometriosis, surgery beforehand may be advisable as oocyte retrieval can be painful and there is an increased risk of bowel perforation because of associated adhesions.

Alternative management protocols

It is increasingly being asked whether it is necessary to perform a laparoscopy in all cases of suspected endometriosis. Hence, the recommendation in the RCOG Green-Top Guideline:

If a woman wants pain symptoms suggestive of endometriosis to be treated without a definitive diagnosis, a therapeutic trial of a hormonal drug to reduce menstrual flow is appropriate.

In other words, there is a role for a therapeutic trial of a COC (monthly or tricycling) or a progestagen to treat pain symptoms suggestive of endometriosis without

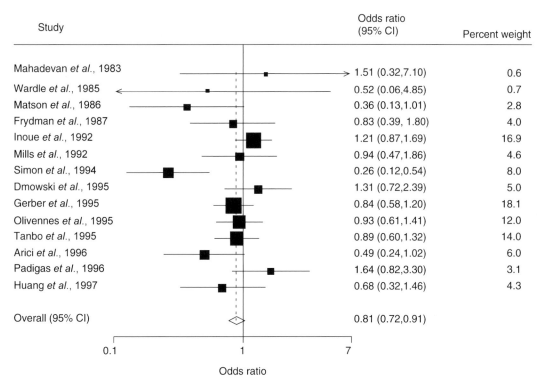

Study		Odds ratio (95% CI)	Percent weight
Mahadevan *et al.*, 1983		1.51 (0.32,7.10)	0.6
Wardle *et al.*, 1985		0.52 (0.06,4.85)	0.7
Matson *et al.*, 1986		0.36 (0.13,1.01)	2.8
Frydman *et al.*, 1987		0.83 (0.39, 1.80)	4.0
Inoue *et al.*, 1992		1.21 (0.87,1.69)	16.9
Mills *et al.*, 1992		0.94 (0.47,1.86)	4.6
Simon *et al.*, 1994		0.26 (0.12,0.54)	8.0
Dmowski *et al.*, 1995		1.31 (0.72,2.39)	5.0
Gerber *et al.*, 1995		0.84 (0.58,1.20)	18.1
Olivennes *et al.*, 1995		0.93 (0.61,1.41)	12.0
Tanbo *et al.*, 1995		0.89 (0.60,1.32)	14.0
Arici *et al.*, 1996		0.49 (0.24,1.02)	6.0
Padigas *et al.*, 1996		1.64 (0.82,3.30)	3.1
Huang *et al.*, 1997		0.68 (0.32,1.46)	4.3
Overall (95% CI)		0.81 (0.72,0.91)	

Fig. 49.5 Unadjusted meta-analysis of odds of pregnancy in endometriosis patients versus controls with tubal subfertility [33].

performing a diagnostic laparoscopy first. Although the recommendation reflects the common practice of using a COC in this way, or even continuously, there is no evidence that one method is better than any other, or that any COCs are better than others.

Since then, other management protocols along similar lines have been produced by North American authors. For example, the clinical practice guideline of the Society of Obstetricians and Gynaecologists of Canada [35] states:

Diagnostic laparoscopy is not required before treatment in all patients presenting with pelvic pain. Although laparoscopy is considered a minimally invasive procedure, it still carries the risks of surgery, including bowel and bladder perforation and vascular injury.

Olive and Pritts [10] recommend the use of a non-steroidal anti-inflammatory drug (NSAID) or COC in the first instance and, if unsuccessful, operative laparoscopy or a therapeutic trial of a GnRH agonist plus add-back can be offered. Operative laparoscopy can also be performed if the GnRH agonist fails to relieve symptoms. The recommendations of Gambone *et al.* [34] are similar: first-line treatment with a NSAID or COC, or both, based upon the nature of the pain, any contraindications and the need for contraception. If first-line treatment fails, the options are operative laparoscopy or a therapeutic trial of danazol, a progestagen or a GnRH agonist with add-back for 2 months, continuing for 6 months if successful. Both protocols acknowledge the value of continuing on maintenance therapy if adequate pain relief is achieved with one or a combination of drugs. It should be acknowledged, however, that these protocols have been at least partially inspired by cost considerations, and perhaps by the realization that not all women with endometriosis-associated pain have access to adequate surgical treatment.

Recommended reading

Berkley KJ, Rapkin AJ, Papka RE. The pains of endometriosis. *Science* 2005;308:1587–1589.

Giudice LC. Clinical practice. Endometriosis. *N Engl J Med* 2010;362:2389–2398.

Rogers PA, D'Hooghe TM, Fazleabas A *et al.* Priorities for endometriosis research: recommendations from an international consensus workshop. *Reprod Sci* 2009;16:335–346.

References

1 Eskenazi B, Warner ML. Epidemiology of endometriosis. *Obstet Gynecol Clin North Am* 1997;24:235–258.

2 Koninckx PR. Is mild endometriosis a condition occurring intermittently in all women? *Hum Reprod* 1994;9:2202–2205.

3 Revised American Society for Reproductive Medicine classification of endometriosis: 1996. *Fertil Steril* 1997;67:817–821.

4 Koninckx PR, Barlow D, Kennedy S. Implantation versus infiltration: the Sampson versus the endometriotic disease theory. *Gynecol Obstet Invest* 1999;47(Suppl. 1):3–9.

5 Nisolle M, Donnez J. Peritoneal endometriosis, ovarian endometriosis, and adenomyotic nodules of the rectovaginal septum are three different entities. *Fertil Steril* 1997;68: 585–596.

6 Donnez J, Nisolle M, Gillerot S, Smets M, Bassil S, Casanas RF. Rectovaginal septum adenomyotic nodules: a series of 500 cases. *Br J Obstet Gynaecol* 1997;104:1014–1018.

7 Koninckx PR, Martin DC. Deep endometriosis: a consequence of infiltration or retraction or possibly adenomyosis externa? *Fertil Steril* 1992;58:924–928.

8 Zondervan KT, Cardon LR, Kennedy SH. The genetic basis of endometriosis. *Curr Opin Obstet Gynecol* 2001;13:309–314.

9 Treloar SA, Wicks J, Nyholt DR *et al.* Genomewide linkage study in 1,176 affected sister pair families identifies a significant susceptibility locus for endometriosis on chromosome 10q26. *Am J Hum Genet* 2005;77:365–376.

10 Olive DL, Pritts EA. The treatment of endometriosis: a review of the evidence. *Ann NY Acad Sci* 2002;955:360–372.

11 Jones G, Kennedy S, Barnard A, Wong J, Jenkinson C. Development of an endometriosis quality-of-life instrument: The Endometriosis Health Profile-30. *Obstet Gynecol* 2001;98: 258–264.

12 Koninckx PR, Meuleman C, Oosterlynck D, Cornillie FJ. Diagnosis of deep endometriosis by clinical examination during menstruation and plasma CA-125 concentration. *Fertil Steril* 1996;65:280–287.

13 Moore J, Copley S, Morris J, Lindsell D, Golding S, Kennedy S. A systematic review of the accuracy of ultrasound in the diagnosis of endometriosis. *Ultrasound Obstet Gynecol* 2002;20: 630–634.

14 Mol BW, Bayram N, Lijmer JG *et al.* The performance of CA-125 measurement in the detection of endometriosis: a meta-analysis. *Fertil Steril* 1998;70:1101–1108.

15 May KE, Conduit-Hulbert SA, Villar J, Kirtley S, Kennedy SH, Becker CM. Peripheral biomarkers of endometriosis: a systematic review. *Hum Reprod Update* 2010;16:651–674.

16 Davis L, Kennedy SS, Moore J, Prentice A. Modern combined oral contraceptives for pain associated with endometriosis. *Cochrane Database Syst Rev* 2007;3:CD001019.

17 Prentice A, Deary AJ, Goldbeck WS, Farquhar C, Smith SK. Gonadotrophin-releasing hormone analogues for pain associated with endometriosis. In: *The Cochrane Library*, Issue 3. Chichester, UK: John Wiley & Sons, Ltd, 2004.

18 Prentice A, Deary AJ, Bland E. Progestagens and anti-progestagens for pain associated with endometriosis. In: *The Cochrane Library*, Issue 3. Chichester, UK: John Wiley & Sons, Ltd, 2004.

19 Selak V, Farquhar C, Prentice A, Singla A. Danazol for pelvic pain associated with endometriosis. *Cochrane Database Syst Rev* 2007;4:CD000068.

20 Vercellini P, Trespidi L, Colombo A, Vendola N, Marchini M, Crosignani PG. A gonadotropin-releasing hormone agonist versus a low-dose oral contraceptive for pelvic pain associated with endometriosis. *Fertil Steril* 1993;60:75–79.

21 Surrey ES, Hornstein MD. Prolonged GnRH agonist and add-back therapy for symptomatic endometriosis: long-term follow-up. *Obstet Gynecol* 2002;99:709–719.

22 Kennedy S, Bergqvist A, Chapron C *et al.* ESHRE guideline for the diagnosis and treatment of endometriosis. *Hum Reprod* 2005;20:2698–2704.

23 Bahamondes L, Petta CA, Fernandes A, Monteiro I. Use of the levonorgestrel-releasing intrauterine system in women with endometriosis, chronic pelvic pain and dysmenorrhoea. *Contraception* 2007;75(6 Suppl.):S134–S139.

24 Hughes E, Brown J, Collins JJ, Farquhar C, Fedorkow DM, Vandekerckhove P. Ovulation suppression for endometriosis. *Cochrane Database Syst Rev* 2007;3:CD000155.

25 Sallam HN, Garcia-Velasco JA, Dias S, Arici A. Long-term pituitary down-regulation before *in vitro* fertilisation (IVF) for women with endometriosis. *Cochrane Database Syst Rev* 2006;1:CD004635.

26 Jacobson TZ, Duffy JM, Barlow D, Koninckx PR, Garry R. Laparoscopic surgery for pelvic pain associated with endometriosis. *Cochrane Database Syst Rev* 2009;4:CD001300.

27 Vercellini P, Aimi G, Busacca M, Apolone G, Uglietti A, Crosignani PG. Laparoscopic uterosacral ligament resection for dysmenorrhoea associated with endometriosis: results of a randomised, controlled trial. *Fertil Steril* 2003;80:310–319.

28 Jacobson TZ, Duffy JM, Barlow D, Farquhar C, Koninckx PR, Olive D. Laparoscopic surgery for subfertility associated with endometriosis. *Cochrane Database Syst Rev* 2010;1:CD001398.

29 Hart RJ, Hickey M, Maouris P, Buckett W. Excisional surgery versus ablative surgery for ovarian endometriomata. *Cochrane Database Syst Rev* 2008;2:CD004992.

30 Tsoumpou I, Kyrgiou M, Gelbaya TA, Nardo LG. The effect of surgical treatment for endometrioma on *in vitro* fertilisation outcomes: a systematic review and meta-analysis. *Fertil Steril* 2009;92:75–87.

31 Yap C, Furness S, Farquhar C. Pre and post operative medical therapy for endometriosis surgery. *Cochrane Database Syst Rev* 2004;3:CD003678.

32 Moen MH, Rees M, Brincat M *et al.* EMAS position statement: Managing the menopause in women with a past history of endometriosis. *Maturitas* 2010;67:94–97.

33 Barnhart K, Dunsmoor-Su R, Coutifaris C. Effect of endometriosis on *in vitro* fertilization. *Fertil Steril* 2002;77:1148–1155.

34 Gambone JC, Mittman BS, Munro MG, Scialli AR, Winkel CA, the Chronic Pelvic Pain/Endometriosis Working Group. Consensus statement for the management of chronic pelvic pain and endometriosis: proceedings of an expert-panel consensus. *Fertil Steril* 2002;78:961–972.

35 Society of Obstetricians and Gynaecologists of Canada. Clinical guideline. Endometriosis: diagnosis and management. *J Obstet Gynaecol Can* 2010;32:S1–S32.

Part 13
Urogynaecology

Chapter 50
Uterovaginal Prolapse

Anthony R.B. Smith
The Warrell Unit, St Mary's Hospital, Manchester, UK

Introduction

Up to half of the normal female population will develop uterovaginal prolapse during their lifetime. Twenty per cent of these women will be symptomatic and need treatment [1]. A North American actuarial analysis revealed that a woman up to the age of 80 years has an 11% risk of needing surgery for pelvic floor weakness. Furthermore, if she has an operation, she has a 29% risk of requiring further surgery [2]. These figures suggest that the current management of pelvic floor dysfunction is less than ideal. Pelvic floor dysfunction increases with advancing age. As the world population increases in age, the prevalence of pelvic floor dysfunction is likely to increase. For most countries the over-eighties age group is the fastest growing segment of the population, so gynaecologists need to improve their understanding of pelvic floor dysfunction and its sequelae to improve the outcomes from treatment.

Structure and function of the pelvic floor

The pelvic floor functions to support the pelvic and abdominal viscera and help maintain control of their contents. It has two major components, which are interdependent: the muscle and fascia.

Muscle

Levator ani muscles consist of pubococcygeus, coccygeus and ileococcygeus muscles on each side, which together form a muscular floor to the pelvis. The striated muscle of levator ani is under voluntary control but is a unique striated muscle in having a resting tone. As with other striated muscles, its strength can be increased by exercise such as pelvic floor physiotherapy. Contraction of the muscles results in a forward elevation of the pelvic floor which is important in their role of continence. This forward elevation helps to increase the angulation between bladder and urethra anteriorly and rectum and anal canal posteriorly. Increase in this angulation is one of the fundamental mechanisms that aid continence. Thus, the healthy pelvic floor muscle will, at rest, provide support and assistance with continence. When the intra-abdominal pressure rises, levator ani muscles contract and provide additional support and outlet resistance to the bladder and rectum. This reflex response to intra-abdominal pressure rise also requires an intact innervation, so damage to the pelvic floor muscle innervation is likely to impair the pelvic floor muscle response in both speed and strength.

Fascia

Fascia envelopes levator ani, attaches it to bone at its origin and holds the two muscles together in the midline. The urethra, vagina and rectum perforate this midline fascia. Thus, the pelvic viscera are supported by both the levator ani muscle and the fascial attachments that are condensed in some areas and are often referred to as ligaments – the uterosacral, cardinal and round ligaments being examples. There has been much debate for over a century about the structure and function of the pelvic fascia. It is generally accepted that the pelvic floor has evolved as man has assumed the upright stature and this evolution has involved replacement of some of the muscular component of the pelvic floor with fascia to provide additional supportive strength to cope with the effect of gravity. Thus, any factor that influences the strength or integrity of pelvic floor fascia will influence the function of the pelvic floor. These factors may be congenital (such as hyperelasticity of the collagenous component of fascia) or environmental, such as stretching or tearing of fascia during childbirth or heavy lifting.

Dewhurst's Textbook of Obstetrics & Gynaecology, Eighth Edition. Edited by D. Keith Edmonds.
© 2012 John Wiley and Sons, Ltd. Published 2012 by John Wiley and Sons, Ltd.

Weakness of the pelvic floor, which may result from impairment of function of either muscle or fascia, can result in uterovaginal prolapse. Prolapse is largely a result of loss of support from the pelvic floor but the pelvic floor weakness may produce other symptoms than those due to the displacement of the pelvic viscera. Incontinence of the bladder or bowel are common examples.

An understanding of the pathophysiology of pelvic floor dysfunction will help to develop an appropriate management strategy.

Pathophysiology of pelvic floor dysfunction

Muscle

The striated muscle of the pelvic floor, in common with other striated muscles throughout the body, undergoes a gradual denervation with age [3]. This denervation will result in a gradual weakening of the muscle over time. While some of the ageing effect can be counteracted by muscle training, the impact of denervation will be to diminish the number of neurones that can stimulate muscle fibres to contract. Pelvic floor muscle denervation is increased by vaginal delivery, particularly if the active second stage of labour is prolonged [4].

Caesarean section may offer some protection from this injury. Following childbirth, some reinnervation will occur, which will result in rehabilitation of the muscle, at least to some degree. Reinnervation results in more muscle fibres being innervated by each remaining nerve fibre. This results in the pelvic floor muscle being more vulnerable to age-related denervation because further nerve loss with age will result in a more marked loss of muscle fibre activity. Thus, the damage to the pelvic floor muscle during childbirth often only becomes evident when age-related changes are superimposed. The site of pelvic floor muscle denervation during childbirth is unclear. It has been proposed that stretching of the pudendal nerve distal to Alcock's canal at the ischial spine results in nerve injury but crushing injury at the neuromuscular junction in the muscle must also be possible.

In neurological diseases such as multiple sclerosis, pelvic floor muscle may behave unpredictably, ranging from inappropriate relaxation causing incontinence to spasm resulting in voiding dysfunction.

Women with ectopia vesicae have incomplete development of the pelvic floor anteriorly. This predisposes them to uterovaginal prolapse, which is an additional surgical challenge partly because of previous surgical procedures and partly because of anatomical distortion from the absence of a normally formed anterior pelvis (bony and soft tissue).

Fascia

Fascia is composed of a number of components including collagen, elastin and smooth muscle embedded in a connective tissue matrix. Each of the components may influence the overall biomechanical properties of the fascia. The following factors have a significant influence on pelvic floor support.

Congenital

Congenital differences in collagen behaviour are clinically evident in women who have increased joint elasticity. Women with hyperextensible joints will also have additional pelvic fascia stretchiness, which may be manifested in the development of uterovaginal prolapse at an earlier age. Such women often excel at sports requiring increased joint elasticity (such as gymnastics) and they develop fewer striae gravidarum during pregnancy because of increased skin elasticity. Labour may be rapid because of reduced obstruction from the pelvic floor fascia. Extreme forms of this are seen in Ehlers–Danlos syndrome but much more commonly seen are milder forms (see Fig. 50.1). It is important for gynaecologists to recognize women who have such problems because their treatment may need to be different from that for women with childbirth or age-related pelvic floor weakness. Recurrence after surgery is more likely and use of prosthetic support materials may be advisable (see Fig. 50.1).

Age

With increasing age fascial tissues become stiffer and more liable to rupture. The elderly adult is invariably stiffer in movement than the young child. The fascia of the pelvic floor will provide weaker support with advancing years. Gynaecologists repairing the pelvic floor often recognize that the tissues used for building a repair are of poor quality and are poorly vascularized. The repair

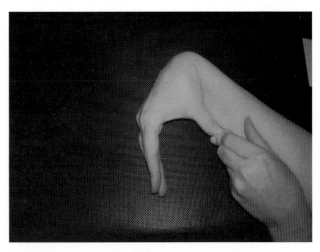

Fig. 50.1 Joint hyperextensibility as an index of fascial stretchiness.

after surgery will heal with less strength and more slowly. The recurrence of prolapse, widely reported after surgery, must in some part be due to a deterioration of fascial strength with age. This is supported by the fact that the longer the follow-up period after surgical treatment, the higher the risk of recurrence.

Childbirth injury

Most women recognize that their pelvic floor is different after vaginal delivery. Similarly, regaining the tone and shape of their anterior abdominal wall is also often a difficult challenge. These changes are because of a combination of muscle and fascial changes. There has been much unresolved debate as to whether pelvic floor fascia stretches or tears during pregnancy and childbirth. Some believe that stretching occurs and therefore repair of the pelvic floor during prolapse surgery should involve fascial plication. Others believe that fascia can only tear and does not stretch and therefore repair should involve determining the site of the tears and repairing them (site-specific repair – see p. 500).

Endocrine

The menstrual cycle, pregnancy and menopause are the most significant endocrine events that can influence pelvic floor fascia. Women often declare that prolapse symptoms are worse around the time of menstruation. This is thought to be secondary to higher progesterone levels increasing fascial elasticity. Recent studies have shown that women examined at the time of menstruation will have a higher stage of prolapse than at other times of the cycle. This has important implications when deciding on treatment. During pregnancy, prolapse symptoms will be more evident in the first trimester but diminish as the pregnant uterus enlarges out of the pelvis. During pregnancy many women develop stress incontinence of urine for the first time. Research has shown that fascial elasticity increases in pregnancy [5] and this probably results in diminished pelvic floor support and a tendency to stress incontinence. Women who develop stress incontinence of urine during pregnancy are more likely to experience the same symptom after childbirth. The prevalence of uterovaginal prolapse increases after the menopause. How secondary this is to endocrine changes rather than age-related changes is not known.

 Summary box 50.1

- Pelvic floor weakness may be congenital or acquired.
- Young women (<35 years of age) who present with prolapse have a significant risk of congenital fascial hyperelasticity. They have a higher risk of surgical failure and recurrence.

Uterovaginal prolapse

Description

Prolapse is normally divided into anterior, uterine/vault and posterior compartments. Although anterior vaginal wall prolapse is still commonly called a cystocoele and posterior prolapse a rectocoele or enterocoele, the difficulty in providing reproducible descriptions for the purpose of research has led to the development of scoring systems. The most frequently used validated method in current literature is a system called the POPQ (Pelvic Organ Prolapse Quantification) [6]. The system is shown diagrammatically in Fig. 50.2. This system may also be used to grade prolapse. Thus, for example, in grade 2 prolapse, the leading part of prolapse presents somewhere between 1 cm above and 1 cm below the introitus.

Symptoms

Prolapse classically produces a sensation of fullness in the vagina or a visible or palpable lump at the introitus. This sensation is always posture dependent, as are many prolapse symptoms. If the symptoms do not resolve when lying down an alternative aetiology should be considered. Research has shown that most women do not become aware of prolapse until the presenting part has reached the introitus. Low backache is a common symptom but is also commonly experienced by women who do not have prolapse. Vaginal atrophy, if present, will exacerbate many prolapse symptoms and should be treated as a first priority with topical oestrogens unless clinically contraindicated.

Urinary symptoms

Anterior vaginal wall prolapse may result in a range of urinary symptoms. While women who have anterior

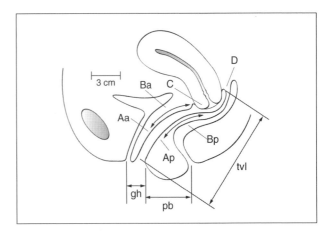

Fig. 50.2 The POPQ system. Aa, anterior wall; Ap, posterior wall; Ba, anterior wall; Bp, posterior wall; C, cervix or cuff; D, posterior fornix; gh, genital hiatus; pb, perineal body; tvl, total vaginal length.

prolapse may have stress incontinence, particularly if the urethra is not well supported, they may also have voiding dysfunction secondary to kinking of the urethra. Voiding dysfunction may result in frequency (due to incomplete bladder emptying), hesitancy and a poor urinary stream. Incomplete bladder emptying may in turn result in recurrent urinary infection with accompanying frequency, urgency and urge incontinence. Prolapse of the bladder may result in congestion of the bladder base, which in turn may cause overactive bladder symptoms. However, it is important to note that anterior vaginal wall prolapse is unlikely of itself to produce detrusor overactivity, which may have an independent pathology. Thus, surgical repair of anterior vaginal wall prolapse may not always resolve urinary symptoms. If the anterior prolapse is kinking the urethra, it may be preventing stress incontinence of urine. Surgical repair, by elevating the bladder base and straightening out the urethrovesical angle, can lead to the development of stress incontinence *de novo*, which will not please the patient. Occasionally, posterior vaginal wall prolapse, if associated with obstructed defaecation, may result in urinary voiding dysfunction.

Bowel symptoms

Posterior vaginal wall prolapse may be associated with a range of bowel symptoms, but not all women who have posterior vaginal wall prolapse have bowel symptoms. It is often difficult to know whether the bowel symptoms are caused by the prolapse or associated with a fascial weakness that may also be affecting the bowel. Slow transit constipation and diverticular disease are bowel disorders more prevalent in women with fascial weakness. Constipation is a common symptom in women and may contribute to obstructed defaecation. The presence of posterior vaginal wall prolapse may not be the cause of the obstructed defaecation but more a symptom of it. Posterior vaginal wall prolapse does not normally result in anorectal incontinence.

Coital symptoms

Uterovaginal prolapse, in all but the most severe cases, retracts when a woman is lying in bed. Prolapse often does not interfere with normal sexual activity. However, many women feel unhappy with the vaginal discomfort experienced through the day and the presence of the prolapse can inhibit couples from continuing normal sexual activity for mainly aesthetic reasons but also from concern about causing harm. Additionally, concern about continence or other urinary and bowel symptoms may be inhibiting. Some couples find that the loss of tone in the vagina leads to sexual dissatisfaction for both parties. The growth of interest in cosmetic vaginal surgery and drugs for male impotence may be influencing this phenomenon.

Summary box 50.2

- A careful history of symptoms must be taken from women with prolapse.
- Asymptomatic prolapse does not need to be treated.
- Women with prolapse may have symptoms of urinary, bowel and sexual dysfunction, which may be of greater significance to the patient than the awareness of a lump.

Investigation of prolapse symptoms
Examination

General examination should include general medical fitness, including fitness for surgery. Chronic chest conditions and obesity increase the risk of prolapse and where possible should be managed before surgery is considered. Abdominal examination should be performed to exclude an intra-abdominal mass. A bimanual pelvic examination or ultrasound should exclude a pelvic mass and delineate the size of the uterus and ovaries if present.

The patient should be examined in the horizontal position, conventionally in the left lateral position with a Sims' speculum. If prolapse is not evident, even with a Valsalva manoeuvre, the patient should be examined in the upright position. It is important to reproduce the symptoms and signs with which the patient presents. If this is not possible a further examination may be required. Many women are aware of their symptoms only after a long period in the upright position. An early morning clinic appointment may preclude detection of the prolapse. An examination may need to be performed later in the day and in the upright position to reveal significant prolapse. Some clinicians examine women in the lithotomy position. This enables closer inspection of vaginal supports, particularly if looking for site-specific defects in the endopelvic fascia. A second retracting instrument will be required to do this to visualize the lateral sulci.

The POPQ examination (see Fig. 50.2) gives an objective record of the prolapse stage.

Urodynamic studies

If there are no urinary symptoms, urodynamic studies are not justified outside the research setting. If a woman has significant urinary symptoms urodynamics may help to define the cause of the symptoms, which will enable the gynaecologist to give some prognosis for treatment. Hence, if urodynamics indicates obstructed voiding then there is a good prognosis for surgical repair of the cystocoele, resolving the voiding dysfunction, whereas if urodynamics suggests that the bladder is atonic then the prognosis is less favourable. If urodynamics indicate that the bladder is overactive then it is less likely that surgery will improve the urinary symptoms. This may influence a woman's decision on whether to proceed with surgery.

The development of stress incontinence is an irritating sequel to anterior vaginal wall repair in some women. Some clinicians perform a urinary stress test with the prolapse reduced digitally with either a sponge forceps or a ring pessary. There is no evidence that this technique reliably predicts which women will develop stress incontinence after surgery.

Proctography

An anterior rectocoele may result in obstructed defaecation. Rectal mucosal prolapse may also result in obstructed defaecation and will not be apparent on vaginal examination though may be felt on rectal examination. Proctography can give some insight into factors that may be contributing to difficulty with defaecation and may help avoid unnecessary, unhelpful vaginal operations. A rectopexy may be required if significant rectal mucosal prolapse is found on proctography.

Magnetic resonance imaging

Magnetic resonance imaging has been used as a research tool to try to identify prolapse not clinically evident. It has not been proven to aid or improve treatment outcome to date.

Treatment

Conservative

Some women elect for non-surgical treatment of their prolapse because they:
- fear an adverse outcome from surgery;
- do not wish to lose time from work;
- are unfit for surgery; or
- they wish to delay surgical treatment for other reasons. Conservative treatment may involve:
- *Lifestyle advice* This may include advice on diet and weight loss including avoidance of drinks with caffeine, water intake, fibre content, laxative use and modification of drug regimes, e.g. diuretics. Avoidance of high-impact exercise and lifting may improve symptoms.
- *Pelvic floor physiotherapy* There have been no studies that have reported on the value of pelvic floor physiotherapy on vaginal prolapse symptoms. Although it is unlikely that advanced prolapse will be helped by pelvic floor exercises, earlier stage prolapse may be improved sufficiently to avoid further intervention.
- *Vaginal pessary* Vaginal pessaries have been available in some form for 4000 years. The first pessaries described were pomegranate skins. Currently in the UK the most frequently used pessary is the polypropylene ring pessary (Fig. 50.3). The most appropriate vaginal anatomical configuration for the ring pessary has not been defined but if there is little or no posterior perineal support the ring pessary will often not be retained. The optimal size is

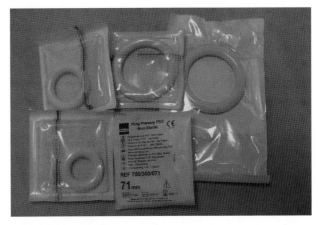

Fig. 50.3 Ring pessaries.

usually determined by trial and error. The optimal time interval for changing pessaries has also not been defined, nor has the role of topical oestrogens. A wider range of vaginal pessaries is now available (see, for example, www.mediplus.co.uk). Some women find that softer, silicone pessaries are more acceptable. Pessaries such as the ring can normally allow sexual intercourse without problems, although a few women prefer to remove the pessary. Vaginal pessaries can be removed and cleaned by the patient, but there is little evidence that this is of any value. Space-occupying pessaries such as the shelf pessary virtually preclude normal sexual relations and are therefore unsuitable for sexually active women. The shelf pessary may be particularly helpful for uterine or vaginal vault prolapse. The shelf pessary may be quite difficult to change and can become embedded in the vaginal wall. Careful examination at least every 6 months is advisable and topical oestrogens may reduce the risk of ulceration and erosion.

Surgical

Over the last 100 years surgery has been considered to be the treatment of choice for uterovaginal prolapse. The surgical techniques employed until recently have differed little from those described by the surgical icons of a century ago. Increasingly, it is being acknowledged that a desirable outcome should include more than a satisfactory anatomical result. Functional outcome may be more important to the patient than the appearance of the vagina. There have been very few robust studies comparing techniques of prolapse surgery performed that define both the anatomical and functional outcomes with some measure of the impact on the patient's quality of life. Further research is urgently needed in this field.

Surgically, the key issues are:

1 Which technique produces the best, long-lasting anatomical result?

2 Is the abdominal approach superior to the vaginal approach?

3 If uterine prolapse is present, should the uterus be removed or conserved?

4 How can adverse functional outcomes be avoided?

5 Should the repair be augmented with an implanted material?

6 Are there relevant comorbidities that should influence the approach to surgery?

Anterior vaginal wall prolapse

In 1909, White [7] described the vaginal paravaginal repair to repair a cystocoele (see Fig. 50.4). Four years later, Kelly [8] described the anterior vaginal repair with a central plication of the pubocervical fascia (see Fig. 50.4). The Kelly operation became the treatment of choice for anterior prolapse partly because of the simplicity of the procedure and partly because of Kelly's high standing in the surgical community.

Debate about the relative merits of the Kelly-type repair and the paravaginal repair continue to this day. A review of over 90 articles between 1966 and 1995 by Weber and Walters [9] illustrated the deficiencies of the literature and found that there was no significant difference in success rate between the paravaginal repair (failure rate 3–14%), whether performed vaginally or abdominally, and the central plication repair (failure rate 0–20%). Beck *et al.* [1] reviewed 246 anterior repairs and noted that 5% of women

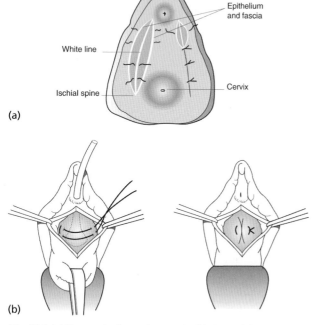

(a)

(b)

Fig. 50.4 (a) Paravaginal anterior repair. (b) Central fascial anterior repair.

developed *de novo* stress incontinence and 5% *de novo* detrusor overactivity postoperatively. Longstanding voiding problems occurred in less than 1%. Postoperative pyrexia developed in 10% of women but the overall morbidity can be described as low.

The anterior vaginal wall repair continues to be the most frequently performed prolapse repair operation. Recurrence of prolapse is most frequent in this compartment.

Posterior vaginal wall prolapse

The classical posterior vaginal repair involves not only plication of the fascia underlying the vaginal skin but also a central plication of the fascia overlying the pubococcygeus muscle, even including the muscle itself. There can be little doubt that inclusion of the pubococcygeus fascia and muscle will create a more solid repair with accompanying intra- and postoperative morbidity, but it is unclear whether the functional outcome is better. Kahn and Stanton [10] performed a 2-year follow-up of their posterior vaginal repairs performed in the conventional manner (including levator plication). They noted that, in addition to one in four of the women having posterior prolapse on examination, more women volunteered functional problems with respect to bowel and dyspareunia than preoperatively. Some have suggested that a transanal approach to rectocoele repair should be more effective for treatment of defaecation difficulty but the limited robust literature available does not support this [11]. Although the site-specific fascial defect repair has been found to be more effective by some surgeons [12], it has not been studied in a robust, systematic manner.

Perineal descent is commonly seen with posterior vaginal wall prolapse. Its clinical relevance is not clear but in anatomical terms it indicates that either the perineum is no longer supported by the pelvic floor or there is weakness of the pelvic floor as a whole. This may be an index of the support of the vaginal vault or the uterus and vaginal apex.

Uterine prolapse

The current conventional approach to uterine prolapse, when a woman no longer wishes to have children, is a vaginal hysterectomy with any additional repair to the vaginal walls as appropriate. The vaginal vault is then supported by reattaching the uterosacral/cardinal ligaments to the vagina with shortening of the ligaments, if required. These ligaments can also be plicated together in the midline to try to prevent the development of enterocoele. The Manchester repair is now less popular but when employed the cardinal ligaments are brought together anterior to the cervix, which was amputated as part of the operation. The use of the uterosacral/cardinal ligaments has the fundamental problem that it is the weakness of these ligaments that has contributed to the development of the prolapse. Use of such weak tissues must make the risk of recurrence a concern. There is increasing interest in other uterine-conserving procedures such as abdominal or laparoscopic sacrohysteropexy or sacrospinous hysteropexy, but to date it is unclear whether this is a real advance in treatment. There is no evidence that routine use of sacrospinous colpopexy performed at the time of hysterectomy reduces the risk of vault prolapse, though the morbidity of the additional procedure is likely to be higher.

This would suggest that, in the absence of evidence to the contrary, for uterine prolapse the gynaecologist should perform a vaginal hysterectomy with the provision of support to the vaginal vault from the uterosacral ligaments. In the absence of defined support tissue a sacrospinous colpopexy or sacrocolpopexy may be required. It is to be hoped that surgical trials will address this area in the near future.

Vaginal vault prolapse

Vaginal vault prolapse occurs in approximately 5% of women after hysterectomy, although lesser degrees of deficient vaginal vault support are more common. Most studies indicate that an equal proportion of women have had an abdominal or a vaginal hysterectomy, which, given that abdominal hysterectomy is performed more frequently than vaginal, suggests that vaginal hysterectomy predisposes to vault prolapse. Vault prolapse is always accompanied by some degree of upper anterior and posterior vaginal prolapse, the latter usually being the predominant component. Frequently extensive vaginal epithelial stretching occurs and this is usually of the posterior vaginal wall (see Fig. 50.5). Failure to treat

extensive vault prolapse may lead to ulceration and, less commonly, bowel extrusion.

Vaginal vault prolapse may be treated surgically by a vaginal sacrospinous colpopexy or an abdominal (or laparoscopic) sacrocolpopexy. A Cochrane review [11] has reported that the sacrocolpopexy has a higher cure rate and recurrence; when it does occur, it does so sooner with a sacrospinous colpopexy. Dyspareunia appears to occur more frequently after sacrospinous colpopexy. The two procedures do not appear to produce any difference in urinary and bowel symptoms postoperatively. Sacrocolpopexy is associated with a longer recovery (when performed as an open procedure) and is therefore more expensive. Adverse events appear to occur with similar frequency and patient satisfaction rates are similar. Both procedures have the potential to cause large-volume haemorrhage (sacrum for sacrocolpopexy and pudendal vessels for sacospinous colpopexy). There is much debate on which procedure produces a more correct anatomical result.

The gap between the vagina and the sacrum can be secured with either an absorbable or a non-absorbable implant material. There is some evidence in the literature to suggest that the non-absorbable material will provide a longer lasting support. The disadvantage of non-absorbable materials is the risk of erosion of the material through the vaginal wall. This complication occurs in 5 to 10% of cases. Erosion may be managed in many cases by a simple trimming of the mesh but on occasions, abdominal removal may be required. Erosion can occur many years after surgery and must always be considered if a patient presents with a discharge or vaginal bleeding after sacrocolpopexy. Laparoscopic sacrocolpopexy is now being performed by an increasing number of surgeons. The reduced morbidity and faster recovery provide obvious advantages for the patient. Robotic laparoscopic surgery is also being employed in a few centres.

Colpocleisis, whereby the vaginal lumen is completely occluded, may be used rarely in women who are unfit for major surgery and in whom conservative measures have failed. Strips of vaginal skin are removed from anterior and posterior vaginal walls and the two are sutured together (Plate 50.1).

Augmentation of vaginal repairs

The high reported risk of failure or recurrence following vaginal repair surgery has led to an increased use in recent years of implants to supplement the fascial repair. The implants employed vary from absorbable to non-absorbable materials and may be synthetic or harvested from animals or humans. Concerns about transmission of infective agents has encouraged surgeons to use the synthetic materials more frequently. A review of the literature

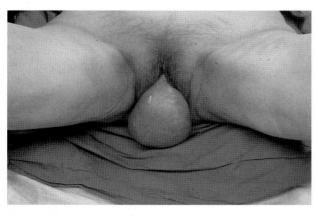

Fig. 50.5 Vaginal vault prolapse.

on prolapse repair concluded that there is as yet insufficient evidence to determine whether it is appropriate to employ implants to augment vaginal repairs [13]. There is some evidence to suggest that augmentation of a repair with mesh reduces the risk of prolapse recurrence. However, there is also evidence that use of mesh increases the risk of dyspareunia after surgery. Furthermore, mesh erosion occurs in approximately 10% of cases, and often further surgery is required to treat the erosion. It would appear that the advantage of reducing the risk of recurrence has to be balanced against the risk of erosion or dyspareunia.

Mesh design has changed significantly over the last 10 years. The meshes now recommended for use in vaginal surgery are of a macroporous, monofilament polypropylene construction with lower material weight and density than previously employed. It is believed by the protagonists of mesh use that this will reduce the risks of erosion and dyspareunia. Multicentre trials are currently being performed to determine whether mesh use is appropriate and beneficial. Until this is clarified, many surgeons are avoiding mesh use or reserving its use for patients with recurrent prolapse.

> **Summary box 50.3**
>
> - The patient should be made aware of all the non-surgical treatment options for prolapse before surgery is offered.

> **Summary box 50.4**
>
> - Prolapse repair may be augmented with mesh.
> - In accordance with National Institute for Health and Clinical Excellence guidelines, patients who are thought to be suitable for mesh augmentation of their prolapse repair should be fully appraised of the risks and potential benefits of the procedure.
> - Surgeons should audit their results.

Conclusions

Pelvic floor weakness can result in prolapse with accompanying mechanical and functional symptoms. Improving our understanding of the aetiology of prolapse should help direct the treatment, including non-surgical and surgical methods. More research is required into treatment and its outcome measures if gynaecologists are to make significant progress in this field. Surgical treatment of prolapse is now being studied in a more critical manner, which should help determine whether the new techniques, including mesh augmentation, produce significant benefit.

References

1 Beck RP, McCormick S, Nordstrom L. A 25-year experience with 519 anterior colporrhaphy procedures. *Obstet Gynecol* 1991;78:1011–1018.
2 Olsen AL, Smith VJ, Bergstrom JO, Colling JC, Clark AL. Epidemiology of surgically managed pelvic organ prolapse and urinary incontinence. *Obstet Gynecol* 1997;89:501–506.
3 Smith AR, Hosker GL, Warrell DW. The role of partial denervation of the pelvic floor in the aetiology of genitourinary prolapse and stress incontinence of urine. A neurophysiological study. *Br J Obstet Gynaecol* 1989;96:24–28.
4 Allen RE, Hosher GL, Smith ARB, Warrell DW. Pelvic floor damage and childbirth: a neurophysiological study. *Br J Obstet Gynaecol* 1990;97:770–779.
5 Landon CR, Smith ARB, Crofts CD, Trowbridge EA. Mechanical properties of fascia in pregnancy: its possible relationship to the later development of stress incontinence of urine. *Contemp Rev Obstet Gynaecol* 1990;2:40–46.
6 Bump RC, Mattiason A, Bo K *et al.* The standardization of terminology of female pelvic organ prolapse. *Am J Obstet Gynecol* 1996;175:10–17.
7 White GR. Cystocele. *J Am Med Assoc* 1909;21:1707–1710.
8 Kelly HA. Incontinence of urine in women. *Urol Cutan Rev* 1913;17:291–293.
9 Weber AM, Walters MD. Anterior vaginal prolapse: review of anatomy and techniques of surgical repair. *Obstet Gynecol* 1997;89:311–318.
10 Kahn MA, Stanton SL. Posterior colporrhaphy: its effects on bowel and sexual function. *Br J Obstet Gynaecol* 1997; 104:82–86.
11 Maher C, Baessler K, Glazener CMA, Adams EJ, Hagen S. Surgical management of pelvic organ prolapse in women (Review). *Cochrane Collaboration* 2005;4:CD004014.
12 Shull BL. Urologic surgical techniques. *Curr Opin Obstet Gynecol* 1991;3:534–540.
13 Jia X, Glazener C, Mowatt G *et al.* Efficacy and safety of using mesh or grafts in surgery for anterior and/or posterior vaginal wall prolapse: systematic review and meta-analysis. *BJOG* 2008;115:1350–1361.

Chapter 51
Urinary Incontinence

Dudley Robinson and Linda Cardozo
King's College Hospital, London, UK

Urinary incontinence is a distressing condition that, although rarely life threatening, severely affects all aspects of a woman's quality of life. Through ignorance, embarrassment and a belief that loss of bladder control is a 'normal' result of childbirth and ageing, many women suffer for years before seeking help [1]. This is unfortunate because with appropriate investigations an accurate diagnosis can be made and many women can be cured, most improved and all helped by various different management strategies.

Urinary incontinence is defined as the complaint of any involuntary loss of urine [2]. Conversely, continence is the ability to hold urine within the bladder at all times except during micturition. Both continence and micturition depend upon a lower urinary tract, consisting of the bladder and urethra, which is structurally and functionally normal. In order to understand urinary incontinence in women it is necessary to have a basic knowledge of the embryology, anatomy and physiology of the lower urinary tract.

Structure of the lower urinary tract

Embryology

In women the lower urinary and genital tracts develop in close proximity. The gut is formed by an invagination of the yolk sac and the most caudal part (hindgut) develops a diverticulum, the allantois (Fig. 51.1a). That part of the hindgut connected to the allantois is the cloaca. At about 28 days after fertilization a mesenchymal wedge of tissue, the urorectal septum, starts to migrate caudally and divides the cloaca into a ventral part, the urogenital sinus and a dorsal part, which will become the anorectal canal (Fig. 51.1b). The two are eventually separated from one another when the septum fuses with the cloacal membrane some 10 days later.

At the same time the pronephros develops within the mesoderm but this undergoes early degeneration. The mesonephros initially forms a primitive kidney draining into the mesonephric duct on each side. The tubules undergo degeneration but the ducts remain and grow caudally to enter the anterior part of the cloaca on each side. This divides the urogenital sinus into two parts: the area lying between the mesonephric ducts and allantois is the vesicourethral canal and the area below the mesonephric ducts is the urogenital sinus (Fig. 51.1c). The ureteric bud develops as an outgrowth from the mesonephric duct by proliferation of cells. It grows towards the caudal end of the nephrogenic ridge and initiates the development of the metanephros (later to become the kidney) between 30 and 37 days after fertilization.

Dilatation of the cranial portion of the vesicourethral canal leads to the development of the bladder. The area of the bladder bounded by the ureteric orifices cranially and the termination of the mesonephric ducts caudally gives rise to the trigone. The caudal part of the vesicourethral canal narrows to form the upper urethra. The urogenital sinus gives rise to the distal part of the urethra and part of the vagina. These developments occur by 42 days after fertilization (Fig. 51.1d).

Anatomy

The bladder is a hollow muscular organ normally situated behind the pubic symphysis and covered superiorly and anteriorly by peritoneum. It is composed of a syncytium of smooth muscle fibres known as the detrusor. Contraction of this meshwork of fibres results in simultaneous reduction of the bladder in all its diameters. The smooth muscle cells within the detrusor contain significant amounts of acetylcholinesterase, representing their cholinergic parasympathetic nerve supply.

The trigone is easily distinguishable from the rest of the smooth muscle of the bladder as it is divided into two layers. The deep trigonal muscle is similar to that of the detrusor, whereas the superficial muscle of the trigone is thin with small muscle bundles; the cells are devoid of acetylcholinesterase and have a reduced cholinergic nerve

Dewhurst's Textbook of Obstetrics & Gynaecology, Eighth Edition. Edited by D. Keith Edmonds.
© 2012 John Wiley and Sons, Ltd. Published 2012 by John Wiley and Sons, Ltd.

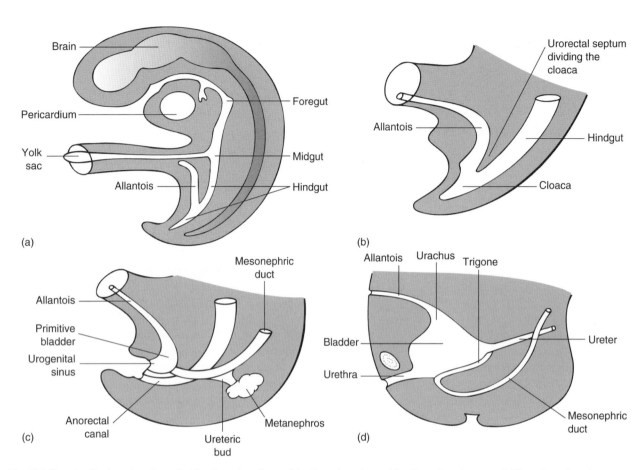

Fig. 51.1 Longitudinal section through (a) a 4-week embryo; (b) a 5-week embryo; (c) a 6-week embryo; and (d) an 8-week embryo.

supply. This superficial trigonal muscle merges into the proximal urethra and into the ureteric smooth muscle. In women the smooth muscle of the bladder neck is also different from that of the detrusor with orientation of the muscle bundles obliquely or longitudinally; they do not form a sphincter in women. The smooth muscle fibres of the detrusor, trigone and urethra have been shown embryonically to be distinct from one another. The urothelium lining the bladder is composed of two or three layers of transitional cells.

The normal adult female urethra is between 3 and 5 cm in length (Fig. 51.2). It is a hollow tubular structure joining the bladder to the exterior and is located under the pubic symphysis, piercing the pelvic diaphragm anterior to the vagina. It is lined with pseudostratified transitional cell epithelium in its proximal half and distally by non-keratinized stratified squamous epithelium. Beneath this is a rich vascular plexus that contributes up to one-third of the urethral pressure and which decreases with age. Beneath this there is longitudinally orientated smooth muscle that is continuous morphologically with the detrusor, but histochemically distinct. Contraction of this

muscle layer leads to shortening and opening of the urethra. The main bulk of striated muscle is located in the middle third of the urethra and is orientated in bundles of circularly arranged fibres, thickest anteriorly, thinning laterally and almost totally deficient posteriorly. This is the rhabdosphincter urethrae, and has also been called the external sphincter or the intrinsic sphincter mechanism. The muscle fibres of the rhabdosphincter consist of small diameter slow-twitch fibres that are rich in acid-stable myosin adenosine triphosphatase (ATPase) and possess a number of mitochondria. This muscle mass is responsible for urethral closure at rest.

The extrinsic sphincter mechanism consists of striated periurethral muscle (levator ani), which has no direct connection with the urethra and is situated at the junction of the middle and lower thirds of the urethra. This muscle consists of large diameter fibres, most of which are rich in alkaline-stable myosin ATPase characteristic of fast-twitch muscle fibres. This extrinsic sphincter mechanism contributes an additional closure force at times of physical effort. Together, the intrinsic and extrinsic sphincter mechanisms of the urethra produce a greater pressure

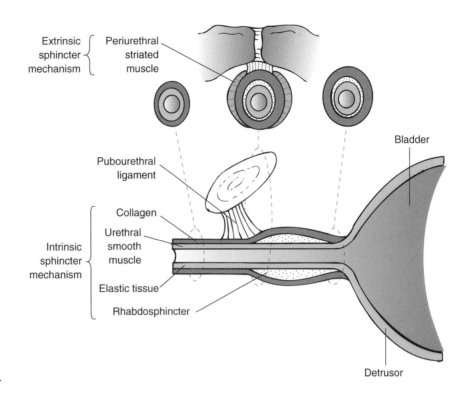

Fig. 51.2 The adult female urethra.

within the urethra than in the bladder. This is known as the positive closure pressure and is partly responsible for the maintenance of continence.

The proximal urethra is supported by the pubourethral ligaments, which attach the proximal urethra to the posterior aspect of the pubic symphysis. These were originally described by Zacharin [3] as consisting of parallel collagen bundles and elastic connective tissue. However, his histological examinations were of cadaveric specimens and Wilson *et al.* [4] have shown in operative specimens that these ligaments contain large numbers of smooth muscle bundles. Gosling *et al.* [5] reported that the pubourethral suspensory ligaments are histochemically identical to the detrusor with an abundant supply of cholinergic nerve fibres. But Wilson *et al.* [4] failed to demonstrate acetylcholinesterase activity in these fibres, and thus their origin remains unclear. DeLancey [6] has described two distinct entities: the pubourethral ligament composed of collagen and a pubovesical ligament containing muscle fibres.

Innervation

The detrusor muscle is innervated primarily by the parasympathetic nerves S2–S4 and receives a rich efferent supply (Fig. 51.3). Adrenergic receptors have also been shown to be present in the lower urinary tract, with β receptors in the dome of the bladder and bladder neck,

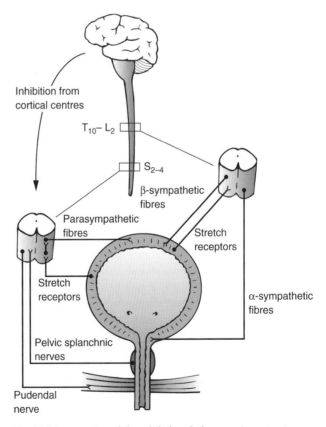

Fig. 51.3 Innervation of the adult female lower urinary tract.

and α receptors in the bladder neck and urethra [7]. Sympathetic outflow is from T10 to L2 but it is unclear whether it acts directly on β receptors in the bladder, causing relaxation, or indirectly via parasympathetic ganglia, causing inhibition of the excitatory parasympathetic supply. Visceral afferent fibres travel with the thoracolumbar and sacral efferent nerves, conveying the sensation of bladder distension.

Urethral smooth muscle is innervated by sympathetic efferent fibres; cholinergic stimulation of these produces contraction. The rhabdosphincter urethrae is supplied via sacral nerve roots (S2–S4), which travel with the pelvic splanchnics to the intrinsic smooth muscle of the urethra. The levator ani is also innervated by motor fibres of S2–S4 origin, but these fibres travel via the pudendal nerve. This explains why electromyographic activity of the pelvic floor and urethral sphincter are not necessarily the same.

The central nervous control of micturition is complex and requires a sacral spinal reflex arc controlled by the cerebral cortex, the cerebellum and subcortical areas, including the thalamus, basal ganglia, limbic system, hypothalamus and pontine reticular formation. There are parasympathetic, sympathetic and somatic afferent and efferent connections from the brainstem. Stretch receptors within the bladder wall pass impulses through the pelvic plexus and via the visceral afferent fibres travelling with the pelvic splanchnic nerves, ending in S2–S4 of the spinal cord. This visceral reflex arc is controlled by both the excitatory and inhibitory centres, which, under normal circumstances, prevent detrusor contractions and maintain urethral sphincter control, thereby inhibiting micturition.

Functioning of the lower urinary tract

Physiology

The main role of the bladder is to store the urine that continuously enters it, in order to achieve convenient intermittent voiding. Thus, the bladder must act as an efficient low-pressure continent reservoir. Urine from the kidneys enters the bladder via the ureters at a rate of 0.5–5 mL/min. Normally, the first sensation of bladder filling is noted at between 150 and 250 mL and there is a strong desire to void at approximately 400–600 mL (bladder capacity). During filling the bladder pressure should not normally rise by more than 10 cm of water to 300 mL or 15 cm of water to 500 mL. In order to maintain continence the maximum urethral pressure must exceed the bladder pressure at all times except during micturition. Thus, for continence to exist it is not only essential that the intravesical pressure remains low but also that the urethral lumen should seal completely. Three essential components of urethral function are required to achieve hermetic closure: (i) urethral inner wall softness; (ii) inner

urethral compression; and (iii) outer wall tension. These three functions are dependent on an intact urothelium, together with a major component from the submucosal vascular plexus as well as the collagen and elastic tissue within the urethra and the striated and smooth muscle.

Storage phase

During this time the urethra remains closed, as previously described. Proprioceptive afferent impulses from the stretch receptors within the bladder wall pass via the pelvic nerves to the sacral roots S2–S4. These impulses ascend the cord via the lateral spinothalamic tracts and the detrusor motor response is subconsciously inhibited by descending impulses from the basal ganglia. Gradually, as the bladder volume increases, further afferent impulses are sent to the cerebral cortex and the first sensation of desire to void is usually appreciated at about half the functional bladder capacity. Inhibition of detrusor contraction becomes cortically mediated. As the bladder fills further, these afferent impulses reinforce the desire to void and conscious inhibition of micturition occurs until a suitable time. When functional capacity is reached, voluntary pelvic floor contraction is initiated to aid urethral closure. This may result in marked variations in urethral pressure as the sensation of urgency develops.

Voiding phase

At a suitable time and place, cortical inhibition is released and relaxation of the pelvic floor occurs, together with relaxation of the intrinsic striated muscle of the urethra. This results in a fall in urethral pressure, which occurs a few seconds prior to the increase in bladder pressure. A few seconds later, a rapid discharge of efferent parasympathetic impulses via the pelvic nerve causes the detrusor to contract and also to open the bladder neck and shorten the urethra. The detrusor pressure rises by a variable amount, normally less than 60 cm of water in women. However, it may not need to rise at all if the fall in urethral resistance is adequate for the urethral pressure to be lower than the intravesical pressure, so that urine is voided.

Once micturition has been initiated the intravesical pressure normally remains constant. The efficiency of detrusor contraction increases as the muscle fibres of the detrusor shorten, therefore decreasing the forces that are required to maintain micturition.

Interruption of micturition is usually achieved by contraction of the extrinsic striated muscle of the pelvic floor, associated with a rise in urethral pressure to exceed the intravesical pressure and thus stop the flow of urine. As the detrusor is composed of smooth muscle, it is much slower to relax and therefore continues to contract against the closed sphincter; this causes an isometric detrusor contraction that will eventually die away to the premicturition detrusor pressure.

When the bladder empties at the end of micturition, the urinary flow stops, the pelvic floor and intrinsic striated muscle of the urethra contract and any urine that is left in the proximal urethra will be milked back into the bladder. As the urethra closes off, subconscious inhibition of the sacral micturition centre is reinstituted and the bladder storage phase begins again.

Pathophysiology of urinary incontinence

Under normal circumstances, in a woman with a healthy lower urinary tract urine will leave the bladder via the urethra only when the intravesical pressure exceeds the maximum urethral pressure. In general terms and in the majority of cases of urinary incontinence, the bladder pressure exceeds the urethral pressure because the urethral sphincter mechanism is weak (urodynamic stress incontinence) or because the detrusor pressure is excessively high (detrusor overactivity; neurogenic detrusor overactivity).

In urodynamic stress incontinence the factors that maintain positive urethral closure pressure at rest may be inadequate when there is an increase in intra-abdominal pressure. This is particularly likely to occur if the bladder neck and proximal urethra are poorly supported or have descended through the pelvic floor, as in cases of concomitant cystourethrocele.

An abnormally high detrusor pressure may occur in detrusor overactivity when there is inability to inhibit detrusor contractions. In cases of a low compliance, incontinence may occur when there is a failure of the bladder to accommodate a large volume of urine for a small rise in pressure.

Epidemiology

Prevalence of urinary incontinence

Urinary incontinence is common. Table 51.1 shows the prevalence of urinary incontinence in women living at home according to a report published by the Royal College of Physicians [8]. Thomas *et al.* [9] have shown that urinary incontinence occurs twice or more per month in at least one-third of the female population over the age of 35 years and, although there is a small rise with increasing age, it is a very common problem in women of all ages. The situation is worst amongst the elderly and in psychogeriatric hospital wards, where up to 90% of female patients are incontinent of urine.

More recently, a large epidemiological study on urinary incontinence of 27 936 women has been reported in Norway [10]. Overall, 25% of women reported urinary incontinence, of which 7% felt it to be significant, and the prevalence of incontinence was found to increase with age. When considering the type of incontinence, 50% of women complained of stress, 11% urge and 36% mixed

Table 51.1 Prevalence of urinary incontinence.

Age (years)	Incontinence (%)
Women living at home	
15–44	5–7
45–64	8–5
65+	10–20
Men living at home	
15–64	3
65+	7–10
Both sexes living in institutions	
Residential homes	25
Nursing homes	40
Hospital	50–70

Data from [8].

incontinence. Further analysis has also investigated the effect of age and parity. The prevalence of urinary incontinence among nulliparous women ranged from 8% to 32% and increased with age. In general, parity was associated with incontinence and the first delivery was the most significant. When considering stress incontinence in the age group 20–34 years the relative risk was 2.7 (95% CI 2.0–3.5) for primiparous women and 4.0 (95% CI 2.5–6.4) for multiparous women. There was a similar association for mixed incontinence, although not for urge incontinence [11].

In a large study of patients assessed after tertiary referral 60% of women were found to have delayed seeking treatment for more than 1 year from the time their symptoms became severe. Of these women, 50% claimed that this was because they were too embarrassed to discuss the problem with their doctor, and 17% said that they thought the problem was normal for their age [1].

The financial burden of incontinence is also considerable with $26 billion being spent per annum in the USA alone [12].

Age

The incidence of urinary incontinence increases with increasing age. Elderly women have been found to have a reduced flow rate, increased urinary residuals, higher filling pressures, reduced bladder capacity and lower maximum voiding pressures. In a large study of 842 women aged 17–64 years the prevalence rates of urinary incontinence increased progressively over seven birth cohorts (1900–1940) from 12% to 25%. These findings agree with those of a large telephone survey in the USA that reported a prevalence of urge incontinence of 5% in the 18–24 age rising to 19% in women over 65 years of age

[13]. Conversely, as mobility and physical exercise decrease with advancing age so does the prevalence of stress urinary incontinence.

Race

Several studies have been performed examining the impact of racial differences on the prevalence of urinary incontinence in women. In general, there is evidence that there is a lower incidence of both urinary incontinence and urogenital prolapse in black women, and North American studies have found a larger proportion of white than African American women reported symptoms of stress incontinence (31% vs. 7%) and a larger proportion were found to have demonstrable stress incontinence on objective assessment (61% vs. 27%). Overall, white women had a prevalence of urodynamic stress incontinence 2.3 times higher than African American women [14]. Although most studies confirm these findings, there is little evidence regarding the prevalence of urge incontinence or mixed incontinence.

Pregnancy

Pregnancy is responsible for marked changes in the urinary tract and consequently lower urinary tract symptoms are more common and many are simply a reflection of normal physiological change. Urine production increases in pregnancy due to increasing cardiac output and a 25% increase in renal perfusion and glomerular filtration rate.

Frequency of micturition is one of the earliest symptoms of pregnancy, affecting approximately 60% of women in the first- and mid-trimester and 81% in the final trimester. Nocturia is also a common symptom, although it was thought to be a nuisance in only 4% of cases. Overall frequency occurs in over 90% of women in pregnancy.

Urgency and urge incontinence have also been shown to increase in pregnancy. Urge incontinence has been shown to have a peak incidence of 19% in multiparous women, while other authors have reported a rate of urge incontinence of 10% and urgency of 60%. The incidence of detrusor overactivity and low compliance in pregnancy has been reported as 24% and 31%, respectively. The cause of the former may be due to high progesterone levels while the latter is probably caused by a consequence of pressure from the gravid uterus.

Stress incontinence has also been reported to be more common in pregnancy, with 28% of women complaining of symptoms, although only 12% remained symptomatic following delivery. The long-term prognosis for this group of women remains guarded. Continent women delivered vaginally have been compared with those who had a Caesarean section. Although there was initially a difference in favour of Caesarean section, this effect was insignificant by 3 months after delivery [15].

Childbirth

Childbirth may result in damage to the pelvic floor musculature as well as injury to the pudendal and pelvic nerves. The association between increasing parity and urinary incontinence has been reported in several studies. Some authorities have found this relationship to be linear whereas others have demonstrated a threshold at the first delivery and some have shown that increasing age at first delivery is significant. A large Australian study has demonstrated a strong relationship between urinary incontinence and parity in young women (18–23 years), although in middle age (45–50 years) there was only a modest association and this was lost in older women (70–75 years) [16].

Obstetric factors themselves may also have a direct effect on continence following delivery. The risk of incontinence increases by 5.7-fold in women who have had a previous vaginal delivery, although a previous Caesarean section did not increase the risk [17]. In addition, an increased risk of urinary incontinence has been associated with increased exposure to oxytocic drugs, vacuum extraction, forceps delivery and fetal macrosomia.

Menopause

The urogenital tract and lower urinary tract are sensitive to the effects of oestrogen and progesterone throughout adult life. Epidemiological studies have implicated oestrogen deficiency in the aetiology of lower urinary tract symptoms occurring following the menopause, with 70% of women relating the onset of urinary incontinence to their final menstrual period. Lower urinary tract symptoms have been shown to be common in postmenopausal women attending a menopause clinic, with 20% complaining of severe urgency and almost 50% complaining of stress incontinence. Urge incontinence in particular is more prevalent following the menopause and the prevalence would appear to rise with increasing years of oestrogen deficiency. Some studies have shown a peak incidence in perimenopausal women whereas other evidence suggests that many women develop incontinence at least 10 years prior to the cessation of menstruation, with significantly more premenopausal than postmenopausal women being affected.

Quality of life

Urinary incontinence is a common and distressing condition known to adversely affect quality of life (QoL) [18]. Research has often concentrated on the prevalence, aetiology diagnosis and management of urinary incontinence, with little work being performed on the effects of this chronic condition, or its treatment, on QoL. Over the last few decades interest in the incorporation of patient-assessed health status or QoL measures into the evaluation of the management of urinary incontinence has increased [19].

The views of clinicians and patients regarding QoL and the effects of treatments differ considerably. Consequently, there is increased recognition of the patient's perception when assessing new interventions in the management of lower urinary tract dysfunction. The measurement of QoL allows the quantification of morbidity and the evaluation of treatment efficacy, and also acts as a measure of how lives are affected and coping strategies adopted. It is estimated that 20% of adult women suffer some degree of life disruption secondary to lower urinary tract dysfunction [20].

The World Health Organization has defined health as 'not merely the absence of disease, but complete physical, mental and social well-being' [21]. QoL has been used to mean a combination of patient-assessed measures of health including physical function, role function, social function, emotional or mental state, burden of symptoms and sense of well-being [22]. QoL has been defined as including

those attributes valued by patients including their resultant comfort or sense of well-being; the extent to which they were able to maintain reasonable physical, emotional, and intellectual function; the degree to which they retain their ability to participate in valued activities within the family and the community [23].

This helps to emphasize the multidimensional nature of QoL and the importance of considering patients' perceptions of their own situation with regard to non-health-related aspects of their life [24].

Although QoL is highly subjective, it has now been acknowledged that it is as important as physical disease state in the management of women with lower urinary tract dysfunction [25]. Consequently, the success of treatment can no longer be judged on clinical parameters alone and QoL needs to be considered in both clinical and research settings [26].

Quality of life assessment

There are many validated questionnaires available, although all have the same structure, consisting of a series of sections (domains) designed to gather information regarding particular aspects of health (Table 51.2). There are two types of QoL questionnaires: generic and disease or condition specific.

More recently, the International Consultation on Incontinence (ICI) has published levels of recommendation for both generic and disease-specific questionnaires [27] (Table 51.3).

Generic quality of life questionnaires

Generic questionnaires are designed as general measures of QoL and are therefore applicable to a wide range of populations and clinical conditions. Many different

Table 51.2 Quality of life domains.

Physical function, e.g. mobility, self-care, exercise
Emotional function, e.g. depression, anxiety, worry
Social function, e.g. intimacy, social support, social contact leisure activities
Role performance, e.g. work, housework, shopping
Pain
Sleep/nausea
Disease-specific symptoms
Severity measures

Table 51.3 Criteria for the recommendation of questionnaires.

Grade of recommendation	Evidence required
Grade A: Highly recommended	Published data indicating that it is valid, reliable and responsive to change on psychometric testing
Grade B: Recommended	Published data indicating that it is valid and reliable on psychometric testing
Grade C: With potential	Published data (including abstracts) indicating that it is valid or reliable or responsive on psychometric testing

Table 51.4 Generic quality of life questionnaires.

Generic quality of life questionnaires (Grade A)
Short form 36 (SF-36) [28]
Generic quality of life questionnaires (Grade B)
Sickness impact profile [29]
Nottingham health profile [30]
Goteborg quality of life [31]

validated generic questionnaires have been developed, although not all are suitable for the assessment of lower urinary tract problems (Table 51.4). They are not specific to a particular disease, treatment or age group, and hence allow broad comparisons to be made. Consequently, they lack sensitivity when applied to women with lower urinary tract symptoms and may be unable to detect clinically important improvement.

Disease-specific quality of life questionnaires

To improve the sensitivity of QoL questionnaires disease-specific tools have been developed to assess particular medical conditions more accurately and in greater detail (Table 51.5). The questions are designed to focus on key aspects associated with lower urinary tract symptoms, and scoring is performed so that clinically important changes can be detected.

Table 51.5 Disease-specific quality of life questionnaires (Grade A).

Urogenital distress inventory (UDI) [32]
Urogenital distress inventory – 6 (UDI-6) [33]
Urge UDI [34]
Incontinence severity index [35]
Quality of life in persons with urinary incontinence (I-QoL) [36]
King's health questionnaire [18]
Incontinence impact questionnaire (IIQ) [37]

Table 51.6 Causes of urinary incontinence in women.

Urodynamic stress incontinence (urethral sphincter incompetence)
Detrusor overactivity (neurogenic detrusor overactivity)
Overactive bladder
Retention with overflow
Fistulae – vesicovaginal, ureterovaginal, urethrovaginal, complex
Congenital abnormalities, e.g. epispadias, ectopic ureter, spina bifida occulta
Urethral diverticulum
Temporary, e.g. urinary tract infection, faecal impaction
Functional, e.g. immobility

Table 51.7 Causes of incontinence in the elderly, many of which may be transient.

Infection (e.g. urinary tract infection)
Confusional states (e.g. dementia)
Faecal impaction
Oestrogen deficiency
Restricted mobility
Depression
Drug therapy (e.g. diuretics)
Endocrine disorder (e.g. diabetes)
Limited independence

In general, perhaps the best solution when assessing women with urinary incontinence is to use a generic and a disease-specific questionnaire in combination, both of which have been validated and used previously.

Classification

Urinary incontinence is best classified according to aetiology, as shown in Table 51.6. There are a number of additional causes of urinary incontinence in elderly woman (Table 51.7), many of which can be reversed by appropriate intervention.

More recently, the term overactive bladder (OAB) has been introduced to describe the symptom complex of urinary urgency, usually accompanied by frequency and nocturia, with or without urgency urinary incontinence, in the absence of urinary tract infection or other obvious pathology [2].

Recent epidemiological studies have reported the overall prevalence of OAB in women to be 16.9%, suggesting that there could be 17.5 million women in the USA who suffer from the condition. The prevalence increases with age: 4.8% in women under 25 years increasing to 30.9% in those over the age of 65 [13]. This is supported by recent prevalence data from Europe in which 16 776 interviews were conducted in a population-based survey [38]. The overall prevalence of OAB in individuals 40 years and older was 16.6% and increased with age. Frequency was the most commonly reported symptom (85%) and 54% complained of urgency and 36% urge incontinence. When considering management, 60% had consulted a physician, although only 27% were currently receiving treatment.

Clinical presentation of urinary incontinence

Symptoms of lower urinary tract dysfunction fall into three main groups: (i) incontinence; (ii) OAB symptoms; and (iii) voiding difficulties.

Stress incontinence is the most common complaint. It may be a symptom or a sign but it is not a diagnosis. Apart from stress incontinence, women may complain of urge incontinence, dribble or giggle incontinence or incontinence during sexual intercourse. Nocturnal enuresis (bed wetting) may occur on its own or in conjunction with other complaints. Symptoms of voiding difficulty include hesitancy, a poor stream, straining to void and incomplete bladder emptying.

Apart from the symptoms of lower urinary tract dysfunction, it is important to take a full history from all women who present with urinary incontinence. Other gynaecological symptoms such as prolapse or menstrual disturbances may be relevant. A fibroid uterus may compress the bladder and can cause urinary frequency and urgency. There is an increased incidence of stress incontinence amongst women who have had large babies, particularly following instrumental vaginal delivery, so an obstetric history may be helpful. Information regarding other urological problems such as recurrent urinary tract infections, episodes of acute urinary retention or childhood enuresis should be sought.

Urinary incontinence is sometimes the first manifestation of a neurological problem (such as multiple sclerosis) so it is important to enquire about neurological symptoms. Endocrine disorders such as diabetes may be responsible for symptoms of lower urinary tract dysfunction and should therefore be recorded.

Some drugs affect urinary tract function, especially diuretics, which increase urine output. In older people they may cause urinary incontinence where only urgency existed previously. Other drugs that affect detrusor function include tricyclic antidepressants, major tranquillizers and α-adrenergic blockers.

Unfortunately, clinical examination is usually unhelpful in cases of female urinary incontinence. General examination should include the subject's mental state and mobility as well as the appearance of local tissues. Excoriation of the vulva will indicate the severity of the problem and atrophic changes may reveal longstanding hormone deficiency. A gynaecological/urological examination should be carried out and, although stress incontinence may be demonstrated, this will only confirm the patient's story; it will not actually indicate the cause. If a neurological lesion is suspected then the cranial nerves and sacral nerve roots S2–S4 should be examined.

The bladder has been described as an 'unreliable witness'. The correlation between clinical diagnosis and urodynamic diagnosis is poor, and therefore it is unusual to be able to make an accurate diagnosis based on history and examination alone. Urodynamic stress incontinence is the commonest cause of urinary incontinence in women and detrusor overactivity is the second most common cause. These two diagnoses account for over 90% of cases of female urinary incontinence. As their treatment differs it is important to make an accurate initial diagnosis. Jarvis *et al.* [39] studied 41 women with urodynamic stress incontinence and 34 women with detrusor overactivity. They found that, although 98% of women with urodynamic stress incontinence complained of the symptom of stress incontinence, so did 25% of those with detrusor overactivity. In addition, 89% of women with detrusor overactivity complained of the symptom of urge incontinence, but so did 37% of those with urodynamic stress incontinence. Thus, it is difficult to separate these two common conditions on history alone. In fact, comparing the initial clinical diagnosis with the accurate urodynamic diagnosis, Jarvis *et al.* [39] found that 68% of those with urodynamic stress incontinence were correctly diagnosed, whereas only 51% of those with detrusor overactivity would have been correctly allocated.

Table 51.8 Investigations of female urinary incontinence.

General practitioner/outpatient
Mid-stream specimen of urine
Frequency/volume chart
Pad test

Basic urodynamics
Uroflowmetry
Cystometry
Videocystourethrography

Specialized
Urethral pressure profilometry
Cystourethroscopy
Ultrasound
Cystourethrography
Intravenous urography
Electromyography
Ambulatory urodynamics

Investigations

Investigations range from the very simple to the highly sophisticated and complex and are outlined in Table 51.8.

Mid-stream urine sample

A mid-stream urine (MSU) specimen should always be sent for culture and sensitivity prior to further investigation. Although the patient's symptoms are unlikely to be caused by a urinary tract infection, they can be altered by one, and catheterization in the presence of an infection could result in septicaemia. In addition, the results of the investigations themselves may be inaccurate in the presence of an infection.

Frequency–volume charts

It is often helpful to ask women to complete a frequency–volume chart or urinary diary (Fig. 51.4). This is informative for the doctor as well as the patient and may indicate excessive drinking or bad habits as the cause of lower urinary tract symptoms. There is a tendency for patients to exaggerate their urinary symptoms when giving a history [40] and their recall of incontinent episodes may not be reliable. The frequency–volume chart (urinary or bladder diary) provides an objective assessment of a patient's fluid input and urine output.

As well as the number of voids and incontinence episodes, the mean volume voided over a 24-h period can also be calculated, as well as the diurnal and nocturnal volumes. Frequency–volume charts have the advantage of assessing symptom severity in the everyday situation.

Self-monitoring techniques may themselves modify the behaviour they are assessing [41]. However, reported micturition frequency and the number of incontinent

Summary box 51.1

Urinary incontinence:
- Defined as the complaint of any involuntary loss of urine.
- Often under diagnosed and under treated.
- The incidence increases with age.
- Known to have a significant effect on quality of life.
- Stress urinary incontinence (SUI), noveractive bladder (OAB) (with or without incontinence) and mixed incontinence are the commonest types of urinary incontinence.

Time	Day 1 In	Out	W	Day 2 In	Out	W	Day 3 In	Out	W	Day 4 In	Out	W	Day 5 In	Out	W
6 am															
7 am							200	150						300	
8 am / 8.30	200 200	350		200	250		200				350		200		
9 am										400	50		200	150	
10 am / 10.45	200	50			75										
11 am								50		200					
12 pm				200	60		200				50			50	
1 pm	200	100						25		200					
2 pm				200	60					200	100			175	
3 pm	100				100					100					
4 pm		75					200	100							
5.30 pm	100			50	150			300		100					
6.15 pm		150									100	40			
7 pm		100			50									100	
8 pm							200	175		200	150				
9 pm		250			100						150		50	100	
10 pm	200				50		200				100				
11.30 pm	200 100							325			100			150	
12 am							100								
1.30 am		100		100	50						100				
2 am								50							
3 am		75													
4 am					150										
5 am											150			200	

Fig. 51.4 King's College Hospital frequency–volume chart. Example of a frequency–volume chart showing frequent small voided volumes.

episodes have been found to be highly reproducible on test–retest analysis [42].

There is ongoing discussion regarding the optimum duration for which the charts should be completed. Clearly there needs to be a balance between asking the patient to complete a diary for a long period of time (and thus increasing the reliability) and the inconvenience this causes. Current practice is to use a 5-day chart, although some authorities would suggest only 3 days. A short urinary diary of only 2 days has also been assessed in 151 asymptomatic women aged 19–81 years [43]. Of these women, only 8% had a micturition frequency of eight times or more in 24 h with a tendency for the number of nocturnal micturitions to increase with age. Unfortunately, in symptomatic women it is not possible to reliably distinguish patients with urodynamic stress incontinence from those with other urodynamic diagnoses using a frequency–volume chart alone [44].

Pad test

Incontinence can be confirmed (without diagnosing the cause) by performing a pad weighing test. Many different types of pad test have been described. The following is just an example. The subject is asked to drink 500 mL of water. She then applies a preweighed perineal pad (sanitary towel) to her perineum and spends the next hour walking around, performing normal household duties. She performs a series of exercises, including coughing and deep knee bending and washes her hands under running water before the pad is reweighed. A weight gain of more than 1 g in 1 h normally represents urinary incontinence. The 24- and 48-h home pad tests have been described and, although they may be more representative, they require greater patient compliance and motivation to perform.

Urodynamics

The term urodynamic studies describes several investigations that are employed to determine bladder function.

Uroflowmetry

Uroflowmetry, the measurement of urine flow rate, is a simple test that can exclude the presence of outflow obstruction, or a hypotonic detrusor, but on its own will not differentiate between the two. Various different types of flowmeter are available and utilize a strain gauge weighing transducer, an electronic dipstick, a rotating disc or ultrasound. In order to obtain a flow rate, the patient is asked to void onto the flowmeter, in private, when her bladder is comfortably full. The maximum flow rate and volume voided are recorded. In women, the normal recording is a bell-shaped curve with a peak flow rate of at least 15 mL/s for a volume of 150 mL of urine voided (Fig. 51.5a). A reduced flow rate in an asymptomatic woman may be important if she is to undergo incontinence surgery as she is more likely to develop voiding difficulties in the postoperative period (Fig. 51.5b).

Cystometry

Cystometry, which measures the pressure–volume relationship within the bladder, can differentiate between urodynamic stress incontinence and detrusor overactivity in the majority of cases (Fig. 51.6). Simple cystometry is easy to perform and can be carried out in all district general hospitals. The bladder is filled with physiological saline via a blood-giving set and urethral catheter (Fig. 51.7). During bladder filling the intravesical (total bladder) pressure is measured using a central venous pressure line water manometer. This type of simple cystometry is subject to two major sources of error. First, the intravesical pressure cannot be measured continuously during bladder filling so sequential bladder filling must be employed.

Second, measurement of the intravesical pressure does not always accurately represent changes in detrusor pressure. As the bladder is an intra-abdominal organ the detrusor is subject to changes in intra-abdominal pressure and therefore subtracted cystometry, which involves

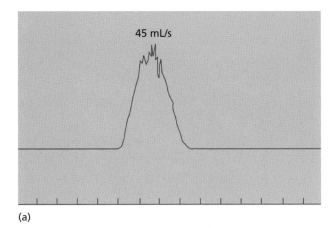

(a)

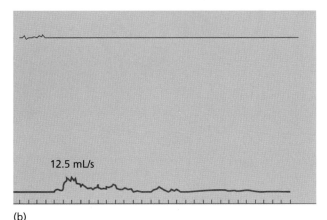

(b)

Fig. 51.5 (a) Normal uroflowmetry (maximum flow 45 mL/s, voided volume 330 mL); (b) reduced flow rate (maximum flow rate 12.5 mL/s, voided volume 225 mL)

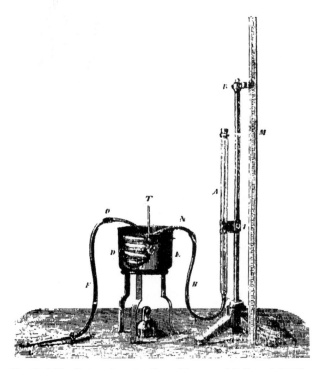

Fig. 51.6 The first cystometer. From Mosso and Pellacani (1882).

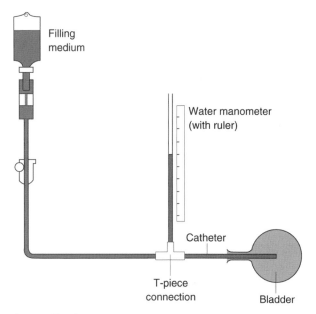

Fig. 51.7 Simple cystometry.

measurement of both the intravesical and the intra-abdominal pressure simultaneously, is more accurate.

Subtracted cystometry

A subtracted cystometrogram can be performed in many different ways, but in the UK the bladder is normally filled with physiological saline at body temperature and the pressure is measured via a narrow fluid-filled catheter using a large external pressure transducer. The rectal (or vaginal) pressure is recorded to represent intra-abdominal pressure and this is subtracted from the bladder (intra-vesical) pressure to give the detrusor pressure (Fig. 51.8). Catheter-mounted solid-state microtip pressure transducers are becoming increasingly popular for bladder and rectal pressure measurements. They are more expensive and less durable than the large external pressure transducers, but have the advantage of reducing the bulk of the urodynamic equipment.

The information that can be obtained from a subtracted cystometrogram includes sensation, capacity, contractility and compliance (Fig. 51.9). The urinary residual volume is normally less than 50 mL, the first sensation of desire to void is normally at 150–250 mL and the cystometric bladder capacity is normally 400–600 mL. Under normal circumstances, the detrusor pressure does not rise by more than 10 cm of water for a volume of 300 mL or 15 cm of water for a volume of 500 mL, and there are no detrusor contractions during bladder filling. When the bladder has been filled to capacity the woman is stood up and the filling catheter removed. She is asked to cough several times and to heel bounce and any rise in detrusor pressure or leakage per urethram is recorded. She is then asked to pass urine and the detrusor pressure is

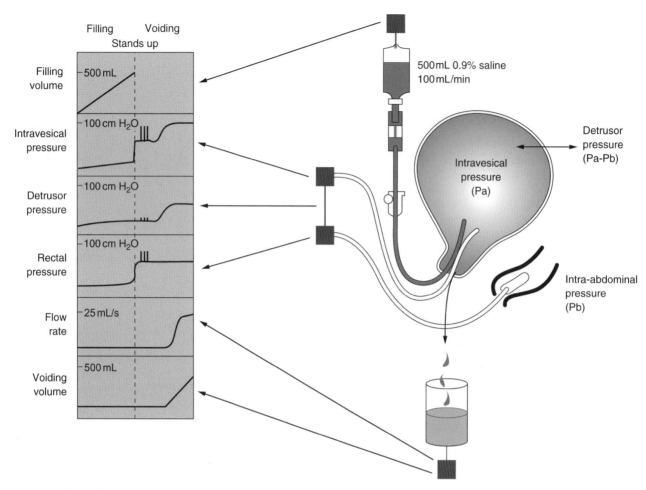

Fig. 51.8 Subtracted cystometry.

measured. At some point during voiding she is told to interrupt her urinary stream. The striated urethral sphincter and pelvic floor will contract immediately, but the smooth muscle of the detrusor will not relax instantaneously and the resulting rise in detrusor pressure is known as the isometric detrusor contraction. When the detrusor pressure has fallen to its premicturition level, the subject is asked to empty her bladder completely and any urinary residual volume can be noted. The normal maximum voiding pressure is not more than 60 cm of water in women (Fig. 51.10).

Videocystourethrography

Videocystourethrography with pressure and flow studies, which combines cystometry, uroflowmetry and radiological screening of the bladder and urethra, is the single most informative investigation (Fig. 51.11). It is relatively expensive and time-consuming and is only available in tertiary referral centres. A radiological contrast medium such as Urografin® (Bayer, Berkshire, UK) is used to fill the bladder instead of saline and a subtracted provocative cystometrogram is performed in the normal way. After

bladder filling the patient is tilted erect on the X-ray screening table and the image intensifier is used to visualize the bladder and urethra. The patient is then asked to cough with a full bladder and the extent of bladder base descent and any leakage of contrast medium are recorded. During voiding abnormal bladder morphology can be assessed as well as the presence of vesicoureteric reflux, trabeculation or diverticula. Occasionally, a urethral diverticulum or vesicovaginal fistula may be identified (Fig. 51.12). In addition, bony abnormalities of the pelvis may occasionally be seen. The whole investigation can be recorded on video tape or computer with a sound commentary for immediate and later replay, in order to facilitate diagnosis, audit, data storage, research and education. Although videocystourethrography has no advantage over subtracted cystometry when differentiating between urodynamic stress incontinence and detrusor overactivity, there are some occasions when videocystourethrography is particularly useful. These include patients in whom previous incontinence surgery has failed, mixed or unusual symptoms and neurological disorders (Fig. 51.13).

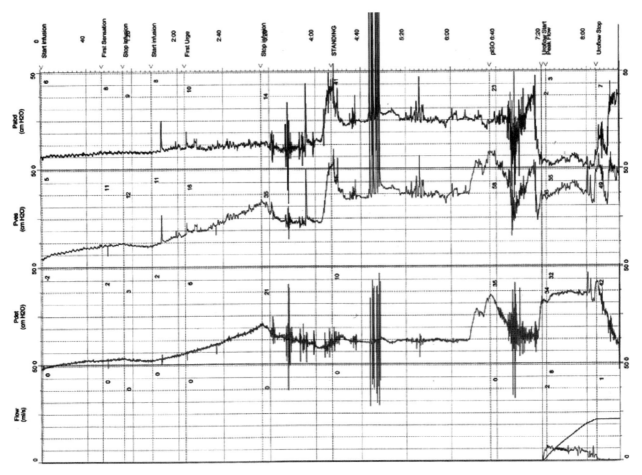

Fig. 51.9 Subtracted cystometrogram trace showing a picture of low compliance.

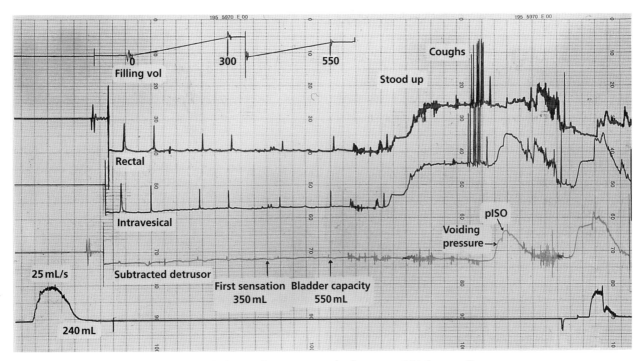

Fig. 51.10 A normal cystometrogram trace (the bottom line represents the flow rate, which is normal).

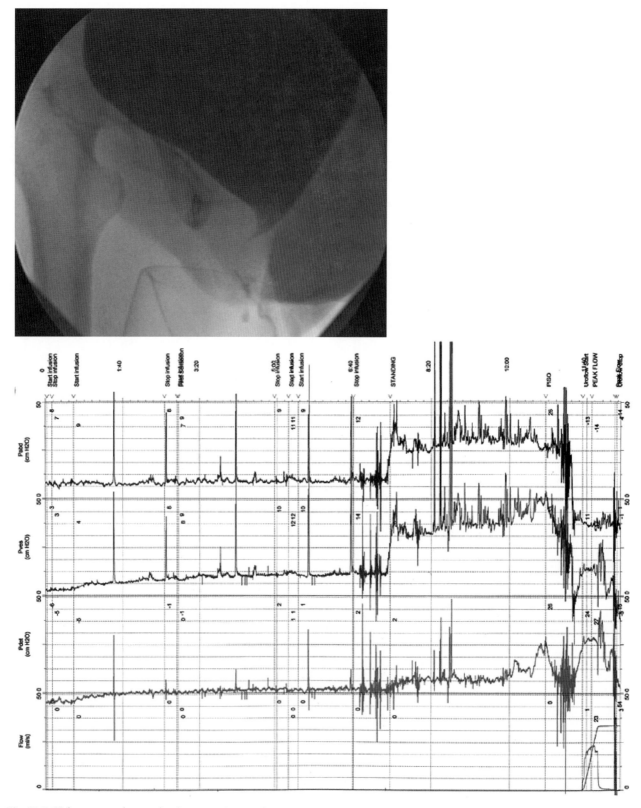

Fig. 51.11 Videocystourethrography demonstrating urodynamic stress incontinence. Subtracted filling cystometry showing no evidence of detrusor overactivity and synchronous screening demonstrating urethral sphincter incompetence on coughing.

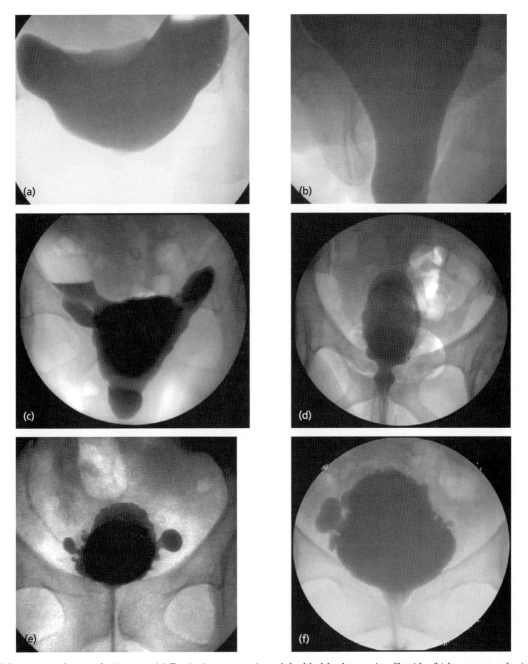

Fig. 51.12 Videocystourethrography images. (a) Extrinsic compression of the bladder by uterine fibroids; (b) large cystocele; (c) multiple bladder diverticulae; (d) neurogenic bladder with uninhibited detrusor contraction and associated leakage; (e) bladder trabeculation, diverticulae and right sided vesico-ureteric reflux; and (f) multiple diverticulae, bladder trabeculation and an unprovoked contraction with leakage.

Voiding cystometry

Following the completion of filling cystometry the filling catheter is removed prior to voiding to prevent any unnecessary urethral obstruction. The intravesical and rectal pressure recording lines are left *in situ*, allowing simultaneous measurement of detrusor pressure along with the urine flow rate (Fig. 51.14). As with uroflowmetry, the patient is asked to void while sitting on a flowmeter in private.

During normal voiding there is a coordinated contraction of the bladder and at the same time relaxation of the urethra, which is sustained until the bladder is empty. Women normally void with a detrusor pressure of less than 60 cm water and a peak flow of >15 mL/s for a voided volume of at least 150 mL [45] (Benness 1997). Some women have an excellent flow of urine with little or no rise in detrusor pressure, which is simply a reflection that the contraction has occurred in the presence of

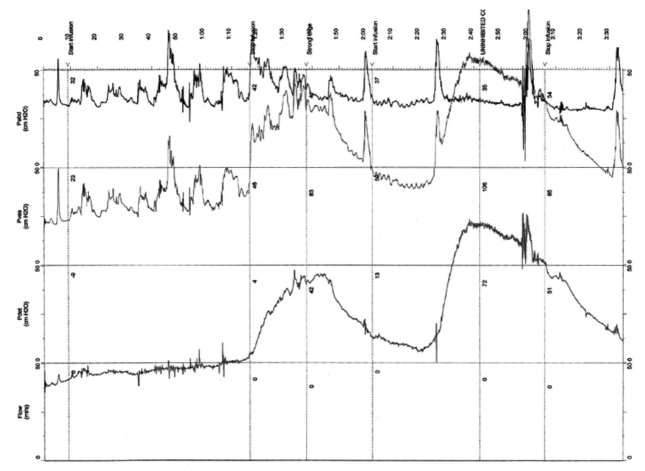

Fig. 51.13 Subtracted cystometrogram showing a picture of severe neurogenic detrusor overactivity in a patient with multiple sclerosis.

low outlet resistance. However, if the detrusor pressure during voiding is reduced with low flow rates and a significant postmicturition residual the patient is classified as having voiding difficulty. In women, voiding problems are rarely due to bladder outflow obstruction and are much more likely to be secondary to impaired detrusor contractility. Bladder outflow obstruction is characterized by a low flow rate and raised detrusor pressure during voiding. The patient may also be seen to use additional abdominal straining to try to improve the intravesical pressure.

The situation is further complicated by the fact that in some women with outflow obstruction the detrusor decompensates with time, resulting in both low detrusor pressure and low flow rate [44]. In some women, and particularly those with overt neurological disease, pathological contraction of the external sphincter occurs during a bladder contraction. This is called detrusor sphincter dyssynergia (DSD). Characteristically, there is a high detrusor pressure during voiding associated with a poor flow rate. In some women urinary retention may occur and catheterization is therefore necessary.

Both relaxation of the urethral sphincter and initiation of voiding are subject to cortical influence, so the results

of urodynamic investigation may be confounded by embarrassment or an unfamiliar testing environment. Most patients are able to pass urine at the end of the investigation but their inability to do so does not necessarily indicate a functional abnormality. Some women will subsequently have free flow rates and residual urine assessments, which indicate normality.

Special investigations

Urethral pressure profilometry

The resting urethral pressure profile (UPP) is a graphical record of pressure within the urethra at successive points along its length. A number of measurements can be taken allowing an objective comparison of urethral function between patients and also before and after treatment. Although the concept of measuring the urethral pressure profile appears physiological, there is considerable uncertainty regarding its use as a measure of urethral function and also as a prognostic tool.

Urethral pressure profilometry has been performed for at least 50 years, initially using balloon catheters and, subsequently, fluid perfusion. However, both these

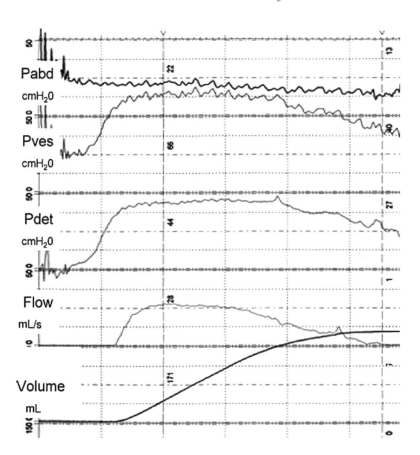

Fig. 51.14 Voiding cystometry.

methods were unsatisfactory as they enabled urethral pressure profile measurements to be made only at rest and not under stress. Solid-state microtransducer catheters are now employed. Two microtransducers are sited 6 cm apart on a size 7 french silicone-coated solid catheter. They are gradually withdrawn at a constant rate along the length of the urethra, enabling the intraurethral and intravesical pressure to be recorded simultaneously. Many different parameters can be measured [46]; of particular interest are the maximum urethral closure pressure and functional urethral length (Figs 51.15 and 51.16). In addition, stress pressure profiles can be performed if the patient coughs repeatedly during the procedure. This enables the pressure transmission ratio (the increment in urethral pressure, on stress, as a percentage of the simultaneously recorded increment in intravesical pressure) to be calculated. Urethral instability or relaxation can also be identified. Although urethral pressure profilometry is not useful in the diagnosis of urodynamic stress incontinence [47,48], it is helpful in women whose incontinence operations have failed and also in those with voiding difficulties.

Cystourethroscopy

Cystourethroscopy is normally carried out under general anaesthesia, but local anaesthesia is adequate if a flexible cystoscope is employed. Cystoscopy is particularly useful when there is a history of haematuria or recurrent urinary tract infections, or when no underlying cause can be found for sensory urgency or the symptoms of frequency, urgency or dysuria with normal urodynamic results. Cystoscopy may reveal abnormalities of the bladder epithelium, such as inflammation suggestive of infection, petechial haemorrhages or shallow ulcers due to interstitial cystitis. Papillomas or other tumours may be seen. Biopsies can be taken to confirm the underlying diagnosis, for example mast cell infiltration in interstitial cystitis or a possible transitional cell carcinoma.

Imaging of the lower urinary tract

Imaging of the lower urinary tract can be informative and, although videocystourethrography and cystoscopy are still the most commonly employed techniques, other forms of radiology, ultrasound and, most recently, magnetic resonance imaging (MRI) are being employed increasingly frequently.

Micturition cystography has largely been replaced by videocystourethrography, as the morphological information it provides is similar. However, it can be used to diagnose an anatomical abnormality such as a fistula or a urethral diverticulum when lower urinary tract dysfunction is not suspected.

Intravenous urography (IVU) has now largely been replaced by ultrasound of the upper urinary tract. However, it is important to perform an intravenous urogram in cases of haematuria, recurrent urinary tract

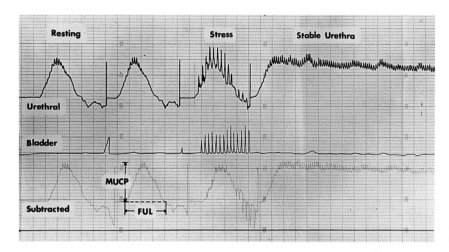

Fig. 51.15 Urethral pressure profilometry – normal trace.

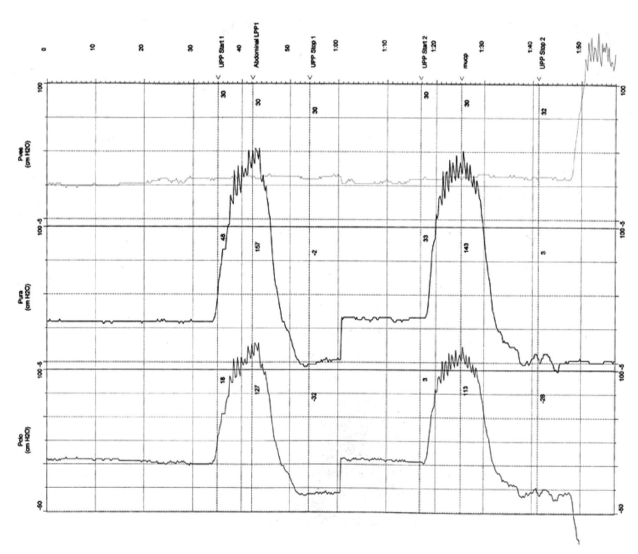

Fig. 51.16 Normal urethral pressure profile trace.

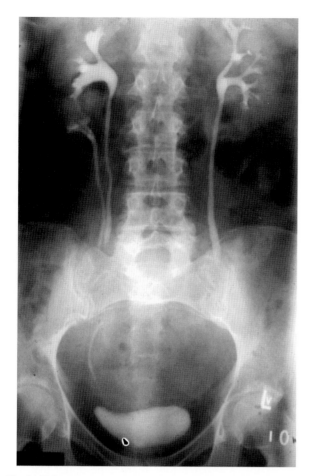

Fig. 51.17 Intravenous urogram showing a right duplex ureter.

infections, voiding difficulties or vesicoureteric reflux (Fig. 51.17). Additional pathology may be diagnosed, such as the presence of a ureteric fistula, a transitional cell carcinoma or calculi.

Ultrasound is now routinely used for assessing bladder volumes [49]. Abdominal, vaginal, rectal, perineal and introital ultrasound have all been employed and are useful for estimating bladder capacity, urinary residual volume and assessing the upper urinary tracts. However, the role of ultrasound in the diagnosis of lower urinary tract dysfunction is still undergoing evaluation. Transvaginal ultrasound does allow clear visualization of the urethra and urethral diverticula. Bladder wall thickness of an empty bladder can be measured transvaginally giving a reproducible, sensitive method of screening for detrusor overactivity (a mean bladder wall thickness of >5 mm gave a predictive value of 94% in the diagnosis of detrusor overactivity) [50]. Measurement of bladder wall thickness has also been shown to have a role as an adjunctive test in those women whose lower urinary tract symptoms are not explained by conventional urodynamic investigations [51].

Rectal ultrasound [52] and perineal ultrasound [53] have been employed to examine the anatomy and mobil-ity of the bladder neck and urethra, but it is important to appreciate that ultrasound cannot be used instead of urodynamic investigations, which assess the function rather than the morphology of the lower urinary tract.

Three-dimensional ultrasound is currently being employed mainly as a research tool. It can be used to estimate the volume of irregularly shaped organs such as the rhabdosphincter urethrae, which has been shown to be smaller in women with urodynamic stress incontinence than those with detrusor overactivity [54] and has also been shown to correlate with maximum urethral closure pressure [55]. Three-dimensional ultrasound has also been used to measure the levator ani hiatus, which is significantly larger in women with prolapse than those with urodynamic stress incontinence or asymptomatic women [56].

Magnetic resonance imaging is non-invasive and non-ionizing and allows tissues to be visualized in great detail. The urethra, bladder neck and pelvic floor have been examined [57] and fast MRI scan has been used to study prolapse [58]. MRI may also be useful in diagnosing urethral diverticulae and imaging the pelvic floor muscles.

Electromyography

Electromyography can be employed to assess the integrity of the nerve supply to a muscle. The electrical impulses to a muscle fibre are measured following nervous stimulation. Two main types of electromyography are employed in the assessment of lower urinary tract dysfunction. Surface electrodes can be placed on the perineum, vagina or anal canal as an anal plug. The pudendal nerve is stimulated and potentials measured via the electrode. This is inaccurate as the muscular activity of the levator ani is not necessarily representative of that of the rhabdosphincter urethrae. Single-fibre electromyography is more accurate as it assesses the nerve latency within individual muscle fibres of the rhabdosphincter. In this way denervation of motor units can be assessed. Research from Manchester has suggested that the occurrence of urodynamic stress incontinence post partum is due to partial denervation of the pelvic floor musculature and rhabdosphincter urethrae and is characterized by increased motor latencies [59].

Electromyography is not useful in the routine clinical evaluation of patients with uncomplicated urinary incontinence. However, it may be useful in the assessment of women with neurological abnormalities or those with voiding difficulties and retention of urine.

Ambulatory urodynamics

All urodynamic tests are unphysiological and most are invasive. Various authors have suggested that long-term ambulatory monitoring may be more physiological as the assessment takes place over a prolonged period of time and during normal daily activities [60].

Ambulatory urodynamic studies are defined as a functional test of the lower urinary tract utilizing natural filling and reproducing the subject's everyday activities [2].

There are three main components to an ambulatory urodynamic system: the transducers, the recording unit and the analysing system (Fig. 51.18). The transducers are solid state and are mounted on size 5 french and size 7 french bladder and rectal catheters. It is our practice to use two bladder transducers in order to reduce artefact. The recording system should be portable in order to allow freedom of movement with a digital memory aiding compression and expansion of the traces that are obtained. An event marker is attached to the recording unit allowing

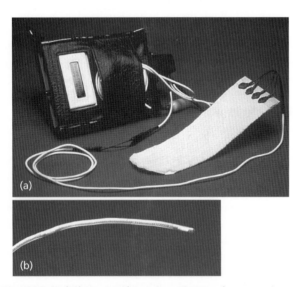

Fig. 51.18 Ambulatory urodynamic equipment demonstrating the (a) digital recording unit and urilos pad and (b) microtip pressure transducer.

the patient to mark episodes of urgency and also to document voids. In addition, the recording unit is attached to an electronic (urilos) pad to document episodes of leakage during the study and should have the facility to attach to a flowmeter so as to record pressure flow voiding studies. The ambulatory protocol at King's College Hospital consists of a 4-h period during which time the patient is asked to drink 200 mL of fluid every 30 min and also to keep a diary of events and symptoms (Fig. 51.19). On completion of the test the trace is then analysed with the patient, using a personal computer and the urinary diary. Detrusor overactivity should be diagnosed only if there is a detrusor contraction noted in both bladder lines in the presence of symptoms (Fig. 51.20).

The clinical usefulness of ambulatory urodynamics is limited by the high prevalence of abnormal detrusor (38–69%) contractions in asymptomatic volunteers [61,62]. However, the diagnosis of detrusor overactivity is highly dependent on interpretation of the results; in a prospective study of 26 asymptomatic women the incidence of detrusor overactivity varied from 11.5% to 76.9% depending on the criteria used [63]. However, if the criteria for defining abnormal detrusor contractions are a simultaneous pressure rise on both bladder lines in addition to patient-reported symptoms of urgency or urge incontinence, the findings are normal in 90% of women, which is similar to that reported in laboratory urodynamics.

Although ambulatory urodynamics is still considered to be mainly a research tool, there is no doubt that it is often exceedingly helpful in cases where the clinical and conventional urodynamic diagnoses differ, or when no abnormality is found on laboratory urodynamics [64]. Ambulatory urodynamics have been shown to be more sensitive than laboratory urodynamics in the diagnosis of detrusor overactivity but less sensitive in the diagnosis of urodynamic stress incontinence [65], although their role in clinical practice remains controversial [66].

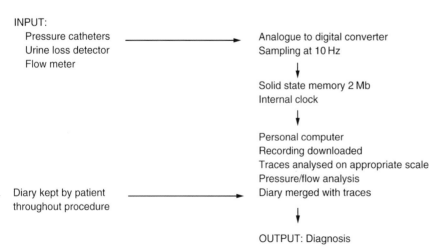

INPUT:
    Pressure catheters ———————→ Analogue to digital converter
    Urine loss detector   Sampling at 10 Hz
    Flow meter
                                                    ↓
                                       Solid state memory 2 Mb
                                       Internal clock
                                                    ↓
                                       Personal computer
                                       Recording downloaded
                                       Traces analysed on appropriate scale
                                       Pressure/flow analysis
    Diary kept by patient ——————→ Diary merged with traces
    throughout procedure
                                                    ↓
                                       OUTPUT: Diagnosis

Fig. 51.19 Schematic flow diagram representing ambulatory urodynamics: 4-h test, standardized fluid intake, instruction sheet.

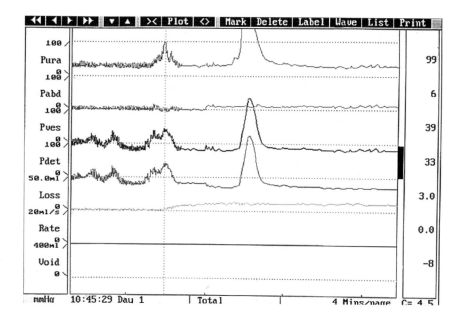

Fig. 51.20 Ambulatory urodynamic trace showing detrusor overactivity, which is associated with urine loss into the urilos pad.

 Summary box 51.2

Investigation of urinary incontinence:
- Diagnosis may be based on symptoms or urodynamic studies.
- All women should have a full history and clinical examination.
- Frequency volume charts are useful in making a diagnosis.
- Infection and voiding difficulties should be excluded.
- Subtracted cystometry should be considered in those patients who fail conservative therapy.
- Women with recurrent incontinence or who may have neurological problems should be investigated with videocystourethrography.
- Ambulatory urodynamics may be useful in women with symptoms not explained by conventional cystometry.
- All women with haematuria and bladder pain require cystoscopy.

Causes of urinary incontinence

Urethral incontinence will occur whenever the intravesical pressure involuntarily exceeds the intraurethral pressure. This may be due to an increase in intravesical (or detrusor) pressure or a reduction in urethral pressure or a combination of the two. Thus, the fault which leads to incontinence may lie in the urethra or the bladder or both.

Urodynamic stress incontinence
Urodynamic stress incontinence is defined as the involuntary leakage of urine during increased abdominal pressure in the absence of a detrusor contraction [2]. There are various different underlying causes that result in weakness of one or more of the components of the urethral sphincter mechanism (Table 51.9).

Table 51.9 Causes of urodynamic stress incontinence.

Urethral hypermobility
Urogenital prolapse

Pelvic floor damage or denervation
Parturition
Pelvic surgery
Menopause

Urethral scarring
Vaginal (urethral) surgery
Incontinence surgery
Urethral dilatation or urethrotomy
Recurrent urinary tract infections
Radiotherapy

Raised intra-abdominal pressure
Pregnancy
Chronic cough (bronchitis)
Abdominal/pelvic mass
Faecal impaction
Ascites
(Obesity)

The bladder neck and proximal urethra are normally situated in an intra-abdominal position above the pelvic floor and are supported by the pubourethral ligaments. Damage to either the pelvic floor musculature (levator ani) or pubourethral ligaments may result in descent of the proximal urethra such that it is no longer an intra-abdominal organ, and this results in leakage of urine per urethram during stress.

It has been postulated that vaginal delivery results in denervation of the urethral sphincter mechanism [59].

Snooks *et al.* [67] employed electromyography to reveal evidence of pelvic floor denervation in women who had delivered vaginally but not those who had undergone Caesarean section. They later compared antenatal with postpartum women and confirmed that vaginal delivery results in pelvic floor denervation [68]. In a study of 96 nulliparous women who delivered vaginally, Allen *et al.* [69] reported electromyographic evidence of denervation of the pelvic floor in postpartum women with urinary incontinence. A long active second stage of labour was the only factor associated with severe damage.

Although pudendal function has been shown to recover with time [67,70], it has also been shown to deteriorate progressively with ageing and subsequent vaginal deliveries [71]. Because of the increased incidence of pelvic floor trauma with vaginal delivery, especially instrumental delivery, it has been proposed that elective Caesarean section should be offered to women who are at increased risk [72].

More recently, the 'mid-urethral theory' or 'integral theory' has been described by Petros and Ulmsten [73]. This concept is based on earlier studies suggesting that the distal and mid-urethra play an important role in the continence mechanism [74] and that the maximal urethral closure pressure is at the mid-urethral point [75]. This theory proposes that damage to the pubourethral ligaments supporting the urethra, impaired support of the anterior vaginal wall to the mid-urethra, and weakened function of part of the pubococcygeal muscles which insert adjacent to the urethra are responsible for causing stress incontinence. Urodynamic stress incontinence is the commonest cause of urinary incontinence in women and represents over half of those referred for a gynaecological opinion. Women usually complain of the symptom of stress incontinence with or without frequency, urgency, urge incontinence or prolapse [76]. Stress incontinence may be demonstrated on clinical examination, but this will only verify the patient's history and will not diagnose the cause of the incontinence. Usually the diagnosis of urodynamic stress incontinence is made by negative rather than positive findings. If cystometry is normal and stress incontinence is observed, a diagnosis of urodynamic stress incontinence can be made. If a woman complains of stress incontinence as her sole symptom and stress incontinence can be demonstrated on coughing, there is a 95% chance that the diagnosis is urodynamic stress incontinence. However, Haylen *et al.* [77] have shown that only 2% of women who present for urodynamic assessment fall into this category.

Conservative treatment

Types of conservative treatment for urodynamic stress incontinence are listed in Table 51.10. Conservative treatment is indicated when the incontinence is mild, the

Table 51.10 Conservative treatment for urodynamic stress incontinence.

Pelvic floor muscle training (PFMT)
Perineometry
Vaginal cones
Maximum electrical stimulation
Duloxetine

patient is medically unfit for surgery or does not wish to undergo an operation, or in women who have not yet completed their families. It may also be useful prior to surgery when the patient's name is on a long waiting list. However, it is unusual for anything more than mild urodynamic stress incontinence to be completely cured by these conservative measures, and most women require surgery eventually [78].

Pelvic floor muscle training

Pelvic floor muscle training (PFMT) and pelvic floor physiotherapy remain the first-line conservative measures since their introduction in 1948 [79]. PFMT appears to work in a number of different ways:
• women learn to consciously pre-contract the pelvic floor muscles before and during increases in abdominal pressure to prevent leakage ('the knack');
• strength training builds up long-lasting muscle volume and thus provides structural support; and
• abdominal muscle training indirectly strengthens the pelvic floor muscles [80].
In addition, during a contraction the urethra may also be pressed against the posterior aspect of the symphysis pubis producing a mechanical rise in urethral pressure [81]. As up to 30% of women with stress incontinence are unable to contract their pelvic floor correctly at presentation [82], some patients may simply need to be retaught the 'knack' of squeezing the appropriate muscles at the correct time [83]. Cure rates varying from 21% to 84% have been reported [79,84,85]. Success appears to depend upon the type and severity of incontinence treated, the instruction and follow-up given, the compliance of the patient and the outcome measures used. However, the evidence would suggest that PFMT is more effective if patients are given a structured programme to follow rather than simple verbal instructions [86].

The success of PFMT may be further enhanced by the use of biofeedback [87]. This technique allows patients to receive visual or audio feedback relating to contraction of their pelvic floor. The most commonly used device in clinical practice is the perineometer, which may give women an improved idea of a pelvic floor contraction and provide an effective stimulus to encourage greater and continued effort.

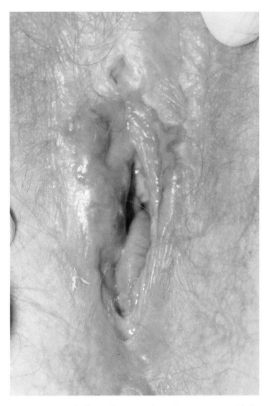

Plate 52.11 Erosive lichen planus – there is scarring with loss of the labia minora. Wickham's striae are seen at the edge of the erosions.

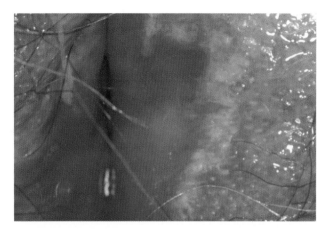

Plate 52.12 The lacy white edge of the eroded area is seen. This is the best site for biopsy.

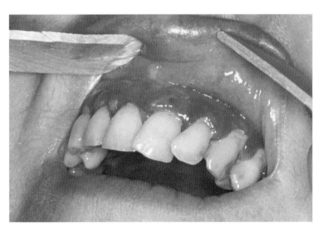

Plate 52.13 Erosive lichen planus with gingival involvement. Erythema and erosions are seen at the gingival margins. Similar lesions may be seen on the buccal mucosa and tongue.

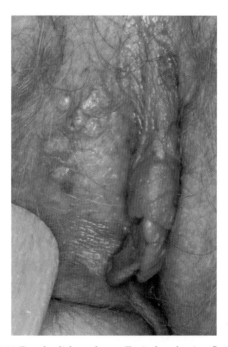

Plate 52.14 Papular lichen planus. Typical coalescing flat-topped papules showing white Wickham's striae. They are blueish in colour and are usually also found on the inner wrist and elsewhere.

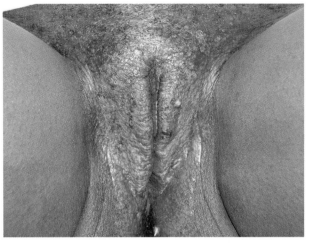

Plate 52.15 Vulval lichen simplex – the outer labia majora are significantly lichenified with accentuated skin markings and loss of hair from rubbing.

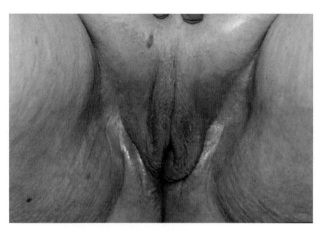

Plate 52.16 Vulval psoriasis – erythema and maceration with extension into the inguinal folds. The edge is still well defined.

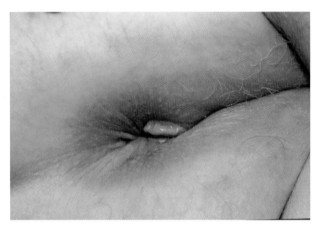

Plate 52.17 Perianal psoriasis – well-demarcated erythema with extension into the natal cleft.

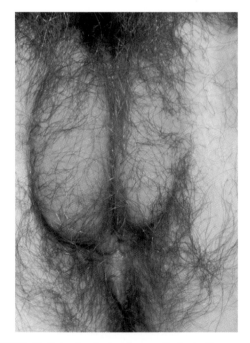

Plate 52.19 Unilateral vulval oedema – Crohn's disease. Sometimes vulval oedema, usually unilateral, can accompany Crohn's disease of the gastrointestinal tract.

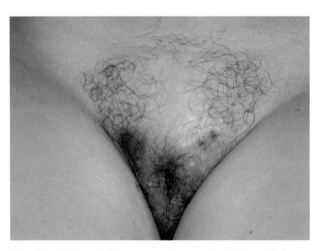

Plate 52.18 Hidradenitis suppurativa – oozing inflamed lesions are seen on the mons pubis with bridged comedones.

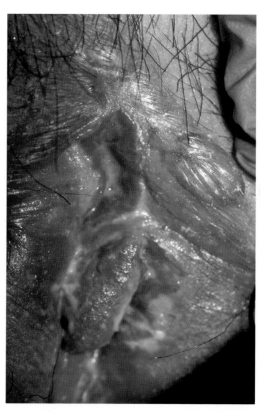

Plate 52.20 Vulval Crohn's disease – deep 'knife-cut' fissures are seen in the inter-labial sulci.

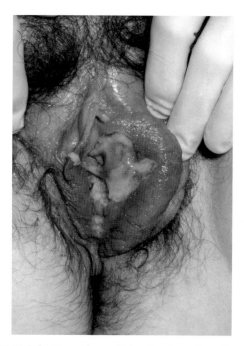

Plate 52.21 Behçet's syndrome. Extensive deep ulcers, here penetrating the labia in a 45-year-old Turkish woman.

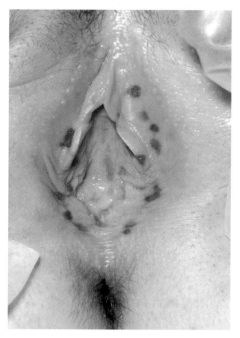

Plate 52.22 Vulval melanosis – irregular areas of pigmentation without any preceding inflammation.

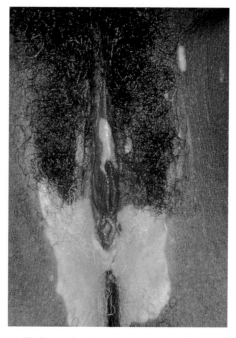

Plate 52.23 Vitiligo – showing symmetrical loss of pigmentation.

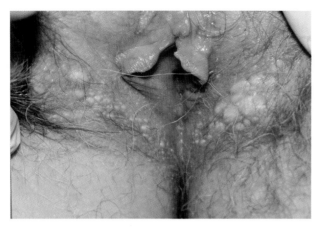

Plate 52.24 Multiple epidermoid cysts on outer labia majora. These are usually asymptomatic.

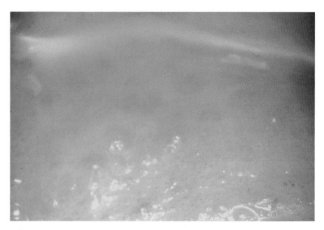

Plate 53.1 Trichomoniasis with 'strawberry' vaginitis.

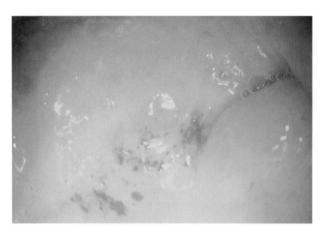

Plate 53.2 Bleeding and adhesions at the vaginal vault.

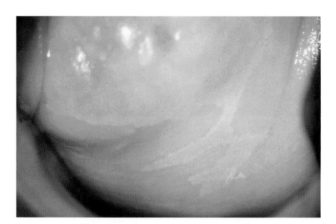

Plate 53.3 Vaginal intraepithelial neoplasia (VAIN) as an extension of a cervical lesion.

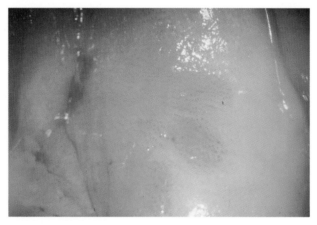

Plate 53.4 Vaginal intraepithelial neoplasia (VAIN) in post-hysterectomy vaginal angle.

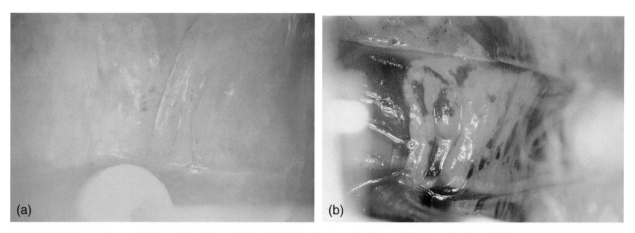

Plate 53.5 (a,b) Area of vaginal intraepithelial neoplasia (VAIN) before an after the application of iodine solution.

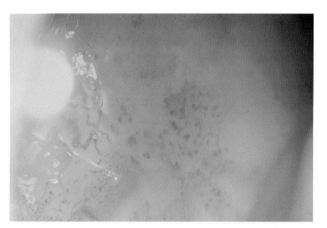

Plate 53.6 Appearance of the vaginal vault after radiotherapy.

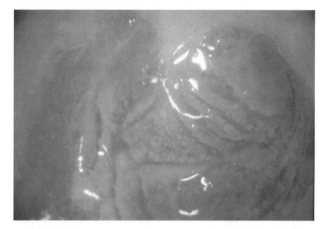

Plate 53.7 Eversion of the cervix during pregnancy.

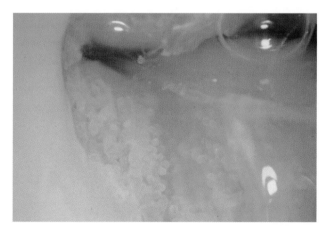

Plate 53.8 Columnar villi at the squamocolumnar junction.

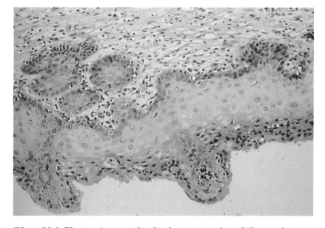

Plate 53.9 Photomicrograph of columnar and multilayered immature metaplastic epithelia.

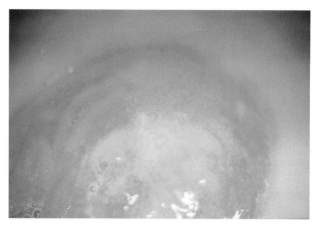

Plate 53.10 Squamous metaplasia of the cervix.

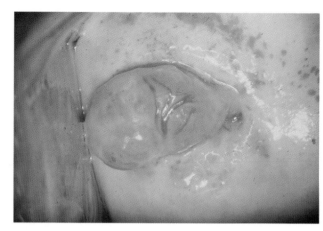

Plate 53.13 A large polyp with adjacent atrophic epithelium and ecchymoses.

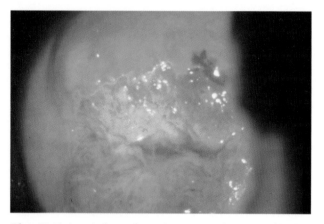

Plate 53.11 A typical transformation zone with a mucus-filled Nabothian follicle at 11 o'clock.

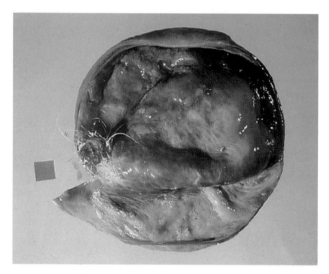

Plate 53.14 A benign cystic teratoma of the ovary showing hair and skin.

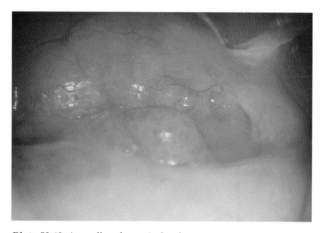

Plate 53.12 A small endocervical polyp.

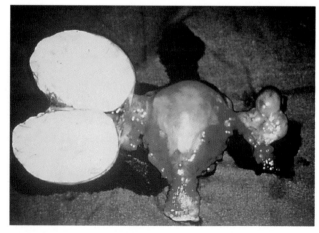

Plate 53.15 An ovarian fibroma.

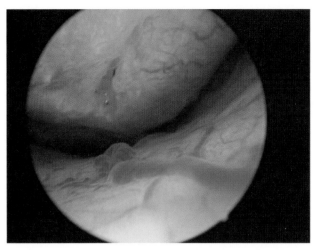

Plate 54.1 A hysteroscopic view of an intrauterine polyp in a woman receiving tamoxifen. By kind permission of Dr Justine Clark, Consultant Gynaecologist, Birmingham Women's Hospital, UK.

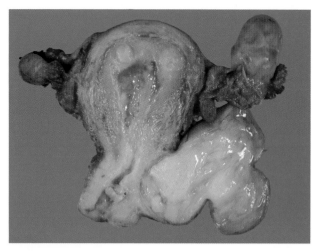

Plate 54.2 Cut surface of fibroid uterus – demonstrates pale appearance of fibroid and line of demarcation between normal myometrium and fibroid tissue.

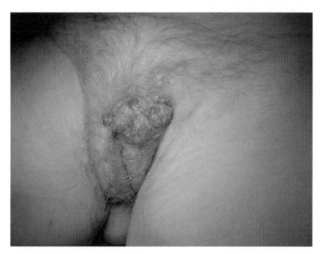

Plate 55.1 Large anterior vulval cancer with satellite skin deposits.

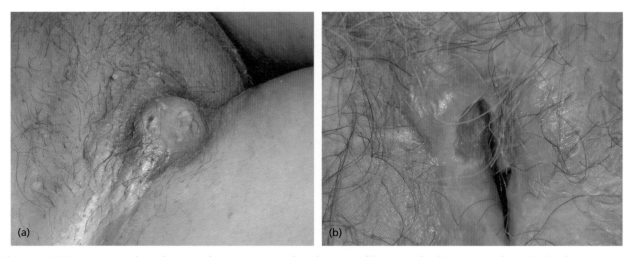

Plate 55.2 (a) Recurrence in the right groin after previous simple vulvectomy. (b) Anterior local recurrence after radical vulvectomy.

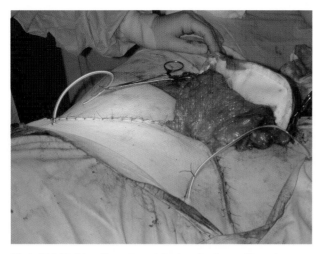

Plate 55.3 En bloc dissection of the inguinofemoral lymph nodes.

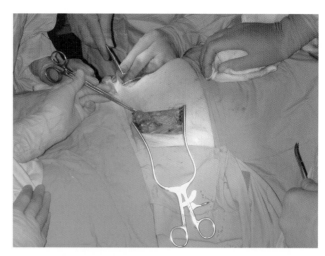

Plate 55.4 Separate groin incisions.

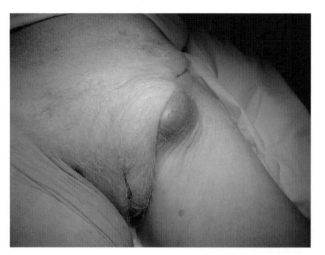

Plate 55.5 Clinically suspicious left groin nodes.

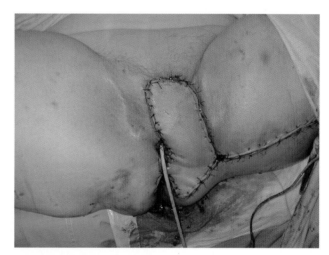

Plate 55.6 Rotation skin flap to fill a large defect.

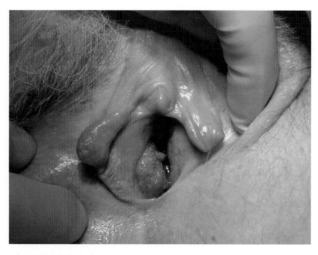

Plate 55.7 Vaginal cancer.

Perineometry

A perineometer is a cylindrical vaginal device that can be used to assess the strength of pelvic floor contractions. It can be used to help an individual to contract her pelvic floor muscles appropriately and is also useful in detecting improvement following pelvic floor exercises. Perineometers are available for both hospital and home use.

Weighted vaginal cones

These are currently available as sets of five or three [88], all of the same shape and size but of increasing weight (20–90 g). When inserted into the vagina a cone stimulates the pelvic floor to contract to prevent it from falling out and this provides 'vaginal weight training'. A 60–70% improvement rate has been reported using this technique [89] and two studies have shown that cones are as effective as more conventional forms of pelvic floor re-education and require less supervision [90,91]. However, longer term studies suggest that initial improvement may not be maintained [92] and their effectiveness in the treatment of urodynamic stress incontinence is limited with a randomized controlled study of conservative treatments showing that only 7.5% of women felt they no longer had a continence problem after using vaginal cones for 6 months. In addition, there was no difference in pelvic muscle strength when compared with the control group [84]. Furthermore, there have been some reports that vaginal cones may produce prolonged isometric contraction of the pelvic floor muscles and muscle injury if overused [93].

Maximal electrical stimulation

Maximal electrical stimulation can be carried out using a home device that utilizes a vaginal electrode through which a variable current is passed. The woman is able to adjust the strength of the stimulus herself and is instructed to use the device for 20 minutes daily initially for 1 month. Maximum electrical stimulation has been employed in both the management of urodynamic stress incontinence and detrusor overactivity, although it has not gained popularity. In a multicentre trial Sand *et al.* (1995) [94] have shown that this type of electrical stimulator is more effective both subjectively and objectively (pad weighing test) than a sham device in the treatment of urodynamic stress incontinence. In addition, a more recent meta-analysis has shown that electrical stimulation is as effective as PFMT for the treatment of urodynamic stress incontinence [95].

Vaginal devices

There are many women who, for various reasons, are not suitable for, or do not wish to undergo, active treatment of their incontinence. They do, however, require some sort of 'containment' of their leakage and vaginal devices

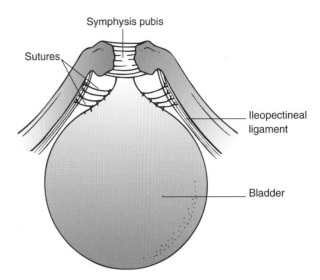

Fig. 51.21 Vaginal continence devices. (a) Contrelle (CCT) and (b) Conveen (CCG).

may be suitable for use during exercise on a short-term basis.

Sanitary tampons are easily available and reduce urinary leakage by elevating the bladder neck and causing a degree of outflow obstruction. The Conveen Continence Guard (CCG) (Coloplast, Peterborough, UK) is a specially shaped vaginal tampon that has been assessed in a multicentre trial of 85 women with urodynamic stress incontinence aged 31–65 years. It was used daily for 4 weeks and assessed both subjectively and objectively using a pad weight test [96]. Overall, 75% of the women were objectively improved while the device was *in situ*. More recently, the CCG has been compared with the Contrelle Continence Tampon (CCT) (Codon, Lenshan, Germany) (Fig. 51.21) in a prospective study of 94 women with urodynamic stress incontinence [97]. Overall, both devices were found to significantly reduce the amount of urinary leakage, but this was significantly greater in the CCT group. In addition, two-thirds of women preferred the CCT to the CCG. There were no serious adverse events and no association with vaginal or lower urinary tract infections.

Medical therapy

Although various agents such as α1-adrenoceptor agonists, oestrogens and tricyclic antidepressants have all been used anecdotally in the past for the treatment of stress incontinence, duloxetine is the first drug to be specifically developed and licensed for this indication.

Duloxetine is a potent and balanced serotonin (5-hydroxytryptamine) and noradrenaline reuptake inhibitor (SNRI) that enhances urethral striated sphincter activity via a centrally mediated pathway [98]. The efficacy and safety of duloxetine (20 mg, 40 mg, 80 mg) has been evaluated in a double-blind randomized parallel-group placebo-controlled phase II dose-finding study in 48 centres in the USA involving 553 women with stress incontinence [99]. Duloxetine was associated with significant and dose-dependent decreases in incontinence episode frequency. Reductions were 41% for placebo and 54%, 59% and 64% for the 20, 40 and 80 mg groups, respectively. Discontinuation rates were also dose dependent: 5% for placebo and 9%, 12% and 15% of 20 mg, 40 mg and 80 mg, respectively, the most frequently reported adverse event being nausea.

A further global phase III study of 458 women has also been reported [100]. There was a significant decrease in incontinence episode frequency and improvement in QoL in those women taking duloxetine 40 mg once daily when compared with placebo. Once again, nausea was the most frequently reported adverse event, occurring in 25.1% of women receiving duloxetine compared with a rate of 3.9% in those taking placebo. However, 60% of nausea resolved by 7 days and 86% by 1 month. These findings are supported by a further double-blind, placebo-controlled study of 109 women awaiting surgery for stress incontinence [101]. Overall, there was a significant improvement in incontinence episode frequency and QoL in those women taking duloxetine when compared with placebo. Furthermore, 20% of women who were awaiting continence surgery changed their minds while taking duloxetine. More recently, the role of synergistic therapy with PFMT and duloxetine has been examined in a prospective study of 201 women with stress incontinence. Women were randomized to one of four treatment combinations: duloxetine 40 mg twice daily, PFMT, combination therapy or placebo. Overall, duloxetine, with or without PFMT, was found to be superior to placebo or PFMT alone whereas pad test results and QoL analysis favoured combination therapy over single treatment [102].

Surgery

Surgery is usually the most effective way of curing urodynamic stress incontinence, and a 90% cure rate can be expected for an appropriate, properly performed primary procedure. Traditional surgery for urodynamic stress incontinence aims to elevate the bladder neck and proximal urethra into an intra-abdominal position, to support the bladder neck and align it to the posterosuperior aspect of the pubic symphysis, and in some cases to increase the outflow resistance. Undoubtedly, the results of suprapubic operations such as the Burch colposuspension or Marshall–Marchetti–Krantz procedure are better than those for the traditional, anterior colporrhaphy with bladder neck buttress [103]. Numerous operations have been described and many are still performed today. Common operations for urodynamic stress incontinence are listed in Table 51.11.

Table 51.11 Operations for urodynamic stress incontinence.

Vaginal
Anterior colporrhaphy ± Kelly/Pacey suture
Urethrocliesis
Urethral bulking agents
Retropubic mid-urethral tape procedures
Transobturator mid-urethral tape procedures

Abdominal
Marshall–Marchetti–Krantz procedure
Burch colposuspension

Laparoscopic
Colposuspension

Combined
Sling
Endoscopic bladder neck suspension, e.g. Stamey, Raz

Complex
Neourethra
Artificial sphincter
Urinary diversion

Anterior colporrhaphy

Anterior colporrhaphy is only rarely performed for urodynamic stress incontinence. Although it is usually the best operation for a cystourethrocele, the cure rates for urodynamic stress incontinence are poor compared with those from suprapubic procedures [104]. As prolapse is relatively easier to cure than stress incontinence, it is appropriate to perform the best operation for incontinence when the two conditions coexist.

Marshall–Marchetti–Krantz procedure

The Marshall–Marchetti–Krantz procedure is a suprapubic operation in which the paraurethral tissue at the level of the bladder neck is sutured to the periostium and/or perichondrium of the posterior aspect of the pubic symphysis. This procedure elevates the bladder neck but will not correct any concomitant cystocele. It has been largely superseded by the Burch colposuspension because its complications include osteitis pubis in 2–7% of cases.

Colposuspension

The Burch colposuspension has been modified by many authors since its original description [105]. Until recently, colposuspension has been the operation of choice in primary urodynamic stress incontinence as it corrects both stress incontinence and a cystocele. It may not be suitable if the vagina is scarred or narrowed by previous surgery. The operation is performed via a low transverse suprapubic incision. The bladder, bladder neck and proximal urethra are dissected medially off the underlying paravaginal fascia and three or four pairs of non-absorbable or

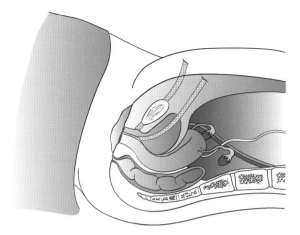

Fig. 51.22 Modified Burch colposuspension.

long-term absorbable sutures are inserted between the fascia and the ipsilateral iliopectineal ligament. Haemostasis is secured and the sutures are tied, thus elevating the bladder neck and bladder base (Fig. 51.22). Simultaneous hysterectomy does not improve results but if there is uterine pathology (menorrhagia or uterovaginal prolapse) then a total abdominal hysterectomy should be performed at the same time. Postoperatively, a suction drain is left in the retropubic space and a suprapubic catheter is inserted into the bladder. Perioperative antibiotics and/or subcutaneous heparin may be employed. In virtually all reported series comparing the results of a Burch colposuspension with any other procedure to cure urodynamic stress incontinence, the results of the colposuspension have been the best.

Although the colposuspension is now well recognized as an effective procedure for stress incontinence, it is not without complications. Detrusor overactivity may occur *de novo* or may be unmasked by the procedure [106], which may lead to long-term urinary symptoms. Voiding difficulties are common postoperatively and although they usually resolve within a short time after the operation, long-term voiding dysfunction may result. In addition, a rectoenterocele may be exacerbated by repositioning the vagina [107]. However, the colposuspension is the only incontinence operation for which long-term data are available. Alcalay *et al.* [108] have reported a series of 109 women with an overall cure rate of 69% at a mean of 13.8 years.

Laparoscopic colposuspension

Minimally invasive surgery is attractive and this trend has extended to surgery for stress incontinence. Although many authors have reported excellent short-term subjective results from laparoscopic colposuspension [109], early studies have shown inferior results to the open procedure [110,111].

More recently, two large prospective randomized controlled trials have been reported from Australia and the UK comparing laparoscopic and open colposuspension. In the Australian study, 200 women with urodynamic stress incontinence were randomized to either laparoscopic or open colposuspension [112]. Overall, there were no significant differences in objective and subjective measures of cure or in patient satisfaction at 6 months, 24 months or 3–5 years. Although the laparoscopic approach took longer (87 versus 42 min; $P < 0.0001$) it was associated with less blood loss ($P = 0.03$) and a quicker return to normal activities ($P = 0.01$).

These findings are supported by the UK multicentre randomized controlled trial of 291 women with urodynamic stress incontinence comparing laparoscopic with open colposuspension [113]. At 24 months, intention-to-treat analysis showed no significant difference in cure rates between the procedures. Objective cure rates for open and laparoscopic colposuspension were 70.1% and 79.7%, respectively, and subjective cure rates were 54.6% and 54.9%, respectively.

These studies have confirmed that the clinical effectiveness of the two operations is comparable, although the cost-effectiveness of laparoscopic colposuspension remains unproven. A cost analysis comparing laparoscopic with open colposuspension was also performed alongside the UK study [114]. Healthcare resource use over the first 6-month follow-up period translated into costs of £1805 for the laparoscopic group versus £1433 for the open group.

It is important that this information is made available to women who are undergoing incontinence surgery as most would prefer their stress incontinence to be cured rather than a have a reduced hospital stay. In addition, it has been well established that the first operation is the one most likely to succeed, and therefore it is unfortunate if a good outcome is prejudiced by an inferior operation.

Sling procedures

Sling procedures are normally performed as secondary operations where there is scarring and narrowing of the vagina. The sling material can be either biological (autologous rectus fascia, porcine dermis, cadaveric fascia) or synthetic (Prolene®, and Mersilene®, Ethicon, New Jersey, USA). The sling may be inserted either abdominally or vaginally, or by a combination of both. Normally, the sling is used to elevate and support the bladder neck and proximal urethra, but not to intentionally obstruct it. Sling procedures are associated with a high incidence of side effects and complications. It is often difficult to decide how tight to make the sling. If it is too loose, incontinence will persist, and if it is too tight, voiding difficulties may be permanent. Women who are going to undergo insertion of a sling must be prepared to perform clean, intermittent self-catheterization postoperatively. In addition, there is a risk of infection, especially if inorganic material is used. The sling may erode into the urethra or vagina, in which case it must be removed, and this can be exceedingly difficult.

Retropubic mid-urethral tape procedures

Tension-free vaginal tape

The tension-free vaginal tape (TVT, Gynecare®, New Jersey, USA), first described by Ulmsten in 1996 [115], is now the most commonly performed procedure for stress urinary incontinence in the UK, and more than two million procedures have been performed worldwide. A knitted 11 mm × 40 cm polypropylene mesh tape is inserted transvaginally at the level of the mid-urethra, using two 5 mm trochars (Fig. 51.23). The procedure may be performed under local, spinal or general anaesthesia. Most women can go home the same day, although some do require catheterization for short-term voiding difficulties (2.5–19.7%). Other complications include bladder perforation (2.7–5.8%), *de novo* urgency (0.2–15%) and bleeding (0.9–2.3%) [116].

A multicentre study carried out in six centres in Sweden has reported a 90% cure rate at 1 year in women undergoing their first operation for urodynamic stress incontinence, without any major complications [117]. Long-term results would confirm durability of the technique with success rates of 86% at 3 years [118], 84.7% at 5 years [119], 81.3% at 7 years [120] and 90% at 11 years [121].

The TVT has also been compared with open colposuspension in a multicentre, prospective, randomized trial of 344 women with urodynamic stress incontinence [122]. Overall, there was no significant difference in terms of objective cure: 66% in the TVT group and 57% in the colposuspension group. However, operation time, post-operative stay and return to normal activity were all longer in the colposuspension arm. Analysis of the long-term results at 24 months using a pad test, QoL assessment and symptom questionnaires showed an objective cure rate of 63% in the TVT arm and 51% in the colposuspension arm [123]. At 5 years there were no differences in subjective cure (63% in the TVT group and 70% in the colposuspension group), patient satisfaction and QoL assessment. However, although there was a significant reduction in cystocele in both groups, there was a higher incidence of enterocele, rectocele and apical prolapse in the colposuspension group [124]. Furthermore, cost–utility analysis has also shown that at 6 months' follow-up TVT resulted in a mean cost saving of £243 when compared with colposuspension [125].

A smaller randomized study has also compared TVT with laparoscopic colposuspension in 72 women with urodynamic stress incontinence. At a mean follow-up of 20 months objective cure rates were higher in the TVT group when compared with the laparoscopic colposuspension group: 96.8% versus 71.2%, respectively (P = 0.056) [126].

SPARC™ – mid-urethral sling suspension system

The SPARC™ sling system (American Medical Systems, Minnesota, USA) is a minimally invasive sling procedure using a knitted 10 mm-wide polypropylene mesh that is placed at the level of the mid-urethra by passing the needle via a suprapubic to vaginal approach (Fig. 51.24) [127]. The procedure may be performed under local, regional or general anaesthetic. A prospective multicentre study of 104 women with urodynamic stress incontinence has been reported from France [128]. At a mean follow-up of 11.9 months the objective cure rate was 90.4% and the subjective cure rate was 72%. There was a 10.5% incidence of bladder perforation and 11.5% of women complained of *de novo* urgency following the procedure. More recently, SPARC has been compared with TVT in a prospective

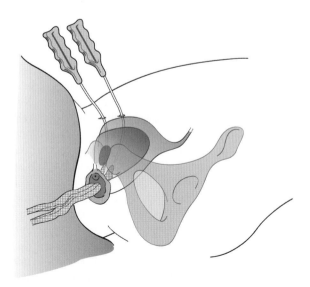

Fig. 51.23 Tension-free vaginal tape (TVT).

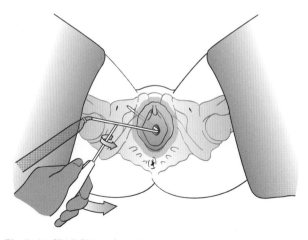

Fig. 51.24 SPARC™ mid-urethral sling suspension system.

randomized trial of 301 women [129]. At short-term follow-up there were no significant differences in cure rates, bladder perforation rates and *de novo* urgency. There was, however, a higher incidence of voiding difficulties and vaginal erosions in the SPARC group.

Transobturator mid-urethral sling procedures

The transobturator route for the placement of synthetic mid-urethral slings was first described in 2001 [130]. As with the retro-pubic sling procedures transobturator tapes may be performed under local, regional or general anaesthetic and have the theoretical advantage of eliminating some of the complications associated with the retropubic route. However, the transobturator route may be associated with damage to the obturator nerve and vessels; in an anatomical dissection model the tape passes 3.4–4.8 cm from the anterior and posterior branches of the obturator nerve, respectively, and 1.1 cm from the most medial branch of the obturator vessels [131]. Consequently, nerve and vessel injury, in addition to bladder injury and vaginal erosion, remain a potential complication of the procedure.

The transobturator approach may be used as an 'inside-out' (TVT-O™, Gynecare, Massachusetts, USA) (Fig. 51.25) or alternatively an 'outside-in' (Monarc, American Medical Systems; Obtryx, Boston Scientific, Massachusetts, USA) technique. Initial studies have reported cure and improved rates of 80.5% and 7.5%, respectively, at 7 months [132] and 90.6% and 9.4%, respectively, at 17 months [133].

More recently, the transobturator approach (TVT-O) has been compared with the retropubic approach (TVT) in an Italian prospective multicentre randomized study of 231 women with urodynamic stress incontinence [134]. At a mean of 9 months, subjectively 92% of women in the TVT group were cured compared with 87% in the TVT-O group. Objectively, on pad test testing, cure rates were 92% and 89%, respectively. There were no differences in voiding difficulties and length of stay, although there were more bladder perforations in the TVT group; 4% versus none in the TVT-O group. A further multicentre prospective randomized trial comparing TVT and TVT-O has also recently been reported from Finland in 267 women complaining of stress urinary incontinence [135]. Objective cure rates at 9 weeks were 98.5% in the TVT group and 95.4% in the TVT-O group (P = 0.1362). Although complication rates were low and similar in both arms of the study, there was a higher incidence of groin pain in the TVT-O group (21 vs. 2; P = 0.0001).

These data are supported by a recent meta-analysis of the five randomized trials comparing TVT-O with TVT and six randomized trials comparing TOT with TVT [136]. Overall, subjective cure rates were identical with the retropubic and transobturator routes. However, adverse events such as bladder injuries [odds ratio (OR) 0.12; 95% confidence interval (CI) 0.05–0.33] and voiding difficulties (OR 0.55; 95% CI 0.31–0.98) were less common, whereas groin pain (OR 8.28; 95% CI 2.7–25.4) and vaginal erosions (OR 1.96; 95% CI 0.87–4.39) were more common after the transobturator approach. Long-term data would also seem to support the durability and efficacy of the transobturator approach. A 3-year follow-up study of a prospective, observational study evaluating the use of TVT-O has recently been reported [137]. Of the 102 patients recruited, 91 (89.2%) were available for follow-up at a minimum of 3 years. The objective cure rate was 88.4%, with an improvement in 9.3% of cases and there was no statistical difference in outcome as compared with the results reported at 1 year. In addition, there was a significant improvement in subjective outcome including incontinence severity and QoL. Although four patients required tape division, there were no cases of erosion or persistent pain.

Minimally invasive tape procedures

Although the development of the mid-urethral retropubic and transobturator tapes has transformed the surgical approach to stress urinary incontinence by offering a minimally invasive day case procedure, there has recently been interest in developing a new type of 'mini-sling', which could offer a truly office-based approach. The TVT Secur™ (Gynecare) is the first of these mini-slings to be introduced, although there are several other devices currently under investigation and development (Fig. 51.26).

The TVT Secur was launched in 2006 and currently there are few long-term data supporting its use, although several short-term studies have been reported. The first published case series reported on a small sample of 15 women with an overall subjective cure rate of 93% at 1- to 3-month follow-up [138]. More recently, a multicentre prospective trial has been reported from Italy in 95 women with primary stress incontinence who had a TVT Secur. Follow-up at 1 year reported subjective and objective cure rates of 78% and 81%, respectively, while

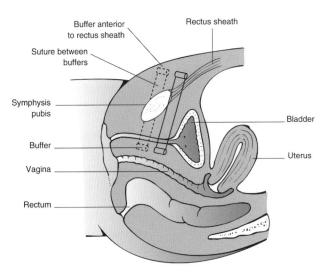

Fig. 51.25 Transobturator tape – 'inside-out' procedure.

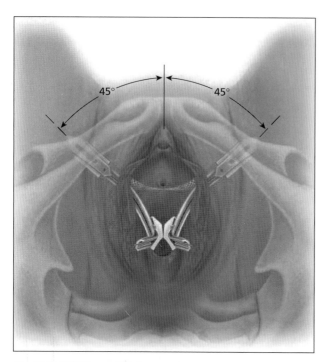

Fig. 51.26 TVT Secur: 'U' placement.

Table 51.12 Urethral bulking agents.

Urethral bulking agent	Application technique
Glutaraldehyde cross-linked bovine collagen (Contigen*)	Cystoscopic
Polydimethylsiloxane (Macroplastique†)	Cystoscopic MIS implantation system
Pyrolytic carbon-coated zirconium oxide beads in β glucan gel (Durasphere‡)	Cystoscopic
Ethylene vinyl co-polymer in dimethyl sulfoxide (DMSO) gel	Cystoscopic
Calcium hydroxylapatite in carboxymethylcellulose gel (Coaptite§)	Cystoscopic
Copolymer of hyaluronic acid and dextranomer	Cystoscopic Implacer system
Polyacrylamide hydrogel (Bulkamid¶)	Cystoscopic

*Bard, Georgia, USA.
†Uroplasty, Minnesota, USA.
‡Coloplast, Peterborough, UK.
§Boston Scientific, Massachusetts, USA.
¶Gynecare, New Jersey, USA.

8% of women complained of voiding difficulties. In addition, there were two cases of mesh erosion [139]. These data are supported by a multicentre prospective observational study in France of 150 patients with 1-year follow-up. Cure and improvement rates were 76.9% in those women with pure stress incontinence, although this fell to 60% in a smaller group with intrinsic sphincter deficiency [140].

The current evidence would appear to suggest that TVT Secur efficacy rates may be slightly inferior to those of the retropubic mid-urethral tapes [141], and current experience would suggest that the procedure is technically different from a retropubic or obturator approach. Initial success rates have been disappointing in some series and the effect of the 'learning curve' has been clearly documented, with objective success rates increasing from 76.2% to 94.7% depending on the experience of the operating surgeon [142].

From the clinical evidence available to date, it would appear that TVT Secur offers an alternative, minimally invasive approach for the treatment of stress urinary incontinence, although more data are required to document the long-term efficacy and safety.

Bladder neck suspension procedures

Endoscopically guided bladder neck suspensions [143–145] are simple to perform but are less effective than open suprapubic procedures and are now seldom used. In all these operations a long needle is used to insert a loop of nylon on each side of the bladder neck; this is tied over the rectus sheath to elevate the urethrovesical junction.

Cystoscopy is employed to ensure accurate placement of the sutures and to detect any damage to the bladder caused by the needle or the suture. In the Stamey procedure buffers are used to avoid the sutures cutting through the tissues, and in the Raz procedure a helical suture of Prolene is inserted deep into the endopelvic fascia lateral to the bladder neck to avoid cutting through. The main problem with all these operations is that they rely on two sutures and these may break or pull through the tissues. However, endoscopically guided bladder neck suspensions are quick and easy to perform. They can be carried out under regional blockade and postoperative recovery is fast. Temporary voiding difficulties are common after long needle suspensions, but these usually resolve and there are few other complications.

Urethral bulking agents

Urethral bulking agents are a minimally invasive surgical procedure for the treatment of urodynamic stress incontinence and may be useful in the elderly and those women who have undergone previous operations and have a fixed, scarred fibrosed urethra.

Although the actual substance injected may differ, the principle is the same. It is injected either periurethrally or transurethrally on either side of the bladder neck under cystoscopic control, and is intended to 'bulk' the bladder neck and mid-urethra in order to stop premature bladder neck opening, without causing outflow obstruction. They may be performed under local, regional or general anaesthesia. There are now several different products available (Table 51.12). The use of minimally invasive implantation

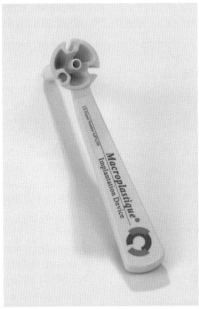
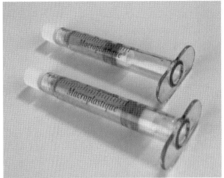

Fig. 51.27 Macroplastique urethral bulking agent and implantation device.

systems (Fig. 51.27) has also allowed some of these procedures to be performed in the office setting without the need for cystoscopy.

In the first reported series 81% of 68 women were dry following two injections with collagen [146]. There have been longer-term follow-up studies, most of which give a >50% objective cure rate at 2 years but a subjective improvement rate of about 70% [147–149]. Macroplastique has recently been compared with Contigen in a recent North American study of 248 women with urodynamic stress incontinence. The outcome was assessed objectively using pad tests and subjectively at 12 months. Overall objective cure and improvement rates favoured Macroplastique over Contigen (74% vs. 65%; $P = 0.13$). Although this difference was not significant, subjective cure rates were higher in the Macroplastique group (41% vs. 29%; $P = 0.07$) [150].

Although success rates with urethral bulking agents are generally lower than those with conventional continence surgery, they are minimally invasive and have lower complication rates meaning that they remain a useful alternative in selected women.

Artificial urinary sphincter

An artificial sphincter is a device that may be employed when conventional surgery fails [151]. It is implantable and consists of a fluid-filled inflatable cuff that is surgically placed around the bladder neck. A reservoir, containing fluid, is sited in the peritoneal cavity and a small finger-operated pump is situated in the left labium majus. The three major components are connected via a control valve. Under normal circumstances the cuff is inflated, and thus obstructing the urethra. When voiding is desired the pump is utilized to empty the fluid in the cuff back into the balloon reservoir so that voiding may occur. The cuff then gradually refills over the next few minutes. Artificial sphincters are associated with many problems. They are expensive, the surgery required to insert them is complicated and the tissues around the bladder neck following previous failed operations may be unsuitable for the implantation of the cuff. In addition, mechanical failure may occur, necessitating further surgery. However, there is a place for these devices and their technology is likely to improve in the future.

Conclusions: stress incontinence

There are a few unfortunate women in whom neither conventional nor even the newer forms of incontinence surgery produce an effective cure. For them, a urinary diversion may be a more satisfactory long-term solution than the continued use of incontinence aids.

It is important to remember that the first operation for stress incontinence is the most likely to succeed. Most suprapubic operations in current use produce a cure rate in excess of 85–90% in patients undergoing their first operation for correctly diagnosed urodynamic stress incontinence. The colposuspension has long been recognized as the 'best' first operation, although mid-urethral tape procedures would now appear to be as efficacious. More recently, the transobturator approach has also been shown to be as effective as the retropubic approach and may be useful in women who have had previous retropubic surgery.

Redo continence surgery is often less efficacious than primary surgery and subsequent surgery may have to be performed on a vagina that is less mobile and in which there is fibrosis of the urethra. In such cases, a urethral bulking agent may be easier to perform and more effective. Ultimately, it is important that the operative procedure performed is tailored to suit the needs of the individual.

Summary box 51.3

Stress urinary incontinence:
- Stress urinary incontinence (SUI) is a symptom.
- Urodynamics stress incontinence is a urodynamic diagnosis.
- SUI is the commonest form of incontinence in women.
- All women should be treated conservatively with pelvic floor muscle training (PFMT) initially.
- Duloxetine may be useful in addition to PFMT.
- Women who fail to improve with conservative measures may be suitable for surgery.
- Mid-urethral tapes are currently the most commonly performed operation for SUI.

National Institute for Health and Clinical Excellence guidelines

The management of stress urinary incontinence has recently been reviewed by the National Institute for Health and Clinical Excellence (NICE) [152]. A trial of supervised PFMT of at least 3 months' duration should be offered as first-line treatment to all women with stress or mixed urinary incontinence.

Retropubic mid-urethral tape procedures using a 'bottom-up' approach with macroporous (type 1) polypropylene meshes are recommended as treatment options for stress urinary incontinence in cases where conservative management has failed.

Open colposuspension and autologous rectus fascial sling procedures are recommended alternatives where clinically appropriate.

Synthetic slings using materials other than polypropylene that are not of a macroporous (type 1) construction are not recommended for the treatment of stress urinary incontinence.

Intramural bulking agents [glutaraldehyde cross-linked (GAX) collagen, silicone, carbon-coated zirconium beads] should be considered for the management of stress urinary incontinence if conservative management has failed, although women should be made aware that repeat injections may be required and that efficacy diminishes with time and is inferior to that of a retropubic suspension or sling.

Laparoscopic colposuspension is not recommended as a routine procedure for the treatment of stress urinary incontinence in women and should only be performed by an experienced laparoscopic surgeon.

Anterior colporrhaphy, needle suspension procedures, paravaginal defect repair and the Marshall–Marchetti–Krantz procedure are not recommended.

Detrusor overactivity

Detrusor overactivity is defined as a urodynamic observation characterized by involuntary contractions during the filling phase, which may be spontaneous or provoked [2]. It is the second commonest cause of urinary incontinence in women and accounts for 30–40% of cases. The incidence is higher in the elderly and after failed incontinence surgery. The cause of detrusor overactivity remains uncertain and in the majority of cases it is idiopathic, occurring when there is a failure of adequate bladder training in childhood or when the bladder escapes voluntary control in adult life. Often emotional or other psychosomatic factors are involved. In some cases detrusor overactivity may be secondary to an upper motor neurone lesion, especially multiple sclerosis. In such cases it is known as neurogenic detrusor overactivity. In men detrusor overactivity may be secondary to outflow obstruction and may be cured when the obstruction is relieved. However, outflow obstruction in women is rare.

Low compliance is said to exist when there is a sustained rise in detrusor pressure without actual detrusor contractions during bladder filling. There are a variety of causes, including radical pelvic surgery, radiotherapy, recurrent urinary tract infections and interstitial cystitis, but the symptoms associated with phasic detrusor overactivity and with low compliance may be indistinguishable without cystometry (Figs 51.28 and 51.29).

Detrusor overactivity and overactive bladder

The symptoms of OAB are due to involuntary contractions of the detrusor muscle during the filling phase of the micturition cycle. These involuntary contractions are termed detrusor overactivity and are mediated by acetylcholine-induced stimulation of bladder muscarinic receptors [153]. However, OAB is not synonymous with detrusor overactivity as the former is a symptom-based diagnosis whereas the latter is a urodynamic diagnosis. It has been estimated that 64% of patients with OAB have urodynamically proven detrusor overactivity and that 83% of patients with detrusor overactivity have symptoms suggestive of OAB [154].

Muscarinic receptors

Molecular cloning studies have revealed five distinct genes for muscarinic acetylcholine receptors in rats and humans and it has been shown that five receptor subtypes (M_1–M_5) correspond to these gene products [155]. In the human bladder the occurrence of mRNA encoding M_2 and M_3 subtypes has been demonstrated, although not for

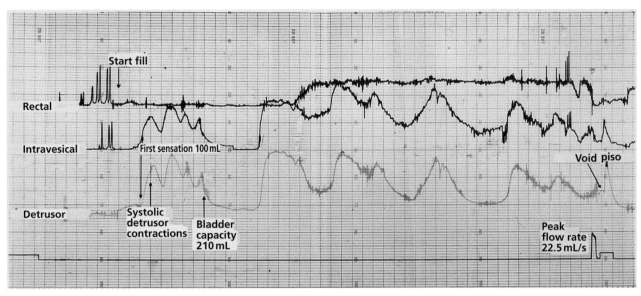

Fig. 51.28 Cystometrogram recording showing phasic detrusor overactivity.

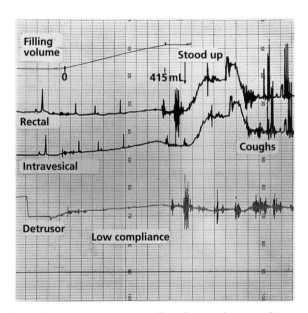

Fig. 51.29 Cystometrogram recording showing low compliance.

M_1 [156]. The M_3 receptor is thought to cause a direct smooth muscle contraction [157]. Although the role of the M_2 receptor has not yet been clarified, it may oppose sympathetically mediated smooth muscle relaxation [158] or result in the activation of a non-specific cationic channel and inactivation of potassium channels [159]. In general, it is thought that the M_3 receptor is responsible for the normal micturition contraction, although in certain disease states, such as neurogenic bladder dysfunction, the M_2 receptors may become more important in mediating detrusor contractions [160].

Pathophysiology of detrusor overactivity

A detrusor contraction is initiated in the rostral pons. Efferent pathways emerge from the sacral spinal cord as the pelvic parasympathetic nerves (S2, S3, S4) and run forwards to the bladder. Although preganglionic neurotransmission is predominantly mediated by acetylcholine acting on nicotinic receptors, transmission may also be modulated by adrenergic, muscarinic, purinergic and peptidergic presynaptic receptors.

Acetylcholine is released by the postganglionic nerves at the neuromuscular junction and results in a coordinated detrusor contraction mediated through muscarinic receptors. However, adenosine triphosphate (ATP) also has a role [161] mediated through non-adrenergic, noncholinergic (NANC) receptors.

Conversely, sympathetic innervation is from the hypogastric and pelvic nerves acting on β-adrenoreceptors, causing relaxation of the detrusor muscle. Thus, a balance between sympathetic and parasympathetic stimulation is required for normal detrusor function.

Outflow obstruction hypothesis

The association of detrusor overactivity with outflow obstruction has been recognized for some time [162], although it is more important in men than women.

Outflow obstruction may lead to partial denervation, and morphological studies have demonstrated a reduction in acetylcholinesterase staining nerves in obstructed human bladder [163]. In addition, pharmacological studies have shown that muscle strips from patients with detrusor overactivity exhibit supersensitivity to acetylcholine [164].

In addition, outflow obstruction may alter the contraction properties of the detrusor muscle [165], leading to changes in cell-to-cell propagation of electrical activity, and this in turn may lead to a higher incidence of instability of membrane potential [166]. These findings suggest that individual cells are more irritable when synchronous activation is damaged.

Outflow obstruction has also been shown to lead to the facilitation of the spinal reflex [167] mediated by C-fibres with increased expression of nerve growth factor (NGF) and tachykinins [168]. The latter have been shown to have an effect on spinal and supraspinal control of the bladder via neurokinin receptors [169].

Neurogenic hypothesis

The pathophysiology of detrusor overactivity remains unclear. *In vitro* studies have shown that the detrusor muscle, in cases of idiopathic detrusor overactivity, contracts more than normal detrusor muscle. These detrusor contractions are not nerve mediated and can be inhibited by the neuropeptide vasoactive intestinal polypeptide [170]. Other studies have shown that increased α-adrenergic activity causes increased detrusor contractility [171].

There is evidence to suggest that the pathophysiology of idiopathic and obstructive OAB is different. From animal and human studies on obstructive overactivity, it would seem that the detrusor develops postjunctional supersensitivity, possibly due to partial denervation [172], with reduced sensitivity to electrical stimulation of its nerve supply but a greater sensitivity to stimulation with acetylcholine [173]. If outflow obstruction is relieved, the detrusor can return to normal behaviour and reinnervation may occur [174].

Urethral reflex

Relaxation of the urethra is known to precede contraction of the detrusor in a proportion of women with detrusor overactivity [175]. This may represent primary pathology in the urethra, which triggers a detrusor contraction or may merely be part of a complex sequence of events that originates elsewhere. It has been postulated that incompetence of the bladder neck, allowing passage of urine into the proximal urethra, may result in an uninhibited contraction of the detrusor. However, Sutherst and Brown [176] were unable to provoke a detrusor contraction in 50 women by rapidly infusing saline into the posterior urethra using modified urodynamic equipment.

Myogenic hypothesis

Brading and Turner [177] have suggested that the common feature in all cases of detrusor overactivity is partial denervation of the detrusor, which may be responsible for altering the properties of the smooth muscle, leading to increased excitability and increased ability of activity to spread between cells, resulting in coordinated myogenic contractions of the whole detrusor [178]. They dispute the concept of neurogenic detrusor overactivity, that is increased motor activity to the detrusor, as the underlying mechanism in detrusor overactivity, proposing that there is a fundamental abnormality at the level of the bladder wall with evidence of altered spontaneous contractile activity consistent with increased electrical coupling of cells, a patchy denervation of the detrusor and a supersensitivity to potassium [179]. Charlton *et al.* [180] suggest that the primary defect in the idiopathic and neuropathic bladders is a loss of nerves accompanied by hypertrophy of the cells and an increased production of elastin and collagen within the muscle fascicles.

Urothelial afferent hypothesis

More recently, the role of afferent activation in the urothelium and suburothelial myofibroblasts has been investigated as a factor in the pathophysiology of detrusor overactivity. C-fibre afferents are known to have nerve endings in the suburothelial layer of the bladder wall as well as in the urothelium. Studies have revealed that ATP is released from the urothelium by bladder distension [181], and this may lead to activation of purinergic receptors on afferent nerve terminals, which in turn evokes a neuronal discharge leading to bladder contraction.

In addition, prostanoids [182] and nitric oxide [183] are synthesized locally in the urothelium and are also released by bladder distension. It is probable that a cascade of stimulatory (ATP, prostanoids, tachykinins) and inhibitory (nitric oxide) mediators are involved in the activation of sensory pathways during bladder filling [184]. The role of C-fibres in the pathophysiology of detrusor contractions is also supported by the use of intravesical vanilloids (capsaicin and resiniferatoxin) in patients with idiopathic detrusor overactivity and hypersensitivity disorders [185].

Clinical symptoms

Most women with an OAB exhibit a multiplicity of symptoms including urgency, urgency incontinence, stress incontinence, enuresis, frequency and especially nocturia and sometimes incontinence during sexual intercourse. There are no specific clinical signs and the diagnosis can only be made urodynamically when there is a failure to inhibit detrusor contractions during cystometry.

Treatment for detrusor overactivity aims to re-establish central control or to alter peripheral control via bladder innervation (Table 51.13). The fact that so many different types of treatment are available for this condition shows that none is universally successful. Various behavioural interventions (habit retraining) have been successfully used to treat idiopathic detrusor overactivity and have been shown to improve symptoms in up to 80% of women [186,187]. Unfortunately, these types of therapy are time-consuming and require the patient to be highly motivated. In addition, there is a high relapse rate and patients

Table 51.13 Treatment of detrusor overactivity.

Psychotherapy
Bladder drill
Biofeedback
Hypnotherapy
Acupuncture

Drug therapy
Inhibit bladder contractions
Anticholinergic agents
Musculotrophic relaxants
Tricyclic antidepressants
Improve local tissues
Oestrogens
Reduce urine production
DDAVP (synthetic vasopressin)

Intravesical therapy
Capsaicin
Resiniferatoxin
Botulinum toxin

Neuromodulation
Peripheral – Posterior Tibial Nerve Stimulation (PTNS)
Central – Sacroneuromodulation (SNS)

Cystoplasty
Clam ileocystoplasty
Detrusor myectomy

Other
Maximum electrical stimulation
Acupuncture

do not seem to respond as well on a second occasion. However, it is always appropriate to instruct patients with detrusor overactivity regarding the use of bladder drill, often as an adjunct to drug therapy. The regimen suggested by Jarvis [188] is commonly employed and is described as follows:

1 Exclude pathology.
2 Explain rationale to the patient.
3 Instruct to void every 1.5h during the day; she must not void between these times, she must wait or be incontinent.
4 Increase voiding interval by half an hour when initial goal achieved, and continue with 2-hourly voiding, and so on.
5 Give normal volume of fluids.
6 Keep fluid balance chart.
7 Give encouragement.

Drug therapy

Drug therapy is the most widely employed treatment for detrusor overactivity (Table 51.14). From the number of preparations studied it is clear that there are no ideal drugs and very often the clinical results have been

Table 51.14 Drugs used in the management of detrusor overactivity.

	Level of evidence	Grade of recommendation
Antimuscarinic drugs		
Tolterodine	1	A
Trospium	1	A
Solifenacin	1	A
Darifenacin	1	A
Fesoterodine	1	A
Propantheline	2	B
Atropine, hyoscamine	3	C
Drugs acting on membrane channels		
Calcium channel antagonists	2	D
Potassium channel openers	2	D
Drugs with mixed actions		
Oxybutynin	1	A
Propiverine	1	A
Flavoxate	2	D
Alpha-antagonists		
Alfuzosin	3	C
Doxazosin	3	C
Prazosin	3	C
Terazosin	3	C
Tamsulosin	3	C
Beta agonists		
Terbutaline	3	C
Salbutamol	3	C
Antidepressants		
Imipramine	3	C
Duloxetine	2	C
Prostaglandin synthesis inhibitors		
Indomethacin	2	C
Flurbiprofen	2	C
Vasopressin analogues		
Desmopressin	1	A
Other drugs		
Baclofen	3	C (Intrathecal)
Capsaicin	2	C (Intravesical)
Resiniferatoxin	2	C (Intravesical)
Botulinum toxin (idiopathic)	3	B (Intravesical)
Botulinum toxin (neurogenic)	2	A (Intravesical)

Table taken from Andersson KE, Chapple CR, Cardozo L *et al.* Pharmacological treatment of urinary incontinence. In: Abrams P, Cardozo L, Khoury S, Wein A (eds) *Incontinence*, 4th edn. Paris, France: Health Publication Ltd, 2009: 631–700.

disappointing, this being partly due to poor efficacy and side effects [189].

Drugs that have a mixed action

Oxybutynin

Oxybutynin is a tertiary amine that undergoes extensive first-pass metabolism to an active metabolite, N-desmethyl oxybutynin [190], which occurs in high concentrations [191] and is thought to be responsible for a significant part of the action of the parent drug. It has a mixed action, consisting of both an antimuscarinic and a direct muscle relaxant effect in addition to local anaesthetic properties. The latter is important when given intravesically, but probably has no effect when given systemically. Oxybutynin has been shown to have a high affinity for muscarinic receptors in the bladder [192] and has a higher affinity for M_1 and M_3 receptors than for M_2 [193].

The effectiveness of oxybutynin in the management of patients with detrusor overactivity is well documented. A double-blind placebo-controlled trial found oxybutynin to be significantly better than placebo in improving lower urinary tract symptoms, although 80% of patients complained of significant adverse effects, principally dry mouth or dry skin [194]. Similar results have also been demonstrated in further placebo-controlled trials [195,196].

The antimuscarinic adverse effects of oxybutynin are well documented and are often dose limiting [197]. Using an intravesical route of administration, higher local levels of oxybutynin can be achieved while limiting the systemic adverse effects. Using this method, oxybutynin has been shown to increase bladder capacity and lead to a significant clinical improvement [198]. Rectal administration has also been shown to be associated with fewer adverse effects when compared with oral administration [199].

A controlled-release oxybutynin preparation using an osmotic system (OROS, Janssen Cilag, Buckinghamshire, UK) has also been developed, which has been shown to have comparable efficacy when compared with immediate-release oxybutynin, although is associated with fewer adverse effects [200].

These findings are in agreement with a further study of controlled-release oxybutynin (Lyrinel XL®, Janssen Cilag), which reported the incidence of moderate to severe dry mouth to be 23% and only 1.6% of participants discontinued the medication because of adverse effects [201].

In order to maximize efficacy and minimize adverse effects alternative delivery systems are currently under evaluation. An oxybutynin transdermal delivery system (Kentera®, Orion Pharma, Berkshire, UK) has been developed and compared with extended-release tolterodine in 361 patients with mixed urinary incontinence. Both agents significantly reduced incontinence episodes, increased volume voided and led to an improvement in QoL when compared with placebo. The most common adverse effect in the oxybutynin patch arm was application site pruritus in 14%, although the incidence of dry mouth was reduced to 4.1% compared with 7.3% in the tolterodine arm [202]. Although transdermal oxybutynin is effective in reducing the number of adverse effects related with antimuscarinic therapy, it may be associated with significant skin site reactions. More recently, the use of oxybutynin topical gel has been investigated in a large North American multi-centre randomized, placebo-controlled study of 789 patients with OAB [203]. Overall, oxybutynin gel was associated with a significant decrease in urge incontinence episodes and urinary frequency when compared with placebo, with a corresponding increase in voided volume. Dry mouth was higher in the oxybutynin arm than the placebo arm (6.9% vs. 2.8%) as were skin site reactions (5.4% vs. 1.0%), although would appear to be lower than those associated with the patch. Consequently, the gel formulation may offer a better combination of reduced local and systemic adverse effects and is an alternative to oral preparations in those women who suffer with intolerable antimuscarinic adverse effects.

Propiverine

Propiverine (Detrumorm®, Amdipharm, Essex, UK) has been shown to combine anticholinergic and calcium channel blocking actions [204] and may be useful in women who have troublesome adverse effects with other antimuscarinic agents. An extended-release preparation has also recently been launched. Open studies in patients with detrusor overactivity have demonstrated a beneficial effect [205] and in a double-blind placebo-controlled trial of its use in neurogenic detrusor overactivity it was shown to significantly increase bladder capacity and compliance in comparison with placebo. Dry mouth was experienced by 37% in the treatment group as opposed to 8% in the placebo group, with drop-out rates being 7% and 4.5% [206].

Antimuscarinic drugs

Tolterodine

Tolterodine is a competitive muscarinic receptor antagonist with relative functional selectivity for bladder muscarinic receptors [207] and, although it shows no specificity for receptor subtypes, it does appear to target the bladder over the salivary glands [208]. The drug is metabolized in the liver to the 5-hydroxymethyl derivative, which is an active metabolite having a similar pharmacokinetic profile and is thought to significantly contribute to the therapeutic effect [209].

Several randomized, double-blind, placebo-controlled trials on patients with both idiopathic detrusor overactivity and neurogenic detrusor overactivity have demonstrated a significant reduction in incontinent episodes and micturition frequency [210–212]. Further studies have confirmed the safety of tolterodine and at the recommended daily dosage the incidence of adverse events was no different to that in patients taking placebo [213].

A pooled analysis of the safety, efficacy and acceptability of tolterodine in 1120 patients in four randomized, double-blind, parallel, multicentre trials found that both tolterodine and oxybutynin significantly decreased incontinent episodes, although tolterodine was associated with fewer adverse events, dose reductions and patient withdrawals than oxybutynin [214].

Tolterodine has also been developed as an extended-release once-daily preparation, Detrusitol XL® (Pfizer, Kent, UK). A double-blind multicentre trial of 1235 women compared tolterodine extended release with immediate-release tolterodine and placebo. Although both formulations were found to reduce the mean number of urge incontinence episodes per week, the extended-release preparation was found to be significantly more effective [215]. In addition to increased efficacy, tolterodine extended release has been shown to have better tolerability. In a double-blind, multicentre, randomized placebo-controlled trial of 1529 patients, tolterodine extended release was found to be 18% more effective in the reduction of episodes of urge incontinence while having a 23% lower incidence of dry mouth [216].

Oxybutynin extended release and tolterodine extended release have also been compared in the OPERA (Overactive bladder: performance of extended release agents) study, which involved 71 centres in the USA. Improvements in episodes of urge incontinence were similar for the two drugs, although oxybutynin extended release was significantly more effective than tolterodine extended release in reducing frequency of micturition. Significantly more women taking oxybutynin were also completely dry (23% vs. 16.8%; $P = 0.03$), although dry mouth was significantly more common in the oxybutynin group [217].

Trospium

Trospium chloride (Specialty European Pharma, London, UK) is a quaternary ammonium compound that is non-selective for muscarinic receptor subtypes and shows low biological availability [218]. It crosses the blood–brain barrier to a limited extent, and hence would appear to have few cognitive effects [219]. In a placebo-controlled, randomized, double-blind, multicentre trial trospium chloride produced significant improvements in maximum cystometric capacity and bladder volume at the first unstable contraction. Clinical improvement was significantly greater in the group receiving trospium, and the frequency of adverse events was similar in both groups [220]. Trospium chloride has also been compared with oxybutynin in a randomized, double-blind, multicentre trial. With both agents there was a significant increase in bladder capacity, a decrease in maximum voiding detrusor pressure and a significant increase in compliance,

although there were no statistically significant differences between the two treatment groups. Those taking trospium had a lower incidence of dry mouth (4% vs. 23%) and were also less likely to withdraw (6% vs. 16%) when compared with the group receiving oxybutynin [221]. More recently, the use of extended-release trospium chloride has been investigated in a large phase III placebo-controlled trial of 601 patients in North America [222]. Overall, trospium chloride was associated with a significant improvement in urinary frequency, incontinence episodes, urgency severity and volume voided when compared with placebo. The most common side effect was dry mouth (trospium 8.7% vs. placebo 3%) and constipation (trospium 9.4% vs. placebo 1.3%). The efficacy and tolerability of once-daily trospium chloride has also been confirmed in a further large study of 564 patients with OAB [223] and has been shown to have a meaningful impact on QoL [224].

Solifenacin

Solifenacin (Astellas, Surrey, UK) is a potent M_3 receptor antagonist that has selectivity for the M_3 receptors over M_2 receptors and has much higher potency against M_3 receptors in smooth muscle than it does against M_3 receptors in salivary glands [225].

The clinical efficacy of solifenacin has been assessed in a multicentre, randomized, double-blind, parallel-group, placebo-controlled study of solifenacin 5 and 10 mg once daily in patients with OAB [226]. The primary efficacy analysis showed a statistically significant reduction of the micturition frequency following treatment with both 5 and 10 mg doses when compared with placebo, although the largest effect was with the higher dose. In addition, solifenacin was found to be superior to placebo with respect to the secondary efficacy variables of mean volume voided per micturition, episodes of urgency per 24 h, number of incontinence episodes and episodes of urge incontinence. The most frequently reported adverse events leading to discontinuation were dry mouth and constipation. These were also found to be dose related. In order to assess the long-term safety and efficacy of solifenacin (5 and 10 mg once daily) a multicentre open-label long-term follow-up study has recently been completed. This was essentially an extension of two previous double-blind placebo-controlled studies in 1637 patients [227]. Overall, the efficacy of solifenacin was maintained in the extension study with a sustained improvement in symptoms of urgency, urge incontinence, frequency and nocturia over the 12-month study period. The most commonly reported adverse events were dry mouth (20.5%), constipation (9.2%) and blurred vision (6.6%) and were the primary reason for discontinuation in 4.7% of patients.

More recently, solifenacin 5 and 10 mg once daily have been compared with tolterodine extended release 4 mg once daily in the solifenacin (flexible dosing) once daily and tolterodine extended release 4mg once daily as an active comparator in a randomized trial (STAR) [228]. This was a prospective double-blind, double-dummy, two-arm, parallel-group, 12-week study of 1200 patients with the primary aim of demonstrating non-inferiority of solifenacin to tolterodine extended release. Solifenacin was non-inferior to tolterodine extended release with respect to change from baseline in the mean number of micturitions per 24h ($P = 0.004$). In addition, solifenacin resulted in a statistically significant improvement in urgency ($P = 0.035$), urge incontinence ($P = 0.001$) and overall incontinence when compared with tolterodine extended release. Furthermore, 59% of solifenacin-treated patients who were incontinent at baseline became continent by the study end-point compared with 49% of those on tolterodine extended release ($P = 0.006$). The most commonly reported adverse events were dry mouth, constipation and blurred vision, and were mostly mild to moderate in severity. The number of patients discontinuing medication was similar in both treatment arms (3.5% in the solifenacin arm vs. 3.0% in the tolterodine arm).

Urgency is now generally regarded to be the driving symptom of the OAB syndrome [229]. Urgency drives the symptoms of daytime frequency and nocturia by reducing the inter-void interval and also may be responsible for causing urgency incontinence. The first study to investigate urgency as the primary outcome measure was SUNRISE (Solifenacin in the treatment of urgency symptoms of OAB in a rising dose, randomized, placebo-controlled double-blind efficacy trial), which was performed in Europe [230]. This was a large, 16-week multicentre study of solifenacin 5mg and 10mg in 863 patients with OAB syndrome. Overall, solifenacin 5mg and 10mg was significantly more effective than placebo in reducing the mean number of episodes of severe urgency with or without incontinence (−2.6 vs. −1.8; $P < 0.001$). In addition, there was a significant effect over placebo in terms of the secondary patient-orientated outcomes, and improvement was seen as early as 3 days after starting active treatment. Interestingly, the rate of dry mouth and constipation reported in this was lower than in those reported previously (15.8% and 6.9%, respectively).

The evidence would appear to suggest that solifenacin may offer superior efficacy to the other currently available antimuscarinic agents and that switching from tolterodine to solifenacin offers improved efficacy rates [231]. Pooled data from the phase III studies have demonstrated equal efficacy in the elderly [232] while phase IV studies have shown little cognitive effect [233], a synergistic effect with conservative therapy [234] and improvement in QoL and patient-reported outcome measures [235].

Darifenacin

Darifenacin (Warner Chilcott, New Jersey, USA) is a tertiary amine with moderate lipophilicity and is a highly selective M_3 receptor antagonist that has been found to have a fivefold higher affinity for the human M_3 receptor relative to the M_1 receptor [236].

A review of the pooled darifenacin data from three phase III, multicentre, double-blind clinical trials in patients with OAB has recently been reported in 1059 patients [237]. Darifenacin resulted in a dose-related significant reduction in median number of incontinence episodes per week. Significant decreases in the frequency and severity of urgency, micturition frequency, and number of incontinence episodes resulting in a change of clothing or pads were also apparent, along with an increase in bladder capacity. Darifenacin was well tolerated. The most common treatment-related adverse events were dry mouth and constipation, although together these resulted in few discontinuations. The incidence of central nervous system and cardiovascular adverse events were comparable to placebo.

Fesoterodine

Fesoterodine (Pfizer, Kent, UK) is a new and novel derivative of 3,3-diphenyl-propylamine, which is a non-selective antimuscarinic agent that has recently been developed for the management of OAB. It is rapidly and extensively converted by ubiquitous estereases to its active metabolite, 5-hydroxymethyl tolterodine (5-HMT) [238]. The pharmacokinetic profile of 5-HMT is dose proportional at doses up to 12mg, and thus allows for flexible dosing [239]. Although tolterodine is also converted to 5-HMT, this occurs primarily in the liver via cytochrome P450 (CYP) 2D6, and hence is more dependent on the metabolizer status of the patient. Consequently, the potential benefit of fesoterodine over tolterodine is that it allows a more predictable dose–effect relationship.

A phase II dose-finding study was conducted in 728 patients at 81 sites throughout Europe and South Africa [240]. Fesoterodine 4mg, 8mg and 12mg were all found to show significantly greater decreases in micturition frequency than placebo. The most commonly reported side effect was dry mouth with an incidence of 25% in the 4mg group, rising to 34% in the 12mg group. Discontinuation rates were 6% and 12%, respectively. Subsequently, a phase III randomized placebo-controlled trial has been reported comparing fesoterodine 4mg and 8mg with tolterodine extended-release 4mg in 1135 patients complaining of OAB at 150 sites throughout Australia, New Zealand, South Africa and Europe [241,242]. Both doses of fesoterodine demonstrated significant improvements over placebo in reduction of daytime frequency and number of urge incontinence episodes per day and were found to be superior to tolterodine. Dry mouth was the most commonly reported adverse effect in 22%, 34% and 17% in the fesoterodine 4mg, 8mg and tolterodine arms, respectively. Further studies have also demonstrated a significant improvement in QoL in women with OAB treated with fesoterodine 4mg and 8mg [243].

Fesoterodine has recently been compared with tolterodine in a large-scale 12-week, double-blind, double-dummy, placebo-controlled randomized head-to-head superiority study involving 1590 patients [244]. Overall, fesoterodine 8 mg was found to significantly improve urinary urge incontinence episodes compared with tolterodine extended-release 4 mg ($P = 0.017$) and placebo ($P < 0.001$). In addition, fesoterodine also produced significantly greater improvements over tolterodine in mean volume voided ($P = 0.005$) as well as leading to a significant improvement in all diary variables over placebo ($P < 0.001$) except for nocturnal voids. Dry rates in patients with urgency incontinence at baseline were significantly higher in the fesoterodine arm compared with the tolterodine arm (64% vs. 57%; $P < 0.001$). Dry mouth and constipation rates were 28% and 5% in the fesoterodine arm compared with 16% and 4% in the tolterodine arm and 6% and 3% with placebo.

The current evidence would suggest that fesoterodine may offer some advantages over tolterodine in terms of efficacy and flexible dosing regimens.

Antidepressants
Imipramine
Imipramine has been shown to have systemic anticholinergic effects [245] and blocks the reuptake of serotonin. Some authorities have found a significant effect in the treatment of patients with detrusor overactivity [246], although others report little effect [247]. In light of this evidence and the serious adverse effects associated with tricyclic antidepressants, their role in detrusor overactivity remains of uncertain benefit, although they are often useful in patients complaining of nocturia or bladder pain.

Prostaglandin synthetase inhibitors
Bladder mucosa has been shown to have the ability to synthesize eicosanoids [248], although it is uncertain whether these contribute to the pathogenesis of uninhibited detrusor contractions. However, they may have a role in sensitizing sensory afferent nerves, increasing the afferent input produced by a given bladder volume. A double-blind controlled study of flurbiprofen in women with detrusor overactivity was shown to have an effect, although it was associated with a high incidence of adverse effects (43%) including nausea, vomiting, headache and gastrointestinal symptoms [249]. Indomethacin has also been reported to give symptomatic relief, although the incidence of adverse effects was also high (59%) [250]. At present, this evidence does not support their use in detrusor overactivity.

Antidiuretic agents
Desmopressin
Desmopressin (1-desamino-8-D-arginine vasopressin; DDAVP) (Ferring Pharmaceuticals, Copenhagen, Denmark) is a synthetic vasopressin analogue. It has strong antidiuretic effects without altering blood pressure. The drug has been used primarily in the treatment of nocturia and nocturnal enuresis in children [251] and adults [252]. More recently, nasal desmopressin has been reported as a 'designer drug' for the treatment of daytime urinary incontinence [253]. Desmopressin is safe for long-term use; however, the drug should be used with care in the elderly owing to the risk of hyponatraemia.

Intravesical therapy
Capsaicin
Capsaicin is the pungent ingredient found in red chillies and is a neurotoxin of substance P containing C nerve fibres. Patients with neurogenic detrusor overactivity secondary to multiple sclerosis appear to have abnormal C-fibre sensory innervation of the detrusor, which leads to premature activation of the holding reflex arc during bladder filling [254]. Intravesical application of capsaicin dissolved in 30% alcohol solution appears to be effective for up to 6 months. The effects are variable [255] and the clinical effectiveness remains undefined.

Resiniferatoxin
This is a phorbol-related diterpene isolated from the cactus and is a potent analogue of capsaicin that appears to have a similar efficacy but with fewer side effects of pain and burning during intravesical instillation [256]. It is 1000 times more potent than capsaicin at stimulating bladder activity [257]. As with capsaicin, the currently available evidence does not support the routine clinical use of the agents, although they may prove to have a role as an intravesical preparation in neurological patients with neurogenic detrusor overactivity.

Botulinum toxin
In 1817 an illness caused by *Clostridium botulinum* toxin was first recorded, when Justinus Kerner described a link between a sausage and a paralytic illness that affected 230 people. He was a district health officer and made botulism (from the Latin *botulus*, meaning sausage) a notifiable disease [258]. In 1897, the microbiologist Emile-Pierre van Ermengen identified a Gram-positive, spore-forming, anaerobic bacterium in a ham from a Belgian restaurant that caused 23 cases of botulism. He termed the bacterium *Bacillus botulinus*; it was later re-termed *Clostridium botulinum* [259].

The bacterium produces its effect by production of a neurotoxin – different strains produce seven distinct serotypes, designated A–G. All seven have a similar structure and molecular weight, consisting of a heavy (H) and a light (L) chain, joined by a disulphide bond [260]. They interfere with neural transmission by blocking the calcium-dependent release of the neurotransmitter acetylcholine, causing the affected muscle to become weak and atrophic. The affected nerves do not degenerate, but as the blockage is irreversible, only the development of new nerve terminals and synaptic contacts allows recovery of function.

The use of intravesical *C. botulinum* toxin was first described in the treatment of intractable neurogenic detrusor overactivity in 31 patients with traumatic spinal cord injury [261]. Subsequently, a larger European study has reported on 231 patients with neurogenic detrusor overactivity [262]. All were treated with 300 units of botulinum-A toxin, which was injected cystoscopically into the detrusor muscle at 30 different sites sparring the trigone. At 12- and 36-week follow-up there was a significant increase in cystometric capacity and bladder compliance. Patient satisfaction was high, the majority stopped taking antimuscarinic medication and there were no significant complications. More recently, the first randomized placebo-controlled trial has been reported in 59 patients with neurogenic detrusor overactivity [263]. At 6 months there was a significant reduction in incontinence episodes in the botox group compared with the placebo group and a corresponding improvement in QoL evaluation.

Although the role of botulinum toxin has been established in the treatment of neurogenic detrusor overactivity, the data regarding its use in intractable idiopathic detrusor overactivity are less robust. A prospective open-label study has recently been reported, assessing the use of botulinum-A toxin in both neurogenic (300 units) and idiopathic (200 units) detrusor overactivity in 75 patients [264]. When considering urodynamic outcome parameters in both groups, there was a significant increase in cystometric capacity and decrease in maximum detrusor pressure during filling in both groups. Clinically, there was also a significant reduction in frequency and episodes of urge incontinence. Interestingly, however, 69% of patients with neurogenic detrusor overactivity required self-catheterization following treatment compared with 19.3% of those with idiopathic detrusor overactivity.

At present, the evidence would suggest that intravesical administration of botulinum toxin may offer an alternative to surgery in those women with intractable detrusor overactivity, although the effect is only temporary and at present there are few long-term data regarding the efficacy and complications associated with repeat injections [265].

Neuromodulation
Peripheral neuromodulation
Stimulation of the posterior tibial nerve in patients with urge incontinence was first reported in 1983 [266] and has also been proposed for pelvic floor dysfunction [267]. The tibial nerve is a mixed nerve containing L4–S3 fibres and originates from the same spinal cord segments as the innervation to the bladder and pelvic floor. Consequently,

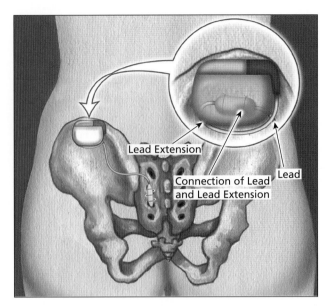

Fig. 51.30 Sacral neuromodulation.

peripheral neural modulation may have a role in the management of urinary symptoms (Plate 51.1).

In a prospective multicentre study 35 patients with urge incontinence underwent 12 weekly sessions of posterior tibial nerve stimulation (PTNS), with 70% of patients reporting a >50% reduction in urinary symptoms and 46% being completely cured [268]. More recently, a prospective randomized multicentre North American study has been reported comparing PTNS with tolterodine 4 mg extended release in 100 patients. Overall, there was an improvement in 75% of patients with PTNS compared with 55.8% with tolterodine extended release, and there was a significant improvement in QoL in both groups [269].

Consequently, peripheral neuromodulation may offer an alternative therapeutic option for those patients with intractable OAB who have failed to respond to medical therapy, although it remains less cost-effective than treatment with antimuscarinic agents [270].

Sacral neuromodulation
Stimulation of the dorsal sacral nerve root using a permanent implantable device in the S3 sacral foramen has been developed for use in patients with both idiopathic and neurogenic detrusor overactivity (Fig. 51.30). The sacral nerves contain nerve fibres of the parasympathetic and sympathetic systems providing innervation to the bladder as well as somatic fibres providing innervation to the muscles of the pelvic floor. The latter are larger in diameter, and hence have a lower threshold of activation meaning that the pelvic floor may be stimulated selectively without causing bladder activity. Prior to implantation, temporary cutaneous sacral nerve stimulation is performed to check for a response and, if successful, a permanent implant is inserted under general anaesthesia.

Initial studies in patients with detrusor overactivity refractory to medical and behavioural therapy have demonstrated that, after 3 years, 59% of 41 urinary urge incontinent patients showed a >50% reduction in incontinence episodes with 46% of patients being completely dry [271].

More recently, a 5-year worldwide multicentre study has been reported in 163 patients (87% female) [272]. Following test stimulation, 11 patients declined implantation and 152 underwent implantation using InterStim® (American Medical Systems, Minnetonka, MN, USA). Voiding diaries were collected annually for 5 years, with success being defined as a >50% improvement in symptoms. At 5 years after implantation 68% of patients with urge incontinence, 56% with urgency frequency and 71% with retention had successful outcomes, although revision rates were reported to be up to 42%, indicating that sacral neuromodulation may be associated with considerable long-term morbidity.

Although neuromodulation remains an invasive and expensive procedure in the future, it offers a useful alternative to medical and surgical therapies in patients with severe, intractable detrusor overactivity.

Surgery

For those women with severe detrusor overactivity that is not amenable to simple types of treatment, surgery may be employed.

Clam cystoplasty

In the clam cystoplasty [273,274] the bladder is bisected almost completely and a patch of gut (usually ileum) equal in length to the circumference of the bisected bladder (about 25 cm) is sewn in place (Fig. 51.31). This often cures the symptoms of detrusor overactivity [275] by converting a high-pressure system into a low-pressure system, although inefficient voiding may result. Patients have to learn to strain to void, or may have to resort to

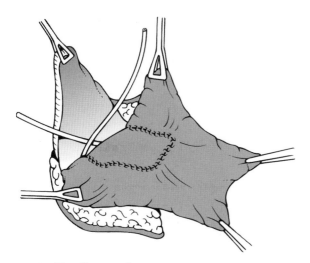

Fig. 51.31 Clam ileocystoplasty.

clean intermittent self-catheterization, sometimes permanently. In addition, mucus retention in the bladder may be a problem, but this can be partially overcome by ingestion of 200 mL cranberry juice each day [276] in addition to intravesical mucolytics such as acetylcysteine. The chronic exposure of the ileal mucosa to urine may lead to malignant change [277]. There is a 5% risk of adenocarcinoma arising in ureterosigmoidostomies, in which colonic mucosa is exposed to *N*-nitrosamines found in both urine and faeces, and a similar risk may apply to enterocystoplasty. Biopsies of the ileal segment taken from patients with 'clam' cystoplasties show evidence of chronic inflammation of villous atrophy, and diarrhoea owing to disruption of the bile acid cycle is common [278]. This may be treated using cholestyramine. In addition, metabolic disturbances such as hyperchoraemic acidosis, B_{12} deficiency and occasionally osteoporosis secondary to decreased bone mineralization may occur.

Urinary diversion

As a last resort for those women with severe detrusor overactivity or neurogenic detrusor overactivity who cannot manage clean intermittent catheterization, it may be more appropriate to perform a urinary diversion. Usually this will utilize an ileal conduit to create an abdominal stoma for urinary diversion. An alternative is to form a continent diversion using the appendix (Mitrofanoff) or ileum (Koch pouch), which may then be drained using self-catheterization.

Detrusor myectomy

Detrusor myectomy offers an alternative to clam cystoplasty by increasing functional bladder capacity without the complications of bowel interposition. In this procedure, the whole thickness of the detrusor muscle is excised from the dome of the bladder, thereby creating a large bladder diverticulum with no intrinsic contractility [279]. Although there is a reduction in episodes of incontinence, there is little improvement in functional capacity, and thus frequency remains problematic [280,281].

National Institute for Health and Clinical Excellence guidelines

The medical management of OAB has recently been reviewed by NICE [9]. In the first instance, bladder retraining lasting for a minimum of 6 weeks should be offered to all women with mixed or urge incontinence. In those women who do not achieve satisfactory benefit from bladder retraining alone the combination of an antimuscarinic agent, in addition to bladder retraining, should be considered.

When considering drug therapy immediate-release non-propriety oxybutynin should be offered to women with OAB or mixed urinary incontinence as first-line drug treatment if bladder retraining has been ineffective. If immediate-release oxybutynin is not well tolerated, darifenacin, solifenacin, tolterodine, trospium or an extended-release or transdermal formulation of oxybutynin should be considered as alternatives. In addition, women should be counselled regarding the adverse effects of antimuscarinic drugs.

Propiverine should be considered as an option to treat frequency of micturition but is not recommended for the treatment of urinary incontinence. Flavoxate, propantheline and imipramine should not be used for the treatment of OAB. Although desmopressin may be considered specifically to reduce nocturia in women, it is currently outside marketing authorization and hence informed consent must be obtained.

When considering the role of oestrogens systemic hormone replacement therapy should not be recommended, although intravaginal oestrogens are recommended for the treatment of OAB in postmenopausal women with urogenital atrophy.

Summary box 51.4

Overactive bladder and detrusor overactivity:
- OAB is a symptomatic diagnosis.
- Detrusor overactivity is a urodynamics diagnosis.
- All women benefit from conservative measures and bladder retraining.
- Antimuscarinics are the most commonly used drugs.
- Patients refractory to drug therapy may benefit from botulinum toxin.
- Neuromodulation may be useful in refractory cases.
- Reconstructive surgery should only be considered when all other therapy has failed.

Mixed incontinence

Although a large proportion of women complain of both stress and urge incontinence, only about 5% suffer from mixed detrusor overactivity and urethral sphincter incompetence. They pose a difficult management problem. A study comparing medical and surgical treatment has shown that of the 27 women who underwent a Burch colposuspension, 59% were cured and 22% improved, whereas of the 25 who received drug therapy (oxybutynin, imipramine and oestrogen), 32% were cured and 28% improved. The authors concluded that combined stress incontinence and detrusor overactivity should be managed medically initially as this will reduce the need for surgical intervention [282]. In such cases, it is our practice to treat the detrusor overactivity with antimuscarinic agents and to repeat the urodynamic assessment while the patient is taking her medication. If she still leaks without significant detrusor activity and her main

Table 51.15 Causes of voiding difficulties leading to overflow incontinence in women.

Neurological
Lower motor neurone lesion
Upper motor neurone lesion

Inflammation
Urethritis, e.g. 'honeymoon cystitis'
Vulvitis, e.g. herpes
Vaginitis, e.g. candidiasis

Drugs
Tricyclic antidepressants
Antimuscarinic agents
Ganglion blockers
Epidural anaesthesia
Patient-controlled analgesia

Obstruction
Urethral stenosis/stricture
Oedema following surgery or parturition
Fibrosis due to repeated dilatation or irradiation
Pelvic mass, e.g. fibroids, retroverted uterus, ovarian cyst, faeces
Urethral distorsion due to large cystocele

Myogenic
Atonic detrusor secondary to over distension
Functional
Anxiety

---

complaint is stress incontinence, we would undertake conventional bladder neck surgery. However, if urge incontinence still predominates, surgery may aggravate her symptoms.

Retention with overflow

In women, chronic retention with resultant overflow incontinence is uncommon and often no cause can be found. It is one manifestation of the wide range of voiding difficulties which may occur, the major causes of which are shown in Table 51.15.

Women with overflow incontinence present in a variety of ways. They may complain of dribbling urine or of voiding small amounts at frequent intervals, or of stress incontinence. Alternatively, they may notice recurrent urinary tract infections. The diagnosis is usually made by the discovery of a large bladder on clinical examination. This can be confirmed by a postmicturition ultrasound scan to assess the residual urine volume or by catheterization, which will reveal a residual volume >50% of her bladder capacity. There may, in addition, be a reduced peak flow rate of <15 mL/s.

Clinical examination will rule out many of the causes, such as a pelvic mass or a cystocele. It is important to investigate cases of urinary retention thoroughly in order to exclude any treatable underlying pathology. A midstream specimen of urine should be sent for culture and sensitivity, and the appropriate swabs (urethral, vaginal and cervical) should be sent. Radiological investigations should include intravenous urography, an X-ray of the lumbosacral spine and an MRI scan where indicated. It is particularly important to identify diabetes so that treatment can be undertaken before permanent damage occurs.

Treatment for overflow incontinence will depend upon the underlying pathology. If the detrusor is hypotonic, cholinergic agents such as bethanechol 25 mg three times a day may be helpful. If there is outflow obstruction, urethral dilatation or urethrotomy may be required. In cases where no cause can be found, clean intermittent self-catheterization is the best long-term method of management for these patients.

If possible, it is far better to avoid urinary retention by implementing prophylactic measures. The human female bladder, once overdistended, may never contract normally again [283]. When bladder neck surgery for urinary incontinence or radical pelvic surgery for malignant disease is undertaken, adequate postoperative bladder drainage (preferably with a suprapubic catheter) should be employed until normal voiding per urethram has resumed. When epidural anaesthesia is used for surgical procedures or childbirth, an indwelling Foley catheter should be left *in situ* for at least 6 h and probably 12 h after normal sensation to the lower limbs is present. Those women who are known to have inefficient voiding (a low flow rate together with a low maximum voiding pressure) should be taught clean intermittent self-catheterization prior to any surgical intervention for urodynamic stress incontinence.

Acute urinary retention needs to be dealt with as an emergency. A catheter, indwelling either urethral or suprapubic, should be inserted immediately and left on free drainage. There is no need for intermittent clamping of the catheter as this can lead to further overdistension and there is no evidence to suggest that sudden decompression of the bladder is harmful. The volume of urine drained should be recorded and if it is over a litre the catheter should be left *in situ* on free drainage for a week or two before initiating a trial of voiding per urethram. It is, of course, easier to do this is if a suprapubic catheter has been inserted. The urinary residuals should be checked regularly once spontaneous micturition has been resumed to ensure that the bladder is emptying adequately. This can be achieved by 'in–out' catheterization, or less invasively by transabdominal ultrasound. Unless there is an obvious cause for the episode of acute retention, investigations should be undertaken. If further episodes of retention occur, it is prudent to teach the woman clean intermittent self-catheterization to avoid damage to the bladder by overdistension should she find herself in the same position again.

Oestrogens in the management of incontinence

Oestrogen preparations have been used for many years in the treatment of urinary incontinence [284,285], although their precise role remains controversial. Many of the studies performed have been uncontrolled observational series examining the use of a wide range of different preparations, doses and routes of administration. The inconsistent use of progestogens is also a further confounding factor, making interpretation of the results difficult.

Systemic oestrogen therapy
The role of systemic oestrogen replacement therapy in the prevention of ischaemic heart disease has recently been assessed in a 4-year randomized trial, the Heart and Oestrogen/progestin Replacement Study (HERS) [286] involving 2763 postmenopausal women younger than 80 years with intact uteri and ischaemic heart disease. In the study, 55% of women reported at least one episode of urinary incontinence each week, and were randomly assigned to oral conjugated oestrogen plus medroxyprogesterone acetate or placebo daily. Incontinence improved in 26% of women assigned to placebo as compared with 21% receiving hormone replacement therapy (HRT) whereas 27% of the placebo group complained of worsening symptoms compared with 39% in the HRT group ($P = 0.001$). The incidence of incontinent episodes per week increased by an average of 0.7 in the HRT group and decreased by 0.1 in the placebo group ($P < 0.001$). Overall, combined HRT was associated with worsening stress and urge urinary incontinence, although there was no significant difference in daytime frequency, nocturia or number of urinary tract infections.

These findings have also been confirmed in the Nurse's Health Study [287], which followed 39 436 postmenopausal women aged 50–75 years over a 4-year period. The risk of incontinence was found to be elevated in those women taking HRT when compared with those who had never taken HRT. There was an increased risk in women taking oral oestrogen [relative ratio (RR) 1.54; 95% CI 1.44–1.65], transdermal oestrogen (RR 1.68; 95% CI 1.41–2.00), oral oestrogen and progesterone (RR 1.34; 95% CI 1.24–1.34) and transdermal oestrogen and progesterone (RR 1.46; CI 1.16–1.84). In addition, although there remained a small risk after the cessation of HRT (RR 1.14; 95% CI 1.06–1.23), by 10 years the risk was identical (RR 1.02; 95% 0.91–1.41) to those women who had never taken HRT.

These data are also supported by the most recent report from the Women's Health Initiative (WHI) group [288]. Overall, 27 347 postmenopausal women aged 50–79 years were assessed in a multicentre, double-blind placebo-controlled trial. Of these, 23 296 were known to complain of lower urinary tract symptoms at baseline and at 1-year follow-up. Women were randomized based on hysterectomy status to active treatment or placebo in either the oestrogen and progestogen or oestrogen-only trials. The oestrogen was conjugated equine oestrogen (CEE) and the progestogen was medroxyprogesterone acetate (MPA). The main outcome measure was the incidence of urinary incontinence at 1 year amongst women who were continent at baseline and the severity of urinary incontinence at 1 year in those who were incontinent at baseline.

Overall, HRT was found to increase the incidence of all types of urinary incontinence at 1 year in those women continent at baseline. The risk was highest for stress incontinence [CEE + MPA: RR 1.87 (1.61–2.18); CEE alone: RR 2.15 (1.77–2.62)] followed by mixed incontinence [CEE + MPA: RR 1.49 (1.10–2.01); CEE alone: RR 1.79 (1.26–2.53)]. However, the effect on urge urinary incontinence was not uniform [CEE + MPA; RR 1.15 (0.99–1.34); CEE alone: RR 1.32 (1.10–1.58)].

When considering those women who were symptomatic at baseline, urinary frequency was found to increase in both arms [CEE + MPA: RR 1.38 (1.28–1.49); CEE alone: RR 1.47 (1.35–1.61)] and the incidence of urinary incontinence was seen to increase at 1 year [CEE + MPA: RR 1.20 (1.06–1.36); CEE alone: RR 1.59 (1.39–1.82)]. In addition, although no formal quality of life assessment was reported, women receiving HRT were more likely to report that urinary incontinence limited their daily activities and bothered and disturbed them.

Oestrogens in the management of stress urinary incontinence

Oral oestrogens have been reported to increase the maximum urethral pressures and lead to symptomatic improvement in 65–70% of women [289,290], although other work has not confirmed this [291,292]. In addition, two placebo-controlled studies have been performed examining the use of oral oestrogens in the treatment of urodynamic stress incontinence in postmenopausal women. Neither CEE and MPA [293] nor unopposed oestradiol valerate [294] showed a significant difference in either subjective or objective outcomes. Furthermore, a review of eight controlled and 14 uncontrolled prospective trials concluded that oestrogen therapy was not an efficacious treatment for stress incontinence but may be useful for symptoms of urgency and frequency [295].

From the available evidence oestrogen alone does not appear to be an effective treatment for stress urinary incontinence.

Oestrogens in the management of overactive bladder

Oestrogens have been used in the treatment of urinary urgency and urge incontinence for many years, although there have been few controlled trials to confirm their efficacy. A double-blind placebo-controlled crossover study using oral oestriol in 34 postmenopausal women produced subjective improvement in eight women with mixed incontinence and 12 with urge incontinence [296]. However, a double-blind multicentre study of the use of oestriol (3 mg/day) in postmenopausal women complaining of urgency has failed to confirm these findings [297], showing both subjective and objective improvement but not significantly better than placebo. Oestriol is a naturally occurring weak oestrogen that has little effect on the endometrium and does not prevent osteoporosis, although has been used in the treatment of urogenital atrophy. Consequently, it is possible that the dosage or route of administration in this study was not appropriate in the treatment of urinary symptoms, and higher systemic levels may be required.

The use of sustained-release 17β-oestradiol vaginal tablets (Vagifem®, Novo Nordisk, West Sussex, UK) has also been examined in postmenopausal women with urgency and urge incontinence or a urodynamic diagnosis of sensory urgency or detrusor overactivity. These vaginal tablets have been shown to be well absorbed from the vagina and to induce maturation of the vaginal epithelium within 14 days [298]. However, following a 6-month course of treatment, the only significant difference between active and placebo groups was an improvement in the symptom of urgency in those women with a urodynamic diagnosis of sensory urgency [299]. A further double-blind, randomized, placebo-controlled trial of vaginal 17β-oestradiol vaginal tablets has shown lower urinary tract symptoms of frequency, urgency, urge and stress incontinence to be significantly improved, although there was no objective urodynamic assessment performed [300]. In both of these studies the subjective improvement in symptoms may simply represent local oestrogenic effects reversing urogenital atrophy rather than a direct effect on bladder function.

More recently, a randomized, parallel-group, controlled trial has been reported comparing the oestradiol-releasing vaginal ring (Estring®, Pfizer) with oestriol vaginal pessaries in the treatment of postmenopausal women with bothersome lower urinary tract symptoms [301]. Low-dose vaginally administered oestradiol and oestriol were found to be equally efficacious in alleviating lower urinary tract symptoms of urge incontinence (58% vs. 58%), stress incontinence (53% vs. 59%) and nocturia (51% vs. 54%), although the vaginal ring was found to have greater patient acceptability.

To try to clarify the role of oestrogen therapy in the management of women with urge incontinence a meta-analysis of the use of oestrogen in women with symptoms of OAB has been reported by the HUT Committee [302]. In a review of 10 randomized placebo-controlled trials oestrogen was found to be superior to placebo when considering symptoms of urge incontinence, frequency and nocturia, although vaginal oestrogen administration was found to be superior for symptoms of urgency. In those taking oestrogens there was also a significant increase in first sensation and bladder capacity as compared with placebo.

Oestrogen therapy: Cochrane review

The most recent meta-analysis of the effect of oestrogen therapy on the lower urinary tract has been performed by the Cochrane group [303]. In total, 33 trials were identified, including 19 313 incontinent women (1262 involved in trials of local administration), of which 9417 received oestrogen therapy.

Overall, systemic administration (of unopposed oral oestrogens) resulted in worse incontinence than on placebo (RR 1.32; 95% CI 1.17–1.48), although this result is heavily influenced by the weight of the WHI study. When considering combination therapy there was a similar worsening effect on incontinence when compared with placebo (RR 1.11; 95% CI 1.04–1.18). There was some evidence suggesting that the use of local oestrogen therapy may improve incontinence (RR 0.74; 95% CI 0.64–0.86) and overall there were one or two fewer voids in 24 h and less frequency and urgency.

The authors conclude that local oestrogen therapy for incontinence may be beneficial, although there was little evidence of long-term effects. The evidence would suggest that systemic hormone replacement using conjugated equine oestrogens may make incontinence worse. In addition, they comment that there are too few data to comment reliably on the dose, type of oestrogen and route of administration.

Fistulas

Urinary fistulas may be ureterovaginal, vesicovaginal, urethrovaginal or complex, and can occur following pelvic surgery or in cases of advanced pelvic malignancy, especially when there has been radiotherapy. The most common varieties in the UK are lower ureteric or bladder fistulas occurring after an abdominal hysterectomy. In developing countries, poor obstetrics with obstructed labour resulting in ischaemic necrosis of the bladder base is more likely to be the cause of a vesico- or urethrovaginal fistula.

Fistulas give rise to incontinence that is continuous, occurring both day and night. They are usually visible on speculum examination but cystoscopy and intravenous urography may be required to confirm the diagnosis.

Treatment is surgical. Ureterovaginal fistulas should be repaired as quickly as possible to prevent upper urinary tract damage. Vesicovaginal fistulas are usually treated conservatively, initially with bladder drainage and antibiotics, during which time some will close spontaneously. Abdominal or vaginal repair is normally performed 2 or 3 months after the initial injury, although there is now a trend towards earlier repair; if a fistula is detected within a very short period of time after the initial operation, it can often be closed immediately.

Congenital abnormalities

Congenital abnormalities are uncommon and are usually diagnosed at birth or during childhood. The most common gross abnormality is ectopia vesicae, which requires surgical reconstruction during the neonatal period. Other less obvious congenital abnormalities include epispadias, which can be diagnosed by a bifid clitoris. This abnormality is difficult to treat and may require reconstruction in the form of a neourethra. An ectopic ureter may open into the vagina and cause urinary incontinence that is not diagnosed until childhood, and spina bifida occulta may present with urinary symptoms during the prepubertal growth spurt.

Urethral diverticulum

Urethral diverticula are becoming more common, presumably because of the increased incidence of sexually transmitted diseases. They are found in women of any age and lead to various complaints including pain, particularly after micturition, postmicturition dribble and dyspareunia. Diagnosis can be made either radiologically on a micturating cystogram or videocystourethrogram or by urethroscopy. In addition, MRI may be useful. Urethral diverticula should be managed conservatively, initially with intermittent courses of antibiotics if necessary; but if there are severe symptoms, then surgical excision of the diverticulum may be required. It is usual to perform a subtotal diverticulectomy in order to avoid urethral stricture formation, and following the procedure a urethral catheter is left in place for 2 weeks, acting as a stent to allow the urethra to heal.

Temporary causes of urinary incontinence

Lower urinary tract infections (cystitis or urethritis) may uncommonly cause incontinence of urine that is temporary and will resolve once treatment with the appropriate antibiotics has been employed. Diuretics, especially in the elderly, may also be responsible for urgency, frequency and incontinence. In older people, anything that limits their independence may cause urge incontinence where only urgency existed before. This applies particularly to immobility, and if an older person is unable to reach the toilet in a short space of time, she may become incontinent. Thus, the provision of appropriate facilities and adequate lighting can alleviate the problem. Faecal impaction may cause urinary incontinence or retention of urine, which will resolve once suitable laxatives or enemas have been effective.

Functional incontinence

In a small proportion of women, no organic cause can be found for incontinence. Some of them have anxiety states that respond well to physiotherapy or to psychotropic drugs such as diazepam. Immobility may prevent a woman from reaching the lavatory in time, and, for her, simple remedies such as a toilet downstairs or the use of a commode may prevent urinary leakage.

General conservative measures

All incontinent women benefit from simple measures such as the provision of suitable incontinence pads and pants. Those with a high fluid intake should be advised to restrict their drinking to a litre a day, particularly if frequency of micturition is a problem. Caffeine-containing drinks (such as teas, coffee and cola) and alcohol are irritant to the bladder and act as diuretics, so should be avoided if possible. Anything that increases intra-abdominal pressure will aggravate incontinence, so patients with a chronic cough should be advised to give up smoking, and constipation should be treated appropriately. Pelvic floor exercises may be particularly helpful in the puerperium or after pelvic surgery. For younger, more active women who have not yet completed their family, a device or sponge tampon may be used during strenuous activity such as sport. Oestrogen replacement therapy for postmenopausal women is often beneficial as it improves quality of life as well as helping with the overactive bladder symptoms. Diuretics, which are often given to older people for fluid retention or mild hypertension, may make their urinary symptoms worse and should be stopped if possible.

Women with long-standing severe incontinence, especially the elderly, may be more comfortable and easier to manage with a regularly changed indwelling suprapubic catheter; and for the young disabled, urinary diversion should be considered earlier rather than later. It is not always possible to cure urinary incontinence but it is usually possible to help the sufferer and thus improve her quality of life.

Other lower urinary tract disorders

Urethral lesions
Urethral caruncle

A urethral caruncle is a benign red polyp or lesion covered by transitional epithelium usually found on the posterior aspect of the urethral meatus. It is commonly seen in postmenopausal women and although usually asymptomatic it may cause pain, bleeding and dysuria. The cause is unknown. Treatment is by excision biopsy followed by local or systemic oestrogens.

Urethral mucosal prolapse

Prolapse of the urethral mucosa also occurs in the postmenopausal woman but, in addition, is sometimes seen in girls (usually black) between the ages of 5 and 10 years. It is a reddish lesion that encompasses the whole circumference of the external urethral meatus, thus differentiating it from the urethral caruncle. Urethral mucosal prolapse is not painful but may cause bleeding, dysuria or urethral discharge. It may be treated by excision or cautery.

Urethral stenosis or stricture

Outflow obstruction due to urethral stenosis or a stricture is rare in women. Such lesions usually present after the menopause and are found in the distal urethra. They are often the result of chronic urethritis or may follow fibrosis from repeated urethral dilatations or other surgery to the urethra. The most common symptoms are of voiding difficulties, but recurrent urinary tract infections may occur. Diagnosis can be made using uroflowmetry in conjunction with cystometry or by videocystourethrography. Urethral pressure profilometry or cystourethroscopy will help to localize the lesion. Urethrotomy, either Otis or open, is the treatment of choice, and local oestrogen therapy may be helpful in postmenopausal women.

Carcinoma of the urethra

Urethral carcinoma is rare and is usually a transitional cell carcinoma located in the proximal urethra. Secondary deposits may arise from adenocarcinoma of the endometrium, transitional cell carcinoma of the bladder or squamous carcinoma of the vulva or vagina. Symptoms include haematuria, vaginal bleeding and discharge, frequency of micturition, dysuria and recurrent urinary tract infections. A mass may be palpable or may be seen on speculum examination. The diagnosis can be confirmed by taking urethroscopically directed biopsies. Treatment consists of radical surgery, usually cystourethrectomy and lymph node dissection followed by radiotherapy.

Urinary frequency and urgency
Definitions [2]

• *Diurnal frequency* The complaint that micturition occurs more frequently during waking hours than previously deemed normal.
• *Nocturia* The complaint of interruption of sleep one or more times because of the need to micturate. Each void is preceded and followed by sleep.
• *Urgency* The complaint of a sudden compelling desire to pass urine, which is difficult to defer.

• *Urgency incontinence* The complaint of involuntary leakage accompanied by or immediately preceded by urgency.

Prevalence

Frequency and urgency are common symptoms in women of all ages. They often coexist and may occur in conjunction with other symptoms such as urinary incontinence or dysuria. It is unusual for urgency to occur alone because once it is present it almost invariably leads to frequency to avoid urge incontinence and to relieve the unpleasant painful sensation. Bungay *et al.* [304] found that approximately 20% of a group of 1120 women aged between 30 and 65 years admitted to frequency of micturition and 15% of women from the same series reported urgency. In this study there was no specific increase in the prevalence of frequency or urgency with age or in relation to the menopause.

Over the age of about 60 years it is common for women to develop 'nocturia'. This increases once per decade of life so that it is not unusual for a woman in her eighties to have to rise four times during the night to void. This represents a relative impairment in cardiovascular function rather than a urological abnormality.

Causes and assessment

There are many different causes of frequency and urgency of micturition; the more common ones are shown in Table 51.16.

Clinical examination will exclude many of the causes. This is important before expensive time-consuming investigations are undertaken. As one of the commonest causes of frequency of micturition is a lower urinary tract infection, it is important to send a midstream specimen of urine for culture and sensitivity. If difficulty is encountered obtaining an uncontaminated midstream specimen of urine suprapubic aspiration should be employed. When urine culture is repeatedly negative in a woman with urgency, frequency and dysuria where no other cause can be found, urine should be sent for culture of fastidious organisms such as *Mycoplasma hominis* and *Ureaplasma urealyticum,* which are being seen with increasing frequency in symptomatic women.

Those women who have an abnormal vaginal discharge, history of sexually transmitted diseases or obvious vulval excoriation should have vaginal, cervical and urethral swabs sent for culture. *Chlamydia trachomatis* may be a causative organism that requires a special culture medium for its detection. If there is a history of haematuria, loin or groin pain, and a urinary tract infection cannot be identified, intravenous urography and cystoscopy should be performed and the patient referred to a urologist. In cases of impaired renal function serum urine electrolyte concentration and urine osmolarity

Table 51.16 Causes of urgency and frequency in women.

Urological
Urinary tract infection
Urethral syndrome
Detrusor overactivity
Bladder tumour
Bladder calculus
Small capacity bladder
Interstitial cystitis
Radiation cystitis/fibrosis
Chronic retention/residual
Urethral diverticulum

Gynaecological
Cystocele
Pelvic mass, e.g. fibroids, ovarian cyst
Previous pelvic surgery

Genital
Urethritis ('honeymoon cystitis')
Vulvovaginitis
Urethral caruncle
Herpes
Warts
Sexually transmitted diseases
Atrophy (hypo-oestrogenism)

Medical
Upper motor neurone lesion
Impaired renal function
Diabetes mellitus
Diabetes insipidus
Hypothyroidism
Congestive cardiac failure
Diuretic therapy
Faecal impaction

General
Excessive drinking habit
Anxiety
Pregnancy

should be estimated. A plain radiograph of the abdomen (kidneys, ureter and bladder) is useful in the diagnosis of a calculus and if a significant urinary residual volume is discovered then an X-ray of the lumbar sacral spine should be obtained.

The investigations performed should be organized around the patient's precise symptomatology. However, a frequency–volume chart is often useful as it may identify excessive drinking as the cause of urinary frequency. In addition, cystourethroscopy may reveal underlying pathology within the bladder or urethra. For women with incontinence in addition to frequency with or without urgency it is best to organize urodynamic studies prior to cystoscopy as the latter is usually unrewarding. Subtracted cystometry detects detrusor overactivity, which is a major cause of urgency and frequency and also reveals chronic retention of urine with an atonic bladder, which may lead to frequency or recurrent urinary tract infections. For women with frequency, urgency and dysuria without incontinence a cystourethroscopy may be more helpful than a urodynamic assessment.

In a large proportion of cases no obvious cause will be found for the symptoms of frequency and urgency. Some patients with negative findings void frequently from habit, which usually develops following an acute urinary tract infection or an episode of incontinence. Alternatively, bad habits may have been present since childhood, especially if one parent voids frequently. It is interesting that often several members of the same family suffer from similar urinary complaints.

Treatment

Treatment should be directed towards the underlying cause if one has been identified. Those women who drink excessively should be advised to limit their fluid intake to between 1 and 1.5 L/day and to avoid drinking at times when their frequency causes the most embarrassment. Certain drinks such as tea, coffee and cola (all of which contain caffeine) and alcohol precipitate frequency, especially nocturia, in some individuals and should therefore be avoided.

Habit retraining (bladder drill) is useful for women without organic disease and can be undertaken by patients at home [187]. Inpatient bladder drill is more effective but often impossible to organize, and the regimen described by Jarvis and Millar [186] is easy to follow and effectively improves symptoms in up to 80% of women initially. Unfortunately, the relapse rate is high [305]. This is mainly due to the underlying factors in the patient's home environment that exacerbate her symptoms.

Sometimes antimuscarinic drug therapy may be helpful. If anxiety or nocturia is a problem then imipramine or amitriptyline 50 mg nightly can be tried. Desmopressin may also be useful in patients who complain of nocturia alone.

Urethral pain syndrome

This is defined as the occurrence of recurrent episodic urethral pain usually on voiding with daytime frequency and nocturia in the absence of infection or other obvious pathology [2]. The urethral pain syndrome can occur at any age. There are believed to be two basic causative factors – a bacterial and a urethral element. The bacterial element is thought to be due to migration of *Escherichia coli* across the perineum and up the urethra for which Smith [306] has recommended perineal hygiene, especially after sexual intercourse. In the case of an acute

attack many authorities suggest a high fluid intake combined with bicarbonate of soda to alter the pH of the urine and short courses of antibiotics such as co-trimoxazole, nitrofurantoin or, more recently, norfloxacin. Prolonged low-dose chemotherapy is sometimes necessary for relapsing and chronic cases. Norfloxacin 400 mg taken at night for 3 months can be employed. *Chlamydia trachomatis* is a possible causative organism [307], in which case doxycycline 100 mg nightly for 3 months is an effective antibiotic.

Various surgical manoeuvres have been tried for resistant cases of urethral pain syndrome. Urethral dilatation has been employed but there is no rationale behind its use as it is rare to find outflow obstruction in these women. Similarly, urethrotomy is sometimes performed. However, it is not indicated and may cause incontinence or a urethral stricture. Rees *et al.* [308] found that less than 8% of 156 women with the urethral syndrome had outflow obstruction and that the results of urethral dilatation or internal urethrotomy were no better than medication alone.

Painful bladder syndrome

Painful bladder syndrome is the compliant of suprapubic pain related to bladder filling accompanied by other symptoms such as increased daytime and night-time frequency, in the absence of proven urinary infection or other obvious pathology [2]. A cause of painful bladder syndrome in women is interstitial cystitis.

Interstitial cystitis

Interstitial cystitis produces severe symptoms that include frequency, dysuria, lower abdominal and urethral pain. It affects individuals of both sexes, although only about 10% of sufferers are men. Although the peak age is 30–50 years [309], it has also been found in children [310]. The aetiology remains obscure but the absence of any detectable bacterial or fungal agent is a prerequisite for the diagnosis [311]. There is growing evidence that interstitial cystitis is an autoimmune disease. Histological changes in bladder wall biopsies are consistent with a connective tissue disorder. The most common marker is mast cell infiltration of the muscularis layer of the bladder. This was first recognized in 1958 by Simmons and Bruce and, although there is no consensus on the role of mast cells and their usefulness as a diagnostic criterion, two papers have investigated degranulation of mast cells [312,313], both showing increased degranulation in patients suffering from interstitial cystitis. Parsons *et al.* [314] proposed that there is a failure of the protective function of the mucosal glycosaminoglycan layer of the bladder, and thus allowing infective agents to attack the underlying epithelium, and subsequently they postulated that patients with interstitial cystitis have an abnormal sensitivity to intravesical potassium [315].

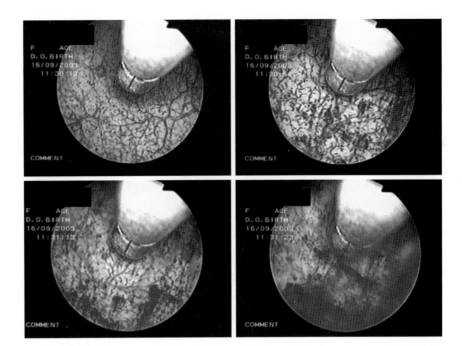

Fig. 51.32 Series of cystoscopic images showing gradual cystodistension with haemorrahage in a young woman with interstitial cystitis.

Diagnosis

The diagnosis of interstitial cystitis can be difficult. Pain is the most common presenting complaint and occurs in 70% of sufferers. This is usually suprapubic, although urethritis, loin pain and dyspareunia are also frequently encountered. A long history of a combination of overactive urinary symptoms (frequency, urgency and dysuria) in the absence of proven infection is often present. Other urinary complaints may coexist. Many of the women have previously undergone hysterectomy, although it is difficult to know if this represents a true relationship or just reflects desperate attempts on the part of the doctor to relieve the patient's symptoms.

Clinical examination is usually unrewarding and the diagnosis is often based on the finding of sensory urgency (painful catheterization, urgency and the absence of a rise in detrusor pressure and a bladder capacity of less than 300 mL) at dual-channel subtracted cystometry. Cystoscopy needs to be undertaken under general anaesthesia in order to obtain a good-sized bladder biopsy. Terminal haematuria at either urodynamic investigation or cystoscopy is suggestive of interstitial cystitis (Fig. 51.32). Characteristically, the cystoscopic findings include petechial haemorrhages on distension, especially second fill, reduced bladder capacity and, classically, although uncommonly, ulceration. There is still confusion due to the lack of conformity in diagnostic parameters commonly used. Bladder capacity in particular is a contentious issue. Hanno [316] states that the bladder capacity must not exceed 350 mL whereas Messing and Stamey [317] demonstrated that the bladder capacity differed significantly between cystoscopies performed under local or no anaesthetic and those performed under general

Table 51.17 Criteria for the exclusion of a diagnosis of interstitial cystitis.

Bladder capacity of >350 mL on awake cystometry

Absence of an intense desire to void at 150 mL during medium-fill cystometry (30–100 mL/min)

Demonstration of phasic involuntary bladder contractions on cystometry

Symptomatology of <9 months' duration

Absence of nocturia

Symptoms relieved by antimicrobials, urinary antiseptics, antimuscarinics or antispasmodics

Urinary diurnal frequency <9 times

A diagnosis of bacterial cystitis within the last 3 months

Bladder calculi

Active genital herpes

Gynaecological malignancy

Urethral diverticulum

Chemical cystitis

Tuberculosis

Radiation cystitis

Bladder tumours

Vaginitis

Age <18 years

anaesthesia, concluding that bladder volumes were not a useful guide to diagnosis. Gillespie [318] states that restricting the maximum bladder capacity excludes patients who may have early interstitial cystitis and may benefit from treatment before an accepted diagnosis can be established. Table 51.17 lists the criteria for excluding a diagnosis of interstitial cystitis.

Treatment

It is likely that the condition we call interstitial cystitis is the final common pathway of a multifactorial disease process, and it is therefore not surprising that many different types of treatment have been proposed (none of which has proved to be completely satisfactory). Both non-steroidal and steroidal anti-inflammatory agents such as azathioprine, sodium chromoglycate and chloroquine have been tried [319]. Sodium pentosanpolysulphate is believed to decrease the bladder wall permeability, and variable success rates have been quoted, from 27% [320] to 83% [321]. It appears to be effective when administered intravesically [322]. Heparin, which is thought to reduce the available cations and have a similar effect to sodium pentosanpolysulphate, has also been employed [315].

Those who prefer an infective hypothesis of causation have employed long-term antibiotics. Norfloxacin can be given 400 mg nightly for 3 months or, alternatively, a bladder antiseptic such as hexamine hippurate may be used.

Dimethylsulphone (DMSO) has also been instilled into the bladder with some success [323]. Many clinicians believe that this gives good symptomatic relief, even if only in the short term, although there are concerns that it may be carcinogenic. Other treatments that have been tried include local anaesthetics, calcium channel blockers and tricyclic antidepressants, which should probably be used as an adjunct to treatment to help to relive pain [316].

Although bladder distension has been used for the treatment of sensory bladder disorders, there is no evidence to support the use of this technique in interstitial cystitis. Short-term benefit may be reported, but repeated distensions can lead to an exacerbation of symptoms. There is still a place for either substitution cystoplasty or urinary diversion in severely affected patients but augmentation cystoplasty is rarely effective as pain continues to be a problem.

Many patients benefit from simple self-help measures [318], and the avoidance of caffeine-containing compounds (tea, coffee and cola). Gillespie [324] has written extensively about the role of diet in the management of interstitial cystitis.

The majority of women who suffer with interstitial cystitis do so for many years until they either find ways of coping with their symptoms or eventually undergo surgery. Fortunately, the symptoms tend to wax and wane and it is often possible to provide support and intermittent therapy until a remission occurs [325].

Sexual problems

Many women develop an urgent desire to pass urine during or immediately after sexual intercourse. This is thought to be caused by the rigid nulliparous perineum, which allows irritation of the posterior bladder wall to occur during intercourse [326]. Postcoital dysuria, commonly known as 'honeymoon cystitis', may be followed by a urinary tract infection. The use of the contraceptive diaphragm may lead to bouts of frequency, urgency and dysuria as well as recurrent urinary tract infections [327]. An alternative method of contraception should be employed. Symptoms of urgency and frequency following sexual intercourse can be helped by simple measures such as perineal hygiene, change of coital technique and voiding a fairly full bladder after sexual intercourse.

For postmenopausal women, failure of adequate lubrication during sexual intercourse may be a problem so a lubricant gel or preferably oestrogen replacement should be prescribed [328]. For those women with a uterus who do not wish to suffer the recurrence of monthly withdrawal bleeds local oestrogen therapy using oestriol pessaries, low-dose sustained-released 17β-oestradiol tablets (Vagifem) or a sustained-release oestradiol-impregnated ring (Estring) may be employed.

Occasionally women who associate attacks of the urethral syndrome with sexual intercourse have a urethral meatus that is situated far back along the anterior vaginal wall where it is vulnerable to trauma during coitus. Symptoms in such women may be relieved by urethrovaginoplasty with freeing and advancement of the urethra or urethrolysis.

For premenopausal women who develop recurrent urinary tract infections associated with sexual intercourse, postcoital antibiotic prophylaxis has been shown to be highly effective. Trimethoprim, nitrofurantoin or cephalexin have all been employed and a more recent highly satisfactory addition is norfloxacin 400 mg taken at around the time of sexual intercourse.

Conclusion

Urinary incontinence is common and, though not life threatening, is known to have a significant effect on QoL. Appropriate investigation and management allows an accurate diagnosis and avoids inappropriate treatment. Although many forms of conservative therapy may be initiated in primary care, continence surgery, and the investigation of more complex and recurrent cases of incontinence, should be performed in specialist secondary and tertiary referral units. Ultimately, an integrated pathway utilizing a multidisciplinary team approach including specialist nurses, continence advisors, physiotherapists, urologists and colorectal surgeons will ensure the best possible outcomes in terms of 'cure' and patient satisfaction.

Appendix: Levels of evidence [329,330]

I   Systematic review of all relevant randomized controlled trials (RCTs)

IIA   One RCT: low probability of bias and high probability of causal relationship

IIB   One RCT

IIIA   Well-designed controlled trials (no randomization)

IIIB   Cohort or case–control studies

IIIC   Multiple time series or dramatic results in uncontrolled experiments

IV   Expert opinion (traditional use)

Grades of recommendations

A   A systematic review of RCTs or a body of evidence consisting principally of studies rated as I directly applicable to the target population and demonstrating overall consistency of results.

B   A body of evidence including studies rated as IIA directly applicable to the target population and demonstrating overall consistency of results *or* Extrapolated evidence from studies rated as I.

C   A body of evidence including studies rated as IIB directly applicable to the target population and demonstrating overall consistency of results *or* Extrapolated evidence from studies rated as II.

D   Evidence level III or IV *or* Extrapolated evidence from studies rated as II.

References

1 Norton P, MacDonald L, Sedgwick P, Stanton SL. Distress and delay associated with urinary incontinence, frequency and urgency in women. *Br Med J* 1988;297:1187–1189.

2 Haylen BT, de Ridder D, Freeman RM *et al*. An International Urogynaecological Association (IUGA)/International Continence Society (ICS) joint report on the terminology for female pelvic floor dysfunction. *Int Urogynaecol J* 2010;21: 5–26.

3 Zacharin R. The suspensory mechanism of the female urethra. *J Anat* 1963;97:423–427.

4 Wilson PD, Dixon JS, Brown ADG, Gosling JA. A study of the pubo-urethral ligament in normal and incontinent women. In: *Proceedings of the 9th International Continence Society Meeting.* Rome, 1979.

5 Gosling JA, Dixon JS, Humpherson JR. *Functional Anatomy of the Lower Urinary Tract.* London: Churchill Livingstone, 1983.

6 DeLancey JOL. Pubovesical ligament: a separate structure from the urethral supports ('pubo-urethral ligaments'). *Neurourol Urodyn* 1989;8:53–61.

7 Khanna OMP. Disorders of micturition: neurophysiological basis and results of drug therapy. *Urology* 1986;8:316–328.

8 Royal College of Physicians. *Incontinence: Causes, management and provision of services.* London, Royal College of Physicians, 1995.

9 Thomas TM, Plymat KR, Blannin J, Meade TW. Prevalence of urinary incontinence. *Br Med J* 1980;281:1243–1245.

10 Hannestad YS, Rortveit G, Sandvik H, Hunskar S. A community-based epidemiological survey of female urinary incontinence: The Norwegian EPINCONT Study. *Clin Epidem* 2000;53:1150–1157.

11 Rortveit G, Hannnestad YS, Daltveit AK, Hunskaar S. Age and type dependent effects of parity on urinary incontinence: the Norwegian EPINCONT study. *Obstet Gynaecol* 2001;98: 1004–1010.

Department of Health (1998) Modernising Health and Social Services; National Priorities Guidance 1999/2000–2001/2002.

12 Smith CP, Chancellor MB. Genitourinary tract patent update. *Exp Opin Ther Patents* 2001;11:17–31.

13 Stewart WF, Corey R, Herzog AR *et al*. Prevalence of overactive bladder in women: results from the NOBLE program. *Int Urogynaecol J* 2001;12:S66.

14 Bump RC. Racial comparisons and contrasts in urinary incontinence and pelvic organ prolapse. *Obstet Gynaecol* 1993;81:421.

15 Viktrup L, Lose G, Rolff M, Farfoed K. The symptom of stress incontinence caused by pregnancy or delivery in primiparas. *Obstet Gynaecol* 1992;79:945.

16 Chairelli P, Brown W, Mcelduff P. Leaking urine: prevalence and associated factors in Australian women. *Neurourol Urodyn* 1999;18:567.

17 Hojerberg KE, Salvig JD, Winslow NA, Lose G, Secher NJ. Urinary incontinence; prevalence and risk factors at 16 weeks of gestation. *Br J Obstet Gynaecol* 1999;106:842.

18 Kelleher CJ, Cardozo LD, Khullar V, Salvatore S. A new questionnaire to assess the quality of life of urinary incontinent women. *Br J Obstet Gynaecol* 1997;104:1374–1379.

19 Fitzpatrick R, Fletcher A, Gore S, Jones D, Spiegelhalter D, Cox D. Quality of life measures in healthcare. 1: Applications and issues in assessment. *Br Med J* 1992;305:1075–1077.

20 Burgio KL, Matthews KA, Engel BT. Prevalence, incidence and correlates of urinary incontinence in healthy, middle-aged women. *J Urol* 1991;146:1255–1259.

21 World Health Organization. *Definition of health from preamble to the constitution of the WHO basic documents*, 28th edn. Geneva: WHO, 1978, p. 1.

22 Coulter A. Measuring quality of life. In: AL Kinmouth, R Jones (eds) *Critical Reading in General Practice.* Oxford: Oxford University Press, 1993.

23 Naughton MJ, Shumaker SA. Assessment of health related quality of life. In: CD Furberg, DL DeMets (eds) *Fundamentals of Clinical Trials*, 3rd edn. St Louis: Mosby Press, 1996, p. 185.

24 Gill TM, Feinstein AR. A critical appraisal of the quality of life measurements. *JAMA* 1974;272:619–626.

25 Murawaski BJ. Social support in health and illness; the concept and its measurement. *Ca Nurs* 1978;1:365–371.

26 Blavis JG, Appell RA, Fantl JA *et al*. Standards of efficacy for evaluation of treatment outcomes in urinary incontinence: recommendations of the urodynamics society. *Neurourol Urodynam* 1997;16:145–147.

27 Staskin D, Kelleher C, Avery K *et al*. Patient-reported outcome assessment. In: P Abrams, L Cardozo, S Khoury, A Wein (eds)

Incontinence, 4th edn. Paris: Health Publication Ltd, Editions 21, 2009. pp. 363–412.

28 Lyons RA, Perry HM, Littlepage BNC. Evidence for the validity of the short form 36 questionnaire (SF-36) in an elderly population. *Age Ageing* 1994;23:182–184.

29 Hunskaar S, Vinsnes A. The quality of life in women with urinary incontinence as measured by the sickness impact profile. *J Am Geriatric Soc* 1991;39:378–382.

30 Grimby A, Milsom I, Molander U, Wiklund I, Ekelund P. The influence of urinary incontinence on the quality of life of elderly women. *Age Ageing* 1993;22:82–89.

31 Sullivan M, Karlsson J, Bengtsson C, Furunes B, Lapidus L, Lissner L. The Goteberg Quality of life instrument – a psychometric evaluation of assessments of symptoms and well being among women in a general population. *Scand J Prim Health Care* 1993;11:267–275.

32 Shumaker SA, Wyman JF, Uebersax JS, McClish D, Fantl JA. Health related quality of life measures for women with urinary incontinence: the Incontinence Impact Questionnaire and the urogenital distress inventory. *Qual Life Res* 1994;3: 291–306.

33 Uebersax JS, Wyman JF, Shumaker SA, McClish DK, Fantl AJ. Short forms to assess life quality and symptom distress for urinary incontinence in women; The incontinence impact questionnaire and the urogenital distress inventory. *Neuourol Urodynam* 1995;14:131–139.

34 Lubeck DP, Prebil LA, Peebles P, Brown JS. A health related quality of life measure for use in patients with urge urinary incontinence: a validation study. *Qual Life Res* 1999;8: 337–344.

35 Sandvik H, Hunskaar S, Seim A, Hermstad R, Vanik A, Bratt H. Validation of a severity index in female urinary incontinence and its implementation in an epidemiological survey. *J Epidemio Commun Health Med* 1993;47:497–499.

36 Wagner TH, Patrick DL, Bavendam TG, Martin ML, Buesching DP. Quality of life of persons with urinary incontinence: development of a new measure. *Urology* 1996;47:67–72.

37 Wyman JF, Harkins SW, Taylor JR, Fantl JA. Psychosocial impact of urinary incontinence in women. *Obstet Gynaecol* 1987;70:378–381.

38 Milsom I, Abrams P, Cardozo L, Roberts RG, Thuroff J, Wein AJ. How widespread are the symptoms of overactive bladder and how are they managed? A population-based prevalence study. *BJU Int* 2001;87:760–766.

39 Jarvis GJ, Hall S, Stamp S, Miller DR, Johnson A. An assessment of urodynamic examination in incontinent women. *Br J Obstet Gynaecol* 1980;87:893–896.

40 Cutner A. Uroflowmetry. In: Cardozo L (ed.) *Urogynaecology*. London: Churchill Livingstone, 1997: 109–116.

41 Verbrugge LM. Health diaries. *Med Care* 1980;18:73.

42 Larsson G, Victor A. Micturition patterns in a healthy female population studied with a frequency volume chart. *Scan J Urol Nephrol Suppl* 1988;4:53–57.

43 Barnick C. Frequency/volume charts. In: L Cardozo (ed.) *Urogynaecology*. London: Churchill Livingstone, 1997, pp. 101–107.

44 Cutner A. Uroflowmetry. In: L Cardozo (ed.) *Urogynaecology*. London: Churchill Livingstone, 1997, pp. 109–116.

45 Benness C. Cystometry. In: Cardozo L (ed.) *Urogynaecology*. London: Churchill Livingstone, 1997: 117–134.

46 Hilton P, Stanton SL. Urethral pressure measurement by microtransducer: the results in symptom free women and in those with genuine stress incontinence. *Br J Obstet Gynaecol* 1983;90:919–933.

47 Versi E, Cardozo LD. Symptoms and urethral pressure profilometry for the diagnosis of genuine stress incontinence. *J Obstet Gynaecol* 1988;9:168–169.

48 Versi E. Discriminant analysis of urethral pressure profilometry data for the diagnosis of genuine stress incontinence. *Br J Obstet Gynaecol* 1990;97:251–259.

49 Haylen BT. Residual urine volumes in a normal female population: application of transvaginal ultrasound. *Br J Urol* 1989;64:347–349.

50 Khullar V, Salvatore S, Cardozo LD, Hill S, Kelleher CJ. Ultrasound bladder wall measurement: a non-invasive sensitive screening test for detrusor instability. *Neurourol Urodyn* 1994;13:461–462.

51 Robinson D, Anders K, Cardozo L, Bidmead J, Toozs-Hobson P, Khullar V. Can ultrasound replace ambulatory urodynamics when investigating women with irritative urinary symptoms? *Br J Obstet Gynaecol* 2002;109:145–148.

52 Richmond DH, Sutherst JR. Clinical application of transrectal ultrasound for the investigation of the incontinent patient. *Br J Urol* 1989;63:605–609.

53 Gordon D, Pearce M, Norton P, Stanton SL. Comparison of ultrasound and lateral chain urethrocystography in the determination of bladder neck descent. *Am J Obstet Gynecol* 1989;160:182–185.

54 Khullar V, Salvatore S, Cardozo LD, Hill S, Kelleher CJ. Three dimensional ultrasound of the urethra and urethral sphincter: a new diagnostic technique. *Neurourol Urodyn* 1994;13: 352–354.

55 Robinson D, Toozs-Hobson P, Cardozo L, Digesu A. Correlating structure and function; three-dimensional ultrasound of the urethral sphincter. *Ultrasound Obstet Gynaecol* 2004;23: 272–276.

56 Athanasiou S, Hill S, Cardozo LD, Khullar V, Anders K. Three dimensional ultrasound of the urethra, peri-urethral tissues and pelvic floor. *Int Urogynecol J* 1995;6:239.

57 Klukte C, Golomb J, Barbaric Z, Raz S. The anatomy of stress incontinence; magnetic resonance imaging of the female bladder neck and urethra. *J Urol* 1990;143:563–566.

58 Yang A, Mostwin JL, Rosenheim NB, Zerhouni EA. Pelvic floor descent in women: dynamic evaluation with fast magnetic resonance imaging and cinematic display. *Radiology* 1991;179:25–33.

59 Smith ARB, Hosker GL, Warrell DW. The role of pudendal nerve damage in the aetiology of genuine stress incontinence in women. *Br J Obstet Gynaecol* 1989;96:29–32.

60 van Waalwijk van Doorn ESC, Zwiers W, Wetzels LLRH, Debruyne FMJ. A comparative study between standard and ambulatory urodynamics. *Neurourol Urodyn* 1987;6: 159–160.

61 Heslington K, Hilton P. Ambulatory urodynamic monitoring. *Br J Obstet Gynaecol* 1996;103:393–399.

62 Robertson AS, Griffiths CJ, Ramsden PD, Neal DE. Bladder function in healthy volunteers: ambulatory monitoring and conventional urodynamic studies. *Br J Urol* 1994;73:242–249.

63 Salvatore S, Khullar V, Cardozo L, Anders K, Zocchi G, Soligo M. Evaluating ambulatory urodynamics: a prospective study

in asymptomatic women. *Br J Obstet Gynaecol* 2001;108: 107–111.

64 Cardozo LD, Khullar V, Anders K, Hill S. Ambulatory urodynamics: a useful urogynaecological service? *Proceedings of the 27th British Congress of Obstetrics and Gynaecology*. London: RCOG, 1995, p. 404.

65 Anders K, Khullar V, Cardozo L *et al.* Ambulatory urodynamic monitoring in clinical urogynaecological practice. *Neurourol Urodyn* 1997;5:510–512.

66 Gorton E, Stanton S. Ambulatory urodynamics: do they help clinical management? *Br J Obstet Gynaecol* 2000;107: 316–319.

67 Snooks SJ, Swash M, Setchell M, Henry MM. Injury to innervation of the pelvic floor sphincter musculature in childbirth. *Lancet* 1984;ii:546–560.

68 Snooks SJ, Swash M, Henry MM, Setchell M. Risk factors in childbirth causing damage to the pelvic floor innervation. *Int J Colorect Dis* 1986;1:20–21.

69 Allen RE, Hosker GL, Smith ARB, Warrell DW. Pelvic floor damage and childbirth: a neurophysiological study. *Br J Obstet Gynaecol* 1990;97:770–779.

70 Tetzschuer T, Sorensen M, Lose G, Christiansen J. Pudendal nerve recovery after a non-instrumental vaginal delivery. *Int Urogynecol J* 1996;7:102–104.

71 Snooks SJ, Swash M, Mathers SE, Henry MM. Effects of vaginal delivery on the pelvic floor: a five year follow-up. *Br J Surg* 1990;77:1358–1360.

72 Sultan A, Stanton SL. Preserving the pelvic floor and perineum during childbirth – elective caesarean section? *Br J Obstet Gynaecol* 1996;103:731–734.

73 Petros P, Ulmsten U. An integral theory of female urinary incontinence. Experimental and clinical considerations. *Acta Obstet Gynaecol Scand* 1990;153(Suppl):7–31.

74 Ingelman-Sundberg A. Urinary incontinence in women, excluding fistulas. *Acta Obstet Gynaecol Scand* 1953;31: 266–295.

75 Westbury M, Asmussen M, Ulmsten U. Location of maximal intraurethral pressure related to urogenital diaphragm in the female subject as studied by simultaneous urethra-cystometry and voiding urethrocystography. *Am J Obstet Gynaecol* 1982;144:408–412.

76 Cardozo LD, Stanton SL. Genuine stress incontinence and detrusor instability – a review of 200 cases. *Br J Obstet Gynaecol* 1980;87:184–190.

77 Haylen BT, Sutherst JR, Frazer MI. Is the investigation of most stress incontinence really necessary? *Br J Urol* 1989;64: 147–149.

78 Tapp A, Cardozo LD, Hills B, Barnick C. Who benefits from physiotherapy? *Neurourol Urodyn* 1988;7:259–261.

79 Kegel AH. Progressive resistance exercise in the functional restoration of the perineal muscles. *Am J Obstet Gynaecol* 1948;56:238–249.

80 Bo K. Pelvic floor muscle training is effective in treatment of female stress urinary incontinence, but how does it work? *Int Urogynaecol J Pelvic Floor Dysfunct* 2004;15:76–84.

81 DeLancey JOL. Anatomy and mechanics of structures around the vesical neck: how vesical position may affect its closure. *Neurourol Urodyn* 1988;7:161–162.

82 Bo K, Larsen S, Oseid S, Kvarstein B, Hagen RH. Knowledge about and ability to correct pelvic floor muscle exercises in

women wit urinary stress incontinence. *Neurourol Urodyn* 1988;7:261–262.

83 Miller JM, Ashton Miller JA, DeLancey JOL. A pelvic muscle precontraction can reduce cough-related urine loss in selected women with mild SUI. *J Am Geriatric Soc* 1998;46:870–871.

84 Bo K, Talseth T, Holme I. Single blind, randomised controlled trial of pelvic floor muscles exercises, electrical stimulation, vaginal cones and no treatment in management of genuine stress incontinence in women. *Br Med J* 1999;318:487–493.

85 Bernstein IT. The pelvic floor muscles: muscle thickness in healthy and urinary incontinent women measured by perineal ultrasonography with reference to the effect of pelvic floor training. Oestrogen receptor studies. *Neurourol Urodyn* 1997;16:237–275.

86 Bo K, Hagen RH, Kvarstein B, Jorgensen J, Larsen S. Pelvic floor muscle exercise for the treatment of female stress urinary incontinence. III: Effects of two different degrees of pelvic floor muscle exercise. *Neurourol Urodyn* 1990;9:489–502.

87 Burgio KL, Robinson JC, Engel BT. The role of biofeedback in Kegel exercise training for stress urinary incontinence. *Am J Obstet Gynacol* 1986;154:58–63.

88 Plevnik S. New methods for testing and strengthening the pelvic floor muscles. In: *Proceedings of the 15th Annual Meeting of the International Continence Society*. London, 1985, pp. 267–268.

89 Peattie AB, Plevnik S, Stanton SL. Vaginal cones: a conservative method of treating genuine stress incontinence. *Br J Obstet Gynaecol* 1988;95:1049–1053.

90 Olah KS, Bridges N, Denning J, Farrar D. The conservative management of patients with symptoms of stress incontinence: a randomised prospective study comparing weighted vaginal cones and interferential therapy. *Am J Obstet Gynecol* 1990;162:87–92.

91 Haken J, Benness CJ, Cardozo LD, Cutner A. A randomised trial of vaginal cones and pelvic floor exercises in the management of genuine stress incontinence. *Neurourol Urodyn* 1991;10:393–394.

92 Kato K, Kondo A, Hasegalera S *et al.* Pelvic floor muscle training as treatment of stress incontinence. The effectiveness of vaginal cones. *Jpn J Urol* 1992;83:498–504.

93 Bo K. Vaginal weighted cones. Theoretical framework, effect on pelvic floor muscle strength and female stress urinary incontinence. *Acta Obstet Gynaecol Scand* 1995;74:87–92.

94 Sand PK, Richardson DA, Staskin DR *et al.* Pelvic floor stimulation in the treatment of geuine stress incontinence: a multicentre placebo controlled trial. *Neurorol Urodyn* 1994;13: 356–357.

95 Berghmans LC, Hendricks HJ, Bo K, Hay-Smith EJ, de Bie RA, van Waalwijk van Doorn ES. Conservative treatment of stress incontinence in women. A systematic review of randomised review of randomised clinical trials. *Br J Urol* 1998;82: 181–191.

96 Thyssen H, Lose G. Long term efficacy and safety of a vaginal device in the treatment of stress incontinence. *Neurourol Urodyn* 1996;15:394–395.

97 Thyssen H, Bidmead J, Lose G, Moller Bek K, Dwyer P, Cardozo L. A new intravaginal device for stress incontinence in women. *BJU Int* 2001;88:889–892.

98 Thor KB, Katofiasc MA. Effects of Duloxetine, a combined serotonin and norepinephrine reuptake inhibitor, on

central neural control of lower urinary tract function in the chloralose-anesthetised female cat. *Pharmacol Exp Ther* 1995; 74:1014–1024.

99 Norton PA, Zinner NR, Yalcin I, Bump RC, Duloxetine Urinary Incontinence Study Group. Duloxetine versus placebo in the treatment of stress urinary incontinence. *Am J Obstet Gynaecol* 2002;187:40–48.

100 Millard R, Moore K, Yalcin I, Bump R. Duloxetine vs. placebo in the treatment of stress urinary incontinence: a global phase III study. *Neurourol Urodynam* 2003;22:482–483.

101 Cardozo L, Drutz HP, Baygani SK, Bump RC. Pharmacological treatment of women awaiting surgery for stress urinary incontinence. *Obstet Gynaecol* 2004;104:511–519.

102 Ghoniem GM, Van Leeuwen JS, Elser DM, Freeman RM, Zhao YD, Yalcin I, Bump RC and Duloxetine/Pelvic Floor Muscle Training Clinical Trial Group. A randomised controlled trial of duloxetine alone, pelvic floor muscle training alone, combined treatment and no active treatment in women with stress urinary incontinence. *Urol* 2005;173:1453–1454.

103 Stanton SL, Tanagho E. *Surgery of Female Incontinence*, 2nd edn. Berlin: Springer-Verlag, 1986.

104 Hilton P. Which operation for which patient? In: J Drife, P Hilton, SL Stanton (eds) *Micturition*. Berlin: Springer-Verlag, 1990.

105 Burch J. Urethrovaginal fixation to Cooper's ligament for correction of stress incontinence, cystocele and prolapse. *Am J Obstet Gynaecol* 1961;81:281.

106 Cardozo LD, Stanton SL, Williams JE. Detrusor instability following surgery for stress incontinence. *Br J Urol* 1979;58: 138–142.

107 Wiskind AK, Creighton SM, Stanton SL. The incidence of genital prolapse following the Burch colposuspension operation. *Neurourol Urodyn* 1991;10:453–454.

108 Alcalay M, Monga A, Stanton SL. Burch colposuspension: 10–20 year follow-up. *Br J Obstet Gynaecol* 1995;102:740–745.

109 Liu CY. Laparoscopic retropubic colposuspension (Burch procedure): a review of 58 cases. *J Reprod Med* 1993;38:526–530.

110 Burton G. A randomised comparison of laparoscopic and open colposuspension. *Neurourol Urodyn* 1994;13:497–498.

111 Su T, Wang K, Hsu C, Wei H, Hong B. Prospective comparison of laparoscopic and traditional colposuspension in the treatment of genuine stress incontinence. *Acta Obstet Gynecol Scand* 1997;76:576–582.

112 Carey MP, Goh JT, Rosamilia A *et al.* Laparoscopic versus open Burch colposuspension: a randomised controlled trial. *BJOG* 2006;113:999–1006.

113 Kitchener HC, Dunn G, Lawton V, Reid F, Nelson L, Smith ARB on behalf of the COLPO study group. Laparoscopic versus open colposuspension – results of a prospective randomised controlled trial. *BJOG* 2006;113:1007–1013.

114 Dumville JC, Manca A, Kitchener HC, Smith ARB, Nelson L, Torgerson DJ, on behalf of the COLPO study group. Cost effectiveness analysis of open colposuspension versus laparoscopic colposuspension in the treatment of urodynamic stress incontinence. *BJOG* 2006;113:1014–1022.

115 Ulmsten U, Henriksson L, Johnson P, Varhos G. An ambulatory surgical procedure under local anesthetic for treatment of female urinary incontinence. *Int Urogynaecol J* 1996;7:81–86.

116 Nilsson CG. Tension free vaginal tape procedure for treatment of female urinary stress incontinence. In: L Cardozo, D Staskin

(eds) *Textbook of Female Urology and Urogynaecology*. Informa Healthcare: Abingdon, UK, 2006:917–923.

117 Ulmsten U, Falconer C, Johnson P, Jones M *et al.* A multicentre study of Tension Free Vaginal Tape (TVT) for surgical treatment of stress urinary incontinence. *Int Urogynecol J* 1998;9: 210–213.

118 Ulmsten U, Johnson P, Rezapour M. A three year follow up of tension free vaginal tape for surgical treatment of female stress urinary incontinence. *BJOG* 1999;106:345–350.

119 Nilsson CG, Kuuva N, Falconer C *et al.* Long term results of the tension free vaginal tape (TVT) procedure for surgical treatment of female stress urinary incontinence. *Int Urogynaecol J* 2001;12(Suppl):5–8.

120 Nilsson CG, Falconer C, Rezapour M. Seven year follow up of the tension free vaginal tape procedure for the treatment of urinary incontinence. *Obstet Gynaecol* 2004;104:1259–1262.

121 Nilsson CG, Palva K, Rezapour M, Falconer C. Eleven years prospective follow up of the tension free vaginal tape procedure for the treatment of stress urinary incontinence. *Int Urogynaecol J Pelvic Floor Dysfunct* 2008;19:1043–1047.

122 Ward K, Hilton P & United Kingdom and Ireland Tension Free Vaginal Tape Trial Group. Prospective multicentre randomized trial of tension free vaginal tape and colposuspension as primary treatment for stress incontinence. *BMJ* 2002; 325:67.

123 Ward KL, Hilton P and UK and Ireland TVT Trial Group. A prospective multicentre randomized trial of tension free vaginal tape and colposuspension for primary urodynamic stress incontinence: two-year follow up. *Am J Obstet Gyanecol* 2004;190:324–331.

124 Ward K, Hilton P. Multicentre randomized trial of tension free vaginal tape and colposuspension for primary urodynamic stress incontinence: five year follow up. *Neurourol Urodynam* 2006;6:568–569.

125 Manca A, Sculpher MJ, Ward K, Hilton P. A cost utility analysis of tension free vaginal tape versus colposuspension for primary urodynamic stress incontinence. *BJOG* 2003;110: 255–262.

126 Paraiso MF, Walters MD, Karram MM, Barber MD (2004) Laparoscopic Burch colposuspension versus tension free vaginal tape: a randomised trial. *Obstet Gyanecol* 2004;104: 1249–1258.

127 Staskin DR, Tyagi R. The SPARC sling system. *Atlas Urol Clinic* 2004;12:185–195.

128 Deval B, Levardon M, Samain E, Rafii A, Cortesse A, Amarenco G, Ciofu C, Haab F. A French multicentre clinical trial of SPARC for stress urinary incontinence. *Eur Urol* 2003;44: 254–258.

129 Lord HE, Taylor JD, Finn JC, Tsokos N, Jeffery JT, Atherton MJ, Evans SF, Bremner AP, Elder GO, Holman CD. A randomised controlled equivalence trial of short term complications and efficacy of tension free vaginal tape and suprapubic urethral support sling for treating stress incontinence. *BJU Int* 2006;98:367–376.

130 Delorme E. [Transobturator urethral suspension: mini-invasive procedure in the treatment of stress urinary incontinence in women.] *Prog Urol* 2001;11:1306–1313.

131 Whiteside JL, Walters MD. Anatomy of the obturator region: relations to a transobturator sling. *Int Urogynaecol J Pelvic Floor Dysfunct* 2004;15:223–226.

132 Costa P, Grise P, Droupy S *et al*. Surgical treatment of female stress urinary incontinence with a transobturator tape (TOT). Uratape: short term results of a prospective multicentric study. *Eur Urol* 2004;46:102–106.

133 Delorme E, Droupy S, De Tayrac R *et al*. Transobturator tape (Uratape): a new minimally invasive procedure to treat female urinary incontinence. *Eur Urol* 2004;45:203–207.

134 Meschia M, Pifarotti P, Bernasconi F, Baccichet R, Magatti F, Cortese P, Caria M, Bertozzi R. Multicentre randomised trial of tension free vaginal tape (TVT) and transobturator tape in out technique (TVT-O) for the treatment of stress urinary incontinence. *Int Urogynaecol J Pelvic Floor Dysfunct* 2006;17: S92–S93.

135 Laurikainen EH, Valpas A, Kiiholma P *et al*. A prospective randomised trial comparing TVT and TVT-O procedures for treatment of SUI: immediate outcome and complications. *Int Urogynaecol J Pelvic Floor Dysfunct* 2006;17:S104–S105.

136 Latthe PM, Foon R, Toozs-Hobson P. Transobturator and retropubic tape procedures in stress urinary incontinence: a systematic review and meta-analysis of effectiveness and complications. *BJOG* 2007;114:522–531.

137 Waltregny D, Gaspar Y, Reul O, Hamida W, Bonnet P, de Leval J. TVT-O for the treatment of female stress urinary incontinence: results of a prospective study after a 3 year minimum follow up. *Eur Urol* 2008;53:401–408.

138 Martan A, Masata J, Svabik K. TVT-Secur system – tension free support of the urethra in women suffering from stress urinary incontinence – technique and initial experience. *Ceska Gynecol* 2007;72:42–49.

139 Meschia M, Barbacini P, Ambroqi V, Pifarotti P, Ricci L, Spreafico L. TVT-Secur: a minimally invasive procedure for the treatment of primary stress urinary incontinence. One year data from a multicentre prospective trial. *Int Urogynecol J Pelvic Floor Dysfunct* 2009;20:313–317.

140 Debodinance P, Lagrange E, Amblard J, Yahi H, Lucot J, Cosson M, Villet R, Jacquetin B. TVT-Secur: Prospective study and follow up to 1 year about 150 patients. *Urogynecol J Pelvic Floor Dysfunct* 2008;19:S11–S12.

141 Molden SM, Lucente VR. New minimally invasive slings: TVT-Secur. *Curr Urol Rep* 2008;9:358–361.

142 Vervest H, van Dessel N, Lammerink E, Hinoul P, Roovers J. TVT-Secur: The learning curve. *Urogynecol J Pelvic Floor Dysfunct* 2008;19:S3–S4.

143 Pereyra A. A simplified surgical procedure for the correction of stress incontinence in women. *West J Surg* 1959;67:223.

144 Stamey T. Endoscopic suspension of the vesical neck for urinary incontinence. *Surg Gynecol Obstet* 1973;136:547–554.

145 Raz S. Modified bladder neck suspension for female stress incontinence. *Urology* 1981;17:82.

146 Appell RA. New developments: injectables for urethral incompetence in women. *Int Urogynaecol* 1990;1:117–119.

147 Harris DR, Iacovou JW, Lemberger RJ. Peri-urethral silicone micro implants (Macroplastiqie) for the treatment of genuine stress incontinence. *Br J Urol* 1996;78:722–728.

148 Khullar V, Cardozo LD, Abbot D, Anders K. GAX collagen in the treatment of urinary incontinence in elderly women: a 2 year follow-up. *Br J Obstet Gynaecol* 1997;104:96–99.

149 Stanton SL, Monga AK. Incontinence in elderly women: is periurethral collagen an advance? *Br J Obstet Gynaecol* 1997; 104:154–157.

150 Ghoniem G, Bernhard P, Corcos J *et al*. Multicentre randomised controlled trial to evaluate Macroplastique urethral bulking agent for the treatment of female stress urinary incontinence. *Int Urogynaecol J* 2005;16: S129–S130.

151 Scott FB, Bradley WE, Tim G. Treatment of urinary incontinence by implantable prosthetic sphincter. *Urology* 1973;1:252.

152 NICE Guideline 40. *The Management of Urinary Incontinence in Women*. London: Department of Health, 2006. Available at: www.nice.org.uk.

153 Anderson KE. The overactive bladder: pharmacologic basis of drug treatment. *Urology* 1997;50:74–89.

154 Hashim H, Abrams P. Is the bladder a reliable witness for predicting detrusor overactivity? *J Urol* 2006;175:191–195.

155 Caulfield MP, Birdsall NJ. International Union of Pharmacology XVII. Classification of muscarinic acetylcholine receptors. *Pharmacol Rev* 1998;50:279.

156 Yamaguchi O, Shisida K, Tamura K *et al*. Evaluation of mRNAs encoding muscarinic receptor subtypes in human detrusor muscle. *J Urol* 1996;156:1208.

157 Harris DR, Marsh KA, Birmingham AT *et al*. Expression of muscarinic M_3 receptors coupled to inositol phospholipid hydrolysis in human detrusor cultured smooth muscle cells. *J Urol* 1995;154:1241.

158 Hedge SS, Chopin A, Bonhaus D *et al*. Functional role of M_2 and M_3 muscarinic receptors in the urinary bladder of rats *in vitro* and *in vivo*. *Br J Pharmacol* 1997;120:1409.

159 Hegde SS, Eglen RM. Muscarinic receptor subtypes modulating smooth muscle contractility in the urinary bladder. *Life Sci* 1999;64:419.

160 Braverman AS, Ruggieri MR. The M_2 receptor contributes to contraction of the denervated rat urinary bladder. *Am J Physiol* 1998;275:1654.

161 Burnstock G. Purinergic signaling in lower urinary tract. In: Abbracchio MP, Williams M (eds) *Purinergic and Pyrimidinergic Signalling I: Molecular, Nervous and Urogenitary System Function*. Berlin: Springer, 2001:423–515.

162 Abrams P. Detrusor instability and bladder outlet obstruction. *Neurourol Urodyn* 1985;4:317.

163 Gosling JA. Decrease in the autonomic innervation of human detrusor muscle in outflow obstruction. *J Urol* 1986;136: 501–504.

164 Harrison SC, Hunnam GR, Farman P *et al*. Bladder instability and denervation in patients with bladder outflow obstruction. *Br J Urol* 1987;60:519–522.

165 Van Koeveringe GA, Mostwin JL, van Mastrigt R *et al*. Effect of partial urethral obstruction on force development of the guinea pig bladder. *Neurourol Urodyn* 1993;12:555–556.

166 Seki N, Karim OM, Mostwin JL. The effect of experimental urethral obstruction and its reversal on changes in passive electrical properties of detrusor muscle. *J Urol* 1992;148: 1957–1961.

167 Steers WD, De Groat WC. Effect of bladder outlet obstruction on micturition reflex pathways in the rat. *J Urol* 1988;140: 864–871.

168 Steers WD, Kolbeck S, Creedon D *et al*. Nerve growth factor in the urinary bladder of the adult regulates neuronal form and function. *J Clin Invest* 1991;88:1709–1715.

169 Ishizuka O, Igawa Y, Lecci A *et al*. Role of intrathecal tachykinins for micturition in unanaesthetised rats with and without bladder outlet obstruction. *Br J Pharmacol* 1994;113:111–116.

170 Kinder RB, Mundy AR. Pathophysiology of idiopathic overactive bladder and detrusor hyperreflexia – an *in vitro* study of human detrusor muscle. *Br J Urol* 1987;60:509–515.

171 Eaton AC, Bates CP. An *in vitro* physiological study of normal and unstable human detrusor muscle. *Br J Urol* 1982;54:653–657.

172 Sibley GN. Developments in our understanding of overactive bladder. *Br J Urol* 1997;80:54–61.

173 Sibley GNA. An experimental model of overactive bladder in the obstructed pig. *Br J Urol* 1985;57:292–298.

174 Speakman MJ, Brading AF, Gilpin CJ, Dixon JS, Gilpin SA, Gosling JA. Bladder outflow obstruction – cause of denervation supersensitivity. *J Urol* 1987;183:1461–1466.

175 Wise BG, Cardozo LD, Cutner A, Benness CJ, Burton G. The prevalence and significance of urethral instability in women with overactive bladder. *Br J Urol* 1993;72:26–29.

176 Sutherst JR, Brown M. The effect on the bladder pressure of sudden entry of fluid into the posterior urethra. *Br J Urol* 1978;50:406–409.

177 Brading AF, Turner WH. The unstable bladder: towards a common mechanism. *Br J Urol* 1994;73:3–8.

178 Brading AF. A myogenic basis for the overactive bladder. *Urology* 1997;50:57–67.

179 Mills IW, Greenland JE, McMurray G, *et al.* 2000 Studies of the pathophysiology of idiopathic overactive bladder: the physiological properties of the detrusor smooth muscle and its pattern of innervation. *J Urol* 2000;163:646–651.

180 Charlton RG, Morley AR, Chambers P, Gillespie JI. Focal changes in nerve, muscle and connective tissue in normal and unstable human bladder. *BJU Int* 1999;84:953–960.

181 Ferguson DR, Kennedy I, Burton TJ. ATP is released from rabbit urinary bladder epithelial cells by hydrostatic pressure changes – a possible sensory mechanism? *J Physiol* 1997;505:503–511.

182 Maggi CA. Prostanoids as local modulators of reflex micturition. *Pharmacol Res* 1992;25:13–20.

183 Birder LA. Adrenergic and capsaicin evoked nitric oxide release from urothelium and afferent nerves in urinary bladder. *Am J Physiol* 1998;275:F226–F229.

184 Andersson KE. Bladder activation: afferent mechanisms. *Urology* 2002;59:43–50.

185 Silva C, Ribero MJ, Cruz F. The effect of intravesical Resiniferatoxin in patients with idiopathic detrusor instability suggests that involuntary detrusor contractions are triggered by C-fibre input. *J Urol* 2002;168:575–579.

186 Jarvis GJ, Millar DR. Controlled trial of bladder drill for detrusor instability. *Br Med J* 1980;281:1322–1323.

187 Frewen WK. Bladder training in general practice. *Practitioner* 1982;266:1874–1879.

188 Jarvis GJ. The management of urinary incontinence due to vesical sensory urgency by bladder drill. In: *Proceedings of the 11th Annual Meeting of the International Continence Society.* Lund, 1981, pp. 123–124.

189 Kelleher CJ, Cardozo LD, Khullar V, Salvatore S. A medium-term analysis of the subjective efficency of treatment for women with detrusor instability and low bladder compliance. *Br J Obstet Gynaecol* 1997;104:988–993.

190 Waldeck K, Larsson B, Andersson KE. Comparison of oxybutynin and it's active metabolite, N-desmethyl-oxybutynin, in the human detrusor and parotid gland. *J Urol* 1997;157:1093–1097.

191 Hughes KM, Lang JCT, Lazare R *et al.* Measurement of oxybutynin and its N-desethyl meatbolite in plasma, and its application to pharmacokinetic studies in young, elderly and frail elderly volunteers. *Xenobiotica* 1992;22:859–869.

192 Nilvebrant L, Andersson KE, Mattiasson A. Characterization of the muscarinic cholinoreceptors in the human detrusor. *J Urol* 1985;134:418–423.

193 Nilvebrant L, Sparf B. Dicyclomine, benzhexol and oxybutynin distinguish between subclasses of muscarinic binding sites. *Eur J Pharmacol* 1986;123:133–143.

194 Cardozo LD, Cooper D, Versi E. Oxybutynin chloride in the management of idiopathic detrusor instability. *Neurourol Urodyn* 1987;6:256–257.

195 Moore KH, Hay DM, Imrie AE, Watson A, Goldstein M. Oxybutynin hydrochloride (3 mg) in the treatment of women with idiopathic detrusor instability. *Br J Urol* 1990;66:479–485.

196 Tapp AJS, Cardozo LD, Versi E, Cooper D. The treatment of detrusor instability in post menopausal women with oxybutynin chloride: a double blind placebo-controlled study. *Br J Obstet Gynaecol* 1990;97:479–485.

197 Baigrie RJ, Kelleher JP, Fawcett DP, Pengelly AW. Oxybutynin: is it safe? *Br J Urol* 1988;62:319–322.

198 Weese DL, Roskamp DA, Leach GE, Zimmern PE. Intravesical oxybutynin chloride: experience with 42 patients. *Urology* 1993;41:527–530.

199 Collas D, Malone-Lee JG. The pharmacokinetic properties of rectal oxybutynin – a possible alternative to intravesical administration. *Neurourol Urodyn* 1997;16:533–542.

200 Anderson RU, Mobley D, Blank B, Saltzstein D, Susset J, Brown JS. Once daily controlled versus immediate release oxybutynin chloride for urge urinary incontinence. OROS Oxybutynin Study Group. *J Urol* 1999;161:1809–1812.

201 Gleason DM, Susset J, White C, Munoz DR, Sand PK. Evaluation of a new once-daily formulation of oxybutynin for the treatment of urinary urge incontinence. Ditropan XL Study Group. *Urology* 1999;54:420–423.

202 Dmochowski RR, Sand PK, Zinner NR, Gittelman MC, Davila GW, Sanders SW, Transdermal Oxybutynin Study Group. Comparative efficacy and safety of transdermal oxybutynin and oral tolterodine versus placebo in previously treated patients with urge and mixed urinary incontinence. *Urology* 2003;62:237–242.

203 Staskin DR, Dmochowski RR, Sand PK *et al.* Efficacy and safety of oxybutynin chloride topical gel for overactive bladder: a randomised, double blind, placebo controlled, multicentre study. *J Urol* 2009;181:1764–1772.

204 Haruno A, Yamasaki Y, Miyoshi K *et al.* (1989) Effects of propiverine hydrochloride and its metabolites on isolated guinea pig urinary bladder. *Folia Pharmacol Jpn* 94:145–150.

205 Mazur D, Wehnert J, Dorschner W, Schubert G, Herfurth G, Alken RG. Clinical and urodynamic effects of propiverine in patients suffering from urgency and urge incontinence. *Scand J Urol Nephrol* 1995;29:289–294.

206 Stoher M, Madersbacher H, Richter R, Wehnert J, Dreikorn K. Efficacy and safety of propiverine in SCI-patients suffer-

ing from detrusor hyperreflexia: a double-blind, placebo-controlled clinical trial. *Spinal Cord* 1999;37:196–200.

207 Ruscin JM, Morgenstern NE. Tolterodine use for symptoms of overactive bladder. *Ann Pharmacother* 1999;33:1073–1082.

208 Nilvebrant L, Andersson K-E, Gillberg P-G, Stahl M, Sparf B. Tolterodine – a new bladder selective antimuscarinic agent. *Eur J Pharmacol* 1997;327:195–207.

209 Nilvebrant L, Hallen B, Larsson G. Tolterodine – a new bladder selective muscarinic receptor antagonist: preclinical pharmacological and clinical data. *Life Sci* 1997;60:1129–1136.

210 Hills CJ, Winter SA, Balfour JA. Tolterodine. *Drugs* 1998; 55:813–820.

211 Jonas U, Hofner K, Madesbacher H, Holmdahl TH. Efficacy and safety of two doses of tolterodine versus placebo in patients with detrusor overactivity and symptoms of frequency, urge incontinence, and urgency: urodynamic evaluation. *World J Urol* 1997;15:144–151.

212 Millard R, Tuttle J, Moore K *et al.* Clinical efficacy and safety of tolterodine compared to placebo in detrusor overactivity. *J Urol* 1999;161:1551–1555.

213 Rentzhog L. Stanton SL, Cardozo LD, Nelson E, Fall M, Abrams P. Efficacy and safety of tolterodine in patients with detrusor instability: a dose ranging study. *Br J Urol* 1998;81: 42–48.

214 Appell RA. Clinical efficacy and safety of tolterodine in the treatment of overactive bladder: a pooled analysis. *Urology* 1997;50:90–96.

215 Swift S, Garely A, Dimpfl T, Payne C and Tolterodine Study Group. A new once daily formulation of tolterodine provides superior efficacy and is well tolerated in women with overactive bladder. *Int J Pelvic Floor Dysfunct* 2003;14:50–54.

216 Van Kerrebroeck P, Kreder K, Jonas U, Zinner N, Wein A and Tolterodine Study Group. Tolterodine once-daily: superior efficacy and tolerability in the treatment of overactive bladder. *Urology* 2001;57:414–421.

217 Diokno AC, Appell RA, Sand PK, Dmochowski RR, Gburek BM, Klimberg IW, Kell SH and OPERA Study Group. Prospective, randomised, double blind study of the efficacy and tolerability of the extended-release formulations of oxybutynin and tolterodine for overactive bladder: results of the OPERA trial. *Mayo Clin Proc* 2003;78:687–695.

218 Schladitz-Keil G, Spahn H, Mutschler E. Determination of bioavailability of the quaternary ammonium compound trospium chloride in man from urinary excretion data. *Arzneimittel Forsch/Drug Res* 1986;36:984–987.

219 Fusgen I, Hauri D. Trospium chloride: an effective option for medical treatment of bladder overactivity. *Int J Clin Pharmacol Ther* 2000;38:223–234.

220 Cardozo LD, Chapple CR, Toozs-Hobson P *et al.* Efficacy of trospium chloride in patients with detrusor instability: a placebo-controlled, randomized, double-blind, multicentre clinical trial. *BJU Int* 2000;85:659–664.

221 Madersbacher H, Stoher M, Richter R, Burgdorfer H, Hachen HJ, Murtz G. Trospium choride versus oxybutynin: a randomised, double-blind, multicentre trial in the treatment of detrusor hyperreflexia. *Br J Urol* 1995;75:452–456.

222 Staskin DR, Sand P, Zinner N, Dmochowski R; Trospium Study Group. Once daily trospium chloride is effective and well tolerated for the treatment of overactive bladder;

results from a multicentre phase III trial. *J Urol* 2007;178: 978–983.

223 Dmochowski RR, Sand PK, Zinner NR, Staskin DR. Trospium 60 mg once daily (QD) for overactive bladder syndrome: results from a placebo controlled interventional study. *Urology* 2008;71:449–454.

224 Dmochowski RR, Rosenberg MT, Zinner NR, Staskin DR, Sand PK. Extended release trospium chloride improves quality of life in overactive bladder. *Value Health* 2010;13: 251–257.

225 Robinson D, Cardozo L. Solifenacin: pharmacology and clinical efficacy. *Expert Rev Clin Pharmacol* 2009;2:239–253.

226 Cardozo L, Lisec M, Millard R *et al.* Randomised, double blind placebo controlled trial of the once daily antimuscarinic agent solifenacin succinate in patients with overactive bladder. *J Urol* 2004;172:1919–1924.

227 Haab F, Cardozo L, Chapple C, Ridder AM and Solifenacin Study Group. Long-term open label solifenacin treatment associated with persistence with therapy in patients with overactive bladder syndrome. *Eur Urol* 2005;47:376–384.

228 Chapple CR, Martinez-Garcia R, Selvaggi L, Toozs-Hobson P, Warnack W, Drogendijk T, Wright DM, Bolodeoku J; for the STAR study group. A comparison of the efficacy and tolerability of solifenacin succinate and extended release tolterodine at treating overactive bladder syndrome: results of the STAR trial. *Eur Urol* 2005;48:464–470.

229 Chapple CR, Artibani W, Cardozo LD, Castro-Diaz D, Craggs M, Haab F, Khullar V, Versi E. The role of urinary urgency and its measurement in the overactive bladder syndrome: current concepts and future prospects. *BJU Int* 2005;95:335–340.

230 Cardozo L, Hebdorfer E, Milani R *et al.* for the SUNRISE study group. Solifenacin in the treatment of urgency and other symptoms of overactive bladder; results from a randomised, double-blind, placebo-controlled, rising dose trial. *BJU Int* 2008;102:1120–1127.

231 Karram MM, Chancellor M. Solifenacin treatment reduces symptoms of overactive bladder in patients with residual urgency on tolterodine treatment: results of the VERSUS study. *Int Urogynaecol J* 2006;17 (Suppl 3):S441.

232 Wagg A, Wyndaele JJ, Sieber P. Efficacy and tolerability of solifenacin in elderly subjects with overactive bladder syndrome: a pooled analysis. *Am J Geriatr Pharmacother* 2006;4: 14–24.

233 Wesnes K, Edgar C, Tretter R, Patel H, Bolodeoku J. Solifenacin is not associated with cognitive impairment or sedation in the elderly; the randomised double-blind SCOPE study. Poster Presentation. *38th Annual Meeting of the International Continence Society, Cairo, Egypt*, 2008.

234 Mattiasson A, Morton R, Bolodeoku J. Solifenacin alone and with simplified bladder retraining in overactive bladder syndrome: the prospective randomised SOLAR study. Poster Presentation. *38th Annual Meeting of the International Continence Society, Cairo, Egypt*. 2008.

235 Garley AD, Kaufman JM, Sand PK, Smith N, Andoh M. Symptom bother and health-related quality of life outcomes following solifenacin treatment for overactive bladder: the Vesicare Open Label Trial. *Clin Ther* 2006;28:1935–1946.

236 Alabaster VA. Discovery and development of selective M3 antagonists for clinical use. *Life Sci* 1997;60:1053–1060.

237 Chapple CR. Darifenacin is well tolerated and provides significant improvement in the symptoms of overactive bladder: a pooled analysis of phase III studies. *Urol* 2004;171(Suppl):130 (abstract 487).

238 Michel MC. Fesoterodine: a novel muscarinic receptor antagonist for the treatment of overactive bladder syndrome. *Expert Opin Pharmacother* 2008;9:1787–1796.

239 Malhotra BK, Guan Z, Wood N, Gandelman K. Pharmacokinetic profile of fesoterodine. *Int J Clin Pharmacol Ther* 2008;46:556–563.

240 Chapple C. Fesoterodine: a new effective and well tolerated antimuscarinic for the treatment of urgency-frequency syndrome: results of a phase II controlled study. *Neurourol Urodyn* 2004;23:598–599.

241 Chapple C, Van Kerrebroeck P, Tubaro A, Millard R. Fesoterodine in non-neurogenic voiding dysfunction – results on efficacy and safety in a phase III trial. *Eur Urol* 2006;5(Suppl):117.

242 Chapple CR, Van Kerrebroeck PE, Junemann KP, Wang JT, Brodsky M. Comparison of fesoterodine and tolterodine in patients with overactive bladder. *BJU Int* 2008;102:1128–1132.

243 Kelleher CJ, Tubaro A, Wang JT, Kopp Z. Impact of fesoterodine on quality of life: pooled data from two randomised trials. *BJU Int* 2008;102:56–61.

244 Herschorn S, Swift S, Guan Z, et al. Comparison of fesoterodine and tolterodine extended release for the treatment of overactive bladder: a head to head placebo controlled trial. *BJU Int* 2009;105:58–66.

245 Baldessarini KJ. Drugs in the treatment of psychiatric disorders. In: Goodman LS, Gilman A, Goodman Gilman A *et al.* (eds) *The Pharmacological Basis of Therapeutics*, 7th edn. New York: MacMillan Publishing Company, 1985:387–445.

246 Castleden CM, Duffin HM, Gulati RS. Double-blind study of imipramine and placebo for incontinence due to bladder instability. *Age Ageing* 1986;15:299–303.

247 Diokno AC, Hyndman CW, Hardy DA, Lapides J. Comparison of action of imipramine (Tofranil) and propantheline (Probanthine) on detrusor contraction. *Urol* 1972;107:42–43.

248 Jeremy JY, Tsang V, Mikhailidis DP, Rogers H, Morgan RJ, Dandona P. Eicosanoid synthesis by human urinary bladder mucosa: pathological implications. *Br J Urol* 1987;59:36–39.

249 Cardozo LD, Stanton SL, Robinson H, Hole D. Evaluation on flurbiprofen in detrusor instability. *Br Med J* 1980;280:281–282.

250 Cardozo LD, Stanton SL. A comparison between bromocriptine and indomethacin in the treatment of detrusor instability. *J Urol* 1980;123:399–401.

251 Norgaard JP, Rillig S, Djurhuus JC. Nocturnal enuresis: an approach to treatment based on pathogenesis. *Pediatr* 1989; 114:705–709.

252 Mattiasson A, Abrams P, Van Kerrebroeck P, Walter S, Weiss J. Efficacy of desmopressin in the treatment of nocturia: a double blind placebo controlled studying men. *BJU Int* 2002; 89:855–862.

253 Robinson D, Cardozo L, Akeson M, Hvistendahl G, Riis A, Norgaard J. Anti-diuresis – a new concept in the management of daytime urinary incontinence. *BJU Int* 2004;93:996–1000.

254 Fowler CJ, Jewkes D, McDonald WI, Lynn B, DeGroat WC. Intravesical capsaicin for neurogenic bladder dysfunction. *Lancet* 1992;339:1239.

255 Chandiramani VA, Peterson T, Beck RO, Fowler CJ. Lessons learnt from 44 intravestial instillations of capsaicin. *Neurourol Urodynam* 1994;13:348–349.

256 Kim DY, Chancellor MB. Intravesical neuromodulatory drugs: capsaicin and resiniferatoxin to treat the overactive bladder. *J Endourol* 2000;14:97–103.

257 Ishizuka O, Mattiasson A, Andersson K-E. Urodynamic effects of intravesical resiniferatoxin and capsaicin in conscious rats wth and without outflow obstruction. *J Urol* 1995;154: 611–616.

258 Kerner J. Vergiftung durch verdobene *Würste*. *Tübinger Blätt Naturwißenschaften Arzenykunde* 1817;3:1–25.

259 van Ermenegen E. Uber einen neuen anaeroben Bacillus und seine Beziehungen zum Botulismus. *Z Hyg Infektionskrankh* 1897;26:1–56.

260 Dolly JO. Therapeutic and research exploitation of Botulinum neurotoxins. *Eur J Neurol* 1997;4(Suppl 2):S5–S10.

261 Schurch B, Stohrer M, Kramer G, Schmid DM, Gaul G, Hauri D. Botulinum-A toxin for treating detrusor hyperreflexia in spinal cord injured pateints: a new alternative to anticholinergic drugs? Preliminary results. *Urol* 2000;164:692–697.

262 Reitz A, Stroher M, Kramer G et al. European experience of 200 cases treated with botulinum-A toxin injections into the detrusor muscle for urinary incontinence due to neurogenic detrusor overactivity. *Eur Urol* 2004;45:510–515.

263 Schurch B, de Seze M, Denys P et al. Botulinum toxin type A is a safe and effective treatment for neurogenic urinary incontinence: results of a single treatment, randomized, placebo controlled 6-month study. Botox Detrusor Hyperreflexia Study Team. *J Urol* 2005;174:196–200.

264 Popat R, Apostolidis A, Kalsi V, Gonzales G, Fowler CJ, Dasgupta P. A comparison between the response of patients with idiopathic detrusor overactivity and neurogenic detrusor overactivity to the first intradetrusor injection of Botulinum-A toxin. *J Urol* 2005;174:984–989.

265 Grosse J, Kramer G, Stoher M. Success of repeat detrusor injections of Botulinum-A toxin in patients with severe neurogenic detrusor overactivity and incontinence. *Eur Urol* 2005;47: 653–659.

266 McGuire EJ, Shi-Chun Z, Horwinski ER et al. Treatment of motor and sensory detrusor instability by electrical stimulation. *J Urol* 1983;129:78.

267 Stoller ML. Afferent nerve stimulation for pelvic floor dysfunction. *Eur Urol* 1999;135:32.

268 Vandoninick V, van Balken MR, Finazzi Agro E, Petta F, Caltragirone C, Heesakkers JPFA, Kierneney LALM, Debruyne FMJ, Bernelmans BLH. Posterior tibial nerve stimulation in the treatment of urge incontinence. *Neurourol Urodyn* 2003; 22:17–23.

269 Peters KM, Leong FC, Shoberi SA, MacDiarmid SA, Rovner ES, Wooldridge LS, Siegel SW, Tate SS, Jarnagin BK, Rosenblatt PL, Feagins BA. A randomised multicentre study comparing percutaneous tibial nerve stimulation with pharmaceutical therapy for the treatment of overactive bladder. Poster presentation. AUA, Orlando, Florida, 2008.

270 Robinson D, Jacklin P, Cardozo L. Is cost the Achilles heal of posterior tibial nerve stimulation: a cost minimisation comparison with antimuscarinic therapy. *Neurourol Urodyn* 2009; 28:879–881.

271 Seigel SW, Cantanzaro F, Dijkema HE et al. Long term results of a multicentre study on sacral nerve stimulation for treatment of urinary urge incontinence, urgency-frequency and retention. *Urology* 2000;56:87–91.

272 van Kerrebroeck PE, van Voskuilen AC, Heesakkers JP *et al.* Results of sacral neuromodulation therapy for urinary voiding dysfunction: outcomes of a prospective, worldwide clinical study. *J Urol* 2007;178:2029–2034.

273 Mast P, Hoebeke, Wyndale JJ, Oosterlinck W, Everaert K. Experience with clam cystoplasty. A review. *Paraplegia* 1995;33: 560–564.

274 Bramble FJ. The clam cystoplasty. *Br J Urol* 1990;66:337–341.

275 McRae P, Murray KH, Nurse DE, Stephenson JP, Mundy AR. Clam entero-cystoplasty in the neuropathic bladder. *Br J Urol* 1987;60:523–525.

276 Rosenbaum TP, Shah PJR, Rose GA, Lloyd-Davies RW. Cranberry juice helps the problem of mucus production in enterouroplastics. *Neurourol Urodynam* 1989;8:344–345.

277 Harzmann R, Weckerman D. Problem of secondary malignancy after urinary diversion and enterocystoplasty. *Scand J Urol Nephrol* 1992;142(Suppl):56.

278 Barrington JW, Fern Davies H, Adams RJ, Evans WD, Woodcock JP, Stephenson TP. Bile acid dysfunction after clam enterocystoplasty. *Br J Urol* 1995;76:169–171.

279 Cartwright PC, Snow BW. Bladder autoaugmentation: partial detrusor excision to augment the bladder without use of bowel. *J Urol* 1989;142:1050–1053.

280 Snow BW, Cartwright PC. Bladder autoaugmentation. *Urol Clin N Am* 1996;23:323–331.

281 Kennelly MJ, Gormley EA, McGuire EJ. Early clinical experience with adult bladder autoaugmentation. *J Urol* 1994;152:303–306.

282 Karram MM, Bhatia NN. Management of co-existent stress and urge incontinence. *Br J Urol* 1989;57:641–646.

283 Shah PJR. Pathophysiology of voiding disorders. In: J Drife, P Hilton, S Stanton (eds) *Micturition*. London: Springer-Verlag, 1990.

284 Salmon UL, Walter RI, Gast SH. The use of oestrogen in the treatment of dysuria and incontinence in postmenopausal women. *Am J Obstet Gynaecol* 1941;14:23–31.

285 Youngblood VH, Tomlin EM, Davis JB. Senile urethritis in women. *J Urol* 1957;78:150–152.

286 Grady D, Brown JS, Vittinghoff E, Applegate W, Varner E, Synder T. Postmenopausal hormones and incontinence: the Heart and Oestrogen/progestin Replacement Study. *Obstet Gynaecol* 2001;97:116–120.

287 Grodstein F, Lifford K, Resnick NM, Curhan GC. Postmenopausal hormone therapy and risk of developing urinary incontinence. *Obstet Gynaecol* 2004;103:254–260.

288 Hendrix SL, Cochrane BR, Nygaard IE *et al.* Effects of oestrogen with and without progestin on urinary incontinence. *JAMA* 2005;293:935–948.

289 Caine M, Raz S. The role of female hormones in stress incontinence. In: *Proceedings of the 16th Congress of the International Society of Urology*, Amsterdam, The Netherlands, 1985.

290 Rud T. The effects of oestrogens and gestagens on the urethral pressure profile in urinary continent and stress incontinent women. *Acta Obstet Gynaecol Scand* 1980;59:265–270.

291 Wilson PD, Faragher B, Butler B, Bullock D, Robinson EL, Brown ADG. Treatment with oral piperazine oestrone sulphate for genuine stress incontinence in postmenopausal women. *Br J Obstet Gynaecol* 1987;94:568–574.

292 Walter S, Wolf H, Barlebo H, Jansen H. Urinary incontinence in postmenopausal women treated with oestrogens: a double-blind clinical trial. *J Urol* 1978;33:135–143.

293 Fantl JA, Bump RC, Robinson D *et al.* Efficacy of oestrogen supplementation in the treatment of urinary incontinence. *Obstet Gynaecol* 1996;88:745–749.

294 Jackson S, Shepherd A, Brookes S, Abrams P. The effect of oestrogen supplementation on post-menopausal urinary stress incontinence: a double-blind, placebo controlled trial. *Br J Obstet Gynaecol* 1999;106:711–718.

295 Sultana CJ, Walters MD. Oestrogen and urinary incontinence in women. *Maturitas* 1995;20:129–138.

296 Samsicoe G, Jansson I, Mellstrom D, Svanberg A. Urinary incontinence in 75 year old women. Effects of oestriol. *Acta Obstet Gynaecol Scand* 1985;93:57.

297 Cardozo LD, Rekers H, Tapp A *et al.* Oestriol in the treatment of postmenopausal urgency: a multicentre study. *Maturitas* 1993;18:47–53.

298 Nilsson K, Heimer G. Low dose oestradiol in the treatment of urogenital oestrogen deficiency – a pharmacokinetic and pharmacodynamic study. *Maturitas* 1992;15:121–127.

299 Benness C, Wise BG, Cutner A, Cardozo LD. Does low dose vaginal oestradiol improve frequency and urgency in post-menopausal women. *Int Urogynaecol J* 1992;3:281.

300 Eriksen PS, Rasmussen H. Low dose 17β-oestradiol vaginal tablets in the treatment of atrophic vaginitis: a double-blind placebo controlled study. *Eur J Obstet Gynaecol Reprod Biol* 1992;44:137–144.

301 Lose G, Englev E. Oestradiol-releasing vaginal ring versus oestriol vaginal pessaries in the treatment of bothersome lower urinary tract symptoms. *Br J Obstet Gynaecol* 2000;107:1029–1034.

302 Cardozo L, Lose G, McClish D, Versi E. Oestrogen treatment for symptoms of an overactive bladder, results of a meta analysis. *Int J Urogynaecol* 2001;12:v.

303 Cody JD, Richardson K, Moehrer B, Hextall A, Glazener CMA. Oestrogen therapy for urinary incontinence in post-menopausal women. *Cochrane Database Syst Rev* 2009;4:CD001405.

304 Bungay G, Vessey MP, McPherson CK. Study of symptoms in middle life with special reference to the menopause. *Br Med J* 1980;281:181–183.

305 Holmes DM, Stone AR, Barry PR, Richards CJ, Stephenson TP. Bladder training – 3 years on. *Br J Urol* 1983;55:660–664.

306 Smith PJ. The urethral syndrome. In: AM Fisher, H Gordon (eds) *Gynaecological Enigmata*. London: WB Saunders, 1981: 161–172.

307 Stamm WE, Running K, McKevitt M, Counts GW, Turck M, Holmes KK. Treatment of the acute urethral syndrome. *N Engl J Med* 1981;304:956–958.

308 Rees DL, Whitfield HN, Islam AK. Urodynamic findings in the adult female with frequency and dysuria. *Br J Urol* 1975; 47:853–860.

309 Oravisto KJ. Interstitial cystitis as an autoimmune disease. *Eur Urol* 1980;6:10–13.

310 Geist RW, Antolak SJ. Interstitial cystitis in children. *J Urol* 1970;138:508–512.

311 Parivar F, Bradbrook RA. Interstitial cystitis. *Br J Urol* 1986; 58:239–244.

312 Lynes WL, Flynn LD, Shortliffe ML, Zipser R, Roberts J, Stamey TA. Mast cell involvement in interstitial cystitis. *J Urol* 1987;138:746–752.

313 Christmas TJ, Rode J. Characteristics of mast cells in normal bladder, bacterial cystitis and interstitial cystitis. *Br J Urol* 1991;68:473–478.

314 Parsons CL, Stanffer C, Schmidt JD. Bladder surface gly-cosaminoglycans. An efficient mechanism of environmental adaptation. *Science* 1980;208:605–607.

315 Parsons CL, Stein PC, Bidair M, Lebow D. Abnormal sensitivity to intravesical potassium in interstitial cystitis. *Neurourol Urodyn* 1994;13:515–520.

316 Hanno PM. Amitriptyline in the treatment of interstitial cystitis. *Urol Clin N Am* 1994;21:89–91.

317 Messing ED, Staney TA. Interstitial cystitis: early diagnosis, pathology and treatment. *Urology* 1978;12:381–391.

318 Gillespie L. *You Don't Have To Live With Cystitis!* New York: Avon Books, 1986.

319 Badenoch AW. Chronic interstitial cystitis. *Br J Urol* 1971;43: 718–721.

320 Mulholland SG, Hanno P, Parsons CL, Sant GR, Staskin DR. Pentosan polysulfate sodium for therapy of interstitial cystitis. A double blind placebo-controlled clinical study. *Urology* 1990; 35:552–558.

321 Parsons CL, Schmidt JD, Pollen JY. Successful treatment of interstitial cystitis with sodium pentosanpolysulphate. *J Urol* 1983;130:51–53.

322 Bade JJ, Laseur M, Nieuwenburg L, van der Weele Th, Mensink HJA. A placebo-controlled study of intravesical pentosan-polysulphate for the treatment of interstitial cystitis. *Br J Urol* 1997;79:168–171.

323 Childs SJ. Dimethyl sulfone (DMSO) in the treatment of interstitial cystitis. *Urol Clin N Am* 1994;21:85–88.

324 Gillespie L. *My Body, My Diet.* Beverley Hills, CA: American Foundation for Pain Research, 1992.

325 Whitmore KE. Self care regimens for patients with interstitial cystitis. *Urol Clin N Am* 1994;21:121–130.

326 Masters WH, Johnson VE. *Human Sexual Response.* London: Churchill Livingstone, 1966.

327 Vessey MP, Metcalf MA, McPherson K, Yeates D. Urinary tract infection in relation to diaphragm use and obesity. *Int J Epidemiol* 1987;16:1–4.

328 Cardozo LD. Sex and the bladder. *Br Med J* 1988;296: 587–588.

329 Hadorn DC, Baker D, Hodges JS, Hicks N. Rating the quality of evidence for clinical practice guidelines. *Clin Epidemiol* 1996;49:749–754.

330 Harbour R, Miller J. A new system for grading recommendations in evidence based guidelines. *BMJ* 2001;323:334–336.

Part 14
Benign Gynaecological Disease

Chapter 52
Benign Diseases of the Vulva

Fiona M. Lewis[1,2] *and Sallie M. Neill*[2]

[1]Wexham Park Hospital, Slough, UK
[2]St John's Institute of Dermatology, St Thomas's Hospital, London, UK

Introduction

The majority of women who present with vulval symptoms have a dermatological problem rather than an infective or gynaecological complaint. However, as many of these patients will be referred to gynaecology clinics, it is very important that gynaecologists learn to recognize the common skin conditions that affect the vulva and to refer them for dermatological advice and management appropriately. Many clinics with a multidisciplinary team have been established to provide a specific service for women with vulval disorders [1], and it is vital that these include a dermatologist.

This chapter gives an overview of the common skin problems that affect the vulva and basic principles of management.

History taking

The importance of a good history is vital to making an accurate diagnosis in any patient who presents with vulval symptoms. A clear method of history taking should be used, and a proforma can be helpful to ensure that the key areas are covered.

The interview should take place in a sympathetic environment and it is helpful initially to enquire about the general dermatological history before moving on to the more personal questions related to vulval disease.

The important areas to cover are as follows:
• Presenting symptoms – does it itch or is there pain? Patients may report irritation but this should always be qualified. It is helpful to ask if they want to scratch to alleviate the symptoms. Is the itching constant or intermittent and are there any triggering factors?
• Previous treatments – what has been used (prescribed and over-the-counter medication) and what was the response?

• Dermatological history – ask about a personal and family history of atopy and psoriasis. Ask about any other skin problems, either present or past, and also specifically about oral and ocular symptoms. Have they any known allergies?
• Gynaecological history – is there any relationship with menstruation? Were there problems conceiving and, if the patient had been pregnant, were there any skin problems? Were deliveries straightforward or complicated resulting in trauma to the vulva? The history relating to cervical smears and any abnormalities or treatment is important, particularly in patients with vulval intraepithelial neoplasia, where cervical intraepithelial neoplasia may be associated.
• Sexual history – any history of sexually transmitted infections, vaginal discharge or dyspareunia? If appropriate, ask about risk factors for human immunodeficiency virus (HIV) infection. Loss of libido is common with any dermatological condition of the vulva.
• General medical history – underlying medical conditions can be relevant to some vulval problems, i.e. inflammatory bowel disease and other autoimmune conditions.
• Medication.
• Social history – details on the smoking history, alcohol intake and travel history where appropriate.

Examination

The examination should always be carried out with a trained chaperone present. Good lighting and appropriate magnification is essential. The vulva can be adequately examined with the patient in the dorsal and left lateral position. Again, the examination should be approached systematically. The vulva is first examined overall but the labia majora need to be separated in order to adequately visualize many of the structures.

Dewhurst's Textbook of Obstetrics & Gynaecology, Eighth Edition. Edited by D. Keith Edmonds.
© 2012 John Wiley and Sons, Ltd. Published 2012 by John Wiley and Sons, Ltd.

General view
• Hair
• Skin colour, texture and surface

Specific areas to be inspected
• Mons pubis
• Labia majora
• Labia minora
• Interlabial sulci
• Clitoris
• Vestibule
• Perianal skin

The vagina and cervix should be examined in all muco-cutaneous diseases and vulval intraepithelial neoplasia, as well as in patients complaining of a vaginal discharge. An examination of the skin at extragenital sites will often give valuable diagnostic information, and inspection of the oral mucosa, eyes, scalp, nails and other flexural sites may also be important.

Normal variants

There are some very common and important normal variants seen on examination of the vulva. These should be easy to recognize and the patient should be reassured. There are also physiological changes that vary with age and hormonal status.

Angiokeratomas
These are common and are usually seen on the labia majora. They are often multiple and appear as small red or purple vascular lesions with overlying hyperkeratosis (Plate 52.1).

Hart's line
This demarcates the junction of the keratinized and non-keratinized epithelia of the labia minora and vestibule, respectively (Plate 52.2). It can be very prominent in some women.

Vestibular papillae
A common finding is the presence of tiny filiform projections on the inner labia minora and vestibule (Plate 52.3). Originally, it was thought that these were human papillomavirus (HPV)-related but there is good evidence that this is not the case. They are a normal variant and do not require any treatment.

Fordyce spots
These are small sebaceous papules found on the inner surfaces of the labia minora (Plate 52.4). They can be very prominent in some women and may be seen on the buccal mucosa as well.

Normal physiological changes

Childhood
In the first few weeks of life, the vulva is under the influence of maternal hormones. The clitoral hood and labia minora are relatively prominent and may be seen without separation of the labia majora. Labial adhesions are common and usually resolve with topical oestrogens.

Puberty
Deposition of fat increases the size of the labia majora and mons pubis, and pubic hair appears. The labia minora may become pigmented. The clitoris enlarges and the vestibular glands become active.

Pregnancy
The vulva can be engorged and varicosities are common. Hyperpigmentation can be significant.

Postmenopause
The labia majora become less rounded and there is a reduction in hair growth.

Investigations

In some cases, a diagnosis may be made on the clinical appearance alone, but in others a variety of investigations may be helpful in confirming the diagnosis.

Biopsy
This is a very simple procedure that can be performed in the outpatient clinic under local anaesthesia. A 6-mm punch biopsy is taken after infiltrating the area with lidocaine. Topical EMLA® (lidocaine 2.5%, prilocaine 2.5%, Asbra Zeneca, London, UK) may be used before the lidocaine, but care must then be taken in interpreting the histological appearances as subepidermal cleavage can be induced by this agent [2]. Good clinical–pathological correlation is vital in all cases of vulval dermatoses.

Microbiological investigation
Appropriate swabs and transport media for bacterial, yeast and viral culture may be needed. If a sexually transmitted infection is suspected, the patient should be referred for investigation in a clinic specializing in genitourinary medicine.

Skin scrapings to look for fungi can be taken in the clinic and examination under Wood's lamp may be helpful. This latter examination is useful in cases of erythrasma, in which the affected skin will fluoresce pink.

Patch testing
This is performed when there is the possibility of an allergic contact dermatitis, either as a primary problem or

where it is a secondary phenomenon caused by an allergy to treatment. Patients will need to be referred to a dermatologist for these tests.

Inflammatory diseases of the vulva

Lichen sclerosus

Lichen sclerosus is an inflammatory dermatosis with a predilection for the anogenital skin. It is significantly more common in women than in men. Extragenital lesions may be seen in about 10% of those with genital involvement. They present as ivory white plaques, often at sites of trauma or friction (Plate 52.5).

Summary box 52.1

Lichen sclerosus:
- Lichen sclerosus is an autoimmune-associated dermatosis that commonly affects the anogenital skin.
- There are two peaks of presentation: pre-pubertal girls and postmenopausal women.
- It presents with itchy white atrophic lesions, often with ecchymosis and oedema.
- Scarring will occur if untreated.
- An ultra-potent topical steroid is the first-line treatment.
- Patients require long-term follow-up as there is a small risk of malignancy developing.
- Any resistant areas, ulcers or hyperkinetic lesiors should be biopsied.

Aetiology

The aetiology remains unclear but it is thought that it is mediated by a lymphocyte reaction. Immunohistochemical alterations of the epidermis and dermis support an autoimmune cause [3], and circulating immunoglobulin G (IgG) antibodies to extracellular matrix protein have been demonstrated [4]. There is an association in both the patient and his or her first-degree relatives with other autoimmune diseases, particularly thyroid disorders [5].

Clinical features

There are two peaks of presentation – in childhood and around or after the menopause. The predominant symptom is that of pruritus, but soreness and dyspareunia will be experienced in the presence of ulceration, erosions and fissures. In children, constipation is a frequent feature if the perianal area is affected.

The early lesions are white ivory papules, which may coalesce to form plaques. Ecchymosis due to rupture of dermal vessels is common, as is oedema (Plate 52.6).

Ecchymosis is common in children and often leads to the erroneous diagnosis of sexual abuse. Extension of disease around the perianal area presents as a 'figure of eight' pattern. As the disease progresses, scarring occurs with loss of the labia minora, which become fused to the labia majora. The clitoral hood can seal over and the clitoris may be buried (Plate 52.7). The vagina is not involved in lichen sclerosus as mucous membranes are spared, which may be a useful distinguishing feature from lichen planus (LP).

Histology shows a thinned epidermis overlying a homogenized band of collagen in the upper dermis. There is a lymphocytic inflammatory cell infiltrate in the dermis under the band of homogenized collagen (Plate 52.8).

Lichen sclerosus and malignancy

Squamous cell carcinoma (SCC) is a rare complication of lichen sclerosus, occurring in about 4–6% of patients [6]. This may present as a small persistent erosion or ulcer, a hyperkeratotic area, or fleshy friable papule or nodule (Plate 52.9). Any suspicious lesions must be biopsied. If vulval intraepithelial neoplasia (VIN) is found in association with lichen sclerosus, it is usually the differentiated form in which there is basal atypia but normal maturation of the epidermis. It is less common to have undifferentiated VIN.

Treatment

The treatment of lichen sclerosus in adults and children is the use of a super-potent topical steroid such as clobetasol propionate 0.05% ointment. This is applied once daily for a month, on alternative days for the second month and then twice weekly for the third month. Emollients are used as a soap substitute. After this, the topical steroid ointment can be used as needed if there is recurrence of symptoms.

There is no role for the use of topical testosterone. Surgery is required only to treat the scarring complications or if there is neoplastic or pre-neoplastic change. Other therapies have been used [7]. Topical calcineurin inhibitors are increasingly popular but should not be used first line as there are concerns about their long-term safety in relation to the development of malignancy.

In those with resistant symptoms, it is important to exclude allergic-contact dermatitis to treatment, irritant dermatitis due to urinary incontinence or an additional problem such as herpes simplex or candidiasis. A proportion of patients will develop a secondary dysaesthesia, for example vulvodynia, after their lichen sclerosus has been controlled. Treatment must be targeted at this rather than increasing the use of topical steroids. Patients with difficult to control disease or those with any history of VIN or SCC need prolonged follow-up in specialized clinics.

Vulval lichen planus

Lichen planus is an inflammatory disorder which can affect both the skin and mucosal surfaces. The characteristic cutaneous lesions are small purplish papules which may exhibit a fine lace-like network over their surface, known as 'Wickham's striae'. These can also be seen on mucosal lesions. The papules commonly occur on flexor surfaces and can koebnerize at sites of trauma. The nails can show pterygium formation, and scalp lesions can result in a scarring alopecia.

Histology shows irregular acanthosis with a 'sawtoothed' pattern, basal cell degeneration and a dense band-like dermal infiltrate of lymphocytes. There is often pigmentary incontinence, which is responsible for the marked hyperpigmentation sometimes seen clinically (Plate 52.10).

Aetiology
The cause is unknown but it is likely that it is a T lymphocyte-mediated inflammatory response to some form of antigenic insult. Lichenoid eruptions can be seen in graft-versus-host disease and secondary to drugs such as non-steroidal anti-inflammatory drugs. Although there has been interest in the association of hepatitis C infection and LP, there is evidence for this only in certain populations. It is not relevant in northern Europe [8]. There is an association of LP and other autoimmune disorders.

There are three major clinical patterns of LP affecting the anogenital skin – erosive, classic and hypertrophic. These may occur in isolation without the presence of disease at other sites.

Erosive lichen planus
Erosive LP is the commonest form to affect the genital skin. There is a specific subtype of erosive mucosal LP, the VVG syndrome, which affects the vulva, vagina and gingival margins [9]. This has been found to be associated with the HLA-DQB1*0201 allele [10]. The lacrimal duct, external auditory meatus and oesophagus can also be involved, and disease at these sites needs a multidisciplinary approach to management.

The vulval lesions mainly affect the inner labia minora and vestibule where erythema and erosions occur (Plate 52.11). A lacy white edge is seen and this is the best site for a confirmatory biopsy (Plate 52.12). There may be marked scarring with significant architectural change, which, in some cases, can be impossible to differentiate from lichen sclerosus. Symptomatically the condition is itchy and painful, and dyspareunia is a common feature. If there is vaginal involvement, there may be a blood-stained discharge and episodes of postcoital bleeding. It is important to recognize vaginal disease because scarring at this site can result in complete vaginal stenosis. Glazed erythema and erosions occur on the gingivae (Plate 52.13), buccal mucosa and also on the tongue.

The disease tends to fluctuate with a relapsing and recurring pattern.

Classic lichen planus
Papules, very similar to the cutaneous lesions, are found on the vulva (Plate 52.14) and perianal skin. They may be asymptomatic in over 50% of patients [11,12]. Wickham's striae can also be seen associated with the lesions. Flexural hyperpigmentation can be significant even many months after the disease has resolved.

Hypertrophic lichen planus
Hypertrophic lesions are less common and mainly affect the perineum and perianal skin. They can become ulcerated and painful. They can be resistant to topical treatment.

Lichen planus and malignancy
Squamous cell carcinoma [13] and SCC *in situ* [14] have been reported in classic and hypertrophic types but not in VVG syndrome. In studies of patients with vulval malignancy, LP has been seen in the surrounding epithelium [15].

Management
The major treatment used is a super-potent topical steroid ointment. In general, clobetasol propionate 0.05% is used daily for the first month and then reduced to be used as needed. Bland emollients can be helpful as a soap substitute. Petroleum jelly used as a barrier will help symptomatically. For vaginal disease, some of the foam preparations used in inflammatory bowel disease can be used, e.g. hydrocortisone acetate. This is inserted via the applicator into the vagina at night. Dilators may also be required to keep the vagina patent.

There is interest in the new topical calcineurin modulators, tacrolimus and pimecrolimus, in the treatment of LP. There are small case series that support their use but there is also concern over the long-term safety, particularly with regard to the development of malignancy. It is therefore recommended that they are not used as first-line treatment but only for short periods of time in those who do not respond to potent topical steroids.

Several systemic treatments have been used in LP but no controlled trials exist [16].

Eczema

The terms eczema and dermatitis are used synonymously for an epidermal inflammation which has many forms. It is characterized histologically by spongiosis in which the keratinocytes lose cohesion and vesicles may form. The dermis is infiltrated by many different inflammatory cells. The skin becomes scaly secondary to parakeratosis and fluid may ooze onto the surface and dry to a crust. In chronic cases, the skin becomes thickened and lichenified. The vulva may be involved in various eczematous processes.

Seborrhoeic eczema

This is a common type of eczema, with peaks in childhood (cradle cap and nappy rash) and early adulthood. There is evidence that it is caused by the yeast *Pityrosporum ovale*. The lesions are erythematous with a greasy scale and particularly affect the naso-labial folds, eyebrows, forehead, scalp and behind the ears. The anogenital skin may be involved together with other flexural sites including the inguinal folds and gluteal cleft. The skin may show erythema and a build up of keratinous debris.

It is often very difficult to distinguish seborrhoeic eczema from flexural psoriasis. Characteristic lesions at other sites may help and the histology may be similar. The management of seborrhoeic eczema is the same as that of psoriasis.

Irritant eczema

The anogenital skin is very susceptible to an irritant eczema as it is a site that is occluded and often exposed to many irritant substances. There is diffuse erythema, fissuring and the skin may become thickened and macerated in areas. Deodorants, bubble baths, soaps and irritant topical treatment, for example wart preparations, are common causes. It is a particular problem in those suffering from urinary or faecal incontinence.

Allergic contact dermatitis

Allergic contact dermatitis is a delayed type IV hypersensitivity reaction and in the genital area is much more likely to occur on perianal skin than on the vulva [17].

Relevant positive patch test reactions are found and the most common culprits are topical medicaments, local anaesthetics, cosmetics and fragrances.

Dermatology advice on patch testing should be sought. In addition to the standard patch test series, extended testing is often necessary to find the allergen.

Lichen simplex

Lichenification is the term used to describe a thickening of the skin with accentuation of the skin lines. It is a response to chronic scratching and rubbing of the skin and is usually seen on a background of eczema or psoriasis. Lichen simplex is the term used to describe an isolated area of lichenification without an obvious background dermatatis. It is common in areas that the patient can easily reach. The thickened plaques may be hypo- or hyperpigmented, and the common sites are the outer labia majora and mons pubis. There may also be a loss of hair from rubbing (Plate 52.15). It is considered to be a sensory problem and treatment needs to be directed towards breaking the itch–scratch cycle.

Management of vulval eczema

The management of all eczematous processes is similar. All potential irritants and allergens should be withdrawn. Bland emollients, for example emulsifying ointment, are used as a soap substitute. A topical steroid, combined with an antimicrobial agent if appropriate, can be used once daily initially and then as needed as the problem improves. If the eczema is acute and the skin is oozing and wet, then potassium permanganate soaks (1:10 000 dilution) are helpful. Gauze is soaked in the solution and applied to the affected areas for 15 minutes once or twice a day. Patients with lichen simplex may require a potent topical steroid to gain control of their symptoms. The frequency of application can slowly be reduced as the lichenification resolves. Antihistamines may help at night to reduce scratching.

Psoriasis

Psoriasis is one of the commonest skin conditions, affecting about 2% of the population in some form. The characteristic lesions are silvery-white scaly plaques on the extensor aspects of the limbs, but generalized disease may occur with scalp and nail involvement. The aetiology is unknown, but there is a genetic predisposition and the disease may be triggered by streptococcal infection and trauma (the Koebner phenomenon). Psoriasis may also be exacerbated by some drugs, for example beta blockers, lithium and chloroquine.

Histology shows marked epidermal thickening (acanthosis) with deep epidermal ridges projecting into the dermis. Spongiosis with a neutrophil infiltrate of the epidermis may be seen.

Genital flexural psoriasis is common and may occur in isolation. There is little scaling because of the moist occluded environment of the anogenital skin. The lesions present on the inner and outer aspects of labia majora as well-demarcated erythema or salmon-pink patches which are usually symmetrical (Plate 52.16). The genitocrural and inguinal folds may also be affected. Perianal involvement is common with extension into the gluteal cleft (Plate 52.17). Itching and burning are common symptoms, but as maceration and fissuring is often seen, women may also complain of soreness. It is helpful to examine the rest of the skin to look for other signs – the scalp may show scaling and the nails in psoriasis display thimble pitting, onycholysis and subungual hyperkeratosis.

The use of an emollient as a soap substitute is helpful. The traditional treatments for psoriasis, for example tar, dithranol and calcipotriol, are usually too irritating to be used in the flexures and therefore a mild-to-potent topical steroid is used. This can be applied once daily and then reduced in frequency to be used as needed. In patients with severe disease, systemic treatment may be required, but these patients should be under specialist dermatological supervision. Oral therapy with methotrexate, ciclosporin and acitretin can be used and the new biological therapies may be considered in very extensive, resistant cases.

Reiter's disease is an inflammatory response to an enteric or lower genital tract infection with arthritis, uveitis and skin lesions which are very similar to psoriasis. The vulva may be affected with a circinate ulcerative vulvitis, similar to the balanitis that commonly occurs in men with this syndrome [18]. The histology is similar to that of pustular psoriasis.

Hidradenitis suppurativa

Hidradenitis suppurativa is an inflammatory disorder affecting areas where apocrine glands are present. The basic pathology is not in the gland itself but in the follicular epithelium [19] where an infundibular inflammation, possibly triggered by antimicrobial peptides produced after injury [20], leads to abscess formation and deep sinus tracts.

Anogenital involvement is common with painful nodules, sinuses and scarring (Plate 52.18). Bridged comedones are characteristic. SCC has been reported in chronic disease.

The management of this condition can be difficult. Topical antibiotics can be used in mild disease together with other measures such as stopping smoking and weight reduction. In moderate-to-severe disease, long-term oral tetracyclines are the first-line treatment. Oral clindamycin has been used in some cases with success. Second-line treatments include surgery, anti-androgen therapies and, more recently, the newer biologicals [21].

Bullous diseases

Genetic causes
Epidermolysis bullosa

Epidermolysis bullosa is used to describe a group of inherited conditions (dominant or recessive) that are characterized by skin fragility and bullae. The junctional and dystrophic types involve the vulva and scarring may result. Affected children must be cared for in specialist centres with access to expert nursing care.

Benign familial chronic pemphigus (Hailey–Hailey disease)

This is a rare autosomal dominant condition in which moist red plaques in the flexures and genital areas develop in the second to fourth decades. Friction worsens the problem and the plaques may fissure and become secondarily infected. Histology shows extensive intra-epidermal acantholysis described as a 'delapidated brick wall'. Treatment is unsatisfactory but topical steroids and prompt treatment of any infection can be helpful. Photodynamic therapy has had limited success in a few patients.

Bullous drug eruptions
Fixed drug eruption

Fixed drug eruptions occur at the same cutaneous or mucosal site each time the causative drug is ingested. Vulval involvement usually presents with swelling that may then form blisters and erode. As this is intermittent, it is not often associated with medication, and challenge tests may be needed. There are many drugs that can cause this problem. The most relevant for the vulva are septrin, fluconazole, aciclovir and non-steroidal anti-inflammatory drugs. Resolution frequently results in post-inflammatory hyperpigmentation.

Erythema multiforme

Erythema multiforme is an acute reaction pattern where mucosal erosions and ulcers occur, often with cutaneous 'target' lesions. Stevens–Johnson syndrome is a severe form of erythema multiforme where bullous lesions, which may scar, occur. Vaginal involvement can lead to stenosis and it is important to do a vaginal examination and treat the site involved, otherwise permanent stenosis can be a postinflammatory sequela. Erythema multiforme and Stevens–Johnson syndrome may be induced by herpes simplex infection or medications, especially antibiotics and non-steroidal anti-inflammatory agents. However, no cause is found in up to 50% of cases.

Toxic epidermal necrolysis (Lyell's syndrome)

This is a dermatological emergency in which severe and widespread epidermal loss occurs. It carries a very significant mortality. Drug hypersensitivity is the usual cause (most commonly antiepileptics, non-steroidal anti-inflammatories and antibiotics), but idiopathic cases may be seen.

There is a sudden onset of painful areas of erythema which rapidly become eroded or blistered, usually the genitalia, mouth and eyes. Vulvo-vaginal scarring and stenosis may occur as erosions heal. The triggering drug must be stopped and the patient transferred to a specialist dermatology centre or burns unit with experience in the management of these cases. Treatment is mainly supportive, with the role of steroids and immunoglobulin still undecided. In the early stages, the differential diagnosis is that of staphylococcal-scalded skin. In this latter condition, there is very superficial desquamation caused by staphylococcal exotoxins. Treatment is with high-dose antibiotics such as flucloxacillin.

Autoimmune bullous disorders
Bullous pemphigoid
Bullous pemphigoid is the commonest autoimmune bullous disorder and mainly affects the elderly, although cases have been reported in children. IgG antibodies are directed against the basement membrane, and these are demonstrated in a linear fashion on direct immunofluorescence studies. Circulating IgG antibodies may be found. Histology shows subepidermal blisters. The mucous membranes may be involved, with tense blisters which rupture to form superficial erosions.

These patients need to be managed by a dermatologist. Potent topical steroids may be used but systemic steroids and immunosuppressive drugs are usually needed.

Mucous membrane pemphigoid (cicatricial pemphigoid)
This is a rare autoimmune bullous disorder, but the mucosal involvement is prominent with the vulva, vagina, eyes, mouth and larynx being affected. Scarring is common and can cause problems with the vulva and eyes. It generally affects older women. The histological and immunofluorescence findings are similar to bullous pemphigoid, but there are often fewer eosinophils present. Treatment can be difficult, but steroids, mycophenolate and other immunosuppressive treatment are used [22]. These patients are at risk of ophthalmological and oesophageal complications, and management should involve dermatologists and any other relevant specialists. These patients share many of the clinical features of the vulvovaginal gingival form of LP (see above).

Pemphigus
Pemphigus vulgaris is a rare bullous disorder affecting the skin and mucous membranes. IgG antibodies are directed against keratinocytes. The bullae are flaccid and erosions are more commonly seen. The patients are often younger and cases have been reported in children.

Histology shows intraepidermal bullae. IgG is seen in the intercellular spaces on direct immunofluorescence and circulating IgG antibodies are seen.

This disease carries a high degree of morbidity and patients should always be under the care of a dermatologist. Treatment includes high-dose systemic steroids, azathioprine cyclophosphamide and mycophenolate mofetil.

Vulval ulceration
Aphthous ulcers
Oral aphthae are common but similar lesions can occur on the vulva and are frequently mistaken for herpetic infection. The vulval ulcers measure a few millimetres and have a yellow base surrounded by an erythematous rim. Histology is non-specific. Treatment is difficult but topical steroids, tetracyclines and local anaesthetic agents can be helpful.

Acute ulcers associated with infection
Lipschutz [23] described acute painful ulcers in young women in 1913 [23]. They are now known to be a reaction to systemic infection and have been reported most commonly in association with Epstein–Barr infection [24]. They typically occur in teenagers and present as rapidly enlarging painful ulcers, often occurring in apposition in a 'kissing' pattern. They usually heal without scarring after a few weeks but a short course of prednisolone can speed resolution. There may be a few episodes of relapse over the ensuing year.

Manifestations of underlying disease
Inflammatory bowel disease
Although anogenital lesions can occur in ulcerative colitis, they are rare. They are commoner in Crohn's disease, affecting up to 30% of patients, and they may precede the onset of bowel disease by some years. The lesions are termed metastatic where there is no continuity with bowel disease or they occur in distant sites, and most vulval lesions are of this type. Typical presentation includes unilateral or bilateral oedema (Plate 52.19), lymphangiectasia and classic 'knife-cut' fissures in the interlabial sulci (Plate 52.20). Sinus tracks and fistulae may also occur. Perianal ulceration or oedematous tags are also often present.

Histology may show granulomatous inflammation but is often non-specific. The main differential diagnosis is hidradenitis suppurativa and the two may coexist.

Treatment can be challenging and ideally should involve a multidisciplinary team. Potent topical steroids may be useful but systemic treatment is often needed, which may include steroids, immunosuppressive agents and antibiotics, especially metronidazole. There have now been several reports that the use of tumour necrosis factor alpha (TNF-α) blockers such as infliximab successfully improves the condition [25,26].

Pyoderma gangrenosum

Pyoderma gangrenosum is an aggressive ulcerative disorder of unknown aetiology but with a strong association with an underlying inflammatory disease such as rheumatoid arthritis, inflammatory bowel disease and myeloproliferative disorders.

Purulent ulcers with a prominent violaceous edge are most commonly seen on the lower limb, but the vulva may be involved. The initial lesion is sometimes pustular, which then ulcerates rapidly to form single or multiple ulcers with an indurated edge.

Histology is inflammatory but non-specific and the diagnosis is usually clinical. Early recognition is important as there is often a prompt response to systemic steroids or ciclosporin [27]. Other agents such as dapsone, azathioprine or minocycline may be needed. Surgery should be avoided at all costs as the lesions koebnerize, and so debridement is often followed by disease progression.

Behcet's syndrome

The original description by Behcet was a triad of oral and genital ulceration with uveitis. It is now known as a multisystem disorder and the diagnostic criteria were refined in 1990. The diagnosis is made when a patient has recurrent oral ulceration with at least two of the following – recurrent genital ulceration, eye lesions, cutaneous lesions (erythema nodosum, folliculitis, pyodermatous plaques) and a positive pathergy test (where pustulation occurs at the site of minor skin trauma, such as venepuncture).

It usually starts before the age of 50 years. The oral ulcers are similar to common aphthae, but the vulval ulcers are usually larger, more painful and tend to heal with scarring. The labia minora are most commonly affected (Plate 52.21). The histology is rather non-specific but thrombosed arterioles may be seen.

The management of these patients should be multidisciplinary as many organ systems may be involved. Neurological and ophthalmological complications can be serious and must be actively treated. Several drugs are used, including steroids, colchicines, dapsone and thalidomide. Topical steroids may be used for the genital ulcers. There may be a role for the use of biological agents [28].

Necrolytic migratory erythema (glucagonoma syndrome)

This is a rare syndrome of unknown cause in which cutaneous changes are seen secondary to a pancreatic islet cell tumour. The eruption is erosive and can migrate with a spreading serpiginous edge. The perineum is most severely affected but peri-oral lesions may also be seen. Glossitis and diabetes are usually associated. The diagnosis is made by finding a raised glucagon level. The rash often responds well to surgical removal of the primary tumour.

Acrodermatitis enteropathica

This is related to zinc deficiency and may be inherited as an autosomal recessive condition or acquired secondary to parenteral nutrition, malabsorption, severe eating disorders or penicillamine. The erythematous and pustular lesions affect the genitalia and also the peri-oral skin. Diagnosis is made on a low zinc level and treatment is with oral supplementation.

Disorders of pigmentation

The pigmentation of the vulval skin can vary widely with ethnicity and hormonal status. Dark areas can result from deposition of haemosiderin or melanin. Haemosiderin pigmentation tends to be red/brown and occurs after an inflammatory dermatosis such as LP. Melanin pigmentation is usually darker brown or black and any new pigmented areas where the diagnosis is not clinically obvious must be biopsied.

Hyperpigmentation

The most common cause of pigmented patches on the vulval skin is postinflammatory hyperpigmentation. It most frequently occurs after LP but can be seen after other inflammatory dermatoses and fixed drug eruptions.

Vulval melanosis

Areas of pigmentation may be seen without any preceding history of inflammation (Plate 52.22). These can be very irregular and must always be biopsied to confirm their benign nature. Histology shows an increased number of melanocytes and some pigmentary incontinence. Similar lesions may be found in the oral cavity and there is no evidence that they become malignant at either site.

Acanthosis nigricans

Velvety, thickened and hyperpigmented plaques are seen symmetrically spreading from the labia majora to the inguinal folds and may extend perianally. Similar lesions can be seen on the neck and in the axillae. Multiple skin tags are often seen on the surface of the plaques. The condition is most frequently seen in overweight individuals and it is associated with insulin resistance. Some cases, particularly those of sudden onset and in thin patients, can be associated with an underlying malignancy and appropriate investigations should be performed.

Hypopigmentation

Hypopigmentation can occur as a postinflammatory change and is most clearly seen in darker skin. It resolves spontaneously after the inflammation is treated.

Vitiligo

This is a common autoimmune disorder in which complete depigmentation of the skin occurs. It is patchy but symmetrical and peri-oroficial sites including the genitalia are often involved. The main differential diagnosis is lichen sclerosus; indeed, the two diseases may coexist. However, in vitiligo, there is no ecchymosis or architectural change and the texture of the skin is normal (Plate 52.23). There is no effective treatment.

Pigmented lesions
Benign pigmented lesions can occur on the vulva. However, any pigmented lesion should be subjected to histological examination to exclude pigmented variants of vulval intraepithelial neoplasia or malignant melanoma of the vulva.

Seborrhoeic keratoses
These may be heavily pigmented and have a 'stuck-on' appearance. They are usually found on the outer labia majora and in the groins. No treatment is generally required but cryotherapy or curettage and cautery are effective if they become troublesome. If there is any suspicion of HPV infection or cervical intraepithelial neoplasia, the lesions should be biopsied to exclude undifferentiated VIN.

Melanocytic naevi
Vulval naevi are not common. Some have atypical features and are regarded as atypical genital naevi [29] rather than variants of 'dysplastic' naevi. The unwary pathologist may report a malignant melanoma as there is cytological atypia but the lesions are symmetrical with normal cellular maturation. Naevi seen with lichen sclerosus can also mimic malignant melanoma clinically and histologically [30], but there are case reports of malignant melanoma developing in association with lichen sclerosus [31].

Benign tumours

Skin tags (acrochordia)
These small lesions are very common, particularly at flexural and frictional sites such as the axillae, eyelids and groins. No treatment is needed, but they can be removed by cryotherapy or cautery if they enlarge and become painful.

Cysts
Epidermoid cysts are the most common type of cyst found on the vulva and are usually seen on the labia majora. They present as small, painless yellow lumps. No treatment is needed but surgical excision is effective if they become symptomatic (Plate 52.24).

Bartholin's cysts occur due to an obstruction in Bartholin's ducts and are therefore seen on the lower third of the inner labia majora. They can become infected and enucleation is the treatment of choice. Rarely, a carcinoma of Bartholin's glands can present as a cyst and any recurrent lesions should be excised to exclude this.

Hidradenoma papilliferum
These arise from anogenital mammary glands and are therefore usually found in the interlabial sulcus or on the perineum. They are painless but excision is needed for histological examination.

Syringomata
These are eccrine duct tumours that are most commonly found on the face. They present as small papules on the genitalia, which may be itchy. They occur most frequently on the labia majora, but the labia minora can be involved. Treatment is unsatisfactory but laser ablation is used in those who are highly symptomatic.

Vascular lesions

Angiokeratoma (see normal variants)
Haemangiomas
Capillary haemangiomas are present at birth and do not fade. They are asymptomatic and cause no functional problems. Although laser treatment can be used, this is done only to improve the cosmetic appearance.

Cavernous haemangiomas (strawberry naevi) develop within the first few weeks of life and may grow rapidly. When present on the vulva, the labia majora are the most common sites involved, but the perianal area and buttocks may also be affected. Occasionally, they break down and cause painful areas of ulceration which often become infected. Early assessment by a paediatric dermatologist is helpful as propranolol or prednisolone may be required to shrink the lesions. They do spontaneously resolve over a period of years but if troublesome may require ablative treatment such as laser or excision.

Varicosities
Vulval varicosities are common during pregnancy and some thrombose spontaneously after delivery. They are usually associated with varicosities on the lower limbs, but if they are isolated to the genitalia the patient should be further investigated to exclude an obstructive pelvic lesion.

Disorders of lymphatics

Acute lymphoedema
Some swelling may occur in diseases such as candidiasis or acute eczema but resolves quickly with appropriate

treatment of the condition. Urticaria and angioedema may involve the vulva, the history is that of acute swelling, sometimes related to intercourse, where it may be pressure-induced.

Type I hypersensitivity contact urticarial reactions to latex are an increasing problem. There is immediate swelling of the labia after using latex condoms and it can also occur if healthcare workers wear latex gloves for examination. In severe cases, the reaction may be life-threatening if full-blown anaphylaxis follows. Contact urticaria to seminal fluid has also been described but is rare. The symptoms are completely abolished if condoms are used. Desensitization may be successful [32] and a successful pregnancy can be achieved by artificial insemination after removing the allergenic components of the seminal fluid [33].

Chronic lymphoedema

Lymphoedema may follow chronic inflammation (such as hidradenitis suppurativa or Crohn's disease), infection, malignancy, surgery or radiotherapy. The vulva becomes thickened and indurated and may be more prone to attacks of cellulitis. Prophylactic penicillin may be required.

Lymphangiectasia

Small lymphatic vesicles (lymphangiectasia) may develop on a background of chronic lymphoedema. They may be primary, due to an inherited defect, or secondary, due to Crohn's disease or following radiotherapy for cervical or vaginal cancer. The lesions have a verrucose appearance and are often incorrectly diagnosed as viral warts.

Treatment with carbon dioxide laser can be used in symptomatic cases where there is leakage of lymph. Congenital lesions may need imaging studies to identify whether there are deeper lymphatic abnormalities.

References

1 Bauer A, Grief C, Vollandt R *et al.* Vulvar diseases need an interdisciplinary approach. *Dermatology* 1999;199:223–226.

2 Cazes A, Prost-Squarcioni C, Boedemer C *et al.* Histologic cutaneous modifications after the use of EMLA cream, a diagnostic pitfall: review of 13 cases. *Arch Dermatol* 2007;143:1074–1076.

3 Farrell AM, Marren P, Dean D, Wojnarowska F. Lichen sclerosus: evidence that immunological changes occur at all levels of the skin. *Br J Dermatol* 1999;140:1087–1092.

4 Chan I, Oyama N, Neill SM *et al.* Characterization of IgG autoantibodies to extracellular matrix protein 1 in lichen sclerosus. *Clin Exp Dermatol* 2004;29:499–504.

5 Meyrick Thomas RH, Ridley CM, McGibbon DH, Black MM. Lichen sclerosus and autoimmunity – a study of 350 women. *Br J Dermatol* 1988;118:41–46.

6 Wallace HJ. Lichen sclerosus et atrophicus. *Trans St John's Dermatol Soc* 1971;57:9–30.

7 Neill SM, Lewis FM, Tatnall FM, Cox NH. British Association of Dermatologists' guidelines for the management of lichen sclerosus 2010. *Br J Dermatol* 2010;163:672–682.

8 Carrozzo M, Pellicano R. Lichen planus and hepatitis C virus infection: an updated critical review. *Minerva Gastroenterol Dietol* 2008;54:65–74.

9 Pelisse M, Leibowitch M, Sedel D, Hewitt J. Un nouveau syndrome vulvo-vagino-gingival. Lichen plan érosif plurimuqueux. *Ann Dermatol Vénéréol* 1982;110:797–798.

10 Setterfield JA, Neill S, Shirlaw P *et al.* The vulvo-vaginal-gingival syndrome: a severe sub-group of lichen planus with characteristic clinical features and a novel association with the class II HLA DQB1*0201 allele. *J Am Acad Dermatol* 2006;55:98–113.

11 Lewis FM, Shah M, Harrington CI. Vulval involvement in lichen planus: a study of 37 women. *Br J Dermatol* 1996;135:89–91.

12 Belfiore P, de Fede O, Cabibi D *et al.* Prevalence of vulval lichen planus in a cohort of women with oral lichen planus; an interdisciplinary study. *Br J Dermatol* 2006;155:994–998.

13 Lewis FM, Harrington CI. Squamous cell carcinoma arising in vulval lichen planus. *Br J Dermatol* 1994;131:703–705.

14 Franck JM, Young AW. Squamous cell carcinoma in situ arising within lichen planus of the vulva. *Dermatol Surg* 1995;21:890–894.

15 Derrick EK, Ridley CM, Kobza-Black A *et al.* A clinical study of 23 cases of female anogenital carcinoma. *Br J Dermatol* 2000;143:1217–1223.

16 Cooper SM, Haefner HK, Abrahams-Gessel S, Margesson LJ. Vulvo-vaginal lichen planus treatment: a survey of current practices. *Arch Dermatol* 2008;144:1520–1521.

17 Goldsmith PC, Rycroft RJ, White IR *et al.* Contact sensitivity in women with anogenital dermatoses. *Contact Dermatitis* 1997;36:174–175.

18 Edwards L Hansen R. Reiter's syndrome of the vulva. *Arch Dermatol* 1992;128:811–814.

19 Boer J, Weltevreden EF. Hidradenitis suppurativa or acne inversa. A clinico-pathological study of early lesions. *Br J Dermatol* 1996;135:721–725.

20 Bardan A, Nizet V, Gallo RL. Antimicrobial peptides and the skin. *Exp Opin Biol Ther* 2004;4:53–59.

21 Alikhan A, Lynch PJ, Eisen DR. Hidradenitis suppurativa: a comprehensive review. *J Am Acad Dermatol* 2009;60:539–561.

22 Bruch-Gerharz D, Hertl M, Ruzicka T. Mucous membrane pemphigoid: clinical aspects, immunopathological features and therapy. *Eur J Dermatol* 2007;17:191–200.

23 Lipschutz B. Uber eine eigenartige Geshwursform des weiblichen Genitales (ulcus vulvae acutum). *Arch Dermatol Res* 1913;114:363–396.

24 Halverson JA, Brevig T, Aas T *et al.* Genital ulcers as initial manifestation of Epstein Barr virus infection: two new cases and review of the literature. *Acta Dermato-venereologica* 2006;86:439–442.

25 Preston PW, Hudson NH, Lewis FM. Treatment of vulval Crohn's disease with infliximab. *Clin Exp Dermatol* 2006;31:378–380.

26 Makhija S, Trotter M, Wagner E *et al.* Refractory Crohn's disease of the vulva treated with infliximab: a case report. *Can J Gastroenterol* 2007;21:835–837.

27 Vidal D, Puig L, Gilaberte M, Alomar A. review of 26 cases of classical pyoderma gangrenosum: clinical and therapeutic features. *J Dermatol Treatment* 2004;15:146–152.

28 Alpsoy E, Akman A. Behcet's disease: an algorithmic approach to its treatment. *Arch Dermatol Res* 2009;301:693–702.

29 Gleason BC, Hirsch MS, Nucci MR *et al.* Atypical genital naevi. A clinicopathological analysis of 56 cases. *Am J Surg Pathol* 2008;32:51–57.

30 Carlson JA, Mu XC, Slominski A *et al.* Melanocytic proliferations associated with lichen sclerosus. *Arch Dermatol* 2002;138:77–87.

31 Rosamilia LL, Schwartz JL, Lowe L *et al.* Vulvar melanoma in a 10-year-old girl in association with lichen sclerosus *J Am Acad Dermatol* 2006;54:S52–53

32 Lee Wong M, Collins JS, Nozad C, Resnick DJ. The diagnosis and treatment of human seminal plasma hypersensitivity. *Obstet Gynaecol* 2008;111:538–539.

33 Feer-Ybarz L, Basagana M, Coroleu B, Bartolome B, Cistero-Bahima A. Human seminal plasma allergy and successful pregnancy. *J Invest Allergy Clin Immunol* 2006;16:314–316.

Chapter 53
Benign Diseases of the Vagina, Cervix and Ovary

D. Keith Edmonds
Queen Charlotte's & Chelsea Hospital, London, UK

Vagina

The vagina is the lowest part of the internal genital tract of the female. Frequently it is ignored by the clinician as it merely allows the passage of the fetus from its *in utero* existence to the outside world, or as it is bypassed with both the speculum and vaginal fingers to gain access to the cervix and uterus during pelvic examination.

The vagina consists of a non-keratinized squamous epithelial lining supported by connective tissue and surrounded by circular and longitudinal muscle coats. The muscle coat is attached superiorly to the fibres of the uterine cervix, and inferiorly and laterally to the pubococcygeus, bulbospongiosus and perineum. The lower end of the epithelium joins, near the hymen, the mucosal components of the vestibule and superiorly extends over the uterine cervix to the squamocolumnar junction. The vaginal epithelium has a longitudinal column in the anterior and posterior wall, and from each column there are numerous transverse ridges or rugae extending laterally on each side. The squamous epithelium during the reproductive years is thick and rich in glycogen. It does not change significantly during the menstrual cycle, although there is a small increase in glycogen content in the luteal phase and a reduction immediately premenstrually. The prepubertal and postmenopausal epithelium is thin or atrophic.

The vagina has a varied bacterial flora in oestrogenized women, and knowledge of what is normal and abnormal is important for determining infection. The main organisms are listed in Table 53.1.

Vaginal infection

Between puberty and the menopause the vaginal lactobacilli maintains a pH level between 3.8 and 4.2. This protects against infection. Before puberty and after the menopause, the higher pH level and urinary and faecal contamination increase the risks of infection. The other time when vaginal atrophy is noted is in the postpartum period, and it is also associated with lactation. Normal physiological vaginal discharge consists of a transudate from the vaginal wall, squames containing glycogen, polymorphs, lactobacilli, cervical mucus and residual menstrual fluid, as well as a contribution from the greater and lesser vestibular glands. Vaginal discharge varies according to oestrogen levels during the menstrual cycle and is a normal physiological occurrence. Vaginal discharge does not normally have an unpleasant odour, and if this occurs in the presence of change in appearance of copiousness, then it may reflect infection. Non-specific vaginitis may be associated with sexual trauma, allergy to deodorants or contraceptives, and chemical irritation from topical antimicrobial treatment. Non-specific infection may be further provoked by the presence of foreign bodies, for example, ring pessary, continual use of tampons and the presence of an intrauterine contraceptive device.

Bacterial vaginosis

Bacterial vaginosis has been previously associated with organisms of the *Corynebacterium* or *Haemophilus* species and more recently with the organism *Gardnerella vaginalis*. It is now believed to be due to a *Vibrio* or comma-shaped organism named *Mobiluncus*. These organisms are believed to be sexually transmitted. Usually the vagina is not inflamed and therefore the term vaginosis is used rather than vaginitis. Nearly half of 'infected' patients will not have symptoms [1]. Examination will reveal a thin grey–white discharge and a vaginal pH level increased to greater than 5, and a Gram stain of collected material will show 'clue cells', which consist of vaginal epithelial cells covered with microorganisms and the absence of lactobacilli. The diagnosis can also be confirmed by adding a drop of vaginal discharge to saline on a glass slide and adding one drop of 10% potassium hydroxide. This releases a characteristic fishy amine

Table 53.1 Normal frequency.

	100%	50%	<5%
Staphylococccus epidermidis	+	–	–
Lactobaccilus	+	–	–
Staphylococcus aureus	–	+	–
Staphylococcus mitis	–	+	–
Enterococcus faecalis	–	+	–
Streptococcus pneumoniae	–	–	+
Streptococcus pyogenes	–	–	+
Neisseria sp.	–	+	–
Neisseria meningitidis	–	+	–
Escherichia coli	–	+	–
Proteus sp.	–	+	–
Bacteroides sp.	–	–	+
Corynebacterium	–	+	–
Mycoplasma	–	+	–
Candida albicans	–	–	+

smell. Bacterial vaginosis may be associated with increased risk of preterm labour [2], pelvic inflammatory disease and postoperative pelvic infection [3,4]. The treatment of bacterial vaginosis is with metronidazole, either as 200 mg three times a day for 7 days or as a single 2-g dose. Alternatively, clindamycin can be used as a vaginal cream.

Trichomoniasis

Trichomoniasis is a sexually transmitted disease caused by the parasite *Trichomonas vaginalis*. Symptoms usually appear 5–28 days after exposure and include a yellow–green vaginal discharge, often foamy, with a strong odour, dyspareunia and vaginal irritation. Ten per cent of women infected also manifest a 'strawberry' cervix on examination (Plate 53.1). *T. vaginalis* is a flagellated organism which can damage the vaginal epithelium, increasing a woman's susceptibility to infection by human immunodeficiency virus (HIV). This is caused by lysis of the epithelial cells. Treatment is with metronidazole 400 mg three times daily for 7 days or tinidazole at 2 mg as a single dose. As this is a sexually transmitted disease, diagnosis should prompt the gynaecologist to refer the patient to a genitourinary medicine clinic for contact tracing.

Vaginal candidiasis

This is a fungal infection commonly referred to as 'thrush'. It is caused by any of the species of *Candida*, of which *Candida albicans* is the most common. This is an infection that causes vaginal irritation and vaginitis, which leads to itching, burning, soreness and a classic whitish or whitish-grey cottage cheese-like discharge. The irritation and inflammation spreads across the vulva. This may also involve the perianal skin. *Candida* can be transmitted to a

sexual partner in whom it can cause red patchy sores near the head of the penis or on the foreskin, causing a severe itching and burning sensation. *C. albicans* usually causes infection when lactobacilli production or lactic acid is interfered with, resulting in a change in the pH level in the vagina and subsequent overgrowth of *Candida*. Diabetics and patients using antibiotics for other infections have an increased incidence of candidiasis. This, in conjunction with other treatments, e.g. steroids or conditions including HIV, leads to a weakening in the immune response system, allowing *Candida* to thrive. *Candida* is infrequently found in the vagina but frequently in part of the intestinal flora. The diagnosis is usually made on inspection, but a swab from the infected area will confirm the diagnosis in culture. Treatment for vaginal candidiasis is primarily with antifungal pessaries or cream inserted high into the vagina. Single-dose preparations offer the advantage of compliance, and imidazole drugs (clotrimazole, econazole) are effective in short courses of 1–14 days according to the preparation. Oral medication is also available in the form of fluconazole or itraconazole and these treatments are usually extremely effective at eradicating the disease. Some 10% of women who contract candidiasis will develop recurrent disease – this is particularly likely if there are predisposing factors, such as pregnancy, diabetes or oral contraceptive use. It is important to consider partner treatment in those patients who get recurrent disease and in those patients who are resistant to two courses of imidazoles. If bacteriological confirmation of recurrent disease is made, a number of long-term treatments can be prescribed. These include fluconazole 100 mg orally every week for 6 months, clotrimazole 500-mg pessary weekly for 6 months or itraconazole 400 mg every month for 6 months. There is extensive alternative medicine literature on the treatment of *Candida* but there is very little scientific evidence to prove its efficacy.

> **Summary box 53.1**
>
> Vaginal infection:
> - It is important to differentiate between infection and normal flora in diagnosing vaginal infection.
> - Bacterial vaginosis may be associated with preterm labour.
> - Recurrent vaginal candidiasis needs systemic investigation prior to long-term treatment.

Syphilitic lesions of the vagina

Syphilis is uncommon among women in the UK. However, unusual vaginal lesions must be considered, particularly if the patient or partner has recently travelled overseas.

The primary lesion may be in the vagina or on the vulva or cervix. There is usually a single, painless, well-demarcated ulcer with indurated edges, associated with lymphadenopathy. Secondary lesions include condylomata lata, mucous patches and snail-track ulcers.

Diagnosis is based on identification of the causative organism, *Treponema pallidum*, on dark-ground microscopy, or by serological examination for syphilis, for example enzyme-linked immunoabsorbent assay (ELISA). For further details and details of treatment with bicillin (i.e. procaine penicillin with benzyl-penicillin sodium) (see Chapter 47) [5].

Gonococcal vaginitis

Gonorrhoea may infect the cervix or Bartholin's gland but not the vaginal epithelium, except in prepubertal girls or postmenopausal women. If there is suspicion of sexual abuse in a young child with a vaginal discharge, a swab for culture for *Neisseria gonorrhoeae* (see Chapter 47) should be taken.

Viral infections

Lesions due to human papilloma and herpes simplex virus can be seen in the vagina. Further information is given in Chapter 47.

Toxic shock syndrome

This topic has been included because it is associated with the use of vaginal tampons during menstruation or less frequently in the puerperium [6]. Although there is a link between this syndrome and certain organisms found within the vagina of affected women, it is not a vaginal infection.

The syndrome was first described by Todd *et al.* [7] in seven children and teenagers (aged 8–17 years) with particular multisystem manifestations and similarities with other conditions produced by staphylococcal toxins. The sudden appearance in the early 1980s of a large number of similar cases in young women led to epidemiological investigation, with the resultant finding that 92% of reported cases were associated with menstruation, and 99% of these were in tampon users [8]. The majority of cases were seen in the USA but also occasionally in the UK or elsewhere.

The characteristics of the syndrome are an abrupt onset of pyrexia equal to or greater than 38.9°C, myalgia, diffuse skin rash with oedema and blanching erythema, like sunburn, and subsequent (1–2 weeks later) desquamation of the palms and soles. Less commonly, vomiting and diarrhoea symptomatic of hypotension are seen. Laboratory results include leukocytosis, thrombocytopenia and increased serum bilirubin, liver enzymes and creatine phosphokinase. *Staphylococcus aureus* can be identified frequently from the vagina but blood cultures are usually negative. It is believed that the syndrome is due to the systemic features of a toxin (TSST-1; toxic shock syndrome toxin) and subsequent release of bradykinin, tumour necrosis factor or other biological response mediators. Group A β haemolytic streptococci have also been implicated because they can release a similar toxin (erythrogenic toxin A) [9].

An initial study [6] could find no association with the brand of tampon used, degree of absorbency as stated on the packet, frequency of tampon change, frequency of coitus or coitus during menstruation, or type of contraception. Subsequent assessment has suggested that the inclusion of synthetic superabsorbent materials in certain brands of tampons was responsible. Removal of these brands from the market in the USA reduced the frequency of the syndrome from 17 per 100 000 menstruating women to only 1 per 100 000. However, this reduction also coincided with increased public education and greater care in tampon use, including insertion.

Mortality rates from the syndrome were initially reported to be as high as 15%, but fell to 3% by 1981 [8]. The high mortality was probably due to earlier underreporting of less severe cases, but mortality fell with increasing awareness of the diagnosis and early effective treatment of the hypervolemia in severe cases. Recommended treatment is as for any septicaemia and includes intravenous fluids and, where necessary, inotropic support. The cause, where possible, should be eliminated and a β lactamase-resistant penicillin given parenterally. Relapse can occur with subsequent menstruation and it is recommended that tampons should not be used until *Staphylococcus aureus* has been eradicated from the vagina. Relapse has been described in the puerperium [10].

Vaginal atrophy

This is seen not only following the menopause, but also prior to puberty and during lactation. Examination shows loss of rugal folds and prominent subepithelial vessels, sometimes with adjacent ecchymoses. The patient may present with vaginal bleeding, vaginal discharge or vaginal dryness and dyspareunia. Superficial infection, with Gram-positive cocci or Gram-negative bacilli, may be associated.

Treatment requires oestrogen to restore the vaginal epithelium and pH level. This is usually by topical oestrogen cream, and some of the oestrogen will be absorbed systemically. The endometrial safety of long-term use is uncertain. Preparations vary in length of recommended treatment, but usually this is administered for 3 months and then the effect is assessed. Repeated applications over time may be needed depending on symptoms returning. Alternatively, in postmenopausal women hormone replacement therapy can be used.

Vaginal trauma

This may follow coitus, with damage to the epithelium or less frequently the vaginal muscle wall, or breaking down of adhesions at the vault following vaginal surgery (Plate 53.2). It may be associated with parturition or be iatrogenic, for example, ulceration associated with the use of a ring pessary. Trauma may be associated with significant haemorrhage and occasionally will leave vesicle or rectal fistulae.

Fistula

A fistula may result from trauma, as described earlier, or it may be due to carcinoma or Crohn's disease. Fistula of the anterior wall is now uncommon in association with childbirth, but rectovaginal fistula may follow an obstetric tear or extension of an episiotomy, and an incomplete or inadequate repair. Fistulae involving ureter, bladder or rectum may follow gynaecological surgery.

Endometriosis

Occasionally, deposits of endometriosis can be found beneath the vaginal epithelium following surgery or episiotomy. They may cause abnormal vaginal bleeding or pain. They are most easily identified while bleeding but have a blueish appearance at other times. Treatment can be by laser vaporization or excision, or by drug therapy as for endometriosis elsewhere.

Vaginal intraepithelial neoplasia

Vaginal intraepithelial neoplasia (VAIN) is seen in 1–6% of patients with cervical intraepithelial neoplasia (CIN) (Plate 53.3). It is almost always in the upper vagina and confluent with the cervical lesion [11]. It is uncommon to find VAIN in the presence of a normal cervix, but Lenehan *et al.* [12] reported that 43% of their patients with VAIN after hysterectomy had a history of negative cervical smears and benign cervical pathology. Imrie *et al.* [13] reported VAIN occurring in an artificial vagina in a woman who had congenital absence of vagina and cervix. VAIN may be present in the vaginal vault or suture line after hysterectomy (Plate 53.4) (this may be residual after CIN has been treated) or may be distant from the vault and associated with multicentric intraepithelial neoplasia. Hummer *et al.* [14] reported a series of 66 patients with VAIN and showed that one-third of cases had developed within 2 years of their previous cervical lesion being treated. The longest time interval between the diagnosis of CIN and VAIN was 17 years; the age of patients with VAIN in that series ranged from 24 to 74 years with a mean age of 52 years.

The aetiology of VAIN is probably similar to that of CIN. Extension of the transformation zone into the fornices would seem to be responsible, even though no abnormality was recognized when the cervical lesion was treated. A higher incidence of VAIN has been noted in patients on chemotherapy or immunosuppressive therapy. The role of radiotherapy for carcinoma of the cervix some 10–15 years prior to the development of VAIN has been noted, particularly when a subsequent lesion is in the lower vagina. It is thought by some [14] that a sublethal dose of radiation may induce tumour transformation and that VAIN or vaginal sarcoma may result.

As for cervical lesions, VAIN I is equivalent to mild dysplasia, VAIN II to moderate dysplasia and VAIN III to severe dysplasia or carcinoma *in situ*. The disease is normally recognized as a result of abnormal cytology seen in a vaginal vault smear specimen. Townsend [15] recommended that vault smears should be performed annually for women after hysterectomy performed for CIN, and every 3 years if the hysterectomy was for benign disease. Current teaching discourages the need for any subsequent smears in this latter group but recommends a follow-up of patients who have had hysterectomy for cervical lesions. Gemmell *et al.* [16] recommend that vault smears should be taken 6 months, 12 months and 2 years after hysterectomy; the patient should then return to 5-yearly screening.

Colposcopic assessment of patients with abnormal vault smears will delineate areas of aceto-white epithelium. Punctuation may be apparent in more that 50%, and areas of abnormality will often fail to stain following the application of Lugol's iodine solution (Plate 53.5). However, atrophic changes within the vagina may lead to extensive areas of non-Lugol's staining and difficulty in defining the limits of lesions. A preliminary 2-week course of oestrogen cream to correct oestrogen deficiency and then colposcopy examination 2 weeks following this will improve the definition of lesions. Problems may be encountered in interpreting or getting access to areas of change disappearing into post-hysterectomy vaginal angles or suture line. Vaginal biopsies from the vault can usually be taken without anaesthesia, but occasionally difficult access into vaginal angles may require the use of general anaesthesia and appropriate vaginal retractors.

No adequate study on the progression of VAIN to invasive disease has been reported. Among the series of patients reported by McIndoe *et al.* [17] were patients who had abnormal smears following hysterectomy; some of these patients were followed up for almost 20 years before developing invasive carcinoma while others progressed more rapidly.

There have been a wide variety of treatments for VAIN. These include excision biopsy for smaller lesions and 5-fluorouracil cream or laser vaporization for more extensive lesions [18–20]. Experience with the use of 5-fluorouracil has been less in the UK than in the USA. Caglar *et al.* [21] claimed that the subsequent denudation of epithelium was specific for only abnormal epithelium. However, sometimes the epithelial ulceration is extensive, accompanied by severe vaginal burning, and subsequent healing may take several months. Treatment failure is common. Use of the carbon dioxide laser is more likely to be successful in treating those women who have not had hysterectomy and where the full extent of the lesion can be demarcated. It must be noted that the vaginal wall may be thin in postmenopausal women and the bladder and rectal mucosa less than 5 mm away. The advantage of the carbon dioxide laser over other forms of selective ablation, for example diathermy or loop excision, is that there should be greater control of the area and depth of laser vaporization. Techniques using high-power density and rapid beam movement minimize carbonization and adjacent thermal necrosis to allow recognition of tissue architecture with removal of lesional epithelium down to the underlying stroma, thereby reducing the risk of bladder or bowel damage.

The difficult patient to treat is the one who has already undergone a hysterectomy for a cervical lesion and returns with an area of abnormality in the suture line. Whether leaving the vault open at the time of hysterectomy avoids sequestration of the vaginal mucosa above the usual suture line has not been proven. Ireland and Monaghan [22] found that 9 of their 32 patients with VAIN had invasive carcinoma in the area of the suture line, and they emphasized both the difficulty in assessing the vaginal vault and the need for obtaining adequate tissue for histological examination. They therefore advocated partial vaginectomy whenever abnormal epithelium is seen at the angles or suture line of the vault. This procedure [23] requires an abdominal approach after packing the vaginal vault and involves the mobilization of the ureters down to their insertion into the bladder, dissection of bladder and rectum from the vagina, and sufficient mobilization to allow removal of the upper 1–2 from the top of the vagina. The definition of just how much to remove is usually best achieved by commencing a mucosal dissection from below prior to packing the vagina. Occasionally, more extensive disease will require total vaginectomy followed by either skin grafting or mobilization of a loop of bowel to reconstruct the neovagina. There are some who advocate a vaginal approach [24], but access may not be easy and occasionally brisk bleeding from vaginal arteries may be encountered [25]. The other option is to use radiotherapy by the intravaginal approach [26,27]. Concerns that such treatment may produce vaginal narrowing and interfere with coitus have not been realized, but some younger women develop radiation-induced menopause and require hormone replacement therapy. The latter authors reported that all of their patients remained cytologically normal and free of disease at a follow-up of more than 2 years; colposcopic appearances after radiotherapy may be complex (Plate 53.6). Soutter [25] suggested the management of VAIN after hysterectomy in young women is better by the surgical approach and recommended radiotherapy in older women. Such treatment may not be simple and referral to a centre with gynaecological oncology expertise is desirable.

Diethylstilboestrol and related vaginal lesions

Diethylstilboestrol (DES) was used from the mid-1940s for the treatment of recurrent or threatened abortion and

Summary box 53.2

- VAIN coexists in up to 6% of patients with CIN.
- Colposcopic assessment and follow-up is mandatory.
- Treatment is either by excision or local ablative therapy.

unexplained fetal loss late in pregnancy, predominantly in the north-eastern states of the USA (where it is estimated that 2 million women were treated) and also Canada, Mexico, Western Australia and Western Europe.

Herbst and Scully [28] reported seven cases of clear cell adenocarcinoma of the vagina seen and treated in Massachusetts General Hospital, Boston, in young women aged between 14 and 22 years. A retrospective study by them linked these carcinomas with the intrauterine exposure of the patients to DES given to their mothers during pregnancy. The more extensive survey [29] looked at 346 cases of clear cell adenocarcinoma of the cervix and vagina. The maternal history was available in 317 patients and it was found that two-thirds of the patients had been exposed *in utero* to DES or a similar non-steroid oestrogen given to the mothers during pregnancy. In a further 10%, drugs of doubtful origin were given but in 25% no history of maternal hormone therapy could be obtained. They found that the age incidence for clear cell adenocarcinoma of the vagina in young women began at 14 years, peaked at 19 years and then subsequently declined. They estimate that the probable risk of development of clear cell carcinoma in women exposed to DES *in utero* is 0.14–1.4 per 1000 women. DES produced various other vaginal and cervical lesions. Vaginal adenosis was often seen in combination with cervical eversion or ectropion. The patients often had a ridge between the vaginal and cervical tissue referred to as a collar, a rim or a 'cock's comb cervix'. Such appearances occurred in approximately 25% of exposed patients. The adenosis can affect the anterior and posterior vaginal walls and lateral vaginal fornices, but is usually restricted to the upper third of the vagina. Sometimes there will be cytological abnormality, extensive immature metaplasia and CIN. Originally it was recommended that women who were known to have been exposed to DES *in utero* should be screened from the age of 14 years with both cytology and colposcopy. DES exposure was uncommon in the UK and associated vaginal changes will be seen infrequently. Such patients should be managed by annual cervical and vaginal cytological surveillance and colposcopic assessment. It is still not known if the risk of adenocarcinoma persists, for example, after the menopause.

Benign vaginal tumours

These are uncommon but occur within the vaginal wall and include myoma, fibromyoma, neurofibroma, papilloma, myxoma and adenomyoma.

Cystic lesions may be found within the vagina, usually laterally and occasionally extending from the fornix down to the introitus. These are usually of Gartner's or Wolffian duct origin. They may increase to such a size as to interfere with coitus or tampon use. They can usually be managed by de-roofing, but care must be taken in the fornices to avoid large uterine and vesicle vessels.

Cervix

Benign lesions

Position of the squamocolumnar junction and changes within the transformation zone

It is known that the uterine cervix increases in size in response to oestrogens; because the cervix is anchored at the fornices, the end result of any enlargement is eversion to expose the columnar epithelium of the endocervical canal. This occurs dramatically in the neonate and under the influence of maternal oestrogens, at puberty under the influence of rising oestrogen levels, during the use of the combined oral contraceptive pill and during the first pregnancy (Plate 53.7). Ectopy is the preferred term for this display of columnar epithelium (rather than 'erosion'); colposcopic examination demonstrates the folding of the epithelium into villi (Plate 53.8). Upon withdrawal of oestrogen, for example in the puerperium or at the menopause, the squamocolumnar junction approaches the external os once more and indeed may be found within the endocervical canal.

In approximately 5% of women there will be extension of the squamocolumnar junction into the anterior and posterior fornices so that on subsequent examination an extensive area of change will be noted – the so-called congenital transformation zone. The presence of this may not be apparent to the naked eye but can be demonstrated following the application of Lugol's iodine. Biopsy will show no evidence of intraepithelial neoplasia but delayed or immature metaplasia.

Cervical metaplasia

Exposure of the columnar epithelium to low pH as found within the vagina promotes a series of physiological changes, known as metaplasia. It is believed that reserve cells lying within the monolayer of columnar epithelium will proliferate giving a multilayered epithelium with the columnar cells left perched on the surface (Plate 53.9). These cells will initially appear immature and undifferentiated, but with the passage of time will show the usual differentiation to resume a squamous epithelium with glycogenation of the superficial squamous cells. This process occurs at the squamocolumnar junction, or transformation zone, starting in the neonate and continuing until well after the menopause. Examination of the endocervix will show a series of longitudinal ridges with columnar cells lining both the tops of the ridges and extending down into the depths or crypts (Plate 53.10). Metaplasia usually occurs initially in the ridges and may well bridge over these, leaving a squamous cover with columnar epithelium remaining within the crypts. If a crypt cannot expel the mucus produced from the columnar epithelium, a retention cyst or Nabothian follicle will occur (Plate 53.11); sometimes these follicles are large and extensive across the transformation zone. They are entirely benign and are not associated with infection, i.e. they are not a sign of cervicitis.

Endocervical polyps

The recognition of endocervical polyps at the time of taking a cervical smear is common and usually increases with age up to the menopause (Plates 53.12 and 53.13). Occasionally these polyps will be symptomatic, producing heavy vaginal discharge or bleeding upon coital contact. Histology of these polyps will show that they consist of columnar epithelium, sometimes with metaplastic squamous epithelium across the tip. Malignant change is most unusual. However, if these polyps are removed, for example by polypectomy, tissue should be sent for histology, recognizing that some 15% of uterine tumours will be polypoidal and occasionally will extrude through the external os.

Chronic cervicitis

There was previous enthusiasm for treating by cautery or diathermy those patients who complained of chronic watery vaginal discharge and were found to have an 'erosion'. As explained earlier, these areas of ectopy or everted columnar epithelium are not pathological and the term cervicitis is not appropriate.

However, some women with *Chlamydia trachomatis* (and rarely with *Neisseria gonorrhoeae*) will present with symptoms of discharge and an abnormal cervix will be noted. Brunham *et al.* [30] described 'mucopurulent cervicitis' in association with *Chlamydia*, and Hare *et al.* [31] described the colposcopy appearances of 'follicular cervicitis'. Providing these organisms have been excluded by appropriate microbiology, 'cervicitis' does not require treatment except by increasing vaginal acidity to promote squamous metaplasia.

Ovaries

Benign disorders

Anatomy

The ovaries are attached to the lateral pelvic side walls by the suspensory ligament containing the ovarian vessels, and to the cornua of the uterus by a ligamentous condensation of the broad ligament. Each ovary is $3 \times 2 \times 1$ cm in size in the resting or inactive state, but will increase in size during physiological stimulus; they will shrink after the menopause. The surface is covered by a flattened monolayer of epithelial cells, and beneath this are the ovarian follicles, with oocyte, granulosa layer and surrounding theca. Beneath this cortical layer are a stromal medulla and a hilum where the vessels enter through the mesovarium. The events that are associated with follicular development and ovulation are described elsewhere (Chapter 39). The size and position of the ovaries varies between puberty and menopause – the mean volume, as assessed by transvaginal ultrasound scan of a premenopausal ovary, is $6.8\,cm^3$ (upper limit of normal $18\,cm^3$) compared with a mean postmenopausal size of $3\,cm^3$ (upper limit $8\,cm^3$) [32].

Ovarian enlargement

Ovarian enlargement will occur in response to follicle-stimulating and luteinizing hormones. Follicular and luteal cysts can occur, and theca lutein cysts up to 15 cm in size will develop in response to very high levels of chorionic gonadotrophin as seen with trophoblastic disease. Hyperstimulation syndrome can occur, with massive enlargement of the ovaries and development of ascites, in response to doses of gonadotrophin injections during fertility treatment.

Polycystic disease

Polycystic enlargement of the ovaries has been described under a variety of names. Stein and Leventhal [33] described seven cases of amenorrhoea or irregular menstruation with enlarged polycystic ovaries demonstrated by 'pneumoroentgenography' and restoration of normal physiological function after wedge resection. Judd *et al.* [34] demonstrated that the mildly elevated androgen levels found in this syndrome were of ovarian origin. The changes in gonadotrophin ratios and androgen levels are not always consistent with the appearances of the ovaries, and increasingly the diagnosis of polycystic ovarian disease is based on ultrasound findings of peripheral distribution of 10 or more follicles of 2–8 mm in diameter, with increased ovarian volume (see Chapter 41).

Ovarian pregnancy

Ovarian ectopic pregnancy is uncommon, with an estimated incidence of 1 per 25 000 of all pregnancies, although Grimes *et al.* [35] reported an incidence of 1 per 7000 deliveries in their Chicago series. There appears to be an association with intrauterine contraceptive device use [36] or tubal pathology and infertility [35]. Patients usually present with features of an extrauterine pregnancy or bleeding from a corpus luteum. The Spiegelberg criteria [37] to fulfil the diagnosis are as follows:
1 that the tube including the fimbria is intact and separate from the ovary;
2 that the gestation sac definitely occupies the normal position of the ovary;
3 that the sac be connected with the uterus by the ovarian ligament; and
4 that unquestionable ovarian tissue be demonstrated in the walls of the sac.

Treatment is surgical removal, which may require removal of the ovary. This can usually be achieved laparoscopically.

Ovarian endometriosis

Ovarian enlargement may be found secondary to endometriosis, that is, endometriomas. Endometriomas of more than 10 cm in diameter will not respond to medical management alone and require laparotomy with the risks of eventually having to perform oophorectomy or laparoscopic cyst aspiration, 3-months' treatment with luteinizing hormone releasing hormone analogue and then laparoscopic dissection of the cyst lining or destruction with, for example, a KTP (potassium-titanylphosphate) laser [38] (see Chapter 49).

Ovarian tumours

There is a large list of benign ovarian tumours (cystic, solid or a mixture of both) contained within the World Health Organization Committee on the Nomenclature and Terminology of Ovarian Tumour Classification. Common benign tumours include mature cystic teratomas (Plate 53.14), epithelial (serous or mucinous) cystadenoma and various soft-tissue tumours not specific to the ovary, for example fibroma (Plate 53.15).

Corpus luteum

The corpus luteum is a physiological development following ovulation, and the corpus luteum in a normal menstrual cycle may reach 3 cm in diameter. Occasionally, the corpus luteum may persist in the absence of pregnancy and may increase in size to up to 5 cm in diameter. It is usual at this point that regression begins and the corpus luteum cyst will disappear. These cysts are often seen incidentally on ultrasound in asymptomatic women or in women who have mild abdominal pain. The management is conservative. In 95% of cases, repeat ultrasound at 6–8 weeks will show that the structure has disappeared and normal ovarian function ensues. It is extremely important that a conservative approach is adopted in these circumstances and these cysts only need to be removed laparoscopically if they persist or increase in size over time.

Mature cystic teratomas (dermoid cyst)

Dermoid cysts are cystic teratomas that contain elements of ectoderm that may include skin, hair follicles and sweat glands, and occasionally hair can be quite prolific. There can also be pockets of sebum, blood, fat, bone, nails, teeth and cartilage and occasionally thyroid tissues. Dermoid cysts usually present with abdominal discomfort or pain in women between the ages of 18 and 25 years. Diagnosis may be made on ultrasound, which has classic features, and if there is any doubt as to the aetiology, a magnetic resonance imaging scan can be performed although is rarely necessary. Dermoid cysts can vary in size and grow over time until diagnosis is made. Occasionally, dermoid cysts may be diagnosed for the first time during pregnancy, and here clinical decisions about whether to adopt a conservative approach with management of the cyst postnatally needs to be made in the light of clinical symptoms and size. Dermoid cysts may be bilateral.

The management of dermoid cysts is removal as they will increase in size and cause increasing symptoms over time. It is difficult to determine whether dermoid cysts have malignant potential as it is normal practice to remove these in all patients in whom they are diagnosed. Surgical removal may either be through laparotomy or laparoscopy, but it is essential that all tissue is removed to prevent recurrence. It is also imperative to ensure that bilateral dermoid cysts are not present during the time of surgery. It is almost always possible to retain the ovary at the time of surgery.

Serous cystadenoma

These account for approximately 25% of all benign ovarian neoplasms and their peak incidences are in the fourth and fifth decade of life. Symptoms are usually rather non-specific but can include pelvic pain or discomfort or occasionally a pelvic mass discovered at routine examination. Approximately 20% of cystadenomas are bilateral and they are benign, and treatment is either by salpingo-oophorectomy or ovarian cystectomy depending on the circumstance. Recurrence is extremely rare.

Mucinous cystadenoma

These comprise 50% of benign ovarian epithelial neoplasms and tend to occur most often between the third and sixth decade of life, with a mean age of around 50 years. Small tumours are often found incidentally, whereas the larger tumours present as an obvious pelvic or abdominal mass. They are rarely bilateral. Treatment is by oophorectomy, which may be performed either laparoscopically or by laparotomy.

Ovarian cyst accidents

Ovarian cysts may present in an acute situation, and here pain may be acute following either rupture or haemorrhage into the cyst. Haemorrhage can be dramatic and severe bleeding can cause hypervolemia and a haematoperitoneum. Patients present in a collapsed state and the differential diagnosis is often of a ruptured ectopic pregnancy. Treatment is by emergency laparotomy to stop the bleeding, and salvage of the ovary can occur if possible. Tortion of an ovarian cyst presents as intermittent acute abdominal pain, usually in the iliac fossa associated with the ovary. The pain is colicky in nature and the pain may be referred to the sacral iliac joint or to the upper medial thigh. Episodes of tortion may be spread over quite long periods of time and it is important for the clinician to recognize the pattern of symptoms of acute presentation if multiple tortion is to be avoided, or it will result in ovarian ischaemia. Sadly, failure to recognize this sequence of events may lead to an acute situation with surgery resulting in a salpingo-oophorectomy as salvage of the ovary is not possible. However, with prudent diagnosis a laparoscopic removal of the ovarian cyst and plication of the infundibulopelvic ligament can salvage the ovary and prevent further tortion.

Summary box 53.4

Benign disease of the ovary:
- Cysts of the corpus luteum should be monitored and will resolve spontaneously in 95% of cases.
- Mature cystic teratomas should be removed surgically.
- Cyst accidents are common and careful diagnosis and management will avoid loss of an ovary.

References

1 Thomason JL, Gelbart SM, Anderson RJ, Watt AK, Osypowski PJ, Broekhuizen FF. Statistical evaluation of diagnostic criteria for bacterial vaginosis. *Am J Obstet Gynecol* 1990;162:155–160.
2 McDonald HM, O'Loughlin JA, Jolley P *et al.* Vaginal infection and preterm labour. *Br J Obstet Gynaecol* 1991;98:427–435.
3 Paavonen J, Teisala K, Heinonen PK *et al.* Microbiological and histopathological findings in acute pelvic inflammatory disease. *Br J Obstet Gynaecol* 1987;94:454–460.
4 Eschenbach DA, Hillier S, Critchlow C, Stevens C, De Rouen T, Holmes KK. Diagnosis and clinical manifestations of bacterial vaginosis. *Am J Obstet Gynecol* 1988;158:819–828.

5 Roberts J. Genitourinary medicine and the obstetrician and gynaecologist. In: MacLean AB (ed.) *Clinical Infection in Obstetrics and Gynaecology*. Oxford: Blackwell Scientific Publications, 1990: 237–254.

6 Shands KN, Schmid GP, Dan BB *et al*. Toxic shock syndrome in menstruating women. Association with tampon use and *Staphylococcus aureus* and clinical features in 52 cases. *N Engl J Med* 1980;303:1436–1442.

7 Todd J, Fishant M, Kapral F, Welch T. Toxic shock syndrome associated with phage-group-1 staphylococci. *Lancet* 1978;ii:1116–1118.

8 Reingold AL, Hargreett NT, Shands KN *et al*. Toxic shock syndrome surveillance in the United States, 1980 to 1981. *Ann Int Med* 1982;96:875–880.

9 Sanderson P. Do streptococci cause toxic shock? *Br Med J* 1990;301:1006–1007.

10 Tweardy DJ. Relapsing toxic shock syndrome in the puerperium. *J Am Med Assoc* 1985;253:3249–3350.

11 Nwabineli NJ, Monaghan JM. Vaginal epithelial abnormalities in patients with CIN: clinical and pathological features and management. *Br J Obstet Gynaecol* 1991;98:25–29.

12 Lenehan PM, Meffe F, Lickrish GM. Vaginal intraepithelial neoplasia: biologic aspects and management. *Obstet Gynecol* 1986;68:333–337.

13 Imrie JEA, Kennedy JH, Holmes JD, McGrouther DA. Intraepithelial neoplasia arising in an artificial vagina. Case report. *Br J Obstet Gynaecol* 1986;93:886–888.

14 Hummer WA, Mussey E, Decker DC, Docherty MB. Carcinoma *in situ* of the vagina. *Am J Obstet Gynecol* 1970;108:1109–1116.

15 Townsend DE. Intraepithelial neoplasia of vagina. In: Coppleson M (ed) *Gynaecologic Oncology*. Edinburgh: Churchill Livingstone, 1981: 339–344.

16 Gemmell J, Holmes DM, Duncan ID. How frequently need vaginal smears be taken after hysterectomy for cervical intraepithelial neoplasia? *Br J Obstet Gynaecol* 1990;97:58–61.

17 McIndoe WA, McLean MR, Jones RW, Mullins PR. The invasive potential of carcinoma *in situ* of the cervix. *Obstet Gynecol* 1984;64:451–458.

18 Petrilli ES, Townsend DE, Morrow CP, Nakao CY. Vaginal intraepithelial neoplasia: biologic aspects and treatment with topical 5-fluorouracil and the carbon dioxide LASER. *Am J Obstet Gynecol* 1980;138:321–328.

19 Woodman CBJ, Jordan JA, Wade-Evans T. The management of vaginal intraepithelial neoplasia after hysterectomy. *Br J Obstet Gynaecol* 1984;91:707–717.

20 Stuart GCE, Flagler EA, Nation JG, Duggan M, Robertson DI. Laser vaporization of vaginal intraepithelial neoplasia. *Am J Obstet Gynecol* 1988;158:240–243.

21 Caglar H, Hertzog RW, Hreschchyshyn MM. Topical 5-fluorouracil treatment in vaginal intraepithelial neoplasia. *Obstet Gynecol* 1981;58:580–583.

22 Ireland D, Monaghan JM. The management of the patient with abnormal vaginal cytology following hysterectomy. *Br J Obstet Gynaecol* 1988;95:973–975.

23 Monaghan JM. Operations on the vagina. In: Monaghan JM (ed) *Bonney's Gynaecological Surgery*. London: Baillière Tindall, 1986: 138–142.

24 Curtis EP, Shepherd JH, Lowe DG, Jobling T. The role of partial colpectomy in the management of persistent vaginal neoplasia after primary treatment. *Br J Obstet Gynaecol* 1992;99:587–589.

25 Soutter WP. The treatment of vaginal intraepithelial neoplasia after hysterectomy. *Br J Obstet Gynaecol* 1988;95:961–962.

26 Hernandez-Linares W, Puthawala A, Nolan JF, Jernstrom PB, Morrow CP. Carcinoma *in situ* of the vagina: past and present management. *Obstet Gynecol* 1980;56:356–360.

27 Woodman CB, Mould JJ, Jordan JA. Radiotherapy in the management of vaginal intraepithelial neoplasia after hysterectomy. *Br J Obstet Gynaecol* 1988;95:976–979.

28 Herbst AL, Scully RE. Adenocarcinoma of the vagina in adolescence; a report of seven cases including six clear cell carcinomas (so-called mesonephromas). *Cancer* 1970;25:745–757.

29 Herbst AL, Norvsis MJ, Rosenow PJ *et al*. An analysis of 346 cases of clear cell adenocarcinoma of the vagina and cervix with emphasis on recurrence and survival. *Gynecol Oncol* 1979;7:111–122.

30 Brunham RC, Paavonen J, Stevens CE *et al*. Muco-purulent cervicitis: the ignored counterpart in women of urethritis in men. *N Engl J Med* 1984;311:1–6.

31 Hare MJ, Toone E, Taylor-Robinson D *et al*. Follicular cervicitis – colposcopic appearances in association with *Chlamydia trachomatis*. *Br J Obstet Gynaecol* 1981;88:174–180.

32 van Nagell JR, Higgins RV, Donaldson ES *et al*. Transvaginal sonography as a screening method for ovarian cancer. *Cancer* 1990;65:573–577.

33 Stein IF, Leventhal ML. Amenorrhea associated with bilateral polycystic ovaries. *Am J Obstet Gynecol* 1935;29:181–191.

34 Judd HL, Barnes AB, Kliman B. Long-term effect of wedge resection on androgen production in a case of polycystic ovarian disease. *Am J Obstet Gynecol* 1971;110:1061–1065.

35 Grimes HG, Nosal RA, Gallagher JC. Ovarian pregnancy: a series of 24 cases. *Obstet Gynecol* 1983;61:174–180.

36 Majumdar DN, Ledward RS. Primary ovarian pregnancy in association with an intra-uterine conceptive device *in situ*. *J Obstet Gynaecol* 1982;3:131–132.

37 Novak ER, Woodruff JD. Ovarian pregnancy. In: Novak ER (ed.) *Novak's Gynecologic and Obstetric Pathology*, 8th edn. Philadelphia: Saunders, 1979: 556–560.

38 Sutton CJG. Minimally invasive surgical approach to endometriosis and adhesiolysis. In: Studd S, Jardine Brown C (eds) *Yearbook of the Royal College of Obstetricians and Gynaecologists*. London: RCOG Press, 1993: 117–125.

Chapter 54
Benign Disease of the Uterus

Aradhana Khaund[1] and Mary Ann Lumsden[2]

[1]Department of Obstetrics and Gynaecology, Southern General Hospital, South Glasgow University Hospitals, Glasgow, UK

[2]University of Glasgow, Royal Infirmary, Glasgow, UK

Introduction

Benign disease of the uterus is a significant problem for many women and their gynaecologists. Uterine fibroids are the commonest condition in this category but adenomyosis and uterine polyps are also of importance. Both fibroids and endometrial polyps occur frequently, and although many women with these pathologies are asymptomatic, they can cause considerable morbidity for others.

This chapter will discuss each of these conditions and consider their aetiology, pathogenesis, presenting symptoms, diagnosis and treatment with inclusion of new developments, particularly in the treatment of symptomatic fibroids.

Adenomyosis

Definition

Adenomyosis is defined as the benign invasion by the endometrium into the myometrium. Both endometrial glands and endometrial stroma must be present and some pathologists also consider that these should be surrounded by hypertrophic hyperplastic musculature. Such features typically result in significant uterine enlargement. Since the endomyometrial border is irregular, the definition usually includes a depth of penetration between 2.5 and 5 mm. Alternatively, it can be determined in terms of microscope fields, with one low-power field being equivalent to 1 cm [1]. Since the symptoms appear to be related to the depth of penetration, it would seem reasonable to include only those with a greater degree of invasion. The result is an enlarged uterus in which the adenomyosis may be either diffuse or present as focal deposits or adenomyomas.

Incidence

Owing to the difficulties in definition as outlined above, the incidence of adenomyosis reported in the literature varies considerably between 8% and 61%, the preoperative diagnosis usually being less than 10%. It is therefore predominantly a post-hysterectomy (in 15–30%) diagnosis and some discrepancy is likely to result from the varying diagnostic methodologies used by different pathologists.

Aetiology

The ectopic endometrium is responsive to steroid hormones. In addition, gene polymorphisms have been identified in the oestrogen receptor with mutations of oestrogen receptor alpha [2]. This ectopic tissue may respond to the cyclical hormone changes of the menstrual cycle which contributes to the symptoms of heavy menstrual bleeding (HMB) and dysmenorrhoea. Abnormal prostaglandin production also occurs and this could exacerbate both pelvic pain and heavy bleeding. These symptoms are associated with a gradually enlarging uterus, a finding which is unlikely to be picked up clinically unless serial vaginal examinations are performed.

Clinical presentation

The commonest presentation is that of HMB associated with significant dysmenorrhoea, the latter being worse in deep infiltrating disease [3]. The condition is characteristic of the fifth decade of life, with 45 years being the commonest age of presentation. It is very rare in nulliparous women [4] and occurs less frequently in smokers.

Diagnosis

The diagnosis is normally made on histological examination of the uterus after hysterectomy. However, magnetic resonance imaging (MRI) has been shown to be more accurate than ultrasound in diagnosing adenomyosis (Fig. 54.1) [5]. This modality enables the clinician to distinguish adenomyosis from other pathologies such as uterine fibroids, which may also present with an enlarged uterus. More often, however, transvaginal ultrasound (TVS) is used as the primary and only investigative tool

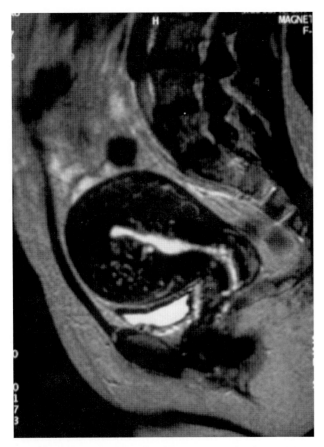

Fig. 54.1 Diffuse adenomyosis of the uterus. By kind permission of Dr Nigel McMillan, Consultant Radiologist, The Western Infirmary, Glasgow, UK.

deeply infiltrating disease, however, tend to have persistent symptoms and ideally should be offered hysterectomy over repeat ablation [7].

The minimally invasive radiological technique of uterine artery embolization (UAE) is used in some centres for the treatment of symptomatic adenomyosis. It has been shown to be effective in the short term, but there is a high rate of symptom recurrence within 2 years of treatment [8].

Optimal treatment of adenomyosis is hysterectomy as this is the only method of permanently curing the problem. Oophorectomy at the same time is not required, unless otherwise indicated.

> **Summary box 54.1**
>
> - Adenomyosis is a cause of menorrhagia, dysmenorrhoea and uterine enlargement.
> - Its true prevalence is unknown, but it is present in 15–30% of hysterectomy specimens.
> - TVS is the primary diagnostic tool, but MRI is often superior in distinguishing adenomyosis from other pathologies such as fibroids.
> - Medical treatment should be first-line management (including the Mirena IUS).
> - Endometrial ablation is also of value, but less so in the presence of deep infiltrating disease.
> - Hysterectomy is the definitive treatment.

for women with suspected adenomyosis. Early diagnosis can impact significantly on the choice of treatment offered to an individual patient.

Treatment

Various medical and minor surgical techniques have been shown to be of some benefit in the short term. Antifibrinolytics, non-steroidal anti-inflammatory drugs, the oral contraceptive pill and high-dose progestins should all be considered as a first-line method of treatment, as occurs in the management of menorrhagia and dysmenorrhoea. The levonorgestrel-releasing intrauterine system (Mirena IUS; Bayer Schering Pharma, Berkshire, UK) has been shown to be effective for the reduction of uterine volume and relief of adenomyosis-related symptoms at 1 year, but the efficacy of this device declines with time [6]. Endometrial ablation is not used as a first-line treatment of adenomyosis as it fails to remove deeply infiltrating endometrial glands. It has been shown to improve menorrhagia and dysmenorrhoea in some women, and those with superficial disease have good results from this treatment option. Those with

Endometrial polyps

Definition

Endometrial polyps are discrete outgrowths of the endometrium that contain a variable amount of glandular tissue, stroma and blood vessels. They are attached to the endometrium by a pedicle and may be either pedunculated or sessile. It would appear that they are relatively insensitive to cyclical hormonal changes and thus are not shed at the time of menstruation. In addition, they may contain hyperplastic foci, particularly in those who are symptomatic in terms of their bleeding pattern.

Epidemiology

The presence of endometrial polyps is being increasingly recognized since the widespread adoption of transvaginal ultrasound and outpatient hysteroscopy. It is probable that they are present in 25% of women with abnormal vaginal bleeding, although at least 10% of asymptomatic women are also likely to have polyps. They are particularly common in women taking hormone replacement therapy (HRT) or preparations such as tamoxifen, which has both oestrogen receptor agonistic (endometrium) and antagonistic (breast) effects.

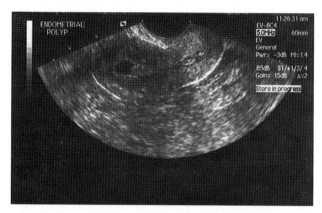

Fig. 54.2 A transvaginal ultrasound scan demonstrating an endometrial polyp. By kind permission of Dr Justine Clark, Consultant Gynaecologist, Birmingham Women's Hospital, UK.

 Summary box 54.2

- Endometrial polyps occur in ~25% of women who present with unscheduled vaginal bleeding.
- They are more common in women using HRT or tamoxifen therapy.
- Diagnosis is usually made using TVS (may be enhanced with the use of saline), hysteroscopy or blind endometrial sampling.
- Treatment involves excision under direct vision (using hysteroscopy) with or without the use of diathermy instruments.

Presentation

Unscheduled vaginal bleeding or spotting is the commonest presentation for endometrial polyps. In women taking tamoxifen, the whole endometrial surface may appear polypoid.

Diagnosis

Endometrial polyps are frequently missed with blind endometrial sampling. Uterine imaging is more sensitive in diagnosing these focal lesions, particularly TVS, which may identify them in isolation or as part of an abnormally thickened endometrium (Fig. 54.2). However, studies have noted marked interobserver variation in interpretation of the ultrasound images. Intrauterine injection of saline can markedly increase the diagnostic performance of transvaginal ultrasound.

Hysteroscopic characteristics

The best method for diagnosing polyps is hysteroscopy, which also facilitates the possibility of concurrent treatment (Plate 54.1). Polyps may be pedunculated, sessile, single or multiple. They can be distinguished from pedunculated fibroids as they have fewer vessels over their surface. Malignant polyps are more likely to be irregular, vascular and/or friable. Biopsy and pathological analysis must be carried out to confirm the diagnosis as visual appearance alone, is insufficient.

Treatment

In symptomatic women, treatment may be performed under either general anaesthesia or in an outpatient setting with or without local anaesthesia. The latter is becoming increasingly popular, although patient selection is of vital importance in the success of this treatment setting [9]. Treatment involves either removal under direct vision or excision with the use of specially developed hysteroscopic instruments.

Uterine leiomyomata (fibroids)

Definition

These are the most common benign tumours of the female genital tract. While they can develop at various sites within the body, they most frequently affect the uterine myometrium, arising from neoplastic transformation of single smooth muscle cells. They usually appear as well-circumscribed firm tumours with a characteristic white-whorled appearance on cross section. Fibroids are paler than the surrounding myometrium and there is usually a very sharp line of demarcation between the tumour and the normal uterine muscle (Plate 54.2).

Histologically, they are typically composed of varying proportions of spindled smooth muscle cells and fibroblasts. The size of fibroids varies greatly and uterine enlargement is equated to the pregnant uterus. Unlike the pregnant uterus, however, it is usually irregular in shape. Fibroids may be single but are commonly multiple and can be further classified according to their location. The vast majority are found in the corpus (body) of the uterus and may be either subserosal, intramural or submucous. These benign growths may also occur in the cervix, uterine ligaments and ovary (Fig. 54.3). Further descriptive classification include pedunculated fibroids, where a fibroid is attached to the normal myometrium of the uterus by a stalk, and the rare parasitic fibroid, where the fibroid has developed an alternative blood supply having separated from the uterus and become attached to another structure in the pelvis.

Incidence

The true incidence of fibroids is uncertain as many women with these tumours are asymptomatic. Prevalence rates tend to be based on rates of diagnosis in symptomatic individuals and following pathological assessments of hysterectomy specimens. While such estimates represent the morbidity associated with fibroids, it is likely that that we significantly underestimate the true prevalence of these uterine lesions. Nonetheless, we are aware that these common tumours are clinically apparent in 20–30%

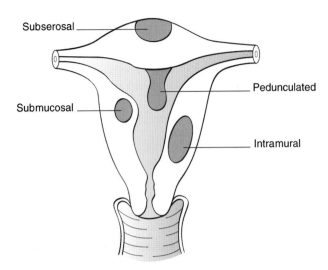

Fig. 54.3 The position of fibroids in the uterus.

of women during reproductive life and may be present in as many as 70% of uterii removed at the time of hysterectomy [4].

There are significant racial differences in the incidence of fibroids, with Afro-Caribbean women having a two- to ninefold greater risk of developing fibroids. In addition, they tend to present at a younger age compared with Caucasian women and have multiple fibroids, higher uterine weights and are more prone to both anaemia and severe pelvic pain [10,11]. These racial characteristics are more likely to be due to a genetic predisposition.

Reproductive factors also influence the risk of fibroids, with a reduction in incidence with increasing parity (beyond 24 weeks' gestation) and the prolonged use of the oral contraceptive pill outwith teenage years [11,12], an effect which is directly proportional to the duration of pill use.

Environmental factors also influence the risk of fibroid development. Independent of body mass index, smoking appears to decrease the risk of fibroid development [13,14].

Aetiology

The pathophysiology of fibroids remains poorly understood. Clonality studies using the homozygosity of glucose-6-phosphate dehydrogenase forms show that multiple tumours in the same uterus are derived from individual myometrial cells rather than occurring through a metastatic process. This, together with their high prevalence, suggests that initial development arises from a frequently occurring event, the nature of which is currently unknown. Growth of fibroids is partly dependent on the ovarian steroids (discussed later) that act through receptors present on both fibroid and myometrial cells. It is likely that the control of growth is due, in part, to

alterations in apoptosis. Bcl-2, an inhibitor of apoptosis, is significantly increased in cultured leiomyoma cells. It is also influenced by the steroid hormone milieu.

Cytogenetic abnormalities occur in 40% of uterine fibroids. Most commonly, these involve translocation within or deletion of chromosome 7, translocations of chromosome 12 and 14, and occasionally structural aberrations of chromosome 6 [15]. These cytogenetic abnormalities are not observed in normal myometrial tissue and may not be present in all the fibroids in a single uterus [16]. In addition, mutations in the gene encoding fumarate hydratase (an enzyme of the tricarboxylic acid cycle) were shown to predispose women to hereditary syndromes involving the presence of multiple uterine fibroids in association with cutaneous leiomyomata and renal cell carcinoma [17]. This is an interesting example of a mutation in a gene with a general function causing disease in a highly restricted range of tissue. However, the incidence of this mutation does not appear to be increased in uterine fibroids.

Malignancy in uterine fibroids is extremely uncommon. Leiomyosarcoma is a disease largely occurring in the seventh decade of life whereas fibroids tend to occur in women 20 to 30 years younger. The cytogenetic profile is completely different between benign and malignant disease and there is the possibility that their origins are separate. Nonetheless, gynaecologists with an interest in this area will all have anecdotal examples of malignancy occurring in younger women; thus, the possibility of a sarcoma must be considered in women with fibroids who differ from the norm in clinical presentation or response to treatment.

Myometrium and fibroids consist of spindled cells arranged in fascicles with abundant eosinophilic cytoplasm and uniform nuclei. In contrast, a malignant leiomyosarcoma is hypercellular and consists of atypical smooth muscle cells with hyperchromatic, enlarged nuclei. Increased mitotic figures and necrosis also commonly occur. However, benign fibroids may also have one or more of these characteristics, making prediction of malignant potential sometimes extremely difficult [17].

Abnormalities in uterine blood vessels and angiogenic growth factors are also involved in the pathophysiology of uterine fibroids. The myomatous uterus has increased numbers of arterioles and venules and is also associated with venule ectasia or dilatation. It was thought that the latter was due to pressure from these large tumours, but it may also simply be due to the presence of increased numbers of vessels. It has been noted that there are no mature vessels running through uterine fibroids despite the fact that they have a well-developed blood supply (Fig. 54.4, pre-embolization). This feature might be useful in trying to distinguish clinically between benign and malignant lesions. Typically, a sarcoma may have large

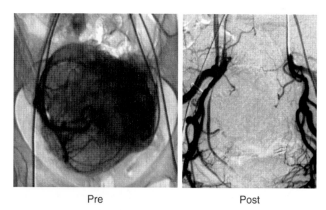

Pre   Post

Fig. 54.4 Uterine artery embolization. The left-hand image shows an angiogram of the uterine arteries illustrating the vascularity of the fibroid. The right-hand image is post uterine artery embolization and little flow is seen.

vessels running through it, which could be identified using colour Doppler ultrasound.

Control of growth

More information is available on the control of uterine fibroid growth than on the aetiology of these benign tumours. Growth factors are of importance in the control of growth of fibroids and their composition. Higher concentrations of the angiogenic fibroblast growth factor have been found in fibroids than in the surrounding myometrium. In addition, the functions of transforming growth factor β, granulocyte–macrophage colony-stimulating factor and epidermal growth factor (EGF), amongst others, have been shown to differ between fibroid and normal myometrial tissue [16].

As fibroids have not been identified in pre-pubertal girls and usually shrink at the time of the menopause, it has long been assumed that these lesions are dependent on the presence of the sex steroids, oestrogen and progesterone. Much of the research relating to fibroids has therefore concentrated on this area and been exploited for the purposes of developing novel medical treatments for these tumours.

The sex steroids act via receptors. The steroid combines with the receptor, which is then translocated to the nucleus of the cell. Studies have identified that steroid receptors are present in higher concentrations in the fibroid than in the surrounding myometrium and that the concentration of receptors is significantly affected by the administration of agents which alter circulating oestradiol concentration. Further work has centred on the relationship between steroid hormones and growth factors such as EGF and insulin-like growth factor, factors which would appear to be important, possibly as mediators for oestrogen action. The role of progesterone, however, is less clear. The number of progesterone receptors is greater in fibroids than in the surrounding myometrium. Like oestrogen, it has an impact on EGF receptor content and also suppresses apoptosis. Studies using antiprogestins, progesterone receptor modulators and the administration of progestogens to hypoestrogenic women suggest that progesterone may stimulate fibroid growth. The relative contribution of oestradiol and progesterone to such growth, however, remains unclear.

Symptoms associated with uterine fibroids

It is estimated that only 20–50% of women with one or more fibroids will experience symptoms which are directly attributable to them. It is, however, not always clear why some produce symptoms and others do not [4]. In the case of small fibroids, the assumption that only those impinging on the uterine cavity cause symptoms is often made. However, data suggest that even subserosal lesions may lead to menstrual problems.

Symptoms associated with fibroids may be variable, ranging from mild to severe, causing distress and impinging significantly on health-related quality of life (QoL). Women commonly present with menstrual problems, particularly heavy menstrual bleeding [18]. In women with dysfunctional uterine bleeding, at least half of those who complain of heavy menstrual loss have a blood loss within the normal range, following objective menstrual blood loss assessment. The vast majority of women with uterine fibroids, however, are likely to have objectively confirmed menorrhagia, sometimes with more than a litre of blood being lost with every period. Not surprisingly, this is likely to be associated with anaemia and has a detrimental effect on QoL. Dysmenorrhoea may be an additional problem leading to a further negative impact on a woman's health. Menorrhagia is not just confined to those who have submucous fibroids but can also be associated with subserosal lesions, as mentioned above. However, it is probable that those with intracavity fibroids are more likely to experience unscheduled bleeding and menorrhagia. This may be a result of the presence of surface vessels on the fibroid and the resultant increased surface area of the uterine cavity. There has been much speculation over the years as to why the heavy bleeding occurs, and abnormalities of endometrial function are also considered to be likely contributing factors [4,11].

Not all women will present with a menstrual problem. Some experience symptoms related purely to the size of the fibroid. This may be a dragging sensation or feeling of pressure in the pelvis, abdominal swelling or urinary symptoms. Other women may be identified as having fibroids incidentally, during routine cervical smear screening or gynaecological assessment for any reason, or simply during pregnancy.

The relationship between fibroids and fertility is discussed in Chapters 45 and 46.

In women who wish to retain their fertility and conceive in the future, the concept of a hysterectomy, which

Table 54.1 Presenting symptoms of uterine fibroids.

Menstrual upset – menorrhagia and/or dysmenorrhoea
Abdominal discomfort
Sensation of pelvic pressure or backache
Abdominal distension
Urinary frequency, difficulty in micturition, incomplete bladder
    emptying or incontinence
Bowel problems such as constipation
Reproductive dysfunction – difficulty in conceiving, pregnancy
    loss, postpartum haemorrhage

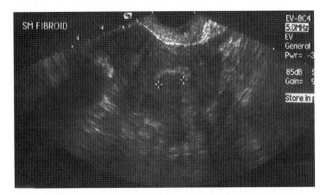

Fig. 54.5 An ultrasound scan showing an intrauterine fibroid. By kind permission of Dr Justine Clark, Consultant Gynaecologist, Birmingham Women's Hospital, UK.

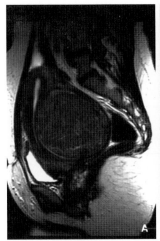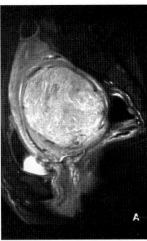

Fig. 54.6 A magnetic resonance image of a uterine fibroid. The fibroid is enhanced in the right-hand image using gadolinium that provides an indication of the vascularity of the lesion. By kind permission of Dr Alan Reid, Consultant Radiologist, Glasgow Royal Infirmary, Glasgow, UK.

guarantees infertility, causes significant distress. Consequently, non-surgical options for the treatment of fibroids have been developed, as will be discussed below, and their impact on fertility is discussed by Olive and colleagues [19].

Table 54.1 highlights the commonly encountered symptoms associated with fibroids.

Diagnosis

The uterus is often found to be enlarged and presents as a pelvic mass (often central and mobile) on both abdominal and vaginal examinations. However, it may be difficult to distinguish between an enlarged uterus and an ovarian mass and so further imaging is mandatory. Ultrasonography, especially transvaginal, is very useful as a first line (Fig. 54.5) unless the uterus is very large or distorted, leading to difficulty in visualizing the ovaries and assessing fibroid location. Under these circumstances, an MRI scan can give excellent visualization of the uterus and ovaries. In addition, enhancement with gadolinium gives an indication of the vascularity of the uterus and fibroids (Fig. 54.6).

Treatment of uterine fibroids

The management of fibroids very much depends on the symptoms that they cause and their effects, if any, on general health and lifestyle. The treatment of these benign tumours has historically been surgical, namely hysterectomy and, less commonly, myomectomy. However, with a shift in emphasis of gynaecological practice towards less invasive techniques and the findings of research over the past 20 or 30 years, a number of medical options and non-surgical techniques have gained popularity. Medical treatments do not eradicate fibroids but are designed to provide symptomatic relief.

Medical treatment of uterine fibroids

Gonadotrophin-releasing hormone agonists

The most established medical option is administration of a gonadotrophin-releasing hormone (GnRH) agonist. These drugs lead to the downregulation of pituitary receptors that result initially in stimulation of gonadotrophin release, followed by gonadotrophin output reduction and consequent reduction in ovarian steroid production within 2–3 weeks of commencing treatment. The decreased output of ovarian steroids continues while treatment is ongoing. These analogues are usually given as 1- or 3-monthly depot injections as the most convenient option, although other methods of administration such as the nasal spray are available. Fibroid shrinkage occurs rapidly in the first 3 months but then tends to slow down with little further decline. The reason for this is likely to be related to the alteration in the blood supply to the uterus that occurs with GnRH agonist administration. Most studies suggest a fibroid volume reduction of 40% [20]. The volume is calculated using the prolate ellipse equation where D_1, D_2 and D_3 are the transverse, oblique and vertical axes measurements of the fibroid. It is worth noting that a large volume reduction of a large fibroid may be associated with only a small decrease in diameter. The principal disadvantages of GnRH analogue administration are that the fibroids re-grow when treatment has stopped. In addition, they are associated with postmenopausal side effects. The latter consist of hot flushing and vaginal dryness, but what is more important from a public health perspective is the significant bone loss which occurs with prologed use. It is possible to counteract these side effects by administering low-dose hormone replacement therapy (HRT). The fibroids do not appear to re-grow, the symptoms are alleviated and side effects are halted. Nonetheless, GnRH agonists are licensed for 6 months and a maximum of 1 year with concurrent HRT or 'addback' therapy. The option should always be considered in women who are unsuitable for surgery, possibly due to either multiple previous abdominal operations, medical problems or morbid obesity.

These agonists are also useful prior to surgery [21,22] and have a licence for use in the UK in women with severe anaemia. Their administration results in amenorrhoea, which is associated with a significant increase in haemoglobin. They also enable more procedures to be carried out vaginally, with or without laparoscopic assistance. Intraoperative blood loss, whatever the major surgical technique used, has been shown to be reduced with the preoperative use of this medication. Consequently, they are often used preoperatively in the cases of large fibroids or those associated with an awkward position. GnRH agonists may also be useful prior to myomectomy for similar reasons, although the chance of recurrence of fibroids after surgery is increased. It is, however, important to note that the plane of cleavage between the fibroid and the surrounding myometrium can be masked with such preoperative use, making the surgery significantly more difficult.

Despite the significant benefits, GnRH agonists are not thought to be cost-effective [23] and therefore should be used in selected women only.

Progesterone receptor modulators

Although antiprogestins have been shown to lead to the shrinkage of uterine fibroids, they are not widely used in clinical practice. However, further development of new preparations that affect the progesterone receptors have led to the testing of the progesterone receptor modulators (PRMs). These drugs are still in the research domain but may potentially become an important treatment option for uterine fibroids. When administered to women, they cause amenorrhoea in a vast majority of cases without causing anovulation. Essentially, they have a direct effect on the endometrium and it is thought that the main site of action is the endometrial vasculature. Preliminary data suggest that fibroid shrinkage occurs with the use of these drugs in association with a significant decrease in vaginal

bleeding. Short-term administration appears to be safe and these preparations may have a profound effect on the way we treat symptomatic fibroids in the future [24]. Asoprisnil, an oral selective PRM, has been shown in the short term to moderately decrease uterine artery blood flow, reduce uterine bleeding and improve health-related QoL in women with symptomatic fibroids prior to hysterectomy [25].

Levonorgestrel-secreting intrauterine system (Mirena IUS)

This device has revolutionized the treatment of dysfunctional uterine bleeding and evidence suggests that it may be one of the reasons why the hysterectomy rate has declined over recent years. However, the use of this system in women with fibroids has not been widely studied as some consider it to be a relative contraindication. This may partly be because the device is more likely to be expelled during a very heavy menstruation. It may also be because the presence of a very distorted uterine cavity, which occurs with some fibroid uterii, may make insertion of the device impossible.

Intuitively, if the cavity is normal and not especially enlarged, then a trial with the Mirena IUS system maybe appropriate. Coil placement should, however, be checked after a very heavy menstruation. It is well known that the Mirena IUS is associated with irregular bleeding for 3–4 months after insertion in many women. However, it is not known if this problem is worsened in those with fibroids.

Other medical treatments used in the treatment of uterine fibroids tend to involve the induction of amenorrhoea or at least a significant reduction in menstrual bleeding. Women who opt for the latter may be satisfied with the relief of menstrual symptoms alone, despite the fact that the fibroids themselves have not actually decreased in size. Data are available to support this in relation to administration of progestogens and the oral contraceptive pill.

Surgical treatment of uterine fibroids

Hysterectomy remains the most popular and hence the most common surgical treatment option for uterine fibroids. It ensures immediate resolution of menstrual upset and other fibroid-associated symptoms as well as permanent removal of fibroids. However, it also guarantees infertility, which may not be an appropriate option for some women, and is associated with significant morbidity, a relatively long inpatient hospital stay and prolonged recovery period. Major complications occur with hysterectomy and data from a large UK audit (the VALUE audit) suggest that complications are all increased in the presence of uterine fibroids [26].

In women who wish to retain their fertility, uterine sparing options must be considered. The first of these is myomectomy, which involves removal of the fibroids only with conservation of normal myometrial tissue. This can be carried out as an open/abdominal, laparoscopic or hysteroscopic procedure. Small pedunculated intracavity fibroids lend themselves to hysteroscopic removal, and this has been documented as being associated with decreased blood loss and improved fertility, although randomized data are lacking in this area. Generally, hysteroscopic resection of submucous (and less commonly, intramural) fibroids is restricted to those lesions less than 5 cm in diameter and those where more than 50% of the fibroid is present within the endometrial cavity. Complications to consider during this method of myomectomy include uterine perforation and the associated potential for visceral damage, haemorrhage, infection and fluid overload.

One of the problems with myomectomy is that fibroids are often multiple, such that it is often extremely difficult to remove them all at surgery. Intraoperative blood loss may also be excessive, and in a small number of cases an emergency hysterectomy may be required to control the bleeding. It is very difficult to achieve perfect haemostasis after myomectomy, and postoperative adhesion formation may also be a major problem in some women, further compromising reproductive potential. Some of these issues are likely to be even more significant when laparoscopic myomectomy is performed. Rupture of the uterus in labour is also a risk after myomectomy if the cavity is breached during the myomectomy. This occurs much less frequently with lower-segment Caesarean section. Myomectomy is thus not the perfect answer for women wishing to maintain their fertility and, not surprisingly, other uterine-sparing modalities have been sought.

Endometrial ablation is a minor surgical technique which may be performed as a day case. It is a popular first-line option amongst women with HMB who have completed their family [27]. Successful outcome is obtained in approximately 75% of women. A number of the studies evaluating ablation have included women with small fibroids of 3 cm or less in diameter, but often the presence of fibroids may not be documented at all. Consequently, it is not possible to separate out the data relating to fibroids alone from those women with normal uterii, although it is likely that ablation is less successful in the presence of fibroids. Overall, provided that the uterine cavity is not too enlarged or distorted, ablation appears to be a successful option. It would seem that microwave endometrial ablation (MEA) may be the best of the second-generation techniques, although once again randomized data looking at fibroids in particular are not available. For reasons stated above, its use can be justified only in women with small fibroids. Endometrial ablation may be performed with or without myomectomy and is associated with a high rate of amenorrhoea.

Uterine artery embolization

Uterine artery embolization (UAE) is a minimally invasive radiological technique that has been offered to women with symptomatic fibroids in specialist units over the last 15 years. Pelvic arterial embolization has been used in the treatment of massive obstetric haemorrhage for more than three decades, but it was not until a French gynaecologist, Ravina [28], published a paper suggesting it as a surgical alternative for uterine fibroids that its use has become reasonably widespread. Under conscious sedation, UAE involves the cannulation of the femoral artery with a small plastic tube which is fed around the aortic arch through the iliac vessels and thereafter into the contralateral internal iliac artery and corresponding uterine artery. Multiple particulate material (usually in the form of polyvinyl alcohol) is then injected down into the circulation to effect embolization and thus cease flow beyond the level of the uterine artery. Visualization of the latter is facilitated by the use of a contrast medium and digital fluoroscopy. Embolization is then carried out on the opposite side. Most procedures take approximately 45 minutes and may be carried out either as a daycase or with an overnight hospital stay. Opiate analgesia is usually required up to 24 hours following treatment and then most women are managed thereafter with oral analgesia, returning to normal activities within 2 weeks of their procedure.

For poorly understood reasons, the blood supply to the normal myometrium renews itself via the rich pelvic collateral circulation with contributions from ovarian and vaginal arteries. However, the fibroids do not usually revascularize to a significant extent. This leads to shrinkage of the fibroids and subsequent relief of fibroid-related symptoms. In contrast to the effects of GnRH agonists, where shrinkage of fibroids is maintained only as long as treatment continues, embolization results in sustained shrinkage for some time after treatment.

There has been much discussion in the literature regarding the pros and cons of uterine artery embolization (UAE) [29]. Observational data suggest that there is a significant beneficial effect on menstrual blood loss and bulk-related symptoms with personal series reporting promising early and midterm results [30,31]. Patient satisfaction rates following the procedure are also high and comparable to those found after hysterectomy. More recent data suggest that in addition to the shorter hospital stay and recovery period associated with UAE, improvements in health-related QoL are also sustained in the long term post UAE [32]. Another significant benefit of embolization is uterine conservation, and thus preservation of fertility.

The average uterine shrinkage is 40%, although in some instances this can be greater (Fig. 54.7). A cervical or submucosal fibroid may also pass vaginally in the weeks or months following treatment, resulting in an anatomically

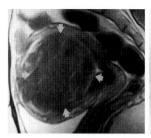
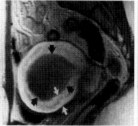
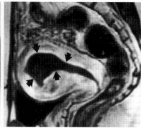

Pre-embolization
(GAD enhanced)

3 months post embolization
(GAD enhanced)
71% vol. reduction

1 year post embolization
(GAD enhanced)
88% vol. reduction

Fig. 54.7 These magnetic resonance images were taken before (left-hand image), 3 months (middle image) and 12 months after uterine artery embolization. Fibroid shrinkage is continuing even up to 1 year. By kind permission of Dr Nigel McMillan, Consultant Radiologist, The Western Infirmary, Glasgow, UK.

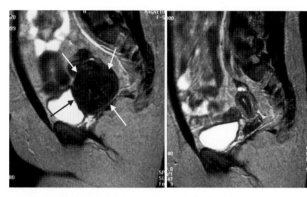

Fig. 54.8 This image illustrates a cervical fibroid that was passed after uterine artery embolization leaving a normal uterus. By kind permission of Dr Nigel McMillan, Consultant Radiologist, The Western Infirmary, Glasgow, UK.

Table 54.2 The complications of uterine artery embolization.

Groin injury – haematoma – infection
Contrast allergy
Radiation exposure to ovaries
Non-target or misembolization – ovary, bowel or bladder
Fibroid expulsion
Persistent vaginal discharge
Amenorrhoea – secondary to premature ovarian failure, endometrial atrophy or intrauterine adhesions
Ovarian failure
Post-embolization syndrome
Infection
Sepsis – requiring emergency hysterectomy (occurs <1%)
Death (rare)
Treatment failure – failed cannulation – revascularization or regrowth of fibroids

normal uterus (Fig. 54.8). Variable recurrence rates for fibroids, however, have been reported after embolization as occurs with myomectomy [33]. Unlike hysterectomy, there is no guarantee that the procedure will eliminate all menstrual symptoms and revascularization with subsequent regrowth of fibroids does occur in some women. Nonetheless, most case series report improvements in HMB of 85–88% at 1 year [33]. More recently, longer term data from randomized trials have been published, stating that health-related QoL measures improve significantly and remain stable at 5-year follow-up evaluation [34].

Some women may require further treatment either with hysterectomy, myomectomy, endometrial ablation or a repeat embolization. Importantly, with increasing long-term follow-up, it appears that such reintervention rates associated with UAE are higher than previously suggested, with rates of 28% being reported at 5 years [34].

A number of complications (Table 54.2) may be associated with embolization and these may be serious, particularly if severe sepsis occurs.

In approximately 10% of women, the post-embolization syndrome occurs 7–10 days after the procedure. It consists of a flu-like illness and is characterized by general malaise and pelvic pain in association with a mild pyrexia and raised white cell count. This is not as a result of infection but is thought to be due to cytokine release at the time of necrosis of the fibroid. The syndrome is often very difficult to distinguish from infection and is treated with a combination of analgesia, adequate hydration, prophylactic antibiotics and reassurance.

Another significant problem resulting from embolization is infection. Most women require a simple course of antibiotics, but, rarely, sepsis may occur, a complication that has led to the death of at least one woman following treatment.

There is a radiation penalty to the ovaries associated with the procedure which occurs during digital fluoroscopy or with non-target embolization. This, in combination with disruption of uterine blood flow, may increase the chance of ovarian failure in some women after the procedure. Rates of ovarian failure are increased in women over the age of 45 years. Reassuringly, however, recent studies demonstrate that there is no evidence for UAE accelerating a decline in ovarian function at 1 year following treatment when compared with surgery, irrespective of age [35,36]. Nonetheless, the issue of ovarian failure is an important area of discussion for women who wish to conceive in the future.

There are some studies reported in the literature of pregnancies. While some suggest that the outcome is not adversely affected [37], others report increased rates of miscarriage, intrauterine growth restriction, preterm delivery, malpresentation and postpartum haemorrhage following embolization [38].

While a few non-randomized studies have assessed UAE versus myomectomy [39], a randomized study suggests that of the two treatment options, myomectomy is associated with superior reproductive outcomes in the first 2 years after treatment in terms of miscarriage, pregnancy and labour rates. Perinatal outcomes were similar [40].

The cost-effectiveness of UAE versus surgery has been studied. Short-term data reported embolization to be more cost-effective at 1 year [41], but more recent unpublished studies suggest that owing to reintervention and return visits to hospital after UAE, both embolization and surgery are cost-neutral in the long term.

It appears that embolization should be offered routinely to all women with symptomatic fibroids. However, it remains clear that studies must continue to be carried out assessing the durability and long-term outcomes of the procedure. In particular, more randomized studies are needed to allow appropriate comparison between embolization and other currently available uterine-sparing techniques for the treatment of symptomatic fibroids.

Other radiological techniques

Laser ablation of fibroids can be carried out at surgery using either a hysteroscope or a laparoscope depending on the position of the fibroids. Laser can also be used with MRI or ultrasound guidance.

These techniques allow target treatment and lead to significant fibroid shrinkage and reduction in menstrual blood loss [42]. MRI-guided laser treatment requires an open MRI machine and few are available in the UK. However, high-intensity focused ultrasound does not require such sophisticated equipment and is an option available in some centres. This treatment induces thermocoagulation and mechanical damage to fibroid tissue but, unlike UAE, is not associated with an infarction-like syndrome. QoL symptom severity scores are similar to those associated with UAE, but the impact of treatment on HMB is less than for embolization [43]. This modality is neither suitable for large fibroids nor large numbers of fibroids, and its impact on the recurrence rate of these benign tumours is unclear.

Alternatively, MRI guidance may be used to focus ultrasound and induce fibroid necrosis without significant adverse outcomes.

Summary box 54.3

- Fibroids occur in 25% of women during reproductive life.
- Aetiology is poorly understood.
- Symptoms include menorrhagia, bulk-related problems and reproductive dysfunction.
- Diagnosis is by clinical examination and TVS.
- Abdominal ultrasound and MRI may be of additional value in the case of larger fibroids or where there is doubt about the nature of the uterine mass.
- MRI with gadolinium enhancement is used prior to UAE.
- Medical treatment is the first line of management in women who present with menstrual upset.
- GnRH analogues with addback therapy may be used in the short term or as a useful adjunct to surgery in the presence of large fibroids or associated anaemia.
- The Mirena IUS or endometrial ablation may considered in the presence of a fibroid uterus which is no more than 14 weeks in size in the absence of significant uterine cavity distortion.
- Myomectomy permits uterine conservation but is associated with fibroid regrowth and subsequent adhesion formation.
- Hysterectomy remains a good treatment option for some women but is associated with significant morbidity, a prolonged hospital stay and recovery, and induces infertility.
- UAE appears to be a promising alternative to surgery for symptomatic fibroids.
- Other uterine-sparing modalities require further evaluation.

Conclusions

Benign gynaecological disease is common and may cause women many problems, some of which can have a significant impact on QoL. Although medical treatments for adenomyosis and endometrial polyps are lacking, new modalities are being sought for uterine fibroids. This, together with work studying the aetiology and pathogenesis of these benign tumours, should lead to progress and the development of new treatment options.

References

1 McElin T, Bird C. Adenomyosis of the uterus. *Obstet Gynaecol Ann* 1974;3:425–441.

2 Villanova FE, Andrade PM, Otsuka AY *et al.* Estrogen receptor alpha polymorphism and susceptibility to uterine leiomyoma. *Steroids* 2006;71:960–965.

3 Bird C, McElin T, Manalo-Estella F. The elusive adenomyosis of the uterus – revisited. *Am J Obstet Gynecol* 1972;112: 583–593.

4 Buttram VC Jr, Reiter RC. Uterine leiomyomata: etiology, symptomatology, and management. *Fertil Steril* 1981;36: 433–445.

5 Ascher SM, Jha RC, Reinhold C. Benign myometrial conditions: leiomyomas and adenomyosis. *Top Magn Reson Imag* 2003;14: 281–304.

6 Cho S, Nam A, Kim H *et al.* Clinical effects of the levonorgestrel-releasing intrauterine device in patients with adenomyosis. *Am J Obstet Gynaecol* 2008;198:373.e1–7.

7 McCausland V, McCausland A. The response of adenomyosis to endometrial ablation/resection. *Hum Reprod Update* 1998;4: 350–359.

8 Bratby MJ, Walker WJ. Uterine artery embolization for symptomatic adenomyosis – midterm results. *Eur J Radiol* 2009;70: 128–132.

9 Marsh FA, Rogerson LJ, Duffy SRG. A randomized controlled trial comparing outpatient versus daycase endometrial polypectomy. *BJOG Int J Obstet Gynaecol* 2006;113:896–901.

10 Kjerulff KH, Langenberg P, Seidman JD, Stolley PD, Guzinski GM. Uterine leiomyomas. Racial differences in severity, symptoms and age at diagnosis. *J Reprod Med* 1996;41: 483–490.

11 Stewart EA, Nowak RA. Leiomyoma-related bleeding: a classic hypothesis updated for the molecular era. *Hum Reprod Update* 1996;2:295–306.

12 Marshall LM, Spiegelman D, Goldman MB *et al.* A prospective study of reproductive factors and oral contraceptive use in relation to the risk of uterine leiomyomata. *Fertil Steril* 1998;70: 432–439.

13 Parazzini F, Negri E, La Vecchia C *et al.* Uterine myomas and smoking. Results from an Italian study. *J Reprod Med* 1996;41: 316–320.

14 Schwartz SM. Epidemiology of uterine leiomyomata. *Clin Obstet Gynaecol* 2001;44:316–326.

15 Andersen J. Factors in fibroid growth. *Baillieres Clin Obstet Gynaecol* 1998;12:225–243.

16 Brosens I, Deprest J, Dal Cin P, Van den BH. Clinical significance of cytogenetic abnormalities in uterine myomas. *Fertil Steril* 1998;69:232–235.

17 Stewart EA. Uterine fibroids. *Lancet* 2001;357:293–298.

18 Lumsden MA, Wallace EM. Clinical presentation of uterine fibroids. *Baillieres Clin Obstet Gynaecol* 1998;12:177–195.

19 Olive DL, Lindheim SR, Pritts EA. Non-surgical management of leiomyoma: impact on fertility. *Curr Opin Obstet Gynecol* 2004;16:239–243.

20 West CP, Lumsden MA, Lawson S, Williamson J, Baird DT. Shrinkage of uterine fibroids during therapy with goserelin (Zoladex): a luteinising hormone-releasing hormone agonist administered as a monthly subcutaneous depot. *Fertil Steril* 1987;48:45–51.

21 Lumsden MA, West CP, Thomas E *et al.* Treatment with the gonadotrophin releasing hormone-agonistgoserelin before hysterectomy for uterine fibroids. *Br J Obstet Gynaecol* 1994;101: 438–442.

22 Lethaby A, Vollenhoven B, Sowter M. Efficacy of pre-operative gonadotrophin hormone releasing analogues for women with uterine fibroids undergoing hysterectomy or myomectomy: a systematic review. *Br J Obstet Gynaecol* 2002;109:1097–1108.

23 Farquhar C, Brown PM, Furness S. Cost effectiveness of pre-operative gonadotrophin releasing analogues for women with uterine fibroids undergoing hysterectomy or myomectomy. *Br J Obstet Gynaecol* 2002;109:1273–1280.

24 Chwalisz K, DeManno D, Garg R, Larsen L, Mattia-Goldberg C. Therapeutic potential for the selective progesterone receptor modulator asoprisnil in the treatment of leiomyomata. *Semin Reprod Med* 2004;22:113–119.

25 Wilkens J, Chwalisz K, Han C *et al.* Effects of the selective progesterone receptor modulator asoprisnil on uterine artery blood flow, ovarian activity, and clinical symptoms in patients with uterine leiomyomata scheduled for hysterectomy. *J Clin Endocrinol Metabol* 2008;93:4664–4671.

26 McPherson K, Metcalfe MA, Herbert A *et al.* Severe complications of hysterectomy: the VALUE study. *Br J Obstet Gynaecol* 2004;111:688–694.

27 National Institute for Health and Clinical Excellence. *Heavy Menstrual Bleeding.* London: NICE, 2007. Clinical guideline 44.

28 Ravina JH, Herbreteau D, Ciraru-Vigneron N *et al.* Arterial Embolization to treat uterine myomata. *Lancet* 1995;346: 671–672.

29 Lumsden MA. Embolization versus myomectomy versus hysterectomy: which is best, when? *Hum Reprod* 2002;17:253–259.

30 Khaund A, Moss JG, McMillan N, Lumsden MA. Evaluation of the effect of uterine artery embolization on menstrual blood loss and uterine volume. *BJOG Int J Obstet Gynaecol* 2004;111: 700–705.

31 Walker WJ, Pelage JP. Uterine artery embolization for symptomatic fibroids: clinical results in 400 women with imaging follow up. *Br J Obstet Gynaecol* 2002;109:1262–1272.

32 Goodwin SC, Spies JB, Worthington-Kirsch R *et al.* Fibroid Registry for Outcomes Data (FIBROID) Registry Steering Committee and Core Site Investigators. Uterine artery embolization for treatment of leiomyomata: long-term outcomes from the FIBROID Registry. *Obstet Gynaecol* 2008;111:22–33.

33 Kim MD, Lee HS, Lee MH, Kim HJ, Cho JH, Cha SH. Long-term results of symptomatic fibroids treated with uterine artery embolization: in conjunction with MR evaluation. *Eur J Radiol* 2010;73:339–344

34 van der Kooij SM, Hehenkamp WJK, Volkers NA, Birnie E, Ankum WM, Reekers JA. Uterine artery embolisation vs hysterectomy in the treatment of symptomatic uterine fibroids: 5-year outcome from the randomized EMMY trial. *Am J Obstet Gynaecol* 2010;105:e1–105.e13.

35 Tropeano G, Di Stasi C, Litwicka K, Romano D, Draisci G, Mancuso S. Uterine artery embolisation for fibroids does not have adverse effects on ovarian reserve in regularly cycling women younger than 40 years. *Fertil Steril* 2004;81: 1055–1061.

36 Rashid S, Khaund A, Murray LS *et al.* The effects of uterine artery embolization and surgical treatment on ovarian function in woman with uterine fibroids. *BJOG Int J Obstet Gynaecol* 2010;117:985–989.

37 Goldberg J, Pereira L, Berghella V *et al.* Pregnancy outcomes after treatment for fibromyomata: uterine artery embolisation versus laparoscopic myomectomy. *Am J Obstet Gynecol* 2004;191: 18–21.

38 Holob Z, Mara M, Kuzel D, Jabor A, Maskova J, Eim J. Pregnancy outcomes after uterine artery occlusion: prospective multicentric study. *Fertil Steril* 2008;90:1886–1891.

39 Broder MS, Goodwin S, Chen G *et al.* Comparison of long-term outcomes of myomectomy and uterine artery embolisation. *Obstet Gynecol* 2002;1005:864–868.

40 Mara M, Maskova J, Fucikova Z, Kuzel D, Belsan T, Sosna O. Midterm clinical and first reproductive results of a randomized controlled trial comparing uterine fibroid embolisation and myomectomy. *CardioVascular Interventional Radiol* 2008;31: 73–85.

41 Beinfeld MT, Bosch JL, Isaacson KB, Gazelle GS. Cost-effectiveness of uterine artery embolisation and hysterectomy for uterine fibroids. *Radiology* 2004;230:207–213.

42 Law P, Gedroyc WM, Regan L. Magnetic-resonance-guided percutaneous laser ablation of uterine fibroids. *Lancet* 1999;354: 2049–2050.

43 Hindley J, Gedroyc WM, Regan L *et al.* MRI guidance of focused ultrasound therapy of uterine fibroids: early results. *AJR* 2004; 183:1713–1719.

Part 15
Gynaecological Oncology

Chapter 55
Malignant Disease of the Vulva and the Vagina

David M. Luesley
University of Birmingham, Birmingham, UK

Background

Cancer of the vulva is rare, and together with cancer of the vagina accounts for less than 1% of all cancers and 7% of all gynaecological cancers diagnosed in women in the UK. The lifetime risk of developing vulval cancer is 1 in 316 for British women. This is the most recent calculation (2009), using incidence and mortality data for 2001–2005 [1–4].

In 2006, 1063 new cases of vulval cancer were diagnosed (Table 55.1) [1–4]. The European age-standardized incidence rate of vulval cancer in the UK is around 2.4 per 100 000 of the female population.

Most vulval cancers occur after the menopause, with the peak incidence between the ages of 65 and 75 years. Rates are around 1 per 100 000 among women aged 25–44 years, rising to around 3 per 100 000 in those aged 45–64 years, and peak at 13.2 per 100 000 in women aged 65 years and over (Fig. 55.1). There has been a significant increase in rates of vulval cancer in younger women. The proportion of cases diagnosed in those under the age of 50 years rose from 6% in 1975 to 15% in 2006 [1–4]. A similar trend has been documented in other countries [5,6]. These tumours appear to be more frequently associated with vulval intraepithelial neoplasia, human papillomavirus (HPV) infection and immunosuppression. In older women they are more frequently associated with non-neoplastic epithelial disorders such as lichen sclerosus. This suggests that there are at least two oncogenic pathways for the development of this cancer.

The overall increase in vulval cancer might be explained by the rise in the average age of the female population and possibly because of an increase in HPV infection in younger women.

Currently, there are 300–400 deaths ascribed to vulval cancer each year (2003–2007) for all age groups, giving a death rate of 1.2 per 100 000 women ($0.6/10^5$ persons) and ranking it the nineteenth most common cause of cancer death in women. The age-standardized death rate

has fallen since the early 1970s. Between 1971 and 2007, the death rate fell by more than half (52%) from 1.3 per 100 000 female population to 0.6 per 100 000, respectively. The most marked fall has been seen in women aged 45–64 years, where a 70% reduction in mortality has been recorded.

Risk factors

The following are recognized as risk factors for developing vulval cancer:
- lichen sclerosus (4–7% risk of developing cancer) [7,8];
- vulval intraepithelial neoplasia (VIN) and multifocal disease (5–90%) [9,10];
- Paget's disease [11];
- melanoma, *in situ* [12,13];
- smoking [14];
- immunosuppression;
- advanced age; and
- history of cervical neoplasia [15].

Aetiology

The aetiology of vulval cancer remains unknown. Oncogenic HPVs are, however, strongly associated with some vulvar cancers [16] and non-neoplastic epithelial disorders (lichen sclerosus) with others. Currently available data suggest two hypotheses. First is the classic *de novo* neoplasm in the elderly that is frequently seen in association with conditions such as lichen sclerosus (but there is no evidence of a direct cause as yet). The second type is more often associated with VIN, particularly multifocal disease and disease elsewhere in the lower genital tract. This 'infectious-like' type is presumed to be HPV-linked [17].

Recently it has been suggested that non-HPV VIN or differentiated VIN might be the precursor lesion

Dewhurst's Textbook of Obstetrics & Gynaecology, Eighth Edition. Edited by D. Keith Edmonds.
© 2012 John Wiley and Sons, Ltd. Published 2012 by John Wiley and Sons, Ltd.

Table 55.1 New cases and incidence of vulval cancer in the UK.

	England	Wales	Scotland	Northern Ireland	UK
Cases	862	76	103	22	1063
Rate per 100 000	3.3	5	3.9	2.5	3.4
Age-standardized rate per 100 000	2.3 (2.2–2.5)	3.3 (2.6–4.1)	2.9 (2.3–3.4)	1.9 (1.1–2.7)	2.4 (2.3–2.6)

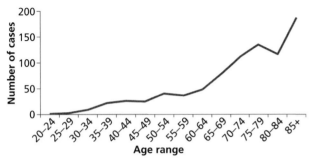

Fig. 55.1 Age distribution of vulval cancer: number of cases in England in 2000.

associated with lichen sclerosus and therefore non-HPV squamous cell cancers. Previously it had been thought that differentiated VIN was found only in association with established cancers, but it has now become clear that this type of VIN can and does occur without contemporaneous cancers but usually with lichen sclerosus. This observation provides additional support for the two oncogenic pathways hypotheses [18].

Histology

The majority of vulvar cancers are squamous in origin. The various histotypes include:
• squamous cell carcinomas (SCCs);
• malignant melanoma;
• Paget's disease;
• Bartholins gland carcinoma;
• adenocarcinomas;
• sarcomas (dermatofibrosarcoma protuberans, Kaposi's sarcoma); and
• metastatic malignant disease and lymphomas.

Verrucous cancer and basal cell cancer are variants of SCCs. Non-squamous cancers of the vulva account for 10% of all vulval cancers. Histology does have a bearing on management, largely because of the different risks of nodal metastases and the predilection for distant spread (Fig. 55.2; Table 55.2).

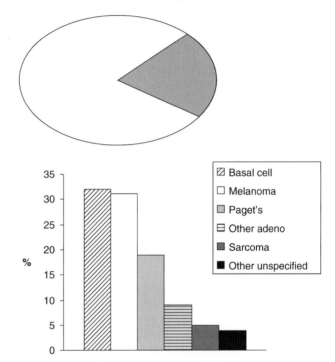

Fig. 55.2 Histological variants of vulval cancer.

Summary box 55.1

• Vulval carcinoma is an uncommon tumour that is most common in the elderly.
• There is evidence suggesting a gradual increase in the number of younger women with this disease.
• There are likely to be two distinct carcinogenic processes, one linked to oncogenic papillomaviruses and the other to conditions such as lichen sclerosus.
• The majority of vulval cancers are squamous.

Presentation

Most squamous cancers primarily involve the medial aspects of the labia majora, with the labia minora being involved only one-third as often. Other sites of predilection include the clitoral and periurethral areas. Small

Table 55.2 Histological types of vulval cancer.

Histotype	Comments
Squamous cell carcinomas	Account for 90% of malignant vulvar neoplasms
	Metastasize to the local lymph nodes, primarily the superficial and deep inguinal nodes, and they may be involved bilaterally
	The risk of nodal disease varies with location and degree of invasion
	Usually present with a nodule or ulcer and may cause pruritus or soreness and pain. Bleeding and an offensive odour may be present with larger lesions
Veruccous and basal cell carcinomas	Squamous variants and rarely, if ever, metastasize locoregionally
	Verrucous carcinomas present as slow-growing wart-like lesions with a tendency to recur locally after excision
	Basal cell carcinomas usually present as an ulcerated nodule on the labia. They do not metastasize and can be managed by local excision or radiation. Up to 20% recur locally after treatment
Malignant melanoma	Has a poor prognosis and is generally managed as for cutaneous melanomas at other sites
	The overall 5-year survival ranges between 8% and 50% and appears to be worse than for cutaneous melanomas elsewhere
	Three patterns of vulval melanoma are identified – mucosal lentinginous (commonest), superficial spreading and nodular. Breslow's thickness of invasion (invasion greater than 1.75 mm has a high risk of recurrence), ulceration and amelanosis are significant prognostic factors. Surgical excision of the lesion with wide margins remains the mainstay of the treatment
Adenocarcinomas	Exceedingly rare and are more likely to represent metastases from another site. There is an association with vulvar Paget's disease
Carcinoma of the Bartholin's gland	Also rare and may be either squamous, adenocarcinoma or an adenoid cystic carcinoma. They occur more often in younger, premenopausal women and overall have a survival rate of about 35% at 5 years
	They usually present as a solid mass in the region of Bartholin's gland with intact overlying skin. Surgical management is similar to squamous cell carcinoma
Sarcomas	Very uncommon and in general are biologically similar to soft-tissue sarcomas at other sites. Generally there is poor prognosis after the appearance of regional or distant relapse. Wide local excision appears to offer the best chance of preventing local recurrence. Elective treatment of the regional nodes is not indicated and there is no advantage in resecting metastatic nodes. The role of adjuvant radiation and chemoradiation has not been assessed largely because of its rarity
Metastatic tumours	Rare and account for about 8% of all vulvar neoplasms. Cervix, endometrium and renal carcinomas have been the most frequently documented primary sites
Paget's disease	Presents as a crusty, erythematous, dark pink/red eczematous 'glazed' area on the vulva. It is an intraepithelial malignancy in 90%. Up to 10–15% of vulval Paget's disease is associated with underlying adenocarcinoma, which may be of the breast, stomach, bowel and bladder. Fluorescein dye has been used to detect the lateral extent of disease spread. Wide local excision with closure of large defects with advancement flaps is required to manage this condition

lesions may be asymptomatic and go unnoticed by the patient, and even now there would appear to be excessive delay in diagnosis for some women. A recent review of practice in the West Midlands suggests that up to one-third of patients apparently report symptoms for over a year. This may reflect patients' attitudes in seeking medical attention or, as suggested by Stroup *et al.* [19], a lack of awareness of the disease in both patients and clinicians. This study also suggested that older patients were more likely to be diagnosed with advanced disease. As SCC of the vulva often progresses slowly, early disease presentation should be feasible and could enable diagnosis to be made at a less advanced stage. Both younger patient age and early disease stage are associated with favourable disease outcome [10,12]. Therefore, efforts should be considered that improve both patient and primary care awareness. This observation is not new – Monagham reported that 32 out of 335 patients delayed seeking medical attention for more than 24 months, and only 35 out of 335 presented within 3 months of noticing symptoms [20]. Similar delays ranging from 1 to 36 months with a mean of 10 months were noted by Hacker *et al.* [21]. Whether this is due to fear or ignorance on the part of the patients or to delay in clinical examination by her primary carer is unknown. The reasons for presenting have been analysed by Podratz *et al.* [22] (see Table 55.3).

Table 55.3 Presenting symptoms in vulvar carcinoma.

Symptoms	Frequency (%)
Pruritus	71
Vulvar lump or swelling	58
Vulvar ulceration	28
Bleeding	26
Pain or soreness	23
Urinary tract symptoms	14
Discharge	13

Assessment

There are two phases of investigation. First, the diagnosis and extent of disease (stage) needs to be confirmed. Second, the patient's fitness needs to be assessed, as does the possibility of concurrent disease, which might influence management.

Examination

The clinical assessment of a vulval malignancy should document both the size and location(s) of all the lesions and the characteristics of the adjacent skin. Care should be taken to assess any involvement of the vagina, urethra, base of bladder or anus. Palpation is important with large tumours to determine whether the tumour is infiltrating deep to the pubic and ischial bone. The integrity of the anal sphincter can only be reliably assessed by a combined rectal and vaginal examination.

Discomfort and tenderness are often associated with large tumours, necessitating examination under general anaesthesia. The presence or absence of groin lymphadenopathy or discrete skin metastases should also be noted.

Diagnosis

Diagnosis is based upon a representative biopsy of the tumour that should include an area where there is a transition of normal to malignant tissue. Biopsies should be of a sufficient size to allow differentiation between superficially invasive and frankly invasive tumours and orientated to allow quality pathological interpretation. Occasionally an alternative strategy might be considered. In certain situations where the clinical diagnosis is apparent and the patient is very symptomatic, that is experiencing heavy bleeding and/or pain, definitive surgery to the vulval lesion may be performed. However, biopsy with

frozen section is recommended before performing any radical procedure.

Because of the potential for other genital tract malignancy, the vagina and cervix should also be thoroughly assessed and biopsied as necessary.

Spread

The tumour spreads both locally and via the lymphatics to the regional lymph nodes. Local spread may involve the vagina, perineum and anal canal, urethra, clitoris and, in late disease, involvement of bone may occur. The sites and extent of spread as well as the involvement of structures where function may be impaired (anal sphincter, urethra, clitoris, etc.) are of extreme importance when planning treatment. Skin beyond the vulva may also become involved (Plate 55.1), particularly over the mons onto the lower abdominal wall and laterally to involve the skin of the thighs. Lymphatic drainage of the vulva is initially to the superficial inguinal nodes, thence to the deep inguinofemoral chain and on to the pelvic (iliac) nodes. In general, central vulvar structures drain bilaterally whereas lateral structures drain to the ipsilateral nodes primarily. Deep pelvic node involvement in the absence of inguinal node disease is rare. Overall, about 30% of operable patients have nodal spread, 10–15% with International Federation of Gynecology and Obstetrics (FIGO) stage I and II tumours and more for higher stage tumours [23–28].

Haematogenous spread can also occur but is uncommon and tends to be associated with large tumours that have already involved the regional nodes.

Premalignant and malignant change in the vagina and cervix is not infrequently seen in association with vulvar cancers. This is not necessarily a metastatic process but may indicate a common aetiological event such as oncogenic HPV infection that can render the whole lower genital tract vulnerable to neoplastic transformation.

Staging

Vulval cancer is staged surgico-pathologically using the FIGO staging system, last updated in 2009 [29]. FIGO staging employs the familiar four categories with substages but now takes into account the number of positive nodes and type of nodal positivity. It also recognizes that tumour size on its own has little discriminatory value in terms of survival, large node-negative tumours having almost as good an outcome as small node-negative tumours (Table 55.4). An alternative is the tumour node metastasis (TNM) system, which is a composite of primary tumour, nodal and metastatic status. Both systems employ nodal status to allocate stage.

Table 55.4 International Federation of Gynecology and Obstetrics (FIGO) staging of vulval cancer (2009).

Stage I	Tumour confined to the vulva
Ia	Lesions ≤2cm in size, confined to the vulva or perineum and with stromal invasion ≤1mm. No nodal metastasis
Ib	Lesions >2cm in size or with stromal invasion >1mm confined to the vulva or perineum. No nodal metastasis
Stage II	Tumour of any size with extension to adjacent perineal structures (lower third of urethra; lower third of vagina; anus) with negative nodes
Stage III	Tumour of any size with or without extension to adjacent perineal structures (lower third of urethra; lower third of vagina; anus) with positive inguinofemoral nodes
IIIa	With one lymph node metastasis (≥5mm), or one or two lymph node metastasis(es) (<5mm)
IIIb	With two or more lymph node metastases (≥5mm), or three or more lymph node metastases (<5mm)
IIIc	With positive nodes with extracapsular spread
Stage IV	Tumour invades other regional (upper two-thirds of urethra; upper two-thirds of vagina) or distant structures
IVa	Tumour invades any of the following: upper urethral and or vaginal mucosa; bladder mucosa; rectal mucosa or fixed to pelvic bone; or fixed or ulcerated inguinofemoral lymph nodes
IVb	Any distant metastasis including pelvic lymph nodes

Table 55.5 Relationship of depth of invasion to risk of nodal disease [28].

Invasion depth (mm)	Per cent node positive
<1	00
1.1–2	07.7
2.1–3	08.3
3.1–5	26.7
>5	34.2

Prognostic factors

The 5-year survival in cases with no lymph node involvement is in excess of 80%, falling to less than 50% if the inguinal nodes are involved and 10–15% if the iliac or other pelvic nodes are involved. Nodal status and primary lesion diameter, when considered together, are the only variables associated with prognosis [30]. Several other factors may also impact on outcome and need to be taken into consideration when formulating a plan of treatment.

Site of the tumour
Central tumours located close to midline structures such as the clitoris, urethra, vagina and anus are at a higher risk of bilateral inguinal nodal spread than tumours located on the lateral surface. In practice, the distance from the midline is somewhat arbitrary, although if the excision margin around the tumour is planned to be 2cm and crosses the midline, then it is defined as a centrally placed tumour. Bilateral groin node dissection is required for invasive tumours, whereas unilateral groin node dissection is required for lateral tumours.

Tumour size
Tumours larger than 2cm in diameter have a greater chance of being frankly invasive and metastasizing to the lymph nodes.

Depth of invasion
Invasion less than 1mm in depth (superficially invasive or stage Ia) is associated with a negligible risk of lymph node involvement, but this rises to 8% for a depth of 1–2mm, 11% for 2–3mm and over 25% for lesions of greater than 3mm depth (Table 55.5) [28].

Lymphovascular space involvement
Although lymphovascular space involvement is not included in the surgico-pathological staging of vulval cancer, it is associated with an increased risk of metastasis, as is tumour border pattern (infiltrating versus pushing) and perineural invasion [31,32].

Lymph node involvement
Lymph node involvement is one of the most important prognostic variables. The number of lymph nodes involved and the type of involvement also influences the prognosis. Metastasis to more than one node, involvement of multiple nodal sites and extracapsular spread of metastasis adversely influence the prognosis.

Lymph node status

The most important feature of vulvar cancer, and that which influences the outcome more than any other, is the histological state of the lymph nodes. The overall survival for all cases of histologically proven groin node-negative vulvar cancers is approximately 70–90%, while that for node-positive is between 25% and 40%. Those with positive pelvic lymph nodes rarely survive. Furthermore, recurrence in the groin is virtually always fatal, whereas local vulvar recurrence may often be amenable to either surgical or non-surgical salvage (Plate 52.2). It is therefore of vital importance that the risk of nodal disease is properly addressed at the outset.

It is well recognized that groin node dissection is associated with significant morbidity. Almost 50% of patients undergoing groin node dissection will suffer postoperative complications, most commonly wound infection, wound breakdown and lymphoedema [33]. For these reasons an investigation that could identify those at least risk could have a significant therapeutic benefit. Assessment by clinical palpation of the groins is inadequate; of patients with clinically normal lymph nodes, 16–24% have metastases, while 24–41% of those with clinically suspicious nodes are negative when examined histologically [34,35]. Even though the majority of vulval cancers are still assessed clinically, there is increasing interest in utilizing additional imaging, particularly of the regional node groups.

Groin node assessment

Magnetic resonance imaging

Magnetic resonance imaging (MRI) allows clear delineation of tissue planes, detailed anatomical assessment and assessment of the depth of the tumour extension, as well as clearly visualizing the involvement of adjacent pelvic structures (e.g. urethra, bladder, vagina and anal sphincters). MRI also allows the assessment of nodal involvement [36], which has a high specificity of 97–100% but low sensitivity of 40–50%. These findings may assist in the preoperative staging of vulval cancer. Identifying nodal involvement is important preoperatively, as this will clearly identify a group of patients who would benefit from groin lymphadenectomy. MRI is also important in recurrent disease to exclude distant metastases before any radical procedure such as exenteration.

Magnetic resonance lymphography

In this technique, ultra-small iron oxide peroxide (USIOP) particles coated with dextran are administered intravenously. These particles are taken up by macrophages in the lymph nodes and effectively reduce the signal intensity on T1 and T2 weighted images. In metastatic nodes, however, where malignant cells have replaced macrophages, the signal intensity is not altered. This technique has improved the sensitivity of detecting involved lymph nodes from 55% to 89% [37].

Ultrasound

Ultrasonography is relatively cheap and widely available [38,39]. It has also been shown to be of use in assessing groin nodes. Suspicious sonographic features include:

- larger than 1 cm in size;
- loss of oval shape;
- hypoechoic cortex;
- loss of echogenic hilar sinus fat;
- irregular margin; and
- increasing low attenuation of the cortex.
- increased peripheral vascularity on colour Doppler (rather than a hilar perfusion in reactive nodes).

Ultrasound assessment of the nodes can be combined with fine-needle aspiration cytology (FNAC) but has a low sensitivity of 58% owing to sampling error. It is also associated with a failure to obtain an analysable sample [38], false-negative histology [40] and a potential risk of metastatic spread.

Computed tomography scan

Computed tomography (CT) scanning has a limited role in the assessment of vulval cancers. The use of CT scanning has some value in determining whether or not there is pelvic or indeed para-aortic nodal enlargement, although it would be unusual to detect enlargement in these nodal groups without evidence of more proximal nodal disease.

Positron emission tomography

Positron emission tomography (PET) is useful for detecting extranodal disease. It is expensive and has limited availability; therefore, is not routinely used. In one prospective evaluation of this non-invasive technique it was found to have relatively poor accuracy rates [41], making it unfeasible for routine use. The reasons for this are unclear but may be related to a reduced metabolic activity associated with tumour necrosis. No robust studies relating to the performance of PET-CT scanning in detecting nodal metastases in vulval cancer have yet been published.

Sentinel node lymphoscintigraphy

The sentinel node is defined as the first node in the lymphatic chain draining an anatomical area. If the sentinel node from the suspected lesion is negative for disease then the remainder of the nodes should also be free of the disease (Fig. 55.3). The sentinel node for vulval lesions can be identified by injecting methylene blue dye into the tumour edge and/or using immunoscintigraphy where a radiolabelled marker (technetium-99) is injected into and around the margins of the lesion. A hand-held gamma camera is used to identify the radioactive tracer uptake in the regional lymph nodes [42,43]. Identification during surgery is further enhanced by the use of blue dye, which, along with the raised radiation count, allows the sentinel node to be clearly seen (Plate 55.2). This technique has

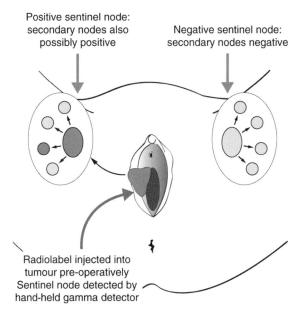

Positive sentinel node: secondary nodes also possibly positive

Negative sentinel node: secondary nodes negative

Radiolabel injected into tumour pre-operatively Sentinel node detected by hand-held gamma detector

Fig. 55.3 Schematic of sentinel node sampling.

Summary box 55.2

- Most vulval cancers present with soreness, pruritus or the presence of a mass or ulcer.
- All suspicious lesions should be subjected to a diagnostic biopsy.
- Primary spread is both local and to the inguinofemoral nodes.
- The status of the lymph nodes has a major bearing on clinical outcome.
- Invasion >1 mm in depth is associated with increasing rates of lymph node involvement.
- Clinical examination of the lymph nodes is unreliable.
- Staging of vulval cancer is surgical and clinical.
- Sentinel node sampling is proving to be the most accurate method of assessing lymph node spread.

Table 55.6 Groin node diagnostic studies.

Test	Pooled sensitivity
Sentinel nodes (technetium)	97% (91–100)
Sentinel nodes (blue dye)	95% (82–99)
Ultrasonography (+FNA)	72% (56–85)
Ultrasonography	45% (35–85)
MRI	86% (57–98)
PET CT	71% (50–86)

FNA, fine-needle aspiration; MRI, magnetic resonance imaging; PET CT, positron emission tomography computed tomography.

gained in popularity over the last 5 years. The first multi-centre observational study using the combined technique was published in 2008 [44]. Over a 6-year period, 403 assessable patients were included and 623 groins were assessed. Only lesions less than 4 cm in diameter were included. The protocol dictated that if the sentinel nodes were negative, no further groin dissection was required. In 259 patients with unifocal vulval disease and negative sentinel nodes, six groin recurrences (2.3%) were diagnosed. Treatment-related morbidity was significantly improved when compared with complete groin dissection. The authors concluded that the sentinel node technique performed within the context of a quality controlled multidisciplinary team (MDT) should become the standard treatment in selected patients with early-stage vulval cancer.

Comparisons of nodal assessment

There has been one meta-analysis published to date that sets out to compare the performance of the above techniques [45]. The analysis included five diagnostic tests in 29 studies (961 groins). Accuracy in excluding node metastasis was defined as the most important performance parameter, and therefore pooled sensitivity was defined as the ability to exclude disease when the test was negative.

As one might expect, sentinel node sampling performed much better than any of the others. This must, however, be set against the relative 'invasiveness' of the technique (Table 55.6).

Management of vulvar cancer

Managing the vulvar lesion

The objectives of managing the primary vulvar lesion are to remove the cancer, minimize the risk of local recurrence and preserve as much function as possible. These objectives have initially been addressed by modifications of the surgical approach and more latterly by considering combined modality management, especially combinations of surgery, radiotherapy and chemoradiation.

Surgical management of the primary vulvar lesion

The site, size and relation of the lesion to important functional structures will determine the most appropriate method for treating the vulvar lesion. Similarly, the clinical presence or absence of nodal or distant disease will affect the strategies designed to manage non-vulvar, and to a certain extent vulvar, disease. It would, for instance, be illogical to embark upon radical local treatment for the primary cancer in the presence of distant untreatable

metastases unless there was no other suitable form of palliation. Two broad categories of patient can be identified at the outset:
• Those who have small unifocal vulvar lesions with no clinical evidence of nodal involvement.
• Those who have more advanced vulvar disease and or have clinical evidence of nodal involvement.
For the purposes of further discussion, these will be termed as early and late disease, respectively.

Surgical management of early vulvar cancer
Radical vulvectomy is excessive treatment for the majority of unifocal and early cancers. Wide local excision is usually sufficient for the majority of lesions between 1 and 10 mm in depth. The most important factor governing local recurrence is the margin of excision. The risk of recurrence increases as the disease-free margins decrease (≥ 8 mm, 0%; 8–4.8 mm, 8%; <4.8 mm, 54%) [31,46]. Because of shrinkage associated with fixing, this margin should be increased. Surgical excision should therefore be at least 15 mm on all the tumour dimensions. The excision should be taken to the depth of the fascia lata, which is coplanar with the fascia of the urogenital diaphragm. Lateral margins should not be compromised even if this would entail excision of a functional midline structure such as the anus, clitoris or urethra. In situations where this pertains, for example in early but midline cancers, radiotherapy may have a role in allowing local control without loss of function. Even if wide excision has been achieved, there may be other variables identified after examination of the specimen that some have suggested indicate a high risk of relapse. These include tumour thickness (or invasiveness) and capillary lymphatic space (CLS) involvement, but this suggestion requires further confirmation. In addition the adjacent epithelium, which may reflect the underlying oncogenic process, may influence recurrence. Differentiated VIN appears to have a higher rate of recurrence than basaloid or warty VIN, although this is based on a very small case series [47].

As one would expect, the local recurrence rate for wide local excision compares favourably with that following radical vulvectomy. Hacker and Van der Velden [46] have collated data from 12 published series including 530 patients, of whom 165 were treated by radical local excision and 365 by radical vulvectomy. The local recurrence rates were 7.2% and 6.3%, respectively.

Although the technique may be appropriate, there is evidence that the drive towards more conservative excision may result in less than appropriate clearances even in situations of centralized care by specialist gynaecological oncologists. An audit on the impact of improving outcomes guidance conducted in the south-west of England suggested adequate margins in only 49% of cases [48].

Surgical management of advanced vulvar lesions
The reader should appreciate that 'advanced' in vulvar terms indicates that wide local excision would either be a radical vulvectomy and/or would compromise function. The same principles apply here as with the smaller unifocal lesions in that the objective is to obtain clearance by at least 15 mm on all of the resection margins. As subsequent function and cosmesis are more likely to be affected, consideration should also be given to adjunctive treatment. It is important to consider the woman and her feelings when constructing the management plan. An elderly woman with extensive or multifocal disease with an associated symptomatic non-neoplastic epithelial disorder such as lichen sclerosus may well gain an overall benefit from radical vulvectomy with subsequent grafting. Conversely, a young woman with a clitoral cancer may be managed initially by radiotherapy, reserving surgery for failed local control. These types of cases form the basis for local management of advanced vulvar lesions. The prime objective is to maximize local control, closely followed by consideration of further function and cosmesis in that particular woman.

Lymph node disease
Patients with superficially invasive vulvar cancer are at minimal risk of nodal disease (Table 55.5). This is defined as a depth of invasion of less than 1 mm. Depth of invasion is closely related to the risk of nodal disease. It should be measured from the most superficial dermal papilla adjacent to the tumour.

Overall, about 30% of vulvar cancers will have inguinofemoral nodal disease and about one-fifth of those with positive inguinofemoral nodes will have positive pelvic nodes (i.e. about 5% overall). It has been known for many years that pelvic nodes are rarely, if ever, involved if the inguinal nodes are negative. The low frequency of pelvic node involvement and the doubts surrounding the ability of surgery to control disease at this site have led most to conclude that the routine application of pelvic node dissection in vulvar cancer should be discontinued.

The following clinical factors can predict for the presence of lymph node disease, although clinical examination of the nodes themselves is unreliable:
• lesion size;
• whether or not the nodes are clinically suspicious; and
• disease that involves both the labia minora and majora has a 50% chance of nodal involvement, whereas when only one of these structures is involved the risk is approximately 20%. Steheman *et al.* [49] also suggested that clitoral or perineal siting of the tumour carried an increased risk of nodal disease.

Other risk factors depend on histopathological assessment of the primary lesion and not surprisingly are similar to the general prognostic factors for outcome. They include:

• tumour grade;
• capillary lymphatic space involvement;
• degree of invasion (tumour thickness); and
• perineural invasion.

Management of the lymph nodes

Types of lymph node dissection

The primary lymphatic drainage of the vulva and distal vagina is to the inguinal (superficial femoral) and the nodes lying along the femoral vein. Efferent vessels from the superficial inguinal nodes drain to the deep inguinal or femoral nodes. The most cephalad femoral lymph node is the node of Cloquet. This is not a constant anatomical finding and has been noted to be absent in 54% of cadavers. The femoral nodes also receive some direct afferents, particularly from the clitoris and anterior vulva, thus explaining the observation of involved femoral nodes with uninvolved inguinal nodes. One prospective study [50] has suggested that superficial lymphadenectomy alone may be associated with a higher risk of groin relapse, although the relatively low relapse rate in early disease renders any conclusion somewhat unreliable.

Laterality

Extensive crossover of lymphatic channels of the vulva may result in nodal involvement of the contralateral groins in addition to the ipsilateral groin nodes. Because of this, bilateral groin node dissection is usually required. However in small (<2 cm) lateral tumours, only an ipsilateral groin node dissection need initially be performed. A lateralized lesion, agreed by consensus, is defined as one in which wide excision, at least 1 cm beyond the visible tumour edge, would not impinge upon a midline structure [consensus statement of the European Organization for Research and Treatment of Cancer (EORTC) Vulva Group]. If the ipsilateral nodes are subsequently shown to be positive for cancer, the contralateral nodes should also be excised or irradiated as the nodes are more likely to be positive in this scenario.

Andrews *et al.* [51] noted that this was also the case for T2 lesions despite a relatively high ipsilateral positivity rate of 34%. Exceptions have, however, been reported. For larger lateralized lesions the picture is more confused and, until further data become available, bilateral node dissection would be advisable.

En bloc and separate groin incisions

The need for en bloc removal of the lymph nodes has received much attention, largely because it has been felt that this type of procedure accounts for a significant pro-

portion of the morbidity (Plate 55.3) and that the technique employing separate groin incisions (Plate 55.4) results in a better cosmetic outcome. The triple incision technique was first described in 1965, although it only became popular in the 1980s. Those who have reported on its use have not shown any disadvantages in terms of survival or local relapse for early-stage carcinomas, and there have been quite marked improvements in the morbidity.

The anxiety relating to the triple incision is the possibility of relapse in the bridge of tissue left between the vulvectomy or local excision and the groin nodes. This tissue will contain lymphatic channels, but whether lymphatic metastasis is an intermittent or embolic event or a continuous or permeation event remains uncertain. Certainly if the lymphatic channels contain malignant cells at the time of resection, then recurrence would seem to be a real possibility.

Current consensus would suggest that en bloc dissection of the nodes is probably best retained for large vulvar lesions and in situations where there is gross involvement of the groin nodes (Plate 55.5).

Management of involved lymph nodes

Resection of the groin lymph nodes provides prognostic information and might also confer some survival benefit. There are varying degrees of positivity from microscopic deposits in one of many nodes to gross extracapsular spread in the entire group of nodes. As with overall stage, this spectrum is also associated with a spectrum of outcomes (Table 55.7) and requires different approaches to management. The most important variable influencing survival is extracapsular spread from the lymph nodes, and for patients who have only one node involved the most important prognostic factor is the greatest dimension of the metastasis within the node (Table 55.8). These

Table 55.7 Survival in relation to nodal status and size of vulvar lesion [30].

Node status	Primary size	Survival (%)
Negative (N = 385)	≤2 cm	97.9
	2–3 cm	90.5
	>3 cm	75–80
	All	90.9
Positive (N = 203)	All	57.2
1 or 2 positive nodes	–	75
3 or 4	–	36
5 or 6	–	24
7 or more	–	0

Table 55.8 Management in relation to lymph node status

Groin nodes negative	No further treatment
Groin nodes positive after surgery	–
One node only involved*	Observation only
Two or more nodes involved	Inguinal and pelvic radiation
Clinically positive before surgery	Resection followed by radiation
	Radiation followed by resection
	Radiation only

*In the situation where there is only one node involved but the node is either completely replaced by tumour or there is extracapsular spread, the author feels that adjuvant radiotherapy is justifiable.

Table 55.9 Complications of surgery.

Groin dissection
Wound breakdown/cellulitis
Lymphocyst
Lymphoedema

Vulvar resection
Wound breakdown/cellulitis
Rectocoele
Urinary problems
Psychological

observations explain and underpin the recent revisions in FIGO staging.

In the past, pelvic lymphadenectomy was considered to be appropriate if the inguinal femoral nodes were involved. This practice has become increasingly uncommon as it has been well demonstrated in Gynecologic Oncology Group (GOG) protocol 37 [52] that in this situation pelvic radiation confers a better outcome than pelvic node dissection. Interestingly, the survival difference appeared to reflect better control of disease in the groin than pelvic or distant disease.

A final observation in regard to the lymph nodes is that all the available data are based upon what is considered to be standard pathological evaluation of the groin nodes (standard sections stained with haematoxylin and eosin). In other tumour systems it has been possible to define a group of patients with micrometastases by using complete serial sectioning and immunohistochemical (IHC) staining. These micrometastasis-positive nodes would have been negative on standard assessment. There are no studies available as yet indicating what, if any, clinical significance of such findings might be in vulval cancer, but this issue is being addressed in the ongoing GROINS V2 study.

Complications of surgical treatment

The complications of vulval and groin surgery are listed in Table 55.9. Any major cancer procedure carries immediate morbidity risks such as haemorrhage, thromboembolism and infection, and vulvar procedures are no exception to this. Prophylactic antiembolic strategies are of value and should be used in all cases. Reducing the length of hospitalization and early mobilization indirectly enhances such prophylaxis and may result from modifications of the radical approach.

Radical en bloc dissection (radical vulvectomy and bilateral node dissection) results in lymphoedema in between 8% and 69% of cases. Wound breakdown is very common, occurring in anything between 27% and 85% of cases, and can become secondarily infected, resulting in cellulitis. The average hospital stay in days for this radical procedure varies from 17 to 33. The triple incision technique has yielded significant improvements in operative blood loss and length of stay, although high breakdown rates continue to be reported (22–52%) [53,54]. The occurrence of lymphocyst (Plate 55.5) and lymphoedema does not seem to be significantly less than that with the radical en bloc technique. Unilateral groin dissection does appear to lower the incidence of morbidity, but there is no significant difference in morbidity when superficial is compared with deep groin node dissection. Van der Zee *et al.* have reported significant reductions in wound breakdown, cellulitis, length of hospital stay and lymphoedema when sentinel node sampling is compared with inguinofemoral lymphadenectomy [44].

Less radical approaches to the vulva have certainly improved cosmesis and subsequent function. Other surgical modifications [55] to reduce morbidity are sparing the saphenous vein at the time of surgery to reduce wound and lower limb complications, although the data on outcome in terms of lymphoedema are inconclusive [56,57]. It has also been suggested that the tissues most lateral in the groin need not be resected. Sartorius transposition to cover the femoral vessels in thin and emaciated patients also helps to reduce wound morbidity [57]. Wound healing is also improved by avoiding undermining of the skin edges, performing tension-free closures, using wound drainage and administering prophylactic antibiotics. More recently, surgeons have employed grafting techniques either at the time of initial surgery or as a second-stage procedure. The grafts successfully employed have been the gracilis and rectus muscle myocutaneous flaps and rotational full-thickness skin flaps taken from the inner thigh or buttock (Plate 55.6). The use of these flaps to fill considerable defects and a more conservative approach to excision have resulted in less scarring and more functional vulvas. As yet it has not been possible to demonstrate that this translates into improved psychological well-being, although the psychological trauma of radical excision without reconstruction is well documented [58].

Management of complications

For lymphoedema, compression hosiery is prescribed along with rest and exercise, avoidance of trauma (skin care), simple gravity drainage and manual lymphatic drainage (MLD). For lymphocyst, a conservative approach is adopted and drainage under antibiotic cover is recommended only for symptomatic cases, but they tend to reform.

Wound healing can be promoted with manuka honey dressing [59]. Recently there have been anecdotal reports of using tissue sealant to promote healing in groin wounds that have broken down [60].

Radiotherapy and chemotherapy

The role of radiotherapy and chemotherapy in the treatment of vulvar cancer is less defined than that for surgery. There are, however, data quite clearly indicating that squamous vulvar cancers are sensitive to both radiotherapy and chemotherapy.

Basal cell cancers are well recognized as being radiosensitive, and radiotherapy may be the treatment of choice if surgery is likely to result in either functional or cosmetic impairment. Melanomas have not been shown to respond and verrucous cancers have been reported as becoming much more aggressive as a result of radiotherapy.

Adjuvant radiotherapy

The factors influencing the need for adjuvant radiotherapy are:
• surgical margins; and
• groin node positivity.

There is insufficient evidence to recommend adjuvant local therapy routinely in patients with suboptimal surgical margins (<8mm). Adjuvant treatment for positive margins is associated with improved survival when compared with observation alone [61].

Adjuvant radiotherapy should be considered when two or more lymph nodes are involved with microscopic metastatic disease or there is complete replacement and or extracapsular spread in any node [50,62,63]. Treatment should be to the groins and the pelvic nodes, although there is no evidence to show whether treatment should be directed at both sides or to the involved side only. The increasing use of the sentinel node technique may require a re-evaluation of this strategy. The current GROINS 2

protocol dictates that patients should be offered adjuvant radiation therapy if the sentinel node is positive. This, of course, could represent overtreatment in current terms as the sentinel node might be the only positive node and as such would not result in adjuvant treatment if all other nodes were negative. What the current GROINS protocol cannot answer, however, is whether or not the effect of adjuvant radiotherapy to the groins is additive to surgical resection. The outcome in people who are sentinel node-positive and treated with radiation is eagerly awaited, and one would hope that it will compare favourably (in terms of disease control) with those receiving adjuvant radiation after complete lymphadenectomy.

Primary treatment

Radiotherapy with or without concurrent or sequential chemotherapy is being used more frequently in the management of advanced vulval cancer. Radiotherapy may, in certain circumstances, be the sole treatment, but more usually it is used preoperatively with a view to allowing for sphincter-preserving surgery. Radiotherapy may also be of use in place of surgery for histologically proven involved groin lymph nodes. Whether such irradiated nodes require removal after treatment remains unknown.

Radiotherapy and chemotherapy schedules

Most schedules are based upon those developed by the Toronto Group [64]. Fraction size is important, with 1.7Gy being close to tolerance although it is recognized that some centres may use slightly larger fractions (1.8Gy). Doses will have to be reduced for radical treatment if fractions greater than 1.7Gy are employed.

Radical treatment usually requires that a prophylactic dose (45–50Gy) is delivered to the primary and nodal sites and the tumour is then boosted by a second phase of treatment using electrons, conformal radiotherapy or brachytherapy to a total dose of 65Gy. The total prescribed dose is determined by the clinical context.

A Cochrane review suggests that there is no evidence that prophylactic groin irradiation should be used in preference to surgery [65]. With regard to the use of concurrent chemotherapy and radiation therapy, there are no robust prospective data. Several small retrospective studies have suggested that there may be some improvement in local control with regimens employing cisplatinum and 5-fluorouracil, Mitomycin C and 5-fluorouracil, and 5-fluorouracil alone.

When there is no obvious macroscopic disease and the sole intention is adjuvant treatment, the total dose is 45–50Gy with no concurrent chemotherapy.

Complications of radiotherapy

The reason for the limited application of radiotherapy in this disease lies in the poor record of tolerance and high levels of complications reported in the older series. This almost certainly relates to the type of treatments and techniques available in these series. More modern equipment and a greater understanding of its potential and applications have resulted in a marked improvement in tolerance and morbidity.

Most women will note erythema and some moist desquamation as a result of radiotherapy. With appropriate care and attention to local hygiene, such problems rarely result in a premature discontinuation of treatment. Radiation-induced cystitis requires bladder irrigation and treatment of any infection. Proctitis is managed with steroid [Predfoam (prednisolone)], normacol and loperamide.

More severe side effects include necrosis of bone (symphysis and femoral heads) and fistula formation. Careful planning of field sizes, dose and fractionation minimize such risks.

Recurrent disease

Between 15% and 30% of cases will develop recurrence. The most common site is the residual vulva (70%), with the groin nodes accounting for almost 20% and the remainder of relapses occurring in the pelvis or as distant metastases [66].

Up to 80% of recurrences occur 2 years after primary treatment, and close surveillance every 3 months in the first 2 years is usually practised. This is reduced to 6-monthly surveillance for a further 2–3 years and annually thereafter [67]. Additionally, patients are encouraged to self-inspect and report any symptoms of pain, bleeding or discharge. It should be stated that this schedule for follow-up is empirical and not evidence-based.

Survival is poor following regional relapse, hence the efforts to prevent this at the outset. Skin bridge recurrence has been reported to be more likely to occur in patients with positive lymph nodes [68].

Treatment

The management of relapsed disease will depend on the site and extent of the recurrence [66]. Wide excision of local recurrences can result in a 5-year survival rate of 56% if the inguinal nodes are negative [69]. If excision would risk sphincter function, radiotherapy should be considered as the first choice. If radiotherapy has already been given to maximum dose, then excision should be considered.

Groin recurrence has a much poorer prognosis and is difficult to manage. In patients who have not been treated previously with groin irradiation, radiotherapy (with or without additional surgery) would be the preferred option. The options are much more limited in those who have already been irradiated and palliation, which may include surgery, should be considered. There is no standard chemotherapy or other systemic treatment effective in patients with metastatic disease.

Summary box 55.3

- Radical excision of the primary lesion(s) should aim to achieve disease-free margins of at least 8 mm after fixation.
- All lesions with invasion greater than 1 mm should be considered for either ipsilateral or bilateral lymph node dissection.
- Adjuvant radiotherapy or re-excision should be considered if the excision margins are suboptimal.
- One lymph node replaced or breached by a tumour or two with microscopic deposits should prompt adjuvant radiotherapy.
- Advanced tumours or tumours where excision may cause functional compromise should have treatment individualized (surgery, radiotherapy and chemotherapy) to maximize cure and minimize functional compromise.
- Local recurrence may be managed by either re-excision or radiotherapy, whichever would be associated with the least functional compromise.
- Groin recurrences are difficult to treat and the outcome is poor.

Vaginal cancer

Background

Vaginal cancer is rare and accounts for only 1–2% of all gynaecological malignancies. They arise as primary squamous cancers or are the result of extension from the cervix or vulva. Most authors report a wide age range (18–95 years), with the peak incidence in the sixth decade of life and a mean age of approximately 60–65 years. There would appear to be no relationship with race or parity.

Aetiology

The cause of vaginal cancer is unknown, although several predisposing and associated factors have been noted. These include:

- previous lower genital tract intraepithelial neoplasia and neoplasia [mainly cervical intraepithelial neoplasia (CIN) and/or cervical carcinoma];
- HPV infection (oncogenic subtypes); and
- previous gynaecological malignancy.

Several authors report that approximately one of four or as high as one of three of patients have had a previous gynaecological malignancy. Large case-control studies have not been able to confirm pelvic radiotherapy, previous hysterectomy, long-term use of a vaginal pessary and chronic uterovaginal prolapse as causative factors.

Presentation

The symptoms at presentation will depend on the stage of tumour at presentation. The most common presenting features are:

- vaginal bleeding, which accounts for more than 50% of presentations;
- vaginal discharge;
- urinary symptoms;
- abdominal mass or pain; and
- asymptomatic – approximately 10% of tumours will be asymptomatic at the time of diagnosis.

Vaginal tumours may be overlooked during vaginal examination, particularly when a bivalve speculum is used. Careful inspection of the vaginal walls while withdrawing the speculum is necessary to avoid this otherwise the blades of the speculum may obscure a tumour on the anterior or posterior vaginal wall.

Pathology

Eighty to ninety per cent of tumours in the larger series are squamous. Other carcinomas include adenocarcinomas, adenosquamous carcinomas and clear cell adenocarcinomas. Other rarer primary vaginal cancers are discussed separately.

Site and size

Tumours can occur at any site in the vagina. The upper third of the vagina is the site most frequently involved, either alone or together with the middle third in approximately two of three of cases. Approximately one in six will be found to involve the entire length of the vagina. There is no predilection for any particular wall of the vagina. Plate 55.7 demonstrates a well-localized lesion in the lower vagina that does not originate from the vulva.

As with site, the size of tumour shows great variation at presentation, ranging from small ulcers less than a centimetre in diameter to large pelvic masses, although the majority of tumours are a maximum of 2–4 cm in diameter.

Staging and assessment

Any tumour classified as a primary vaginal carcinoma should not involve the uterine cervix. There should be no clinical evidence that the tumour represents metastatic or recurrent disease. Staging should be carried out according to the FIGO classification. This classification is summarized in Table 55.10.

The staging process itself can present problems since it may be difficult to differentiate one stage from another. This applies particularly to stage I and II disease that may be hard to separate clinically, and similarly it is difficult to separate stage IIa and IIb on purely clinical grounds. Differences also exist in interpretations of the significance of positive inguinal nodes and their effect on staging. The current staging does not indicate in which group such patients should be placed, and some authors would assign these patients to stage III with others preferring IVa or IVb.

Table 55.10 International Federation of Gynecology and Obstetrics (FIGO) clinical staging of primary vaginal carcinoma.

FIGO	
Stage	Definition
0	Vaginal intraepithelial neoplasia III (carcinoma *in situ*)
I	Invasive carcinoma limited to vaginal wall
IIa	Carcinoma involves subvaginal tissue but does not extend to parametrium
IIb	Carcinoma involves parametrium but does not extend to pelvic sidewall
III	Carcinoma extends to pelvic sidewall
IVa	Involvement of mucosa of bladder or rectum (bullous oedema does not qualify for stage IV) or direct extension beyond true pelvis
IVb	Spread to distant organs

The majority of series report that stage II disease is most commonly found at presentation (approximately 50% of all cases). Stages I and II combined consistently constitute 70–80% of cases.

Assessment

The assessment is best performed under general anaesthesia.

- The site and limits of the tumour can be accurately determined and a full-thickness biopsy taken for histological analysis.
- Combined rectal and vaginal examination is helpful to determine whether there is any extension of the tumour beyond the vagina and the extent of any spread.
- Cystoscopy and sigmoidoscopy are required to exclude or confirm the involvement of bladder or rectum.
- Chest X-rays or intravenous urograms can be used for the assessment.
- More complex radiological investigations such as rectal ultrasound scanning or MRI may be helpful in selected instances to define the dimensions and extension of the tumour.

Treatment

The majority of cases of vaginal carcinoma are treated using pelvic radiotherapy, although surgical excision is an appropriate form of management in selected cases. Experimental chemotherapeutic regimes are being developed both alone and in conjunction with radiotherapy for advanced cases or recurrent disease.

Radiotherapy

The proximity of the bladder and rectum means that, except in early cases, salvage of normal bladder and rectal

function can only be achieved using radiotherapeutic techniques. Radiotherapy is certainly effective in treating vaginal cancer and survival rates have improved throughout the century as techniques have developed and improved. Techniques utilized have included:
- external beam radiotherapy (teletherapy);
- brachytherapy (e.g. interstitial implants, intravaginal cylinders or vaginal ovoids); and
- a combination of the two.

There is little place for using external beam therapy alone and the majority of tumours should be treated in combination with brachytherapy, with small early-stage tumours being suitable for treatment by brachytherapy alone. The optimal dose remains unclear but the mid-tumour dose should be at least 75 Gy. Above this dose any survival benefit must be weighed against the increased toxicity of therapy, and doses of 98 Gy or more have been shown to cause a higher incidence of severe side effects. Complication rates reported for radiotherapy vary according to dosage and techniques used and to the different grading systems used by different authors. Most report complications as occurring in 10–20% of patients. Life-threatening complications have been reported to occur in 6% of those undergoing radiotherapy for gynaecological malignancies, and vaginal carcinoma is no exception.

Acute complications include:
- proctitis;
- radiation cystitis; and
- vulvar excoriation or ulceration and even vaginal necrosis.

Significant long-term complications reported include:
- vesico-vaginal or recto-vaginal fistulae;
- rectal stricture; and
- vaginal stenosis.

In younger women, vaginal stenosis may be a long-term complication of great significance.

Surgery

There are relatively few reports of the use of surgery in vaginal cancer. Given what little information does exist, there are three general situations where surgery might be considered as first-line management. These are:

1 patients presenting with a stage I tumour in the upper third of the vagina, particularly on the posterior wall where resection may be technically straightforward. These patients can be treated with radical hysterectomy (if uterus *in situ*), pelvic lymphadenectomy and vaginectomy;

2 patients with small mobile stage I tumours low down in the vagina, which if amenable to excision can be treated by vulvectomy with inguinal lymphadenectomy; and

3 bulky lesions that are unlikely to be cured by primary radiotherapy may be considered for exenteration in a few carefully selected cases.

It is undoubtedly possible in many instances to remove a vaginal carcinoma by surgical means, and there is little evidence to suggest that survival is improved following either treatment modality. The choice of treatment will depend on the potential toxicity of the proposed treatment in relation to an individual patient and an individual tumour. Surgery is problematic in this respect because, to achieve adequate margins around tumour, important structures (e.g. bladder or rectum) may be compromised.

The addition of lymphadenectomy would appear important as Stock *et al.* [70] reported that 10 (34%) of 29 patients undergoing pelvic node dissection and all three of their patients subjected to inguinal lymphadenectomy had positive nodes. High rates of metastasis to inguinal nodes from tumours of the lower third of the vagina have been noted. Early reports suggested that morbidity after surgical treatment of vaginal cancer was both frequent and serious.

However, the majority of complications were seen in patients undergoing surgical management of post-irradiation recurrence or following exenterative surgery for advanced disease. Serious complications include urinary problems (stress and/or urge incontinence) and fistulae. Lastly, any procedure requiring removal of the entire vagina will render the patient apareunic, although lesser degrees of vaginal excision usually allow subsequent sexual function.

Chemotherapy

There is little published work regarding the use of chemotherapy in vaginal cancer. Reports that exist concern combined chemoradiation as first-line treatment of advanced disease and the palliative use of chemotherapy for recurrent disease. In squamous vaginal cancer the use of chemotherapy should be regarded as experimental.

Survival

Overall 5-year survival rates are now in the region of 50%, with rates of 39–66% reported. Survival is much higher in early-stage disease. However, there is some inconsistency in the allocation of cases to stages I and II. Survival rates for stage I disease are consistently reported at between 70% and 80%.

Prognostic factors

Stage, size, site, histological grade and type have all been proposed as factors that may influence survival. Only tumour stage and site, however, are consistently reported as being directly related to survival.

Recurrence

Recurrence occurs locally or within the pelvis in most instances, with about 20% relapsing with distant metastasis. The majority of relapses occur soon after primary therapy. Stock *et al.* [70] found a median time to relapse of 0.7 years. The outlook after failure of primary therapy is poor and in the majority further treatment is unlikely to be successful. As with cervical carcinoma, those patients with purely pelvic recurrence are sometimes suitable for salvage surgery by anterior and posterior exenteration.

Uncommon vaginal tumours

Sarcomas

Leiomyosarcomas are most frequently diagnosed, with other types reported including adenosarcoma and angiosarcoma. Primary therapy is surgical involving wide local excision of the tumour with free margins. Adjuvant radiotherapy has been advocated for high-grade tumours or in recurrent disease. Adjuvant chemotherapy has been utilized by some but has not been shown to confer a survival advantage in soft-tissue sarcomas of the extremities. The majority of women present with discomfort or bleeding.

Rhabdomyosarcoma (sarcoma botryroides)

Rhabdomyosarcoma accounts for <2% of vaginal sarcomas. It is the most common soft-tissue tumour in the genitourinary tract during childhood. About 90% of cases occur in children under 3 years of age and almost two out of three occur in the first 2 years of life, although rare cases are reported in older women. Presentation is classically with a vaginal mass composed of soft 'grape-like' vesicles, but others may present with vaginal bleeding, discharge, a single small polyp or, occasionally, a black haemorrhagic mass.

Treatment involves conservative surgery (aimed at preserving function of the female pelvic organs) but depends largely on combination chemotherapy using vincristine, actinomycin-D and cyclophosphamide. Adjuvant surgery or radiotherapy may be added dependent on response to chemotherapy. Survival has been greatly improved by the advent of combination chemotherapy and over 90% of individuals have been reported to survive following treatment.

Clear cell adenocarcinoma

As suggested by its name, it displays characteristic histological features that include the presence of solid sheets of clear cells, or of tubules and cysts lined by hobnail cells. The median age at diagnosis is 19 years (range 7–42 years) and approximately 61% of patients have documented exposure to diethylstilboestrol (DES) or to a chemically related non-steroidal oestrogen *in utero*. Although the risk of developing a clear cell adenocarcinoma following exposure to such drugs *in utero* was thought to be considerable, it is now appreciated that the risks are in fact very low at 0.014–0.14%. Highest risks are for exposure which

occurs early in pregnancy, the risk after exposure in the first 12 weeks' gestation being threefold that at 13 weeks. The majority occurs in the upper third of the anterior vaginal wall. Treatment is either by radical surgery or radiotherapy dependent on stage, in a fashion akin to the management of cervical carcinoma.

Although the peak incidence of DES-associated clear cell carcinoma in the USA was in 1975, a recent report suggests that there may also be an association with the development of non-clear cell adenocarcinomas occurring in older DES-exposed women [71].

Melanoma

Primary malignant melanoma of the vagina is an aggressive and rare gynaecological malignancy. Fewer than 200 cases have been reported worldwide to date but it is known that this disease has the worst prognosis of all gynaecological malignancies. Malignant melanoma of the vagina is 100-fold less common than melanoma of non-genital skin. The behaviour of this tumour also differs from that of melanomas found in other sites in that it is more aggressive than cutaneous melanomas (including vulvar melanoma) and that there is no difference in incidence between different races or skin types. The median age at presentation is around 66 years and the incidence increases with advancing age. The commonest presenting complaint is vaginal bleeding, but presentation may also be with a pelvic mass, vaginal discharge or dyspareunia. The optimal mode of treatment remains unclear, but whatever method is used the outlook is bleak. Prognostic factors that have been proposed include age, stage, tumour diameter depth of invasion and mitotic rate. As with squamous vaginal carcinoma, the choice of treatment lies between surgery, radiotherapy or a combined approach. A number of recent articles support the use of radical surgery as a primary approach [72]. Radical surgery refers to either anterior or complete exenteration and it is suggested that although a 5-year survival is not necessarily increased by such measures, the median and disease-free survival may be prolonged.

Endodermal sinus tumour

Endodermal sinus tumours, which more commonly arise in the ovary or testis of infants, are also recognized in the vaginas of very young girls. Approximately 50 cases have been reported, with no patients aged over 3 years. Presentation will usually follow an episode of vaginal bleeding or discharge in a young girl who at examination is found to have a friable polypoid exophytic tumour.

Immunohistochemistry will reveal positive staining for alpha fetoprotein (αFP), and in some cases serum αFP levels are elevated.

The behaviour of the tumour is locally aggressive but metastasis will also occur via haematogenous or lymphatic spread. Most tumours arise on the posterior vaginal wall and, if untreated, patients are known to die within 2–4 months of diagnosis.

The emphasis for treatment has moved towards limited excisional surgery combined with pre- or postoperative chemotherapy. Multiagent chemotherapy is used and is the same as that used for the successful treatment of ovarian endodermal sinus tumour.

Summary box 55.4

- Vaginal cancer is rare and most are squamous cancers.
- Superficial disease in the upper third may be managed similarly to cervical cancer.
- Superficial disease in the lower third may be managed as for vulval cancer.
- Deeply invasive disease and any disease whose excision would result in functional compromise should first be treated with radiotherapy with or without chemotherapy.
- Stage and tumour site are the most important prognostic variables.

Conclusions

The rarity of vaginal cancer means that many questions regarding its management remain unanswered. Many cases are amenable to treatment by more than one method with comparable results in terms of survival. Choice of treatment may, therefore, often be made in relation to the potential toxicities of different treatments and should be tailored to each individual patient.

References

1 ISD Scotland Online Cancer Registrations in Scotland, 2009.
2 Cancer Registrations in Northern Ireland. Northern Ireland Cancer Registry, 2009.
3 Cancer Registrations in England. Office for National Statistics, 2009.
4 Cancer Registrations in Wales. Welsh Cancer Intelligence and Surveillance Unit, 2009.
5 Jones RW, Baranyai J, Stables S. Trends in squamous cell carcinoma of the vulva: the influence of vulvar intraepithelial neoplasia. *Obstet Gynecol* 1997;90:448–452.
6 Joura EA, Lösch A, Haider-Angeler MG, Breitenecker G, Leodalter S. Trends in vulvar neoplasia. Increasing incidence of vulvar intraepithelial neoplasia and squamous cell carcinoma of the vulva in young women. *J Reprod Med* 2000;45:613–615.
7 MacLean AB, Buckley CH, Luesley D *et al*. Squamous cell carcinoma of the vulva: the importance of non-neoplastic epithelial disorders. *Int J Gynecol Cancer* 1995;5:70.
8 Meffert JJ, Davis BM, Grimwood RE. Lichen sclerosus. *J Am Acad Dermatol* 1995;32:393–416.
9 Jones RW, Baranyai J, Stables S. Trends in squamous cell carcinoma of the vulva: the influence of vulvar intraepithelial neoplasia. *Obstet Gynecol* 1997;90:448–452.
10 Herod JJO, Shafl MI, Rollason TP, Jordan JA, Luesley DM. Vulvar intraepithelial neoplasia: long term follow up of treated and untreated women. *Br J Obstet Gynaecol* 1996;103:446–452.
11 Fishman DA, Chambers SK, Shwartz PE, Kohorn EL, Chambers JT. Extramammary Paget's disease of the vulva. *Gynecol Oncol* 1995;56:266–270.
12 Ragnarssonolding B, Johanson H, Rutgvist LE, Ringborg U. Malignant melanoma of the vulva and vagina: trends in incidence, age distribution and long term survival among 245 consecutive cases in Sweden 1960–1984. *Cancer* 1993;71:1893–1897.
13 Bradgate M, Rollason TP, McConkey CC, Powe UJ. Malignant melanoma of the vulva: a clinico-pathological study of 50 cases. *Br J Obstet Gynaecol* 1990;97:124–133.
14 Daling JR, Sherman KJ, Hislop TG *et al*. Cigarette smoking and the risk of anogenital cancer. *Am J Epidemiol* 1992;135:180–189.
15 Ansink AC, Heintz AP. Epidemiology and etiology of squamous cell carcinoma of the vulva. *Eur J Obstet Gynecol Reprod Biol* 1993;48:111–115.
16 Tate JE, Mutter GL, Prasad CJ, Berkowitz R, Goodman H, Crum CP. Analysis of HPV-positive and -negative vulvar carcinomas for alterations in c-myc, Ha-, Ki-, and N-ras genes. *Gynecol Oncol* 1994;53:78–83.
17 Crum CP, McLachlin CM, Tate JE, Mutter GL. Pathobiology of vulvar squamous neoplasia. *Curr Opin Obstet Gynecol* 1997;9:63–69.
18 Eva LJ, Ganesan R, Chan KK, Honest H, Luesley DM. Differentiated-type vulval intraepithelial neoplasia has a high risk association with vulval squamous cell carcinoma. *Int J Gynecol Cancer* 2009;19:741–744.
19 Stroup AM, Harlan LC, Trimble EL. Demographic, clinical and treatment trends among women diagnosed with vulvar cancer in the United States. *Gynecol Oncol* 2008;108:577–583.
20 Monagham JM. Management of vulval carcinoma. In: Shepherd JH, Monaghan JM (eds) *Clinical Gynaecological Oncology*. Oxford: Blackwell Scientific Publications, 1990:145.
21 Hacker NF, Leucher RS, Berek JS, Casaldo TW, Lagasse LD. Radical vulvectomy and inguinal lymphadenectomy through separate groin incisions. *Obstet Gynecol* 1981;58:574–579.
22 Podratz KC, Symmonds RE, Taylor WF, Williams TJ. Carcinoma of the vulva: analysis of treatment and survival. *Obstet Gynecol* 1983;61:63–74.
23 Ross M, Ehrmann RL. Histologic prognosticators in stage I squamous cell carcinoma of the vulva. *Obstet Gynecol* 1987;70:774–784.
24 Parker RT, Duncan I, Rampone J, Creasman W. Operative management of early epidermoid carcinoma of the vulva. *Am J Obstet Gynecol* 1975;123:349–355.
25 Magrina JF, Webb MJ, Gaffey TA, Symmonds RE. Stage I squamous cell cancer of the vulva. *Am J Obstet Gynecol* 1979;134:453–459.
26 Iversen T, Abeler V, Aalders J. Individualised treatment of stage I carcinoma of the vulva. *Obstet Gynecol* 1981;57:85–89.
27 Boyce J, Fruchter RG, Kasambilides E, Nicastri AD, Sedlis A, Remy JC. Prognostic factors in carcinoma of the vulva. *Gynecol Oncol* 1985;20:364–377.
28 Hacker NF, Berek JS, Lagasse LD, Leuchter RS, Moore JG. Management of regional lymph nodes and their prognostic influence in vulvar cancer. *Obstet Gynecol* 1983;61:408–412.

29 Pecorelli S. Revised FIGO staging for carcinoma of the vulva, cervix and endometrium. *Int J Gynecol Obstet* 2009;105: 103–104.

30 Homesley HD, Bundy BN, Sedlis A *et al.* Assessment of current International Federation of Gynaecology and Obstetrics staging of vulvar carcinoma relative to prognostic factors for survival (a Gynecologic Oncology Group study). *Am J Obstet Gynecol* 1991;164:997–1003; discussion 1003–1004.

31 Heaps JM, Fu YS, Montz FJ, Hacker NF, Berek JS. Surgical–pathologic variables predictive of local recurrence in squamous cell carcinoma of the vulva. *Gynecol Oncol* 1990;38:309–314.

32 Hopkins MP, Reid GC, Vettrano I, Morley GW. Squamous cell carcinoma of the vulva: prognostic factors influencing survival. *Gynecol Oncol* 1991;43:113–117.

33 Gaarenstroom KN, Kenter CG, Trimbos JB *et al.* Postoperative complications after vulvectomy and inguinofemoral lymphadenectomy using separate groin incisions. *Int J Gynecol Cancer* 2003;13:522–527.

34 Sedlis A, Homesley H, Bundy B. Positive groin lymph nodes in superficial squamous vulvar cancer. *Am J Obstet Gynecol* 1987;156:1159–1164.

35 Homesley H, Bundy B, Sedlis A. Prognostic factors for groin node metastasis in squamous cell carcinoma of the vulva. *Gynecol Oncol* 1993;49:279–83.

36 Barton DP, Shepherd JH, Moskovic EC, Sohaib SA. Identification of inguinal lymph node metastases from vulval carcinoma by magnetic resonance imaging: an initial report. *Clin Radiol* 2003;58:409.

37 Sohaib SA, Moskovic EC. Imaging in vulval cancer. *Best Pract Res Clin Obstet Gynaecol* 2003;17:543–556.

38 Hall TB, Barton DP, Trott PA *et al.* The role of ultrasound-guided cytology of groin lymph nodes in the management of squamous cell carcinoma of the vulva:5-year experience in 44 patients. *Clin Radiol* 2003;58:367–371.

39 Mohammad DKA, Uberoi R, Lopes ADB, Monaghan JM. Inguinal node status by ultrasound in vulval cancer. *Gynecol Oncol* 2000;77:93–96

40 Moskovic EC, Shepherd JH, Barton DP, Trott PA, Nasiri N, Thomas JM. The role of high resolution ultrasound with guided cytology of groin lymph nodes in the management of squamous cell carcinoma of the vulva: a pilot study. *Br J Obstet Gynaecol* 1999;106:863–867

41 Cohn DE, Dehdashti F, Gibb RK *et al.* Prospective evaluation of positron emission tomography for the detection of groin node metastases from vulvar cancer. *Gynecol Oncol* 2002;85:179–184.

42 Boran N, Kayikcioglu F, Kir M. Sentinel lymph node procedure in early vulvar cancer. *Gynecol Oncol* 2003;90:492–493.

43 Hullu JA, van der Zee AG. Groin surgery and the sentinel lymph node. *Best Pract Res Clin Obstet Gynaecol* 2003;17: 571–589.

44 Van Der Zee AGJ, Oonk MH, De Hullu JA *et al.* Sentinel node dissection is safe in the treatment of early stage vulvar cancer. *J Clin Oncol* 2008;26:884–889.

45 Selman TJ, Luesley DM, Acheson N, Khan KS, Mann CH. A systematic review of the accuracy of diagnostic tests for inguinal lymph node status in vulvar cancer. *Gynecol Oncol* 2005;99:206–214

46 Hacker, NF, Van der Velden, J. Conservative management of early vulvar cancer. *Cancer* 1993;71(Suppl 4):1673–1677.

47 Yang B, Hart WR. Vulvar intraepithelial neoplasia of the simplex (differentiated) type: a clinicopathological study including analysis of HPV and p53 expression. *Am J Surg Pathol* 2000;24:429–441.

48 Falconer AD, Hirschowitz L, Weeks J, Murdoch J: Southwest Gynaecology Tumour Panel. The impact of improving outcomes guidance on surgical management of vulval squamous cell cancer in Southwest England. *BJOG* 2007;114: 391–397.

49 Stehman FB, Look KY. Carcinoma of the vulva. *Obstet Gynecol* 2006;107:719–733

50 Stehman FB, Ali S, DiSaia PJ. Node count and groin recurrence in early vulvar cancer: A Gynecologic Oncology Group study. *Gynecol Oncol.* 2009;113:52–56.

51 Andrews SJ, Williams BT, DePriest PD *et al.* Therapeutic implications of lymph nodal spread in lateral T1 and T2 squamous cell carcinoma of the vulva. *Gynecol Oncol* 1994;55:41–46.

52 Homesley HD, Bundy BN, Sedlis A, Adcock L. Radiation therapy versus pelvic node resection for carcinoma of the vulva with positive groin nodes. *Obstet Gynecol* 1986;68:733–740.

53 Berman M, Soper J, Creasman W, Olt G, DiSaia P. Conservative surgical management of superficially invasive stage I vulval carcinoma. *Gynecol Oncol* 1989;35:352–357.

54 Burke T, Stringer A, Gershenson D, Edwards C, Morris M, Wharton J. Radical wide excision and selective inguinal node dissection for squamous cell carcinoma of the vulva. *Gynecol Oncol* 1990;38:328–332.

55 Rouzier R, Haddad B, Dubernard G, Dubois P, Paniel BJ. Inguinofemoral dissection for carcinoma of the vulva: effect of modifications of extent and technique on morbidity and survival. *J Am Coll Surg* 2003;196:442–450.

56 Lin JY, DuBeschter B, Angel C, Dvoretsky PM. Morbidity and recurrence with modifications of radical vulvectomy and groin dissection. *Gynecol Oncol* 1992;47:80–86.

57 Paley PJ, Johnson PR, Adcock LL *et al.* The effect of sartorius transposition on wound morbidity following inguinal femoral lymphadenectomy. *Gynecol Oncol* 1997;64:237–241.

58 Andersen BL. Sexuality and quality of life for women with vulvar cancer. In: Luesley DM (ed) *Cancer and Pre-cancer of the Vulva*. London: Arnold, 2000: 202–206.

59 Barton DP. The prevention and management of treatment related morbidity in vulval cancer. *Best Pract Res Clin Obstet Gynaecol* 2003;17:683–701.

60 Han LY, Schimp V, Oh JC, Ramirez PT. A gelatin matrix-thrombin tissue sealant (FloSeal®) application in the management of groin breakdown after inguinal lymphadenectomy for vulval cancer. *Int J Gynecol Oncol* 2004;14:621–624.

61 Faul CM, Mirmow D, Huang Q *et al.* Adjuvant radiation for vulvar carcinoma: improved local control. *Int J Radiat Oncol Biol Phys* 1997;38:381.

62 Paladini D, Cross P, Lopes A, Monaghan JM. Prognostic significance of lymph node variables insquamous cell carcinoma of the vulva. *Cancer* 1994;74:2491–2496.

63 van der Velden J, van Lindert ACM, Lammes FB *et al.* Extracapsular growth of lymph node metastases in squamous cell carcinoma of the vulva. The impact on recurrence and survival. *Cancer* 1995;75:2885–2890.

64 Thomas G, Dembo A, DePetrillo A *et al.* Concurrent radiation and chemotherapy in vulvar carcinoma. *Gynecol Oncol* 1989;34:263–267.

65 van Der Velden J, Ansink A. Primary groin irradiation vs primary groin surgery for early vulvar cancer [Update in *Cochrane Database Syst Rev* 2001;4:CD002224; PMID:11687151]. *Cochrane Database Syst Rev* 2000:2001;3:CD002224.

66 Piura B, Masotina A, Murdoch J, Lopes A, Morgan P, Monaghan J. Recurrent squamous cell carcinoma of the vulva: a study of 73 cases. *Gynecol Oncol* 1993;48:189–95.

67 Oonk MH, de Hullu JA, Hollema H *et al.* The value of routine follow-up in patients treated for carcinoma of the vulva. *Cancer* 2003;98:2624–2629.

68 Rose PG. Skin bridge recurrences in vulvar cancer: frequency and management. *Int J Gynecol Cancer* 1999;9:508–511.

69 Hopkins MP, Reid GC, Morley GW. The surgical management of recurrent squamous cell carcinoma of the vulva. *Obstet Gynecol* 1990;75:1001–1005.

70 Stock RG, Chen ASJ, Seski JA. 30-year experience in the management of primary carcinoma of the vagina: Analysis of prognostic factors and treatment modalities. *Gynecol Oncol* 1995;56:45–52.

71 Hatch E, Herbst A, Hoover R *et al.* Incidence of squamous neoplasia of the cervix and vagina in des-exposed daughters. *Ann Epidemiol* 2000;10:467.

72 Miner TJ, Delgado R, Zeisler J *et al.* Primary vaginal melanoma: a critical analysis of therapy. *Ann Surg Oncol* 2004;11:34–39.

Chapter 56
Premalignant and Malignant Disease of the Cervix

Mahmood I. Shafi
Addenbrookes Hospital, Cambridge, UK

Introduction

Carcinoma of the cervix is the second commonest cancer among women worldwide, with only breast cancer occurring more commonly. Worldwide, cervical cancer accounts for about 500 000 new diagnoses and 273 000 deaths every year. Of the new cases, 80% occur in the underdeveloped countries, and in some of these countries cervical cancer is the commonest cancer in women. This situation is compounded by the fact that in underdeveloped countries 75% of affected women present with an advanced stage, which is the opposite to presentations in developed countries, where 75% of affected women present early and a cure can be realistically expected. Cervical cancer contributes over 2.7 million years of life lost among women between the ages of 25 and 64 years worldwide, some 2.4 million of which occur in developing areas and only 0.3 million in developed countries. This is partly a result of education and empowerment of women, so that in developed countries they present early because of recognition of symptoms or as part of screening programmes for cervical cancer. There continues to be a disparity between deprivation and the risk for cervical cancer (Fig. 56.1).

While the natural history of breast cancer is poorly understood, cervical cancer is a preventable condition and considerable effort goes into detecting and treating the pre-invasive disease, primarily in developed countries. This should have a direct effect on incidence and mortality from this condition.

The National Health Service Cervical Screening Programme (NHSCSP), established in 1988, has made significant inroads into reducing occurrences of cervical cancer in the UK. Cervical cancer incidence rates in the UK have almost halved in the last 20 years. In 2006, there were 2873 new cases of cervical cancer in the UK. The lifetime risk of a female of developing cervical cancer is 1 in 136 in the UK. In 2006, the age-standardized (European) annual incidence rate of cervical cancer in the UK is 8.5 per 100 000 females. Cervical cancer is the second most common cancer after breast cancer in the females aged under 35 years, with 686 new cases diagnosed in the UK in 2006. Around 940 women die from cervical cancer each year in the UK, almost 80% of these deaths occur in women aged 45 years and over. One anticipates that the falling incidence and mortality will continue, but several areas of the screening programme could be refined further (Fig. 56.2).

One of the areas that has greatly contributed to the overall success of the programme has been the wide coverage of the at-risk population. In England and Wales, women between the ages of 25 and 64 years are offered cervical cytology screening every 3–5 years (Table 56.1) [1]. Before the introduction of the national programme, the target age coverage was 42%, which increased to 82% in 1989 and has since fallen slightly to 79% during 2008/9. High coverage rates are vital in a prevention strategy for cervical cancer.

The introduction of vaccines against human papillomavirus (HPV), the causal agent in cervical cancer, has been a major advance in cervical cancer prevention. These have been introduced widely in developed countries, with high coverage in the UK.

Summary box 56.1

With well-organized cervical screening programmes, a major impact can be made on the incidence of and mortality from cervical cancer.

Historical perspective

Pre-invasive lesions of the cervix have been recognized for over 100 years. In 1886, Sir John Williams presented the Harveian Lectures, in which he described eight cases of cervical cancer, one of which was equivalent to

Dewhurst's Textbook of Obstetrics & Gynaecology, Eighth Edition. Edited by D. Keith Edmonds.
© 2012 John Wiley and Sons, Ltd. Published 2012 by John Wiley and Sons, Ltd.

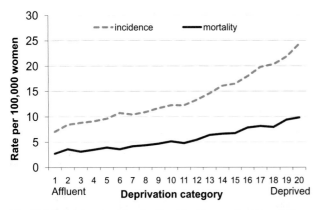

Fig. 56.1 European age-standardized incidence of and mortality, cervical cancer by deprivation category, England and Wales, 1990–93.

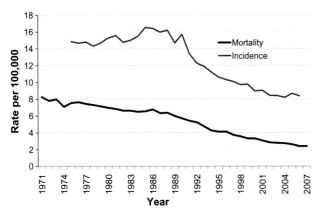

Fig. 56.2 Age-standardized (European) incidence of, and mortality from, cervical cancer, UK, 1971–2007.

Table 56.1 Screening intervals for national cervical screening programme [11].

Age group (years)	Frequency of screening
25	First invitation
25–49	3 yearly
50–64	5 yearly
65+	Only screen those who have not been screened since age 50 years or those who have had recent abnormal tests

carcinoma *in situ* or cervical intraepithelial neoplasia (CIN) 3 [2]. In his lecture he stated that 'this is the earliest condition of undoubted cancer of the portio vaginalis that I have met with, and it is the earliest condition which is recognizable as cancer. It presented no distinct symptoms, and was discovered accidentally'.

In the mid-1920s the basic principles of colposcopy were described by Hinselmann [3]. A system of low-power magnification and illumination of the cervix was developed. Hinselmann hoped that with this system he would be able recognize the earliest lesions of the cervix that were invisible to the naked eye. Schiller [4] described the Schiller iodine test a few years later. When applied to the cervix, Schiller's iodine solution stained normal squamous epithelium rich in glycogen but failed to stain columnar epithelium and abnormal epithelium, which contained little or no glycogen. The colposcopic technique was further developed by the introduction of a green filter, which enhanced recognition of vascular patterns. Colposcopy went into decline when cervical cytology was first described for the screening and detection of premalignant lesions of the cervix [5]. The realization that the techniques were complementary rather than competitive led to the resurgence of colposcopy and its widespread introduction worldwide.

Cervical cytology classification

The NHSCSP has developed guidance on laboratory reporting for cervical cytology [6]. The cytology report should consist of a concise description of cells in precisely defined and generally accepted cytological terms. This may be followed, if appropriate, by a prediction of the histological condition based on the overall picture and should include a recommendation for further management of the patient. In North America and many other countries, the Bethesda reporting system has been adopted [7]. The classification consists of a statement of adequacy, general categorization (normal, epithelial cell abnormality or other) and descriptive diagnoses (organisms, other). The classification uses the term 'squamous intraepithelial lesion' (SIL) to encompass all grades of CIN. SIL is further subdivided into two categories – low grade, which includes cellular changes associated with HPV infection and CIN 1, and high grade, which includes CIN 2 and 3. The atypical squamous cells have two subcategories – atypical squamous cells of undetermined significance (ASC-US) and atypical squamous cells that cannot exclude high-grade SIL (ASC-H).

Management of abnormal cervical smears

Ideally, all women with abnormal cervical cytology should have colposcopic assessment (Fig. 56.3). The aim of colposcopy is first to exclude an invasive process and secondarily to identify the extent of the abnormality and its likely grade, which may allow a more conservative approach to management. For adequate colposcopy, the whole of the transformation zone (TZ) needs to be visualized. If the TZ is not fully visualized, then colposcopy is

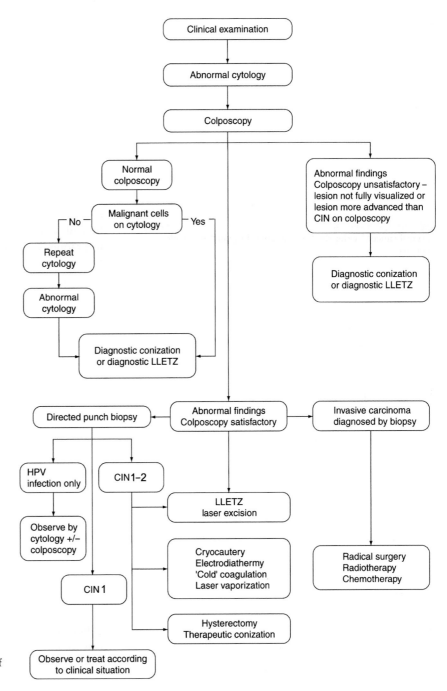

Fig. 56.3 Flow diagram for management of abnormal cervical cytology.

deemed unsatisfactory. This inability to visualize the squamocolumnar junction (SCJ) may be an indication for excisional biopsy of the cervical transformation zone.

Classification of CIN

The CIN classification has almost universally replaced the World Health Organization classification, with CIN 1, 2 and 3 corresponding to mild, moderate and severe dysplasia/carcinoma *in situ*, respectively. A revised classification has been introduced with high-grade lesions (CIN 2 and 3) that are likely to behave as cancer precursors and low-grade lesions (CIN 1 and HPV-associated changes) with unknown but a likely low-progressive potential [8]. Whichever classification is used, there is intra- and interobserver variation in the histopathological reporting.

Progressive potential of cervical intraepithelial neoplasia

The progressive potential of high-grade lesions or CIN 3 is not questioned [9]. The progressive potential has been calculated to be 18% at 10 years and 36% at 20 years. Women with continuing abnormal cytology after initial management of carcinoma *in situ* of the cervix were almost 25 times more likely to develop invasive carcinoma than women who have normal follow-up cytology. When compared with the population at large, the chances of women with normal follow-up cytology developing invasive cervical or vaginal vault carcinoma increase threefold over women who have never had carcinoma *in situ* of the cervix. As a result, there appears to be complete unanimity for the immediate treatment of CIN 3 lesions once diagnosed.

Colposcopy

Various parameters of the colposcopic assessment are studied, including the vascular patterns, the degree of aceto-white epithelium, the border characteristics, the surface pattern and the surface area of the lesion under study. Using these variables an assessment of the likely nature of the lesion can be gauged. Various grading systems are advocated and one of these has been developed [10] using clinical and colposcopic parameters (Table 56.2). Using the Clinico-colposcopic Index (CCI) to devise a score for each individual patient helps in predicting the histological abnormality and management options. The CCI takes

Table 56.2 Clinico-colposcopic Index (CCI) – Shafi and Nazeer [9] – maximum score = 10.

Variable	Score		
	Zero points	One point	Two points
Index cytology	Low grade	–	High grade
Smoking status	No	–	Yes
Age	30 years	>30 years	–
Aceto-whitening	Slight	Marked	–
Surface area of lesion	1 cm² (small lesion)	>1 cm² (large lesion)	–
Intercapillary distance	350 µm (fine/no mosaic or punctation)	>350 µm (coarse mosaic or punctation)	–
Focality of lesion	Unifocal or multifocal	Annular	–
Surface pattern	Smooth	Irregular	–

into account the important prognostic factors and for each patient a maximum score of 10 can be achieved. Those scoring 0–2 on this scale invariably have insignificant lesions. Those scoring 6–10 on this scale generally have high-grade disease present. In those scoring between 3 and 5, the histological pattern is mixed with a tendency of the lesion to harbour CIN grade 1 or 2.

If the TZ is fully visualized, biopsy of the worst atypical epithelium may be undertaken. Excisional methods such as laser excision or diathermy loop provide considerably more histopathological material than a punch biopsy. If the whole of the TZ is not visualized, then colposcopy is deemed to be unsatisfactory, making a colposcopically directed punch biopsy of the worst area impossible. In this situation, recourse to a cone biopsy or an extended diathermy loop procedure is recommended.

Summary box 56.2

Colposcopic assessment of women with abnormal cervical cytology should be undertaken before any treatment.

If the woman is pregnant at the time of colposcopic assessment, a conservative approach is usually employed and treatment is undertaken after delivery. If cancer is suspected, then a large biopsy, usually with an appropriately sized diathermy loop, is taken in the operating room with ready recourse to haemostatic techniques as there is a risk for significant haemorrhage.

Treatment of cervical intraepithelial neoplasia

In an ideal world, all women with truly premalignant lesions destined to develop cancer could be selected and treated with a simple, rapid, non-morbid and effective office technique. The two main methods of treatment are ablative or excisional techniques (Table 56.3). Cure rates for both ablative and excisional techniques are in excess of 90% [11]. Recently there has been a trend towards using excisional methods. This allows better histopathological interpretation of the excised specimen, and in certain circumstances allows a 'see and treat' strategy if the colposcopic assessment is consistent with a lesion requiring local treatment and the patient is agreeable to treatment under local anaesthetic at the initial visit. This policy can lead to overtreatment of insignificant lesions [12], and with this realization a 'select and treat' strategy is employed in most colposcopy units. The CCI scoring system described is a useful aid in this management strategy.

Table 56.3 Methods for treatment of cervical intraepithelial neoplasia (CIN).

Excisional methods	Ablative methods
LLETZ/LEEP	Cryocautery
NETZ/SWETZ	Electrodiathermy
Laser TZ excision	Cold coagulation
Knife cone biopsy	Carbon dioxide laser
Laser cone biopsy	–
Loop cone biopsy	–
Hysterectomy	–

LLETZ, large loop excision transformation zone; LEEP, loop electrosurgical excision procedure; NETZ, needle excision of transformation zone; SWETZ, straight-wire excision of transformation zone; TZ, transformation zone.

The treatment method used is subjectively influenced. An important aspect is the depth of destruction of any local treatment modality. Studies to assess the depth of crypt involvement with CIN suggest that a depth of destruction to 3.8 mm would eradicate premalignant disease in 99.7% of cases. However, some gland crypts with involvement by CIN to 5 mm in depth were observed, and therefore a destructive depth greater than this is desirable. Ablation to a depth of 5–8 mm has been recommended. If depth of destruction is inadequate, then this deep-seated component may be a source of residual or recurrent disease. Meta-analyses of treatment methods show no superior method for eliminating pre-cancerous lesions. Cryocautery, however, was associated with a somewhat higher failure rate compared with other methods especially with larger and high-grade lesions.

Ablative techniques

Cryocautery destroys tissue by freezing using probes of various shapes and sizes and is probably best reserved for small lesions. Although lesion size is important in determining success or failure using any of the treatment modalities [13], it is especially important with cryocautery. When using cryocautery, a double freeze–thaw–freeze technique is advocated to minimize failure rates. With larger lesions, multiple applications may be necessary. The depth of destruction is approximately 4 mm and this may be inadequate for some of the CIN lesions. Depth of destruction cannot be accurately gauged and incomplete eradication of disease may lead to regenerating epithelium covering the residual disease.

While electrodiathermy destroys tissue more effectively than cryocautery, it does require general, regional or local anaesthesia. Under colposcopic control, it is pos-sible to destroy up to a depth of 1 cm using a combination of needle and ball electrodes. An extension of this technique using a wire loop allows electrodiathermy to be used in an excisional mode.

Cold coagulation was a term coined by Kurt Semm, the inventor of the instrument in 1966. Heat is applied to tissue using a Teflon-coated thermosound. Using overlapping applications of the thermosound for 20 seconds at 100°C, the whole of the TZ may be treated. The procedure does not usually require analgesia. Measurement of the depth of destruction is difficult. Depth of destruction is approximately 2.5–4 mm or more after treatment at 100°C for 30 seconds and always exceeds 4 mm after treatment at 120°C for 30 seconds.

Laser is an acronym for light amplification by stimulated emission of radiation. A micromanipulator attached to the colposcope is used to manipulate the laser and treatment is conducted under direct vision. As the technique is precise, it allows good control of the depth of destruction, good haemostasis and excellent healing as there is minimal thermal damage to the adjacent tissue. The technique is particularly useful for treating premalignant disease with vaginal involvement. As there are no gland crypts in the vaginal epithelium, destruction to 2–3 mm depth is adequate for vaginal involvement.

Excisional methods

Transformation zone excision has been developed as a conservative excisional technique. Both the laser and diathermy loop have been used for this purpose. Laser excision is technically more demanding than laser vaporization and requires a high-power density beam with a small spot size that can function in a cutting mode. Both methods can also be used to fashion cone biopsies of the cervix. Diathermy loop excision using low-power voltage apparatus is now widely practised [14]. The technique is referred to as large loop excision of transformation zone (LLETZ) in Europe and as loop electrosurgical excision procedure (LEEP) in North America. Using this technique, a 'see and treat' management strategy for women with abnormal cervical smears can be adopted, whereby women are treated at their first visit to the colposcopy clinic. Strict guidelines need to be adhered to as this policy will undoubtedly lead to overtreatment in some women and will also result in an increased histopathological workload compared with processing punch biopsies. While histopathology workload is increased, this also results in excisional techniques, providing considerably more material for assessment allowing a more reliable interpretation. Needle or straight-wire excision of transformation zone (NETZ/SWETZ) is a recent modification that uses a straight wire rather than a loop. This technique allows individualization of the procedure and aims to eradicate the lesion without removing redundant healthy cervical tissue.

Success rates following local excisional techniques are similar to those quoted for laser ablation and cold coagulation. There appears to be no adverse effect on fertility.

Cone biopsy and hysterectomy still retain a place in the management of CIN. Hysterectomy may need to be contemplated if CIN is present in a woman with other gynaecological conditions such as fibroids, menorrhagia or prolapse. Before operation, colposcopy will identify the extent of the lesion and avoid incomplete excision, which may result in vaginal intraepithelial neoplasia (VAIN). If the lesion is seen to extend onto the vagina, this may be excised as part of the hysterectomy procedure. An alternative is to ablate the vaginal extension of CIN (using laser or diathermy) and then proceed to excision or hysterectomy as indicated.

The size and shape of the cone biopsy is governed by the colposcopic findings. As much of the internal os and the endocervical canal are left intact as is possible within the confines of disease eradication. This limits haemorrhagic morbidity, and fertility will be little compromised.

Histological incomplete excision at the time of cone biopsy represents a management dilemma. Cervical cytology may in fact be a more useful prognostic guide to residual disease than excision cone margins. The risk of invasive disease following incomplete excision is related to the presence of cytological abnormality following treatment. A persistent cytological abnormality after cone biopsy is a good indicator of residual disease; such women warrant further treatment.

Summary box 56.3

- Whichever local method is used for treatment, the depth of destruction should be at least 5–8 mm as gland crypts may be involved with CIN.
- Success rates for local ablative and local excisional techniques are similar after a single-treatment episode (90–95%).

Obstetric implications

Recent meta-analyses and large linkage studies reveal that excisional methods of treatment, namely cold knife cone biopsy, laser conization and LLETZ, are related to an increased risk of preterm delivery and low birthweight [15,16]. LLETZ was also significantly associated with increased risk of premature rupture of membranes. Laser conization and knife conization were also related to an increased risk of perinatal mortality and severe prematurity. Laser ablation and other destructive techniques have no adverse effect. Adverse outcomes are most likely related to the proportion of the cervical volume and

endocervical canal that is removed rather than the actual depth of the excision or the individual treatment method. Caution is recommended in the treatment of young women with mild cervical abnormalities and women should be counselled about the risks accordingly. Every effort should be made to eradicate the lesion without removing excess healthy cervical tissue.

Summary box 56.4

Although the treatment methods have similar efficacy in eradicating pre-cancerous lesions, increasing emphasis is being placed on minimizing morbidity associated with the treatment methods.

Treatment failures

The primary objective of treating women with CIN is to prevent invasive cervical cancer. If invasive disease develops or indeed if there is residual CIN, the initial treatment is deemed a failure.

Women who have undergone treatment of CIN remain at higher risk for invasive cervical disease. Those women who have abnormal cervical cytology following treatment are at a much increased risk compared with those with normal cytology after treatment [9]. Therefore, women who have been treated for CIN need long-term follow-up. Reports of invasive disease after local destructive therapy have been reviewed and many, but not all, of the invasive carcinomas are a result of inappropriate selection for treatment and a failure to recognize early invasive disease at the time of initial assessment. Invasive disease following TZ excision has also been reported. It is suggested that the use of excisional procedures should further reduce the small risk of invasive carcinoma developing after treatment for CIN. Cytological abnormality following treatment, no matter how minor, should be regarded as an indication for colposcopic reassessment.

Colposcopic assessment is technically more difficult in those who have undergone previous treatment and islands of CIN, and indeed invasive disease can be buried under an apparently normal surface epithelium. For failures of initial treatment, it is generally recommended that an excisional method of treatment be used in preference to ablative techniques.

Summary box 56.5

After local treatment for CIN, women remain at higher risk for development of invasive disease than the general population. Those women who have continuing abnormal cervical cytology following treatment are at greatest risk of developing an invasive lesion.

Human papillomavirus

Cervical cancer is a rare outcome of HPV infection. HPV is a common and mainly sexually transmitted infection. It can be found in almost all cases of cervical cancer. However, most HPV infections will not progress to CIN or cancer. The invasive disease does not develop unless there is persistence of HPV DNA and it has been proposed as the first ever identified 'necessary cause' of a human cancer. Out of the 80 known HPV genotypes, 30 are known to infect the genital tract. Of these, 20 have been identified as carcinogenic with types 16 and 18 found most commonly in malignant lesions.

The common types are classified according to their oncogenic potential as follows:
- low risk: 6, 11, 41, 44;
- intermediate risk: 31, 33, 35; and
- high risk: 16, 18, 45, 56.

After the recognition that HPV infection is a necessary cause of cervical cancer, an HPV DNA test has been developed that aims to detect the viral genome. There are three potential clinical applications of HPV DNA testing:

1 In primary screening: The evidence appears to show that HPV testing with or without cytology is significantly more sensitive but also significantly less specific than cytology in primary screening. Perhaps by restricting its use to women over 30 years of age and by increasing the screening interval, it might achieve improved specificity in a cost-effective manner. Current evidence from large randomized trials, including the ARTISTIC trial in the UK, suggests that the combination of HPV test and cytology allows earlier detection of high-grade lesion [17].

2 In the triage of minor cytological abnormalities: Women with smears classified as atypical squamous cells of undetermined significance (ASCUS) or low-grade squamous intraepithelial lesion (LSIL) or their British terminology equivalents of borderline and mild dyskaryosis constitute, roughly, 7% of all the smears performed in the UK every year. These minor abnormalities are more common in younger women and present a difficult problem with regards to their management, with important implications as they consume a disproportionate amount of clinical and health resources with their significance still debatable. However, despite a low-grade cytological phenotype, a considerable proportion of these women have an underlying high-grade lesion and HPV test appears to have a role in the triage of those women who need referral to colposcopy. Evidence in the literature reports a significantly better sensitivity and similar specificity for HPV test in comparison to repeat cytology for the detection of high-grade lesions for ASCUS/borderline cytology (55% positivity). However, this does not appear to be true for low-grade/mild dyskaryosis lesions as the high positivity rate of HPV in this group (85%) fails its use as a triage tool. The management options of mild dyskaryosis smears remain to be either immediate referral to colposcopy or cytological surveillance with repeat smears. The TOMBOLA study in the UK showed that, compared with cytological surveillance, a policy of immediate colposcopy detects more high-grade lesions, but might lead to overtreatment [18]. In order to reduce that, the authors suggested that a policy of targeted punch biopsies with subsequent treatment for CIN 2 and 3 and cytological surveillance for CIN 1 or less provides the best balance between benefits and harms for the management of these women; immediate loop excision results in overtreatment and more after effects and should not be recommended.

3 In the follow-up after treatment: Data from clinical trials but also the cumulative data critically appraised in a series of systematic reviews and meta-analyses report that HPV testing with or without cytology has the potential to enhance the detection of treatment failures. HPV DNA testing predicts that residual or recurrent CIN with higher sensitivity than cytology or histology of the resection margins can pick up a treatment failure earlier and can be used as a 'test of cure'. A large prospective trial from the UK recently reported that the combination of HPV test with cytology has high negative predictive value and women who test negative for both at 6 months can safely return to 3-year recall [19].

Human papillomavirus vaccination

Out of more than 100 subtypes, HPV 16 and 18 account for up to 72% of cervical cancers, whereas HPV 6 and 11 cause 90% of anogenital warts. To date, two vaccines have been developed and clinically evaluated, the quadrivalent (HPV 16/18/6/11 – Gardasil®) and the bivalent vaccine (HPV 16/18 – Cervarix®). Results from trials indicate that the vaccine is safe, well tolerated and highly efficacious in HPV-naive women [20–22]. The optimal target age is in pre-pubertal women before first intercourse, and it will remain an individual decision for older women. Vaccination and screening are complementary strategies, and synergy in a cost-effective manner will be required for the next few decades. The UK HPV immunization programme was initiated in the NHS with the bivalent vaccine from September 2008.

 Summary box 56.6

Human papillomavirus vaccination, ideally before sexual debut, provides an opportunity to impact on cervical cancer and needs to be implemented with wide coverage, especially in those countries where the lifetime risk is highest.

Non-treatment and serial colposcopy

The progressive potential of low-grade lesions is unknown and cannot be predicted from cytological, colposcopic or histological criteria. Many of these low-grade lesions will regress, but others will persist or progress. National recommendations for the UK allow CIN 1 lesions to be treated or kept under close surveillance [12]. However, some women are unlikely to accept even a low risk of malignancy and would prefer treatment. Also, in a transient population, early intervention may be the preferred option as women are unlikely to adhere to a surveillance programme. The use of digital imaging colposcopy and video colposcopy allows scope for close surveillance and will allow serial colposcopy to be performed with comparison of the colposcopic images easily undertaken [23,24].

Cervical cancer presentation

Women may present asymptomatically when their disease is detected as a result of abnormal cervical cytology. In more advanced lesions, there are usually symptoms that raise the possibility of cervical cancer. These include postcoital bleeding, postmenopausal bleeding and offensive blood-stained vaginal discharge. If there is abnormal bleeding during pregnancy, then a cervical lesion needs to be excluded. In some women presenting with late disease, there may be backache, leg pain/oedema, haematuria, bowel changes, malaise and weight loss.

Diagnosis

A full history and clinical examination is undertaken. If the referral is a result of cervical cytology suspicious of invasion, then a colposcopic examination should be performed. Suspicious features at colposcopy include intense aceto-whiteness, atypical vessels, raised/ulcerated surface, contact bleeding and atypical consistency on bimanual examination. Diagnosis is based on histology and appropriate biopsies should be taken. This biopsy should be either wedge- or cone-shaped to obtain sufficient material for histological assessment. Once cancer has been diagnosed, it is important to stage the disease so that treatment can be planned appropriately. The staging will also give an idea of prognosis and facilitates exchange of information between treatment centres.

Staging

Staging should include an assessment of disease extent and sites of spread (Table 56.4). Staging of cervical cancer

Table 56.4 FIGO staging of cervical cancer (2009).

Stage	Description
0	Carcinoma *in situ*, intraepithelial carcinoma
I	The carcinoma is strictly confined to the cervix (extension to the corpus should be disregarded)
IA	Invasive carcinoma which can be identified only by microscopy, with deepest invasion ≤5mm and largest extension ≤7mm
IA1	Measured stromal invasion of ≤3.0mm in depth and extension of ≤7.0mm
IA2	Measured stromal invasion of >3.0mm and not >5.0mm with an extension of not >7.0mm
IB	Clinically visible lesions limited to the cervix uteri or preclinical cancers greater than IA
IB1	Clinically visible lesion ≤4.0cm in greatest dimension
IB2	Clinically visible lesion >4.0cm in greatest dimension
II	Cervical carcinoma invades beyond the uterus, but not to the pelvic wall or to the lower third of the vagina
IIA	Without parametrial invasion
IIA1	Clinically visible lesion ≤4.0cm in greatest dimension
IIA2	Clinically visible lesion >4.0cm in greatest dimension
IIB	With obvious parametrial invasion
III	The tumour extends to the pelvic wall and/or involves the lower third of the vagina and/or causes hydronephrosis or non-functioning kidney
IIIA	Tumour involves lower third of the vagina, with no extension to the pelvic wall
IIIB	Extension to the pelvic wall and/or hydronephrosis or non-functioning kidney
IV	The carcinoma has extended beyond the true pelvis or has involved (biopsy proven) the mucosa of the bladder or rectum. A bullous oedema, as such, does not permit a case to be allotted to stage IV
IVA	Spread of the growth to adjacent organs
IVB	Spread to distant organs

is clinical, although early cancers are staged according to the surgical specimen. All women with stage Ib or worse should have a chest X-ray (CXR) and an intravenous urogram (IVU) to exclude distant metastasis and complete the staging process by looking for obstructive uropathy and therefore disease extending to the pelvic side wall.

Staging should include:
• examination under anaesthetic which should include a combined recto-vaginal assessment;
• biopsy of the suspicious area. This should be suitably large to make a definitive diagnosis;
• cystoscopy should be considered;
• sigmoidoscopy should be considered;
• CXR and IVU; and
• other imaging as indicated and according to facilities available. These might include a computerized axial tomography (CT) scan and a magnetic resonance imaging (MRI) scan.

In the UK, it has become common practice to omit the IVU and place more reliance on MRI assessment.

Survival

Survival is stage dependent and the advanced stages are associated with a poor outlook. Age-standardized 1-year relative survival rate is 83% for the period 2004–6. The age-standardized 5-year relative survival is 64% for the period 2001–6 [25].

Histology

The majority of cervical cancers are squamous (80–85%) and the remainder have an adenocarcinoma element. The proportion containing adenocarcinoma elements has been rising. Rarer histological types include clear cell, lymphomas and sarcomas.

Management

The management options to be considered include surgery, radiotherapy, chemotherapy and combinations of these modalities (Fig. 56.4). Age in itself is not a barrier to full assessment and definitive treatment. The women should be divided into two groups – those in whom the treatment is curative and those in whom the treatment is palliative. For those with early-stage cervical cancer, curative intent with surgery or radiotherapy needs to be contemplated. In those with more advanced disease, chemoradiotherapy is the optimal method of management, but surgery may have a role in a palliative setting.

 Summary box 56.7

Survival for cervical cancer is stage specific and the volume of disease has a major influence on outcomes.

Stage Ia

Stage Ia disease presents a paradox, in that the disease breaches the basement membrane yet is rarely associated with metastasis. It is now considered appropriate for such cases to be managed by simple hysterectomy or even cone biopsy in the majority of cases. This dilemma is pertinent only in those young women wishing to retain fertility. A suitably planned cone biopsy may be both diagnostic and therapeutic. The entire abnormality must be included in the pathological specimen. If the cone biopsy margins are

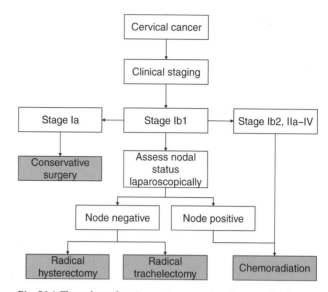

Fig. 56.4 Flow chart showing management options available with suspicion of cervical cancer incorporating minimal access surgery.

positive for CIN or invasive disease, this is a significant risk factor for finding residual invasive disease in the re-excision specimen. The risk of distant spread is <1% in stage Ia1 and <5% in stage Ia2 disease. Some authorities recommend a more aggressive surgical procedure with pelvic node dissection and a modified radical hysterectomy depending on the volume of the tumour. Tumours of less than 420 mm^3 have virtually no risk of metastases. Lesions that invade beyond 5 mm in depth should be considered to be stage Ib carcinoma and require radical surgery or radiotherapy.

No generally accepted definition exists for microinvasive adenocarcinoma. At present, the preferred term for a small invasive adenocarcinoma is 'early invasive adenocarcinoma'. It is very difficult to differentiate extensive high-grade cervical glandular intraepithelial neoplasia (CGIN) from early invasive disease, so borderline cases should probably be treated as invasive.

Stage Ib1

For those with stage Ib1 disease, the options lie between radical surgery (radical hysterectomy with bilateral pelvic lymphadenectomy with or without oophorectomy) or radical radiotherapy. Radical surgery can be classified (Table 56.5) according to the extent of surgery undertaken [26]. The optimal therapy is that which has the highest cure rates with the least associated morbidity. For young women, surgery also offers the opportunity to preserve the ovaries, reduces the risk of sexual dysfunction and is not associated with the late sequelae seen with

Table 56.5 Querleu and Morrow's classification of radical hysterectomy [25]. This classification can be applied to fertility-sparing surgery and can be adapted to open, vaginal, laparoscopic or robotic surgery.

Type	Description
A	Minimum resection of paracervix – this is an extrafascial hysterectomy. The paracervix is transacted medial to the ureter but lateral to the cervix. The uterosacral and vesicouterine ligaments are not transacted at a distance from the uterus. Vaginal resection is generally at a minimum, routinely less than 10 mm, without removal of the vaginal part of the paracervix (paracolpos)
B	Transection of the paracervix at the ureter – partial resection of the uterosacral and vesicouterine ligaments, ureter is unroofed and rolled laterally, permitting transaction of the paracervix at the level of the ureteral tunnel. At least 10 mm of the vagina from the cervix or tumour is resected
C	Transection of paracervix at junction with internal iliac vasculature system – transection of the uterosacral ligament at the rectum and vesicouterine ligament at the bladder. The ureter is mobilized completely. 15–20 mm of vagina from the tumour or cervix and the corresponding paracolpos is resected routinely, depending on vaginal and paracervical extent
D	Laterally extended resection – rare operations feature additional ultraradical procedures. The most radical corresponds to the laterally extended endopelvic resection (LEER) procedure

Lymph node dissection

Level	Description
1	External and internal iliac
2	Common iliac (including presacral)
3	Aortic inframesenteric
4	Aortic infrarenal

radiotherapy. The small but definite risk of radiation carcinogenesis is also avoided. The nodal status impacts long-term survival – the 5-year survival rate is approximately twice as good in node-negative patients (90%) as in node-positive patients (46%). If surgical treatment is offered to women, it should be undertaken by appropriately trained doctors in the context of full support services.

Radical radiotherapy is preferred in those centres where surgical expertise is not available or in women who are not medically fit for surgery. Contraindications to surgery are relative, and some of the factors may also compromise delivery of the radiotherapy schedule (e.g. obesity). Radical radiotherapy aims to control the primary

tumour and also to treat any lymphatic spread. Usually, a combination of intracavitary (to treat the primary tumour) and external beam therapy (to treat pelvic lymph nodes) is used. Planned combinations of radiotherapy and surgery are not advocated as this increases morbidity with no attendant gain in cure or survival rates. As a general rule, intracavitary brachytherapy is given with the addition of external beam therapy. Using modern afterloading techniques with the high-dose regimens (HDR) reduces both the patient morbidity and exposure of staff.

Adjuvant chemoradiotherapy is not routinely indicated but should be offered to those with pelvic lymph node spread, tumour at the excision margins and other risk factors that make a recurrence likely. Neither the overall response rate nor the complete response rate has been reproducibly improved by adding other drugs to cisplatinum. The attendant morbidity is highest when surgery is combined with chemoradiotherapy.

While the incidence of ovarian involvement is <1% in squamous cell cancers, the incidence rises to 5–10% in adenocarcinomas. In the latter, bilateral salpingo-oophorectomy should be discussed if the surgical option is taken.

Summary box 56.8

- There needs to be close cooperation between the clinical and surgical oncologists to make appropriate treatment plans for women with cervical cancer. Treatment needs to be delivered by those individuals and centres with the necessary expertise and support structures.
- For early-stage invasive disease (Ib1) there appears to be no difference in survival outcomes between radical surgery and radical radiotherapy.

Stage Ib2–IVa

For those with stage Ib2–IVa disease, chemoradiotherapy is preferred [27]. Several studies indicate an overall survival advantage for cisplatin-based chemotherapy in conjunction with radiotherapy.

Radiotherapy may be given in either a radical or palliative setting. Radical radiotherapy is given with the intent of cure, whereas palliative radiotherapy does not prolong survival but can control symptoms, especially pain.

Summary box 56.9

For locally advanced cervical cancers (Ib2–IVa), chemoradiotherapy is the preferred management.

Stage IVb

No 'standard' therapeutic protocol applies. The treatment is individualized according to location and extent of disease.

Minimal access surgery

An important factor in outcome for women with cervical cancer is whether there is lymphatic spread at the time of diagnosis. This has a significant effect on survival figures, and current imaging modalities are unable to identify accurately those individuals with metastatic disease to the lymph nodes. Several surgical centres now routinely assess the lymph nodes surgically before planning treatment. This can be done using either minimal access surgery or an extraperitoneal approach. Lymph node yield at laparoscopy is certainly equivalent to the open approach. Lymph nodes that are removed are submitted for histological and immunohistochemical assessment and further management is planned. In those with negative nodes, surgical cure is feasible and these individuals proceed with radical or fertility-sparing surgery. In those with metastatic disease, cure from surgery is not possible, and these women are offered chemoradiotherapy as their best option to attain cure (Fig. 56.4).

Radical procedures, including radical hysterectomy, may be performed using minimal access surgery. These can be undertaken either laparoscopically or using robotic surgery.

Fertility-sparing surgery

In those women who wish to preserve fertility options, radical trachelectomy is a surgical option. This technique has evolved from the radical vaginal hysterectomy and involves removing the cervix, parametrium and upper third of the vagina in those with histologically negative pelvic lymph nodes [28]. Cervical cerclage with a non-absorbable suture is inserted at the end of the surgical procedure to maintain closure of the uterine isthmus in the event of future pregnancy. Caesarean section is advocated for delivery.

Trachelectomy is not appropriate for those women that have completed their family, as long-term data are still being accrued. Those women with tumours of 2-cm depth are most suitable for this treatment. In those achieving a pregnancy, preterm labour is a significant risk factor [29]. Some centres preferentially undertake trachelectomy using an abdominal approach.

Recurrent cervical cancer

Women with recurring cervical cancer should be referred to those with expertise in managing this situation. This may involve the gynaecological, radiation or medical oncologist (Fig. 56.5). If further treatment is planned, it should be conducted in centres suitably equipped and with appropriate support facilities, including an intensive care unit.

Cases of pelvic recurrence are considered for a modality of treatment that has not previously been utilized. Recurrence after surgery is generally treated with radiotherapy (with some protocols including chemotherapy). In postradiation failures where the disease is confined to the pelvis, pelvic exenteration is offered to those women who are surgical candidates. This should be undertaken only by those with the appropriate training in surgical gynaecological oncology who are working in centres with a multidisciplinary team. Positron emission tomography computed tomography (PET-CT) may be useful in excluding distant metastatic disease.

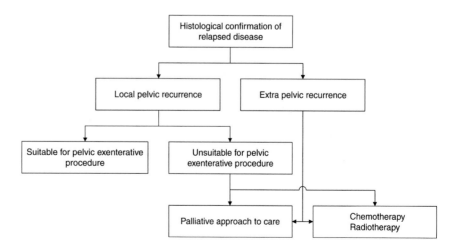

Fig. 56.5 Flow chart of management options with recurrence of cervical cancer.

No single treatment protocol exists for recurrent disease beyond the pelvis or in those women who have failed radiotherapy and are not candidates for further surgery. In those where palliation is appropriate, early involvement of clinicians specializing in palliative care and Macmillan cancer-relief nurses can be extremely beneficial, not only for the patient but also for the family concerned.

Cervical cancer in pregnancy

The presentation is usually abnormal bleeding, though some 20% are asymptomatic. The survival figures are stage for stage the same as those for women who are not pregnant. It is now believed that the route of delivery does not affect the ultimate 5-year survival.

Cone biopsy can result in excessive bleeding and spontaneous abortion. The absolute indications for cone biopsy include a Papanicolaou (Pap) smear suspicious for invasive cancer with no colposcopic proof, and colposcopic suspicion or directed biopsy indicating an invasive lesion.

Before 24 weeks' gestation, the treatment recommended is the same as for women who are not pregnant. If the treatment is radiotherapy, patients in the first trimester usually abort during the external beam therapy. In the second trimester, spontaneous abortion often is not the case, and the fetus must be surgically removed before radiation.

Radical hysterectomy and pelvic lymphadenectomy can be accomplished at any gestational age. When cancer is detected at the time of fetal viability, radical Caesarean hysterectomy can be offered or the fetus can be delivered and therapy instituted thereafter. The route of delivery has traditionally been Caesarean section, though this is more related to the possibility of increased bleeding, rather than the older concept of spread of disease if the vaginal route is chosen.

Patients diagnosed a few weeks before fetal viability, or those who refuse abortion based on moral or religious views, present the greatest challenge. In such cases, with appropriate counselling, the fetus is carried to earliest viability and therapy then undertaken. Antenatal steroids may be used to help with fetal lung maturity.

References

1 Sasieni P, Adams J, Cuzick J. Benefits of cervical screening at different ages: evidence from the UK audit of screening histories. *Br J Cancer* 2003;89:88–93.

2 Williams J. *Cancer of the Uterus. Harveian Lectures for 1886*. London: HK Lewis, 1886.

3 Hinselmann H. Verbesserung der inspektionsmoglichkeit von vulva, vagina und portio. *Munchener Medizinische Wochenschrift* 1925;77:1733.

4 Schiller W. Early diagnosis of carcinoma of the cervix. *Surg Gynaecol Obstet* 1933;56:210–222.

5 Papanicolaou GN, Traut HF. The diagnostic value of vaginal smears in carcinoma of the uterus. *Am J Obstet Gynecol* 1941;42: 193–206.

6 Johnson J, Patnick J. *Achievable Standards, Benchmark for Reporting, and Criteria for Evaluating Cervical Cytopathology*, 2nd edn. NHSCSP publication no. 1. London: Stationery Office, London, 2000.

7 Solomon D, Davey D, Kurman R *et al.* The Forum Group Members & The Bethesda 2001 Workshop. The 2001 Bethesda System: terminology for reporting results of cervical cytology. *JAMA* 2002;287:2114–2119.

8 Richart RM. A modified terminology for cervical intraepithelial neoplasia. *Obstet Gynecol* 1990;75:131–133.

9 McIndoe WA, McLean MR, Jones RW, Mullins PR. The invasive potential of carcinoma in situ of the cervix. *Obstet Gynecol* 1984; 64:451–458.

10 Shafi MI, Nazeer S. Grading system for abnormal colposcopic findings. In: Bosze P, Luesley D (eds) *EAGC Course Book on Colposcopy*. Budapest: Primed-X Press, 2004.

11 Martin-Hirsch PL, Parakevaidis E, Kitchener H. Surgery for cervical intraepithelial neoplasia. *Cochrane Database Syst Rev* 2000;2:CD001318.

12 Luesley DM, Leeson S. *Colposcopy and Programme Management: Guidelines for the NHS Cervical Screening Programme*. NHSCSP publication no. 20. London: Stationery Office, London, 2004.

13 Shafi MI, Dunn JA, Buxton EJ, Finn CB, Jordan JA, Luesley DM. Abnormal cervical cytology following large loop excision of the transformation zone: a case controlled study. *Br J Obstet Gynaecol* 1993;100:145–148.

14 Prendiville W, Davies R, Berry PJ. A low voltage diathermy loop for taking cervical biopsies: a qualitative comparison with punch biopsy forceps. *Br J Obstet Gynaecol* 1986;93: 773–6.

15 Kyrgiou M, Kolioupoulos G, Martin-Hirsch P, Arbyn M, Prendiville W, Paraskevaidis E. Obstetric outcomes after conservative treatment for intra-epithelial or early invasive cervical lesions: a systematic review. *Lancet* 2006;367:489–498.

16 Arbyn M, Kyrgiou M, Simoens C *et al.* Perinatal mortality and other severe adverse pregnancy outcomes associated with treatment of cervical intraepithelial neoplasia: meta-analysis. *BMJ* 2008;337:1284–1295.

17 Kitchener HC, Almonte M, Wheeler P *et al.* HPV testing in routine cervical screening: cross sectional data from the ARTISTIC trial. *Br J Cancer* 2006;95:56–61.

18 Tombola Group. Options for managing low grade cervical abnormalities detected at screening: cost effectiveness study. *BMJ* 2009;339:2549–2556.

19 Kitchener HC, Walker PG, Nelson L *et al.* HPV testing as an adjunct to cytology in the follow up of women treated for cervical intraepithelial neoplasia. *BJOG* 2008;115:1001–1007.

20 Koutsky LA, Ault KA, Wheeler CM *et al.* Proof of Principle Study Investigators. A controlled trial of a human papillomavirus type 16 vaccine. *N Engl J Med* 2004;347:1645–1651.

21 Harper DM, Franco EL, Wheeler C *et al.*, GlaxoSmithKline HPV Vaccine Study Group. Efficacy of a bivalent L1 virus-like particle vaccine in prevention of infection with human papillomavirus types 16 and 18 in young women: a randomized controlled trial. *Lancet* 2004;364:1757–1765.

22 Harper DM. Currently approved prophylactic HPV vaccines. *Exp Rev Vaccines* 2009;8:1663–1679.

23 Shafi MI, Dunn JA, Chenoy R, Buxton EJ, Williams C, Luesley DM. Digital imaging colposcopy, image analysis and quantification of the colposcopic image. *Br J Obstet Gynaecol* 1994;101: 234–238.

24 Etherington IJ, Dunn J, Shafi MI, Smith T, Luesley DM. Video colpography: a new technique for secondary cervical screening. *Br J Obstet Gynaecol* 1997;104:150–153.

25 Cancer Research UK, 2010. Available at: www. cancerresearchuk.org.

26 Querleu D, Morrow CP. Classification of radical hysterectomy. *Lancet Oncol* 2008;9:297–303.

27 Thomas GM. Improved treatment for cervical cancer – concurrent chemotherapy and radiotherapy. *N Engl J Med* 1999;340: 1198–1200.

28 Dargent D, Brun JL, Roy M, Mathevet P, Remy I. La Trachelectomie Elargie (TE). Une alternative a l'hysterectomie radicale dans le traitement de cancers infiltrants developpes sur la face externe du col uterin. *J Obstet Gynaecol* 1994;2: 285–292.

29 Gien LT, Covens A. Fertility-sparing options for early stage cervical cancer. *Gynecol Oncol* 2010;117:350–357.

Further reading

Shafi MI, Earl H, Tan LT. *Gynaecological Oncology*. Cambridge: Cambridge University Press, 2009.

Shafi MI, Nazeer S. *Colposcopy – A Practical Guide*. Salisburg, Fivepin Publishing Ltd, 2006.

Luesley DM, Leeson S. Colposcopy and Programme Management: Guidelines for the NHS Cervical Screening Programme. NHSCSP publication no. 20, 2004.

http://bethesda2001.cancer.gov/
www.cancerresearchuk.org/
www.cancerscreening.nhs.uk/cervical
www.nci.nih.gov/

Chapter 57
Epithelial Ovarian Cancer

Hani Gabra and Sarah Blagden
Ovarian Cancer Action Research Centre, Imperial College London Hammersmith Campus, London, UK

Epithelial ovarian cancer (EOC) is the second leading cause of death from gynaecological cancer, and the fifth most common cancer in women overall. It is a serious disease, particularly in advanced stages with a course that is punctuated by frequent tumour recurrences, and has a negative impact on quality and length of life.

Disease progression typically occurs via locoregional peritoneal dissemination and its consequences rather than via visceral metastatic disease; patients commonly develop recurrent ascites and bowel obstruction.

Some patients are cured completely even of advanced ovarian cancer with first-line multimodality therapy and therefore research interest into reducing the incidence of recurrence and improving the prognosis of the disease is intense.

Aetiology, epidemiology and genetics

The current lifetime risk is 1 per 70 women, the incidence being approximately 22 per 100 000 population. Epithelial ovarian cancer is a disease of older women, the incidence peaking at the age of 67 years [1,2].

There are about 7000 new cases of ovarian cancer diagnosed in the UK annually with about 4370 deaths, and in most centres the overall survival at 5 years is around 40%. Incessant ovulation is thought to be an important factor and in large case–control studies, factors that interfere with ovulation are found to affect the incidence of ovarian cancer [3]. Use of the oral contraceptive pill has been linked to a 40% reduction in risk of ovarian cancer in some studies [4]. Other protective factors include early menarche, late menopause, pregnancy, childbirth and breastfeeding. Within the UK, the 5-year survival rate is improving and the incidence of ovarian cancer has recently started to fall, perhaps reflecting better treatment and the impact of factors such as more widespread use of the oral contraceptive pill [5]. These are balanced against lifestyle factors that increase risk of the disease, such as women opting to conceive later in life and having smaller families. Other aetiological factors may also contribute to a lesser extent such as obesity and use of hormone replacement therapy (HRT) [6,7].

There is geographic variation of ovarian cancer, it is commoner in northern Europe and the USA and less common in developing countries and Japan [8]. However, the risk of ovarian cancer is seen to be reduced by mechanical sterilization and by hysterectomy, and there is an increased risk associated with inflammatory conditions such as pelvic inflammatory disease (PID) and endometriosis [9]. This suggests that chronic inflammation has an important role in the aetiology of ovarian cancer with the deployment of cytokine and inflammatory signalling pathways [10,11].

Genetic factors in ovarian cancer are also important. Approximately 5–10% of ovarian cancers are associated with an autosomal dominant syndrome where there is an inherited defect in one of three known genes: BRCA1 and BRCA2 (site-specific ovarian cancer syndrome and breast–ovarian cancer syndrome) and the mismatch repair genes [identified in the type II Lynch syndrome or hereditary non-polyposis colorectal cancer (HNPCC)] [12]. It is likely that other hereditary gene mutations will be identified in the future. It has recently become apparent that a significant proportion (perhaps even the majority) of patients with sporadic high-grade serous ovarian cancer (i.e. who have not inherited a genetic mutation) have somatic alteration to either BRCA genes or their pathways (also described as 'BRCAness') by a variety of mechanisms, for example somatic mutations of genes involved in the DNA repair pathway, somatic methylation or other epigenetic mechanisms, as well as downstream pathway alterations [13,14]. Drugs designed to target BRCA deficiency (either inherited or somatic), known as poly (ADP-ribose) polymerase (PARP) inhibitors, have shown exciting results in early clinical trials and are likely to be introduced into the routine management of hereditary ovarian cancer [15,16]. Recently, studies of PARP inhibitors have been extended to combine with cytotoxics and are being evaluated in patients with somatic ovarian cancer. We are awaiting results.

Dewhurst's Textbook of Obstetrics & Gynaecology, Eighth Edition. Edited by D. Keith Edmonds.
© 2012 John Wiley and Sons, Ltd. Published 2012 by John Wiley and Sons, Ltd.

Sporadic ovarian cancer is increasingly described as a diverse group of tumours rather than a single disease, and has recently been classified by a molecular rather than a histological profile. Type I ovarian cancers comprise low-grade serous, low-grade endometrioid, clear cell, mucinous and transitional carcinomas. Apart from clear cell and mucinous cancers, these tumours behave in an indolent fashion, lack TP53 mutations, are confined to the ovary at presentation and are relatively genetically stable. They are believed to originate from a benign lesion such as endometriosis or a cystic ovarian neoplasm, sometimes via an intermediate step of borderline disease. In contrast, type II tumours comprise high-grade serous, undifferentiated and malignant mixed mesodermal tumours (carcinosarcomas). These are highly aggressive and usually present at an advanced stage with a high frequency of P53 mutations. It has been proposed that serous ovarian cancers could emanate from implantation of adenocarcinoma cells arising from the adjacent fallopian tube. This is supported by clonality observed between P53 mutations carried by tumour and by intraepithelial fallopian tube lesions [17].

Screening and prophylactic oophorectomy

As over 75% of ovarian cancer cases present with advanced stage disease, when cure rates are <30%, a case can clearly be made for pursuing the aim of screening to try to identify the disease when it is at stage I, where cure rates are higher. However, effective screening methods have not yet been demonstrated although a number of clinical trials are ongoing.

According to World Health Organization (WHO) criteria, successful screening programmes should result in a reduction in the mortality of the screened population relative to the unscreened population, and the screening tools used must have high sensitivity and specificity with a high positive predictive value (defined as the number of true positives divided by the sum of true and false positives). High sensitivity maximizes the potential for picking up the disease, whereas high specificity reduces the chances of false positives that result in unnecessary interventions. Ovarian cancer is a relatively rare condition; thus, around 99.6% specificity is required to detect one case of ovarian cancer in every 10 women who test positive (10% positive predictive value) [18].

UKCTOCS study
The UK Collaborative Trial of Ovarian Cancer Screening (UKCTOCS) study recruited over 200 000 postmenopausal women on a population basis from centres within the UK. Patients were randomized to no treatment, annual CA-125 with subsequent transvaginal ultrasound (TVU) or annual TVU alone. A Bayesian CA-125 risk algorithm was incorporated into this study, each CA-125 was compared with the patient's preceding values and the likelihood that the CA-125 profile reflected that of ovarian cancer, even if still within the reference range. The aim of this algorithm was to improve the positive predictive value of CA-125, particularly in the detection of early-stage disease. For patients with abnormal results, combined CA-125 and TVU were performed within 8 weeks which, if again abnormal, resulted in a referral to a gynaecological oncologist. Although the primary end-point of this study was ovarian cancer mortality, other measured outcomes were the psychosocial, physical and economic cost of ovarian cancer screening. The trial closed to recruitment and initial results were published in 2009 [19]. Results were encouraging in the CA-125 plus TVU or 'multimodal screening' arm of the trial, with sensitivity, specificity and positive predictive values of 89.5%, 99.8% and 43.3%, respectively. Of the 32 invasive ovarian cancers identified in this arm, 47% were early stage, although these were not necessarily stage Ia. Final data including mortality in comparison with the control arm will be available after the trial is completed in 2014.

Confining screening to patients with a higher risk of ovarian cancer (such as those with a strong family history of the disease) would theoretically increase specificity. For women at higher risk of a genetic ovarian cancer predisposition, the UK Familial Ovarian Cancer Screening Study (UKFOCSS) is currently evaluating 4-monthly CA-125 (including algorithm) and annual TVU. The study aims to recruit a total of 5000 women [20]. Final results of the American Prostate, Lung, Colorectal and Ovarian Cancer Screening (PLCO) study are also awaited. In this trial, 150 000 patients were recruited from across the USA and underwent annual CA-125 and TVU tests [21]. Currently, ovarian cancer screening is not routine practice within the USA or UK.

For patients carrying BRCA1 or BRCA2 germline mutations, prophylactic oophorectomy reduces the incidence of subsequent ovarian and breast cancer by 96% and 53%, respectively [22]. For many women in BRCA families this is considered the approach of choice. In general, where it is recommended, prophylactic bilateral salpingo-oophorectomy is performed with completion of childbearing and HRT is commenced thereafter until a point that appropriately corresponds to natural menopause, that is, around the age of 50 years [23].

Clinical presentation

Epithelial ovarian cancer has often been described as a 'silent killer', with 75% patients being diagnosed with late-stage (stage III/IV) disease with a 5-year survival rate of 30–40%, rather than in stage I when survival is 84–94%. This is largely because the symptoms of early-stage ovarian cancer are thought to be subtle or absent, making many patients unsure of whether to seek help and the diagnosis difficult in those that do. However, Goff *et al.* [24] demonstrated that symptoms of EOC are present in 90% of affected women, even with early-stage disease, and that these symptoms are often dismissed, so that for 37% of women with the disease there is a delay of at least 6 months from presentation until a diagnosis is made. Goff *et al.* developed a 'symptom index' (more than 12 episodes of at least one of the following symptoms: pelvic or abdominal pain, urinary urge or frequency, or difficulty with eating/early satiety present for less than a year), which has been shown to accurately predict the presence of ovarian cancer when used in combination with serum tumour markers [25]. As well as the symptoms described by Goff *et al.*, ovarian cancer can also cause pelvic pain due to torsion or haemorrhage of the ovary and rectosigmoid symptoms such as constipation or diarrhoea.

Signs include gaseous abdominal distension, a pelvic mass, abnormal bowel sounds, ascites, palpable abdominal masses, lymphadenopathy, pleural effusion, an umbilical mass (Sister Joseph's nodule) and, rarely, intra-abdominal organomegaly.

Increased awareness of the symptoms of ovarian cancer amongst women and their primary care providers may lead to a quicker diagnosis of EOC, with a subsequent reduction in treatment-related morbidity and possibly increased survival.

Pathology of epithelial ovarian cancer

Most ovarian cancers have serous histology reminiscent of fallopian tube origin, often with characteristic psam-

Table 57.1 International Federation of Gynecology and Obstetrics (FIGO) staging for ovarian cancer.

Stage	
I	Growth limited to the ovaries
Ia	Tumour in one ovary; no ascites, capsule intact, no tumour on surface
Ib	As in Ia but tumour in both ovaries
Ic	Tumour either as in Ia or Ib, but ascites with cancer cells, or capsule ruptured or tumour on surface, or positive peritoneal washings
II	Growth on one or both ovaries with peritoneal implants within the pelvis
IIa	Extension or metastases to uterus or fallopian tubes
IIb	Extension to other pelvic organs
IIc	Tumour either IIa or IIb, but with findings as in Ic
III	Tumour in one or both ovaries with peritoneal implants outside the pelvis, or retroperitoneal node metastases
IIIa	Tumour grossly limited to the true pelvis; negative nodes, but microscopic implants on abdominal peritoneal surfaces
IIIb	As in IIIa, but abdominal implants are <2 cm in diameter
IIIc	Abdominal implants >2 cm or retroperitoneal lymph node metastases
IV	Tumour involving one or both ovaries with distant metastases, e.g. malignant pleural fluid, parenchymal liver metastases

moma bodies. Endometrioid adenocarcinomas and clear cell carcinomas are the next commonest histological type, and mucinous carcinomas are less common still. Uncommonly, ovarian carcinosarcomas do present and are epithelial tumours with sarcomatous differentiation. There is evidence that clear cell and mucinous ovarian cancers are far less responsive to chemotherapy than serous and endometrioid ovarian cancers. An important feature of histological classification is the grade of the cancer, ranging from well-differentiated (grade 1) to moderately differentiated (grade 2) to poorly differentiated (grade 3). Borderline tumours are not regarded as cancers and in general have an excellent prognosis.

Patterns of spread of ovarian cancer

The International Federation of Gynecology and Obstetrics (FIGO) classification for ovarian cancer is shown in Table 57.1 and is based on surgical staging. Like other malignant neoplasms, ovarian cancer can disseminate along locoregional, lymphatic and blood-borne routes. However, there are patterns of dissemination that are characteristic of ovarian cancer, and also patterns that are characteristic of histological subtypes of ovarian cancer.

In the common serous ovarian carcinomas, the dominant pattern is that of transperitoneal locoregional dissemination often resulting in bulky intra-abdominal disease, particularly involving the omentum as well as other peritoneal surfaces. This is often accompanied by malignant ascites. With the exception of malignant unilateral or bilateral pleural effusion, and involvement of the umbilicus owing to tumour spread along the remnant of the umbilical vein (Sister Joseph's nodule), it is unusual to present with visceral metastatic disease, for example visceral hepatic metastases, pulmonary, cerebral or bone metastases that are so common in other gynaecological tumours such as breast or cervical cancer. Lymph node involvement (which stages the patient as IIIc) is relatively common. An exception to this situation is the rare BRCA1/2 familial ovarian cancers that have a very high (73%) incidence of visceral metastatic disease [26].

Diagnosis

The diagnosis of ovarian cancer is histopathological, and most large centres require a detailed histopathological analysis in order to manage the patient rationally. Histopathological type, tumour grade and FIGO stage are all determined by biopsy obtained using radiological or laparoscopic guidance or during formal staging laparotomy. Other markers such as oestrogen receptor status can provide useful information for the later management of the patient. Cytological diagnosis, such as from a sample of ascites, is considered inadequate for diagnosis and management.

CA-125 is a glycoprotein serum marker of ovarian cancer. As a stand-alone test, it is neither adequate for diagnosis nor for screening as it is elevated in a variety of benign and malignant conditions. In addition, CA-125 is elevated in only 80% of known ovarian cancers and in 50% of those with early-stage disease. In patients whose CA-125 is elevated at diagnosis, serial CA-125 measurement provides a means of assessing response to subsequent chemotherapeutic treatment. Patients with an early fall in CA-125 during front-line chemotherapy have been shown to have a more durable response to treatment [27]. Routine evaluation of CA-125 (in those who express the marker) is also performed in patients at completion of treatment as a means of detecting relapse, although the results of the recently reported Medical Research Council (MRC) OVO5/European Organisation for Research and Treatment of Cancer (EORTC) 55955 trials suggest that routine sequential CA-125 measurement after completion of therapy may be unnecessary because waiting until symptoms develop confers no survival disadvantage compared with early treatment on marker rise [28]. It is therefore not clinically disadvantageous if women with EOC refuse serial CA-125 assessment.

> ### Summary box 57.2
>
> MRC-OVO5/EORTC 55955 trial:
> - Of 1442 women registered, 529 had a rise in CA-125 following a complete serological remission after front-line chemotherapy.
> - A total of 254 were randomized to immediate re-treatment with chemotherapy while 233 were randomized to continued blinding of CA-125, and thus were re-treated only on symptomatic relapse.
> - Those randomized to receive early intervention started second-line treatment a median of 4.8 months earlier and third-line treatment 4.6 months earlier than the delayed treatment group.
> - At 2 years' cut-off, there was no difference in overall survival between the two groups [hazard ratio (HR) 1.00, confidence interval (CI) 0.82–1.22, $P = 0.98$] or in quality of life.
> - Although mature data are awaited, this suggests that routine tracking of CA-125 in patients who have completed chemotherapy alongside early intervention may not confer a survival advantage over re-treating at the point of symptomatic relapse.

Prognostic factors

Unfortunately, the majority of patients with ovarian cancer will relapse and ultimately die from their disease. While the prognosis in stage I ovarian cancer is excellent, with earlier lower-grade stages having a cure rate of greater than 90%, prognosis, despite evidence of recent improvement, overall leaves much room for improvement, with 1-year survival of 71%, 5-year survival of 40% and 10-year survival of 33% (CRUK website) [29].

The main factors that predict for survival include FIGO stage of disease, tumour grade, surgical debulking status, histological subtype and sensitivity of disease to platinum-based chemotherapy. Ongoing research is now applying whole genome molecular profiling analysis as well as individual characterized molecular targets to the refinement of predictive and prognostic models.

Treatment of newly diagnosed ovarian cancer

The standard management of stage Ic–IV EOC is to perform primary debulking surgery with the explicit aim of total macroscopic clearance and to enable complete surgical staging. This is followed by adjuvant carboplatin-containing chemotherapy for all patients other than those with FIGO stage Ia and Ib lower-grade tumours for whom surgery is sufficient and chemotherapy can be omitted [30]. Interval debulking surgery can improve survival in suboptimally debulked patients after three cycles of chemotherapy when initial surgery is not performed by a gynaecological oncology surgeon [31], and there has recently been much debate regarding the use of neoadjuvant chemotherapy followed by delayed primary surgery [32]. Recent data suggest that in the context of high surgical quality, there is no disadvantage to neoadjuvant chemotherapy followed by delayed primary surgery [33]. First-line chemotherapy comprises either carboplatin alone or carboplatin in combination with paclitaxel. These standards of care have been defined by international randomized clinical trials [Gynecologic Oncology Group (GOG)111 [34], OV-10 [35], GOG132 [36] and ICON3 [37]).

Integrated multidisciplinary care of ovarian cancer

Ovarian cancer is best managed by centralized integrated multidisciplinary teams. This has been shown to improve outcomes in this disease. In general, the team consists of a surgical oncologist, a non-surgical oncologist, a radiologist and a pathologist specialized in ovarian cancer management. The team crucially also requires a specialist nurse who acts as a conduit between the patient and the multidisciplinary team and is available for the patient throughout her journey. Palliative care specialist input may be required in all phases of the disease. Increasingly, multidisciplinary teams are developing integrated care pathways for patients with ovarian cancer that bring together hospital and community services within one framework. Most recently, survivorship programmes are beginning to become integrated into standard care.

Surgery

The aim of surgery is total macroscopic debulking of tumour as the volume of residual disease remaining after surgical cytoreduction inversely correlates with survival [38]. The GOG defines optimal cytoreduction as leaving residual disease of less than 1 cm in maximum diameter. Complete cytoreduction is defined as no residual disease or total macroscopic clearance. The extent of cytoreduction is variably feasible according to surgical effort and experience as well as tumour biology, with the proportion of patients optimally debulked in various chemotherapy studies varying from 30% (ICON3) up to 85%, with apparently acceptable operative morbidity. Tumour debulking is one of the most important prognostic factors. Complete cytoreduction offers the best improvement in survival,

then optimal cytoreduction (removal of disease to less than 1 cm maximum diameter) as compared with suboptimal cytoreduction (residual disease greater than 1 cm maximum diameter) [39].

Where the surgeon regards debulking surgery as a realistic objective for a patient, a midline incision is performed. After evaluation, the surgeon performs bilateral salpingo-oophorectomy, total abdominal hysterectomy and omentectomy. Removal of all visible deposits is also undertaken. If the surgeon is not able to achieve complete macroscopic debulking, it may nevertheless be possible to achieve optimal debulking.

Is surgery important?

There has been no randomized trial of surgery versus no surgery; however, the survival of patients with advanced ovarian cancer receiving no surgery in the pre-chemotherapy era was of the order of 12–14%. The significance of surgery was explored in the SCOTROC1 chemotherapy trial. In SCOTROC1, all postoperative patients received carboplatin and were randomized to either paclitaxel or docetaxel, with progression-free survival as an end-point. Surgical data were collected from this trial, with two out of three patients from the UK and one out of three from non-UK centres. This allowed comparison of surgical practice and of the relationship between surgery and outcome since the case mix and chemotherapy was identical in all countries. In the UK, although similar rates of total abdominal hysterectomy, bilateral salpingo-oophorectomy and omentectomy were performed, there were significantly fewer bowel resections and para-aortic/pelvic lymphadenectomy procedures performed than in non-UK countries, particularly in those patients who were optimally debulked. Furthermore, the UK had significantly less operating time per patient and complete debulking rates compared with non-UK centres. As an independent prognostic variable with respect to progression-free survival, residual disease (>2 cm) carries an adverse hazard ratio of 1.6; however, this depends on the extent of pre-surgical disease. In less extensive disease, optimal debulking was associated with a large survival benefit, whereas with more extensive disease the benefit was much less. However, UK patients who were completely debulked (as opposed to optimally) did much worse than those who were completely debulked in non-UK centres (HR 2). However, in those optimally debulked, the adverse effect of being operated on in the UK was obviated [40].

Lymphadenectomy in ovarian cancer
Systematic lymphadenectomy (SL) is a procedure performed during primary debulking surgery and comprises

resection of pelvic and para-aortic lymph nodes. Although there is an established association between pelvic or para-aortic node involvement and adverse prognosis, the survival advantage of performing SL in patients with ovarian cancer remains debatable. In some centres within the UK, SL is routinely performed for early-stage ovarian cancer but not for advanced disease.

Lymphadenectomy in early-stage ovarian cancer

Although SL carries additional morbidity to the patient, in the USA, Australia and Europe it is generally the rule that SL is undertaken only for patients with early-stage disease. This provides better staging information and in three studies was shown to improve overall survival [41–43]. In the ICON1/ACTION studies of immediate versus delayed carboplatin in early ovarian cancer, it was found that no subgroup overall failed to benefit from chemotherapy, which was initially interpreted to mean that all patients (whatever the stage of their disease) should be offered chemotherapy, making SL a superfluous and unnecessary procedure [44]. However, chemotherapy carries significant morbidity and mortality risks also. In subgroup analysis of the ACTION study (which was a parallel European study to ICON1), it was found that those who had complete debulking including SL appeared not to benefit from chemotherapy [45]. Therefore, there is an argument to be made that patients with low-grade stage Ia and Ib EOC which is surgically fully staged (i.e. including SL) can be spared chemotherapy.

Lymphadenectomy in advanced ovarian cancer

The use of SL for advanced ovarian cancer is more controversial, although retrospective meta-analysis studies have demonstrated a survival advantage proportional to the number of nodes removed [41]. In 2005, the results of a prospective trial were published in which patients with advanced disease were treated with optimal debulking surgery plus SL or lymph node sampling. Although an improvement in progression-free survival was observed in the SL group (31.2 vs. 21.6%, respectively), there was no change in overall survival [46].

Delayed primary debulking surgery

In patients considered unsuitable for surgery, delayed primary debulking surgery is performed once they have completed three cycles of neoadjuvant chemotherapy. A number of retrospective studies have explored whether patient outcome is better if surgery or chemotherapy is administered first [47–50], and there are mixed results.

Two prospective phase III trials have addressed this question: chemotherapy or upfront surgery (CHORUS) and EORTC 55971. These showed a similar overall and progression-free survival in patients treated with initial or delayed chemotherapy, although there were fewer postoperative deaths and morbidities in patients in the delayed primary surgical debulking arm of the trial [51]. Final results from CHORUS are awaited.

Interval debulking surgery

In patients who have been suboptimally debulked at primary surgery, a second or interval debulking procedure can be performed with the aim of improving survival once the patient has received three cycles of chemotherapy. This was investigated in three prospective randomized trials [52–54], only one of which demonstrated a survival advantage in the interval debulking arm [54]. However, patients on this trial did not receive paclitaxel chemotherapy and did not have primary surgery performed by a specialist gynaecological oncologist. Surgery performed by a trained gynaecological oncologist has been shown to increase survival [55] and therefore it is likely that with the appropriate persons undertaking primary surgery, interval debulking surgery is not required [56].

Advanced ovarian cancer

Front-line chemotherapy post-surgery: benefit and toxicity

It has been demonstrated in a number of clinical trials that systemic platinum agents given after surgery are the best and most important drugs in ovarian cancer either alone or in combination. Systemic therapy with carboplatin and paclitaxel as a chemotherapy regime is at least as good if not marginally better than carboplatin alone, and the addition of a third cytotoxic given alongside carboplatin and paclitaxel has failed to demonstrate an advantage over the doublet. Preliminary results of the GOG218 trial exploring the role of the vascular endothelial growth factor (VEGF) antibody bevacizumab given alongside front-line chemotherapy and as subsequent maintenance have been recently reported in abstract form [57]. This showed a 3.8-month improvement in progression-free survival in patients receiving combined followed by maintenance bevacizumab compared with those receiving chemotherapy alone (or chemotherapy with combined but not maintenance bevacizumab), but no difference at this analysis in overall survival. Mature data from GOG218 are awaited, along with the results of a similar European study, ICON7.

Carboplatin and paclitaxel as front-line therapy

The current standard of care following surgery is a combination of carboplatin and paclitaxel, given for six cycles at 3-weekly intervals. The evidence for this is based on various seminal studies. The GOG111 and OV10 studies demonstrated that cisplatin with cyclophosphamide was inferior to cisplatin and paclitaxel [34,35]. The GOG132 study showed that there was no difference in survival for cisplatin given alone as compared with cisplatin given alongside paclitaxel [36], and in the ICON3 trial, carboplatin plus paclitaxel was compared with the hitherto standard treatment options of carboplatin alone or CAP (cyclophosphamide, doxorubicin and cisplatin) [37]. Although ICON3 showed no difference between progression-free and overall survival between the single-agent carboplatin and carboplatin/paclitaxel arms, a combination of paclitaxel and carboplatin has been widely adopted in patients who are fit, lacking in comorbidities (especially those exacerbated by the treatment or its supportive therapies) and able to cope with combination chemotherapy. More recently, the Japanese Gynecologic Oncology Group (JGOG) undertook a randomized study where in addition to standard 3-weekly carboplatin, paclitaxel was given as either 3 weekly or weekly dose-dense therapy. In this trial there was a significant 11-month improvement in progression-free survival in the dose-

dense arm, with significant improvement in overall survival also [58]. Repetition of this study is awaited and if confirmed will result in a change in standard of care.

It is important to note that there are differences in response rate between histological types. In serous and endometrioid ovarian cancers, the response rates are relatively high (70–80%) with carboplatin and paclitaxel. However, for advanced clear cell and mucinous cancers, the response rate to carboplatin–paclitaxel is in the order of 22% and 14%, respectively [59,60]. In these latter two cancers, response to single-agent platinum is also considerably lower and therefore combination treatment is preferred for patients with these unusual and prognostically poorer histologies in advanced disease.

The toxicities of carboplatin–paclitaxel combination chemotherapy

There are significant toxicities from this standard combination.

Alopecia occurs early and is inevitable but reversible. Some patients retain their hair using the pre-chemotherapy 'cold cap' which reduces scalp temperature and thus hair follicle blood supply.

Neutropaenic sepsis is also a significant risk of this combination chemotherapy, with neutrophil counts reaching a nadir at days 10–14 following treatment. Granulocyte colony-stimulating factor (GCSF) can be administered to neutropaenic patients to reduce the duration of the event. Patients who develop a pyrexia following treatment are advised to immediately seek help and most hospitals have 'neutropaenic sepsis' protocols advising immediate intravenous (i.v.) antibiotics (usually tazocin and gentamycin) for pyrexial patients with neutrophils $<1.0 \times 10^9/L$. In patients who have experience neutropaenic sepsis, prophylactic use of GCSF and/or chemotherapy dose reduction can be introduced for subsequent treatment cycles.

Hypersensitivity due to the Cremophor vehicle that is used as a paclitaxel diluent necessitates the use of dexamethasone, causing potentially significant steroid-induced weight gain for the patient and worsening of diabetic control (if a concurrent comorbidity) that may have significant consequences when combined with the risk of neutropaenic sepsis.

Neurotoxicity occurs with the use of paclitaxel, mainly comprising peripheral sensory neuropathy in fingers and toes which occurs in about one-third of patients but is usually mild and generally settles after the end of chemotherapy. In patients who develop persistent signs of neuropathy during treatment, omission or dose reduction of subsequent paclitaxel is advised. In a small proportion of patients neurotoxicity is severe and may substantially interfere with function, and in some cases is permanent and does not resolve with time.

Joint-pain syndrome typically occurs 3 days after paclitaxel chemotherapy and lasts approximately 3 days. This usually affects knee joints as well as the small joints of the hands and feet. It can be severe and sometimes lasts beyond 3 days. Its severity may necessitate the pre-emptive use of analgesics such as paracetamol and ibuprofen at full dose or require subsequent chemotherapy dose reduction.

Emesis is unusual with this regimen, although *nausea* can be a problem, particularly with younger patients. Prophylactic use and rapid upscaling (if required) of antiemetics such as metoclopromide, domperidone, cyclizine, dexamethasone and ondansetron can minimize this unpleasant side effect.

Other toxicities include ototoxicity, renal impairment and changes to bowel habit.

Are higher-dose intensities or more cycles of chemotherapy better than standard treatment?

Several studies have been conducted utilizing conventional scheduling of greater versus fewer numbers of cycles of chemotherapy (greater total dose) and higher versus lower doses (greater dose intensity) and in general these studies have shown no benefit for either greater total dose or dose intensity. In terms of total dose, Bertelsen *et al.* [61] showed no difference in outcome measures for 6 versus 12 cycles and Lambert and colleagues in 1997 [62] showed no difference for five versus eight cycles. More recently, a study comparing six additional courses of single-agent paclitaxel (vs. control) in patients in complete remission following first-line paclitaxel plus carboplatin failed to show an advantage of prolonged treatment [63]. With respect to dose intensity, seven trials have compared differing dose intensities of first-line chemotherapy, all of these essentially comparing one dose intensity with double that dose intensity, and with the exception of two trials there was no difference in survival [64–69]. Findings from the JCOG trial (described above) and response to dose-dense treatment in relapsed disease suggests that this issue is not entirely closed. High-dose chemotherapy with stem cell transplantation has also been investigated in ovarian cancer. Data from these studies show little difference in survival for standard versus high-dose chemotherapy [70–72].

Neoadjuvant chemotherapy

The gold standard for treating ovarian cancer has long been held to include upfront surgery. However, there is still some controversy as to the optimal timing of surgery and whether the use of neoadjuvant chemotherapy would make the subsequent delayed primary operation easier and more complete. This is currently the subject of the CHORUS and EORTC trials (see above). However, a note of caution is indicated, which is to say that wholesale adoption of neoadjuvant chemotherapy should not be undertaken until these trials report. There are theoretical considerations that neoadjuvant chemotherapy may select resistant disease in a high tumour-burden environment, necessitating a focused approach to surgical quality in the delayed primary debulking setting; and conversely that primary surgical debulking may enhance the chemotherapy effect by debulking chemoresistant clones at an early stage, and these potential consequences need to be considered [73].

Intraperitoneal chemotherapy

Ovarian cancer is principally a disease of locoregional peritoneal dissemination within the abdominal cavity. Control of locoregional dissemination is the top priority for the control of advanced ovarian cancer. The idea of intraperitoneal (i.p.) therapy is not new, having been performed for 30 years or more. Over the last 20 years there have been seven randomized trials comparing i.p. with i.v. chemotherapy for the first-line treatment of patients with stage III ovarian cancer (reviewed in reference 74). The common factor is that all have included platinum, and most have added a second drug. Meta-analyses of these trials showed a significant reduction in hazards of 0.88 with CIs of 0.81–0.95 and an improvement in survival (in the three largest studies) of 8, 11 and 16 months over i.v. chemotherapy beyond an expected median survival of this optimally debulked group of 4 years [74].

The most recent of the three large trials, GOG172 [75], showed the largest difference ever in a randomized ovarian cancer trial with median overall survival of 67 months against the i.v. control arm of 49 months, the improvement being 17.4 months with an HR of 0.71. This regimen utilized i.v. paclitaxel on day 1, i.p. cisplatin on day 2 and i.p. taxol on day 8 on a 21-day cycle for six cycles. However, i.p. chemotherapy was associated with enhanced toxicities including neuropathy, gastrointestinal toxicity and myelotoxicity. Despite encouragement to adopt i.p. chemotherapy as standard of care by the National Cancer Institute (NCI), clinicians are reluctant to adopt it into routine practice until further randomized trials have been performed because of concerns over insertion and maintenance of i.p. catheters and fear of excessive toxicity [76].

Recurrent ovarian cancer

Recurrent ovarian cancer is currently an incurable clinical state, although improved survival can still be realized by utilizing appropriate chemotherapy and overall multidisciplinary clinical effort. Nevertheless, palliation and optimization of quality of life are important considerations in this clinical scenario, including aggressive symptom management, chemotherapy, radiotherapy and surgery.

Community palliative care and hospice provision are important components in this phase of disease. Selecting treatments with minimal treatment toxicities are also a major aim for patients in this clinical scenario.

The timing of reintroduction of therapy was addressed in the MRC-OVO5/EORTC 55955 trials [28]. As described above, patients who were in complete remission with a normal CA-125 after primary treatment were monitored for CA-125 levels and results were blinded to physician and patient. When CA-125 levels reached twice the upper limit of normal, the patients were randomized to either immediate treatment by informing the physician or not informing the physician until clinical recurrence demanded re-treatment. The results of the trial confirmed that there was no patient benefit to early intervention (see Summary box 57.2). Current policy is to try and avoid treatment until early symptomatic progression, but this demands fairly intensive watchful waiting and can generate considerable anxiety for patients. Upon early symptomatic progression, or if there is evidence that the recurrence may cause significant anatomical damage if unchecked ('prophylactic palliation'), palliative treatment can be instituted and this typically consists of chemotherapy, although sometimes multimodality therapy including surgery or radiotherapy may be required.

Chemotherapy

Depending on the time interval between primary platinum-based treatment and relapse, recurrent ovarian cancer may be considered as platinum refractory, resistant or potentially sensitive. Disease that has relapsed after more 12 months is defined as platinum-sensitive, between 6 and 12 months is defined as partially platinum sensitive and under 6 months or during treatment is described as platinum-resistant or refractory. Platinum-refractory ovarian cancer represents primary non-response to chemotherapy and implies that it is unlikely that these patients will respond to further standard chemotherapy agents. These patients often have aggressive disease and poor prognosis. They can be considered for phase I trials, and some phase II trials if sufficiently fit.

Platinum-sensitive recurrence

Platinum-sensitive recurrence has several definitions. A pragmatic definition is that of recurrence of ovarian cancer requiring treatment occurring more than 6 months after last chemotherapy. These patients are potentially platinum-sensitive, and the likelihood of overall response to re-challenge with platinum-based chemotherapy is a function of time, and as Blackledge [77] showed, those relapsing more than 18 months after previous chemotherapy have up to a 94% chance of response to subsequent platinum-based therapy (as compared with a 10% response rate in those relapsing within 6 months of last platinum therapy).

Eisenhauer and colleagues [78] looked at factors predicting response to subsequent chemotherapy in platinum pretreated ovarian cancer using data from 13 randomized trials of six chemotherapy agents (not just platinum). They found that serous histology, tumour bulk (<5 cm) and number of disease sites (<3) were significant factors; yet treatment-free interval was not a feature at first sight at odds with Blackledge's findings. These biological predictors were the main determinants of subsequent response, with the treatment-free interval correlating closely with tumour size.

A seminal randomized clinical trial, MRC ICON4, was conducted in patients relapsing more than 6 months after last chemotherapy requiring additional chemotherapy. This trial asked if the addition of paclitaxel to carboplatin improved survival in platinum-resistant disease. This study was extremely important because the MRC ICON3 study had shown no improvement in survival for carboplatin and paclitaxel as front-line chemotherapy in advanced ovarian cancer. In the ICON4 trial, addition of paclitaxel significantly improved survival in platinum-sensitive recurrent ovarian cancer with an HR of 0.82, an absolute survival advantage at 2 years of 7% and an improvement to median survival of 5 months, in other words, a benefit of similar magnitude to the addition of platinum to front-line chemotherapy for ovarian cancer. There were no real differences in patient-perceived toxicity and, in general, where there are not reasons to avoid paclitaxel (e.g. previous severe neuropathy, concurrent medical comorbidity especially advanced diabetes, etc.) it can be recommended for patients relapsing more than12 months after last chemotherapy [79].

Outside the trial setting, current strategy is to offer combination chemotherapy to all platinum-sensitive recurrent patients if it is not medically contraindicated. Patients are re-treated with platinum alone or platinum in combination with paclitaxel. Patients with partially platinum-sensitive disease are re-treated with platinum alongside paclitaxel or pegylated liposomal doxorubicin hydrochloride (PLDH). Patients who are allergic to platinum are offered single agent PLDH, topotecan or weekly chemotherapy with paclitaxel, although new strategies of replacing platinum with novel cytotoxics in combination with these agents have yielded promising results [80].

Platinum-resistant recurrence

There are various definitions of platinum-resistant recurrence; however, a pragmatic definition is one of recurrent disease requiring treatment within 6 months of completing last chemotherapy. These patients appear to benefit (or fail to benefit) equally from all conventionally dosed and scheduled chemotherapeutic agents. These monotherapies all have a 10–20% overall response rate. Agents that can be considered in this indication include PLDH, topotecan, oral etoposide, paclitaxel and gemcitabine. In this clinical scenario, however, dose-dense treatment with weekly paclitaxel and carboplatin has been shown to improve response rates in platinum-resistant patients. Combination studies using carboplatin and paclitaxel have been explored in non-randomized trials with impressive results. This includes the Rotterdam regimen [two courses (every 28 days) of weekly paclitaxel ($90\,mg/m^2$) and carboplatin given on days 1, 8 and 15, followed by six courses of 3-weekly paclitaxel ($175\,mg/m^2$) and carboplatin (AUC6)] [81] and the Leuven regimen [six courses of paclitaxel ($90\,mg/m^2$) and carboplatin (AUC 4) on days 1 and 8 every 3 weeks] [82]. These regimens were generally well tolerated with low haematological toxicity but prospective randomized trials comparing them to standard treatment are awaited.

Surgery and radiotherapy

The use of secondary surgery in recurrent ovarian cancer is controversial and lacking in a strong evidence base. Patients with malignant bowel obstruction should not be given chemotherapy in general, although these patients may benefit from a palliative surgical procedure to correct their bowel obstruction and enable them to continue with chemotherapy. If patients relapse with solitary recurrences, these can occasionally be completely resected and in these cases individual outcomes can be good. The German AGO group validated a model of three factors, the DESKTOP I Criteria, that predicted for successful secondary debulking: good performance status (ECOG 0), complete resection at primary surgery (or alternatively early FIGO stage at first diagnosis) and absence of ascites. In patients in whom all of these three features were present, complete resection was possible in 79%, conferring a median survival of 45.2 months versus 19.7 months in those who did not undergo complete resection [83]. In the ongoing DESKTOP II trial, this prognostic score is being prospectively validated in platinum-sensitive patients undergoing surgery, and in DESKTOP III patients will be prospectively randomized to surgery or no surgery on the basis of their score. These trials aim to definitively answer the question of whether repeat surgery is beneficial to patients with recurrent disease.

Radiotherapy is in general reserved for palliation of symptomatic disease particularly symptomatic pelvic recurrence, cutaneous and intracerebral disease.

Rarer cancers

Adult granulosa cell tumours

Granulosa cell tumours (GCTs) are sex cord-stromal tumours and represent 5% of all ovarian malignancies. They arise from stromal cells surrounding oocytes and typically present in patients with a mean age of 50–52 years. Presenting features may mimic those of epithelial ovarian cancer: bloating, abdominal pain, weight loss and postmenopausal bleeding (concurrent endometrial hyperplasia or endometrial adenocarcinoma occurs in 5–10% cases). Ovarian rupture can occur in 10–35% cases causing acute, severe abdominal pain. GCTs are of low malignant potential, the majority (60–90%) present at an early stage, with a 5-year survival (for stage I disease) of 90%. For those presenting at a more advanced stage, prognosis is poorer, the 5-year survival rates for stage II and stage III/IV are 55–75% and 22–50%, respectively [84]. Initial surgical staging is similar to that performed for EOC, the only caveat is that fertility-preserving surgery is more frequently considered in young patients with early-stage unilateral tumours in view of their good prognosis. The benefit of adjuvant chemotherapy is controversial, and postoperative chemotherapy is usually confined to those with advanced (stage IV) or inoperable disease or for whom surgery or radiotherapy is contraindicated. Chemotherapy is usually platinum-containing, such as PVB (cisplatin/vinblastine/bleomycin) or the better tolerated BEP (bleomycin, etoposide and cisplatin). Overall response to BEP (complete response plus partial response) in a series of three small studies was approximately 80% [85–87]. Taxanes have also been used with success in a small number of patients, with similar efficacy to BEP, suggesting that carboplatin and paclitaxel is a feasible chemotherapeutic alternative.

Granulosa cell tumours are oestradiol-producing, especially when confined to the ovary, so oestradiol and the follicle stimulating hormone (FSH) inhibitory substance, inhibin B, can act as tumour markers. More reliable markers are sought such as Müllerian inhibitory substance [88]. Late recurrence can occur in patients with GCTs, sometimes up to 25 years after their initial diagnosis. Histological factors in primary tumours that are predictive of recurrence include nuclear atypia, high mitotic index (≥ 4 mitoses per 10 high-power fields) and (controversially) tumour aneuploidy. Where possible, recurrent disease is managed surgically or using radiotherapy. Chemotherapy using BEP can be given for recurrent inoperable disease or hormonal therapy comprising tamoxifen or GnRH analogues.

Carcinosarcoma/mixed malignant Müllerian tumours of the ovary

Carcinosarcoma [also known as mixed malignant Müllerian tumours (MMMTs)] of the ovary comprises 1–5% of ovarian tumours in total, the majority presenting in postmenopausal women aged 50–70 years. The FIGO staging of these tumours adopts that used for ovarian epithelial tumours (see Table 57.1). Carcinosarcomas comprise mixed tumour tissue: an epithelial component (such as serous, endometrioid, undifferentiated or rarely clear cell, or squamous cell carcinoma) and a sarcomatous element. If the sarcomatous component appears to be native to the ovary, it is described as homologous (e.g. endometrial stromal sarcoma, fibrosarcoma or leiomyosarcoma), heterogeneous examples include rhabdomyosarcoma, chondrosarcoma or osteosarcoma. It is still contentious whether both elements arise from a similar source or converge from two different sources [89–91]. Sood *et al.* found that cancers with homologous sarcomatous elements had a better outcome than those that were heterologous [91], and patients bearing tumours in which the sarcomatous elements predominate have been shown to have a worse survival outcome [92]. Other negative prognostic indices include advanced stage at presentation, suboptimal debulking and older age. Patients typically present with abdominal distension and bloating, with >75% having stage III or IV disease at presentation.

Overall, stage-by-stage prognosis is worse than for EOC, with 50%, 100%, 90% and 100% recurrence rates for stage I, II, III and IV, respectively, and a median survival of 75 and <10 months for stage I and stages II–IV, respectively [93,94]. According to data collected in small retrospective studies, optimal cytoreduction followed by platinum-based chemotherapy results in improved progression-free survival. Chemotherapy consisting of carboplatin plus paclitaxel or cisplatin plus ifosfamide is given postoperatively, the latter regimen reporting a better overall survival rate, albeit with greater toxicity [95]. Given the generally poor response to chemotherapy, alternatives are being sought, such as trabectadin which is already licensed for use in advanced soft-tissue sarcomas.

Borderline ovarian cancer

Borderline ovarian tumours (BOTs) account for approximately 10–15% of all ovarian tumours, occur in patients aged 50–60 years and in 50–80% are confined to the ovary (stage I). The early stage at presentation and cellular characteristics of BOTs (they lack infiltrative destructive growth or stromal invasion) gives them an excellent prognosis. The most common histological type is serous (50% of cases), followed by mucinous (46% of cases) and mixed, endometrioid, clear cell or Brenner tumours (3.9% of cases). The epithelial ovarian FIGO staging is adopted for BOTs, which traditionally have been staged surgically in a similar way to that employed for epithelial ovarian cancer (with the addition of appendectomy in cases of mucinous BOTs). Serous BOTs are bilateral in 30% of cases and are associated with extraovarian lesions ('implants') in 35% of cases.

Implants are defined as non-invasive (with papillary structure) or invasive (with structure similar to that of a well-differentiated adenocarcinoma), serous BOTs with non-invasive implants have a lower relapse and mortality rate (18% and 6%, respectively) than those with invasive implants (36% and 25%, respectively). Mucinous BOTs are classified as intestinal (85%) or endocervical/Müllerian

(15%) depending on the histological characteristics of the cystic epithelial cells. In 10% of cases, mucinous BOTs can be associated with pseudomyoxoma peritonei, necessitating a thorough investigation of the gastrointestinal tract and appendix as a source of primary tumour.

The 5-year survival for serous and mucinous BOTs is 98.4 ± 1.1% and 97 ± 1.5%, respectively. For advanced (stage III/IV) disease, survival is 92.3 ± 3% and 85.5 ± 9% for serous and mucinous BOTs, respectively [96]. BOTs have traditionally been surgically managed in a similar way to EOC, with total abdominal hysterectomy, bilateral salpingo-oophrectomy, infracolic omentectomy, resection of macroscopic lesions, peritoneal biopsies and appendicetomy (if mucinous histology). Sytematic lymphadenectomy is now largely avoided owing to similar outcome for patients with or without lymph node involvement [97,98]. Owing to the excellent prognosis of patients with stage I disease, many surgeons now prefer to opt for more conservative fertility-sparing surgery in younger patients, comprising unilateral salpingo-oophrectomy, infracolic omentectomy, peritoneal biopsies and cytology.

There is no proven benefit for adjunctive radiotherapy or chemotherapy following surgery for BOTs, even with advanced disease. Risk factors for recurrence include DNA ploidy, stage, histological type and age. Recurrence occurs at a median time of 3.1 years and is treated surgically. Conservative surgery can again be considered in patients wishing to retain their fertility. In patients who recur with the presence of invasive implants, extensive surgery must be performed with the aim of optimally or completely debulking the tumour. A small percentage of patients with an initial diagnosis of BOT develop invasive ovarian/primary peritoneal cancer after a median time interval of 8.3 years. It is probable that this represents a new primary cancer rather than recurrence. The incidence of invasive malignancy is between 1% and 7% [99–102], although one study containing a high proportion of advanced stage or unstaged patients reported an incidence of 73% [103]. These patients should be treated with a combination of surgery and chemotherapy, as in primary invasive ovarian cancer.

Future developments

Developments in chemotherapy

The further development and refinement of cytotoxic chemotherapy combinations continues. A number of studies have addressed the benefit of adding an additional drug to the standard first-line treatment of carboplatin and paclitaxel. So far, none have demonstrated superiority. An example is the GOG182/ICON5 study, a five-arm phase III randomized trial in which treatment with paclitaxel and carboplatin was compared with paclitaxel and carboplatin given alongside gemcitabine, PLDH or topotecan in patients with advanced-stage disease. Progression-free and overall survival were similar in all arms, suggesting that the addition of another cytotoxic did not warrant the extra toxicity observed [104].

Increasingly, it is becoming clear that the histological heterogeneity of ovarian cancer has therapeutic importance with significantly inferior response outcomes observed for clear cell and mucinous carcinomas of the ovary. The same is also true for carcinosarcoma of the ovary. The JCOG has commenced a phase III clinical trial comparing cisplatin and irinotecan with paclitaxel–carboplatin in advanced clear cell carcinoma of the ovary. The Gynecologic Cancer Intergroup (GCIG) mEOC trial of chemotherapy for the first-line treatment of mucinous carcinoma of the ovary is also under way, utilizing a bowel cancer-type chemotherapy of oxaliplatin plus capecitabine in a randomized setting against paclitaxel–carboplatin.

The MITO-2 study addressed whether carboplatin and PLDH was as effective as carboplatin–paclitaxel as first-line chemotherapy for ovarian cancer and showed that there was non-superiority between the two regimens in terms of progression-free and overall survival [105]. The CALYPSO study looked at the combination of PLDH–carboplatin versus carboplatin–paclitaxel in patients with platinum-sensitive relapse. Preliminary results showed that the PLDH–carboplatin arm offered a superior therapeutic index (benefit/risk ratio) than carboplatin–paclitaxel. Although final results are awaited, this trial suggests that agents other than paclitaxel can be used along with carboplatin at platinum-sensitive relapse, particularly relevant for patients suffering from paclitaxel-induced neurotoxicity [106].

Novel cytotoxic agents have shown efficacy in relapsed ovarian cancer, such as trabectadin, which in the OVA-301 trial was used in combination with PLDH versus PLDH alone in patients who had progressed or recurred after first-line chemotherapy [80]. Interestingly, patients who derived most benefit from the trabectadin combination had relapsed within a 6–12-month time frame, normally considered a fairly treatment-resistant group [107]. Although more myelo- and hepatic toxicity was observed in the trabectadin-containing arm, this trial demonstrates that a non-platinum-containing regimen can be used in patients who are partially platinum-sensitive. It also raises interesting questions about the biological activity of this naturally derived substance, particularly as patients treated with trabectadin demonstrated a more durable response to carboplatin on subsequent relapse.

Biotherapeutic targets

PI3 kinase pathway
The phosphatidylinositol 3′-kinase (PI3K) cell-signalling pathway appears to be highly relevant in ovarian cancer. Mutation or amplifications in *PIK3CA*, the gene encoding PI3K, are found in approximately 30% of ovarian cancers. In addition, the tumour-suppressor gene and PI3K inhibitor, phosphatase and tensin homologue (PTEN) has been shown to be mutated in 20% of endometrioid ovarian cancers resulting in activation of the PI3K pathway via phosphorylation of an effector protein, Akt/protein kinase B (PKB). As a result, this pathway forms an attractive target for ovarian cancer treatment, particularly in chemotherapy resistance [108]. As a result, early clinical trials are currently under way using Akt and PI3K inhibitors in patients with relapsed ovarian cancer.

Angiogenesis inhibitors
Although GOG218 showed that the addition of bevacizumab gave only moderate progression-free survival advantage [57], other antiangiogenic agents are currently being assessed, such as the triple [VEGF, fibroblast growth factor (FGF) and platelet-derived growth factor (PDGF)] angiokinase inhibitor BIBF1120 (Vargatef™). In the AGO-OVAR12 study, BIBF1120 is given alongside and then after carboplatin and paclitaxel in the first-line treatment for ovarian cancer. In ICON 6, the VEGF inhibitor cediranib is given alongside and after chemotherapy for patients with platinum-sensitive relapse and, in AGO-OVAR 16, maintenance use of the multi-tyrosine kinase inhibitor pazopanib is trialled following first-line therapy. Along with results from ICON7, these trials will go some way to defining the role of angiogenesis inhibitors in the treatment of ovarian cancer.

Other targeted therapies
The impressive activity of the PARP inhibitor olaparib in patients with high-grade serous ovarian cancer has led to a number of studies using this and other PARP inhibitors either as single agents or in combination with cytotoxics [16].

Other therapeutic targets are emerging, such as the alpha folate receptor, which is overexpressed in the majority of patients with advanced ovarian cancer. Farletuzumab, a monoclonal antibody against this receptor, has demonstrated impressive activity in phase II clinical trials and phase III trials are under way [109]. Inhibitors of Src (sarcoma protein), the first tyrosine kinase to be identified have also shown impressive pre-clinical activity in ovarian cancer and clinical trials using the small molecule Src inhibitor dasatinib (Sprycel™), are currently ongoing [110]. Other targeted strategies to overcome antiapoptosis mechanisms in ovarian cancer are also being investigated, such via the tumour necrosis factor-related apoptosis-inducing ligand (TRAIL) pathway (reviewed in reference 111).

Summary

The management of ovarian cancer is complex by virtue of its insidious presentation, heterogeneous histology and often rapid development of chemotherapy resistance mechanisms. Despite this, improvements have been made in the 5-year survival over the last 20 years, reflecting advances in surgical technique and the use of more effective chemotherapeutic treatments, both upfront and in recurrence. However, ovarian cancer still remains the most lethal of gynaecological cancers, thus warranting exploration into novel therapeutic strategies. These include personalization of treatment according to histology and genetic profile (such as BRCA status) and the use of novel cytotoxics and targeted therapies. Underpinning these and future developments is an ongoing commitment to unravelling the basic cellular biology of ovarian cancer. Only then can therapies be rationally designed or improved to make a significant impact on the outcome of this most deadly of cancers.

References

1 Boyle P, Ferlay J. Cancer incidence and mortality in Europe, 2004. *Ann Oncol* 2005;16:481–488.

2 Parkin DM, Bray F, Ferlay J, Pisani P. Global cancer statistics, 2002. *CA Cancer J Clin* 2005;55:74–108.

3 Fathalla MF. Incessant ovulation – a factor in ovarian neoplasia? *Lancet* 1971;27716:163.

4 Berchuck A, Schildkraut J. Oral contraceptive pills. Prevention of ovarian cancer and other benefits. *N C Med J* 1997;58: 404–407.

5 CRUK website, 2010. Available at: http://info. cancerresearchuk.org/.

6 Beral V; Million Women Study Collaborators, Bull D, Green J, Reeves G. Ovarian cancer and hormone replacement therapy in the Million Women Study. *Lancet* 2007;369:1703–1710.

7 Reeves GK, Pirie K, Beral V, Green J, Spencer E, Bull D; Million Women Study Collaboration. Cancer incidence and mortality in relation to body mass index in the Million Women Study: cohort study. *BMJ* 2007;335:1134.

8 Parazzini F, Franceschi S, La Vecchia C, Fasoli M. The epidemiology of ovarian cancer. *Gynecol Oncol* 1991;43:9–23.

9 Ness RB. Endometriosis and ovarian cancer: thoughts on shared pathophysiology. *Am J Obstet Gynecol* 2003;189:280–294.

10 Quirk JT, Kupinski JM. Chronic infection, inflammation, and epithelial ovarian cancer. *Med Hypotheses* 2001;57:426–428.

11 Ness RB, Cottreau C. Possible role of ovarian epithelial inflammation in ovarian cancer. *J Natl Cancer Inst* 1999;91: 1459–1467.

12 Sogaard M, Kjaer SK, Gayther S. Ovarian cancer and genetic susceptibility in relation to the BRCA1 and BRCA2 genes. Occurrence, clinical importance and intervention. *Acta Obstet Gynecol Scand* 2006;85:93–105.

13 Turner N, Tutt A, Ashworth A. Hallmarks of 'BRCAness' in sporadic cancers. *Nat Rev Cancer* 2004;4:814–819.

14 Press JZ, De Luca A, Boyd N *et al*. Ovarian carcinomas with genetic and epigenetic BRCA1 loss have distinct molecular abnormalities. *BMC Cancer* 2008;22:17.

15 Fong PC, Yap TA, Boss DS *et al*. Poly(ADP)-ribose polymerase inhibition: frequent durable responses in BRCA carrier ovarian cancer correlating with platinum-free interval. *J Clin Oncol* 2010;28:2512–2519.

16 Audeh MW, Carmichael J, Penson RT *et al*. Oral poly(ADP-ribose) polymerase inhibitor olaparib in patients with BRCA1 or BRCA2 mutations and recurrent ovarian cancer: a proof-of-concept trial. *Lancet* 2010;376:245–251.

17 Kurman RJ, Shih IEM. The origin and pathogenesis of epithelial ovarian cancer: a proposed unifying theory. *Am J Surg Pathol* 2010;34:433–443.

18 Guidozzi F. Screening for ovarian cancer. *Obstet Gynecol Surv* 1996;51:696–701.

19 Menon U, Gentry-Maharaj A, Hallet R *et al*. Sensitivity and specificity of multimodal and ultrasound screening for ovarian cancer, and stage distribution of detected cancers: results of the prevalence screen of the UK Collaborative Trial of Ovarian Cancer Screening (UKCTOCS). *Lancet Oncol* 2009;10:327–340.

20 Rosenthal A, Jacobs I. Familial ovarian cancer screening. *Best Pract Res Clin Obstet Gynaecol* 2006;20:321–338.

21 Grubb RL 3rd, Pinsky PF, Greenlee RT *et al*. Prostate cancer screening in the Prostate, Lung, Colorectal and Ovarian cancer screening trial: update on findings from the initial four rounds of screening in a randomized trial. *BJU Int* 2008;102:1524–1530.

22 Olopade OI, Artioli G. Efficacy of risk-reducing salpingo-oophorectomy in women with BRCA-1 and BRCA-2 mutations. *Breast J* 2004;10(Suppl 1):S5–S9.

23 Armstrong K, Schwartz JS, Randall T, Rubin SC, Weber B. Hormone replacement therapy and life expectancy after prophylactic oophorectomy in women with BRCA1/2 mutations: a decision analysis. *J Clin Oncol* 2004;22:1045–1054.

24 Goff BA, Mandel LS, Melancon CH, Muntz, HG. Frequency of symptoms of ovarian cancer in women presenting to primary care clinics. *JAMA* 2004;291:2705–2712.

25 Andersen MR, Goff BA, Lowe KA *et al*. Use of a Symptom Index, CA125:and HE4 to predict ovarian cancer. *Gynecol Oncol* 2010;116:378–383.

26 Gourley C, Michie CC, Roxburgh P *et al*. Increased incidence of visceral metastases in Scottish patients with BRCA1/2-defective ovarian cancer: an extension of the ovarian BRCAness phenotype. *J Clin Oncol* 2010;28:2505–2511.

27 Rocconi RP, Matthews KS, Kemper MK, Hoskins KE, Hih WK, Straughn JM Jr. The timing of normalization of CA-125 levels during primary chemotherapy is predictive of survival in patients with epithelial ovarian cancer. *Gynecol Oncol* 2009;11: 242–245.

28 Rustin GJ, van der Burg ME, on behalf of MRC and EORTC collaborators. A randomized trial in ovarian cancer (OC) of early treatment of relapse based on CA125 level alone versus delayed treatment based on conventional clinical indicators (MRC OV05/EORTC. 55955 trials). *J Clin Oncol* 2009;27(Suppl): 18s, Abstract 1.

29 CRUK website 2010; CancerStats: Key Facts Ovarian Cancer. Available at: http://info.cancerresearchuk.org/cancerstats/types/ovary/.

30 Junor EJ, Hole DJ, McNulty L, Mason M, Young J. Specialist gynaecologists and survival outcome in ovarian cancer: a

Scottish national study of 1866 patients. *Br J Obstet Gynaecol* 1999;106:1130–1136.

31 van der Burg ME, Vergote I. The role of interval debulking surgery in ovarian cancer. *Curr Oncol Rep* 2003;5:473–481.

32 Dewdney SB, Rimel BJ, Reinhart AJ *et al*. The role of neoadjuvant chemotherapy in the management of patients with advanced stage ovarian cancer: Survey results from members of the Society of Gynecologic Oncologists. *Gynecol Oncol* 2010 [Epub ahead of print].

33 Van Gorp T, Amant F, Neven P, Berteloot P, Leunen K, Vergote I. The position of neoadjuvant chemotherapy within the treatment of ovarian cancer. *Minerva Ginecol* 2006;58:393–403.

34 McGuire WP, Hoskins WJ, Brady MF *et al*. Cyclophosphamide and cisplatin compared with paclitaxel and cisplatin in patients with stage III and stage IV ovarian cancer. *N Engl J Med* 1996;334:1–6.

35 Piccart MJ, Bertelsen K, James K *et al*. Randomized intergroup trial of cisplatin-paclitaxel versus cisplatin-cyclophosphamide in women with advanced epithelial ovarian cancer: three-year results. *J Natl Cancer Inst* 2000;92:699–708.

36 Muggia FM, Braly PS, Brady MF *et al*. Phase III randomized study of cisplatin versus paclitaxel versus cisplatin and paclitaxel in patients with suboptimal stage III or IV ovarian cancer: a Gynecologic Oncology Group study. *J Clin Oncol* 2000;18:106–115.

37 The International Collaborative Ovarian Neoplasm (ICON) Group. Paclitaxel plus carboplatin versus standard chemotherapy with either single-agent carboplatin or cyclophosphamide, doxorubicin, and cisplatin in women with ovarian cancer: the ICON3 randomized trial. *Lancet* 2002;360:505–515.

38 Bristow RE, Tomacruz RS, Armstrong DK, Trimble EL, Montz FJ. Survival effect of maximal cytoreductive surgery for advanced ovarian carcinoma during the platinum era: a meta-analysis. *J Clin Oncol* 2002;20:1248–1259.

39 du Bois A, Reuss A, Pujade-Lauraine E, Harter P, Ray-Coquard I, Pfisterer J. Role of surgical outcome as prognostic factor in advanced epithelial ovarian cancer: a combined exploratory analysis of 3 prospectively randomized phase 3 multicenter trials: by the Arbeitsgemeinschaft Gynaekologische Onkologie Studiengruppe Ovarialkarzinom (AGO-OVAR) and the Groupe d'Investigateurs Nationaux Pour les Etudes des Cancers de l'Ovaire (GINECO). *Cancer* 2009;115:1234–1244.

40 Crawford SC, Vasey PA, Paul J, Hay A, Davis JA, Kaye SB *et al*. Does aggressive surgery only benefit patients with less advanced ovarian cancer? Results from an international comparison within the SCOTROC-1 Trial. *J Clin Oncol* 2005;23: 8802–8811.

41 Chan JK, Urban R, Hu JM *et al*. The potential therapeutic role of lymph node resection in epithelial ovarian cancer: a study of 13918 patients. *Br J Cancer* 2007;96:1817–1822.

42 Maggioni A, Beneditti Panici P, Dell'Anna T *et al*. Randomised study of systematic lymphadenectomy in patients with epithelial ovarian cancer macroscopically confined to the pelvis. *Br J Cancer* 2006;95:699–704.

43 Suzuki S, Kajiyama H, Shibata K *et al*. Is there any association between retroperitoneal lymphadenectomy and survival benefit in ovarian clear cell carcinoma patients? *Ann Oncol* 2008;19:1284–1287.

44 Trimbos JB, Parmer M, Vergote I *et al*. International Collaborative Ovarian Neoplasm trial 1 and Adjuvant Chemotherapy In Ovarian Neoplasm trial: two parallel randomized phase III trials of adjuvant chemotherapy in patients with early-stage ovarian carcinoma. *J Natl Cancer Inst* 2003;95: 105–112.

45 Trimbos B, Timmers P, Pecorelli S *et al*. Surgical staging and treatment of early ovarian cancer: long-term analysis from a randomized trial. *J Natl Cancer Inst* 2010;102:982–987.

46 Panici PB, Maggioni A, Hacker N *et al*. Systematic aortic and pelvic lymphadenectomy versus resection of bulky nodes only in optimally debulked advanced ovarian cancer: a randomized clinical trial. *J Natl Cancer Inst* 2005;97:560–566.

47 Colombo PE, Mourregot A, Fabbro M *et al*. Aggressive surgical strategies in advanced ovarian cancer: a monocentric study of 203 stage IIIC and IV patients. *Eur J Surg Oncol* 2009;35: 135–143.

48 Le T, Faught W, Hopkins L, Fung-Kee-Fung M. Can surgical debulking reverse platinum resistance in patients with metastatic epithelial ovarian cancer? *J Obstet Gynaecol Can* 2009;31:42–47.

49 Rafii A, Deval B, Geay JF *et al*. Treatment of FIGO stage IV ovarian carcinoma: results of primary surgery or interval surgery after neoadjuvant chemotherapy: a retrospective study. *Int J Gynecol Cancer* 2007;17:777–783.

50 Vergote IB, De Wever I, Decloedt J, Tjalma W, Van Gramberen M, van Dam P. Neoadjuvant chemotherapy versus primary debulking surgery in advanced ovarian cancer. *Semin Oncol* 2000;27(3 Suppl 7):31–36.

51 Vergote IB, Tropé CG, Amant F *et al*. EORTC-GCG/NCIC-CTG Randomized trial comparing primary debulking surgery with neoadjuvant chemotherapy in stage IIIC-IV ovarian, fallopian tube and peritoneal cancer (OVCA). *IGCS* 2008; Abstract 1767

52 Rose PG, Nerenstone S, Brady MF *et al*; Gynecologic Oncology Group. Secondary surgical cytoreduction for advanced ovarian carcinoma. *N Engl J Med* 2004;351:2489–2497.

53 Redman CW, Warwick J, Luesley DM, Varma R, Lawton FG, Blackledge GR. Intervention debulking surgery in advanced epithelial ovarian cancer. *Br J Obstet Gynaecol* 1994;101: 142–146.

54 van der Burg ME, van Lent M, Buyse M *et al*. The effect of debulking surgery after induction chemotherapy on the prognosis in advanced epithelial ovarian cancer. Gynaecological Cancer Cooperative Group of the European Organisation for Research and Treatment of Cancer. *N Engl J Med* 1995;332: 629–634.

55 Kehoe S, Powell J, Wilson S, Woodman C. The influence of the operating surgeon's specialization on patient survival in ovarian carcinoma. *Br J Cancer*. 1994;70:1014–1017.

56 Martinek IE, Kehoe S. When should surgical cytoreduction in advanced ovarian cancer take place? *J Oncol* 2010.

57 Burger R, Brady MF, Bookman JL *et al*. Phase III trial of bevacizumab (BEV) in the primary treatment of advanced epithelial ovarian cancer (EOC), primary peritoneal cancer (PPC), or fallopian tube cancer (FTC):A Gynecologic Oncology Group study. *J Clin Oncol* 2010;28:18s.

58 Katsumata N, Yasuda M, Takahashi F *et al*; Japanese Gynecologic Oncology Group. Dose-dense paclitaxel once a week in combination with carboplatin every 3 weeks for advanced ovarian cancer: a phase 3, open-label, randomized controlled trial. *Lancet* 2009;374:1331–1338.

59 Hess V, A'Hern R, Nasiri N et al. Mucinous epithelial ovarian cancer: a separate entity requiring specific treatment. J Clin Oncol 2004;22:1040–1044.

60 Sirichaisutdhikorn D, Suprasert P, Khunamornpong S. Clinical outcome of the ovarian clear cell carcinoma compared to other epithelial ovarian cancers when treated with paclitaxel and carboplatin. Asian Pac J Cancer Prev 2009;10:1041–1045.

61 Bertelsen K, Jakobsen A, Strøyer J et al. A prospective randomized comparison of 6 and 12 cycles of cyclophosphamide, adriamycin, and cisplatin in advanced epithelial ovarian cancer: a Danish Ovarian Study Group trial (DACOVA). Gynecol Oncol 1993;49:30–36.

62 Lambert HE, Rustin GJ, Gregory WM, Nelstrop AE. A randomized trial of five versus eight courses of cisplatin or carboplatin in advanced epithelial ovarian carcinoma. A North Thames Ovary Group Study. Ann Oncol 1997;8:327–333.

63 Pecorelli S, Favalli G, Gadducci A et al; After 6 Italian Cooperative Group. Phase III trial of observation versus six courses of paclitaxel in patients with advanced epithelial ovarian cancer in complete response after six courses of paclitaxel/platinum-based chemotherapy: final results of the After-6 protocol 1. J Clin Oncol 2009;27:4642–4648.

64 McGuire WP, Hoskins WJ, Brady MF et al. Assessment of dose-intensive therapy in suboptimally debulked ovarian cancer: a Gynecologic Oncology Group study. J Clin Oncol 1995;13:1589–1599.

65 Kaye SB, Paul J, Cassidy J et al. Mature results of a randomized trial of two doses of cisplatin for the treatment of ovarian cancer. Scottish Gynaecology Cancer Trials Group. J Clin Oncol 1996;14:2113–2119.

66 Jakobsen A, Bertelsen K, Andersen JE et al. Dose-effect study of carboplatin in ovarian cancer: a Danish Ovarian Cancer Group study. J Clin Oncol. 1997;15:193–198.

67 Gore M, Mainwaring P, A'Hern R et al. Randomized trial of dose-intensity with single-agent carboplatin in patients with epithelial ovarian cancer. London Gynaecological Oncology Group. J Clin Oncol 1998;16:2426–2434.

68 Cocconi G, Bella M, Lottici R et al. Mature results of a prospective randomized trial comparing a three-weekly with an accelerated weekly schedule of cisplatin in advanced ovarian carcinoma. Am J Clin Oncol 1999;22:559–567.

69 Conte PF, Bruzzone M, Carnino F et al. High-dose versus low-dose cisplatin in combination with cyclophosphamide and epidoxorubicin in suboptimal ovarian cancer: a randomized study of the Gruppo Oncologico Nord-Ovest. J Clin Oncol 1996;14:351–356.

70 Cure H, Legros M, Fleury J et al. High-dose chemotherapy and autologous stem cell transplantation in advanced epithelial ovarian cancer. Bone Marrow Transplant 1996;18(Suppl 1):S34–S35.

71 Ledermann JA, Herd R, Maraninchi D et al. High-dose chemotherapy for ovarian carcinoma: long-term results from the Solid Tumour Registry of the European Group for Blood and Marrow Transplantation (EBMT). Ann Oncol 2001;12:693–699.

72 Legros M, Dauplat J, Fleury J et al. High-dose chemotherapy with haematopoietic rescue in patients with stage III to IV ovarian cancer: long-term results. J Clin Oncol 1997;15:1302–1308.

73 Lim MC, Song YJ, Seo SS, Yoo CW, Kang S, Park SY. Residual cancer stem cells after interval cytoreductive surgery following neoadjuvant chemotherapy could result in poor treatment outcomes for ovarian cancer. Onkologie 2010;33:324–330.

74 Elit L, Oliver TK, Covens A et al. Intraperitoneal chemotherapy in the first-line treatment of women with stage III epithelial ovarian cancer: a systematic review with metaanalyses. Cancer 2007;109:692–702.

75 Armstrong DK, Bundy B, Wenzel L et al; Gynecologic Oncology Group. Intraperitoneal cisplatin and paclitaxel in ovarian cancer. N Engl J Med 2006;354:34–43.

76 Rowan K. Intraperitoneal therapy for ovarian cancer: why has it not become standard? J Natl Cancer Inst 2009;101:775–777.

77 Blackledge G, Lawton F, Redman C, Kelly K. Response of patients in phase II studies of chemotherapy in ovarian cancer: implications for patient treatment and the design of phase II trials. Br J Cancer. 1989;59:650–653.

78 Eisenhauer EA, Vermorken JB, van Glabbeke M. Predictors of response to subsequent chemotherapy in platinum pretreated ovarian cancer: a multivariate analysis of 704 patients. Ann Oncol 1997;8:963–968.

79 Parmar MK, Ledermann JA, Colombo N et al; ICON and AGO Collaborators. Paclitaxel plus platinum-based chemotherapy versus conventional platinum-based chemotherapy in women with relapsed ovarian cancer: the ICON4/AGO-OVAR-2.2 trial. Lancet. 2003;361:2099–2106.

80 Kaye SB, Colombo N, Monk BJ et al. Trabectedin plus pegylated liposomal doxorubicin in relapsed ovarian cancer delays third-line chemotherapy and prolongs the platinum-free interval. Ann Oncol 2010 [Epub ahead of print].

81 van der Burg ME, van der Gaast A, Vergote I et al. What is the role of dose-dense therapy? Int J Gynecol Cancer 2005;15(Suppl 3):233–240.

82 Cadron I, Leunen K, Amant F, Van Gorp T, Neven P, Vergote I. The 'Leuven' dose-dense paclitaxel/carboplatin regimen in patients with recurrent ovarian cancer. Gynecol Oncol 2007;106:354–361.

83 Harter P, du Bois, Hahmann M et al; Arbeitsgemeinschaft Gynaekologische Onkologie Ovarian Committee; AGO Ovarian Cancer Study Group. Surgery in recurrent ovarian cancer: the Arbeitsgemeinschaft Gynaekologische Onkologie (AGO) DESKTOP OVAR trial. Ann Surg Oncol 2006;13:1702–1710.

84 Pectasides D, Pectasides E, Psyrri A. Granulosa cell tumour of the ovary. Cancer Treat Rev 2008;34:1–12.

85 Savage P, Costenla D, Fisher C et al. Granulosa cell tumours of the ovary: demographics, survival and the management of advanced disease. Clin Oncol (R Coll Radiol) 1998;10:242–245.

86 Pectasides D, Alevizakos N, Athanassiou AE. Cisplatin-containing regimen in advanced or recurrent granulosa cell tumours of the ovary. Ann Oncol 1992;3(4):316–318.

87 Colombo N, Sessa C, Landoni F, Sartori E, Pecorelli S, Mangioni C. Cisplatin, vinblastine, and bleomycin combination chemotherapy in metastatic granulosa cell tumour of the ovary. Obstet Gynecol 1986;67:265–268.

88 La Marca A, Volpe A. The anti-Müllerian hormone and ovarian cancer. Hum Reprod Update 2007;13:265–273.

89 Jin Z, Ogata S, Tamura G et al. Carcinosarcomas (malignant mullerian mixed tumours) of the uterus and ovary: a genetic study with special reference to histogenesis. Int J Gynecol Pathol 2003;22:368–373.

90 Schipf A, Mayr D, Kirchner T, Diebold J. Molecular genetic aberrations of ovarian and uterine carcinosarcomas – a CGH and FISH study. *Virchows Arch* 2008;452:259–268.

91 Sood AK, Sorosky JI, Gelder MS *et al*. Primary ovarian sarcoma: analysis of prognostic variables and the role of surgical cytoreduction. *Cancer* 1998;82:1731–1737.

92 Nayha V, Stenback F. Angiogenesis and expression of angiogenic agents in uterine and ovarian carcinosarcomas. *APMIS* 2008;116:107–117.

93 Cantrell LA, Van Le L. Carcinosarcoma of the ovary a review. *Obstet Gynecol Surv* 2009;64:673–680.

94 Brown E, Stewart M, Rye T *et al*. Carcinosarcoma of the ovary: 19 years of prospective data from a single centre. *Cancer* 2004;100:2148–2153.

95 Rutledge TL, Gold MA, McMeekin DS *et al*. Carcinosarcoma of the ovary – a case series. *Gynecol Oncol* 2006;100:128–132.

96 Cadron I, Leunen K, Van G pT, Amant F, Neven P, Vergote I. Management of borderline ovarian neoplasms. *J Clin Oncol* 2007;25:2928–37.

97 Camatte S, Morice P, Thoury A *et al*. Impact of surgical staging in patients with macroscopic 'stage I' ovarian borderline tumours: analysis of a continuous series of 101 cases. *Eur J Cancer* 2004;40:1842–1849.

98 Desfeux P, Camatte S, Chantallier G, Blanc B, Querleu D, Lécuru F. Impact of surgical approach on the management of macroscopic early ovarian borderline tumors. *Gynecol Oncol* 2005;98:390–395.

99 Silva EG, Tornos C, Zhuang Z, Merino MJ, Gershenson DM. Tumour recurrence in stage I ovarian serous neoplasms of low malignant potential. *Int J Gynecol Pathol* 1998;17:1–6.

100 Camatte S, Morice P, Atallah D *et al*. Clinical outcome after laparoscopic pure management of borderline ovarian tumours: results of a series of 34 patients. *Ann Oncol* 2004;15:605–609.

101 Crispens MA, Bordurka D, Deavers M, Lu K, Silva EG, Gershenson D. Response and survival in patients with progressive or recurrent serous ovarian tumors of low malignant potential. *Obstet Gynecol* 2002;99:3–10.

102 Kehoe S, Powell J. Long-term follow-up of women with borderline ovarian tumours. *Int J Gynaecol Obstet* 1996;53:139–143.

103 Zanetta G, Rota S, Chiari S, Bonazzi C, Bratina G, Mangioni C. Behavior of borderline tumors with particular interest to persistence, recurrence, and progression to invasive carcinoma: a prospective study. *J Clin Oncol* 2001;19:2658–2664.

104 Bookman MA. GOG0182-ICON5: 5-arm phase III randomized trial of paclitaxel (P) and carboplatin (C) vs combinations with gemcitabine (G), PEG-lipososomal doxorubicin (D), or topotecan (T) in patients (pts) with advanced-stage epithelial ovarian (EOC) or primary peritoneal (PPC) carcinoma. *J Clin Oncol* 2006;24:No. 18S, Abstract 5002

105 Pignata S, Scambia G, Savarese A *et al*. Carboplatin and pegylated liposomal doxorubicin for advanced ovarian cancer: preliminary activity results of the MITO-2 phase III trial. *Oncology* 2009;76:49–54.

106 Pujade-Lauraine E, Mahner S, Kaern J *et al*. A randomized, phase III study of carboplatin and pegylated liposomal doxorubicin versus carboplatin and paclitaxel in relapsed platinum-sensitive ovarian cancer (OC):CALYPSO study of the Gynecologic Cancer Intergroup (GCIG). *J Clin Oncol* 2009; 27:18s.

107 Poveda A, Vergote I, Tjulandin S *et al*. Trabectedin plus pegylated liposomal doxorubicin in relapsed ovarian cancer: outcomes in the partially platinum-sensitive (platinum-free interval 6–12 months) subpopulation of OVA-301 phase III randomized trial. *Ann Oncol* 2011;22:39–48.

108 Dent P, Grant S, Fisher PB, Curiel DT. PI3K: A rational target for ovarian cancer therapy? *Cancer Biol Ther* 2009;8: 27–30.

109 White AJ, Coleman RL, Armstrong DK *et al*. Efficacy and safety of farletuzumab, a humanised monoclonal antibody to folate receptor alpha, in platinum-sensitive relapsed ovarian cancer subjects: Final data from a multicenter phase II study. *J Clin Oncol* 2010;28:15s.

110 Le XF, Mao W, Lu Z, Carter BZ, Bast RC Jr. Dasatinib induces autophagic cell death in human ovarian cancer. *Cancer* 2010; 116:4980–4990.

111 Bevis KS, Buchsbaum DJ, Straughn JM Jr. Overcoming TRAIL resistance in ovarian carcinoma. *Gynecol Oncol* 2010;119: 157–163.

Chapter 58
Endometrial Cancer

Sean Kehoe

Oxford Gynaecological Cancer Centre, Churchill Hospital, Oxford, UK

Introduction

Endometrial cancer is becoming the most common of the gynaecological malignancies in the developed world (Fig. 58.1). In the UK, the indications are that within the next 2–3 years, the numbers of cases will exceed those of ovarian cancer. Some plausible explanations include the overall increased life expectancy, obesity and also the reduction in death rates from other related malignancies – breast cancer in particular. While the disease affects mainly postmenopausal women, approximately 20% of cases occur in pre-menopausal women. Because of these factors, there has been greater attention paid to endometrial cancer, and in recent years pivotal randomized controlled trials in the surgical and non-surgical approaches to care have been reported. Another major event has been the updated International Federation of Gynecology and Obstetrics (FIGO) staging, which was introduced in late 2009 [1] and has inevitably required a certain transitional time of accommodation to clinical practice while the information from trials using the old staging is transferred to the new system. This chapter will endeavour to overview present day evidence-based care and possible future challenges.

Aetiology

There are recognized risk factors for endometrial cancer, shown in Table 58.1. Besides these, there are other environmental factors which influence the disease, as suggested by the variation in the disease in different countries (Fig. 58.2). The main relationship to risk is excess exposure of the endometrium to oestrogen – which has a direct association with both obesity and diabetes. The other factors such as older age and hypertension are interrelated with the above. Age remains the main risk factor, with most cases occurring in women over the age of 50 years.

Genetics

There is only one condition specifically identified with a genetic hereditary relationship with the development of endometrial carcinoma. Known both as hereditary non-polyposis colonic carcinoma, or Lynch type II syndrome, which is an autosomal dominant condition. The main associated primary malignancy is colonic carcinoma – normally developing in women under the age of 40 years. The Amsterdam criteria are used to define those families who conform to the definition of this condition, with the final diagnosis genetically a variety mutations, of which MSH2 and MLH1 are the commonest [2].

In such families, the lifetime risk of developing endometrial carcinoma is about 40%, and relevant is the fact that the life-time risk of developing ovarian cancer is 12%, nearly 10 times the population risk. In such women, the role of screening remains unknown. A small series of women with this condition did undergo annual scans and endometrial sampling, with the final conclusion that such an approach seemed to detect earlier cancers, suggesting that screening may be beneficial. However, the paucity of cases makes this very much an assumption, although the approach is an acceptable manner of managing these patients when there is a desire to retain reproductive function. An alternative strategy is to use preventative modalities. A possible alternative undergoing evaluation is the potential protective effect of progesterones – in the form of the Mirena intrauterine system [3,4]. This is within the context of clinical trials and the results will be awaited with interest. When the woman's family is completed, a hysterectomy is a reasonable course of action. This removes any need for ongoing screening for endometrial cancer. The increased risk of ovarian cancer may also justify removal of the ovaries, although each situation must be managed in accordance with the patient's needs and situation.

Dewhurst's Textbook of Obstetrics & Gynaecology, Eighth Edition. Edited by D. Keith Edmonds.

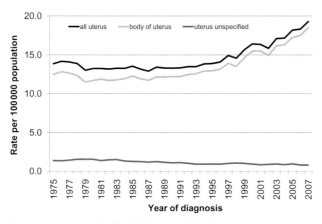

Fig. 58.1 Age-standardized (European) incidence rates, uterus cancer, by sex, UK, 1975–2007.

Table 58.1 Risk factors for endometrial cancer.

High levels of oestrogen/endometrial hyperplasia
Obesity/hypertension/diabetes
Polycystic ovary syndrome [3]
Nulliparity (never having carried a pregnancy)
Tamoxifen use/breast cancer
Postmenopausal
Hereditary non-polyposis colonic carcinoma

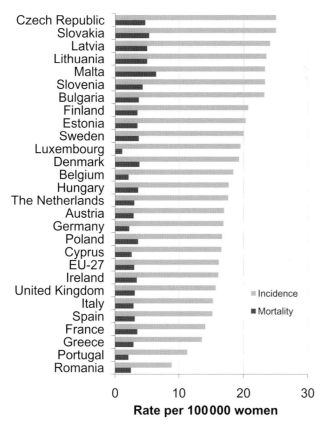

Fig. 58.2 Age-standardized (European) incidence and mortality rates, body of uterus cancer, EU-27, 2008 estimates.

Nulliparity

Nulliparity is associated with the risk of endometrial cancer. However, this may also be a multifactorial factor and have some relationship to the individual's hormonal profile during life. Nulliparous women have a significantly increased number of endometrial shedding events during their menstrual lives compared with parous women. In ovarian cancer, the direct association of the life-time number of ovulatory cycles and ovarian cancer risk (the higher the ovulatory cycles the greater the risk) could be also applied to endometrial cancer risk. The follicular phase of the cycle, increasing proliferation (which increases the probability of abnormal cellular development) and strategies which reduce this may protect against abnormal mitosis. While this is a theory still to be proven in endometrial cancer, it is a reasonable hypothesis. Of course, the use of the combined oral contraceptive – even with menstruation – affords some long-term protection (a risk reduction of 50%), lending support to the theory.

Obesity

Obesity is thought to be related to the development of about 30% of cancers in humans. In obese women, excess oestrogen is produced by the conversion of androgens in the fat, and thus the endometrial tissue has increased oestrone exposure. This is particularly pertinent considering the increased incidence of obesity in the Western world and the concomitant increased rates of endometrial cancer.

Endometrial hyperplasia

Hyperplasia is defined as excessive proliferation of normal cells. There are three types – simple, complex and atypical. Both simple and complex are premalignant conditions and the rate of developing invasive malignancy is less than a 3%. Atypical hyperplasia is more sinister. In a number of series, the risk of underlying malignancy has been shown to be higher than expected. A Gynecologic Oncology Group (GOG) study of 348 women diagnosed with atypical hyperplasia on sampling were eventually found to have a frank malignancy in 46.8% of cases. Specimens from around the world were centralized, with evaluation of the endometrial and hysterectomy specimens performed by independent expert histopathologists. So, it may be preferable to consider these patients as having endometrial cancer and thus expedite surgery.

Clinical presentation

Most women with endometrial cancer present in the postmenopausal years, with postmenopausal bleeding being the initial clinical symptom. Up to 10% of these women will have a diagnosis of endometrial cancer, and as such their access to diagnostics must be deemed urgent. The final diagnosis is confirmed by histology. Based on the UK NICE (National Institute of Clinical Evidence) guidelines, all women who have postmenopausal bleeding should have transvaginal ultrasound and an endometrial thickness greater than 5 mm should undergo sampling of the endometrium. However, many use a cut-off of 4 mm based on the cost-efficacy and detection rates. Sampling can be undertaken in three ways – pipelle, outpatient hysteroscopy or hysteroscopy, and curettage under a general anaesthetic. All methods of sampling will miss some cancers, but the rate of failure is not significantly different between outpatient sampling and hysterectomy. Naturally, avoiding a general anaesthetic is preferable where possible.

Abnormal bleeding in premenopausal women, particularly intermenstrual bleeding in those aged over 45 years, should prompt endometrial sampling. While the overall incidence of malignancy in this group is small, around 20–25% of all endometrial cancers occur in this age group.

Table 58.2 Endometrial cancer types.

Type I	Pre- and perimenopausal women
	History of unopposed oestrogen exposure
	Endometrial hyperplasia
	Minimally invasive
	Low-grade endometrioid type
Type II	Postmenopausal women
	Not associated with increased exposure to oestrogen
	High-grade tumours
	Poorer prognosis
	Good prognosis

Table 58.3 Histological subtypes in endometrial cancer.

Type	% of cases
Endometrioid adenocarcinoma	50–60
Adenosquamous	6–8
Serous papillary	18
Sarcomas/leiomyosarcomas	3–5
Carcinosarcomas	2–3
Clear cell	1–6

Summary box 58.1

- Endometrial cancer is primarily a disease of postmenopausal women, usually presenting with vaginal bleeding.
- A total of 20–25% of cancers will occur in the premenopausal population, usually presenting with erratic vaginal bleeding.
- A transvaginal scan is mandatory to assess endometrial thickness and triage of patients for endometrial sampling.
- Patients with endometrial hyperplasia have about a 50% chance of an underlying malignancy.

Types of endometrial cancer

Recently, endometrial cancers have been categorized into two cohorts –type I and type II disease. The factors associated with these are shown in Table 58.2.

The main histological subtypes are shown in Table 58.3 and some of these conditions may well be related to certain agents. In particular, the use of adjuvant tamoxifen in breast cancer has been proposed to be associated with some of the rarer tumours such as mixed Müllerian tumours – now called carcinosarcomas. There are no specific indicators regarding the other subtypes. Leiomyosarcomas are normally an unexpected finding following removal of a fibroid uterus. The mitotic activity of these tumours relates to their metastatic potential, with mitotic counts of <5 per high-power field associated with a very good outcome, whereas when the count is >10 per high power field the prognosis worsens. Other subtypes

recognized as more aggressive include papillary serous and clear cell tumours, accounting for 10–15% of all tumour types. In most cases, adjuvant therapies (after surgery) would be considered.

In some rare cases of sarcomas, preoperative diagnosis, normally cannon-ball metastases, may be suspected where the endometrial sampling indicates or a preoperative chest X-ray shows evidence of metastatic disease. The differentiation of the disease is also important in that grade will influence with other factors the recommendation for adjuvant therapy (or not).

Management

Preoperative investigations

The FIGO staging for endometrial cancer is shown in Table 58.4. This was redefined in 2009, with positive cytology, previously allocated to stage III disease, now abandoned as part of the staging process. It is, though, recommended to continue to collect peritoneal washings for cytological evaluation. As part of staging, there are agreed preoperative investigations which can be performed. A chest X-ray is mandatory. Magnetic resonance imaging/computed tomography (MRI/CT) scans can be undertaken and in some situations may be of value to ascertain any extrauterine disease. The value of MRI in

Table 58.4 Carcinoma of the endometrium, International Federation of Gynecology and Obstetrics (FIGO) staging 2010.

Stage	Description	5-year survival
IA	Tumour confined to the uterus, no or < ½ myometrial invasion	80–90% (I)
IB	Tumour confined to the uterus, > ½ myometrial invasion	–
II	Cervical stromal invasion, but not beyond uterus	60–70% (II)
IIIA	Tumour invades serosa or adnexa	50–60% (III)
IIIB	Vaginal and/or parametrial involvement	–
IIIC1	Pelvic node involvement	–
IIIC2	Para-aortic involvement	–
IVA	Tumour invasion bladder and/or bowel mucosa	10–20%(IV)
IVB	Distant metastases including abdominal metastases and/or inguinal lymph nodes	–

Table 58.5 Lymph node metastases in endometrial cancer.

Variable	Pelvic/para-aortic nodal disease (%)
<50% uterine invasion and grade 1	0–3
<50% uterine invasion and grade II/III	2–6
>50% uterine invasion and grade I	15–18
>50% uterine invasion and grade II/III	Up to 30

defining the depth of tumour invasion has been examined (which could be useful information regarding the need to excise lymph nodes) but have proved too inaccurate to be of clinical value.

Besides these investigations, cystoscopy, sigmoidoscopy and an examination under anaesthetic are all permitted as staging procedures. Notably, endometrial cancer can be staged both clinically and surgically, with surgical staging been most commonly employed.

Surgical interventions

Surgery remains the main primary intervention in endometrial cancer. While radiotherapy is an alternative, from retrospective case–control studies it would seem that surgery affords a better survival outcome. It is unlikely that there will ever be an RCT comparing primary radiotherapy to surgery, and thus such analyses will remain the basis of care.

The removal of the uterus and (normally) the ovaries is the recommended basic surgical procedure. This may be performed by open laparotomy or a laparoscopic approach. Studies have shown the advantages regarding short- and long-term recovery when the laparoscopic approach is taken, which may entail either a laparoscopic-assisted vaginal hysterectomy or a laparoscopic total hysterectomy [5,6]. Obviously, it is recommended not to insert any instruments into the uterine cavity during such surgery. Also clamping/ligating the fallopian tubes at commencement of surgery would seem a reasonable action to prevent any disease dissemination when moving or handling the uterus.

In some circumstances, the procedure could be performed vaginally, and indeed, this is acceptable as long as the ovaries can be removed, and some peritoneal washing obtained. However, a vaginal-only approach will not permit access to the pelvic lymphatics, thus limiting this type of surgery to selected patients.

Lymphadenectomy in endometrial cancer

The risk of lymphatic spread in endometrial cancer is influenced by the tumour grade, type and the depth of invasion into the uterine wall (Table 58.5). Knowledge of lymphatic disease forms part of the staging process and can influence adjuvant therapy. However, debate still surrounds the value of routine pelvic and para-aortic lymphadenectomy, and randomized trials are required to resolve this issue.

There has only been one prospective randomized trial reported on lymphadenectomy in endometrial cancer. This study, called ASTEC (A Surgical Trial in Endometrial Cancer), randomized over 1400 women with clinically early-stage disease [7]. The study included two parts: (i) patients randomized to pelvic lymphadenectomy or not, and (ii) patients randomized to adjuvant pelvic radiotherapy or not in high-risk cases. The use of brachytherapy [8] was permitted and the decision about whether this was used was made locally. The patient cohort receiving radiotherapy were not necessarily those recruited to the surgical aspects of the study. The conclusions were interesting in that the use of lymphadenectomy did not alter survival rates, and indeed there was the suggestion that it may have a negative impact on outcome, for reasons yet to be explained. Also, the number of lymph nodes retrieved did not influence outcome. Although the study was confined to patients with disease localized to the uterus (based on clinical examination and imaging in some cases), it does indicate that lymphadenectomy should not be undertaken in this group of patients.

Lymphadenectomy and non-randomized studies

There are many non-randomized reports on the role of pelvic and para-aortic lymphadenectomy nodes in endometrial cancer. All these studies naturally suffer from the fact that there are not randomized controlled trials. From some groups, the proposal is that para-aortic nodal excision in particular has a therapeutic effect, based on the fact that those who undergo this therapy have longer survival and a notable reduction in relapsed disease affecting the para-aortic regions [9]. Also, such resection permits either the avoidance of adjuvant radiotherapy in some cases, and identifies those in whom the radiotherapy field can be extended to incorporate the para-aortic region. The main problem with these debates remains the lack of appropriate high-level evidence base that such lymphadenectomy has a real therapeutic effect in relation to survival, and indeed that extension of the field of radiotherapy also enhances survival. Without doubt, both these procedures will entail an increase in morbidity. There is an urgent need to address this issue and ensure that patients are being managed in a manner whereby the morbidity of the intervention can be justified by the improved patient outcome. It can be anticipated that such trials will be undertaken in the near future.

Debulking in advanced disease

When the disease has obvious macroscopic spread beyond the uterus or indeed the pelvis, then multimodal therapy will be required, be this surgery to alleviate symptoms followed by radiotherapy with or without chemotherapy. The combination of chemoradiotherapy increases morbidity, and in endometrial cancer this poses major challenges as many patients have other comorbidities whereby such a combination may be deemed inappropriate. Debulking surgery, an approach taken in ovarian cancer for some decades, has been reported in some small series in endometrial cancer with a suggestion that a smaller residual tumour load correlated with a better survival outcome. This is based primarily on retrospective data or small case–control studies, and the evidence for this is very poor. There is no agreement that this should be considered in the accepted therapy for endometrial cancer at present. However, even in advanced disease, removal of the uterus may yield immediate alleviation of symptoms such as persistent vaginal bleeding, which could justify the intervention.

Fertility-sparing surgery

As women are increasingly delaying having children, the issue regarding fertility-sparing options have become more common, and this is relevant to many other malignancies. There are limited publications relating to such management and the number of cases is small, making it difficult to form firm conclusions. Longer-term outcomes are equally lacking and as such, before embarking on this therapeutic option, it is imperative to provide the patient with counselling about the present information and the 'unknown' risks, particularly as this is a deviation from the normal recommended intervention, which could potentially exclude the patient from a recommended curative therapy.

In those cases reported, the disease was always well differentiated and on clinical and imaging evaluations was confined to the uterus, that is FIGO stage I. Women were then exposed to various progestagenic agents, with careful evaluation of response by curettage, at 6 weeks, 3 months and 6 months from commencement of therapy [10]. Evidence of non-response resulted in immediate surgery and in those with response some pregnancies are reported. A hysterectomy was normally performed following a successful pregnancy.

Radiotherapy

Primary

Radiotherapy can be used either as a primary or adjuvant therapy. In primary therapy, this is normally where disease spread renders surgery impossible or inappropriate. It is not considered to be superior to surgical intervention, with an estimated reduction in 5-year survival of about 5% when compared with surgery in early-stage disease, although this is based on retrospective series.

Adjuvant

The use of radiotherapy in an adjuvant setting continues to be modified. Original studies indicated that the use of brachytherapy with external beam pelvic radiotherapy may be beneficial in those with high-grade disease. This original study from the 1980s by Aalders *et al.* [11] randomized 540 patients with early-stage disease to brachytherapy versus brachytherapy and external beam therapy after undergoing surgery. The relapse rates in the latter group was reduced, although overall 5-year survival was equivalent in both groups. Further analysis suggested that patients with grade III tumours infiltrating >50% of the myometrium might benefit from the addition of pelvic radiotherapy.

Two recent trials, the Postoperative Radiotherapy in Endometrial Cancer (PORTEC) and ASTEC trials, have changed the role of adjuvant radiotherapy [8,12]. In the PORTEC study, 715 women with stage I disease were recruited and randomized to pelvic radiotherapy versus

---

> ### Summary box 58.2
>
> - FIGO staging was revised in recent years [1].
> - Surgery remains the main primary intervention in early-stage endometrial cancer.
> - Routine pelvic lymphadenectomy in early-stage endometrial cancer does not alter outcome [7].
> - Fertility-sparing surgery is feasible in a highly selected patient group with early-stage grade I disease.

no treatment after undergoing a hysterectomy and bilateral salpingo-oophorectomy. The 5-year survival rates were 81% and 85%, respectively. The recurrence rates were lower in the radiotherapy groups (4% vs. 14%), but in those relapsing and then receiving radiotherapy the survival was the same. Analysis showed that radiotherapy was not necessary in women with stage I endometrial cancer who were under 60 years of age with Grade I or II tumours and with <50% myometrial invasion.

The ASTEC study had two parts where patient were randomized and then received external beam therapy to the pelvis. All had undergone surgery consisting of at least a total hysterectomy and bilateral salpingo-oophorectomy. The conclusions were that the routine use of external beam with brachytherapy reduced the incidence of recurrent disease and increased the disease-free survival, but did not have any positive impact on overall survival. The authors also suggested that there may possible a survival benefit in those with high-grade disease.

Chemotherapy

When distant metastatic disease is present, systemic treatments are required. For endometrial cancer, chemotherapeutic agents or hormonal therapies are used. Cisplatin and doxorubin are the commonest cytotoxics used, with medroxyprogesterons the most used hormonal therapy [13–15]. Many trials reporting systemic therapies are small phase II studies, and the overall response rates range from 7% to 69% depending on the study. As previously stated, the comorbidities within this patient cohort often means that hormonal therapy is the best option owing to its ease of administration and lack of adverse side effects.

Many smaller series have suggested that the combination of radiotherapy with chemotherapy may improve outcome by reducing local pelvic recurrences and also extrapelvic disease relapse. Such effects have been proven in chemoradiotherapy as used in cervical tumours. PORTEC 3 is an ongoing prospective randomized trial which compares standard radiotherapy with combination treatment, and the results should hopefully give guidance to the best option.

Summary box 58.3

- Radiotherapy after surgery in high-risk patients is considered to improve outcome [11].
- In patients <60 years old, with grade I or II tumour and <50% myometrial invasion, adjuvant radiotherapy is not necessary [12].
- Radiotherapy after surgery does reduce recurrence rates, but not overall survival.
- Combining chemotherapy with radiotherapy may improve outcome, although ongoing trials are assessing this approach.

Relapsed endometrial cancer

The main issues with respect to deciding the best therapy for patient with relapsed endometrial cancer are (i) previous exposure to non-surgical interventions, (ii) the site of disease relapse, whether localized or multiple sites and (iii) the patients physical condition. Thus, investigations used are similar to those within the staging system, although where available PET scanning can be useful in selected situations.

The commonest site of relapse is the vaginal vault, and if the disease is localized and the area is radiotherapy-naive, radiation is the first course of intervention. If the disease is localized but has previously undergone radiation and then surgical excision, a partial vaginectomy can be performed. If there are distant metastases then a systemic therapy is necessary, and depending on the patient's physical condition either chemotherapy or hormonal therapies can be used. The response rates are variable, but never very high, and the effect is poorer for disease relapsed within a field of radiotherapy.

Exenterative surgery [16], whereby the bladder, vagina and rectum are excised, is only undertaken in very carefully selected patients, and may be occasionally justifiable as a palliative procedure. In the main, many patients have such comorbidities that such surgery is generally deemed unsuitable.

Summary box 58.4

- Disease recurrence in early-stage disease is 14%, but in those given adjuvant radiotherapy it is only 4% [8].
- Disease relapse commonly occurs in the vaginal vault.
- Relapse within the field of prior radiotherapy is difficult to manage.
- Exenterative surgery has a limited role in the management of relapsed disease.

Conclusion

Endometrial cancer is a disease with a reasonably good prognosis that is increasing in incidence. Primary intervention is mainly surgical in nature, with selected patients having adjuvant therapies. Advances in surgical techniques continue to reduce the surgically associated morbidity. Equally, randomized trials are redefining the role of adjuvant therapies. Prevention is inevitably the ultimate goal, and can be partially achieved through educational health policies for reducing the incidence of obesity. Screening is another tool that may either detect premalignant or downstage the disease at presentation, and thus also improve survival rates. However, the latter still requires much more investigation as to the optimum modalities to employ. Inevitably, the future will also include a greater understanding of the disease and greater individualization of therapy focused more on the actual disease biology rather than based purely on the disease stage and histological subtype.

References

1 Pecorelli S. Revised FIGO staging for carcinoma of the vulva, cervix, and endometrium. *Int J Gynaecol Obstet* 2009;105: 103–104.

2 Lynch HT, Lynch PM, Lanspa SJ, Snyder CL, Lynch JF, Boland CR. Review of the Lynch syndrome: history, molecular genetics, screening, differential diagnosis, and medicolegal ramifications. *Clin Genet* 2009;76:1–18.

3 Rice LW. Hormone prevention strategies for breast, endometrial and ovarian cancers. *Gynecol Oncol* 2010;118:202–207.

4 Chin J, Konje JC, Hickey M. Levonorgestrel intrauterine system for endometrial protection in women with breast cancer on adjuvant tamoxifen. *Cochrane Database Syst Rev* 2009;4: CD007245.

5 Mourits MJ, Bijen CB, Arts HJ *et al.* Safety of laparoscopy versus laparotomy in early-stage endometrial cancer: a randomised trial. *Lancet Oncol* 2010;11:763–771

6 de la Orden SG, Reza MM, Blasco JA, Andradas E, Callejo D, Pérez T. Laparoscopic hysterectomy in the treatment of endometrial cancer: a systematic review. *J Minim Invasive Gynecol* 2008;15:395–401

7 Kitchener H, Swart AM, Qian Q, Amos C, Parmar MK. Efficacy of systematic pelvic lymphadenectomy in endometrial cancer (MRC ASTEC trial): a randomised study. *Lancet* 2009;373: 125–136.

8 Blake P, Swart AM, Orton J *et al.* Adjuvant external beam radiotherapy in the treatment of endometrial cancer (MRC ASTEC and NCIC CTG EN.5 randomised trials): pooled trial results, systematic review, and meta-analysis. *Lancet* 2009;373: 137–146.

9 Todo Y, Kato H, Kaneuchi M, Watari H, Takeda M, Sakuragi N. Survival effect of para-aortic lymphadenectomy in endometrial cancer (SEPAL study): a retrospective cohort analysis. *Lancet* 2010;375:1165–1172.

10 Gadducci A, Spirito N, Baroni E, Tana R, Genazzani AR. The fertility-sparing treatment in patients with endometrial atypical hyperplasia and early endometrial cancer: a debated therapeutic option. *Gynecol Endocrinol* 2009;25:683–691.

11 Aalders J, Abeler V, Kolstad P, Onsrud M. Postoperative external irradiation and prognostic parameters in stage I endometrial carcinoma: clinical and histopathologic study of 540 patients. *Obstet Gynecol* 1980;56:419–427.

12 Creutzberg CL, van Putten WL, Koper PC *et al.* Surgery and postoperative radiotherapy versus surgery alone for patients with stage-1 endometrial carcinoma: multicentre randomised trial. PORTEC Study Group. Post Operative Radiation Therapy in Endometrial Carcinoma. *Lancet.* 2000;355:1404–1411.

13 Kokka F, Brockbank E, Oram D, Gallagher C, Bryant A. Hormonal therapy in advanced or recurrent endometrial cancer. *Cochrane Database Syst Rev* 2010;12:CD007926.

14 Brown J, Smith JA, Ramondetta LM *et al.* Combination of gemcitabine and cisplatin is highly active in women with endometrial carcinoma: results of a prospective phase 2 trial. *Cancer* 2010;116:4973–4979.

15 Geller MA, Ivy JJ, Ghebre R *et al.* A phase II trial of carboplatin and docetaxel followed by radiotherapy given in a 'Sandwich' method for stage III, IV, and recurrent endometrial cancer. *Gynecol Oncol* 2011;121:112–117.

16 Awtrey CS, Cadungog MG, Leitao MM *et al.* Surgical resection of recurrent endometrial carcinoma. *Gynecol Oncol* 2006;102: 480–488.

Part 16
Miscellaneous Topics

Chapter 59
Sexual Dysfunction

Claudine Domoney
Institute of Psychosexual Medicine, Chelsea and Westminster Hospital, London, UK

Introduction

As changes in society and fertility control increase the social and economic power of women, there is a greater expectation of 'a state of physical, emotional, mental and social well-being in relation to sexuality . . . not merely the absence of disease, dysfunction or infirmity' and 'pleasurable and safe sexual experiences, free of coercion, discrimination and violence' [1]. Sexology has become an academic discipline with greater understanding of the themes of difference and equality between male and female sexuality. This allows for an improved comprehension of the ultimate psychosomatic activity – sex – and therefore of sexual difficulties or dysfunction. However, to approach these difficulties from a purely physical or psychological perspective is unlikely to be helpful. An overview of female sexuality, the impact of life events and an introduction to sexual therapeutic interventions will provide the foundation for understanding the impact of sexuality on quality of life. Our patients require more expertise from health professionals as they expect more from their sexual lives.

Female sexuality

Female sexuality is a complex interaction of physical, psychological and interpersonal factors. An understanding of sexuality requires a perspective on both male and female sexual behavioural patterns, yet there are some crucial differences between both sexes. An older model of human sexuality from Masters and Johnson [2] in the 1960s incorporates the linear stepwise progression from sexual excitement leading to arousal then orgasm and a period of resolution (Fig. 59.1). They facilitated the idea that orgasm was an important response for women and that some had the capacity for multiple orgasms, yet others would not achieve it. Specific impairment could arise within these phases. Kaplan [3] revised this with the addition of sexual desire replacing sexual excitement. The more recent model of female sexuality from the

International Consensus Conference [4] allows for a better understanding of the different motivators for sexual activity and responsivity (Fig. 59.2). Feelings of arousal may elicit feelings of desire and occur concurrently, rather than desire being the motivating feature of sexual activity (compared with men, in whom it is more likely to be preceded by desire). The motivating factors are more likely to be a drive for physical and emotional intimacy than innate desire in a longer lasting relationship.

Female sexual dysfunction

Presentation in obstetrics and gynaecology

Women may present with overt or covert sexual problems within a gynaecology or obstetric clinic. One study indicated that 90% of women presenting for gynaecological care had at least one sexual concern [5]. In this study, up to 40% of women described sexual coercion during their lifetime. Another paper reported sexual dysfunction in up to 40% [6]. It is not known what proportion of these problems are physical, psychological, interpersonal or a combination, but it does indicate the high prevalence amongst this population.

Women are frequently reluctant to broach sexual subjects in consultations and therefore it is crucial that the physician is able to introduce this line of questioning. Patients are more likely to respond to a physician who appears comfortable and is concerned with a professional demeanour [7,8]. Direct questioning significantly increases the reporting of sexual difficulties, from 3% to 16% in a gynaecology clinic [9].

Although some women may refer themselves directly with sexual problems, others may reveal their difficulties at some other point during their interactions with an observant health professional. Smear taking, difficulty with examination, difficult historians, vague clinical symptoms and signs may all be 'calling cards'. When it is not clear what the patient's agenda is, a pertinent question can be a turning point during a consultation. Recognition of these issues is likely to have significant impact on

Dewhurst's Textbook of Obstetrics & Gynaecology, Eighth Edition. Edited by D. Keith Edmonds.
© 2012 John Wiley and Sons, Ltd. Published 2012 by John Wiley and Sons, Ltd.

therapeutic success and a reduction in unnecessary investigations such as diagnostic laparoscopy for pelvic pain.

Prevalence

Epidemiological studies have indicated a female sexual dysfunction (FSD) prevalence rate of 30–55% [10,11]. An often-cited article [12] from the USA regarding men and women aged 18–59 years indicated a sexual dysfunction rate of 43% in women and 31% in men. However, there has been much discussion regarding the duration and degree of distress required to label these sexual problems as a dysfunction. There is also significant overlap of these disorders, with a wide spectrum of normal functioning. British studies have indicated that prevalence of sexual problems in primary care is high, with 22% of men and 40% of women having a diagnosis of sexual dysfunction, although this was poorly recognized or documented – only 3–4% had an entry in their medical notes [13]. Another reported that 54% of women had a sexual problem lasting at least 1 month over a 2-year period [11]. However, as John Bancroft [14] argues, much of this may be adaptive responses to other life stressors and therefore part of typical behaviours.

Loss of libido is the most common complaint of younger and older women, probably being a final common pathway of many sexual disorders, with estimates ranging from 30% to 45% depending on the population sampled, increasing in the postmenopausal age group [15]. However, the degree of distress associated with this may be minimal. Arousal disorders are found in approximately 20%, increasing in those with hormonal deficiencies [16]. Orgasmic disorders are reported in a quarter of women of reproductive age and up to 45% postmenopausally [17]. Sexual pain disorders are common, with two-thirds of a group of women in their thirties complaining of dyspareunia, half of whom reported it as chronic [18]. The older age group complain of dyspareunia less frequently and report more specific difficulties with lubrication and sensitivity [19]. Vulval pain syndrome may occur in 2–10% [20]. The true prevalence of vaginismus is difficult to ascertain owing to its subjectivity and reliance on physical examination. The rates of sexual problems in specific groups will be discussed later.

Categorization of female sexual disorders

The Diagnostic and Statistical Manual of Mental Disorders IV (DSM-IV) of the American Psychiatric Association [21] has categorized female sexual dysfunction from a psychiatric perspective but reflects the newer Basson model of the female sexual response cycle when compared with the World Health Organization (WHO) International Classification of Diseases (ICD-10) [22]. These are listed in Summary box 59.1 and described below. However, in most sexual disorders, there is an overlap with areas of dysfunction as they do not occur in isolation. This is commonly the

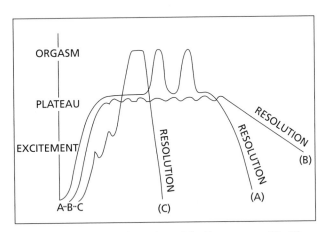

Fig. 59.1 Masters and Johnson's model of human sexuality [2].

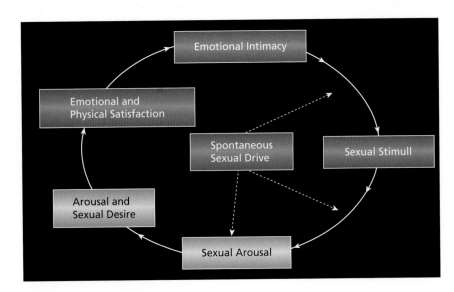

Fig. 59.2 International Consensus Model [4]. (With permission from Wiley.)

case for all sexual pain disorders, where lack of desire and arousal may be common defence mechanisms, whether the pain is physical, psychological or a combination. The DSM-V may re-categorize the sexual pain disorders as a pain disorder rather than a sexual disorder [23].

The DSM definition currently includes causation of 'marked distress and interpersonal difficulty' to be categorized as a dysfunction. DSM-V may stipulate a duration of at least 6 months to be classified as a disorder [24]. Currently, these conditions are further categorized as lifelong or acquired and generalized or situational.

 Summary box 59.1

DSM-IV categories of FSD [21] sexual desire disorders:
- Hypoactive sexual desire disorder (HSDD)
- Sexual aversion disorder
- Female sexual arousal disorder
- Persistent arousal disorder
- Female orgasmic disorder
- Sexual pain disorder
- Dyspareunia
- Vaginismus
- Non-coital sexual pain disorders
- Sexual dysfunction due to a general medical condition
- Substance-induced sexual dysfunction
- Sexual dysfunction not otherwise specified
- Paraphilias
- Gender identity disorders

Definitions of main sexual disorders in women

Desire disorders

Hypoactive desire disorder (HSDD) is the persistent or recurrent deficiency or absence of sexual desire or sexual fantasies or thoughts, and/or the desire for, or receptivity to, sexual activity, which causes distress. The emphasis on causing distress and focus on sexual thoughts allows the flexibility of definition to include those who are not in a relationship or have lost their relationships secondary to their HSDD. Sexual aversion disorder is the persistence of phobic aversion to, and avoidance of, sexual activity, which causes personal distress.

Sexual arousal disorder is defined as the persistent or recurrent inability to attain or maintain sexual excitement, causing personal distress, which may be described as subjective feelings and/or lack of physical changes. As there is a lack of correlation between subjective and genital arousal in women, these are separated into genital, subjective or combined arousal disorders. Persistent sexual arousal syndrome is persistent, involuntary genital congestion in the absence of sexual desire and not relieved by orgasm.

Orgasmic disorder is defined as the persistence or recurrent difficulty or absence of achieving orgasm following sufficient stimulation and arousal. It may follow from both desire and arousal disorders or be truly independent. It may be primary or secondary, i.e. the inability to reach climax under any circumstances or with intercourse only, respectively.

Sexual pain disorders include dyspareunia, defined as persistent or recurrent genital pain associated with sexual intercourse. This may be physical and/or psychological, i.e. psychosomatic in origin. It is important not to dismiss this as non-organic pain without sufficient exploration, although this may not always require physical investigations. Vaginismus has been described by the International Consensus Group as recurrent or persistent involuntary spasm of the pelvic musculature that interferes with intercourse. However, it may be situational, i.e. with only certain partners or just at speculum examination. This should be more often interpreted as a sign, not a symptom of pelvic symptoms, and not considered a diagnosis alone.

Non-coital sexual pain disorders are genital pain disorders induced by non-sexual stimulation, most commonly vulval pain disorders. These frequently cause secondary desire and arousal difficulties or apareunia with a consequential significant impact on relationships and self-esteem.

Sexual dysfunction due to a general medical condition and substance-induced sexual dysfunction are specified as a direct result of the physical effects of the medical condition from history, examination or laboratory findings.

Sexual addiction is rare amongst women.

Male sexual dysfunction

It is clear that male sexual dysfunction is more likely to reduce sexual activity in older couples [25] as female partners may collude with their partner, developing their own sexual problems to protect their partner. However, the use of phosphodiesterase inhibitors has prolonged the potency of men and changed the management of male sexual dysfunction significantly. Erectile dysfunction is the most common problem (experienced by 20% of the male population aged 40–70 years), but desire and ejaculatory disorders are also prevalent [26]. Loss of early morning erections is more likely to indicate an organic aetiology. Erectile disorder may indicate the onset of cardiovascular disease and therefore assessment of blood pressure, pulse, weight, genital and prostate examination are mandatory in addition to assessing serum lipids, glucose and early morning testosterone levels. Identifying comorbid factors, optimizing their management, sexual education and addressing lifestyle issues are all important steps in the treatment of male sexual problems. In addition to phosphodiesterase inhibitors, there are other interventions including testosterone, injectable and urethral prostaglandins, apomorphine, penile pumps and prostheses available. The psychosexual component of male sexual difficulties must be assessed despite the success of physical therapies.

Management

Consultation

The most basic questions that should be incorporated into a general gynaecological consultation regarding sexual function should be a variation on the following:

• Do you have a partner? Are you in a sexual relationship?
• Do you have any difficulties? Do you have pain during intercourse?
• Are these difficulties a problem for you?

Previous work has indicated that three questions (regarding desire, discomfort and satisfaction) were as efficacious for screening as a 30-minute therapist interview [27]. The consultation should address the medical, surgical, psychological, obstetric and gynaecological, and social history. This is directed towards eliciting the patient's understanding of her sexual problem, its origin, its maintaining factors and her wishes for treatment. The techniques of psychosexual medicine use the consultation as a therapeutic event. Questions should be open ended and non-directive, with pause for reflection. Sexual problems are frequently a manifestation of pain and distress that can be explored safely in a supportive consultation. The patient is the expert in her symptoms and the set of circumstances that has enabled them to develop. Knowledge of her sexual biography is not always necessary but understanding when the problem developed and why she has presented it now will be important to the overall evaluation. The features of the history that may be important are listed in Summary box 59.2.

Summary box 59.2

Sexual history – key components:
• Feelings about genitals and perceived abnormalities
• Fears
• Effect of medical complaint
• Effect of treatment
• Feelings about body
• Understanding of condition and its treatment
• Psychosexual problems exacerbating physical symptoms
• Previous experiences
• Key events
• Understanding of 'hidden agenda'
• Partner's feelings and problems

The language used for anatomy and sexual practices is varied, and care must be taken to understand the patient's communications. This includes not making assumptions about the gender of their partner. Any attempt to be unclear about any details can indicate that they are an area for further exploration. Active listening – noticing what is not said as well as what is – is more fruitful than a list of questions that do not address the fears and fantasies of the patient.

There is disagreement amongst many health professionals seeing women with sexual problems about whether couple therapy is essential. Although sexual activity reflects that of both parties, female sexuality and responsivity may relate to her feelings about herself, her genitals as well as her relationship. Within gynaecology clinics, we are likely to review women alone, but if the patient brings her partner with her, it is likely that she wishes to share the consultation with him (or her). Frequently, women will admit to more negative feelings that impact on their sexual lives without a partner present. Occasionally it is clear that the sexual issue is a reflection of relationship difficulties and therefore should be directed to more appropriate agencies or therapists. Dealing with what is brought to the clinician during the consultation is most important as if neglected, this may reinforce the patient's feelings of worthlessness and lack of solution.

Questionnaires

Questionnaires can be useful in clinical practice as they introduce the subject of sex for those who find it uncomfortable – the clinician and/or patient. They may extract information with time efficiency and in a more reproducible manner for research activity. Use also indicates to the patient that clinicians are interested in sexual issues and may be able to provide help and guidance. However, many questionnaires are unwieldy tools designed by psychologists and for some people may be intrusive – there are those with up to 35 'items' or questions so for many practical purposes. Short-form questionnaires have been validated for clinical use. Within a research setting, they may also be useful to monitor the sexual effects of new interventions in a population, rather than for individuals.

Questionnaires can be generic or disease- or condition-specific. Generic questionnaires such as the Female Sexual Function Index (FSFI) are accepted by most patients [28] and can be downloaded from the internet, including analysis instructions. An example of a disease-specific questionnaire is the Prolapse and Incontinence Sexual Questionnaire (PISQ) [29], which comes in a long and short form. The most common condition-specific instruments investigate sexual desire, such as the Profile of Female Sexual Function [30]. There are strengths and weaknesses of every questionnaire and it is important to know in which population they have been validated. Some are not sensitive enough to deal with difficulties in those who are not sexually active. This can have clinical implications depending on why they are not active, secondary to their own difficulties, health or disease status, their partner's or personal preference. In women who are not sexually active owing to another process, the Sexual Distress Scale may be useful [31]. Questionnaires that may be useful in clinical practice or research in obstetrics and gynaecology are listed in Summary box 59.3.

Examination

Attention to the presentation of the patient can reflect many feelings about her body and sexual life: her confidence, appearance and delivery of verbal and non-verbal communication. Body image has a significant impact on sexuality and routine measurement of body mass index may be helpful. General examinations can reveal other conditions that contribute to sexual functioning, including the musculoskeletal and neurological systems. Genital examinations uncover not only physical abnormalities but also the psychological impact that the genitals may have on the patient. The detection of feelings such as disgust, fear and remoteness from the genitals exhibited by the patient can be a representation of attitudes to sex – the patient's body may be expressing feelings that she cannot express verbally.

Pelvic examination should follow according to the tolerance of the patient. She may not be able to allow vaginal examination at a first consultation, particularly where there has been sexual abuse or assault. Careful examination of the skin for dermatoses and cotton bud testing for pain mapping in vulval pain syndrome is performed initially. Atrophy is very common in lactating and post- and perimenopausal women – this should be excluded as a cause of pain or its contribution noted. Digital examinations can be more valuable than speculum examinations as it allows for the ability to make an assessment of pelvic floor tone and the ability to locate the pelvic floor on command (both contraction and relaxation). Swab tests and pH testing also may be of value. Palpation for pain and reproduction of discomfort during sex may delineate the need to pursue further investigations such as diagnostic laparoscopy. Areas of point tenderness may be more indicative of a specific physical problem. Incontinence and prolapse may require an examination in the left lateral position, but some women find it a very vulnerable position to be in and may be disinclined to undergo such an examination. Postoperative or post-childbirth changes should be addressed and incorporated into the woman's

---

💡 Summary box 59.3

Questionnaires/patient-reported outcome measures for assessing sexual function:

Patient-reported outcome	N items (N questions in short forms of questionnaire)	Domains	Brief form available for clinical use	Diagnostic use
Brief Index of Sexual Functioning for Women (BISF-W)	22	Desire, arousal, frequency of sexual activity, receptivity, pleasure, satisfaction, sexual problems	No	No
Changes in Sexual Functioning Questionnaire (CSFQ)	35 (14)	Desire – frequency, desire – interest, pleasure, arousal, orgasm	Yes	Yes
Female Sexual Function Index (FSFI)	19	Desire, arousal, lubrication, orgasm, pain, satisfaction	No	Yes
Short form of the Personal Experience Questionnaire (SPEQ)	9	Desire, arousal, dyspareunia, partner's sexual problems	Yes	Yes
Sexual Function Questionnaire (SFQ)	28	Desire, arousal – lubrication, arousal – cognitive, arousal – sensation, orgasm, pain, enjoyment, partner	Yes	Yes
Profile of Female Sexual Function (PFSF)	37	Desire, arousal, orgasm, self-image, concerns, responsiveness, pleasure	Yes	No
Monash Female Sexual Satisfaction Questionnaire (MFSSQ)	12	Receptivity, arousal, lubrication, orgasm, sexual pleasure, sexual satisfaction	No	Yes (total score only)
Prolapse and Incontinence Sexual Questionnaire (PISQ 31 or 12)	31 (12)	Behavioural – emotive, physical, partner-related	Yes	No
Sexual Distress Scale	12	Distress	No	No

understanding of the change in her genitals. Palpation of the perineum for tenderness and suture material detects pain and the reaction to it. Neurological examinations are also important, but the complaint of lack of sensation is more likely to be a defence against sexual pain or other deep rooted issues.

Physical examinations must obviously exclude physical abnormalities, although vaginismus and adductor spasm may prevent full examination. Any concern that there is a physical abnormality with non-consummation would be an indication for an examination under anaesthesia (EUA), but otherwise is unlikely to be helpful.

Investigations

In the vast majority of women, few investigations are required. Baseline tests that may be considered are listed in Summary box 59.4.

Summary box 59.4

- Follicle-stimulating hormone
- Leuteinizing hormone
- Oestradiol
- Androgen profile
- Testosterone and sex hormone binding globulin (SHBG) to calculate free androgen index (FAI): a reflection of biologically active testosterone
- FAI = TT (in nmol/L) × 100 (ng/L)
- SHBG (in nmol/L): normal range 0.4–0.8 ng/L
- Prolactin
- Blood sugar

In practice, hormone levels are of little value as they do not correlate directly with sexual activity or function. In women of reproductive age, hormone levels are rapidly fluctuating and therefore any sample would only reflect a snapshot in time. There is no current evidence that women's sexual reactions are different at varying times of the menstrual cycle. However, a young woman with premature ovarian failure may have a low free androgen index, reflected in low libido or other symptoms of the menopause. Frequently perimenopausal women may have androgen levels in the low–normal range, but overall there is no significant correlation valuable for clinical use [32]. The measurement of hormone levels may be useful for those who have been prescribed oestrogen and/or androgen therapy to little therapeutic effect. It is important to measure SHBG as this will alter the free levels of other sex steroids. Only 1–2% of testosterone is free in the circulation: 66% is bound to SHBG and 31% to albumin (which is also bioavailable). Peripheral conversion occurs in adipose and muscle tissue. Androgens fall by 50% after the menopause, halve between the third and fifth decade of life and are even more dramatically lowered after bilateral oophorectomy, and therefore may cause significant

symptoms of sexual dysfunction in those who are already menopausal. The symptoms of the female androgen deficiency syndrome are considered to be a reduction in energy and libido. SHBG is altered by other interventions and may impact on free circulating androgens and therefore female sexual response. Most importantly in a gynaecological context, oral hormone replacement therapy (HRT) and the combined oral contraceptive pill (COCP) increase SHBG and therefore reduce free testosterone levels. Some progestogens within the COCP, progestogen-only pill or the levonorgestrel intrauterine system also impact negatively on mood and libido.

An ultrasound scan may detect physical abnormalities or exclude congenital malformations of the genital tract if there is any degree of concern, particularly in women who present with non-consummation.

Treatment

There are many differing approaches to the management of sexual problems. All should involve recognition of the powerful effect of the mind on the body, which is so marked in sexuality. Recognition of sex as a biopsychosocial activity has encouraged a plethora of varying therapists to offer treatment options based on their particular training. Many will use cognitive behavioural techniques targeted at sexual problems. These involve techniques such as sensate focus (see Fig. 59.3) and desensitization using vaginal dilators/trainers. Other therapists will use psychological approaches. It is rare that long-term psychoanalytic therapy will be necessary for most sexual difficulties, although there may be a place for those with other longstanding issues, when sexual problems are a reflection thereof.

The advantage doctors have, particularly gynaecologists, is the use of the genital examination to detect physical abnormalities but also the psychosexual examination, which can act as the 'moment of truth' where the reaction of the patient to their genitals is witnessed. This should be used as a major part of the consultation and can be a therapeutic event. Various interventions including drug treatments and surgery may of value for some women and will be detailed below.

Psychosexual medicine

Many patients are resistant to psychosexual exploration until the mind–body link is explained. There is always a psychological reaction to a physical illness, and in the arena of sexuality, physical problems can be accentuated by the psychological consequences. The reverse somatization of psychological problems into sexual and physical problems is a very powerful sequence of processes. This in part explains the lack of treatment success in those who refuse to acknowledge a psychological component. For instance, patients presenting with non-consummation

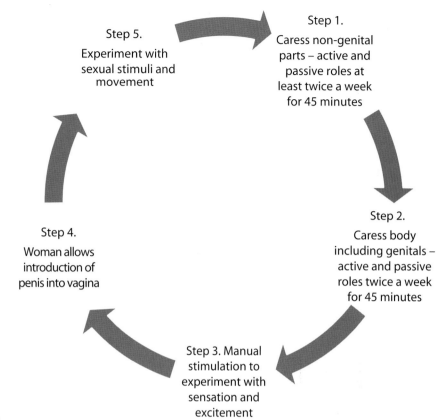

Fig. 59.3 Sensate focus management plan.

may have deep-seated issues that have been suppressed. Non-consummation may in these circumstances be protective and an EUA will not cure these difficulties.

Behavioural therapists can work with individuals or couples. Many prefer to work with couples as the problem may be between two partners. Those involved in women's healthcare may discover sexual problems in women who are not involved in a relationship and it is important to deal with these as they present. The mainstay of gynaecologists who are trained in psychosexual medicine is the analysis of the doctor–patient relationship, reflecting the dynamics of the patient's sexual relationships. The basic tenets of the psychosexual consultation are listed in Summary box 59.5.

Summary box 59.5

Psychosexual medicine principles:
- **Listen** to the patient's story and view of the problem.
- **Observe** the effect of the patient and their presentation on the doctor and understand the patient's body language.
- **Feel** the effect of the doctor's questions and interventions on the patient.
- **Think** about the feelings generated during the consultation and/or examination.
- **Interpret** the observations back into the patient's sexual life.

The patient is central to the process – she is the 'expert' – and the clinician helps to reveal the causative and maintaining factors, understanding, and then facilitating change and hopefully improvement. The empathic consultation may enable the exposure of subconscious feelings and fantasies as a reflection of the physical symptoms and sexual problems. Psychosexual medicine uses consultation, counselling and psychodynamic skills in addition to the psychosomatic examination to manage these difficulties. Consultations should always be sensitive to the patient's mood, although observations can be made that reflect the anxiety/aggression/defensiveness, etc. felt. This may be non-verbal communication rather than verbal but is part of the representation of this patient. Connections may be made with these communications and the difficulties in sexual behaviour. Lifelong or primary disorders are more likely to require long-term therapy than acquired problems. Revelations of sexual abuse may need alternative approaches, occasionally by a psychotherapist, depending on the level of general disturbance.

One of the most important parts of the consultation is the genital examination. It has been described as 'the moment of truth', frequently revealing feelings otherwise hidden. It may mirror the vulnerability of sex. Many guarded women who appear in perfect control yet present with a non-specific gynaecological complaint such as pelvic pain become very emotional at the genital examination. Vaginismus with thigh adductor spasm and the woman becoming a metaphorical 'little girl', trying to escape from the couch, may reveal much about her sexual feelings. The woman disconnected from her examination may also be 'disconnected' from sex, not able to feel or react to desire or arousal. She may have had many investigations, reinforcing a perception that her genitals do not belong to her. The woman with persistent discharge who tells the clinician what an awful job they have is reflecting her disgust with her genital tract. Is her discharge physiological? Requests for labial reduction are becoming more common – are they a response to the trend of increased shaving and therefore exposure to adult female vulva rather than the physiologically exposed prepubescent vulva or an individual reaction to their 'abnormal' genitalia? The vagina that is too small and perceived as too painful with any penetration, the vagina that is blocked and cannot tolerate anything inside, or the vagina that is sharp and will damage any penis put inside – all these are common fantasies that need to be understood before the genitals can become associated with pleasure.

Cognitive behavioural techniques focusing on modification of underlying factors and strategies to improve emotional and physical closeness in addition to erotic techniques are the mainstay of many sex therapists. The PLISSIT (permission, limited information, specific suggestions and intensive therapy) model of sexual counselling [33] aims to give the patient permission to discuss the problem, give limited information and then move onto therapy and more specific instructions before finally receiving intensive therapy from a specialist.

Many therapists will make use of education and bibliotherapy to help patients with sexual problems, but at some point during the therapeutic relationship the patient needs to become the 'adult', owning her own sexual life and using the techniques and understanding she has gained. Excessive reliance on teaching may hamper the ability of the patient to make that transition.

Physical

Various physical therapies are available to gynaecologists. The simplest yet most ubiquitous are lubricants. Water-based lubricants used for medical examination are less useful for intercourse as their effect does not last and they will increase friction. There are a number of commercially available products (oil/silicon based) that are likely to be helpful, or the use of vegetable oils may be acceptable (the compatibility of oils with condoms must be checked). Almond oil is a good option.

Vaginal trainers or dilators are frequently used by doctors and therapists. However, encouraging the use of fingers, tampons and vibrators may give women more ownership of their pelvis. A programme of gradually increasing dilator size (or more fingers) can teach a woman with vaginismus to accept entrance to the vagina with eventual penile penetration. Dilators may be essential for women post-radiotherapy and occasionally after vaginal surgery to maintain vaginal capacity for intercourse. Physiotherapists use pelvic floor modification to assist with sexual difficulties and are able to facilitate behavioural adaptation.

Other devices may be useful for some women. A suction clitoral vacuum device is licensed in the USA and has been shown to have an impact on sexual satisfaction. A concern that vibrators may reduce sensitivity has not been proven.

Pharmacological

The success of phosphodiesterase inhibitors for male erectile disorders has propagated a search for the equivalent medication to treat female sexual disorders. However, the complexity of the female sexual response cycle and the wide overlap in the areas of dysfunction make it much less plausible that a universal pill or potion will be found. A wider reaching political debate is emerging regarding the 'medicalization' of female sexual dysfunction and 'disease mongering' to manipulate populations needing to be medicated for conditions that are part of the normal spectrum [34]. Definitions of female sexual dysfunction (FSD) are controversial and explain the wide range of prevalence rates. Therefore, drug-regulating authorities appear to have an inconsistent approach to licensing products for these indications.

Hormonal

Evidence for the use of oestrogen, progesterone and androgens in women of reproductive age and normal hormonal status is limited. Oestrogen replacement therapy in deficient women may improve the ability to be aroused and genital tissue response. Testosterone is linked to sexual drive and ability to orgasm. There are convincing data for the use of oestrogen and testosterone replacement in women who have been hysterectomized and oophorectomized [35]. The current licence in the UK for testosterone replacement patches are in these women with a diagnosis of hypoactive desire disorder (HSDD) who are receiving adequate oestrogen replacement (300 mg twice weekly). Gels are an unlicensed alternative (one-fifth of the male dose, 10 mg per day). There has been more recent work suggesting a benefit of testosterone for premenopausal women [36] and postmenopause for women not taking oestrogen replacement [37]. These are physiological doses rather than pharmacological doses. The improvement in sexual function may be considered modest by some and involvement in a trial (part of the placebo response) appears to have a beneficial impact on sexual activity. A study of trial subjects reported that 53% had a clinically meaningful improvement [38]. Pharmacological doses of oestrogen and testosterone in implant form may have a higher risk of side effects but no proven advantage over physiological dosing.

It is important to understand that oral oestrogens can increase SHBG levels and therefore reduce free testosterone. Transdermal oestrogen therapies may therefore be more valuable. The lack of long-term safety data with testosterone use for cardiovascular disease and hormone-sensitive cancers have limited the licence for these products in many countries. Dihydroepiandrostenedione (DHEA), a non-licensed prohormone, could have a beneficial effect on female sexual drive, arousal and orgasmic potential but the data are not conclusive at present.

The use of topical oestrogen therapy in the form of vaginal pessaries, creams or rings, is of paramount importance. Changes in the genital mucosa secondary to oestrogen deficiency after the menopause or postpartum during lactation lead to reduced lubrication, increased vaginal irritation and pain. Atrophic vaginitis may lead to postmenopausal bleeding, which can also have a profound impact on sexual function owing to fear of cancer. Up to one-quarter of women using systemic HRT may have residual local symptoms [39]. The use of topical agents should be acceptable to most women and healthcare professionals and a new low-dose form of pessary delivers only 1.4 mg of oestradiol over a year when used twice weekly. Therefore, its use for women who have had hormone-sensitive cancers can be considered. Current topical preparations do not stimulate the endometrium and can be used long term. A vaginal remoisturizer (Replens MD®) used in a similar dosing pattern to vaginal oestrogens can be effective for those who wish to avoid all hormones.

Non-hormonal

There is little evidence that phosphodiesterase inhibitor use is of value for FSD. There is some evidence that the increase in genital engorgement may be of value for women with genital arousal disorder [40], although there are also contradictory trial data [41]. Some interest has indicated a possible use for women with spinal injuries and those on selective serotonin re-uptake inhibitors for treatment of depression (although this psychiatric disorder will have its own direct effect on sexual function).

Pain disorders require interventions targeting the likely pathology if the aetiology is thought to be physical. Vulval pain disorders are frequently treated with medications for chronic pain management such as amitryptilline, gabapentin and local anaesthetic injections or nerve/ganglion blocks. Steroid and anaesthetic injections for point tenderness have a role, particularly postsurgery or postchildbirth. Others are advocating the use of botulinum toxin for levator spasm and vaginismus. Anaesthetic gels suitable for genital skin can be useful to decrease sensitivity and may be valuable for some. However, it is important to recognize the possibility that pain may be a somatization of deep distress which protects the individual. Physical therapies alone in these circumstances will be limited.

There are many other drugs under investigation including sublingual arginine, topical prostaglandins, phentolamine and more recently flibanserin, which may have an impact on satisfaction and the number of satisfying sexual episodes in line with that of testosterone replacement for FSD or HSDD. To date, none of these drugs are licensed for these indications in the UK or USA.

Sexual problems in general obstetrics and gynaecology

It is common for sexual problems to present in the gynaecology clinic setting (see Table 59.1) and some of the more frequent difficulties and associations are detailed below.

Childhood and adolescence

Childhood is an influential time in the formation of relationships, with many theories of bonding eluding to the establishment of healthy, intimate relationships in future life. Events from childhood can evoke strong emotional reactions that impact on sexual responses later in life. Adolescence is a time of massive hormonal upheaval, peer group pressure and evolving self-realization. Prior education with respect to genital function, menstrual cycles, sexual behaviour, contraception and functional relationships are significant throughout this period, in addition to family attitudes to sex. There is scope for further research into the sexuality of children and adolescents.

Pregnancy and childbirth

During pregnancy, research suggests that overall there is a decline in libido and intercourse frequency in the first and third trimesters, with a slight improvement in the middle trimester [42]. The lack of adequate information and fears for the pregnancy have been cited as reasons for the pregnancy decline, but for some women there is heightened sensation, possibly related to oxytocin-induced effects on orgasm and bonding. If there is a decline, it may persist for 3–6 months after delivery and is partially related to postpartum pelvic floor problems

Table 59.1 Common presentations of sexual problems in the gynaecology clinic.

Overt presentation	Covert presentation
Loss of libido	Pelvic pain
Loss of sensation	Prolapse symptoms
Non-consummation	Vulval pain
Vaginismus	Vaginismus
Coital urinary leak	Difficulty with smear taking
Vaginal dryness	Requests for labial reduction
Dyspareunia	Dyspareunia

including perineal pain, breastfeeding and problems of oestrogen deficiency.

Pregnancy and childbirth herald major changes for a couple, with their primary role as partner and lover changing to include that of mother/parent. There is no good evidence to suggest that vaginal delivery decreases postnatal sexual health compared with Caesarean section [43], despite claims to the contrary. Episiotomy, however, does increase the persistence of superficial dyspareunia. In one study, women who breast fed their babies were significantly less interested in sex than those who bottle fed, irrespective of tiredness or depression, although this was not maintained long term [44]. By 6 weeks post partum, 30–60% of women have resumed activity, increasing to 80% by 6 months, yet sexual problems vary between 20% and 86%. Care of these women by open discussion with primary carers and by trained individuals is paramount to prevent long-lasting consequences.

Contraception and termination of pregnancy

Dissatisfaction with contraception is a common 'calling card' for sexual issues in a consultation. Aside from the psychosexual component of fertility control, there have been a number of studies that directly link sexual problems with specific methods of contraception. A recent report from medical students found the risk of dysfunction was highest with non-oral hormonal contraception followed by oral hormonal contraception. The lowest risk was in women using non-hormonal contraception [45]. Synthetic progestogens may have a negative impact on sexual drive and even low doses in sensitive women may be detrimental.

Surprisingly little research has focused on the impact of termination of pregnancy (TOP) on sexuality. A review reported that one prospective study with a control group found no difference in negative psychosexual effects at 1 year post-TOP, but other observational studies reported up to 30% dysfunction with one-quarter of all couples separating [46]. This warrants further investigation.

Sexually transmitted infections

There is a high rate of sexual problems associated with the acquisition of sexually transmitted infections (STIs) (up to 55% in women) [47] but with little understanding of the interactions to date.

Infertility

Sexual function in couples with sub- and infertility are of such significance that most fertility clinics will employ counsellors with experience in psychosexual work. It is not uncommon to encounter couples who are not having penetrative intercourse, either consciously or not. The demands of performing to specific menstrual cycle dates and maintaining celibacy at other times takes its toll on couples. Sex becomes goal-orientated and spontaneity

may disappear. The financial, physical and psychological impact of fertility alters the relationship between the couple, and for some raises questions regarding their motivation and wishes at odds with their previous desires.

Menopause

The time of the menopause and thereafter is one of physical and psychological change. A longitudinal prospective study of Australian women from early menopause to postmenopause demonstrated a change in the FSD rate from 42% to 88% [48]. Yet more recent work measuring the degree of distress associated with low sexual functioning calculated FSD to be 17% in women aged 56–67 [49].

These changes were correlated with oestradiol but not androgen levels, and distress was associated with current and prior negative feelings towards the partner. Continued activity was dependent on the presence of a functioning partner and increased with hormone therapy use. Other work from this group indicates that sexual responsivity is related to ageing, but libido, frequency of intercourse and dyspareunia are associated with oestrogen deficiency. Another study reported that 32% of women aged over 60 years were sexually active, 56% of whom were married women [50]. Activity varies according to the population studied, and there is evidence that the rates are increasing in the elderly population as expectations alter and health is preserved [51].

Simple measures can improve the physical sequelae of hormone deficiency and tissue ageing, such as topical oestrogen, non-hormonal vaginal remoisturizers and suitable lubricants. These should be complemented by a psychosexual approach to these issues.

Gynaecological surgery: hysterectomy, incontinence and prolapse

The relationship between surgery for a variety of gynaecological conditions and sexual dysfunction is not clear. Hysterectomy was previously thought to have an adverse effect on sexual pleasure, particularly when the cervix was removed [52], yet work over the last two decades has indicated that this is not the case. A large prospective trial that followed 1101 women who had hysterectomies up to 24 months postoperatively demonstrated an improvement in sexual function [53], and another study comparing total versus subtotal (conservation of the cervix) hysterectomy showed no difference between the two groups preoperatively in pain, orgasm or satisfaction scores, although both groups had an improvement in perceived sexual function postoperatively [54]. Oophorectomy and inadequate oestrogen with or without testosterone replacement may account for the discrepancies with some earlier studies. Overall, women appropriately listed for the operation and given suitable HRT have increased general and sexual health scores owing to relief of the symptoms warranting the operation, with no significant anatomical impact of removal of the reproductive parts. However, those who had preoperative sexual problems or depression may report a deterioration.

Urinary incontinence and prolapse are common complaints among women, particularly after child bearing, with up to 50% of those presenting for specialist care experiencing a negative sexual impact [55]. Overactive bladder symptoms are more likely to cause worsening sexual problems, and greater degrees of prolapse are associated with less activity [56]. The combination of incontinence and prolapse may have an even greater negative effect [57]. However, surgical correction of stress incontinence or prolapse may not guarantee an improvement in all areas of pelvic floor functioning, including sexual. More studies are under way to find a sensitive-enough tool to measure these changes and reassess the operations currently offered for pelvic floor dysfunction.

Colposcopy and cancer

An abnormal smear and consequent investigations can cause significant anxiety, and without sufficient information patients can experience feelings of blame and shame. There is evidence that abnormal smear results cause a negative impact on sexual responses and feelings towards partners [58]. The misunderstanding of the role of human papillomavirus as a causative agent for cervical intraepithelial changes through sexual transmission also increases psychosexual problems. This reinforces the need for good, supportive information at the time of cervical screening, before an abnormal result is reported.

Gynaecological cancers significantly increase psychosexual morbidity in addition to the direct physical effects of surgery, chemotherapy and radiation therapy. The 'castration' involved in the treatment of many cancers diminishes the self-esteem and sexuality of many sufferers. Any genital symptom may be feared as a harbinger of recurrence, particularly bleeding. The role of the partner as carer may not sit well with the role of sexual partner. A cross-sectional study of mixed gynaecological cancers found that although activity continued in half of the women, a reduction in desire was found in 75% and dyspareunia in 40% [59]. Radical pelvic surgery caused sexual problems in 66% of women 6 months after surgery, increasing to 82% in women who had received radiotherapy. This was worse in the younger group of women, particularly single women, as a relationship tended to be protective [60]. Further data confirm the psychosexual and physical impact on women who have cervical carcinoma, with vaginal changes and dyspareunia compounding lower desire, arousal and subsequent lower quality of life [61,62]. Support with specialist nurses and health professionals trained in sexual medicine is vital to ongoing quality of life in these individuals.

Conclusion

Female sexuality is complex, with a wide range of normal functioning. Dysfunction can be difficult to classify and may be a normal, adaptive variant which is often dependent on the sexual partner. Changes over a women's lifetime will be associated with alteration of sexual function and it is important for all health professionals to be aware of these factors and the interventions that can help alleviate distress.

References

1 Declaration of Alma-Ata. International Conference of Primary Healthcare, Alma-Ata, USSR, 1978. Available at: http://www.who.int/hpr/archive/docs/almaata.html.

2 Masters WH, Johnson VE. *Human Sexual Response*. Boston: Little Brown, 1966.

3 Kaplan HS. *The Sexual Desire Disorders*. New York: Brunner-Routledge, 1995.

4 Basson R, Althof S, Davis S *et al*. Summary of the recommendations on sexual dysfunctions in women. *J Sex Med* 2004;1:24.

5 Nusbaum MR, Gamble G, Skinner B *et al*. The high prevalence of sexual concerns among women seeking routine gynaecologic care. *J Fam Pract* 2000;49:229–232.

6 Rosen RC, Taylor JF, Leiblum SR *et al*. Prevalence of sexual dysfunction in women: results of a survey study of 329 women in an outpatient gynaecological clinic. *J Sex Marital Ther* 1993; 19:171–188.

7 Nusbaum MM, Helton MR, Ray N. The changing nature of women's sexual health concerns through the midlife years. *Maturitas* 2004;49:283–291.

8 Berman L, Berman J, Felder S *et al*. Seeking help for sexual function complaints: what gynaecologists need to know about the female patient's experience. *Fertil Steril* 2003;79:572–576.

9 Bachmann GA, Leiblum SR, Grill J. Brief sexual inquiry in gynecologic practice. *Obstet Gynecol* 1989;73:425–427.

10 Laumann EO, Nicolosi A, Glasser DB *et al*. GSSAB Investigators Group. Sexual problems among women and men aged 40–80 y: prevalence and correlates identified in the Global Study of Sexual Attitudes and Behaviours. *Int J Impot Res* 2005;17:39–57.

11 Mercer CH, Fenton KA, Johnson AM *et al*. Sexual function problems and help seeking behaviour in Britain: national probability sample survey. *BMJ* 2003;327:426–427.

12 Laumann E, Paik A, Rosen R. Sexual dysfunction in the United States: prevalence and predictors. *JAMA* 1999;281:537–544.

13 Nazareth I, Boynton P, King M. Problems with sexual function in people attending London general practitioners: cross sectional study. *BMJ* 2003;327:423–426.

14 Bancroft J, Loftus J, Long JS. Distress about sex: a national survey of women in heterosexual relationships. *Arch Sex Behav* 2003;32:193–208.

15 Hayes RD, Bennett CM, Fairley CK, Dennerstein L. What can prevalence studies tell us about female sexual difficulty and dysfunction? *J Sex Med* 2006;3;589–595.

16 Lewis RW, Fugl-Meyer KS, Corona G *et al*. Definitions/epidemiology/risk factors for sexual dysfunction. *J Sex Med* 2010;7:1598–1607.

17 Sarrel PM, Whitehead MI. Sex and menopause: defining the issues. *Maturitas* 1985;7:217–224.

18 Glatt AE, Zinner SH, McCormack WM. The prevalence of dyspareunia. *Obstet Gynecol* 1990;75:433–436.

19 Sarrel PM. Sexuality and menopause. *Obstet Gynecol* 1990;75: 26s–30s.

20 Munday P, Green J, Randall C *et al.* Vulval vestibulitis: a common cause of dyspareunia? *BJOG* 2005;112:500–503.

21 American Psychiatric Association. *Diagnostic and Statistical Manual of Mental Disorders*, 4th edn. Washington DC: American Psychiatric Association, 2000.

22 The ICD-10 Classification of Mental and Behavioural Disorders. Clinical descriptions and diagnostic guidelines. Geneva: World Health Organization, 1992.

23 Binik YM. Should dyspareunia be retained as a sexual dysfunction in DSM-V? A painful classification. *Arch Sex Behav* 2005; 34:11–21.

24 Balon R, Segraves RT, Clayton A. Issues for DSM-V: sexual dysfunction, disorder, or variation along normal distribution: towards rethinking DSM criteria of sexual dysfunctions. *Am J Psych* 2007;164:198–200.

25 Kleinplatz PJ. Sexuality and older people. *BMJ* 2008;337: 121–122.

26 Saigal CS, Wessels H, Pace J, Schonlau M, Wilt T. Urologic Diseases in America Project. Predictors and prevalence of erectile dysfunction in a racially diverse population. *Arch Intern Med* 2006;166:207–212.

27 Plouffe L. Screening for sexual problems through a simple questionnaire. *Am J Obstet Gynecol* 1985;151:166–169.

28 Rosen R, Brown C, Heiman J, Leiblum S. 'The Female Sexual Function Index (FSFI): a multidimensional self-report instrument for the assessment of female sexual function.' *J Sex Marital Ther* 2000;26:191–208.

29 Rogers RG, Kammerer-Doak D, Villarreal A, Coates K, Qualls C. A new instrument to measure sexual function in women with urinary incontinence and pelvic organ prolapse. *Am J Obstet Gynecol* 2001;184:552–558.

30 McHorney CA, Rust J, Golombok S *et al.* 'Profile of Female Sexual Function: a patient-based, international, psychometric instrument for the assessment of hypoactive sexual desire in oophorectomized women.' *Menopause* 2004;11:474–483.

31 Derogatis LR, Rosen R, Leiblum S, Burnett A, Heiman J. The Female Sexual Distress Scale (FSDS): Initial validation of a standardised scale for assessment of sexually related personal distress in women. *J Sex Mar Ther* 2002;28:4317–4330.

32 Wierman ME, Basson R, Davis SR *et al.* Androgen therapy in women: an Endocrine Society Clinical Practice guideline. *J Clin Endocrinol Metab* 2006;91:3697.

33 Annon JS. The PLISSIT model: a proposed conceptual scheme for the behavioural treatment of sexual problems. *J Sex Educ Ther* 1976;2:1–15.

34 Moynihan R. Merging of marketing and medical science: female sexual dysfunction. *BMJ* 2010;341:c5050.

35 Somboonporn W, Davis S, Seif MW, Bell R. Testosterone for peri- and postmenopausal women. *Cochrane Database Syst Rev* 2005;4:CD004509.

36 Davis S, Papalia MA, Norman RJ *et al.* Safety and efficacy of a testosterone metered-dose transdermal spray for treating decreased sexual satisfaction in premenopausal women: a randomized trial. *Ann Intern Med* 2008;148:569–577.

37 Panay N, Al-Azzawi F, Bouchard C *et al.* Testosterone treatment of HSDD in naturally menopausal women: the ADORE study. *Climacteric* 2010;13:121–231.

38 Kingsberg S, Shifren J, Wekselman K, Rodenberg C, Koochaki P, Derogatis L. Evaluation of the clinical relevance of benefits associated with transdermal testosterone treatment in postmenopausal women with hypoactive sexual desire disorder. *J Sex Med* 2007;4:1001–1008.

39 Suckling J, Lethaby A, Kennedy R. Local oestrogen for vaginal atrophy in postmenopausal women. *Cochrane Database Syst Rev* 2006;18:CD001500.

40 Kaplan SA, Reis RB, Kohn IJ *et al.* Safety and efficacy of sildenafil in postmenopausal women with sexual dysfunction. *Urology* 1999;53:481–486.

41 Basson R, McInnes R, Smith MD *et al.* Efficacy and safety of sildenafil citrate in women with sexual dysfunction associated with female sexual arousal disorder. *J Womens Health Gend Based Med* 2002;11:367–377.

42 Serati M, Salvatore S, Siesto G *et al.* Female sexual function during pregnancy and after childbirth. *J Sex Med* 2010;7: 2782–2790.

43 Barrett G, Peacock J, Victor CR, Manyonda I. Cesarean section and postnatal sexual health. *Birth* 2005;32:306–311.

44 Glazener CM. Sexual function after childbirth: women's experiences, persistent morbidity and lack of professional recognition. *Br J Obstet Gynaecol* 1997;104:330–335.

45 Wallwiener CW, Wallwiener LM, Harald Seeger H, Muck AO, Bitzer J, Wallwiener M. Prevalence of sexual dysfunction and impact of contraception in female German medical students. *J Sex Med* 2010;7:2139–2148.

46 Bianchi-Demichelli F, Kulier R, Perrin E, Campana A. Induced abortion and psychosexuality. *J Psychosom Obstet Gynaecol* 2000;21:213–217.

47 Sadeghi-Nejad H, Wasserman M, Weidner W, Richardson D, Goldmeier D. Sexually transmitted infection and sexual function. *J Sex Med* 2010;7:389–413.

48 Dennerstein L, Alexander JL, Kotz K. The menopause and sexual functioning: a review of the population-based studies. *Ann Rev Sex Res* 2003;14:64–82.

49 Dennerstein L, Guthrie JR, Hayes RD, DeRogatis LR, Lehert P. Sexual function, dysfunction, and sexual distress in a prospective, population-based sample of mid-aged, Australian-born women. *J Sex Med* 2008;5:2291–2299.

50 Diokno AC, Brown MB, Herzog AR. Sexual function in the elderly. *Arch Int Med* 1990;150:197–200.

51 Beckman N, Waern M, Gustafson D, Skoog I. Secular trends in seld reported sexual activity and satisfaction in Swedish 70 year olds: cross sectional survey of four populations, 1971–2001. *BMJ* 2008;337:151–154.

52 Kilkku P, Grönroos M, Hirvonen T, Rauramo L. Supravaginal uterine amputation vs. hysterectomy. Effects on libido and orgasm. *Acta Obstet Gynecol Scand* 1983;62:147–152.

53 Rhodes JC, Kjerulff KH, Langenberg PW, Guzinski GM. Hysterectomy and sexual functioning. *JAMA* 1999;282:1934–1941.

54 Thakar R, Ayers S, Clarkson P, Stanton S, Manyonda I. Outcomes after total versus subtotal abdominal hysterectomy. *N Engl J Med* 2002;347:1318–1325.

55 Geiss IM, Umek WH, Dungl A *et al.* Prevalence of female sexual dysfunction in gynecologic and urogynecologic patients

according to the international consensus classification. *Urology* 2003;62:514–518.

56 Novi JM, Jeronis S, Morgan MA *et al.* Sexual function in women with pelvic organ prolapse and those without pelvic organ prolapse. *J Urol* 2005;173:1669–1672.

57 Ozel B, White T, Urwitz-lane R *et al.* The impact of pelvic organ prolapse on sexual function in women with urinary incontinence. *Int J Urogynecol J Pelvic Floor Dysfunct* 2006;17:14–17.

58 Campion MJ, Brown JR, McCance DJ *et al.* Psychosexual trauma of an abnormal smear. *Br J Obstet Gynaecol* 1998;95:175–181.

59 Thranov I, Klee M. Sexuality among gynaecologic cancer patients- a cross sectional study. *Gynecol Oncol* 1994:52:14–19.

60 Corney RH, Crowther ME, Everett H, Howells A, Shepherd JH. Psychosexual dysfunction in women with gynaecological cancers following radical pelvic surgery *Br J Obstet Gynaecol* 1993;100:73–78.

61 Bergmark K, Avall-Lundquist E, Dickman PW *et al.* Vaginal changes and sexuality in women with a history of cervical cancer. *N Engl J Med* 1999;340:1383–1389.

62 Jensen PT, Groenveld M, Klee MC *et al.* Early stage cervical carcinoma, radical hysterectomy and sexual function. *Cancer* 2004;100:97–106.

Chapter 60
Domestic Violence and Sexual Assault

Maureen Dalton
Royal Devon and Exeter Hospital, Exeter, UK

The effects of domestic violence, rape and child sexual abuse are seen daily in the practice of the obstetrician and gynaecologist. Thus, it is important to be aware of the problems and the correct care of victims.

Domestic abuse

Domestic violence is better considered to be domestic abuse as it is not just physical violence that is involved. The threat of financial and psychological controls are also forms of domestic violence [1]. Domestic abuse is a major cause of maternal mortality and morbidity, and one in four women is a victim of domestic violence [2]. It is not just accident and emergency (A&E) that manages the aftermath – it is now being recognized that the consequences of domestic abuse are commonly seen in obstetrics and gynaecology. It is not always possible to spot a victim, but it is important to try.

Identification

The first step to identifying a victim is to be aware of the possibility that she is being abused. In the past, professionals were either unaware of the problem or thought that domestic abuse was nothing to do with them, being between the patient and her partner or family. However, the consequences of domestic abuse affect health and, if the underlying abuse is missed, the victim may repeatedly re-present and be inappropriately investigated and treated. Therefore, domestic abuse has become a part of the 'diagnostic' aspect of medicine.

Domestic abuse can occur in any social class and affects people of all educational abilities. However, those of lower socioeconomic status generally do not have as much opportunity to remove themselves from the situation and so are more likely to turn to drink or drugs to numb the pain.

The importance of domestic abuse has been stressed in the latest Confidential Enquires into Maternal and Child Health (CEMACE) [3] report *Saving Mothers' Lives*, and in the Royal College of Obstetricians and Gynaecologists (RCOG) publication *Violence Against Women* [1].

The abused woman usually has very low self-confidence and esteem. She feels ashamed of her situation and finds it difficult to ask for help. During their care, all women should have the opportunity to have at least one consultation alone, without partner, friends or relatives present, to allow inquiries about domestic abuse to be made. This may be very difficult to arrange in practice. There are standard questionnaires that can be handed out to women, but they must be given when the woman is alone, filled out when she is alone and handed in when she is alone.

A simple but effective extra way of helping victims to come forward is the 'red spot' system. Notices are placed in women's toilets in the clinics and wards such as that displayed in Summary box 60.1.

Summary box 60.1

Are you living in fear? You are not alone. 1 in 4 women are living with domestic abuse. If you would like to talk to someone about your situation put a red spot on your urine sample and we will find a time to talk to you in confidence about this.

Plastic bags and some adhesive red spots must also be provided. It is unlikely that anyone with the woman is going to realize that there was not a red spot on the sample before. The staff then have to find the time to see the woman alone and help her.

The victims need to be asked specific questions, not generalizations such as 'are things all right at home?'. Women may be desperate to reveal what is going on but

---

only if asked directly and with privacy. The woman needs to be seen in a room with closed windows and doors, in the absence of relatives or friends. Interpreters may be part of the same community even if not members of the family and so may inhibit the revelations. The use of a telephone interpreting service can be useful.

Drawing the curtains around a bed on a ward is definitely not a way to create privacy. Evidence suggests that repeated questioning helps, so it does not matter if someone else has already asked about domestic abuse.

The government equalities office has recently published a guide to good communication with victims of violence [4].

Action when domestic abuse is revealed

- Acknowledge how difficult it has been for the woman to tell another person about it.
- Reassure her that what has been done to her is absolutely wrong and that she did not 'deserve it'.
- Assure her about confidentiality, about who will know and how much, and show her or agree what is written in the notes to demonstrate trust. Remember that she has a right of access to her notes but that in reality within a hospital set-up many people have access to these notes. It is possible that someone who is connected to the perpetrator may be able to read what is in the notes.
- Ask her what she wants to do. Figure 60.1 shows a possible plan of management once a woman has revealed domestic abuse. She may wish to return to her home despite what is happening. She may be worried about her children or afraid of her partner or she may hope he will change.

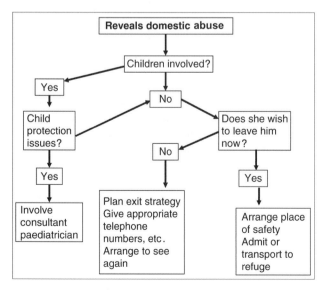

Fig. 60.1 Diagram of management of domestic abuse.

- The woman should *not* be forced to leave home as this would be another form of bullying, controlling behaviour and would contribute to the abuse.
- Advice on leaving the perpetrator should be given if she wishes to receive it, e.g. to give her the telephone numbers of national helplines and local women's refuge, the names of local solicitors interested in family law can be given. Reassure her that the police now take domestic abuse seriously and changes in the law have strengthened what they can do.
- *Write careful notes.*

> **Summary box 60.2**
>
> - One in four women is a victim of domestic abuse.
> - Domestic abuse is a major cause of maternal morbidity and mortality.
> - Children of mothers who are abused are also likely to be abused.
> - Every opportunity must be taken to ask a women seen in both obstetrics and gynaecology departments whether she is a victim. This needs to be when she is alone.
> - Repeated asking aids disclosure.

Child protection issues

If there are children involved, there is a legal obligation to consider whether the children are significantly at risk. If this seems to be the case, the woman's wishes can be overruled. Often she will agree to some form of compromise if there are significant child protection issues. It is vital at this point to follow the agreed child protection protocols drawn up for the local area. Involve the consultant paediatrician on call (safeguarding protocols). Hospital social work departments should also be contacted for advice. It is not appropriate or necessary to follow child protection protocols in every case of domestic abuse, but the possibility should always be considered.

Support for staff

Staff should be reassured that they have made successful use of their communication skills if they have uncovered upsetting levels of abuse. The woman trusted them enough to tell them the situation and was given a choice. Staff may find that they went back to the perpetrator, was severely injured or even murdered but *it was not their fault*. At least the woman had been given a chance to talk about changing her situation. On the other hand, never asking about domestic abuse and never giving the victim an opportunity to reveal what was happening would be a definite failure.

Health consequences

Research in this area is difficult. It is not possible to perform double-blind randomized control trials and even cohort studies in this area rely on the 'non-abused' cohort being genuinely non-abused rather than just too scared to reveal. The number of times that the woman is seen by the researcher in privacy will increase the chance that she will reveal domestic abuse. Therefore, there is conflicting evidence on the effects. The following generalizations can probably be made.

Obstetrics

Pregnancy is a time when domestic abuse often starts or increases, as summarized in Table 60.1. It is highest among teenage pregnancies. There is an association with increased risk of:

- miscarriage;
- low birthweight;
- unintended pregnancy and increased termination of pregnancy (TOP) requests;
- preterm labour; and
- chorioamnionitis.

The *Saving Mothers' Lives* [3] report confirms the tendency of women who were subsequently murdered to present late or to be frequent non-attendees. It must be remembered that this vulnerable group may not be able to attend hospital appointments because they are not allowed to. It is important to consider why a woman has failed to attend a clinic and give further appointments. A 'one strike and you are out' policy will only victimize women who are possibly experiencing abuse.

Partners who perpetrate violence are often with their victim the whole time with a noticeable controlling and dominating attitude.

Summary box 60.3

- The long-term consequences of domestic abuse will affect the woman's visits to the obstetrician and gynaecologist.
- Recurrent failure to keep appointments may reflect past or current abuse rather than fecklessness.

Gynaecology (Table)

It is now being recognized that the consequences of domestic abuse are commonly seen in gynaecology as well as obstetrics. Women who are victims of domestic abuse are more likely to present complaining of the following:

- pelvic pain;
- menstrual disturbances;
- dyspareunia;
- vaginal discharge;
- sterilization;

Table 60.1 Presentation of domestic abuse.

Obstetrics
Miscarriage
Low birthweight
Unintended pregnancy and increased termination of pregnancy requests
Preterm labour
Chorioamnionitis

Gynaecology
Pelvic pain
Menstrual disturbances
Dyspareunia
Vaginal discharge
Sterilization
Top requests
Pelvic inflammatory disease

General
Psychiatric problems
Irritable bowel syndrome
Asthma
Chest pain
Headache

- TOP requests; and
- pelvic inflammatory disease (PID).

The list is similar to that seen in a routine gynaecology clinic but they are also more likely to have the following:

- psychiatric problems;
- irritable bowel syndrome (IBS);
- asthma;
- chest pain;
- headache; and
- alcohol or drug abuse problems.

Sexual assault

Any woman who is seen in obstetric and gynaecology clinics could have been a victim of sexual assault (Fig. 60.2). The British Crime Survey [5] found that 1 in 20 women had been sexually assaulted. This means a woman is more likely to be a victim if sexual assault than have diabetes or a stroke [6]. After they have been assaulted, women are more likely to perceive their health as poor or fair rather than good. They become heavy users of the health service, presenting more frequently than others with vaginal discharge, psychiatric problems, menstrual disorders, dyspareunia, abdominal pain, IBS and headache. It is therefore important to provide good initial care for a victim, that does not necessarily involve the police, to help with her long-term healthcare. This must be done sensitively and accurately to maximize possible forensic evidence.

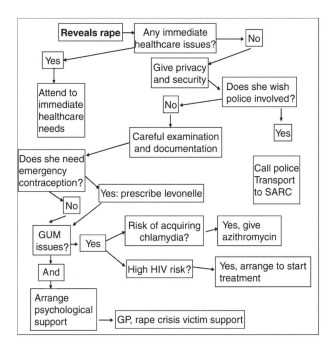

Fig. 60.2 Diagram of management of acute sexual assault. SARC, Sexual Assault Referral Centre; GUM, genitourinary medicine; HIV, human immunodeficiency virus; GP, general practitioner.

They will often not have gone to the police for many reasons, including:

- fear of not being believed;
- fear of the court process;
- fear of the assailant (especially as the assailant is usually known to the victim); and
- embarrassment and fear of further examinations.

The development of post-traumatic stress disorders and the fear of damage from the assault results in frequent visits to healthcare providers.

Initial action following a revelation of an acute sexual assault

The victim may reveal during a consultation for a supposed other problem that she has been recently assaulted.

Immediate health needs must obviously be checked first. If she is bleeding heavily, she needs a drip and appropriate resuscitation. When she is stable, move her into a room where she can have some privacy and then ask if she wishes the police to be involved. Save any urine that is passed before the police arrive (they may wish to screen for drugs).

Check briefly whether there was forced oral sex. If yes, no drinks should be offered until the police can provide an early evidence kit that provides a mouth sample for sperm.

Sexual assault referral centres

Police forces around the country are being encouraged to collaborate with health services to develop Sexual Assault Referral Centres (SARCs) such as the long-standing

Table 60.2 Management of sexual assault victims.

Management of rape victim
Assess immediate health needs
Arrange privacy
Ask if he or she wishes police involvement
Consent to examine
Examine from head to toe
Careful documentation
Swabs if appropriate
Emergency contraception
Infection prophylaxis
Psychological support

centres at St Mary's in Manchester and REACH in the northeast of England. The victim can go to a SARC for examination but counselling and support can also be arranged. Most SARCs do not require that the victim has been to the police. Table 60.2 shows the management of a victim.

When initially seen in a SARC, the doctor has first to consider if the victim can consent to examination. If she has been drugged or is very drunk she may need more time before the examination can take place. A general history, including asking for bleeding problems and psychiatric problems should be taken initially. The doctor's role is not to be the detective and decide whether the woman has or has not been raped. The doctor must appear to believe her for the sake of her long-term recovery, *but* if a written statement is required for the court, it should be independent and *not* written on her behalf or that of the defendant.

The doctor will be seeing the woman before she has given a statement to the police and so should not ask too many questions about the incident in order to avoid inadvertent suggestions being made that effect the memories of the event.

The examination

The advantage of examining in a SARC is that they are specially designed to minimize DNA contamination. If there is no alternative to examining the victim in a ward or emergency department, any human contact before examination should be minimized. Gloves and theatre clothes or gowns should be worn as they are less contaminated than ordinary clothes. A careful head-to-toe examination looking for bruises, scratches and grazes should be performed. Swabs dampened with sterile water taken from areas the perpetrator has kissed such as face and nipples, and even from areas where he has gripped if taken soon enough after the event, can reveal his DNA.

Most normally sexually active victims do not have genital injuries but may have other injuries, e.g. where they have been forcibly held down. Careful, accurate documentation is one of the most important parts of the examination; it is helpful to use body diagrams to show where the injuries are. Bruises need the size, shape and colour recorded. It is not possible to accurately age bruises.

The size and shape of abrasions (scratches and grazes) also need to be recorded. It is often possible to tell the direction of the force in a scratch and if fresh the loops of skin are present. These rub off once they have dried.

From April 2004, the Royal College of Paediatrics and Child Health & Association of Forensic Physicians (RCPCH&AFP) guidelines [7] for the examination of victims of sexual assault under the age of 18 years recommend the use of a colposcope for genital examination. This should still be considered best practice for all female victims as the injuries can be better visualized. All examinations in children should be totally recorded, but for adults, when the majority do not have genital injuries, it is appropriate to use it to record injuries so that they can be discussed with another medical expert. A colposcope also allows intimate examination without invading the victim's personal space too much when looking and taking swabs. Using a magnifying glass and light close in between her knees is intrusive for the victim. In addition, more injuries can be identified using a colposcope.

There must be consent for any photographs or videos taken and access must be restricted. They become part of the medical records, not the police notes. Photographs relating to an assault should only be revealed to a medical expert who must confirm that they will not show them to anyone else without the victim's permission or on the direction of a judge.

Unfortunately there have been occasions when these pictures have fallen into the wrong hands, and if care is not taken women will not allow these useful records to be taken.

Swabs should be taken during the genital examination from outside in, that is, starting with the vulua (including the perineum), then the lower vagina (including the introitus), higher vagina and then the cervix.

The time since the assault and the details of the assault are important in deciding which swabs to take (see Table 60.3).

Aftercare

Once the examination is complete, the woman may take a shower or bath, as she is likely to feel dirty.
There are then the other issues to be discussed:
* emergency contraception if appropriate;
* infection – azithromycin should be offered if there is any possibility of Chlamydia infection.

Table 60.3 Persistence of sperm.

Persistence of sperm	Duration
Vagina	7 days
Anal canal/rectum	3 days
Mouth	Usually 6 h to 2 days
Cervix	7–10 days
Skin/hair	Unknown but may persist after cleaning

* human immunodeficiency virus (HIV) prophylaxis – is the perpetrator likely to have HIV? Is he an intravenous drug abuser or does he come from a high-risk area for HIV, were there multiple assailants, anal intercourse or many bleeding injuries? If so, HIV prophylaxis may be appropriate and most hospitals have a protocol for how to access the start of treatment out of hours so that it can begin as soon as possible. Encourage victims to visit their local genitourinary medicine (GUM) clinic within the following few days where HIV risk and hepatitis vaccination can be discussed further; and
* psychological support – if the local SARC does not have access to counselling services, early involvement of the general practitioner (GP) should be encouraged as initial careful management reduces long-term health risks and it is the GP who will be in the first-line when these problems arise.

Everyone benefits from helping the victim initially.

Guilt feelings are part of a victim's psychological response, so it is useful to stress to her that she has done nothing wrong – the guilt and the shame lie with the perpetrator.

The statement

There is a duty to provide a statement to the court, even if it is the police that ask for it. If a doctor is found to have misled the court with his or her evidence or statements, this is taken seriously by the General Medical Council.

In a 'professional' statement it should be made clear to the police, Crown Prosecution Service and, if necessary, the judge that the doctor has acted as a professional without the expertise to interpret the injuries.

An expert view considers the cause but must remember all reasonable possible alternative causations for each injury. Certainty of causation can be expressed on a scale of one to five where 1 represents no suggestion that the injury is explained by (or relates to) any particular causation and 5 represents certainty of what the injury has been caused by. Any statement must be accurate and look professional. Qualifications and experience should be stated. Conclusions should consider both causation and consistency with the history.

The statement should end with a phrase such as 'based on information given to me to date' as new information may come to light that means conclusions need to be reviewed. Help and advice in writing a statement may be available from the nurse or doctor designated for child protection in your hospital or area.

Child sexual abuse

Many women attending gynaecology clinics were sexually abused as children. Like victims of rape, they present more commonly with gynaecological problems than non-abused women. They may find pelvic examinations difficult. It is helpful to allow the woman to feel in control. She may find it easier to pass the speculum herself. She may find a male doctor more frightening and get flashbacks to her abuse. This may result in her feeling violated and reluctant to return for further treatment. She may not be suitable for outpatient procedures so day case admission and anaesthetic may be a better option for her.

There is evidence that child sex abuse (CSA) is another area that is underdiagnosed currently. When a gynaecologist sees any child, it is appropriate to consider CSA. Clearly this does not mean that every child seen by the gynaecologist is abused, but many of the presentations are similar and so it will frequently be part of the differential diagnosis. Has the child seen in the emergency department really fallen astride a bicycle or is the injury a result of abuse. What about the child with a vaginal discharge?

A child who is old enough to talk will do so, if they feel safe in the environment, and are allowed to use their own terms to give a relevant history. Often the right privacy for disclosure is not provided. Unlike physical abuse of a child, sexual abuse rarely presents acutely and the medical examination findings are usually only a small part of the evidence that decides whether a child has been abused. Often there are no clear indications of abuse on examination.

 Summary box 60.4

All examinations of children where there is a possibility of sexual assault should be combined with a paediatrician and involve two doctors.

If a gynaecologist has any concerns about the possibility of sexual abuse, it is essential to discuss this with a paediatrician who has expertise in this area or the on-call paediatric consultant. A joint examination with a paediatrician is best practice [7] so that there are two people independently assessing the injuries.

The initial examination should be the same as for any forensic examination. A head-to-toe examination looking for bruising, scratches and other injuries that may support the allegation must be performed. The stage of puberty must always be noted.

If the genitalia of a child in whom there may have been a history of abuse needs to be examined. It should be a joint examination and a colposcope is recommended best practice for recording the findings.

A young child may feel more secure sitting on her mother's knee. The interpretation of a normal hymen is difficult. Minor clefts or bumps may be normal and redundant folds of the hymen may hide significant tears. The hymen must be gently inspected all around. Posterior–lateral traction of the labia may improve visualization, as may gently 'floating' the hymen with warmed normal saline or water. Passing a small catheter into the vagina, then blowing up the balloon and gently retracting may also allow the whole hymen to be visualized. It is now appreciated that the size of the hymenal orifice varies considerably, especially in obese children, and so great significance should not be placed on measurements of its size.

When examining the anus, care must be taken to avoid too much pressure for too long or venous suffusion by the separation process can be produced.

Many children who have been sexually abused do not have abnormalities, even when the perpetrator has admitted full penetration. As in adult assault, the finding of no injury does not mean that nothing has happened.

Summary

The gynaecologist will see a number of women who have been sexually assaulted as children or as adults and this must be remembered as it may have a significant influence on the presenting problem and how she should be examined and managed. Domestic abuse is common and victims may not attend clinics but are high-risk patients who should not be rapidly discharged. When they are pregnant, they are at a greater risk of complications and maternal death.

References

1 Bewley S, Friend J, Mezey G (eds) *Violence against Women*. London: RCOG Press, 1997.
2 Dalton M (ed) *Forensic Gynaecology*. London: RCOG Press, 2004.
3 Lewis G. Deaths apparently unrelated to pregnancy from coincidental and late causes including domestic abuse in Centre for Maternal and Child Enquiries (CMACE). Saving Mothers' Lives: reviewing maternal deaths to make motherhood safer: 2006–2008. The eighth report on confidential enquiries into maternal deaths in the United Kingdom. *BJOG* 2011;118(Suppl 1):1–203.

4 Government Equalities Office. Tackling Violence against Women and Girls – A Guide to Good Practice Communications. Available at: http://www.equalities.gov.uk/pdf/297847%20Tackling%20 Violence%20women%20hyperlinked_V3.pdf.

5 Walby S, Allen J. Domestic violence, sexual assault and stalking: findings from the British Crime Survey. Home Office, 2004.

6 Alberti G, responding to violence against women and children – the role of the NHS. Available at: www.dh.gov.uk/prod_ consum_dh/groups/dh_digitalassets/@dh/@en/@ps/ documents/digitalasset/dh_113824.pdf.

7 The Royal College of Paediatrics & Child Health and the Faculty of Forensic and Legal Medicine. Guidelines on Paediatric Forensic Examinations in Relation to Possible Child Sex Abuse. Available at: https://fflm.ac.uk/upload/documents/ 1233931978.pdf.

Chapter 61
Ethical Dilemmas in Obstetrics and Gynaecology

Sheila McLean

Institute of Law and Ethics in Medicine, University of Glasgow, Glasgow, UK

Introduction

It is probably no overstatement to say that obstetrics and gynaecology is amongst the most ethically, and sometimes legally, complex areas of medicine. The ability to create, monitor, manipulate and deliver new lives alone is sufficient to explain why this discipline is so challenging. Advances in fetal medicine have contributed to the range of vital, yet highly sensitive, decisions that professionals are able – and sometimes required – to make on a regular basis.

At the core of these decisions is the relationship between healthcare professionals and those whom they serve – most notably their pregnant female patients. While all good patient/doctor relationships demand trust, what is at stake in this area requires a level of trust that is heightened by the consequences of a poor or failed relationship. Women seeking to become pregnant, women faced with decisions about continuing a pregnancy and women confronted with choices about the welfare of the embryo or fetus are uniquely in need of the best possible advice and treatment, and a relationship firmly grounded in trust with those caring for them is essential to the protection of the women themselves. However, even when that kind of relationship exists, there can sometimes be serious tensions between women's own interests and those of the embryo/fetus they are carrying or hope to carry, and no consensus on the way forward can be achieved.

Although there are many areas which could be the focus of this chapter – not least assisted reproductive technologies and pregnancy termination – the problems that are associated with decisions in pregnancy or labour are arguably those that are the most difficult, as well as the least regulated, and will therefore be the focus of what follows. While legislation covers the activities involved in assisted reproduction, and pregnancy termination is constrained by legislative requirements, decisions about the management of pregnancy and labour must be negotiated with only the common law – and of course, ethics – as a guide. Particularly when women resist medical advice, the loyalties and obligations of doctors to their pregnant patients can stand in direct conflict with their efforts to attain the optimal outcome for the 'child' who is yet to be born.

While undoubtedly beneficial in many ways, the vast progress in the technology and options available to doctors in this specialism has seen some consequences that are by no means universally welcomed. The ability to visualize the fetus in the womb, for example, has been said to change the relationship between doctors and their patients. Squier says that nowadays '. . . the different stages of embryonic/fetal life are increasingly mediated by – and thus constructed by – ultrasound and other fetal visualization technologies . . . ' [1]. Annas also cautions against the potential consequences of fetal imaging, arguing that, '. . . [o]ne of the major consequences of antenatal diagnosis of the fetus has been to view the fetus as a patient, often termed the doctor's 'second patient . . . ' [2].

Summary box 61.1

Advances in technology have changed the perception of pregnancy; this has an effect on both pregnant women's decisions and on the healthcare team caring for her.

Perhaps for this reason, although probably not solely because of this, some clinicians have come to see their responsibilities as extended. No longer is the pregnant woman their sole patient, but – morally, if not legally – the ability to see what was previously hidden, coupled with the (albeit relatively limited) ability to intervene *in utero*, challenges doctors to prioritize their commitments. For this reason, the relationship between the healthcare professional and the pregnant woman can be uncomfortably charged as well as uniquely important.

Moreover, the visualization of the fetus and acceptance of perceived responsibilities towards it have consequences

Dewhurst's Textbook of Obstetrics & Gynaecology, Eighth Edition. Edited by D. Keith Edmonds.
© 2012 John Wiley and Sons, Ltd. Published 2012 by John Wiley and Sons, Ltd.

that go beyond the medical relationship. As Ikenotos [3] has said:

In the past few years, the state has begun stepping in to reinforce the idea that a woman should act in particular ways and for particular reasons during pregnancy. The message used to justify state intervention is that a pregnant woman is a mother who should think and act first and foremost to protect the health of the fetus she carries.

While it is indisputable that the state – like the vast majority of pregnant women and, of course, their doctors – has an interest in ensuring the best possible outcome of a pregnancy, achieving a balance between that interest and any competing ones and adjudicating on where that balance lies is ethically problematic and was, for some time, legally unclear. As we will see in what follows, while the law may now be reasonably settled, at least in the UK, this does not resolve the ethical dilemmas experienced by those who must implement the rules. While we can agree with Purdy [4] that '. . . [r]espect for our right, as moral agents, to control our bodies, is a keystone of liberal society . . . ', others suggest that this assertion of the dominance of individual autonomy sits uneasily with pregnancy, because 'The relationship of pregnancy does not fit easily into the liberal conceptualizations of individuality and separateness . . . While pregnancy is about connectedness, the language of rights and autonomy is about separation . . . ' [5].

On this view, the traditional claim to have the right to make one's own decisions must be tempered by our need to take account of the others who will be affected by our choices, and a truly autonomous decision can only be achieved when we recognize ourselves as embedded in a community (however small or large) and not simply as atomized independent actors. What is clear is that as medicine continues to advance, the way in which we address the problems that can arise from the interplay of women's rights and interests in the fetus will take on increasing significance for the autonomy of pregnant women and the fate of the embryos/fetuses they carry. As Robertson and Shulman [6] say:

Developments in obstetrics, genetics, fetal medicine and infectious diseases will continue to provide knowledge and technologies that will enable many disabled births to be prevented. While most women will welcome this knowledge and gladly act on it, others will not. The ethical, legal, and policy aspects of this situation require a careful balancing of the offspring's welfare and the pregnant woman's interest in liberty and bodily integrity.

The ethical and legal responses to this need for 'careful balancing' will be considered in more depth in what follows.

The fetus, law and morals/ethics

Although both 'morals' and 'ethics' have been used in the heading for this section of the chapter, a distinction should be made between the two which is important for this discussion, although it is contentious. However, even if it does not commend itself to the reader, this is not fatal to the analysis that follows. Morals, here, are taken to mean that in which we believe inherently and personally. They may be shaped by the way we are brought up, our life experiences, our faith and so on. Ethics, on the other hand, is the framework within which we make decisions. While the two may often coincide, they can also be divergent. For example, if my ethic is that the decisions of others are worthy of respect, this may conflict with my moral intuition that what they have chosen to do is fundamentally 'wrong'; the question is, which of these – morals or ethics – should guide my behaviour? As we will see, this is by no means an idle question and it has confronted doctors and courts on a number of occasions.

One of the fundamental questions that must be addressed early in this discussion is, of course, the status to be accorded to the parties most intimately concerned here – the embryo/fetus and the pregnant woman. The second of these is more easily resolved, but the former is the subject of divergent, sometimes polarized, views. For some, the embryo/fetus, irrespective of its stage of development, is not fully morally relevant; for others, it is a person (or perhaps a potential person) and therefore entitled to full status and the rights that go with that. It is obviously not possible to resolve that question here, and it will be conceded with McCullogh and Chervenak [7] that:

All accounts about whether or not the fetus possesses independent moral status commit a common error: they seek to find or reject some time, prior to or at delivery, during which the fetus possesses some intrinsic characteristic that in turn generates independent moral status. This matter is endlessly disputed because . . . it is endlessly disputable.

For the purposes of this chapter, then, the approach taken by the Report of the Committee of Inquiry Into Human Fertilisation and Embryology (Warnock Report) [8] will be adopted; namely that 'the embryo of the human species ought to have a special status . . . ', and that 'although the human embryo is entitled to some added measure of respect beyond that accorded to other animal subjects, that respect cannot be absolute . . . ' [8]. This position, known as the 'gradualist approach', also entails that the respect to be accorded to the embryo increases as it matures towards birth. However, it also implies that, although the respect due to the fetus is greater than that due to the early embryo, it is not equivalent to a born person.

Whereas ethically the status of the embryo/fetus is often the subject of debate, the legal position is rather more clear, although as we will see it has not always been applied in an unequivocal manner in court decisions. However, it now seems to be settled by law that the embryo/fetus does not have legal status unless and until it is born alive.[1] This position has been clearly stated in a number of cases. For example, in the case of *Paton v Trustees of BPAS* [9], the court said, '[t]he fetus cannot, in English law ... have any right of its own at least until it is born and has a separate existence from its mother' [9, at *p*. 989]. In this case, the European Commission of Human Rights was ultimately asked to consider whether the existing abortion law in England and Wales violated rights under Articles 2 (the right to life) and 8 (the right to private and family life) of the European Convention on Human Rights.[2] The first question, therefore, was whether a fetus was owed a right to life under Article 2. The Commission rejected the argument that Article 2 confers a 'strong' right to life on a fetus. The other options open to it were either that Article 2 did not cover a fetus at all or that it conferred a 'weak' right to life on the fetus, a right that, in the early stages of pregnancy, gives way to the interests of the pregnant woman. Although the Commission declined to choose between these two options, it is clear that the fetus is not accorded rights under Article 2 and is consequently not deemed to be 'another' for the purposes of Article 8.

In the later case of *Re MB* [10], the court affirmed that:

The fetus up to the moment of birth does not have any separate interests capable of being taken into account when a court has to consider an application for a declaration in respect of a Caesarean section operation. The court does not have the jurisdiction to declare that such medical intervention is lawful to protect the interests of the unborn child even at the point of birth [11].

Lord Mustill in the House of Lords attempted what might be seen as a compromise proposal, saying:

The mother and the fetus were two distinct organisms living symbiotically, not a single organism with two aspects ... I would, therefore, reject the reasoning which assumes that since (in the eyes of English law) the fetus does not have the attributes which make it a 'person' it must be an adjunct of the mother. Eschewing all religious and political debate, I would say that the fetus is neither. It is a unique organism. To apply to such an organism the principles of a law evolved in relation to autonomous beings is bound to mislead [12].

While these judgements resolve the legal position, they leave untouched the moral position of a number of individuals, including some healthcare professionals, and the position adopted by the law will not commend itself to them as an appropriate approach. In addition, it will clearly be distressing for healthcare professionals to be confronted with a situation in which a fetus could be saved, yet the pregnant woman refuses to act in accordance with clinical recommendations. The problem is that, for as long as fetuses are not accorded legal rights, it is the rights of the pregnant woman that prevail, and, like it or not, there are good reasons why this is the case. First, reproductive liberty is a right for which women (and men) have fought for many years, through periods of compulsory eugenic sterilizations and denial of access to contraception, to name but two inroads into reproductive freedom. As Mary Anne Warren [13] points out: '... the right of individual women and men to make their own decisions about the highly personal matter of reproduction is particularly vulnerable, and must be defended with special care'.

Second, were embryos/fetuses to be accorded rights, the restrictions on (particularly) women's lifestyle would conceivably be incalculable, relegating them to the status of fetal container rather than a full citizen with equal rights to others. Not only would this be politically and socially unacceptable, it would also conflict with the rights that women are accorded by international agreements and, in the case of the UK, specifically by the European Convention on Human Rights. Most particularly, Article 8 of the Convention protects the right to private and family life – often referred to as the 'autonomy' article. While there are some derogations from this right permitted by Article 8(2), these do not include pregnancy. And as we have seen, while Article 2 of the Convention refers to the right to life, it has never been interpreted as applying to the life of an entity not yet born [14].

Further articles of the Convention may also be used in support of women's rights to make decisions even if they may harm their embryos/fetuses. Article 3 offers protection against inhuman or degrading treatment and states that '[*n*]o one shall be subjected to torture or to inhuman or degrading treatment or punishment.' In the case of *Herczegfalvy v Austria* [15], the patient, amongst other things, endured forcible intramuscular injection of sedatives, the use of handcuffs and a security bed. The court held that:

Measures taken out of therapeutic necessity cannot be regarded as inhuman or degrading treatment. However, the court must satisfy itself based upon the evidence that the medical necessity has been convincingly shown to exist [15].

Treatment without the consent of the patient may therefore be permissible where there is a provable 'therapeutic necessity', but in the case of pregnancy and labour would require two pieces of evidence to be established. First, it would have to be shown that the proposed intervention over the protests of the pregnant woman is, indeed, therapeutic. Given that the recommended intervention may in fact be therapeutic for the embryo/fetus rather than the woman, and given that the fetus is not covered by the Convention, it would be extremely difficult to establish this. Second, even if the proposed treatment is to save the life of the pregnant woman, and could therefore be said to be 'therapeutic', the law is clear that when an individual is competent they can reject even optimal treatment recommendations. In the case of *Denmark, Norway, Sweden and the Netherlands v Greece* [16], the European Court of Human Rights (ECHR) stated that 'treatment or punishment of an individual may be said to be degrading if it grossly humiliates him before others or drives him to act against his will or conscience' [16, at *p*. 186]. Being forced to submit, for example to a Caesarean section, would surely qualify as degrading in these terms, even although this particular point has not been directly considered by the European Court of Human Rights.

The case of *R.(on the application of W) v Broadmoor Hospital* [17] provides an insight into the way in which UK courts have addressed the application of Article 3. In this case, W was a psychiatric patient who raised an appeal against the refusal of his application for medical witnesses to attend for cross-examination in judicial review proceedings, which he raised in respect of a decision to administer non-consensual treatment using force. He argued that such forced treatment infringed his human rights as enshrined in Articles 2, 3 and 8 of the ECHR. Having considered his claim, Lord Justice Brown stated that:

. . . the forcible injection of an unwilling patient must constitute at the very least degrading treatment and, if the appellant is properly to be regarded as capacitated, it clearly violates his fundamental rights to autonomy and bodily inviolability. Even if Article 3 is not breached, runs the argument, article 8 is, there being no sufficient justification under Article 8.2 for so fundamental an invasion of the appellant's autonomy and inviolability, basic ingredients of his right to privacy [10].

Lady Justice Hale also referred to the guidance that could be obtained from the *Herczegfalvy* case, mentioned

above, concluding that, '. . . forcible measures inflicted upon an incapacitated patient which are not a medical necessity may indeed be inhuman or degrading. The same must apply to forcible measures inflicted upon a capacitated patient' [18].

The legal position, then, can be summed up as follows:

[a] mentally competent patient has an absolute right to refuse to consent to medical treatment for any reason, rational or irrational, or for no reason at all, even where that decision may lead to his or her own death. . . . [19]

This also includes the death of a fetus, even if it is viable. As the court said in the case of *Re F (in utero)* [20], if that position were to change, it would need to be at the initiative of Parliament – it is not for judges to change the law. It may seem counter-intuitive – even distasteful – that a developing or viable fetus is not accorded protection against the risks taken by the pregnant woman with its life (and perhaps her own), but this is a moral position rather than a legal one. As Judge LJ said in the case of *St. George's Healthcare N.H.S. Trust v S* [21]:

When a human life is at stake the pressure to provide an affirmative answer authorising unwanted medical intervention is very powerful. Nevertheless, the autonomy of each individual requires continuing protections even, perhaps particularly, when the motive for interfering with it is readily understandable, and indeed to many would appear commendable [21].

It is, therefore, one thing to be offended by, or disapproving of, a pregnant woman's decisions, but it is quite another to force her to choose differently using the vehicle of the law.

 Summary box 61.3

The embryo/fetus has no legal status until live birth.
  The pregnant woman has the legal right to reject any medical intervention, even if it puts the embryo or fetus at risk of injury or even death.

Managing pregnancy and childbirth

As mentioned elsewhere:

Even if we are all agreed that an embryo or fetus should have the best possible start on the path towards birth, and even if we do not wish to discount it as merely a mass of unimportant and morally neutral cells, there are very strong reasons for being concerned about the development of foetal rights [22].

The potentially negative impact of developing fetal rights is most clearly demonstrated by what has happened – and continues to happen – in the USA, where a powerful 'pro-life' lobby has had considerable influence on policy makers and courts alike. Concern for the developing embryo/fetus has led to the prosecution of women because of their behaviour during pregnancy, particularly, although not exclusively, where they were using drugs – licit or illicit. The human cost of this behaviour is not doubted. In fact, it has been estimated that 'as many as eleven per cent of babies born in the U.S. (375 000 annually) are born to mothers who have used illicit drugs during their pregnancies . . . Fetal alcohol syndrome, in which babies can suffer growth retardation, microcephaly, facial abnormalities and malformations of the limbs and organs appears once in every 1000 births in the U.S.' [23]. This kind of evidence led to 'a new prosecutorial trend', which saw the prosecution of women who gave birth to babies who had been exposed to drugs during the pregnancy [24]. Not only does this directly challenge women's rights to act in a self-determining manner, it is also of dubious effectiveness. There is no evidence that prosecuting pregnant women with a drug problem, particularly addiction, prevents such behaviour in the future. In addition, programmes to help these women and wean them off drugs (or alcohol) are few and far between. It is an abandonment of social responsibility to deny access to treatment and then punish for behaviour which is difficult, if not impossible, to change without help. Indeed, it may even be counter-productive, as some research suggests that 'when pregnant women fear that they will be prosecuted for their drug use, they do not seek prenatal care and will even choose to deliver their babies at home' [25].

The ugly face of compulsion, is clearly outlined in what follows:

In the name of foetal rights, women across the US have been dragged bleeding from hospitals into prison cells hours after giving birth, charged with homicide following stillbirths, pinned to hospital beds and forced to have Caesareans against their will, or had their babies removed at birth after a single positive test for alcohol or drugs. Since the mid-70s around 300 women have been arrested for these transgressions, and 30 states now have foetal homicide laws [26].

And it is not only women who have abused drugs and/ or alcohol in the course of their pregnancy who have been affected by the recognition of fetal rights. Some have found themselves prosecuted primarily for failing to behave in a manner recommended by their physicians [27]. In addition, in one case, 'a lower court ordered a pregnant woman's cervix sewn up against her will to prevent a possible miscarriage' [28]. Although the state's supreme court eventually vacated this order, the very fact that it was supported by *any* court is troubling. This is not an isolated incident – there are other examples that are equally resistant to the claims of women's rights, and that actively pursue the fetal rights agenda to the detriment of the living person [29].

In addition, by the authority of the law, and sometimes at the initiative of the physicians caring for the pregnant woman, a pattern of forced obstetrical interventions has also emerged. While this is a problem that has arisen most frequently in the USA, it is by no means unheard of in the UK. Because of the particularly egregious nature of the practice in the USA, however, a brief consideration of the situation there will be undertaken before moving to consider the UK position. As long ago as 1987, Kolder *et al.* [30], investigating forced Caesarean sections in the USA, reported that court orders had been obtained for Caesarean sections in 11 states, for hospital detentions in two states and intrauterine transfusions in one state. Among 21 cases in which court orders were sought, they were awarded in 86%. In 88% of these cases, the orders were issued within 6 hours. In a further example, reported by CBS news, a woman was initially charged with murder after repeatedly refusing to undergo a Caesarean section and was finally sentenced to 18 months imprisonment for child endangerment [31]. Similarly, in *Jefferson v Griffin Spaulding County Hospital Auth.* [32], the court upheld the right of doctors to perform a non-consensual Caesarean section, as they did in *Re Madyyun* [33]. In *Taft v Taft* [28] on the other hand, the court reversed an earlier court order compelling a pregnant woman to submit to a surgical procedure to prevent the likelihood of miscarriage. However, in this case it would appear that the critical factor was that the fetus was pre-viable; in other words, it could not in any event have been saved.

Perhaps the best known, and arguably the most distressing, example from the USA can be found in the case of Angela Carder [34]. Mrs Carder had suffered from cancer on two previous occasions, but was currently in remission. When she was about 26 weeks pregnant, it was discovered that her cancer had returned and that her death was imminent. She agreed to a treatment regime that gave her the best chance of surviving until the fetus had a better chance for its own survival, but eventually her condition deteriorated further. The hospital administrators applied for a court order to gain authority to perform a Caesarean section, over Mrs Carder's objections. When she was told that this had been granted, she continued to protest. Her lawyer attempted to have the order blocked even as she was being prepared for surgery, but the Washington D.C. Court of Appeals upheld the original order, and the Caesarean section was duly performed. The baby died after a couple of hours, and Mrs Carder survived for two days (the Caesarean section was listed on the death certificate as a contributing cause of death). The American Civil Liberties Union describes this case in this way: '[i]n Washington, DC, a young pregnant woman, severely ill with cancer, several times mouthed the words "I don't want it done" when told that a court had ordered her to undergo a cesarean and that she likely would not survive the operation' [35]. Although the court's decisions were successfully appealed [36], this obviously came too late for Mrs Carder, whose emotions and distress in her final days can only be imagined.

Similar cases have also arisen in the UK, although perhaps none in quite the dramatic circumstances of Angela Carder [36]. The first reported case is that of *Re S (adult: refusal of medical treatment)* [37], where an English judge authorized a forced Caesarean section on a woman who had refused it on religious grounds. The case was heard as an emergency, and the judgement was delivered in around 20 minutes. The judge took account of the interests of both the woman and the fetus, but it is clear that fetal interests were given considerable weight.

In an earlier case, Lord Donaldson had said that '[a]n adult patient who...suffers from no mental incapacity has an absolute right to choose whether to consent to medical treatment, to refuse it or to choose one rather than another of the treatments being offered' [37]. However, at the end of this statement he inserted a qualification, which is particularly relevant for this discussion, saying '[t]he only possible qualification is a case in which the choice may lead to the death of a viable fetus' [37]. Arguably, it is this caveat that encouraged doubt about the respective status of pregnant women and fetuses in subsequent judgements. Indeed, in *Re F* [20], a local authority attempted to make a fetus a ward of court to protect it from the behaviour of its mother. This application was refused on the basis that 'until the child was actually born, there would be an inherent incompatibility between any projected exercise of the wardship jurisdiction and the rights and welfare of the mother' [38]. In *D (a minor) v Berkshire County Council* [39], it was held competent to make a care order in respect of a child who had been born suffering from drug dependency. In doing so, the court felt able to take into account conditions existing during pregnancy, as well as those existing after birth, but it should be noted that it would not have been possible to act *before* birth. The law was finally clarified by Butler-Sloss [40] in the case of *Re MB*, where she restated that a competent woman has an absolute right to make her own decisions, even if they put her life and that of her fetus at risk of death.

Perhaps the most important UK case is that of *St George's Healthcare N.H.S. Trust v S* [21]. Its importance lies primarily in the fact that it seemed to reverse the trend of forced obstetrical interventions. This case laid down guidelines, which it was anticipated would be followed in the future. Broadly, they were that everyone is presumed to be competent to make medical decisions unless the contrary can be proved and a competent

woman can make her own decisions, even if this results in her own death or that of the fetus. This brings the law in this area broadly into line with that in other areas of law. For example, in the case of *NHS Trust A v M, NHS Trust B v H* [41], Butler-Sloss made it clear that 'Article 8 protects the right to personal autonomy, otherwise described as the right to physical and bodily integrity. It protects a person's right to self-determination and an intrusion into bodily integrity must be justified under Article 8(2)' [41, at *p.* 136].

 Summary box 61.4

The development of so-called fetal rights has historically, and in some cases contemporaneously, threatened the rights of women to make their own decisions.

Courts and healthcare professionals have sometimes been complicit in seeking to use the law to reinforce their moral positions.

Competence/capacity

What has gone before, of course, relates to the competent adult person. In the case of *Airedale NHS Trust v Bland*, Lord Mustill put the legal position in this way [42]:

If the patient is capable of making a decision on whether to permit treatment and decides not to permit it his choice must be obeyed, even if on any objective view it is contrary to his best interests. A doctor has no right to proceed in the face of objection, even if it is plain to all, including the patient, that adverse consequences and even death will or may ensue [42, at *p.* 136].

However, not all pregnant women may be legally competent, although it must be kept in mind that rejection of medical advice is not the same as being incompetent. Nor does the pain associated with labour necessarily negate competence, even if women change their minds, for example about pain relief, as labour progresses. Obviously, good communication between patient and doctor in discussing how labour is to be managed and a good, trusting doctor/patient relationship may serve to avoid any problems of this sort. Nonetheless, these situations aside, pregnant women may on occasion lack the competence to make self-determining decisions about themselves or their fetuses.

A couple of cases highlight a different issue as to the competence of pregnant women. In *Tameside and Glossop Acute Services Trust v CH* [43], for example, a schizophrenic patient was deemed incapable of understanding that without intervention her fetus, which she wanted to survive, would die. A Caesarean section was approved. Interestingly, this decision has been regarded as somewhat odd, since it seems to suggest that '. . . the performance of a Caesarean section on a schizophrenic woman could be 'treatment' of her mental disorder within the terms of the Mental Health Act 1983' [38]. Equally, as we know from the case of *Re C* [44], the presence of diagnosed mental illness does not in and of itself prevent someone from being legally competent.

In *Norfolk and Norwich Healthcare (NHS) Trust v W* [45], a woman arrived at hospital in labour, although she continued to deny that she was even pregnant. Although a psychiatrist said that she was not suffering from a mental disorder, it was apparently not possible to say whether or not she was capable of meeting the usual tests for competence – for example, whether she could comprehend and retain information about the proposed treatment and was capable of believing and using it [46]. In the circumstances of her undoubtedly strange refusal to accept that she was pregnant, the court deemed her not to be competent and agreed that if necessary surgical intervention could proceed.

These two cases may, in some sense, be regarded as unexceptional, because at least there was some reason to doubt whether or not the women concerned were truly competent. The courts in the end took it upon themselves to decide what was in the best interests of the women (and by implication the fetuses) in each of these cases.

One final topic for consideration here concerns refusal of treatment on religious grounds. As we have seen, the patient in the case of *Re S* declined surgical intervention on religious grounds. She and her husband were described as 'born-again Christians', although it is not clear which branch of Christianity actually does prohibit surgery. However, one religion that may cause refusal of certain kinds of treatment is that held to by Jehovah's Witnesses. For them, a central tenet of faith, derived they say directly from certain biblical passages, is that they should abstain from blood – including by transfusion. Unsurprisingly, there has been considerable legal activity on this subject in the USA [47], but it is impossible to give a clear picture of the US position given that decisions on these matters are generally made at state level and each state's attitude to women's and fetal rights may differ.[3]

What is clear, however, is that for some, if not all, Jehovah's Witnesses, their faith is ultimate. No personal concerns can or should intrude into the prohibition on transfusion that is fundamental to their faith. So, for example, in 2007, a 22-year-old woman required a life-saving transfusion following the birth of her twins. She refused to agree and died shortly after giving birth, with her husband and parents – also Jehovah's Witnesses – in full agreement with her decision [47] In 2010, a 15-year-old Jehovah's Witness, Joshua McAuley, died following a conscientious refusal of blood transfusion following a car crash [48].

The major case on blood refusal on the grounds of religion in the UK is probably that of *Re T (adult) (refusal of medical treatment)* [49]. In this case, a pregnant woman had been involved in a car crash, and after speaking with her mother – who was a Jehovah's Witness – signed a 'no blood' form. Following a Caesarean section, her condition deteriorated and transfusion was needed. A court authorized the transfusion, and this was upheld on appeal. Two grounds were used to override her apparent choice – first, that 'if there was doubt as to how the patient was exercising her right of self-determination, that doubt should be resolved in favour of the preservation of life' [50]. Second, was the question as to the voluntariness of her refusal. The patient was not a practising Jehovah's Witness, and it seemed that her mother had exerted undue influence over her decision. As we have seen, if capacity or the voluntariness of the patient's decision is in doubt, then there is reason to question whether or not a truly autonomous decision has been made. While, therefore, *Re T* does not offer broad guidelines as to how the law would respond where a patient is not unduly influenced by others, and where their capacity is not in doubt, it does raise fascinating questions about the role of religion.

There can be no doubt that religious faith can have a profound influence on people's decisions, but it is probably a step too far to regard that influence as 'undue'. If so, then it would be appropriate to accept that religion influences individual choice, but not that it renders faith-based decisions non-voluntary or non-autonomous. Moreover, freedom of religion and the right to express it are clearly covered by Article 9 of the European Convention on Human Rights, meaning that '[w]hen . . . the decision to refuse consent is a consequence of the patient's religious beliefs, Article 9 issues may arise' [51]. Wicks suggests that the decision in the case of *Hoffman v Austria* [52] could permit the conclusion that the refusal of blood by a Jehovah's Witness would be covered by the protections offered by Article 9. However, she notes that the earlier case of *Arrowsmith v U.K* [53] made it clear that 'the term "religious practice" does not cover every act which is motivated or influenced by a religion' [51]. Nonetheless, she also suggests that 'the refusal to consent to blood transfusions is so central to the beliefs of Jehovah's Witnesses that it is difficult to regard it as anything other than a manifestation of their religion' [51].

Like most articles in the Convention, derogation is permissible from Article 9, but only 'provided that the limitations are prescribed by law and necessary in a democratic

---

[3]For example, in the case of *In re Fetus Brown*, 689 N.E.2d 397 (Ill. App. Ct. 1997) a pregnant woman's right to refuse blood transfusion was upheld, even although it was indicated to save her life and that of the fetus. In other states, however, child welfare provisions have been extended to cover and protect fetuses.

society for one of four legitimate aims: public safety, public order, health and morals, or the rights of others.' [54]. Since embryos/fetuses are not 'others' for the purposes of the Convention, no derogation from Article 9 to protect the fetus would be permissible. In the absence of a case entirely on point, it can reasonably safely be deduced that a refusal by a competent person that is true to the tenets of their faith should not be overridden. Quite apart from anything else, in the case of Jehovah's Witnesses, the consequences for the woman who has a forced blood transfusion can be profound and may include being barred from the Fellowship, losing friends, family and social networks. These are by no means trivial nor inconsequential matters.

Conclusion

There are important interests at stake when women and the healthcare professionals caring for them cannot agree on how pregnancy and/or labour should be managed. As we have seen, some commentators argue that these issues have in part arisen – perhaps paradoxically – as a result of the progress that medicine has made. This, it has been suggested, has resulted in a situation where doctors see themselves as having two patients, the fetus and the pregnant woman, rather than only one, the woman herself. The ability to identify the fetus visually, according to Zechmeister, means that 'the focus of surveillance will be less on the mother but increasingly on the fetus. For the profession it becomes *'their'* patient rather than the mother's baby' [55].

Of course, with or without modern techniques and technology, it is not unsurprising that women, doctors and the state have an interest in the embryos and fetuses that might be born. The question is, how should any conflicts between the interests of these individuals and groups be managed? It is not necessary entirely to discount the fetus to see why the development of fetal 'rights' is problematic, however. In the course of pregnancy, and bearing in mind that the gradualist approach to the embryo/fetus is the one most commonly adopted, the interests of the embryo – and even the developed fetus – while worthy of respect cannot trump the rights of the pregnant woman. There are a number of reasons for this, and one does not have to be a radical feminist to understand them. First, is the question of respect for persons an ethical principle that needs to be treated as superior to moral intuitions to the contrary? This concept of respect for persons, however it is phrased, is a constant feature in human rights declarations and is a foundational pillar of liberal western democracies. Second, discrimination on any basis is widely regarded as unacceptable. When women are treated as if their reproductive capacities place them in a weaker (or different) place on the human rights scales, then this institutionalizes and legitimizes discrimination against women [56]. As Johnsen [57] says, '[g]ranting rights to fetuses in a manner that conflicts with women's autonomy reinforces the tradition of disadvantaging women on the basis of their reproductive capability'.

Third, 'policing pregnancy' by penalizing women for their behaviour in the course of pregnancy is both discriminatory and likely to be counter-productive. The perceived imperative to protect the welfare of embryos and fetuses, while understandable, is highly problematic. Take, for example, the case of women who misuse legal or illegal substances during pregnancy – substances (amongst others) that may harm the developing embryo. Marcellus [18] points out that, '[t]he issue of perinatal substance use highlights the difficulty policy-makers face in attempting to balance the autonomy and bodily integrity of pregnant women with society's interest in ensuring the birth of healthy children'. However difficult this may be, in the ultimate, the individual's rights to self-determination must prevail. The alternative is that, to avoid the attribution of legal responsibility, all sexually active women of child-bearing age should act at all times as if they might be pregnant – something that would surely be untenable.

Finally, it seems unlikely that threatening women with deprivation of liberty or other punishment allegedly in the interests of their embryo/fetus would encourage them to present for antenatal care. Paradoxically, then, the measures allegedly designed to protect the embryo/fetus might discourage women – even those who are trying to behave responsibly – from seeking proper care, especially when the kinds of events that trigger intervention can be as trivial as not getting enough rest [27].

When in labour, as we have seen, women may also find themselves threatened – this time with forced surgical interventions. Annas [58] says that, '[t]he forced-cesarean cases . . . illustrate the potential 'dark-side' of technology. The lesson these cases teach is that technology untempered by human rights can lead to brutal dehumaization of pregnant women'. One need only reflect briefly on the fate of Angela Carder to understand precisely what he means. Moreover, we hold autonomy – the right to make self-determining decisions – as being of vital importance. Even though being pregnant means that the woman is largely responsible for the fate of her embryo/fetus, as Jackson [59] says, '. . . acknowledging the unparall[el]ed intimacy of pregnancy does not necessarily render the concept of autonomy redundant or meaningless'. It is worth also reflecting on one further truth – by justifying the imposition of Caesarean sections on unwilling women, we also are holding them to a higher standard than would be expected of them if the child had already been born (and would then have become a legal person with the full range of human rights). In other words:

No mother has ever been legally required to undergo surgery or general anaesthesia . . . to save the life of her dying child. It would be ironic and unfair if she could be forced to submit to more invasive surgical procedures for the sake of her fetus than of her child [60].

Morals, ethics and the law are all in play when we compel women to accept treatment in situations such as those described in this chapter. For those whose morality respects the embryo of the human species as a person (or potential person) from the moment of conception, some of the decisions that have been critiqued here will seem to be either correct or at least a necessary evil. Those whose ethics demand respect for other persons and their decisions may nonetheless struggle with the concept that they should respect the choices of women who put their future children at risk. For the law, a somewhat schizophrenic approach can be identified as it has struggled to juggle interests, rights and good old-fashioned disapproval. Resolving the tensions between the urge to protect the fetus, while still respecting women, is obviously difficult, not least because '[c]onflicts between a woman's needs and those of her fetus are vexing because they pit powerful cultural norms against one another; the ideal of autonomy and the ideal of maternal self-sacrifice' [61]. That UK law has now been clarified is to be welcomed even if we disapprove of some women's choices. As Draper [62] says, 'it is one thing to show what a woman ought to do in relation to her unborn child and quite another thing to say that this obligation ought to be enforced'.

The legal ambivalence identified in this discussion may be a reflection of the law's attempt to accommodate particular moral views, but this is not an appropriate role for the law, which has a bigger task. It must ensure that human rights are respected without prejudice or discrimination. Doubtless, many will regret that these rights do not extend to the embryo/fetus but, a few states excepted, they do not. When the law conspires to subjugate women's rights to the future rights of their potential children this, I would suggest, 'is a monumental misunderstanding of the concept of respect and a perverse interpretation of the value of human rights' [63].

References

1 Squier S. Fetal subjects and maternal subjects: reproductive technology and the new fetal/maternal relation. *J Med Phil* 1996;21:515–535.

2 Annas GJ. The impact of medical technology on the pregnant woman's right to privacy. *Am J Law Med* 1987;13:213–232.

3 Ikenotos LC. Code of perfect pregnancy. 1992;53:1205–1306.

4 Purdy LM. Are pregnant women fetal containers? *Bioethics* 1990;4:273–291.

5 Bennett B. *Health Law's Kaleidoscope: Health Law Rights in a Global Age*. Aldershot: Ashgate, 2008.

6 Robertson J, Shulman J. Pregnancy and prenatal harm to offspring: the case of mothers with PKU. *Hastings Centre Rep* 1987; 17:23.

7 McCullogh LB, Chervenak FA. *Ethics in Obstetrics and Gynaecology*. Oxford: Oxford University Press, 1994: 100–101.

8 Report of the Committee of Inquiry into Human Fertilisation and Embryology (Warnock Report). London: Her Majesty's Stationer's Office, 1984.

9 Paton v Trustees of BPAS, 2 All ER 987 (1978); see also the case of Vo v France, 40 EHRR 12 (2005). Also available at: http://www.moznostvolby.sk/Vo%20v%20France%20written%20comments.pdf [accessed on 12 September 2008].

10 Re MB, 8 Med L R 217 (1997).

11 per Butler-Sloss, at *p*. 227.

12 A-G's Reference (No 3 of 1994), 3 All ER 936 943 (1997).

13 Warren MA. *Gendercide: The Implications of Sex Selection*. New Jersey: Rowman & Allanheld, 1985: 179–180

14 Plomer A. A foetal right to life? The case of *Vo v France*. *Human Rights Law Rev* 2005;5:311–338

15 Herczegfalvy v Austria, 15 EHRR 437 (1992).

16 Denmark, Norway, Sweden and the Netherlands v Greece, 12 YB 1 (1969).

17 R (on the application of W) v Broadmoor Hospital, EWCA Civ 1545 (2001).

18 Marcellus L. Feminist ethics must inform practice: interventions with perinatal substance users. *Health Women Int* 2004;25: 730–742.

19 Re MB, 38 BMLR 175 182 (1997).

20 Re F (in utero), 2 All ER 193 (1998).

21 St. George's Healthcare NHS Trust v S, 3 All ER 673 (1998).

22 McLean SAM. *Old Law, New Medicine*. London: RiversOram/Pandora, 1999: 49.

23 Coutts MC. 'Maternal-Fetal Conflict: Legal and Ethical Issues', ScopeNote 1990. Available at: http://bioethics.georgetown.edu [Accessed on 02 September 2008].

24 McGinnis DM. Prosecution of mothers of drug-exposed babies: constitutional and criminal theory. *U Pa L Rev* 1990;139: 505–539.

25 American Civil Liberties Union, 'Policing Pregnancy: Ferguson v City of Charleston' 11 January 2000. Available at: http://www.aclu.org/reproductiverights/lowincome/12511res20001101.html [Accessed on 12 September 2008].

26 Taylor D. 'The Guardian', Friday April 23 2004. Available at: http://www.guardian.co.uk/society/2004/apr/23/health.genderissues [Accessed on 12 September 2008]; see also Advocates for Pregnant Women paper. Available at: http://www.arcc-cdac.ca/action/LessonsfromUS.pdf [Accessed on 12 September 2008].

27 For example, see People v Stewart (Docket No. M508197). California, San Diego: Municipal Court (1987).

28 Taft v Taft, 446 NE 2d 395:396:397 (Mass 1983).

29 For further examples, see American Civil Liberties Union, 'Policing Pregnancy: Ferguson v City of Charleston' 11/1/2000. Available at: http://www.aclu.org/reproductiverights/lowincome/12511res20001101.html [Accessed on 12 September 2008]; see also, Paltrow L. Pregnant drug users, fetal persons, and the threat to *Roe v Wade*. *Albany Law Rev* 1999;62:999–1054; Paltrow LM. *Criminal Prosecutions Against Pregnant Women*

National Update And Overview April 1992. Available at: http://advocatesforpregnantwomen.org/file/1992%20State-by-State%20Case%20Summary.pdf [Accessed on 16 September 2008].

30 Kolder VE, Gallagher J, Parsons MT. Court-ordered obstetrical interventions. *New Engl J Med* 1987;316:1192–1196.

31 CBC News 'Woman who refused C-section sentenced to 18 months', 29 April 2004. Available at: http://www.cbc.ca/world/story/2004/04/29/csect040429.html [Accessed on 12 September 2008].

32 Jefferson v Griffin Spaulding County Hospital Auth., 274 SE 2d 457 (Ga 1981).

33 Re Madyyan, 114 Daily Wash L 2233 (DC Super Ct 1986).

34 Re AC, 573 A.2d 1235:1241 (DC 1990).

35 The American Civil Liberties Union. Available at: http://www.aclu.org/reproductiverights/gen/16529res19970930.html [Accessed on 17 September 2008].

36 McLean SAM, Ramsey J. Human rights, reproductive freedom, medicine and the law. *Med Law Int* 2002; 5:239–258.

37 Re T (adult: refusal of medical treatment) 9 BMLR 46 50 69 (1992).

38 Mason JK, Laurie GT. *Mason and McCall Smith's Law and Medical Ethics* (7th edn). Oxford: Oxford University Press, 2006.

39 D (a minor) v Berkshire County Council, 1 All ER 20 (1987).

40 8 Med L R 217 (1997).

41 NHS Trust A v M, NHS Trust B v H, 2 WLR 942 (2001).

42 Airedale NHS Trust v Bland, 12 BMLR 64 (1993).

43 Tameside and Glossop Acute Services Trust V CH, 31 BMLR 93 (1996).

44 Re C (adult: refusal of medical treatment), 1 All ER 819 (1994).

45 Norfolk and Norwich Healthcare (NHS) Trust v W, 34 BMLR 16 (1996).

46 Levy JK. Jehovah's Witnesses, pregnancy, and blood transfusions: a paradigm for the autonomy rights of all pregnant women. *J Law Med Ethics* 1999; 27:171–189.

47 Britten N. 'Mother Dies after refusing blood transfusion'. *The Telegraph*, 06 September 2007.

48 'Jehovah's Witness teenager dies after refusing blood transfusion'. *The Guardian*, 18 May 2010.

49 Re T (adult: refusal of medical treatment), 9 BMLR 46 (Court of Appeal 1992).

50 Mason JK, Lauire GT. *Mason and McCall Smith's Law and Medical Ethics* (7th edn). Oxford: Oxford University Press, 2006.

51 Wicks E. The right to refuse medical treatment under the European Convention on Human Rights. *Med Law Rev* 2001;9: 17–40.

52 Hoffman v Austria, Series A, No. 255 (1993).

53 Arrowsmith v UK, 19 DR 5 (1978).

54 Wicks E. Religion, law and medicine: legislating on birth and death in a Christian state. *Med Law Rev* 2009;17:410–437.

55 Zechmeister I. Foetal images: the power of visual technology in antenatal care and the implications for women's reproductive freedom. *Health Anal* 2001;9:387–400.

56 For further discussion see Meredith S. *Policing Pregnancy: The Law and Ethics of Obstetric Conflict.* Aldershot: Ashgate, 2005.

57 Johnsen DE. The creation of fetal rights: conflicts with women's constitutional rights to liberty, privacy, and equal protection. *Yale Law J* 1986;95:599–625.

58 Annas GJ. The impact of medical technology on the pregnant woman's right to privacy. *Am J Law Med* 1987;13:213–232.

59 Jackson E. *Regulating Reproduction: Law, Technology and Autonomy.* Oxford: Hart Publishing, 2001: 3.

60 Annas G. *Judging Medicine.* New York: Humana Press, 1988: 122.

61 Lew JB. Terminally ill and pregnant: state denial of a woman's right to refuse a Caesarean section. *Buffalo Law Rev* 1990;38: 621–622.

62 Draper H. Women, Forced Caesareans and Antenatal Responsibilities, Working Paper no 1, Feminist Legal Research Unit, University of Liverpool, 1992;1:13.

63 McLean SAM. *Old Law, New Medicine.* London: RiversOram/Pandora, 1999: 69.

Chapter 62
The Law and the Obstetrician and Gynaecologist

Bertie Leigh
Hempsons, London, UK

One plausible approach to the predicament of the law in managing society's expectations of your profession is to see it as a by-product of clinical success. The achievements of obstetrics over the last 60 years have been remarkable. The decline of maternal and infant mortality would have astonished our grandparents. The virtual elimination of mortality from anaesthesia and the achievement of safe and predictable remedies for a wide range of gynaecological diseases has naturally brought with it a process of adjustment. Where it used to be the case that a doctor sheltered behind the threat of disease and offered a possible but unreliable bridge over distinctly troubled surgical waters, now that the threat of the disease and the troubles of the waters has largely been eliminated there is inevitably a revaluation of the clinician. Paradoxically, the provision of a safe and predictable service has been associated with diminished confidence in the provider. Where safe and predictable clinical excellence can be produced, the fallible human agency delivering the service is more frequently weighed in the balance and more regularly found wanting.

The rise of autonomy

Because the service is expected to be safe and predictable, society also demands that it be delivered on the patient's own terms. Where the survival of mother and child is a hazardous matter, the clinician responsible for the delivery may insist that it takes place on his own terms and at a place and in circumstances determined by him. The patient who refuses to take medical advice used to be regarded as eccentric, whereas if it is safe and easy to deliver a child, then it readily comes to be viewed as a 'lifestyle choice' in which the pleasure to be derived from the occasion takes a higher priority than the reduction of an already modest risk. Although society is more risk-averse than ever before, it is also predisposed to doubt risks described by experts. The first generation to embrace

evidence-based medicine and to limit the ability of clinicians to introduce new therapies that have not been subjected to a double-blind trial is oddly more willing now than in the past to embrace complementary medicine and to advocate the woman's right to home birth when neither has been subjected to any such evidence-based assessment of risk.

When a 2010 meta-analysis based on over 550 000 deliveries reported that home deliveries involved a significant increase in the risk of infant mortality, *The Lancet* editorial [1] suggested that 'women have the right to choose how and where to give birth, but they do not have the right to put their baby at risk' [2].

It was not exactly clear whether the 'right' in question was legal or ethical. In law, women do have the right, broadly speaking, to do whatever they like in this regard, as the unborn child has no legally enforceable rights against her, in England at least. In ethics, the distinction between the right of the parent to do as she wishes before the birth and the obligation to act in her child's best interests thereafter is certainly less clear, because the parent has the same obligation to act in her child's best interests whether the child has separate legally enforceable rights or not. However, the ethicist also recognizes the parental right and duty to take various decisions on their children's behalf, and the acceptance of certain risks is part of that duty. Thus, the parent is permitted in ethics and law to take reasonable risks on behalf of the child and as a result parents do seem to have the right, for example, to take their children on a sailing dinghy provided they do not stray too far from land, that it is not too stormy and there is a life jacket. It is a question of degree, but clearly some degree of risk is permissible.

The meta-analysis found that the risk of mortality from home birth was increased from 0.09% to 0.2% and the question that *The Lancet* editorial ignored was whether the increased risk of about 0.11% was reasonable or not. There were a number of other questions that arose that will have to be resolved: how far is a meta-analysis based

Dewhurst's Textbook of Obstetrics & Gynaecology, Eighth Edition. Edited by D. Keith Edmonds.

on events in six different countries of any relevance to any of them when it is a reflection of the organization of care, which is not standardized? Since 88% of the deliveries took place in the Netherlands, where one-third of deliveries start at home and 40% of primigravidas transfer to hospital during the first stage, it looks more like a test of the safety of the decision to try home delivery in one compact country set up to transfer in case of difficulty. Indeed, in adding numerous smaller trials to one massive study, it succeeded in blunting the original study's value of the Dutch experience without adding anything of value about other countries. Nevertheless, the true incidence of increased risk is unlikely to be lower, because the Dutch system is so well set up and swift to transfer.

What may raise more troubling ethical questions is the associated demand for an increased share of scarce resources. We already face a shortage of midwives in the UK as we enter an era of rapidly increasing austerity in the National Health Service (NHS). How far is it ethical for a woman to exercise her autonomy at the expense of her sisters who can be handled by far fewer midwives in hospital? How far are the advantages of home delivery that were acknowledged by *The Lancet* editorial – shorter recovery time, fewer lacerations, postpartum haemorrhages, retained placentae and infections – attributable to more intensive 1:1 or even 2:1 care by more senior midwives in an effort to make the home birth safer?

This development spreads beyond obstetrics and gynaecology. Most aspects of medicine have become safer and more predictable, and as a consequence the relative importance of different ethical obligations upon the doctor has changed. Thirty years ago, when medical ethics was first recognized as having practical implications for mainstream clinicians, it was accepted that there were four different ethical obligations that the doctor needed to balance. The primary obligation was to do good, and that obligation preoccupied the thoughts of the clinicians of the 1970s. They might say 'first of all do not harm', but in reality that usually meant take reasonable care and the aspiration to non-maleficience took second place since it appeared to be of less practical importance in most circumstances. Third was the obligation to act justly, since it was crucial in circumstances where doctors were more responsible for the management of the NHS and therefore the allocation of resources. The modern reader of a textbook such as Ian Donald's *Practical Obstetric Problems* (1976) will be surprised by the extent of the advice on how to manage the labour ward effectively. That obligation could cause the accoucheur to hesitate before leaving the labour ward as part of what was then called the Flying Squad. The idea that the patient's autonomy should be respected came fourth. It was seen as an important part of good manners, but hardly a fundamental aspiration of the service rendered by the doctor. Women in the 1970s took themselves to a doctor for the treatment of an ailment rather than the exercise of her autonomy.

Today, respect for the patient's autonomy has grown like a cuckoo in the nest and threatens to drive all other considerations to the margins. A vivid illustration of this was seen in the case of *Chester vs. Afshar* involving spinal surgery which came to the House of Lords in 2004 [3]. The court found that Miss Chester was not told that there was a 1% risk of significant morbidity associated with spinal surgery. The defence accepted that every reasonable surgeon would have warned of this risk, which is in itself a striking change since the *Sidaway vs. Bethlem Royal Hospital's Governors* case [4] failed on precisely that issue in 1985. Miss Chester said that if she had been told of the risk, she might well have undergone the surgery in any event and very likely in the hands of the same surgeon, but only after obtaining a second opinion. On a conventional analysis this meant that Miss Chester could not prove that her surgeon had caused her any damage. However, the House of Lords felt that in these circumstances the plain meaning of the English language needed some trifling adjustment. It did so on a twofold basis.

First, that it was of vital importance that Miss Chester's autonomy be respected, and in circumstances where she was contemplating spinal surgery this demanded that she must be told the risks that she was letting herself in for, otherwise she would be stripped of her dignity as a human being when she disrobed on admission. Second, that if it was not held that the erring doctor became the insurer of the patient's damage, the duty would be emptied of its content. The law would not be upholding the duty. Thus, in order to enforce the duty the law should hold that in these circumstances the doctor has caused the patient damage. Some felt that there would have been more logic about it if the House of Lords had invented a new tort of Showing Disrespect, or *Dis* as modern slang would have it, and said that in these circumstances they would order the surgeon to compensate the patient for the complete tort of advising and treating with disrespect; that would have the advantage of forcing the surgeon to compensate the patient for the insult he had rendered, whether or not she was unlucky enough to get a complication which sounded in damages. A minor solatium of £500 would uphold the duty and reflect society's real evaluation of the insult. Since he had not really caused the complication, it seems illogical to pretend that the law is enforcing a duty to advise that is equally important whether the complication results or not.

Another oddity of the case was that Miss Chester was at no less risk if she opted for conservative therapy. The evidence was conflicting, but some experts thought that she was at greater risk of long-term disability if she did not undergo surgery. As she was in significant pain preoperatively, she would need to persuade the court that she would have undergone surgery or recovered spontaneously to recover full compensation when her quantum was assessed.

The controversy surrounding the judgement in *Chester vs. Afshar* was not diminished a month later when the House of Lords had to deal with a member of the bar who had failed to mention that there was a 50% chance that an application to get in a medical report might be turned down. Jacqueline Perry [5] advised a claimant in a medical negligence case to turn down an offer of damages because she thought that she had a 50% chance of persuading the court to admit a crucial but negligently overdue medical report into evidence and that she thought that he could probably sue his solicitors afterwards if she failed, that is if he could find the resources and stomach for a further bout of litigation. She did not trouble him with these details, simply advising him to turn down the payment into court. The House said that there was a respectable body of opinion that held that a client still paid an advocate for her advice and her opinion rather than her doubts – that it would be a sad day if an advocate in the heat of battle had to watch her own back. This demonstrates how the member of the bar is still seen as delivering an uncertain service, one that cannot be based in evidence. In subsequent cases, the law has held that the doctrine that benefited Miss Chester is not available to those counselled by other professionals, such as solicitors or financial advisers. It remains to be seen whether physicians prescribing pills will be responsible for complications they should have mentioned but which would not have affected the decision of the patient. The crux is that the respect due to the individual's right to decide what is done to their body diminishes the flexibility accorded to the doctor.

The problem is more acute for obstetricians and gynaecologists than it is for other specialties for a number of different reasons. In gynaecology, apart from cancer, most procedures are designed primarily to enhance the woman's comfort or reproductive choices. They are truly elective procedures, which the woman must be free to accept or reject on her own terms. In obstetrics, the reduction of maternal mortality and the marginalization of infant mortality have meant that the woman feels that she should be put in a more powerful position. However, it is in abortion that matters have reached the most unfortunate predicament.

Abortion

Doctors have been in the front line of the legal control of abortion since *R vs. Bourne* in 1938 [6]. There has been thrust upon them a dual role in which they are seen as the servants of the law as well as their patients. Until the Abortion Act 1967 was passed, the doctor who performed an abortion in most circumstances committed a professional offence as well as a crime and would be struck off on conviction. The day the Act came into force, the medical abortionist ceased to be a criminal and such prosecutions before the General Medical Council (GMC) ceased just as abruptly. This struck no-one as odd because the law had been changed by the Queen in Parliament and if abortions were going to be performed lawfully then the GMC had to permit them. The professional offence had been to break the law. Yet the change in GMC policy as a result of the change in the law served to emphasize the fact that the GMC did not impose any distinct medical ethic or code of behaviour, it simply reflected the law. In this respect at least there was no separate stream of doctor-made laws controlling the profession. The Oath of Hippocrates might prohibit abortion but it proved to be subordinate to the general law of the land, perhaps a litmus test for much else that has happened in medicine over the 70 years since *R vs. Bourne*.

Yet the change in abortion law went far beyond that foreseen by Parliament. When Parliament decided that it should be lawful to perform an abortion when the doctor believed that continuation of the pregnancy would be more hazardous to the health of the mother or other children in the family than the termination of the pregnancy, few realized that this in effect legalized abortion on demand since enough doctors honestly believed that such a continuation would always be more hazardous. No doctor has ever been prosecuted before the GMC for exploring the limits of this envelope.

The predicament of the obstetrician who is asked to treat a woman for an unwanted pregnancy was made more complicated in 1990. In essence, Members of Parliament (MPs) faced a widespread doubt about the wisdom of the existing law when the new Human Fertilisation and Embryology Act was being debated. A sizeable group of MPs wished to bring down the upper limit for abortion, which was then when the fetus would be capable of being born alive. Others took a more liberal view. The compromise agreed upon was that until the pregnancy has exceeded its twenty-fourth week, abortion should be available on the existing criteria, which effectively meant abortion on demand. Since women do not become pregnant before they ovulate, which on average is not before the fourteenth day of the cycle, this means that a doctor who believes in good faith that the social ground is satisfied may lawfully terminate a pregnancy until 26 weeks from the last menstrual period. I stress that this is untested in court and the conventional view within medicine is that the limit has been set at 24 weeks. After that limit, apart from where it is necessary to save the mother's life or health, abortion is lawful only when the doctor believes there was a substantial risk that the child, if born, would suffer from a serious handicap. The meaning of neither 'substantial' nor 'serious' was defined by the Act. In essence, MPs who could not agree amongst themselves decided to leave matters to doctors and women. The doctor was given the power to decide in consultation with the patient when it would be appropriate to perform an abortion. A substantial risk is generally speaking regarded as something of substance, to be taken into account in the organization of one's affairs. Usually this means less than the balance of probabilities. If that were right, it is lawful at any point up to delivery to abort a fetus who, on the balance of probabilities, would be born healthy.

Parliament did not consider such questions as whether the child had to be abnormal at birth or destined to remain handicapped permanently. So we do not know if it is lawful to terminate in the case of Huntingdon's chorea, which does not usually afflict a person until the fourth decade of life, or the person with a surgically remediable lesion.

The intervening years have not been kind to a compromise based upon deference to the judgement of an individual clinician. With the rise of personal autonomy and the decline of medical authority there is little role for a doctor to decide what is best for a patient and there is much less of a role for a doctor to tell a patient what they must and must not do. If a medical service is available, the assumption is that the doctor must provide it if the patient demands it and it is clinically appropriate. Something of a crunch point was reached in 2004 when a Curate of the Church of England recognized in the statistics issued by the Department of Health that a pregnancy had been terminated at 26 weeks where the indication given was a cleft palate. If the lesion was a part of a broader syndrome that was not apparent in the information published by the Department of Health. The Curate complained to the Police, who sought guidance from the Royal College of Obstetricians and Gynaecologists (RCOG). The Police decided not to investigate further and an application was made for Judicial Review of that decision. The Police agreed to reconsider matters and did investigate with a view to prosecution. Eventually they decided that the evidence available did not enable them to conclude that a prosecution would have a better than 50% chance of persuading a Jury that the doctors did not have the bona fide belief that the circumstances of the Act were satisfied.

However, the case triggered a debate around several issues. The first is whether the compromise decided by Parliament was far more liberal than can be defended in view of intervening medical developments. Where advances in ultrasound have made it possible to visualize the unborn child more clearly than ever before, the difficulty in defending a decision to terminate on grounds of cleft lip and palate is harder to justify. As advances in neonatology have brought the age of viability down still further, the fetus who is being killed is more often capable of being born alive and of surviving than ever before.

This is something about which obstetricians may provide expert advice to the legislature but must remain essentially neutral. It is not the role of the RCOG or any other professional body to advance a corporate view as to the circumstances in which it should be lawful to perform an abortion. Doctors may express individual views as citizens and have a statutory right to decide whether they are prepared to be involved in this work, but the corporate view that society seeks from the profession should be rendered in neutral professional terms, simply explaining what is and what is not practical and helping the rest of society to understand the implications of a given decision. Thus, the RCOG has published the Reports of Working Parties on the extent to which a fetus may experience pain [8] and provided guidance on the termination of pregnancy for fetal abnormality [9], but in neither case is it articulating a moral view to its fellows and members in the fashion in which the Hippocratic Oath bound all doctors not to procure abortion until comparatively recently.

There is a second underlying debate about the role of the clinician. Is the doctor expected to exercise a judgement about whether the procedure is in the patient's best interests? If so, on what basis? If the indication for the procedure is choice, how can or should the doctor second guess the patient? When Parliament said that it wanted the decision to be taken by doctors and patients together, did it mean that the patient should have complete freedom to decide if the doctor believed that the unborn child would suffer from any recognizable handicap? What is the extent to which it is proper to expect obstetricians to be put in the guise of judges at all in such circumstances? The assessment of the degree of handicap should be undertaken by those appropriately trained for the purpose. Often they will be members of another speciality: in some places such patients are referred to paediatric surgeons for advice, and the RCOG Working Party [9] in 2010 suggested referring to a paediatrician with experience of affected children. I wonder if we will not go further in the future: sometimes the assessment of long-term handicap might be enhanced by a multidisciplinary assessment involving specialists in neurological disability, physiotherapists, speech therapists or occupational therapists. The effect of a given physical lesion will vary greatly from case to case, depending on the personality of the victim and the resources available, as well as the severity of the lesion. The difficulty is that it is hard to see how such an assessment can be organized swiftly enough when the pregnancy is advancing.

The law here has to balance society's interest in protecting the autonomy of the pregnant woman and ensuring that she is not forced to carry to term a baby which she does not want. That right has to be balanced against the right of the unborn child. Few think it appropriate to provide women with an unqualified right to demand the destruction of a normal third trimester fetus. The need to balance these issues calls for a political and judicial assessment. Although doctors were placed in the front line, it is increasingly hard to understand what role society allots to them or how it expects them to perform this task. In few other areas of medicine are doctors asked to legislate between conflicting interests in this fashion; and where they have been granted a broad margin of discretion hitherto, as in end of life decisions, that flexibility is being curtailed.

In these circumstances the individual clinician needs to be aware of the conflicting obligations which are imposed by the law and the demands of patients. My own advice now is that, so far as possible, obstetricians should ensure that they have written objective advice from appropriate specialists on which to base their decisions. In contentious cases I suspect that we will soon advise obstetricians to transfer the decision to the place where it should properly be made – Her Majesty's Judiciary. At least that way we will get some guidelines. It will be very unfortunate if the first time that any guidelines as to the law's assessment of the meaning of substantial risk of serious handicap comes to be decided is in the context of a criminal prosecution. Under the law, until 1990 the reluctance of the Police to intervene meant that no-one attempted to find out what 'capable of being born alive' meant between its passage into law in 1929 [10] and the advent of a negligence action in respect of an obstetrician's failure to advise a woman of the failure of an alphafetoprotein (AFP) test. The Court ducked the question then and was forced to determine it in 1989 when a radiologist was sued in respect of his failure to recognize spina bifida [11]. Only then was it established that 'capable of being born alive' meant capable of maintaining life by means of one's own breathing, even though 60 years had elapsed since the Act was passed.

In the meantime I advise obstetricians to cover themselves by seeking to buttress their decisions by obtaining the sort of written evidence that a court would demand. That evidence should explicitly answer the statutory questions: is the risk substantial and would the handicap be serious? The RCOG has recently reiterated its advice of 1996, and until we have guidance from a court on the meaning of the word 'substantial' in this Act, it would be wise to err on the side of caution [9]. How a court would interpret the meaning of 'substantial' could well determine on the context in which the question was posed. We could get almost any answer from 20% – on the basis that a substantial risk is one that sensible people would take into account in ordering their affairs – to beyond all reasonable doubt, on the basis that a mature fetus should not be killed unless you are sure it will be handicapped. The latter is perhaps an extreme and unlikely view, but the court could easily demand the balance of probabilities.

Professional discipline

Another feature of the landscape of which clinicians need to be aware is the changing role of the GMC. After the profession suffered body blows in public esteem through a series of scandals in the 1990s, the GMC was reformed so as to make it much tougher on the under-performing doctor. The standard of proof was reduced from the criminal to the civil standard: it was emphasized that the civil standard does not simply mean the balance of probabilities but the panels tend to take a confident approach to issues of fact. The innovations were surrounded with honeyed words about reform and rehabilitation, but in practice those doctors who have been identified as underperforming through the GMC processes have rarely found their way back into mainstream practice again. The National Clinical Assessment Service also grapples with the problem of the under-performing doctor, but its hit rate for getting doctors back into practice once they have been identified as under-performing has not been good. These processes usually lead to the end of the clinician's career. The GMC now has a minority of doctors on its panels and the people who are there sometimes have a critical view of the profession.

It was also agreed by the profession that it should embark on some formal system of revalidation. Continuing professional education was instigated in the 1990s in response to the minimal-access surgery furore, and as a result the RCOG was the first College to instigate a system of formal recorded continuing professional education in the UK. It was agreed that revalidation needed to be something more, involving not only evidence of learning but also evidence of continuing ability, but the more ambitious programmes of revalidation seem at the time of writing in 2010 to have fallen on the stony ground of the unaffordable.

Postgraduate training

Another issue that is concerning for the future of the profession arises from the developments in professional training over the last 15 years. The introduction of the Working Time Directive in the UK has halved the number of hours per week that the junior hospital doctor works. The introduction of the Calman Reforms and the Specialist Registrar Grade has reduced the number of years of experience in training grades that a newly appointed consultant can be expected to have achieved by a similar proportion. The result is that the newly minted consultant will acquire about 20% of the clinical hours of experience of his or her predecessor 20 years ago.

In dealing with junior hospital doctors over the last 30 years, one feels that the profession has squandered a monastic tradition of devotion and apprenticeship. The

BMJ reports, for example, that junior surgical trainees are unable to tie knots, a basic skill that used to be acquired by medical students [12]. As a result, trainees cannot be entrusted, even under supervision, with the simplest procedures that their recent predecessors could manage alone. Seniors report occasions when assistants have walked out at 17.00 sharp although the operation has reached a critical point. The sense is that doctors are there to do a job within the hours for which they are paid, rather than to undertake a commitment to patients throughout the clinical pathway.

The result is a decline in continuity of care and an attitude to handover that depends upon written records rather than real communication to another doctor who will accept the same responsibility. Far more time is devoted to handover so that the proportion of junior time available for the management of the sick has fallen still further.

Worst of all, the exposure of the junior doctor in each hour of experience that is gained is markedly reduced. One understands the need to protect patients and to ensure that the service they receive is safe and consistent, but the effects have been extreme. A newly appointed senior registrar of the 1970s would be likely to have performed more surgical procedures alone and to have experienced significant complications more frequently than the newly appointed consultant of today. These events were good for neither patient nor doctor. The emphasis on using the hours of training for that very purpose is all to the good, in the sense that the juniors are well taught in a procedure-specific sense. But it is no way to acquire an understanding of the natural history of disease in man, or the flexibility to recognize when things are going wrong.

At the moment, the position is still being mitigated by the presence of senior consultants who benefited from the old-fashioned model of training. We are pedalling backwards to protect this year's patients at the expense of the experience of next year's consultants; thus, the last three NCEPOD (National Confidential Enquiry into Perioperative Outcome and Death) case studies have advised that all acute admissions should be seen by a consultant within 12 hours.

Every year these consultants retire and are replaced by colleagues who simply do not have the same sort of training. To some extent the problems can be mitigated in elective surgery by increasing subspecialty and higher training in courses post-appointment as consultant, but we are encountering a brave new world in more and more hospitals where there is no consultant who benefited from the old-fashioned sort of training. The idea that junior consultants are going to acquire the experience and training that they need in the course of their early consultant years overlooks the fact that they are not in a training grade and that increasingly there is no-one there to train

them if they do have the modesty to ask for help and guidance.

For a time it looked as if the newly appointed young consultants would take on the attitudes of their seniors when appointed and accept the notion of 24-hour responsibility necessary to provide continuity of care for those they regarded as their patients. The NHS decided in 2003, apparently in ignorance of the fact that most consultants still maintained the same standards of dedication they had acquired as juniors and worked way beyond the hours for which they were paid, that it would pay consultants for the hours they worked. The result was a massive bill that that threatened to cripple many Trusts and there had to be some firm negotiation. This change represented a turning point: the older doctors continue to provide the service their patients need despite the nominal fact that they are not being paid for it, but their attitudes already appear old fashioned and are being replaced by a new respect for an appropriate work–life balance. There is a new generation coming up, shaped in the fashion conjured up by the managers of the service rather than their clinical seniors.

The conflict between the lack of training and the hostile environment

The combination of this crisis in professional training and the less-forgiving professional environment in which doctors work means that the prospects for the individual doctor are ever gloomier. The basic premise of the reforms proposed by the Shipman Inquiry is that there is a plentiful supply of newly minted doctors available to replace those who are found not to have kept their professional skills up to date. This premise is profoundly mistaken and the unprincipled attempt to entice doctors to quit poorer countries cannot provide a sustainable solution. In defending doctors before the GMC, we already find an unforgiving atmosphere and an assumption that someone must have done something wrong whenever a patient has died. The notion of being just to the doctor who is the respondent to a complaint is low down on a set of priorities which are headed by making sure that the service is 'safe' and giving satisfaction to somebody simply because they have complained.

Outside the portals of the GMC the complaints system within hospitals has been reformed and made similarly more hostile to the profession. The advice that one gives to professionals in these circumstances is much the same as it has always been – spend time with patients, talk to them and listen to them; explain in detail what is proposed; recognizing that the purpose of the consultation is to put your knowledge at the patient's disposal so that she can make her decision about what she wants to do. This explicitly involves an acceptance of the proposition that sometimes patients will make decisions which the doctor thinks are surprising, if not profoundly misconceived. The patient has an unfettered right to refuse surgery for good reason, bad reason or no reason. The doctor must make sure that the risks of inaction are spelled out as clearly as the risks of the intervention in question. The doctor's role is to advise and to recognize that while their skills are for their patient, their notes are for themselves and their own protection. It is as important to make detailed records of what is said to and by the patient as it is to make records of the clinical history that is elicited and the signs that are found.

It must also be recognized that the patient's right to choose in effect must sometimes mean a right to demand therapy which the doctor thinks is contraindicated. This is an issue with which the profession and the NHS is only beginning to grapple. It found its first utterance in the National Institute for Health and Clinical Excellence (NICE) guidelines concerning Caesarean section [13]. The patient who demands an unfair share of resources in the form of a Caesarean section that the doctor thinks is not medically indicated is not in the same position as the woman who insists on home delivery against medical advice. Both are demanding a share of medical resources that seems to exceed the clinical indication in the eyes of the medical attendant, but the woman who demands an operation is demanding that her doctor does something that appears to be inappropriate. She should be offered referral to a colleague where practical, but the doctor should never find themselves doing an operation that they believe is contrary to their patient's best interests.

In other areas, the Service operates on the premise that patients will not demand surgery which is not in their interests. How far that premise is well founded is unclear. We do have some experience of professionals being sued for unnecessary procedures in the context of dentistry. There is a long-established line of cases in which patients have demanded extravagant, conservative restoration of teeth whose roots are unsuitable. The smile may be attractive at first but the life expectancy of the bridge is short. The same thing happens even more often in cosmetic surgery. The courts almost invariably criticize the dentist or the cosmetic surgeon for having performed a procedure contrary to the patient's best interests as the professional saw them. The conventional advice to a professional is that when a patient demands a procedure which appears to be contrary to their best interests, the professional should decline to perform it and offer to refer to someone else. That conventional advice must still be good in 2005, but as professional autonomy advances the question must arise as to whether the patient's right to choose will sooner or later entitle them to demand surgery which the doctor thinks is contraindicated, with the same freedom as the waiter should accept an order for an unsuitable combination of dishes. If the autonomy of the patient is paramount and the playing field of knowledge

of the implications of medical procedures becomes ever more level, it is difficult to understand how the status quo can be preserved indefinitely.

Cerebral palsy

All this is a long way from the core of the issues which were at the forefront of professional concern when this chapter's first predecessor was written in 1999. Then, the concern of the obstetrician with the law was as it had been since 1980 when the House of Lords gave judgement in *Jordan vs. Whitehouse* [14] that the doctors involved would be sued by children suffering from cerebral palsy who sought to blame their disability on the doctor. Although Mr Jordan's case resulted in a victory for the defence, the experience of the Defence organizations was that the public remembered only that a claim had been brought in respect of a brain-damaged child, not that it was lost. Although the Defence witness who gave evidence that the damage could not have been caused by the actions of which complaint was made, Professor Ronald Illingworth found his evidence rejected at trial. He subsequently wrote an influential article in the *BMJ* '*Why Blame the Obstetrician?*' [15], which drew on work already being done by neonatologists in America, and over the succeeding 30 years we have become used to a much more measured assessment of causation in these cases.

To date it is still true that two-thirds of the expenditure of the NHS Litigation Authority, which deals with claims against the NHS, is devoted to cases of this sort. It is also true that the number of children in the population suffering from cerebral palsy has remained roughly constant despite improvements in obstetrics and paediatrics that have transformed the rates of infant mortality and the prospects of survival of the child once delivered. This is probably due to the increased age of the parturient woman since the introduction of *in vitro* fertilization: this is has been associated with increased rates of maternal obesity, diabetes and associated complications. EPICure II [16] has found that advances in neonatology have brought more survivors from the extremes of prematurity, but still many suffer from the associated disability. It is also true that social expectations for a perfect result have made it difficult for us to defend such cases, even where the extremity of prematurity makes it clear that survival at all is astonishing.

Yet the problem is no longer at the forefront of professional thinking. There are a number of reasons for this. First and foremost, the advent of NHS indemnity in 1990 has taken the financial burden of these sort of cases off the shoulders of the medical profession. Claims handling was centralized under the Clinical Negligence Scheme for NHS Trusts in 2002 and the claims experience of the Trusts do not so far affect the premium that hospitals pay to be members of the scheme, so that there is an additional level of insulation between the individual doctor and the damage. Risk management and clinical governance demand ever higher and more intolerant standards, but the purely financial impact of these claims is well removed from the services delivered in the individual Trust. There was a period when a multimillion pound claim against the Trust would or could cause cashflow problems which sent the Chief Executive cap in hand to the Regional Office of the Department of Health. That at least has gone.

References

1 *Lancet* 2010;376:303.
2 Wax JR, Lucas FL, Lamont M *et al*. Maternal and newborn outcomes in planned home birth vs planned hospital births: a metaanalysis. *Am J Obstet Gynecol* 2010;203:x.ex–x.ex.
3 Chester vs. Afshar [2004] UKHL. 41.
4 Sidaway vs. Board of Governors of Bethlem Royal Hospital and Maudsley Hospital [1985] AC. 871.
5 Moy vs. Pettman Smith [2005] UKHL. 7; [2005].
6 R vs. Bourne [1938].
7 RCOG Website Fetal Awareness – Review of Research and Recommendations for Practice (Pdf). Available at: http://www.rcog.org.uk/fetal-awareness-review-research-and-recommendations-practice.
8 RCOG Website Termination of Pregnancy for Fetal Abnormality in England, Scotland and Wales (pdf). Available at: http://www.rcog.org.uk/termination-pregnancy-fetal-abnormality-england-scotland-and-wales.
9 Infant Life Preservation Act 1929.
10 Rance vs. Storr [1993] 4 Med LR l17 CA.
11 Chikwe J, de Souza AC, Pepper JR. No time to train the surgeons. *BMJ* 2004;328:418–419; doi:10.1136/bmj.328.7437.418.
12 See NICE Website: Caesarean Section Clinical Guideline 13 April 2004. Available at: http://www.nice.org.uk/nicemedia/live/10940/29331/29331.pdf.
13 [1981] 1 All ER. 261.
14 Illingworth R. Why blame the obstetrician? *Br Med J* 1979; 797–801.
15 Hall D. Birth asphyxia and cerebral palsy. *Br Med J* 299: 279–83.
16 EPICure II. Available at: www.epicure.ac.uk.

Index

Notes: Page numbers in *italics* refer to figures, those in **bold** refer to tables. The following abbreviations have been used:
ART – assisted reproductive techniques
CIN – cervical intraepithelial neoplasia
HRT – hormone replacement therapy
PCOS – polycystic ovary syndrome
PMS – premenstrual syndrome

MULTI-SULFUR AND SULFUR AND OXYGEN

FIVE- AND SIX-MEMBERED HETEROCYCLES

In Two Parts
PART ONE

This is Part One of the twenty-first volume in the series
THE CHEMISTRY OF HETEROCYCLIC COMPOUNDS

THE CHEMISTRY OF HETEROCYCLIC COMPOUNDS

A SERIES OF MONOGRAPHS

ARNOLD WEISSBERGER, *Consulting Editor*